Unleashing the Power of Functional Foods and Novel Bioactives

Unleashing the Power of Functional Foods and Novel Bioactives

Edited by

Tanmay Sarkar
Malda Polytechnic, West Bengal State Council of Technical Education, Government West Bengal, Malda, West Bengal, India

Slim Smaoui
Laboratory of Microbial, Enzymes Biotechnology and Biomolecules (LMEBB), Centre of Biotechnology of Sfax (CBS), University of Sfax, Sfax, Tunisia

Anka Trajkovska Petkoska
Faculty of Technology and Technical Sciences - Veles, University St. Kliment Ohridski - Bitola, North Macedonia

ELSEVIER

ACADEMIC PRESS
An imprint of Elsevier

Academic Press is an imprint of Elsevier
125 London Wall, London EC2Y 5AS, United Kingdom
525 B Street, Suite 1650, San Diego, CA 92101, United States
50 Hampshire Street, 5th Floor, Cambridge, MA 02139, United States

ISBN: 978-0-443-28862-3

For Information on all Academic Press publications
visit our website at https://www.elsevier.com/books-and-journals

Publisher: Mara Conner
Acquisitions Editor: Nicole Denis
Editorial Project Manager: Dan Egan
Production Project Manager: Sruthi Satheesh
Cover Designer: Greg Harris

Typeset by MPS Limited, Chennai, India

Dedication

Dr. Tanmay Sarkar wants to dedicate the book to his beloved mother, Arati Sarkar, his father, Bholanath Sarkar, and his sister, Tanusree Sarkar.

Dr. Slim Smaoui wants to dedicate the book to his deceased father, Mohamed Nejib Smaoui, beloved mother, Raoudha, wife, Hajer, and his children, Mohamed Yassine and Yassmine.

Dr. Anka Trajkovska Petkoska wants to dedicate this book to Alexander Mario, Anna Maria and Vlado Petkoski.

And to God, for the strength and guidance throughout every step of the way.

Contents

21. Sustainable farming practices: nurturing the future of functional foods

Anka Trajkovska Petkoska, Biljana Trajkovska, Hyrije Koraqi, Nishant Kumar and Anita T. Broach

22. The importance of labeling and certification: ensuring quality and transparency

Muskan Kumari Gupta, Vinay Balodi, Abhishek Dutt Tripathi, Rizwana, Aparna Agarwal and Nilesh Prakash Nirmal

23. Educating consumers: making informed choices for better health impact

Sofiane Boudalia, Abderrahmane Aït-Kaddour, Maria Perez-Jimenez, Fernando Capela e Silva, Anissa Zergui and Elsa Lamy

List of contributors

Ahmadreza Abedinia Department of Food Engineering, Inonu University, Malatya, Turkey; Department of Food Science and Technology, Damghan Branch, Islamic Azad University, Damghan, Iran

Aparna Agarwal Department of Food & Nutrition and Food Technology, Lady Irwin College, University of Delhi, New Delhi, Delhi, India

Rinku Sudarshan Agrawal MIT School of Food Technology, MIT Art, Design and Technology University, Pune, Maharashtra, India

Abderrahmane Aït-Kaddour Université Clermont Auvergne, INRAE, VetAgro Sup, UMRF, Lempdes, France; Department of Food Industrial Technology, Universitas Padjadjaran, Bandung, Indonesia

Sarra Akermi Laboratory of Microbial Biotechnology, Enzymatic and Biomolecules, Center of Biotechnology of Sfax (CBS), University of Sfax, Sfax, Tunisia; Laboratory of Microbial Biotechnology and Engineering Enzymes (LMBEE), Center of Biotechnology of Sfax (CBS), University of Sfax, Sfax, Tunisia

Samira Alahyaribeik Food Chemistry and Technology Research Centre, Department of Molecular Biotechnology, Environmental Technology, and Food Technology, Ghent University Global Campus, Yeonsu-gu, Incheon, South Korea

Diyar Salahuddin Ali Department of Chemistry, College of Science, Salahaddin University-Erbil, Erbil, Kurdistan Region, Iraq; Department of Pharmacy, College of Pharmacy, Knowledge University, Erbil, Kurdistan Region, Iraq

Elham Azarpazhooh Agricultural Engineering Research Department, Khorasan Razavi Agricultural and Natural Resources Research and Education Center, AREEO, Mashhad, Iran

Sena Bakir Tourism Faculty, Department of Gastronomy and Culinary Arts, Recep Tayyip Erdogan University, Ardesen, Rize, Türkiye; Blueberry Application and Research Center, Recep Tayyip Erdogan University, Pazar, Rize, Türkiye

Vinay Balodi G. B. Pant University of Agriculture and Technology, Pantnagar, Uttarakhand, India

Esila Bayar Faculty of Health Sciences, Nutrition and Dietetics Department, Istanbul Aydin University, Istanbul, Türkiye; Faculty of Health Sciences, Nutrition and Dietetics Department, Hacettepe University, Sıhhiye, Ankara, Türkiye

Homa Behmadi Agricultural Engineering Research Institute, Agricultural Research, Education and Extension Organization (AREEO), Karaj, Iran

Prabina Bhattarai Department of Health and Human Development, Montana State University, Bozeman, MT, United States

Sofiane Boudalia Université 8 Mai 1945, Département d'Écologie et Génie de l'Environnement, Guelma, Algeria; Laboratoire de Biologie, Eau et Environnement, Université 8 Mai 1945 Guelma BP 4010, Guelma, Algeria

Fernando Capela e Silva MED-Mediterranean Institute for Agriculture, Environment and Development & CHANGE-Global Change and Sustainability Institute, Pólo da Mitra, University of Évora, Apartado 94, Évora, Portugal; Department of Medical and Health Sciences, School of Health and Human Development, University of Évora, Évora, Portugal

Moufida Chaari Laboratory of Microbial Biotechnology, Enzymatic and Biomolecules, Center of Biotechnology of Sfax (CBS), University of Sfax, Sfax, Tunisia; Laboratory of Microbial Biotechnology and Engineering Enzymes (LMBEE), Center of Biotechnology of Sfax (CBS), University of Sfax, Sfax, Tunisia

Altaf Choudhary Pharma Department, Dr APJ Abdul Kalam Technical University, AKTU CDRI RD, Lucknow, Uttar Pradesh, India

Merina Dahal College of Health Solutions, Downtown Phoenix Campus, Arizona State University, Tempe, AZ, United States

Eduarda Silva de Azevedo Institute of Food Science and Technology, Federal University of Rio Grande do Sul, Av. Bento Gonçalves, Porto Alegre, RS, Brazil

Burcu Saygıdeğer Demir Department of Biotechnology, Insititute of Natural and Applied Sciences, Cukurova University, Sarıcam, Adana, Türkiye

Gitanjali S. Deokar MET's Institute of Pharmacy, Bhujbal Knowledge City, Adgaon, Nashik, Maharashtra, India

Abira Dey Moldoc Biotech Private, SINE Limited Business Center, IIT Bombay, Mumbai, Maharashtra, India

Teresa D'Amore Laboratory of Preclinical and Translational Research, IRCCS CROB, Centro di Riferimento Oncologico della Basilicata, Rionero in Vulture, Italy

Khaoula Elhadef Laboratory of Microbial Biotechnology, Enzymatic and Biomolecules, Center of Biotechnology of Sfax (CBS), University of Sfax, Sfax, Tunisia; Laboratory of Microbial Biotechnology and Engineering Enzymes (LMBEE), Center of Biotechnology of Sfax (CBS), University of Sfax, Sfax, Tunisia

Zahra Emam-Djomeh Functional Food Research Core (FFRC), Transfer Phenomena Laboratory (TPL), College of Agriculture & Natural Resources, University of Tehran, Karaj Campus, Tehran, Iran

Burcu Ersoy Faculty of Health Sciences, Department of Nutrition and Dietetics, Istanbul Aydin University, Kucukcekmece, Istanbul, Türkiye

N. A. Michael Eskin Department of Food and Human Nutritional Sciences, University of Manitoba, Winnipeg, MB, Canada

Yan Fang Food Chemistry and Technology Research Centre, Department of Molecular Biotechnology, Environmental Technology, and Food Technology, Ghent University Global Campus, Yeonsu-gu, Incheon, South Korea

Roberto Festuccia Department of Ecological and Biological Sciences, Tuscia University, Viterbo, Italy

Sara Gashtasbi Functional Food Research Core (FFRC), Transfer Phenomena Laboratory (TPL), College of Agriculture & Natural Resources, University of Tehran, Karaj Campus, Tehran, Iran

Pantea Ghalambor Department of Food Science and Technology, Science and Research Branch, Islamic Azad University, Tehran, Iran

Busra Goz Faculty of Health Sciences, Department of Nutrition and Dietetics, Istanbul Aydin University, Kucukcekmece, Istanbul, Türkiye

Zehra Gulsunoglu-Konuskan Faculty of Health Sciences, Department of Nutrition and Dietetics, Istanbul Aydin University, Kucukcekmece, Istanbul, Türkiye

Muskan Kumari Gupta Department of Food & Nutrition and Food Technology, Lady Irwin College, University of Delhi, New Delhi, Delhi, India

Mahdieh Nadali Hazaveh Food Chemistry and Technology Research Centre, Department of Molecular Biotechnology, Environmental Technology, and Food Technology, Ghent University Global Campus, Yeonsu-gu, Incheon, South Korea

Anuruddika Hewage Department of Food and Human Nutritional Sciences, University of Manitoba, Winnipeg, MB, Canada; Richardson Centre for Food Technology and Research, Winnipeg, MB, Canada

Hajer ben Hlima Laboratory of Enzymatic Engineering and Microbiology, Algae Biotechnology Unit, Biological Engineering Department, National School of Engineers of Sfax, 3038, University of Sfax, Sfax, Tunisia

Elahesadat Hosseini Department of Chemical Engineering, Payame Noor University, Tehran, Iran; Department of Food Science and Technology, National Nutrition Sciences and Food Technology Research Institute, Faculty of Nutrition Sciences and Food Technology, Shahid Beheshti University of Medical Sciences, Tehran, Iran

Meetha James Kraft Heinz, Glenview, IL, United States

Zeynep Begum Kalyoncu-Atasoy Faculty of Health Sciences, Department of Nutrition and Dietetics, Istanbul Aydin University, Kucukcekmece, Istanbul, Türkiye

Atefeh Karimidastjerd Yildiz Technical University, Faculty of Chemical and Metallurgical Engineering, Food Engineering Department, Istanbul, Türkiye

Zakir Showkat Khan Department of Food Science & Technology, Guru Nanak Dev University, Amritsar, Punjab, India; Department of Food Technology, School of Applied and Life Sciences, Uttaranchal University, Dehradun, Uttarakhand, India

Anandu Chandra Khanashyam Department of Food Science and Nutrition, University of Minnesota, St Paul, MN, United States

Chamali Kodikara Department of Food and Human Nutritional Sciences, University of Manitoba, Winnipeg, MB, Canada; Richardson Centre for Food Technology and Research, Winnipeg, MB, Canada; Agriculture Agri-Food Canada, Morden Research and Development Centre, Morden, MB, Canada

Hyrije Koraqi Food Science and Biotechnology, University for Business and Technology-UBT, Prishtina, Kosovo

Sanjay J. Kshirsagar MET's Institute of Pharmacy, Bhujbal Knowledge City, Adgaon, Nashik, Maharashtra, India

Kapil S. Kulkarni MET's Institute of Pharmacy, Bhujbal Knowledge City, Adgaon, Nashik, Maharashtra, India

Nishant Kumar National Institute of Food Technology Entrepreneurship and Management (NIFTEM), Kundli, Haryana, India

Elsa Lamy MED-Mediterranean Institute for Agriculture, Environment and Development & CHANGE-Global Change and Sustainability Institute, Pólo da Mitra, University of Évora, Apartado 94, Évora, Portugal

Jorge Luís School of Design, Management and Production Technologies Northern Aveiro, University of Aveiro, Estrada do Cercal, 449, 3720-511, Oliveira de Azeméis, Portugal; EMaRT Group—Emerging Materials, Research, Technology, University of Aveiro, Aveiro, Portugal; CICECO Aveiro—Institute of Materials, University of Aveiro, Campus Universitário de Santiago, Aveiro, Portugal

Lotfi Mellouli Laboratory of Microbial Biotechnology, Enzymatic and Biomolecules, Center of Biotechnology of Sfax (CBS), University of Sfax, Sfax, Tunisia; Laboratory of Microbial Biotechnology and Engineering Enzymes (LMBEE), Center of Biotechnology of Sfax (CBS), University of Sfax, Sfax, Tunisia

Niloofar Mirdamadi School of Medicine, Tehran University of Medical Sciences, Tehran, Iran

Mahta Mirzaei Department of Food Technology, Safety and Health, Faculty of Bioscience Engineering, Ghent University, Ghent, Belgium; Food Chemistry and Technology Research Centre, Department of Molecular Biotechnology, Environmental Technology, and Food Technology, Ghent University Global Campus, Yeonsu-gu, Incheon, South Korea

Ruchira Nandasiri Department of Food and Human Nutritional Sciences, University of Manitoba, Winnipeg, MB, Canada; Division of Neurodegenerative Disorders (DND), St. Boniface Hospital Albrechtsen Research Centre, Winnipeg, MB, Canada; Canadian Centre for Agri-Food Research in Health and Medicine (CCARM), St. Boniface Hospital Albrechtsen Research Centre, Winnipeg, MB, Canada

Nilesh Prakash Nirmal Institute of Nutrition, Mahidol University, Salaya, Nakhon Pathom, Thailand

Kritee Niroula School of Nutrition and Food Sciences, Louisiana State University, Baton Rouge, LA, United States

Caciano Pelayo Zapata Noreña Institute of Food Science and Technology, Federal University of Rio Grande do Sul, Av. Bento Gonçalves, Porto Alegre, RS, Brazil

J.M. Oliveira School of Design, Management and Production Technologies Northern Aveiro, University of Aveiro, Estrada do Cercal, 449, 3720-511, Oliveira de Azeméis, Portugal; EMaRT Group—Emerging Materials, Research, Technology, University of Aveiro, Aveiro, Portugal; CICECO Aveiro—Institute of Materials, University of Aveiro, Campus Universitário de Santiago, Aveiro, Portugal

Azime Özkan Karabacak Bursa Uludag University, Gemlik Asim Kocabiyik Vocational School, Food Technology Program, Gemlik, Bursa, Türkiye; Bursa Uludag University, Science and Technology Application and Research Center, Bursa, Türkiye

Vaishnavi A. Pathak MET's Institute of Pharmacy, Bhujbal Knowledge City, Adgaon, Nashik, Maharashtra, India

Maria Perez-Jimenez MED-Mediterranean Institute for Agriculture, Environment and Development & CHANGE-Global Change and Sustainability Institute, Pólo da Mitra, University of Évora, Apartado 94, Évora, Portugal

Hosahalli S. Ramaswamy Department of Food Science, Macdonald Campus, McGill University, Ste Anne de Bellevue, QC, Canada

Bharathi Ramesh Icahn School of Medicine at Mount Sinai, New York, NY, United States

Rizwana Department of Food Technology, Bhaskaracharya College of Applied Sciences, New Delhi, Delhi, India

Salma Samieitousi Functional Food Research Core (FFRC), Transfer Phenomena Laboratory (TPL), College of Agriculture & Natural Resources, University of Tehran, Karaj Campus, Tehran, Iran

Yasemin Saygideger Department of Pulmonary, Department of Translational Medicine, Faculty of Medicine, Cukurova University, Adana, Türkiye

Kartik Shah Sargento Foods, Elkhart Lake, WI, 53020, United States

Parisa Shamsaie Department of Food Science and Technology, Science and Research Branch, Islamic Azad University, Tehran, Iran

M. Anjaly Shanker Department of Agriculture and Environmental Sciences, National Institute of Food Technology Entrepreneurship and Management (NIFTEM), Sonepat, Haryana, India

Ashwani Sharma Insight Biosolutions, Biopole Rennes, Rennes, France

Pooja A. Shinde MET's Institute of Pharmacy, Nashik, Maharashtra, India

Subrata Sinha Department of Computational Sciences, Brainware University, Kolkata, West Bengal, India

Slim Smaoui Laboratory of Microbial, Enzymes Biotechnology and Biomolecules (LMEBB), Centre of Biotechnology of Sfax (CBS), University of Sfax, Sfax, Tunisia

Liliana R. Sousa School of Design, Management and Production Technologies Northern Aveiro, University of Aveiro, Estrada do Cercal, 449, 3720-511, Oliveira de Azeméis, Portugal; EMaRT Group—Emerging Materials, Research, Technology, University of Aveiro, Aveiro, Portugal; CICECO Aveiro—Institute of Materials, University of Aveiro, Campus Universitário de Santiago, Aveiro, Portugal

Özge Süfer Food Engineering Department, Osmaniye Korkut Ata University, Osmaniye, Türkiye

Yasmina Sultanbawa Centre for Nutrition and Food Sciences, Queensland Alliance for Agriculture and Food Innovation (QAAFI), The University of Queensland Elkhorn Building (#1024), Indooroopilly, QLD, Australia

Anita T. Broach CSI: Create.Solve.Innovate. LLC, Christiansburg, VA, United States

Canan Ece Tamer Department of Food Engineering, Faculty of Agriculture, Bursa Uludag University, Gorukle, Bursa, Türkiye

Loleny Tavares School of Design, Management and Production Technologies Northern Aveiro, University of Aveiro, Estrada do Cercal, 449, 3720-511, Oliveira de Azeméis, Portugal; EMaRT Group—Emerging Materials, Research, Technology, University of Aveiro, Aveiro, Portugal; CICECO Aveiro—Institute of Materials, University of Aveiro, Campus Universitário de Santiago, Aveiro, Portugal

Priyamvada Thorakkattu Department of Animal Sciences and Industry, Food Science Institute, Kansas State University, Manhattan, KS, United States

Kiran Tiwari School of Business and Hospitality, Food and Nutrition Management, Algonquin College, Ottawa, ON, Canada

Biljana Trajkovska Faculty of Biotechnical Sciences, University St. Kliment Ohrdiski, Bitola, North Macedonia

Anka Trajkovska Petkoska Faculty of Technology and Technical Sciences - Veles, University St. Kliment Ohridski - Bitola, North Macedonia

Abhishek Dutt Tripathi Department of Dairy Science and Food Technology, Institute of Agricultural Sciences, Banaras Hindu University, Varanasi, Uttar Pradesh, India

Sayna Zahedinia Yildiz Technical University, Faculty of Chemical and Metallurgical Engineering, Food Engineering Department, Istanbul, Türkiye

Rafael Audino Zambelli Food Engineering Department, Federal University of Ceará, Fortaleza, Brazil

Anissa Zergui Department of Toxicology, University Hospital of Oran, Oran, Algeria; Department of Pharmacy, Faculty of Medicine, University of Oran 1 Ahmed Ben Bella, Oran, Algeria

Zyta M. Ziora Institute for Molecular Bioscience, The University of Queensland-Saint Lucia Campus, Brisbane, QLD, Australia

About the editors

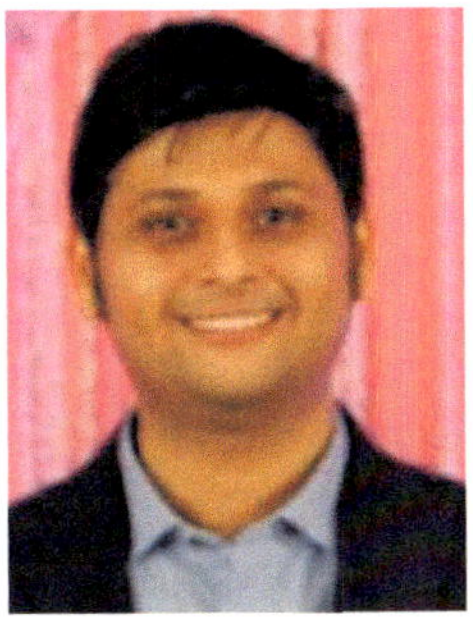

Dr. Tanmay Sarkar is currently working as a Lecturer in the Government of West Bengal. He has received his Bachelor of Technology, Master of Technology, and PhD in Engineering from Jadavpur University, Kolkata, India. With 7 years of experience in both teaching and research, his areas of interest include bioactive components from natural sources, ethnic foods, mathematical modeling, and phytochemicals. He is an editor for several SCI, SCIE, and Scopus-indexed journals and has edited numerous books.

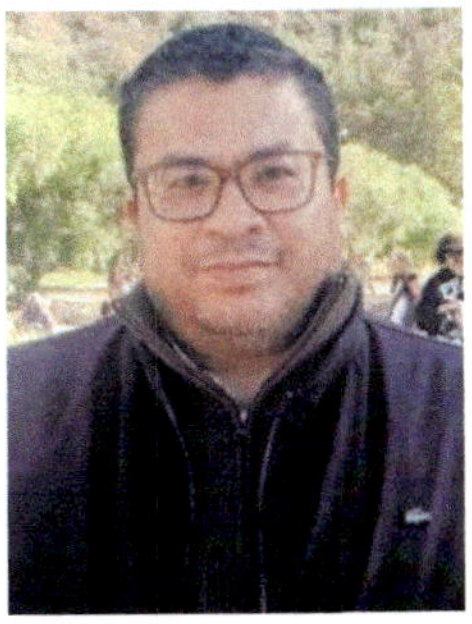

Dr. Slim Smaoui works as an Associate Professor in the Centre of Biotechnology of Sfax. He supervises research for the development of new healthier meat products, the use of agro-food industry by-products as potential sources to obtain valuable and bioactive compounds, and the development of functional foods. He deals with meat quality and safety, analytical chemistry applied to food analysis, and research and development and analytical method validation by the application of chemometric techniques.

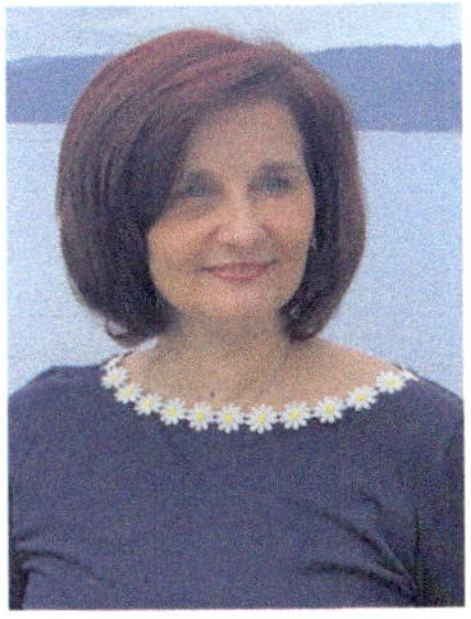

Dr. Anka Trajkovska Petkoska is a Professor at St. Kliment Ohridski University, Bitola (N. Macedonia) and an Adjunct Professor at Korea University, Seoul (South Korea). She has been actively involved in developing novel products, material formulations and cutting-edge technologies in fields related to polymer (nano) composites, antimicrobial materials and compositions, thin films and coatings, nutri-cosmetics, food contact materials, liquid crystals and their applications, etc. She has a strong academic background with a Doctor of Philosophy degree in Chemical Engineering from the University of Rochester, Rochester, NY (United States), and an MSc/BSc from St. Cyril and Methodius University, Skopje (N. Macedonia).

Preface

In recent years, the interest in functional foods and bioactive compounds has grown rapidly. These foods, beyond their basic nutritional value, have shown potential to offer significant health benefits, helping to prevent and manage chronic diseases while also enhancing overall wellness. The integration of new bioactive compounds into food systems represents an exciting new chapter in nutrition science, health, and innovation.

This book, *Unleashing the Power of Functional Foods and Novel Bioactives*, was created to explore this evolving area in detail. It brings together top researchers, scientists, and experts from a variety of fields, sharing their insights into how functional foods can benefit human health. Beyond simply explaining the science behind these foods, this book also provides practical advice on how they can be applied across different sectors, addressing areas such as heart and digestive health, cognitive function, aging, and cancer prevention.

The development of functional foods and novel bioactives is a collaborative effort, involving advances in food technology, biochemistry, nutrition, and medicine. In this book, we examine how these fields come together to offer solutions to modern health issues such as metabolic disorders, inflammation, and immune system support. As the global health focus shifts toward prevention, functional foods have emerged as a key strategy to promote health and wellness through everyday diets.

The chapters cover a broad range of subjects, including the role of functional foods in weight management, sports nutrition, antiaging, and disease prevention. Special attention is given to emerging trends in bioactive compounds, nutraceuticals, and personalized nutrition, which open up new pathways for health improvement. This book's contributors are pioneers in their fields, offering cutting-edge research, deep analysis, and future-focused perspectives on the role of functional foods and bioactives in shaping the future of food science.

While the focus remains on health benefits, this book also addresses important issues like sustainable farming practices, labeling, certification, and consumer education. It underscores the need for ensuring the quality, safety, and transparency of functional foods, empowering consumers to make informed health choices.

We are at a crucial turning point in the food industry, where scientific breakthroughs, sustainability, and consumer awareness are driving the creation of new functional products. In addressing today's complex health challenges, functional foods and bioactives present a promising way forward, harnessing both innovation and the richness of nature's resources to improve human health.

We hope this book will be a valuable tool for researchers, professionals, and anyone interested in the connection between food and health. It provides a comprehensive overview of where the field stands and where it is headed, showcasing the incredible potential that functional foods have to transform human well-being.

This journey would not have been possible without the dedication of our esteemed authors and researchers, whose work highlights the growing importance of this field. As we explore this emerging landscape, we hope this book inspires further research and innovation in the world of functional foods and bioactives.

Dr. Tanmay Sarkar
Dr. Slim Smaoui
Dr. Anka Trajkovska Petkoska

Chapter 1

Introduction: the evolution of functional foods and novel bioactives

Özge Süfer
Food Engineering Department, Osmaniye Korkut Ata University, Osmaniye, Türkiye

1.1 Introduction to functional foods

Over the last two decades, significant academic research has focused on the classification and analysis of various types of foods, particularly those designed for specific dietary purposes such as light, diet, and low-fat options, as well as functional foods. The term "functional foods" is widely used in social and scientific media, leading to increased investment by food producers in the creation of processed foods that offer additional functional benefits for consumers' health. However, due to varying regulations and interpretations in different countries, the exact meaning and definition of this term remain uncertain globally (Granato et al., 2020). Functional foods, as defined by The International Life Sciences Institute, are characterized by their inclusion of various components that aim to enhance health status or mitigate the risk, rather than prevent diseases. Furthermore, these foods must offer advantages that surpass those solely related to basic nutrition. Scientific substantiation is a prerequisite for the classification of food as functional (Ashwell, 2004; Küster-Boluda & Vidal-Capilla, 2017).

The notion of functional food, initially introduced in Japan in 1984, pertains to food items containing health-enhancing components that have been scientifically validated for their positive impact on human physiology. While the United States embraced this concept in the 1990s, it lacked an official definition. Subsequently, European nations embraced functional food in 2006 following the implementation of regulations governing nutritional and health claims, albeit without a formal definition (Alongi & Anese, 2021; Martirosyan & Singh, 2015). The water-soluble extract derived from tomatoes, which was later branded as Fruitflow, achieved the distinction of being the inaugural product in Europe to receive a validated, exclusive health claim pursuant to Article 13(5) of the European Health Claims Regulation 1924/2006, concerning assertions made about the nutritional and health benefits of food products (Duttaroy, 2019).

According to Web of Science database, a total of 149,472 papers were published between the years 1980 and 2023, containing the "functional food" keyword (Fig. 1.1). Nearly, 70% of the articles were published in the gap of

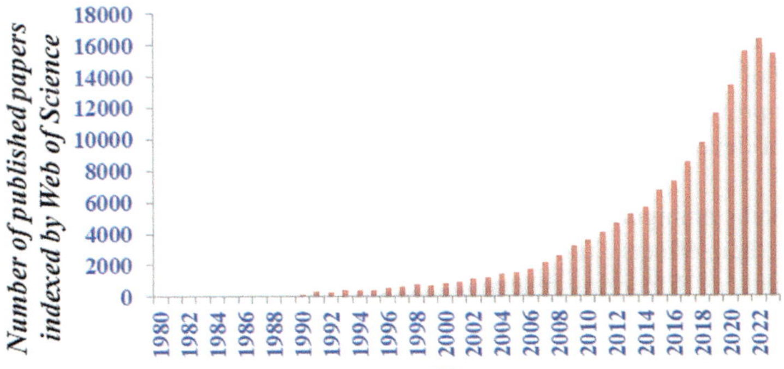

FIGURE 1.1 The number of scholarly articles that were published within the time frame of 1980–2023, which encompass the utilization of the term "functional food."

Unleashing the Power of Functional Foods and Novel Bioactives. DOI: https://doi.org/10.1016/B978-0-443-28862-3.00001-7

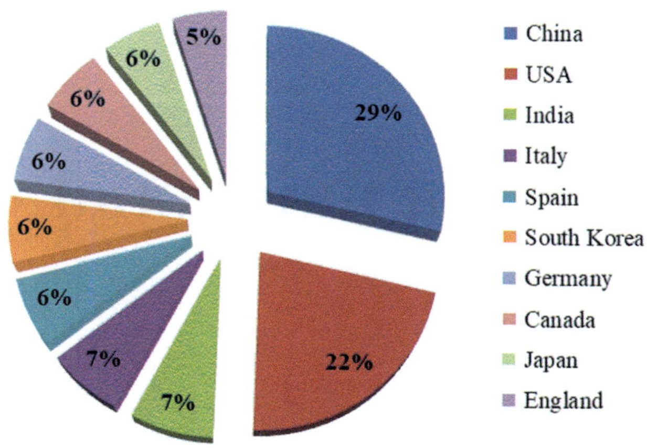

FIGURE 1.2 Distribution of papers by country.

2015–2023, and the maximum number of studies was conducted in 2023. As shown in Fig. 1.2, the leading countries in functional food research are China and the United States.

Functional foods encompass a range of advantageous substances that occur naturally in food or are added to regular diets. These substances include secondary metabolites, prebiotics, probiotics, vitamins, minerals, and amino acids. Within these foods, one can find biologically beneficial compounds such as carotenoids, fatty acids, flavonoids, phenols, phytosterols, alkaloids, and dietary fiber. The consumption of functional foods has been linked to various health benefits, including disease prevention, maintenance of healthy skin, joints, and bones, improved digestion, immune system enhancement, and promotion of longevity. Furthermore, certain functional foods have been shown to possess antioxidant, antidiabetic; cardio-, hepato-, and neuro-protective; and antimicrobial properties. It is generally acknowledged that, consuming bioactive compounds at physiological levels is safe (Motohashi et al., 2017).

1.2 Bioactive compounds in functional foods

Scientists are currently placing their attention on the significance of natural bioactive compounds, which refer to secondary metabolites obtained from seeds, food, and fermentation-based metabolic products. Various factors such as the composition of the food, the size of the molecules, environmental circumstances, and the presence of gastrointestinal material can impede the bioavailability and absorption of bioactive compounds within host cell systems and target locations. Natural bioactive compounds like flavonoids, carotenoids, and phenolic acids play a crucial role in the production of functional foods and medicinal products that hold industrial significance. Nevertheless, it is imperative to gather sufficient evidence to substantiate health claims and market functional foods on an international scale (Banwo et al., 2021).

In Fig. 1.3, the classes of bioactive molecules from different food and/or microorganism origins were illustrated. Phenolic compounds represent a significant category of partially water-soluble compounds derived from fruits and vegetables, characterized by the presence of one or more benzene rings and typically occurring in nature as glycosides (Rasouli et al., 2017). Polyphenols can be found in various plant-based foods and drinks such as berries, citrus fruits, tea, broccoli, and cocoa. These dietary polyphenols include flavonols (like quercetin found in onions), flavanones (such as hesperidin in citrus fruits), flavanols (found in cocoa, and broad beans), hydroxycinnamates (present in coffee and many fruits), and anthocyanins (commonly found in berries) (Fig. 1.4). Numerous studies, in vitro experiments, and epidemiological research provide evidence that, polyphenols play a significant role in preventing chronic diseases. For instance, flavanols regulate energy metabolism and improve reduce blood pressure and cholesterol levels. Moreover, both coffee and tea have been shown to lower the risk of developing type 2 diabetes, due to the presence of polyphenols (Williamson, 2017).

The precise mechanism of action of carotenoids remains ambiguous, although their antioxidant properties and ability to regulate gene expression have been associated with their effects. These compounds are absorbed and stored in the liver and various tissues, where they exert positive influences. Emerging research indicates that a higher intake of carotenoids may lower the susceptibility to liver diseases such as nonalcoholic fatty liver disease, characterized by dysregulated lipid metabolism resulting in lipid accumulation, lipoperoxidation, oxidative stress, and inflammatory processes (Elvira-Torales et al., 2019). Vitamin E is made up of four tocopherols and four tocotrienols, known as tocochromanols

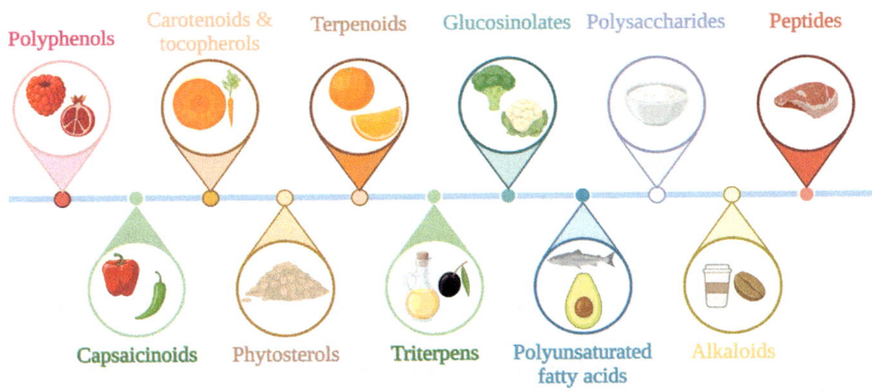

FIGURE 1.3 Food bioactive compounds from plant, animal, fungi, and bacteria origin. *Adapted from Câmara et al. (2021) and created with Biorender.com.*

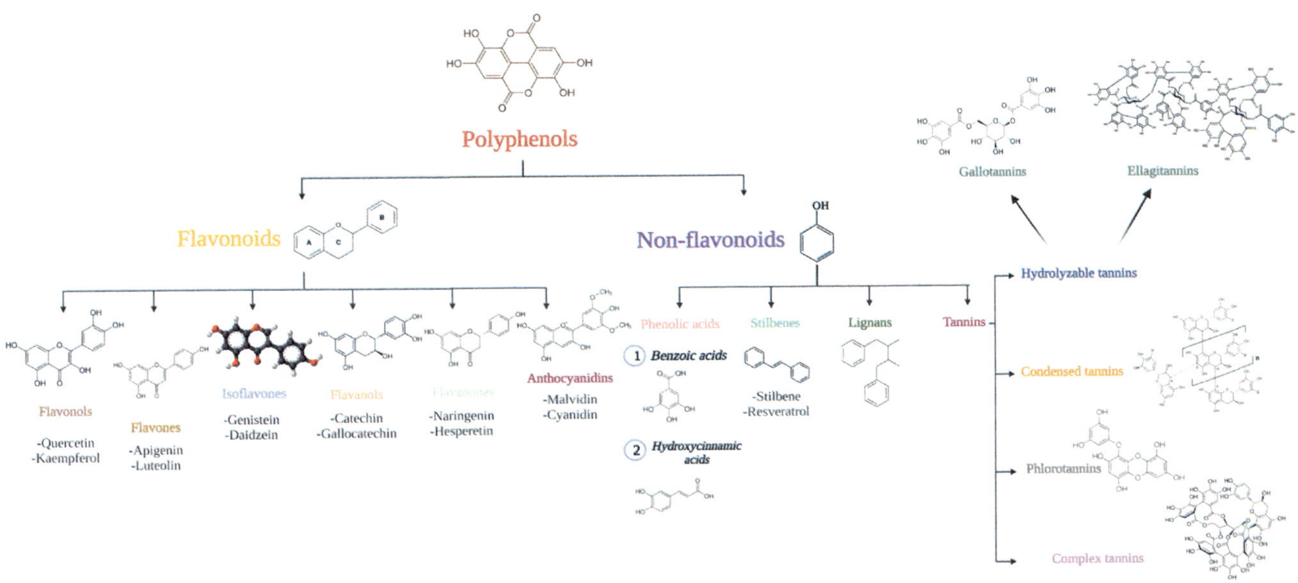

FIGURE 1.4 Categorization of polyphenols and some examples. *Adapted from Câmara et al. (2021) and created with Biorender.com.*

or tocols. These compounds are recognized for their powerful antioxidant, anticancer, immuno-stimulatory, and nephroprotective effects (Saini & Keum, 2016). Edible oils serve as the primary reservoirs of tocopherols and tocotrienols. Plant-based foods with low lipid content generally possess negligible amounts of tocols. However, seeds and byproducts obtained from the processing of plant-based foods can be employed as substitutes. Tocopherols, being vital lipid-soluble antioxidants, are primarily found in lipid-rich areas of cells, fat stores, and lipoproteins, such as low-density lipoprotein (LDL) cholesterol (Shahidi & de Camargo, 2016).

Terpenoids, also known as isoprenoids, constitute the most expansive and varied category of compounds produced by plants, fungi, sponge, and algae. These metabolites serve numerous fundamental purposes in the growth and development, while primarily being utilized for specific chemical interactions and safeguarding against abiotic and biotic factors. Historically, humans have utilized plant-derived terpenoids in the realms of food, pharmaceuticals, and chemicals. Notably, the aromatic leaves of Eucalyptus trees serve as a plentiful reservoir of these compounds (Jaeger & Cuny, 2016; Tholl, 2015).

Cruciferous vegetables have been associated with enhanced health advantages, such as shielding against cancer and cardiovascular disease. These vegetables comprise sulfur-containing plant compounds known as glucosinolates, which can be broken down into isothiocyanates by either plants or the human digestive system. The glucosinolates derived from methionine, and aromatic sources are the most frequently consumed. Research indicates that, these glucosinolates disrupt crucial mechanisms that drive the development of cancer and its spread, while also safeguarding cells against imbalances in redox that contribute to chronic inflammatory ailments (Traka, 2016).

Polysaccharides play a significant role in the composition of higher plant structures, animal cell membranes, and microbial cell walls, and they have a vital position in numerous industries, because of their therapeutic properties and minimal toxicity. They serve as an optimal foundational matrix for enhancing the functionality of foods, owing to their intricate structure and distinct capabilities (Lu et al., 2019; Shi, 2016; Yu et al., 2018). On the other hand, bioactive peptides are a category of biological compounds typically embedded within the structure of larger proteins, only becoming functional upon the enzymatic cleavage of the parent molecule. Additionally, there exists a subset of peptides that are naturally synthesized and present in various microorganisms and organisms. They are recognized for their positive effects on health, have attracted considerable attention, because of their strong affinity for tissues and targeted action. Researchers from various fields are increasingly dedicating their efforts to generate bioactive and functional peptides from various sources, including plants, animals, and by-products of the food industry. Currently, numerous bioactive peptide groups are commercially available through chemical synthesis or recombinant technology (Akbarian et al., 2022; Daliri et al., 2017; Hajfathalian et al., 2018).

Capsaicinoids are secondary compounds present in the fruits of *Capsicum* plants, which contribute to their spiciness and various health advantages. While five cultivated *Capsicum* species exist, their level of pungency may differ due to environmental factors. The *Capsicum* genus is a member of the Solanaceae family, and recent advancements in genome sequencing have unveiled the presence of inactive genes involved in capsaicinoid synthesis. The discovery of the *Capsicum annuum* genome has generated interest in biotechnological approaches to manipulate pungency. Spicy dishes hold significance in traditional cuisine across many nations, and capsaicinoids have been linked to numerous health benefits and industrial applications (Naves et al., 2019). Capcaicin activates the sympathoadrenal system which is responsible for the thermogenic and anorexigenic properties of capsaicinoids. The presence of capsaicinoids has been observed to enhance the influence of caloric restriction on the reduction of body weight (Tremblay et al., 2016).

Phytosterols, which are bioactive compounds derived from plants, have demonstrated a range of health advantages, when consumed through plant-based foods. These benefits encompass the ability to lower cholesterol levels, mitigate the risk of cardiovascular disease, and exhibit antiobesity, antidiabetic, and immunomodulatory properties. Furthermore, they hold promise as potential agents against cancer, as diets abundant in phytosterols could potentially decrease the likelihood of developing cancer by 20% (Nattagh-Eshtivani et al., 2022). Phytosterols are key players in creating crucial bioactive substances like steroidal saponins, phytoecdysteroids, and steroidal glycoalkaloids (Moreau et al., 2018).

Triterpenes, a type of secondary metabolite found in medicinal plants, have immune-boosting properties that can help protect against diseases and improve health. These compounds, found in everyday plants, can help alleviate symptoms and improve overall well-being by regulating the immune system (Renda et al., 2022). Also, related molecules have been identified as possessing multiple mechanisms for combatting diabetes, such as the inhibition of enzymes involved in glucose metabolism, the mitigation of insulin resistance, and the regulation of plasma glucose and insulin levels. Additionally, they demonstrate hypolipidemic and antiobesity effects. Furthermore, triterpenes are effective in averting diabetic complications by virtue of their potent antioxidant properties and their ability to impede the formation of advanced glycation end products, which are associated with conditions such as neuropathy and impaired wound healing (Nazaruk & Borzym-Kluczyk, 2015).

Essential fatty acids such as linoleic acid and α-linolenic acid are essential for maintaining balance within the human body. These fatty acids give rise to compounds like arachidonic acid, eicosapentaenoic acid, and docosahexaenoic acid, which are related to regulate various physiological processes. Eicosanoids, which are derived from these fatty acids, are involved in the regulation of homeostasis. Higher intake of $n-3$ polyunsaturated fatty acids may offer protection against conditions such as inflammatory diseases, cancer, cardiovascular diseases, and other chronic illnesses (Saini & Keum, 2018). Moreover, omega-3 polyunsaturated fatty acids encompass a range of essential nutrients, including α-linolenic acid, eicosapentaenoic acid, stearidonic acid, docosahexaenoic acid, and docosapentaenoic acid (Shahidi & Ambigaipalan, 2018), and are commonly found in foods such as fish, nuts, and seeds (Fig. 1.5).

Alkaloids are a class of nitrogen-containing heterocyclic compounds that are commonly extracted from plants. They are considered significant within the realm of natural products due to their abundance, varied structures, and intricacy. Alkaloids are categorized into subgroups such as isoquinolines, quinolines, indoles, and piperidine alkaloids, based on their fundamental chemical structures (Yan et al., 2021). Many alkaloids extracted from medicinal plants and herbs have been found to possess antiproliferative and anticancer properties against a diverse range of cancer types. Several alkaloids, namely vinblastine, vincristine, and vindesine, have already been effectively formulated into anticancer medications (Mondal et al., 2019).

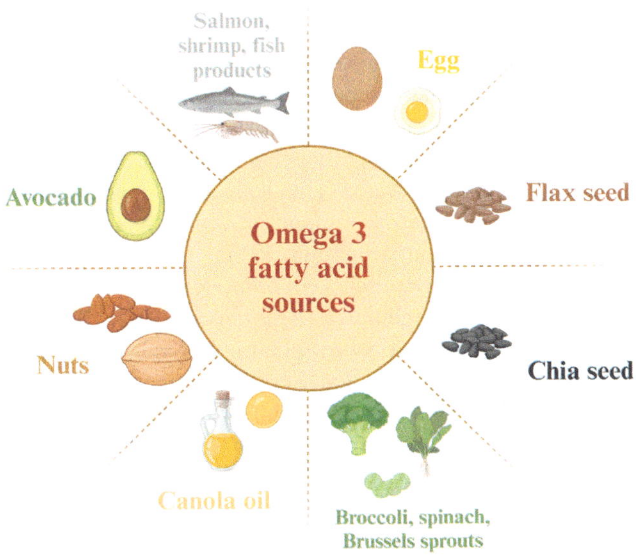

FIGURE 1.5 Several foods that contain omega-3. *Created with Biorender.com.*

Also, prebiotics, probiotics, synbiotics, and dietary fiber can be accepted as a functional food or bioactive ingredients. Extensive research conducted in recent decades has explored the health benefits of probiotics, prebiotics, and synbiotics. These functional food supplements have shown the ability to modify and restore the natural balance of intestinal flora, leading to improved intestinal function. Commonly utilized probiotic strains include *Saccharomyces boulardii*, *Bifidobacterium*, *Bacillus coagulans,* and *Lactobacilli*, while prebiotics such as galactooligosaccharides, fructooligosaccharides, and inulin are commonly used fibers that, when combined with probiotics, form synbiotics that enhance the survival of probiotics (Pandey et al., 2015).

1.3 Evolution of functional foods

Numerous research studies conducted in the 1980s identified certain food substances with tertiary physiological functions. These substances are no longer solely consumed to fulfill basic nutritional requirements, but also to prevent diet-related illnesses and enhance overall physical and mental health (Tarabella et al., 2019). Within this context, the emergence of the concept of "functional food" in Japan can be traced back to the 1980s, when the increasing healthcare costs resulting from an aging population became a concern for institutions. To address this issue, the Japanese Ministry of Education, Science and Culture took the initiative in 1984 to launch the first National Project on Functional Foods, which provided support for both basic and applied research conducted in universities. In parallel, the Ministry of Agriculture, Forestry and Fisheries also sponsored various research projects in its own institutes. In 1991, the Ministry of Health and Welfare issued a decree on "Food for Specific Health Use" (FOSHU), further emphasizing the importance of these research efforts. As a result of the findings generated from these studies, Japan subsequently established a regulatory system aimed at validating certain foods that have been shown to provide documented health benefits, with the ultimate goal of enhancing the well-being of the country's aging population (Farr, 1997; Hasler, 2002; Henry, 2010; Kubomura, 1998; Tarabella et al., 2019; Swinbanks & Obrien, 1993). Probiotics were frequently associated with enhancing gastrointestinal well-being, with claims centered on the reduction of triglycerides, hypertension, LDL cholesterol, and blood sugar levels in related years. Following the market saturation in 2007, a novel regulatory framework known as "Foods with Function Claims" was implemented in 2015, modeled after the Dietary Supplement Health and Education Act in the United States. Key assertions within this framework pertain to fatigue, cognitive function, stress management, sleep quality, circulation, body temperature regulation, and body mass index (Iwatani & Yamamoto, 2019).

Each society and/or region possesses its unique set of traditional and functional foods and dishes. The traditional foods of Türkiye, such as ayran, tarhana, bulgur, kefir, and yogurt, are rich in functional components such as phenolic compounds, vitamins, and essential oils. Many of these foods are fermented products containing probiotic lactic acid bacteria. These foods have the potential to provide various health benefits, such as reducing the risk of cardiovascular disease, lowering cholesterol and low-density lipoprotein levels, regulating intestinal function, and demonstrating antioxidant and antimicrobial properties (Göğüş et al., 2016).

Indian traditional cuisine primarily consists of plant-based foods such as vegetables, dairy products, whole grains, legumes, fruits, spices, and fermented foods. These culinary choices are rich in phytochemicals and possess substantial nutraceutical value, making them a valuable component of a balanced diet. Furthermore, the diverse cultures, languages, climates, religions, and communities in India contribute to the inclusion of these bioactive compounds in their traditional food, further enriching their dietary benefits (Gokhale et al., 2021). For instance, *Rasam*, a traditional South Indian soup, is prepared using a combination of spices including tamarind juice, chili pepper, sesame oil, mustard, tomato, garlic, cumin, turmeric, curry leaves, coriander, sea salt, asafoetida, and water. This soup holds significance as a functional food in the region, with medicinal properties attributed to it for treating a range of ailments. These claims are backed by both preclinical and clinical research studies (Devarajan & Mohanmarugaraja, 2017).

Sri Lanka possesses a plethora of leafy greens (*Aerva lanata* Linn, *Astercantha longifolia*, *Hemidesmus indicus* Linn, etc.), spices (gamboge, nutmeg, cardamom, etc.) and unique fruits and vegetables (*Benincasa hispida*, *Xanthium strumarium*, *Anacardium occidentale* L., etc.), and starch and tuber crops (cassava, sweet potato, and yam) play a vital role in the nation's food production, offering a variety of beneficial compounds. The local population consumes bioactive cereals known for their health-promoting properties. Sri Lanka presents a wealth of opportunities in the global functional food market, with untapped areas that warrant further scientific exploration to uncover their combined effects (Waisundara, 2020).

Southeast Asia is known as the food hub of Asia and is made up of 11 countries. These countries, such as Indonesia and Thailand, mainly eat rice or noodles, fruits, vegetables, fish, and herbs. Their cooking is influenced by Chinese, Indian, and Malay traditions, resulting in a mix of rich and spicy dishes. The diet in Southeast Asia is characterized by an abundance of seafood, fruits, vegetables, and the use of herbs and spices, which add flavor and nutritional advantages. Fish is a popular protein choice, while fruits and vegetables provide essential nutrients. The use of spices not only enhances taste but also adds health benefits. Overall, Southeast Asian food is considered healthy, with lower rates of obesity and heart disease, compared to Western diets. Furthermore, fermented foods high in protein, such as soybean and milk products, are commonly consumed in Asian cultures. These foods undergo fermentation with different types of starter cultures, including lactic acid bacteria, *Bacillus* species, and yeast. Through this fermentation process, a diverse range of bioactive peptides are produced, which offer various health advantages such as lowering blood pressure, combating bacterial infections, managing diabetes, and potentially preventing cancer (Kumari et al., 2022).

Numerous research studies have explored the potential predictors of consumer acceptance of functional foods, revealing a diverse array of influential factors. Nevertheless, the variability in study contexts presents obstacles to achieving a comprehensive understanding of these factors (Baker et al., 2022). Sociodemographic factors, including age, education, income levels, gender, and pricing, played a significant role in influencing consumer awareness and consumption patterns of functional foods. It is crucial to enhance consumer knowledge about the health benefits of these foods through educational initiatives. Approximately 60% of individuals lacked any awareness of functional food, with women being the most informed and engaged user demographic (Gok & Kaan Ulu, 2019). A study conducted by Siegrist et al. (2015) stated that, Chinese consumers exhibit a greater inclination towards purchasing functional foods compared to their German counterparts, with a notable portion of the German population displaying a diminished interest in these products. Individuals displaying heightened health motivation and confidence in the food industry demonstrated a heightened propensity to purchase functional foods. In China, the acceptance of functional foods is hindered by food neophobia, whereas no such correlation was identified in Germany.

1.4 Innovation in functional foods

The market for functional ingredients and foods has expanded, as a result of heightened consumer awareness regarding healthy dietary choices. Challenges persist in maintaining the activity and bioavailability of these ingredients, while postprocessing and during storage, prompting the utilization of encapsulation methods to enhance product quality. Food products have the capability to deliver bioactives and micronutrients in effective quantities, thereby offering health advantages. The choice of encapsulation techniques is influenced by the bioactive properties and desired attributes of the encapsulated and final product. It is crucial to evaluate the physicochemical properties at every stage of food processing (Celli et al., 2015; Day et al., 2009). Nanoencapsulation represents a cutting-edge development in the field of nanoscience, utilized in the food and pharmaceutical sectors to facilitate the precise release of nutrients at specific locations and times. This innovative technique offers a multitude of benefits for targeted nutrient delivery and improved bioavailability within cells (Jafari, 2017). Additionally, the incorporation of bioactive compounds into foods is a complex process, with several factors influencing their bioavailability. These factors include the composition of the matrix, the concentration of the bioactive compound, the food manufacturing process, and storage conditions (Fernandes et al.,

2019). Nevertheless, there is a limited body of research regarding the utilization of bioactive compounds as constituents of food, predominantly centered around the acquisition of said compounds and the assessment of their attributes and bioavailability (Abuajah et al., 2015; Fernandes et al., 2019). Here are the some examples of potential/popular functional food (and/or their ingredients) that can be suitable for novel products.

The concept of "superfruit" has garnered significant interest, due to its perceived health-promoting properties, prompting research into their phytochemical compositions, antioxidant capabilities, and potential health advantages. Notable superfruits encompass maqui, acerola, jaboticaba, açai, camu-camu, jambolão, noni, goji berry, and pitanga. These fruits boast a plethora of phytochemicals and antioxidant properties, positioning them as valuable functional food sources. These phytochemicals are readily absorbed and utilized by the human body, presenting promising health benefits (Chang et al., 2019).

Microalgae are significant and valuable natural reservoirs of bioactive compounds, including vitamins, amino acids, fatty acids, carotenoids, and fiber. These compounds make microalgae a highly promising and innovative resource for the development of novel food and functional products. Additionally, microalgae can be utilized as functional ingredients to augment the nutritional content of food, leading to positive impacts on human health by improving overall well-being, enhancing quality of life, and reducing the risk of diseases and illnesses (Matos et al., 2017). On the other hand, the incorporation of seaweeds, whether in powdered or extracted form, has the potential to enhance the nutritional and textural attributes of food items. They can be utilized to create low-fat products with reduced caloric content and saturated fatty acids, and the inclusion of seaweeds has demonstrated an impact on the health-related characteristics of food products (Roohinejad et al., 2017).

Bamboo, a rapidly growing plant with a significant biomass, has the potential to be utilized as a substitute for the creation of natural antioxidants. The primary antioxidants found in bamboo leaves and shoots include phenols, as well as vitamins C and E, along with essential mineral elements such as selenium, zinc, and manganese (Nirmala et al., 2018).

The research surrounding the *Moringa oleifera* Lam. plant has experienced growth as a result of its widespread usage in traditional cuisines and medicinal treatments. *M. oleifera* is recognized for its abundance of essential nutrients, such as protein, vitamins, and flavonoids. Studies have demonstrated that incorporating *M. oleifera* into diets can enhance health. Additionally, enriching processed foods with *M. oleifera* has been shown to elevate nutritional content, sensory attributes, and oxidative stability (Falowo et al., 2018).

Fenugreek, scientifically known as *Trigonella foenum-graecum*, is classified as a legume and has been historically utilized globally as a culinary spice to improve the taste of dishes. It is renowned for its various medicinal properties, including its potential as an anticarcinogenic, hypocholesterolemic, antidiabetic, antioxidant, and immunological agent. Also, it is valued for its role in creating wholesome and nourishing extruded and bakery products (Wani & Kumar, 2018). Besides that, quinoa, scientifically known as *Chenopodium quinoa* Willd., is a pseudo-grain historically utilized by Andean societies and is gaining global recognition as a functional food. Noteworthy for its rich composition of proteins, fibers, and minerals, as well as its optimal combination of essential amino acids, quinoa has been identified as a source of various phytochemicals such as saponins, phytosterols, phenolics, and bioactive peptides. These bioactive compounds have the potential to offer advantageous effects on metabolic, cardiovascular, and gastrointestinal well-being (Vilcacundo & Hernández-Ledesma, 2017). Black rice contains various phytochemicals that can be beneficial for health and may be used as functional food. These phytochemicals include anthocyanin, oryzanol, and the others. Different types of pigmented rice can help lower the risk of hyperlipidemia and hyperglycemia and prevent cancer (Pratiwi & Purwestri, 2017).

Mushrooms are renowned for their health-enhancing characteristics and substantial nutritional content, attributed to their rich composition of polysaccharides, unsaturated fatty acids, proteins, minerals, and sterols. These components are thought to offer protection against various health concerns such as immunodeficiency, cancer, hypertension, hypercholesterolemia and obesity. Recent studies have indicated a connection between these advantageous effects and the regulation of gut microbiota (Ma et al., 2018).

Goat's milk is renowned for its reduced allergenic properties and superior digestibility in comparison to cow's milk, in addition to containing beneficial compounds for health. It is suitable for use in a diverse range of products and can serve as a vehicle for functional ingredients like prebiotics or probiotics. Several studies have been conducted to investigate the therapeutic properties of goat milk, revealing its impressive biological effects (Verruck et al., 2019).

Postbiotics are substances produced by live bacteria or released, when bacteria break down. These substances include acids, enzymes, peptides and proteins. They are gaining interest, because they contain molecules that may have various health benefits, such as reducing inflammation, boosting the immune system, and fighting against high blood pressure, high cholesterol, and oxidative stress (Aguilar-Toalá et al., 2018). Also, by utilizing lactic acid bacteria, the nutraceutical content of foods can be enhanced through the careful selection of strains. Genetic modification of lactic acid bacteria enables the more effective production of nutraceuticals, leading to positive biological outcomes.

Additionally, lactic acid bacteria can serve as probiotics, delivering health advantages, when consumed in appropriate quantities (De LeBlanc et al., 2018).

3D printing offers significant freedom in design, production, and innovation in a variety of fields, including functional foods. The development of new 3D printers is critical to ensure sanitary quality and control the structure and texture of 3D-printed food products. This makes it possible to create personalized food materials adapted to different categories of the population, such as the elderly or young people (Portanguen et al., 2019).

Functional foods provide additional health benefits beyond just basic nutrition, but the frameworks for their development differ between countries, affecting how food companies approach innovation. In Europe, legal regulations play a significant role in shaping the market for functional foods. Before these products can be brought to market, they must undergo scientific evaluation, and making health cluddaims can give companies a competitive edge. Nevertheless, creating functional food products can be costly and pose various obstacles for food companies to navigate (Villaño et al., 2022). The advancement of innovative bioactive functional food products may necessitate a shift in the innovation strategies of the food industry. Traditional approaches focus on small improvements, but trends like "Health and Wellness" are attracting attention. A product-centric approach could be key in future developments, involving generating analytical knowledge and resources, collaborating with experts, and forming networks of collaboration. Open source development, collaborative research, and new management techniques can help address resource allocation and time constraints. Companies must also cultivate strong partnerships with external organizations and adopt new management techniques to establish effective connections. Successful market launch may require protecting intellectual property, enhancing brand reputation, and fostering an environment conducive to innovation and competition (Khan et al., 2013).

1.5 Health implications and research

Chronic diseases account for around 71% of global mortality. These conditions are characterized by persistent, low-level inflammation and changes in metabolism (Luvián-Morales et al., 2022). The concept of "functional foods" targets key risk factors such as high cholesterol, obesity, metabolic syndrome, diabetes, and elevated LDL cholesterol. Functional foods can help protect the heart by improving blood lipid levels, enhancing endothelial function, managing hypertension, and exerting antioxidant effects (Asgary et al., 2018). Also, these foods have been associated with antiinflammatory effects, as evidenced by experiments on cell cultures and mice; however, evidence from studies conducted on humans remains inconclusive (Luvián-Morales et al., 2022), and there is limited research on how well the active ingredients are absorbed by the body for maximum effectiveness. Baked goods such as bread, biscuits, and cake are a common choice for incorporating these ingredients, but their taste and appeal to consumers can be affected. Mixing different bioactive ingredients could help address this issue. The impact of the microbiome on health also indicates that the benefits of functional foods may vary among individuals (Birch & Bonwick, 2019). Clinical trials can offer substantial and vivid proof to establish a cause-and-effect relationship between the components found in functional foods, and the risks associated with health and disease. Although, these studies must be meticulously planned to maximize the quality of the data obtained. Two commonly utilized experimental designs are parallel and crossover, each with their own benefits. It is crucial to strike a balance between the duration of the studies, ensuring they are short enough to encourage participant compliance and cost-effectiveness, yet long enough to sufficiently assess biological effectiveness. The careful selection of dosage, frequency, and timing of intake throughout the day is of utmost importance. When conducting randomized clinical trials, it is essential to employ validated and emerging surrogate endpoints and employ appropriate statistical tests for accurate data analysis (AbuMweis et al., 2010). On the other hand, the human body possesses the ability to process various chemical substances, including biomarkers, without regard to their source, and "biomarker kinetics" can be widely adopted or recognized in the field of nutrition research focused on functional foods. Presently, decisions regarding sampling times and matrices are largely determined by customary practices and convenience rather than thorough understanding. Instances of biomarker kinetics encompass interleukin-6, malaria, polyphenols, F2-isoprostanes, cholesterol, and plasma triacylglycerides (Verhagen et al., 2004).

1.6 Challenges and opportunities

The functional foods industry is a complex and ever-evolving field, filled with both obstacles and possibilities that greatly impact its current state and future prospects which are listed as follows;

- Given their structural diversity, the methods for isolating and purifying polysaccharides differ from those used for proteins. Nonetheless, attaining uniformity is a fundamental prerequisite for investigating the structure, pharmacology, and structure–activity relationships of polysaccharides, as it is crucial for comprehending their potential applications in healthcare and food production (Shi, 2016).

- Issues such as determining the best conditions for peptide production and a lack of extensive clinical trials persist. Furthermore, considerations such as potential allergies, toxicity, and the ability of peptides to withstand digestion must be carefully examined to establish solid scientific support for health-related assertions (Daliri et al., 2017).
- The extraction and analysis procedures of phytosterols are intricate and have yet to be comprehensively established. The majority of phytosterols are obtained from plant matrices through the utilization of organic solvents, which pose risks to both human health and the environment (Uddin et al., 2018).
- Embracing innovation and harnessing technological advancements will unveil new bioactive compounds, enhancing the nourishing properties of functional foods. But, to substantiate the health proclamations tied to functional foods and their potent bioactive elements, the longing for thorough exploration is required.
- Crafting functional foods that cater to various health concerns and dietary preferences, while also tackling pressing public health issues like obesity, diabetes, and cardiovascular diseases, offers a pathway to create a profound effect.
- Despite the abundance of research on bioactive encapsulation, there remains a notable disparity between academic findings and practical application in the food industry (Celli et al., 2015).
- The integration of bioactive molecules into mainstream food items presents a significant challenge due to their limited stability and low solubility. Hence, new methods are being devised to enhance the solubility of poorly water-soluble natural products with bioactive properties. Nanotechnology has emerged as a promising solution to this issue, offering innovative means to significantly improve the solubility and bioavailability of bioactive ingredients (Fernandes et al., 2019; Recharla et al., 2017).
- The commercialization of mushroom products remains limited, with the majority of mushrooms and their compounds being consumed in their natural state or as dietary supplements. While there has been a growing interest in these products over time, their prevalence in Western countries is not as widespread as in Asia. Therefore the implementation of legislation is necessary to facilitate an increase in the consumption of mushroom products in Western markets (Reis et al., 2017).
- The main challenge in the coming years will be to develop meat products or products that combine alternative protein sources without additives, and to gain consumer acceptance of 3D printed products (Portanguen et al., 2019).
- Because of rising above the veil of ignorance and confusion that shrouds consumers, they should be enlightened on the virtues and correct application of functional foods.
- By capitalizing on the burgeoning market for functional foods, which is propelled by a rising awareness towards health and a steadily increasing elderly demographic, there exists considerable opportunity for significant market expansion and penetration.

1.7 Conclusions and future remarks

The progression of functional foods, transitioning from culturally significant traditional products to technologically advanced items, exemplifies a rapidly changing environment influenced by consumer preferences and market patterns. To ascertain the toxicological impact, therapeutic dosage, and physicochemical, chemical, and sensory attributes of a newly created food product, it is imperative for researchers to conduct an extensive range of in vitro and in vivo experiments. Moreover, it is not sufficient for food scientists to solely focus on evaluating the in vivo functionality of the food; instead, a strong and dynamic collaboration with other relevant disciplines is indispensable (Granato et al., 2017). In the future, the integration of innovative bioactive substances and the impact of biotechnology in their production have the potential to transform the health advantages offered by functional foods, although adherence to regulatory requirements will be crucial. The industry's progression and ability to meet consumer demands and public health goals will depend on seizing opportunities and overcoming challenges. To fully unlock the benefits of functional foods and new bioactive ingredients, ongoing research, partnerships, and innovative strategies are crucial. These efforts are necessary for promoting health and adapting to changing trends in nutrition and wellness.

References

Abuajah, C. I., Ogbonna, A. C., & Osuji, C. M. (2015). Functional components and medicinal properties of food: A review. *Journal of Food Science and Technology*, *52*(5), 2522–2529. Available from https://doi.org/10.1007/s13197-014-1396-5.

AbuMweis, S. S., Jew, S., & Jones, P. J. H. (2010). Optimizing clinical trial design for assessing the efficacy of functional foods. *Nutrition Reviews*, *68*(8), 485–499. Available from https://doi.org/10.1111/j.1753-4887.2010.00308.x.

Aguilar-Toalá, J. E., Garcia-Varela, R., Garcia, H. S., Mata-Haro, V., González-Córdova, A. F., Vallejo-Cordoba, B., & Hernández-Mendoza, A. (2018). Postbiotics: An evolving term within the functional foods field. *Trends in Food Science & Technology*, *75*, 105–114. Available from https://doi.org/10.1016/j.tifs.2018.03.009.

Akbarian, M., Khani, A., Eghbalpour, S., & Uversky, V. N. (2022). Bioactive peptides: Synthesis, sources, applications, and proposed mechanisms of action. *International Journal of Molecular Sciences*, *23*(3), 1445. Available from https://doi.org/10.3390/ijms23031445.

Alongi, M., & Anese, M. (2021). Re-thinking functional food development through a holistic approach. *Journal of Functional Foods*, *81*, 104466. Available from https://doi.org/10.1016/j.jff.2021.104466.

Asgary, S., Rastqar, A., & Keshvari, M. (2018). Functional food and cardiovascular disease prevention and treatment: A review. *Journal of the American College of Nutrition*, *37*(5), 429–455. Available from https://doi.org/10.1080/07315724.2017.1410867.

Ashwell, M. (2004). Concepts of functional food. *Nutrition & Food Science*, *34*(1), 47. Available from https://doi.org/10.1108/nfs.2004.34.1.47.3.

Baker, M. T., Lu, P., Parrella, J. A., & Leggette, H. R. (2022). Consumer acceptance toward functional foods: A scoping review. *International Journal of Environmental Research and Public Health*, *19*(3). Available from https://doi.org/10.3390/ijerph19031217.

Banwo, K., Olojede, A. O., Adesulu-Dahunsi, A. T., Verma, D. K., Thakur, M., Tripathy, S., Singh, S., Patel, A. R., Gupta, A. K., Aguilar, C. N., & Utama, G. L. (2021). Functional importance of bioactive compounds of foods with Potential Health Benefits: A review on recent trends. *Food Bioscience*, *43*. Available from https://doi.org/10.1016/j.fbio.2021.101320.

Birch, C. S., & Bonwick, G. A. (2019). Ensuring the future of functional foods. *International Journal of Food Science and Technology*, *54*(5), 1467–1485. Available from https://doi.org/10.1111/ijfs.14060.

Câmara, J. S., Albuquerque, B. R., Aguiar, J., Corrêa, R. C. G., Gonçalves, J. L., Granato, D., . . . Ferreira, I. (2021). Food bioactive compounds and emerging techniques for their extraction: Polyphenols as a case study. *Foods*, *10*(1), 37. Available from https://doi.org/10.3390/foods10010037.

Celli, G. B., Ghanem, A., & Brooks, M. S. L. (2015). Bioactive encapsulated powders for functional foods—A review of methods and current limitations. *Food and Bioprocess Technology*, *8*(9), 1825–1837. Available from https://doi.org/10.1007/s11947-015-1559-z.

Chang, S. K., Alasalvar, C., & Shahidi, F. (2019). Superfruits: Phytochemicals, antioxidant efficacies, and health effects—A comprehensive review. *Critical Reviews in Food Science and Nutrition*, *59*(10), 1580–1604. Available from https://doi.org/10.1080/10408398.2017.1422111.

Daliri, E. B. M., Oh, D. H., & Lee, B. H. (2017). Bioactive peptides. *Foods*, *6*(5), 1–21. Available from https://doi.org/10.3390/foods6050032.

Day, L., Seymour, R. B., Pitts, K. F., Konczak, I., & Lundin, L. (2009). Incorporation of functional ingredients into foods. *Trends in Food Science and Technology*, *20*(9), 388–395. Available from https://doi.org/10.1016/j.tifs.2008.05.002.

De LeBlanc, A. M., Luerce, T. D., Miyoshi, A., Azevedo, V., & LeBlanc, J. G. (2018). Functional food biotechnology: The use of native and genetically engineered lactic acid bacteria. In *Omics Technologies and Bio-engineering: Volume 2: Towards Improving Quality of Life*, (pp. 105–128). Argentina: Elsevier. Available from https://doi.org/10.1016/B978-0-12-815870-8.00007-3.

Devarajan, A., & Mohanmarugaraja, M. K. (2017). A comprehensive review on Rasam: A South Indian traditional functional food. *Pharmacognosy Reviews*, *11*(22), 73. Available from https://doi.org/10.4103/phrev.phrev_13_17.

Duttaroy, A. K. (2019). Regulation of functional foods in European Union: Assessment of health claim by the European food safety authority. In *Nutraceutical and Functional Food Regulations in the United States and around the World*, (pp. 267–276). Elsevier. Available from https://doi.org/10.1016/B978-0-12-816467-9.00019-8.

Elvira-Torales, L. I., García-Alonso, J., & Periago-Castón, M. J. (2019). Nutritional importance of carotenoids and their effect on liver health: A review. *Antioxidants*, *8*(7), 229. Available from https://doi.org/10.3390/antiox8070229.

Falowo, A. B., Mukumbo, F. E., Idamokoro, E. M., Lorenzo, J. M., Afolayan, A. J., & Muchenje, V. (2018). Multi-functional application of *Moringa oleifera* Lam. in nutrition and animal food products: A review. *Food Research International*, *106*, 317–334. Available from https://doi.org/10.1016/j.foodres.2017.12.079.

Farr, D. R. (1997). Functional foods. *Cancer Letters*, *114*(1–2), 59–63. Available from https://doi.org/10.1016/s0304-3835(97)04626-0.

Fernandes, S. S., Coelho, M. S., & Salas-Mellado, M. d. l. M. (2019). Bioactive compounds as ingredients of functional foods: polyphenols, carotenoids, peptides from animal and plant sources new. In *Bioactive compounds*, (pp. 129–142). Elsevier. Available from https://doi.org/10.1016/B978-0-12-814774-0.00007-4.

Göğüş, F., Ötles, S., Erdoğdu, F., & Özçelik, B. (2016). Functional and Nutritional Properties of Some Turkish Traditional Foods. In K. Kristbergsson, & S. Ötles (Eds.), *Functional Properties of Traditional Foods* (pp. 87–104). Springer Nature. Available from https://doi.org/10.1007/978-1-4899-7662-8_6.

Gok, I., & Kaan Ulu, E. (2019). Functional foods in Turkey: Marketing, consumer awareness and regulatory aspects. *Nutrition & Food Science*, *49*(4), 668–686. Available from https://doi.org/10.1108/nfs-07-2018-0198.

Gokhale, J. S., Lele, S. S., & Ananthanarayan, L. (2021). Indian traditional foods and diets: combining traditional wisdom with modern science of nutraceuticals and functional foods. In S. I. S. Rattan, & G. Kaur (Eds.), *Nutrition, Food and Diet in Ageing and Longevity. Healthy Ageing and Longevity, vol 14* (pp. 357–392). Springer, Cham Science and Business Media LLC. Available from https://doi.org/10.1007/978-3-030-83017-5_18.

Granato, D., Barba, F. J., Bursać Kovačević, D., Lorenzo, J. M., Cruz, A. G., & Putnik, P. (2020). Functional foods: Product development, technological trends, efficacy testing, and safety. *Annual Review of Food Science and Technology*, *11*, 93–118. Available from https://doi.org/10.1146/annurev-food-032519-051708.

Granato, D., Nunes, D. S., & Barba, F. J. (2017). An integrated strategy between food chemistry, biology, nutrition, pharmacology, and statistics in the development of functional foods: A proposal. *Trends in Food Science and Technology*, *62*, 13–22. Available from https://doi.org/10.1016/j.tifs.2016.12.010.

Hajfathalian, M., Ghelichi, S., García-Moreno, P. J., Moltke Sørensen, A. D., & Jacobsen, C. (2018). Peptides: Production, bioactivity, functionality, and applications. *Critical Reviews in Food Science and Nutrition*, *58*(18), 3097–3129. Available from https://doi.org/10.1080/10408398.2017.1352564.

Hasler, C. M. (2002). Functional foods: Benefits, concerns and challenges - A position paper from the American Council on Science and Health. *Journal of Nutrition*, *132*(12), 3772–3781. Available from https://doi.org/10.1093/jn/132.12.3772.

Henry, C. J. (2010). Functional foods. *European Journal of Clinical Nutrition*, *64*(7), 657–659. Available from https://doi.org/10.1038/ejcn.2010.101.

Iwatani, S., & Yamamoto, N. (2019). Functional food products in Japan: A review. *Food Science and Human Wellness*, *8*(2), 96–101. Available from https://doi.org/10.1016/j.fshw.2019.03.011.

Jaeger, R., & Cuny, E. (2016). Terpenoids with special pharmacological significance: A review. *Natural Product Communications*, *11*(9), 1373–1390. Available from https://doi.org/10.1177/1934578x1601100946.

Jafari, S. M. (2017). An overview of nanoencapsulation techniques and their classification. In *Nanoencapsulation Technologies for the Food and Nutraceutical Industries*, (pp. 1–34). Elsevier. Available from https://doi.org/10.1016/B978-0-12-809436-5.00001-X.

Khan, R. S., Grigor, J., Winger, R., & Win, A. (2013). Functional food product development - Opportunities and challenges for food manufacturers. *Trends in Food Science and Technology*, *30*(1), 27–37. Available from https://doi.org/10.1016/j.tifs.2012.11.004.

Kubomura, K. (1998). Japan redefines functional foods. *Prepared Foods*, *167*(5).

Kumari, R., Sanjukta, S., Sahoo, D., & Rai, A. K. (2022). Functional peptides in Asian protein rich fermented foods: Production and health benefits. *Systems Microbiology and Biomanufacturing*, *2*(1), 1–13. Available from https://doi.org/10.1007/s43393-021-00040-0.

Küster-Boluda, I., & Vidal-Capilla, I. (2017). Consumer attitudes in the election of functional foods. *Spanish Journal of Marketing - ESIC*, *21*, 65–79. Available from https://doi.org/10.1016/j.sjme.2017.05.002.

Lu, X., Chen, J., Guo, Z., Zheng, Y., Rea, M. C., Su, H., Zheng, X., Zheng, B., & Miao, S. (2019). Using polysaccharides for the enhancement of functionality of foods: A review. *Trends in Food Science and Technology*, *86*, 311–327. Available from https://doi.org/10.1016/j.tifs.2019.02.024.

Luvián-Morales, J., Varela-Castillo, F. O., Flores-Cisneros, L., Cetina-Pérez, L., & Castro-Eguiluz, D. (2022). Functional foods modulating inflammation and metabolism in chronic diseases: a systematic review. *Critical Reviews in Food Science and Nutrition*, *62*(16), 4371–4392. Available from https://doi.org/10.1080/10408398.2021.1875189.

Ma, G., Yang, W., Zhao, L., Pei, F., Fang, D., & Hu, Q. (2018). A critical review on the health promoting effects of mushrooms nutraceuticals. *Food Science and Human Wellness*, *7*(2), 125–133. Available from https://doi.org/10.1016/j.fshw.2018.05.002.

Martirosyan, D. M., & Singh, J. (2015). A new definition of functional food by FFC: What makes a new definition unique? *Functional Foods in Health and Disease*, *5*(6), 209–223. Available from https://doi.org/10.31989/ffhd.v5i6.183.

Matos, J., Cardoso, C., Bandarra, N. M., & Afonso, C. (2017). Microalgae as healthy ingredients for functional food: A review. *Food & Function*, *8* (8), 2672–2685. Available from https://doi.org/10.1039/c7fo00409e.

Mondal, A., Gandhi, A., Fimognari, C., Atanasov, A. G., & Bishayee, A. (2019). Alkaloids for cancer prevention and therapy: Current progress and future perspectives. *European Journal of Pharmacology*, *858*, 172472. Available from https://doi.org/10.1016/j.ejphar.2019.172472.

Moreau, R. A., Nyström, L., Whitaker, B. D., Winkler-Moser, J. K., Baer, D. J., Gebauer, S. K., & Hicks, K. B. (2018). Phytosterols and their derivatives: Structural diversity, distribution, metabolism, analysis, and health-promoting uses. *Progress in Lipid Research*, *70*, 35–61. Available from https://doi.org/10.1016/j.plipres.2018.04.001.

Motohashi, N., Gallagher, R., Anuradha, V., & Gollapudi, R. (2017). Functional foods and their importance in geriatric nutrition. *Journal of Clinical Nutrition and Metabolism*, *1*(1), 2.

Nattagh-Eshtivani, E., Barghchi, H., Pahlavani, N., Barati, M., Amiri, Y., Fadel, A., ... Ghavami, A. (2022). Biological and pharmacological effects and nutritional impact of phytosterols: A comprehensive review. *Phytotherapy Research*, *36*(1), 299–322. Available from https://doi.org/10.1002/ptr.7312.

Naves, E. R., de Ávila Silva, L., Sulpice, R., Araújo, W. L., Nunes-Nesi, A., Peres, L. E. P., & Zsögön, A. (2019). Capsaicinoids: Pungency beyond capsicum. *Trends in Plant Science*, *24*(2), 109–120. Available from https://doi.org/10.1016/j.tplants.2018.11.001.

Nazaruk, J., & Borzym-Kluczyk, M. (2015). The role of triterpenes in the management of diabetes mellitus and its complications. *Phytochemistry Reviews*, *14*(4), 675–690. Available from https://doi.org/10.1007/s11101-014-9369-x.

Nirmala, C., Bisht, M. S., Bajwa, H. K., & Santosh, O. (2018). Bamboo: A rich source of natural antioxidants and its applications in the food and pharmaceutical industry. *Trends in Food Science and Technology*, *77*, 91–99. Available from https://doi.org/10.1016/j.tifs.2018.05.003.

Pandey, K. R., Naik, S. R., & Vakil, B. V. (2015). Probiotics, prebiotics and synbiotics—A review. *Journal of Food Science and Technology*, *52*(12), 7577–7587. Available from https://doi.org/10.1007/s13197-015-1921-1.

Portanguen, S., Tournayre, P., Sicard, J., Astruc, T., & Mirade, P. S. (2019). Toward the design of functional foods and biobased products by 3D printing: A review. *Trends in Food Science and Technology*, *86*, 188–198. Available from https://doi.org/10.1016/j.tifs.2019.02.023.

Pratiwi, R., & Purwestri, Y. A. (2017). Black rice as a functional food in Indonesia. *Functional Foods in Health and Disease*, *7*(3), 182–194. Available from https://doi.org/10.31989/ffhd.v7i3.310.

Rasouli, H., Farzaei, M. H., & Khodarahmi, R. (2017). Polyphenols and their benefits: A review. *International Journal of Food Properties*, *20*, 1700–1741. Available from https://doi.org/10.1080/10942912.2017.1354017.

Recharla, N., Riaz, M., Ko, S., & Park, S. (2017). Novel technologies to enhance solubility of food-derived bioactive compounds: A review. *Journal of Functional Foods*, *39*, 63–73. Available from https://doi.org/10.1016/j.jff.2017.10.001.

Reis, F. S., Martins, A., Vasconcelos, M. H., Morales, P., & Ferreira, I. C. F. R. (2017). Functional foods based on extracts or compounds derived from mushrooms. *Trends in Food Science and Technology*, *66*, 48–62. Available from https://doi.org/10.1016/j.tifs.2017.05.010.

Renda, G., Gökkaya, İ., & Şöhretoğlu, D. (2022). Immunomodulatory properties of triterpenes. *Phytochemistry Reviews*, *21*(2), 537–563. Available from https://doi.org/10.1007/s11101-021-09785-x.

Roohinejad, S., Koubaa, M., Barba, F. J., Saljoughian, S., Amid, M., & Greiner, R. (2017). Application of seaweeds to develop new food products with enhanced shelf-life, quality and health-related beneficial properties. *Food Research International*, *99*, 1066–1083. Available from https://doi.org/10.1016/j.foodres.2016.08.016.

Saini, R. K., & Keum, Y. S. (2018). Omega-3 and omega-6 polyunsaturated fatty acids: Dietary sources, metabolism, and significance—A review. *Life Sciences*, *203*, 255–267. Available from https://doi.org/10.1016/j.lfs.2018.04.049.

Saini, R. K., & Keum, Y. S. (2016). Tocopherols and tocotrienols in plants and their products: A review on methods of extraction, chromatographic separation, and detection. *Food Research International*, *82*, 59–70. Available from https://doi.org/10.1016/j.foodres.2016.01.025.

Shahidi, F., & Ambigaipalan, P. (2018). Omega-3 polyunsaturated fatty acids and their health benefits. *Annual Review of Food Science and Technology*, *9*(9), 345–381. Available from https://doi.org/10.1146/annurev-food-111317-095850.

Shahidi, F., & de Camargo, A. C. (2016). Tocopherols and tocotrienols in common and emerging dietary sources: Occurrence, applications, and health benefits. *International Journal of Molecular Sciences*, *17*(10), 1745. Available from https://doi.org/10.3390/ijms17101745.

Shi, L. (2016). Bioactivities, isolation and purification methods of polysaccharides from natural products: A review. *International Journal of Biological Macromolecules*, *92*, 37–48. Available from https://doi.org/10.1016/j.ijbiomac.2016.06.100.

Siegrist, M., Shi, J., Giusto, A., & Hartmann, C. (2015). Worlds apart. Consumer acceptance of functional foods and beverages in Germany and China. *Appetite*, *92*, 87–93. Available from https://doi.org/10.1016/j.appet.2015.05.017.

Swinbanks, D., & Obrien, J. (1993). Japan explores the boundary between food and medicine. *Nature*, *364*(6434), 180.

Tarabella, A., Varese, E., & Buffagni, S. (2019). Functional Foods. In *Food Products Evolution: Innovation Drivers and Market Trends*, (pp. 117–142). Springer, International Publishing Science and Business Media LLC. Available from https://doi.org/10.1007/978-3-319-23811-1_9.

Tholl, D. (2015). Biosynthesis and biological functions of terpenoids in plants. In J. Schrader, & J. Bohlmann (Eds.), *Biotechnology of Isoprenoids. Advances in Biochemical Engineering/Biotechnology* (148, pp. 63–106). Springer, Cham Science and Business Media LLC. Available from https://doi.org/10.1007/10_2014_295.

Traka, M. H. (2016). Health benefits of glucosinolates. *Advances in Botanical Research*, *80*, 247–279. Available from https://doi.org/10.1016/bs.abr.2016.06.004.

Tremblay, A., Arguin, H., & Panahi, S. (2016). Capsaicinoids: A spicy solution to the management of obesity? *International Journal of Obesity*, *40*(8), 1198–1204. Available from https://doi.org/10.1038/ijo.2015.253.

Uddin, M. S., Ferdosh, S., Akanda, J. H., Ghafoor, K., Rukshana, A. H., Ali, E., ... Sarker, Z. I. (2018). Techniques for the extraction of phytosterols and their benefits in human health: a review. *Separation Science and Technology*, *53*(14), 2206–2223. Available from https://doi.org/10.1080/01496395.2018.1454472.

Verhagen, H., Coolen, S., Duchateau, G., Hamer, M., Kyle, J., & Rechner, A. (2004). Assessment of the efficacy of functional food ingredients—Introducing the concept "kinetics of biomarkers". *Mutation Research/Fundamental and Molecular Mechanisms of Mutagenesis*, *551*(1-2), 65–78. Available from https://doi.org/10.1016/j.mrfmmm.2004.01.013.

Verruck, S., Dantas, A., & Prudencio, E. S. (2019). Functionality of the components from goat's milk, recent advances for functional dairy products development and its implications on human health. *Journal of Functional Foods*, *52*, 243–257. Available from https://doi.org/10.1016/j.jff.2018.11.017.

Vilcacundo, R., & Hernández-Ledesma, B. (2017). Nutritional and biological value of quinoa (*Chenopodium quinoa* Willd). *Current Opinion in Food Science*, *14*, 1–6. Available from https://doi.org/10.1016/j.cofs.2016.11.007.

Villaño, D., Gironés-Vilapana, A., García-Viguera, C., & Moreno, D. A. (2022). Development of functional foods. In *Innovation strategies in the food industry*, (pp. 193–207). Elsevier.

Waisundara, V. Y. (2020). Traditional functional food of Sri Lanka and their health significance. In *Nutritional and Health Aspects of Food in South Asian Countries*, (pp. 143–158). Sri Lanka: Elsevier. Available from https://doi.org/10.1016/B978-0-12-820011-7.00020-4.

Wani, S. A., & Kumar, P. (2018). Fenugreek: A review on its nutraceutical properties and utilization in various food products. *Journal of the Saudi Society of Agricultural Sciences*, *17*(2), 97–106. Available from https://doi.org/10.1016/j.jssas.2016.01.007.

Williamson, G. (2017). The role of polyphenols in modern nutrition. *Nutrition Bulletin*, *42*(3), 226–235. Available from https://doi.org/10.1111/nbu.12278.

Yan, Y., Li, X., Zhang, C., Lv, L., Gao, B., & Li, M. (2021). Research progress on antibacterial activities and mechanisms of natural alkaloids: A review. *Antibiotics*, *10*(3), 318. Available from https://doi.org/10.3390/antibiotics10030318.

Yu, Y., Shen, M., Song, Q., & Xie, J. (2018). Biological activities and pharmaceutical applications of polysaccharide from natural resources: A review. *Carbohydrate Polymers*, *183*, 91–101. Available from https://doi.org/10.1016/j.carbpol.2017.12.009.

Chapter 2

The science behind functional foods: unraveling the nutritional secrets

Khaoula Elhadef[1], Sarra Akermi[1], Moufida Chaari[1], Elahesadat Hosseini[2,3], Diyar Salahuddin Ali[4,5], Hajer ben Hlima[6], Teresa D'Amore[7], Lotfi Mellouli[1] and Slim Smaoui[8]

[1]*Laboratory of Microbial Biotechnology and Engineering Enzymes (LMBEE), Center of Biotechnology of Sfax (CBS), University of Sfax, Sfax, Tunisia,* [2]*Department of Chemical Engineering, Payame Noor University, Tehran, Iran,* [3]*Department of Food Science and Technology, National Nutrition and Food Technology Research Institute, Faculty of Nutrition Science and Food Technology, Shahid Beheshti University of Medical Sciences, Tehran, Iran,* [4]*Department of Chemistry, College of Science, Salahaddin University-Erbil, Erbil, Kurdistan Region, Iraq,* [5]*Department of Pharmacy, College of Pharmacy, Knowledge University, Erbil, Kurdistan Region, Iraq,* [6]*Laboratory of Enzymatic Engineering and Microbiology, Algae Biotechnology Unit, Biological Engineering Department, National School of Engineers of Sfax, 3038, University of Sfax, Sfax, Tunisia,* [7]*Laboratory of Preclinical and Translational Research, IRCCS CROB, Centro di Riferimento Oncologico della Basilicata, Rionero in Vulture, Italy,* [8]*Laboratory of Microbial, Enzymes Biotechnology and Biomolecules (LMEBB), Centre of Biotechnology of Sfax (CBS), University of Sfax, Sfax, Tunisia*

2.1 Introduction

Growing public awareness regarding the impact of food on human health has led to a notable trend toward the consumption of high-quality, value-added food products, specifically those offering significant health benefits, commonly known as functional foods (Mirzapour-Kouhdasht et al., 2023). There has been a shift in the demand for food as people's living levels rise, prioritizing health and diversity over quantity and taste. This development highlights the urgent need for novel food products that can address a variety of dietary requirements and health problems (Ashraf et al., 2021; Liu et al., 2024). For this reason, the relationship between food's bioactive substances and health has been the focus of a lot of study in recent years. Customers are looking for food products that not only meet their nutritional needs but also provide extra health advantages as they become more conscious of the importance of nutrition for overall wellbeing (Ali & Ali, 2020; Vlaicu et al., 2023). These bioactivity-enhanced functional foods have shown potential in increasing well-being, minimizing the risk of many diseases, and increasing physical performance (Banwo et al., 2021). Functional foods are produced in both marine and terrestrial settings. However, a lot of research has been done on terrestrial resources such as fruits, vegetables, grains, probiotics, and mushrooms. Products derived from marine organisms are becoming more and more popular because of their particular biochemical substances, which set them apart from terrestrial metabolites (Ghosh et al., 2022; Ullah & Khan, 2023). The wide range of bioactive substances found in functional food, each with unique physiological effects, has been demonstrated by recent research. Probiotics, phytochemicals, omega-3 fatty acids, antioxidants, and polyphenols are a few other examples of substances that are essential for maintaining and preventing illness (Adetuyi et al., 2022; Aziz et al., 2024). Furthermore, there is strong evidence from recent research that functional foods can help prevent chronic illnesses, promote general wellness, and improve quality of life (Munekata et al., 2021).

The goal of this study is to investigate the physiological and biochemical properties of functional foods. This chapter also looks at how they affect particular aspects of human health, like the immune system, the gastrointestinal system, the cardiovascular system, and the brain (Fig. 2.1). In addition, the regulatory framework controlling functional foods in the United States, Japan, and Europe was examined, offering a thorough grasp of the norms and regulations established in these countries. For certain items, a specific, harmonized rule is required. Nutraceuticals and functional foods all have health-promoting qualities and may be useful in the treatment of chronic illnesses.

Unleashing the Power of Functional Foods and Novel Bioactives. DOI: https://doi.org/10.1016/B978-0-443-28862-3.00002-9

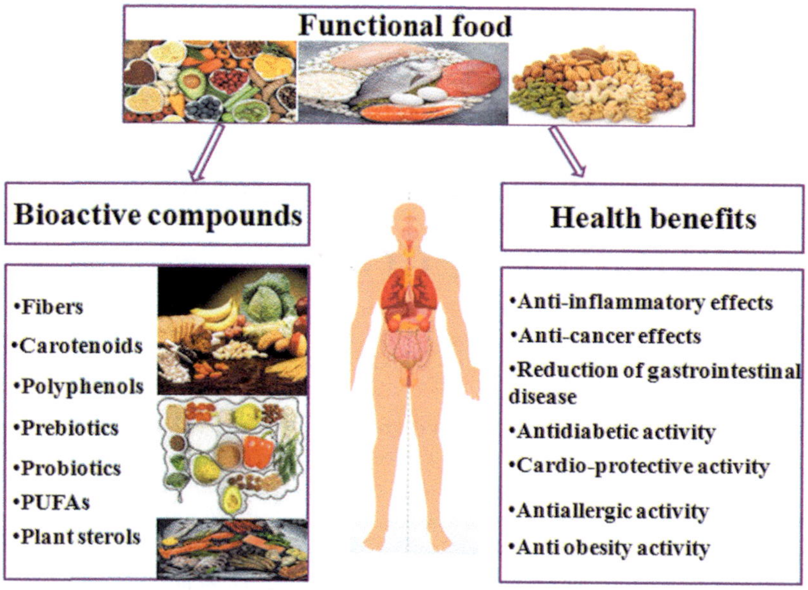

FIGURE 2.1 Bioactive compounds and health benefits in functional food.

TABLE 2.1 Functional food definitions.

Functional food definition	References
Foods that could be healthier than what is required for basic nutrition	Bailey (1999)
"If it is satisfactorily demonstrated to affect beneficially one or more target functions in the body, beyond adequate nutritional effects," a food can be considered functional.	Saher et al. (2004)
Functional foods are natural or industrially processed foods that, when regularly consumed at efficacious levels within a diverse diet, have potentially positive effects on health beyond basic nutrition	Granato et al. (2020)
A food product is only considered functional if every one of its attributes improves overall physical and/or general conditions for humans, or lowers the likelihood that infectious diseases will develop	Luvián-Morales et al. (2022)

2.2 Functional foods

Functional foods, often referred to as nutraceuticals, are foods that are rich in bioactive substances that improve the health of their consumers (Onoruoiza, 2024). Japan is the first nation that has developed a distinct regulatory approval procedure for functional foods to date. Food products to which functional elements have been added to elicit specific health benefits are referred to as "Foods for Specified Health Use" (FOSHU) by the Japanese (Bailey, 1999). Different definitions of functional food have emerged over time as a result of global research activities. These definitions have been put forth by different authorities (Table 2.1).

Functional food was defined by Saher et al. (2004) as any food product that goes beyond simple nutritional impacts and has been convincingly shown to positively influence one or more specific processes within the body. Recently, Granato et al. (2020) defined functional foods as industrially processed or natural foods regularly consumed with a diverse diet and linked with positive health effects. The following requirements are the primary conditions for an ingredient or product meeting a certain functional claim on a food label (Granato et al., 2020): (1) food security, (2) accessible without a prescription (or guidance from a doctor), and (3) proof that consuming it on a regular basis in a balanced diet has health benefits. According to Luvián-Morales et al. (2022), a food product is only considered functional if every one of its attributes improves overall physical and/or general conditions for humans or lowers the likelihood that infectious diseases will develop.

2.3 Health benefit associated with functional foods

Due to an increasing amount of scientific data, our comprehension of the health advantages associated with functional foods has grown dramatically in recent years. Although the idea of choosing foods based on their ability to promote health has long been understood, functional foods are only just beginning to be acknowledged as a separate category with unique health benefits (Knaggs & Lephart, 2023). This change in perception is a result of developments in epidemiology and nutritional science that have clarified the function of bioactive substances in maintaining health and avoiding disease (Laguna et al., 2021).

Numerous research studies have exhibited the diverse health-promoting attributes of functional foods, underscoring their significance in preserving human well-being across different stages of life.

2.3.1 Dietary fiber

Dietary fiber (DF) constitutes a diverse spectrum of bioactive compounds found abundantly in various fruits and vegetables. It comprises lignans and plant polysaccharides resistant to hydrolysis by human digestive enzymes (Table 2.2). While definitions may vary, the American Association of Cereal Chemists characterizes fiber as the edible components of plants or similar carbohydrates resistant to digestion and absorption in the human small intestine, undergoing partial or complete fermentation in the large intestine (Yegin et al., 2020). Its consumption as part of a balanced diet holds the potential to mitigate certain health conditions such as diabetes, hypertension, and coronary diseases. Consequently, DF is considered a promising avenue for the creation of novel food products, supplements, and functional ingredients. Its consumption as part of a balanced diet holds the potential to mitigate certain health conditions such as diabetes, hypertension, and coronary diseases. Consequently, DF is increasingly considered as a promising avenue for the creation of novel food products, supplements, and functional ingredients (Subiria-Cueto et al., 2021). It also encompasses extending the product's shelf life in storage by preventing oxidation and microbiological growth, as noted by Das et al. (2021). In meat food processing, these useful additives enhance the nutritional and functional value of meat products in addition to influencing their physicochemical properties. For instance, Madane et al. (2019) observed a decrease in pH levels in chicken nuggets over a span of 20 days with the utilization of drumstick (*Moringa oleifera*) flower extracts as DF. In addition, drumstick flower extracts enhance emulsion stability and result in higher cooking yields compared to the control, with percentages of 97.83% and 97.26%, respectively, versus 96.79% for the control. DF is also added to meat products to increase the cooking yield owing to greater water and fat retention properties. When added to meat, DF prevents a significant loss of fat and water during cooking which aids in improving the texture of food products (Ferdaus et al., 2024). Soleimanian et al. (2022) reported that the addition of an oat-bran ingredient blended into ground beef and pork sausages resulted in increased cooking yield. Moreover, different sources of DFs influence the gut microbiota in different ways.

Citrus pectin increased the abundance of Bacteroidetes, but apple pectin boosted the population of Clostridiales and decreased that of *Bacteroides* spp. in the gut (Cui et al., 2019). Additionally, water-soluble fiber components, including pectins and β-glucans, are linked to a positive health effect that lowers blood cholesterol levels (Vuksan et al., 2011).

A diet high in soluble fiber reduces the incidence of obesity, type 2 diabetes, and cardiovascular disease (Grube et al., 2013). For instance, soluble fiber from oats decreased blood cholesterol concentration and its accessibility for lipoprotein formation (Whitehead et al., 2014). In individuals with hypercholesterolemia, a daily dose of 3 g of soluble DF from oats reduced total blood cholesterol content by 10.5 mg/dL, whereas in individuals without lipid problems, it fell by 3.4 mg/dL (Earnshaw et al., 2017). Moreover, it has been demonstrated that β-glucans produced from bacteria, yeasts, and oats can improve immunity and control diabetes (Bai et al., 2019; Bozbulut & Sanlier, 2019; Ishimoto et al., 2018). Chronic constipation is caused by a low-fiber diet and affects about 30% of persons 65 years of age and older; women are more likely to have this condition. Furthermore, the fecal abundance of *Bacteroides, Prevotella*, and *Porphyromonas* was considerably raised by broccoli fiber, inulin, potato fiber, potato-resistant starch, garlic (*Allium sativum),* Jerusalem artichoke (*Helianthus tuberosus*), and onions (Shoaib et al., 2016).

2.3.2 Carotenoids

Carotenoids, versatile isoprenoids crucial for both food quality and health promotion, underscore the necessity to establish recommended dietary intakes or nutritional reference values. The three hydrocarbon carotenes (lycopene, α-carotene, and β-carotene) and the three oxygenated xanthophylls (β-cryptoxanthin, zeaxanthin, and lutein) are the main carotenoids found in food and the ones that have been investigated in relation to human health

TABLE 2.2 Major bioactive compounds present in functional food and their physiological impact on human health.

	Sources	Food matrix	Benefits	References
Fibers	Fibers	Chicken nuggets fortified by drumstick flower (*Moringa oleifera*)	Lowering the pH level in meat products enhances emulsion stability and results in higher cooking yields compared to the control, with percentages of 97.83% and 97.26%, respectively, versus 96.79% for the control	Madane et al. (2019)
	Pectin	Citrus	Prebiotic effect: increased the abundance of *Bacteroidetes*	Zhang et al. (2018)
		Apple	Prebiotic effect: increased the population of *Clostridiales* and decreased the abundance of *Bacteroides spp.* in the rat gut	Lopez-Siles et al. (2012)
	β-Glucans from yeast		Modulates the immune system	Ishimoto et al. (2018)
	β-Glucans	Oats	Reduces the probability of cardiovascular disease, obesity, and type 2 diabetes	Jędrusek-Golińska et al. (2020)
	β-Glucans	Oats	Manages diabetes and immune system modulating	Bozbulut and Sanlier (2019), Bai et al. (2019)
	Inulin	Garlic (*Allium sativum*) Jerusalem artichoke (*Helianthus tuberosus*) Onions (red and white)	Prebiotic effect, reduction in risk of gastrointestinal diseases, enhance absorption of calcium, magnesium, and iron	Shoaib et al. (2016)
Carotenoids	β-Carotene	Raw carrot (*Daucus carota*)	Antimutagenic, antitumoral, and antiulcer effect on human health	López-Romero et al. (2018)
		Carrot, orange mango	Precursor of vitamin A, antioxidant activity, chemotherapeutic potential, etc.	Dias and Paulo Silva Cunha (2018), Meléndez-Martínez (2019), Kim (2016)
	Curcumin	Curcuma	Antiinflammatory activity, hepatoprotective effects, etc.	Salehi et al. (2019)
	Lutein	Present in vegetables fruits, cereals and egg yolk	Antioxidant activity, antiinflammatory properties, improve eye health	Buscemi et al. (2018)
	Zeaxanthin	Fruits and vegetables, human milk	Improved ocular and cognitive health in humans	Conboy Stephenson et al. (2021)

Polyphenols	Flavonoids such as anthocyanins, catechins, flavanols, flavones, flavanones, and isoflavones	Red wine, pomegranate, cranberry, grapefruit juice, and dark bitter chocolate	Neutralize free radicals and decrease cancer risk by arresting cellular growth in tumors	Perez-Gregorio and Simal-Gandara (2017)
	Anthocyanins	Red and blue fruits and vegetables, in particular red grapes, blueberries, cherries, and raspberries	Antiinflammatory properties and produce positive vascular effects	Cassidy (2018)
	Anthocyanin from Schott fruits (*Rubus ulmifolius*)	Bakery product	Potential antimicrobial and antitumor effects observed in certain tumor cell lines	Silva et al. (2019)
	Flavan-3-ols	Tea, nuts, cocoa (chocolate), grapes (wine), and legumes	Reduce the risk for diabetes, and cardiovascular-related outcomes	Kelm et al. (2006), Larsson et al. (2016)
	Stilbenes	Grapes, red wine, and berries	Antiinflammatory and antioxidant actions	Tome-Carneiro et al. (2013), Bonkowski and Sinclair (2016)
	Catechin	Green tea	Antioxidant, antidiabetic, antiobesity, antiinflammatory, anticancer, antimicrobial, and antiallergic activities	Xiong et al. (2017), Rashidinejad et al. (2021)
	Luteolin	Fruits and vegetables	Antiinflammatory activity	Fei et al. (2019)
	Caffeic acid and chlorogenic acid	Fruits and vegetables	Cardio-protective and antioxidant properties	Agunloye et al. (2019)
	Kaempferol	Fruits and vegetables	Antidiabetic activity	Sharma et al. (2019)
Prebiotics	Oligofructose, lactulose, inulin, proteins, functional peptides, lipids	Onions, whole grains, garlic, honey, banana	Converted by gut microbes to release other bioactive metabolites; selectively promote the growth of beneficial bacteria	Peng et al. (2020)
	Lactulose, mannitol, Oligosaccharides (inulin), fibers	Chicory root, *Jerusalem artichokes*, raw garlic, onions, and whole wheat products	Improve intestinal health may be able to counteract several metabolic disorders linked to obesity, may modulate the gut endocrine function, affecting satiety, and may act in the prevention of colonic cancer risk	Guimarães et al. (2020)

(*Continued*)

TABLE 2.2 (Continued)

	Sources	Food matrix	Benefits	References
Probiotics	Lactic acid bacteria		Treatment of gastrointestinal disorders	Dahiya and Nigam (2022)
	Lactobacillus spp. *Bifidobacterium spp.* *Bacillus subtilis* *Pediococcus acidilactici* *Bacillus clausii* *Streptococcus thermophilus*	Orange juice, cheese, Ice cream	Provide beneficial effects for the reduction of gastrointestinal disease, exert different immunomodulatory activity, support heart health, prevent carcinogenesis, improve depression symptoms	Guimarães et al. (2020)
Polyunsaturated fatty acids	Omega-3s	Fatty fish such as salmon, tuna, fish oil supplements, ground flax seeds, ground chia seeds, walnuts	Brain development, antiinflammatory effects	Kapoor et al. (2021).
	Omega-6s	Vegetable oil, sunflower seeds	Required for normal blood flow and healthy inflammation	
	omega-3 FA	Varieties of fish, including herring, mackerel, bluefish, salmon, sardines, trout, tuna, and anchovy oil, alongside plant-based sources like chia seeds, flaxseeds, canola oil, walnuts, soybean oil, and algae	Reducing the risk of certain heart and circulatory problems	Jędrusek-Golińska et al. (2020)
Plant sterols	β-Sitosterol, stigmasterol and campesterol	Plant oils, soy seeds, nuts, fruits, and vegetables	Lowering of LDL cholesterol levels in the bloodstream	Trautwein et al. (2018)

(Meléndez-Martínez, 2019). The most prevalent and significant provitamin A carotenoid is β-carotene. Dark green leafy vegetables like kale, spinach, and lettuce, as well as orange and yellow vegetables like carrots and several pepper kinds, are common fruits with high or extremely high concentrations of β-carotene (López-Monterrubio et al., 2021). Among vegetables, the top contributors are carrots (both raw and cooked), providing 573 mg/day, and offering antimutagenic, antitumoral, and antiulcer effects beneficial to human health (López-Romero et al., 2018). Moreover, β-carotene found in carrots, oranges, and mangoes serves as a precursor to vitamin A, a vital nutrient. Consequently, products rich in provitamin A carotenoids play a pivotal role in addressing vitamin A deficiency, offering antioxidant properties, and exhibiting chemotherapeutic potential (Dias & Paulo Silva Cunha, 2018; Kim, 2016; Meléndez-Martínez, 2019). Numerous clinical trials have been conducted to assess curcumin's bioactive effects in a range of inflammatory disorders. Curcumin is widely known for its hepatoprotective and antiinflammatory properties. One of the most often studied diseases is arthritis, a chronic illness that usually causes inflammation in the joints, leading to joint degeneration and disability (Salehi et al., 2019). Establishing recommended dietary intakes for bioactives such as carotenoids, particularly lutein and zeaxanthin, is crucial. These dietary carotenoids play a vital role in maintaining eye health and preventing age-related cataracts and macular degeneration, thanks to their anti-inflammatory and antioxidant properties. They are naturally synthesized and can be found abundantly in corn, specific wheat species, as well as in orange, yellow, and green leafy vegetables, with smaller quantities present in some fruits (Buscemi et al., 2018; Conboy Stephenson et al., 2021).

2.3.3 Polyphenols

Plants produced secondary metabolites known as polyphenolic chemicals, which are a broad class of molecules with various structural variations. Apart from their numerous health benefits as antihypertensive, antimicrobial, antiobesity, and antidiabetic effects in both humans and animals, polyphenols are also known for their antioxidant properties, which, when taken in moderation, inhibit the production of reactive oxygen species (ROS) and avert a host of diseases, including cancer.

Plant-based polyphenols are highly significant functional ingredients in our diet. A broad class of bioactive phytochemicals known as polyphenols is made up of several subclasses, including lignans, flavonoids, stilbenes, and phenolic acids (Fig. 2.2). The flavonoids, which are based structurally on a 15-carbon skeleton of a chromane ring connected to a second aromatic ring, are one of the most researched classes of polyphenols. Flavonoids can be further categorized into distinct subgroups based on their chemical structures, such as isoflavones, flavanones, flavan-3-ols, flavonols, flavones, and anthocyanins.

The majority of flavonoids come from different foods, including fruits, vegetables, grains, and spices. Notably, pomegranate, cranberry, grapefruit juice, red wine, and dark bitter chocolate with a cacao level higher than 70% are significant sources of flavonoids (Bahari et al., 2024). Flavonoids can affect oxidative stress by preserving the hemodynamic and biochemical functions of the cell. They indirectly chelate copper and iron ions, which prevents the formation of hydroxyl radicals, interrupts the free radical reactions cascade in enzymatic and nonenzymatic lipid peroxidation, and protects low molecular weight antioxidants (e.g., ascorbate in the cytosol and α-tocopherol in biological membranes) against oxidation. Thusflavonoids could potentially decrease the risk for CVD, neurological diseases, some

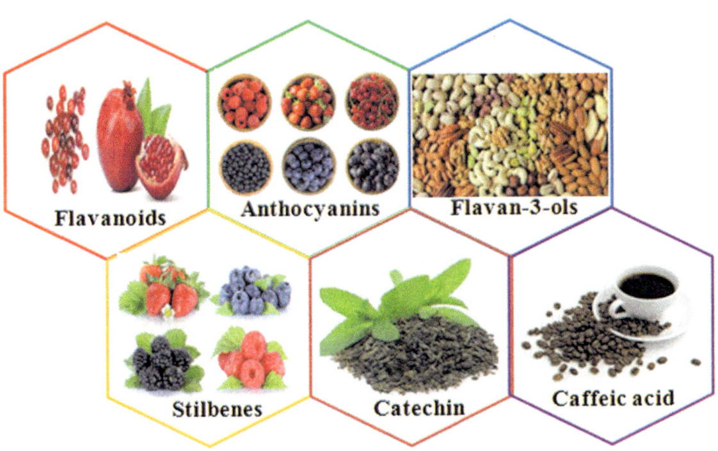

FIGURE 2.2 Major sources and classification of phenolic compounds.

cancers, and diabetes type 2. Flavonoids have been observed to modulate oxidative stress by safeguarding the hemodynamic and biochemical integrity of cells. Their mechanism involves the indirect chelation of iron ions and copper, consequently inhibiting the generation of hydroxyl radicals.

Additionally, flavonoids shield low molecular weight antioxidants, such as ascorbate in the cytosol and α-tocopherol in biological membranes, from oxidation. Consequently, their potential extends to mitigating the risk of neurological disorders, cardiovascular diseases, type 2 diabetes, and certain cancers (Perez-Gregorio & Simal-Gandara, 2017).

Red and blue fruits and vegetables, including blueberries, eggplant, cherries, strawberries, and black grapes, are the primary sources of anthocyanins. Like other polyphenols, anthocyanins are transformed into active metabolites with antiinflammatory and beneficial vascular effects by the host and microbiome after ingestion (Cassidy, 2018). Large consumption of anthocyanins has been associated with a lower incidence of myocardial infarction in men and women, as well as positive effects on a number of cardiovascular risk factors, according to Cassidy et al. (2016). Moreover, when incorporated into bakery products, the anthocyanin-rich extract from Schott fruits exhibited potential antibacterial and anticancer effects in certain tumor cell lines (Silva et al., 2019). Observational studies have demonstrated that the consumption of flavan-3-ols from a variety of dietary sources, such as almonds, tea, grapes (wine), cocoa (chocolate), and legumes, contributes to favorable cardiometabolic outcomes. One of these benefits is a decreased chance of developing diabetes and heart-related illnesses (Larsson et al., 2016).

In addition, the main sources of stilbene include berries, red wine, and grapes. Stilbene has been studied extensively and has drawn interest due to its suggested modes of action, which include cytokine release inhibition, resulting in antioxidant and antiinflammatory actions. One noteworthy mode of action is stilbene's stimulation of sirtuins, which is associated with delaying the aging process (Bonkowski & Sinclair, 2016; Tome-Carneiro et al., 2013). Green tea, the least processed variety, is renowned for having a high concentration of antioxidants, which are derived from polyphenols, especially catechins. Of them, epigallocatechin-3-gallate stands out as the most effective catechin in green tea, attributed to its numerous health advantages, including its ability to fight cancer and diabetes as well as reduce inflammation. Because green tea catechins are very labile in both gastrointestinal and environmental settings, their chemical stability and bioavailability are mostly dependent on the conditions of processing and formulation (Rashidinejad et al., 2021; Xiong et al., 2017).

A number of epidemiological studies have suggested that eating foods high in luteolin on a regular basis is associated with a lower risk of developing chronic diseases. Moreover, numerous studies have revealed the anti-inflammatory characteristics of luteolin, which are especially noticeable in ailments like acute pancreatitis, acute lung damage, and autoimmune thyroiditis (Fei et al., 2019). Also, two significant components of hydroxycinnamic acid are caffeic acid and chlorogenic acid (CHA). They are taken out of vegetables and fruits. According to Agunloye et al. (2019), caffeic and chlorogenic acids have antihypertensive qualities that are typified by their capacity to lower blood pressure, their ability to reduce the activity of some important enzymes involved in the pathophysiology of hypertension, and their ability to protect cells from oxidative damage.

Kaempferol, as shown in Table 2.2, is a natural flavonol found abundantly in different fruits, vegetables, wine, and tea varieties. It is sourced from various plants such as grapefruit, broccoli, propolis, witch-hazel, and others. For decades, plants rich in kaempferol have been utilized for their beneficial properties, including antiinflammatory, antioxidant, lipolytic, and anticancer effects.

Polyphenols derived from diverse plant sources exhibit a protective influence against specific types of cancer (Fig. 2.2). They not only hinder tumor growth but also exert cytotoxic effects on cancer cells, prompting apoptosis and enhancing the activity of various enzymes involved in combating cancer (Oteiza et al., 2018). Nevertheless, elevated doses of certain polyphenols may demonstrate a pro-oxidant effect, along with cytotoxic and apoptotic effects, particularly targeting cancer cells. This scenario also presents an opportunity for utilizing polyphenols in the treatment of such diseases.

2.3.4 Prebiotics

Prebiotics are described as food ingredients, such as nondigested starch, oligosaccharides, and nonstarch polysaccharides, that can specifically promote the growth and/or activity of intestinal bacterial strains capable of digesting those (Ángeles Stegmayer et al., 2023). Prebiotics are similarly ingested to enable bacteria to specifically use them and boost the host's health (Gibson et al., 2017). Prebiotics have the power to enhance probiotics' capacity for survival, development, metabolism, and other health-promoting functions within the digestive tract. The most well-known dietary examples are nonactive food ingredients that are preferentially fermented in the colon, including their hydrolysates and the polymers galactooligosaccharides, xylooligosaccharides, lactulose, inulin, and fructooligosaccharides (Peng et al., 2020).

Nondigestible oligosaccharides, such as fructooligosaccharides (inulin), galactooligosaccharides, xylooligosaccharides, cyclodextrins, and lactulose, are recognized as prebiotics. Oligosaccharides can be found in common foods such as chicory root, Jerusalem artichokes, raw garlic, onions, and whole wheat products. They play a role in improving intestinal health, potentially mitigating various metabolic disorders associated with obesity, modulating gut endocrine function to influence satiety, and may contribute to the prevention of colorectal cancer risk (Guimarães et al., 2020).

2.3.5 Probiotics

Single or mixed cultures of living bacteria are known as probiotics, and when consumed in sufficient proportions, they can change the gut microbiota and offer some health advantages to the host. Live bacteria in probiotic products are present in higher quantities 5×10^{9}CFU/day for 5 days to get health benefits (Jędrusek-Golińska et al., 2020).

The most popular probiotics are found in yogurts, kefir, buttermilk, acidophilus milk, fermented cabbage, pickles, tempeh, miso, and kombucha. They also include strains of Lactobacillus and/or *Bifidobacterium* and, less frequently, Escherichia, Enterococcus, or Bacillus (Zawistowska-Rojek et al., 2016)

Probiotics, such as lactic acid bacteria, have been linked to enhanced immune function. They are also used to treat gastrointestinal diseases like diarrhea, constipation, and diverticular disease by inhibiting pathogens in the intestine. Additionally, probiotics have demonstrated the ability to enhance microbiota composition (Dahiya & Nigam, 2022). The health advantages linked to a particular probiotic strain may not automatically extend to another strain. Hence, it is crucial to specify which strain has been incorporated into fermented products. Achieving the health benefits associated with probiotics necessitates maintaining a proper balance of microflora in the digestive system (Clements & Carding, 2018; Stavropoulou & Bezirtzoglou, 2019). Additionally, according to Guimarães et al. (2020), probiotics such as *Bifidobacterium spp., Lactobacillus spp., Bacillus subtilis, and Streptococcus thermophilus* have demonstrated the capacity to reduce gastrointestinal illness, exert various immunomodulatory activities, support heart health, prevent carcinogenesis, and alleviate symptoms of depression.

Additionally linked to a lower incidence of colon cancer, hypertension, and urinary tract infections, probiotics help lower cholesterol and may shield against allergies (Jędrusek-Golińska et al., 2020).

2.3.6 Polyunsaturated fatty acids

Omega-3 and omega-6 FAs are the two main kinds of polyunsaturated fats (PUFAs). Supplementing with omega-3 FAs is beneficial to the cardiovascular system in both healthy individuals and patients with CVD. More precisely, α-linolenic acid from plant-based meals and omega-3 FA from oily fish marginally decreased serum triglyceride and increased HDL concentration (Fig. 2.3) (Abdelhamid et al., 2018). Significant sources of omega-3 fatty acids such as fish, including herring, bluefish, mackerel, sardines, salmon, tuna, trout, and anchovy oil, were described (Cetin et al., 2024). On the other hand, flaxseeds, chia seeds, canola and soybean oil, walnuts, algae, sea buckthorn, camelina, and avocados are some of the main plant sources of alpha-linolenic acid (Koeder & Perez-Cueto, 2024). During infancy and old age, PUFAs are essential for the growth and operation of the heart, brain, and other organs (Jędrusek-Golińska

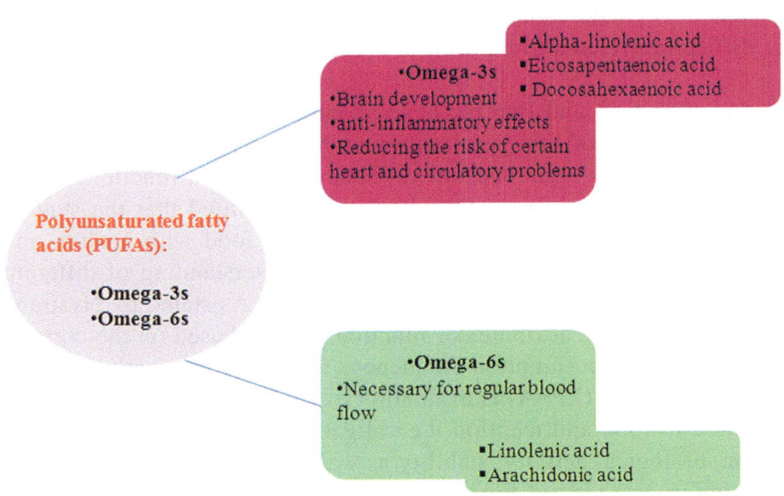

FIGURE 2.3 Polyunsaturated fatty acids types and their functions.

et al., 2020; Kapoor et al., 2021; Nestel et al., 2015). Moreover, according to research by Kapoor et al. (2021), omega-6s from sunflower seeds and vegetable oil are necessary for both good inflammation and regular blood flow. Furthermore, increased consumption of alpha-linolenic acid (such as from enriched margarine or walnuts) may lead to a slight reduction in the risk of certain heart and circulatory diseases. However, it appears to have minimal to no impact on all-cause mortality, cardiovascular or coronary deaths, coronary incidents, and metaregression or subgrouping analyzes have not confirmed any effects related to duration or dose (Abdelhamid et al., 2018). The ratio of omega-3 to omega-6 FA in the diet is the subject of further dietary guidelines. A balanced diet should include a 4:1 to 5:1 ratio of necessary omega-6 to omega-3 FA, according to FAO/WHO (Gogus & Smith, 2010). Supplementing the diet with PUFAs may promote health and regeneration of the nerve cell membrane in older individuals (over 50) with minor memory impairment or Alzheimer's disease, thereby potentially slowing down the aging processes affecting the brain (Yurko-Mauro et al., 2015).

2.3.7 Plant sterols

Potentially effective alternative therapeutics for decreasing total plasma cholesterol and preventing CVDs have drawn a lot of attention to functional foods with cholesterol-lowering potential. Consuming foods high in plant sterols, such as phytostanols (Ogbe, 2015) and phytosterols (such as β-sitosterol, campesterol, and stigmasterol), which have the structure of steroid alcohols, is one alternative (Chanioti et al., 2021). Major sources of plant sterols in the diet include plant oils, soy seeds, nuts, fruits, and vegetables. An average serving of vegetables typically provides between 100 and 350 mg of phytosterols and 20 and 50 mg of phytostanols (Baumgartner et al., 2013). Phytosterols distinguish themselves from cholesterol by featuring an additional methylene group (as in campesterol and campestanol) or an ethylene group (as in sitosterol and sitostanol). Additionally, they may contain one or two double bonds in their chain, leading to slower absorption in the digestive tract. Research by Trautwein et al. (2018) demonstrated that an intake of plant sterols (2 g/day) resulted in a reduction in LDL cholesterol levels in patients aged 58.7 $\pm$ 10.4 years with or at risk of type 2 diabetes. Phytosterols have been added to manufacture food products by a number of regulatory authorities worldwide, including the Food and Drug Administration (FDA) in the United States, in an effort to lower blood cholesterol levels (AbuMweis et al., 2014). Nevertheless, there is no conclusive evidence supporting the notion that plant sterols and stanols reduce the risk of CVDs. Additionally, some investigations suggest a potential increased risk of atherosclerosis with rising concentrations of phytosterols in serum (Cabral & Klein, 2017). It is noteworthy that plant stanols, which are saturated forms of plant sterols, appear to be more effective than sterols in lowering total blood cholesterol levels. Table 2.2 summarizes some recent examples of functional properties with their physiological health impact.

2.4 Regulatory framework of functional food

The increase in global population density has led to an expansion of food consumption and a shortage of resources in some other countries. This situation created a serious challenge and a competitive state in food industry and market to meet the needs of consumers and to fulfill the intensive demand of functional foods that have health promoting benefits and a preventive impact against nutrition-related diseases (Domínguez Díaz et al., 2020). For that reason, new legislations and robust regulations were suggested and applied to create certainties between both manufacturers and consumers. However, legislative authorities faced many difficulties related to the lack of a dedicated category for functional foods (Martirosyan & Alvarado, 2023).

In this regard, different countries, including Japan, America, and Europe, have adopted various regulation strategies and models related to functional food. Taking the example of European countries, Norway applied the theory of planned behavior (TPB) framework to predict and evaluate Norwegian consumers' behaviors toward functional food. This strategy aimed to explain individual intentions and attitudes especially when it was admitted that the studied population is highly doubtful toward manufactures that claims the production of proceeded food with healthy and high nutritional values (Nystrand & Olsen, 2020). In fact, the TPB model facilitates the understanding of different norms related to consumers' motivation to consume functional food by using a hedonic scale. As stated by Nystrand and Olsen (2020), the food industry could better enhance hedonic attributes of functional foods based on the correlation between several factors such as attitudes, self-efficacy, consumption frequency, and utilitarian eating values. Moreover, the main purpose of European Food Safety Authority (EFSA) is evaluation of health claim applications. In this regard, it made many rules and instructions related to food and mention the obligation of including information about the source, chemical structure and composition, biological activity, stability as well as the manufacturing treatment and process. On this basis, the European regulation categorized functional food based on different norms and general food laws. In this context, fortifying food and the existent nutrients with other ingredients that have beneficial characteristics (e.g., the enrichment of juice with vitamins or milk with calcium) falls under the European Regulation (EC) 1925/2006. This latter dictated the list of the approved herbal extracts, vitamins, and minerals that could be incorporated into foodstuffs. The regulation (EU) 2015/2283 described the functional foods that was treated by a novel processes or other elements (Duttaroy, 2019). In addition, the USA adopted only the requirements described by the Federal Food, Drug and Cosmetic Act (1938) (last amendment was in 2018). Concerning Japan, it was the first country that invented the Food with Health Claims (FHC) system to impose interesting and specific approval process and rules for functional foods. In this basis, FHC aimed to categorize functional food in two major groups. The first one is known as FOSHU, and the second one is called Foods with Nutrient Function Claims (FNFC). Article 21 of the Ordinance for Enforcement of the Food Sanitation Act defined the essential rules and requirements to follow by manufacturers to guarantee the approvement of their products by the Minister of Consumer Affairs Agency. These requirements should meet the healthy and hygienic conditions by ensuring the effectiveness, high quality, and safety of the offered food for human consumption to improve the quality of the population's diet and health (Shimizu, 2019). The second direction is related to FNFC which specified the standards that allow the marketing of the food product without filling an application or registration (Inbathamizh et al., 2022). Therefore regulatory guidelines set by the governments is imperatively crucial which guarantee the safety and quality standards for consumers resulting in industry growth and the decrease in food related diseases (Namdeo, 2020).

2.5 Future perspectives

Within the quickly developing field of nutritional science, scientists are exploring foods with bioactive substances that provide unique health benefits above and beyond those of basic nutrition. These foods are known as functional foods. Interdisciplinary cooperation, modern technologies, and a better comprehension of the complex interplay linking health and diet. Personalized nutrition is becoming more and more popular in healthcare approaches. Research shows that dietary interventions can be tailored to each person's genetic profile, metabolic phenotype, and lifestyle choices, greatly improving their overall health (Bakrim et al., 2023). This individualized strategy for eating functional foods provides an opportunity to decrease the risk of illness and meet the nutritional requirements for each individual.

Furthermore, the development of Omics technologies, including proteomics, metabolomics, and genomes, is transforming our knowledge of the molecular processes that underlie the health advantages of functional foods (Hernández-Alonso et al., 2019). Through the identification of complex relationships between dietary elements and biological systems, systems biology methodologies are facilitating the creation of focused functional food treatments. Furthermore, nutrigenomics and epigenetics provide insights into how dietary choices might impact gene expression and epigenetic alterations, influencing individuals' health paths (Caradonna et al., 2020). Subsequent investigations will concentrate on pinpointing the epigenetic indicators of dietary intervention reactions and creating specific functional food plans for illness prevention and control.

The creation of sustainable functional foods is becoming more and more important as worries about ethical food production and environmental sustainability grow (Wezel et al., 2020). To secure the long-term viability of functional food sources, future initiatives will concentrate on streamlining food production systems, cutting waste, and encouraging biodiversity protection. Simultaneously, the incorporation of digital health methods, including sensors and smartphone apps, is revolutionizing the management of health and dietary tracking (Khalil et al., 2023). With the help of these instruments, people may monitor their diets, metabolic processes parameters, and health consequences throughout, giving them the power to choose functional foods and make educated dietary decisions.

In conclusion, the field of functional food science has a bright future ahead of it thanks to developments in nutrigenomics, digital health, omics technologies, personalized nutrition, and sustainability. We may create the foundation for a future that is healthier and more robust by discovering the nutritional secrets of functional foods and utilizing their therapeutic potential.

2.6 Conclusion

The greatest strategy to prevent nutrient shortages and keep good health is to eat a balanced diet. This work is challenging due to physiological alterations brought on by dreams and an elevated risk of chronic illnesses. Therefore taking functional foods and/or dietary supplements that have been altered or enhanced in their nutritional or other bioactive chemical content presents an alluring alternative that may help prevent or treat chronic illnesses. Omega-3 PUFA, carotenoids, phytosterols, and dietary fiber are all enhanced in functional food products. A number of recently developed functional food categories aim to prevent or reduce the risk of noncommunicable diseases like cancer, diabetes type 2, and cardiovascular disease (CVD). Other functional foods target hypercholesterolemia as a particular condition. The fast-growing group is foods supplemented with prebiotics and probiotics, associated with gut health and well-being of population.

Nevertheless, functional food product labels have the ability to include health-related statements, which is a crucial way to educate customers about the connections between nutrition and health. Certain regulations must be in place to control it, as these claims seem to affect customers' food choices.

References

AbuMweis, S. S., Marinangeli, C. P. F., Frohlich, J., & Jones, P. J. H. (2014). Implementing phytosterols into medical practice as a cholesterol-lowering strategy: Overview of efficacy, effectiveness, and safety. *Canadian Journal of Cardiology*, *30*(10), 1225–1232. Available from https://doi.org/10.1016/j.cjca.2014.04.022.

Adetuyi, B., Oluwafemi, G. O., Odine., Olajide, P. A., Adetuyi., Atanda., & Oloke. (2022). Nutraceuticals: Role in metabolic disease, prevention and treatment. *World News of Natural Sciences*, *42*, 1–27.

Ángeles Stegmayer, M., Sirini, N., Frizzo, L. S., Fernández-López, J., Pérez Álvarez, J. Á., Rosmini, M. R., & Soto, L. P. (2023). *Enrichment of foods with prebiotics Strategies to Improve the Quality of Foods* (pp. 171–201). Argentina: Elsevier. Available from https://www.sciencedirect.com/book/9780443153464, https://doi.org/10.1016/B978-0-443-15346-4.00007-0.

Ashraf, S. A., Siddiqui, A. J., Elkhalifa, A. E. O., Khan, M. I., Patel, M., Alreshidi, M., Moin, A., Singh, R., Snoussi, M., & Adnan, M. (2021). Innovations in nanoscience for the sustainable development of food and agriculture with implications on health and environment. *Science of The Total Environment*, *768*(May), 144990. Available from https://doi.org/10.1016/j.scitotenv.2021.144990.

Abdelhamid, A. S., Brown, T. J., Brainard, J. S., Biswas, P., Thorpe, G. C., Moore, H. J., Deane, K. H. O., AlAbdulghafoor, F. K., Summerbell, C. D., Worthington, H. V., Song, F., & Hooper, L. (2018). Omega-3 fatty acids for the primary and secondary prevention of cardiovascular disease. *Cochrane Database of Systematic Reviews*, *2018*(7). Available from https://doi.org/10.1002/14651858.cd003177.pub3.

Agunloye, O. M., Oboh, G., Ademiluyi, A. O., Ademosun, A. O., Akindahunsi, A. A., Oyagbemi, A. A., Omobowale, T. O., Ajibade, T. O., & Adedapo, A. A. (2019). Cardio-protective and antioxidant properties of caffeic acid and chlorogenic acid: Mechanistic role of angiotensin converting enzyme, cholinesterase and arginase activities in cyclosporine induced hypertensive rats. *Biomedicine & Pharmacotherapy*, *109*, 450–458. Available from https://doi.org/10.1016/j.biopha.2018.10.044.

Ali, T., & Ali, J. (2020). Factors affecting the consumers' willingness to pay for health and wellness food products. *Journal of Agriculture and Food Research*, *2*, 100076. Available from https://doi.org/10.1016/j.jafr.2020.100076.

Aziz, T., Hussain, N., Hameed, Z., & Lin, L. (2024). Elucidating the role of diet in maintaining gut health to reduce the risk of obesity, cardiovascular and other age-related inflammatory diseases: Recent challenges and future recommendations. *Gut Microbes*, *16*(1), 2297864. Available from https://doi.org/10.1080/19490976.2023.2297864.

Bahari, H., Pourreza, S., Goudarzi, K., Mirmohammadali, S. N., Asbaghi, O., Hosseini Kolbadi, K. S., Naderian, M., & Hosseini, A. (2024). The effects of pomegranate consumption on obesity indices in adults: A systematic review and meta-analysis. *Food Science & Nutrition*, *12*, 641–660. Available from https://doi.org/10.1002/fsn3.3739.

Bai, J., Ren, Y., Li, Y., Fan, M., Qian, H., Wang, L., Wu, G., Zhang, H., Qi, X., Xu, M., & Rao, Z. (2019). Physiological functionalities and mechanisms of β-glucans. *Trends in Food Science & Technology*, *88*, 57–66. Available from https://doi.org/10.1016/j.tifs.2019.03.023.

Bailey, R. (1999). Foods for specified health use (FOSHU) as functional foods in Japan: Japan has a regulatory framework for the growing area of "Functional Foods.&quot. *Canadian Chemical News*, *51*(5), 18–20, 1999.

Bakrim, S., Aboulaghras, S., Aanniz, T., Benali, T., El Omari, N., El-Shazly, M., Lee, L.-H., et al. (2023). Effects of Mediterranean diets and nutrigenomics on cardiovascular health. *Critical Reviews in Food Science and Nutrition*, 1–20. Available from https://doi.org/10.1080/10408398.2023.2187622.

Banwo, K., Olojede, A. O., Adesulu-Dahunsi, A. T., Verma, D. K., Thakur, M., Tripathy, S., Singh, S., Patel, A. R., Gupta, A. K., Aguilar, C. N., & Utama, G. L. (2021). Functional importance of bioactive compounds of foods with Potential Health Benefits: A review on recent trends. *Food Bioscience*, *43*, 101320. Available from https://doi.org/10.1016/j.fbio.2021.101320.

Baumgartner, S., Mensink, R. P., Husche, C., Lütjohann, D., & Plat, J. (2013). Effects of plant sterol- or stanol-enriched margarine on fasting plasma oxyphytosterol concentrations in healthy subjects. *Atherosclerosis*, *227*, 414–419. Available from https://doi.org/10.1016/j.atherosclerosis.2013.01.012.

Bonkowski, M. S., & Sinclair, D. A. (2016). Slowing ageing by design: The rise of NAD + and sirtuin-activating compounds. *Nature Reviews. Molecular Cell Biology*, *17*(11), 679–690. Available from https://doi.org/10.1038/nrm.2016.93.

Bozbulut, R., & Sanlier, N. (2019). Promising effects of β-glucans on glyceamic control in diabetes. *Trends in Food Science & Technology*, *83*, 159–166. Available from https://doi.org/10.1016/j.tifs.2018.11.018.

Buscemi, S., Corleo, D., Di Pace, F., Petroni, M. L., Satriano, A., & Marchesini, G. (2018). The effect of lutein on eye and extra-eye health. *Nutrients*, *10*, 1321. Available from https://doi.org/10.3390/nu10091321.

Cabral, C. E., & Klein, M. R. S. T. (2017). Phytosterols in the treatment of hypercholesterolemia and prevention of cardiovascular diseases. *Arquivos Brasileiros de Cardiologia 109 (November): 475–82*. Available from https://doi.org/10.5935/abc.20170158.

Caradonna, F., Consiglio, O., Luparello, C., & Gentile, C. (2020). Science and healthy meals in the world: Nutritional epigenomics and nutrigenetics of the Mediterranean diet. *Nutrients*, *12*(6), 1748. Available from https://doi.org/10.3390/nu12061748.

Cassidy, A. (2018). Berry anthocyanin intake and cardiovascular health. *Molecular Aspects of Medicine, Bioactives and their Impact on Human Health*, *61*(June), 76–82. Available from https://doi.org/10.1016/j.mam.2017.05.002.

Cassidy, A., Bertoia, M., Chiuve, S., Flint, A., Forman, J., & Rimm, E. B. (2016). Habitual intake of anthocyanins and flavanones and risk of cardiovascular disease in men. *The American Journal of Clinical Nutrition*, *104*(3), 587–594. Available from https://doi.org/10.3945/ajcn.116.133132.

Cetin, I., Carlson, S. E., Burden, C., da Fonseca, E. B., di Renzo, G. C., Hadjipanayis, A., Harris, W. S., et al. (2024). Omega-3 fatty acid supply in pregnancy for risk reduction of preterm and early preterm birth. *American Journal of Obstetrics & Gynecology MFM*, *6*, 101251. Available from https://doi.org/10.1016/j.ajogmf.2023.101251.

Chanioti, S., Katsouli, M., & Tzia, C. (2021). Chapter 9 - β-Sitosterol as a Functional Bioactive. In M. Mushtaq, & F. Anwar (Eds.), *A centum of valuable plant bioactives* (edited by, pp. 193–212). Academic Press. Available from https://doi.org/10.1016/B978-0-12-822923-1.00014-5.

Clements, S. J., & Carding, S. R. (2018). Diet, the intestinal microbiota, and immune health in aging. *Critical Reviews in Food Science and Nutrition*, *58*, 651–661. Available from https://doi.org/10.1080/10408398.2016.1211086.

Conboy Stephenson, R., Ross, R. P., & Stanton, C. (2021). Carotenoids in milk and the potential for dairy based functional foods. *Foods*, *10*, 1263. Available from https://doi.org/10.3390/foods10061263.

Cui, J., Lian, Y., Zhao, C., Du, H., Han, Y., Gao, W., Xiao, H., & Zheng, J. (2019). Dietary fibers from fruits and vegetables and their health benefits via modulation of gut microbiota. *Comprehensive Reviews in Food Science and Food Safety*, *18*, 1514–1532. Available from https://doi.org/10.1111/1541-4337.12489.

Dahiya, D., & Nigam, P. S. (2022). The gut microbiota influenced by the intake of probiotics and functional foods with prebiotics can sustain wellness and alleviate certain ailments like gut-inflammation and colon-cancer. *Microorganisms*, *10*, 665. Available from https://doi.org/10.3390/microorganisms10030665.

Das, A., Baidya, R., Chakraborty, T., Samanta, A. K., & Roy, S. (2021). Pharmacological basis and new insights of taxifolin: A comprehensive review. *Biomedicine & Pharmacotherapy*, *142*(October), 112004. Available from https://doi.org/10.1016/j.biopha.2021.112004.

Dias, D., & Paulo Silva Cunha, J. (2018). Wearable health devices—Vital sign monitoring, systems and technologies. *Sensors*, *18*, 2414. Available from https://doi.org/10.3390/s18082414.

Domínguez Díaz, L., Fernández-Ruiz, V., & Cámara, M. (2020). The frontier between nutrition and pharma: The international regulatory framework of functional foods, food supplements and nutraceuticals. *Critical Reviews in Food Science and Nutrition*, *60*, 1738–1746. Available from https://doi.org/10.1080/10408398.2019.1592107.

Duttaroy, A. K. (2019). Chapter 19 - Regulation of Functional Foods in European Union: Assessment of Health Claim by the European Food Safety Authority. In D. Bagchi (Ed.), *Nutraceutical and functional food regulations in the United States and around the World (Third Edition)* (edited by, pp. 267–276). Academic Press. Available from https://doi.org/10.1016/B978-0-12-816467-9.00019-8.

Earnshaw, S. R., McDade, C. L., Chu, Y. F., Fleige, L. E., & Sievenpiper, J. L. (2017). Cost-effectiveness of maintaining daily intake of oat β-glucan for coronary heart disease primary prevention. *Clinical Therapeutics*, *39*, 804–818.e3. Available from https://doi.org/10.1016/j.clinthera.2017.02.012.

Fei, J., Liang, B., Jiang, C., Ni, H., & Wang, L. (2019). Luteolin inhibits IL-1β-induced inflammation in rat chondrocytes and attenuates osteoarthritis progression in a rat model. *Biomedicine & Pharmacotherapy*, *109*(January), 1586–1592. Available from https://doi.org/10.1016/j.biopha.2018.09.161.

Ferdaus, M. J., Barman, B., Mahmud, N., & da Silva, R. C. (2024). Oleogels as a promising alternative to animal fat in saturated fat-reduced meat products: A review. *Gels*, *10*(2), 92. Available from https://doi.org/10.3390/gels10020092.

Ghosh, S., Sarkar, T., Pati, S., Kari, Z. A., Edinur, H. A., & Chakraborty, R. (2022). Novel bioactive compounds from marine sources as a tool for functional food development. *Frontiers in Marine Science*, *9*(February). Available from https://doi.org/10.3389/fmars.2022.832957.

Gibson, G., Hutkins, R., Sanders, M., Prescott, S., Reimer, R., Salminen, S., Scott, K., et al. (2017). The International Scientific Association for Probiotics and Prebiotics (ISAPP) consensus statement on the definition and scope of prebiotics. *Department of Food Science and Technology: Faculty Publications*, January. Available from https://digitalcommons.unl.edu/foodsciefacpub/234.

Gogus, U., & Smith, C. (2010). N-3 omega fatty acids: A review of current knowledge. *International Journal of Food Science & Technology*, *45*, 417–436. Available from https://doi.org/10.1111/j.1365-2621.2009.02151.x.

Granato, D., Barba, F. J., Bursać Kovačević, D., Lorenzo, J. M., Cruz, A. G., & Putnik, P. (2020). Functional foods: Product development, technological trends, efficacy testing, and safety. *Annual Review of Food Science and Technology*, *11*, 93–118. Available from https://doi.org/10.1146/annurev-food-032519-051708.

Grube, B., Chong, P.-W., Lau, K.-Z., & Orzechowski, H.-D. (2013). A natural fiber complex reduces body weight in the overweight and obese: A double-blind, randomized, placebo-controlled study. *Obesity*, *21*, 58–64. Available from https://doi.org/10.1002/oby.20244.

Guimarães, J. T., Balthazar, C. F., Silva, R., Rocha, R. S., Graça, J. S., Esmerino, E. A., Silva, M. C., et al. (2020). Impact of probiotics and prebiotics on food texture. *Current Opinion in Food Science, Sensory Science & Consumer Perception • Food Physics and Material Science*, *33*(June), 38–44. Available from https://doi.org/10.1016/j.cofs.2019.12.002.

Hernández-Alonso, P., Giardina, S., Cañueto, D., Salas-Salvadó, J., Cañellas, N., & Bulló, M. (2019). Changes in plasma metabolite concentrations after a low-glycemic index diet intervention. *Molecular Nutrition & Food Research*, *63*, 1700975. Available from https://doi.org/10.1002/mnfr.201700975.

Inbathamizh, L., Prabavathy, D., & Sudha, S. (2022). *Quality assurance of nutraceuticals and their approval, registration, marketing. Handbook of nutraceuticals and natural products* (pp. 337–360). John Wiley & Sons, Ltd. Available from https://doi.org/10.1002/9781119746843.ch27.

Ishimoto, Y., Ishibashi, K.-ichi, Yamanaka, D., Adachi, Y., Kanzaki, K., Iwakura, Y., & Ohno, N. (2018). Production of low-molecular weight soluble yeast β-glucan by an acid degradation method. *International Journal of Biological Macromolecules*, *107*(February), 2269–2278. Available from https://doi.org/10.1016/j.ijbiomac.2017.10.094.

Jędrusek-Golińska, A., Górecka, D., Buchowski, M., Wieczorowska-Tobis, K., Gramza-Michałowska, A., & Szymandera-Buszka, K. (2020). Recent progress in the use of functional foods for older adults: A narrative review. *Comprehensive Reviews in Food Science and Food Safety*, *19*, 835–856. Available from https://doi.org/10.1111/1541-4337.12530.

Kapoor, B., Kapoor, D., Gautam, S., Singh, R., & Bhardwaj, S. (2021). Dietary polyunsaturated fatty acids (PUFAs): Uses and potential health benefits. *Current Nutrition Reports*, *10*, 232–242. Available from https://doi.org/10.1007/s13668-021-00363-3.

Kelm, M. A., Johnson, J. C., Robbins, R. J., Hammerstone, J. F., & Schmitz, H. H. (2006). High-performance liquid chromatography separation and purification of cacao (*Theobroma cacao* L.) procyanidins according to degree of polymerization using a diol stationary phase. *Journal of Agricultural and Food Chemistry*, *54*, 1571–1576. Available from https://doi.org/10.1021/jf0525941.

Khalil, N. M. A., Mohd Mydin, F. H., & Moy, F. M. (2023). Healthy adults' views and experiences on behavior change strategies in mobile applications for diet monitoring: A single centre qualitative study. *PLoS One*, *18*, e0292390. Available from https://doi.org/10.1371/journal.pone.0292390.

Kim, J. K. (2016). An update on the potential health benefits of carotenes. *EXCLI Journal*, *15*. Available from https://doi.org/10.17179/EXCLI2015-664, *Doc1; ISSN 1611-2156*.

Knaggs, H., & Lephart, E. D. (2023). Enhancing skin anti-aging through healthy lifestyle factors. *Cosmetics*, *10*, 142. Available from https://doi.org/10.3390/cosmetics10050142.

Koeder, C., & Perez-Cueto, F. J. A. (2024). Vegan nutrition: A preliminary guide for health professionals. *Critical Reviews in Food Science and Nutrition*, *64*, 670–707. Available from https://doi.org/10.1080/10408398.2022.2107997.

Laguna, J. C., Alegret, M., Cofán, M., Sánchez-Tainta, A., Díaz-López, A., Martínez-González, M. A., Sorlí, J. V., et al. (2021). Simple sugar intake and cancer incidence, cancer mortality and all-cause mortality: A cohort study from the PREDIMED trial. *Clinical Nutrition*, *40*, 5269–5277. Available from https://doi.org/10.1016/j.clnu.2021.07.031.

Larsson, S. C., Åkesson, A., Gigante, B., & Wolk, A. (2016). Chocolate consumption and risk of myocardial infarction: A prospective study and meta-analysis. *Heart (British Cardiac Society)*, *102*, 1017–1022. Available from https://doi.org/10.1136/heartjnl-2015-309203.

Liu, B., Yang, H., Zhu, C., Xiao, J., Cao, H., Simal-Gandara, J., Li, Y., Fan, D., & Deng, J. (2024). A comprehensive review of food gels: Formation mechanisms, functions, applications, and challenges. *Critical Reviews in Food Science and Nutrition*, *64*, 760–782. Available from https://doi.org/10.1080/10408398.2022.2108369.

Lopez-Siles, M., Khan, T. M., Duncan, S. H., Harmsen, H. J. M., Garcia-Gil, L. J., & Flint, H. J. (2012). Cultured representatives of two major phylogroups of human colonic faecalibacterium prausnitzii can utilize pectin, uronic acids, and host-derived substrates for growth. *Applied and Environmental Microbiology*, *78*, 420–428. Available from https://doi.org/10.1128/AEM.06858-11.

Luvián-Morales, J., Varela-Castillo, F. O., Flores-Cisneros, L., Cetina-Pérez, L., & Castro-Eguiluz, D. (2022). Functional foods modulating inflammation and metabolism in chronic diseases: A systematic review. *Critical Reviews in Food Science and Nutrition*, *62*, 4371–4392. Available from https://doi.org/10.1080/10408398.2021.1875189.

López-Monterrubio, D. I., Lobato-Calleros, C., Vernon-Carter, E. J., & Alvarez-Ramirez, J. (2021). Influence of β-carotene concentration on the physicochemical properties, degradation and antioxidant activity of nanoemulsions stabilized by whey protein hydrolyzate-pectin soluble complexes. *LWT*, *143*(May), 111148. Available from https://doi.org/10.1016/j.lwt.2021.111148.

López-Romero, D., Izquierdo-Vega, J. A., Morales-González, J. A., Madrigal-Bujaidar, E., Chamorro-Cevallos, G., Sánchez-Gutiérrez, M., Betanzos-Cabrera, G., Alvarez-Gonzalez, I., Morales-González, Á., & Madrigal-Santillán, E. (2018). Evidence of some natural products with antigenotoxic effects. Part 2: Plants, vegetables, and natural resin. *Nutrients*, *10*, 1954. Available from https://doi.org/10.3390/nu10121954.

Madane, P., Das, A. K., Pateiro, M., Nanda, P. K., Bandyopadhyay, S., Jagtap, P., Barba, F. J., Shewalkar, A., Maity, B., & Lorenzo, J. M. (2019). Drumstick (Moringa Oleifera) flower as an antioxidant dietary fibre in chicken meat nuggets. *Foods*, *8*, 307. Available from https://doi.org/10.3390/foods8080307.

Martirosyan, D., & Alvarado, A. (2023). Functional foods regulation system: Proposed regulatory paradigm by functional food center. *Functional Food Science - Online*, *3*, 275–287. Available from https://doi.org/10.31989/ffs.v3i11.1265, *ISSN: 2767-3146*.

Meléndez-Martínez, A. J. (2019). An overview of carotenoids, apocarotenoids, and vitamin A in agro-food, nutrition, health, and disease. *Molecular Nutrition & Food Research*, *63*, 1801045. Available from https://doi.org/10.1002/mnfr.201801045.

Mirzapour-Kouhdasht, A., Shaghaghian, S., & Garcia-Vaquero, M. (2023). *Production of nutraceuticals or functional foods using sourdough microorganisms. Sourdough innovations*. CRC Press.

Munekata, P. E. S., Pateiro, M., Zhang, W., Dominguez, R., Xing, L., Fierro, E. M., & Lorenzo, J. M. (2021). Health benefits, extraction and development of functional foods with curcuminoids. *Journal of Functional Foods*, *79*(April), 104392. Available from https://doi.org/10.1016/j.jff.2021.104392.

Namdeo, A. (2020). 'CURRENT REGULATORY REQUIREMENTS FOR REGISTRATION OF NUTRACEUTICALS IN INDIA AND JAPAN', March, 183–205. https://doi.org/10.20959/wjpps20204-15477.

Nestel, P., Clifton, P., Colquhoun, D., Noakes, M., Mori, T. A., Sullivan, D., & Thomas, B. (2015). Indications for omega-3 long chain polyunsaturated fatty acid in the prevention and treatment of cardiovascular disease. *Heart, Lung and Circulation*, *24*, 769–779. Available from https://doi.org/10.1016/j.hlc.2015.03.020.

Nystrand, B. T., & Olsen, S. O. (2020). Consumers' attitudes and intentions toward consuming functional foods in Norway. *Food Quality and Preference*, *80*(March), 103827. Available from https://doi.org/10.1016/j.foodqual.2019.103827.

Ogbe, R. (2015). A review of dietary phytosterols: Their occurences, metabolism and health benefits. *Asian Journal of Plant Science and Research*, *5* (July), 10–21.

Onoruoiza, M. A. (2024). 'International Journal of Probiotics and Dietetics'.

Oteiza, P. I., Fraga, C. G., Mills, D. A., & Taft, D. H. (2018). Flavonoids and the gastrointestinal tract: Local and systemic effects. *Molecular Aspects of Medicine, Bioactives and their impact on human health*, *61*(June), 41–49. Available from https://doi.org/10.1016/j.mam.2018.01.001.

Peng, M., Tabashsum, Z., Anderson, M., Truong, A., Houser, A. K., Padilla, J., Akmel, A., Bhatti, J., Rahaman, S. O., & Biswas, D. (2020). Effectiveness of probiotics, prebiotics, and prebiotic-like components in common functional foods. *Comprehensive Reviews in Food Science and Food Safety*, *19*, 1908–1933. Available from https://doi.org/10.1111/1541-4337.12565.

Perez-Gregorio, R., & Simal-Gandara, J. (2017). A critical review of bioactive food components, and of their functional mechanisms, biological effects and health outcomes. *Current Pharmaceutical Design*, *23*, 2731–2741. Available from https://doi.org/10.2174/1381612823666170317122913.

Rashidinejad, A., Boostani, S., Babazadeh, A., Rehman, A., Rezaei, A., Akbari-Alavijeh, S., Shaddel, R., & Jafari, S. M. (2021). Opportunities and challenges for the nanodelivery of green tea catechins in functional foods. *Food Research International*, *142*(April), 110186. Available from https://doi.org/10.1016/j.foodres.2021.110186.

Saher, M., Arvola, A., Lindeman, M., & Lähteenmäki, L. (2004). Impressions of functional food consumers. *Appetite*, *42*, 79–89. Available from https://doi.org/10.1016/j.appet.2003.07.002.

Salehi, B., Stojanović-Radić, Z., Matejić, J., Sharifi-Rad, M., Anil Kumar, N. V., Martins, N., & Sharifi-Rad, J. (2019). The therapeutic potential of curcumin: A review of clinical trials. *European Journal of Medicinal Chemistry*, *163*(February), 527–545. Available from https://doi.org/10.1016/j.ejmech.2018.12.016.

Sharma, D., Gondaliya, P., Tiwari, V., & Kalia, K. (2019). Kaempferol attenuates diabetic nephropathy by inhibiting RhoA/Rho-kinase mediated inflammatory signalling. *Biomedicine & Pharmacotherapy*, *109*(January), 1610–1619. Available from https://doi.org/10.1016/j.biopha.2018.10.195.

Shimizu, M. (2019). Chapter 22 - History and current status of functional food regulations in Japan. In D. Bagchi (Ed.), *Nutraceutical and functional food regulations in the United States and around the World (Third Edition)* (edited by, pp. 337–344). Academic Press. Available from https://doi.org/10.1016/B978-0-12-816467-9.00022-8.

Shoaib, M., Shehzad, A., Omar, M., Rakha, A., Raza, H., Sharif, H. R., Shakeel, A., Ansari, A., & Niazi, S. (2016). Inulin: Properties, health benefits and food applications. *Carbohydrate Polymers*, *147*(August), 444–454. Available from https://doi.org/10.1016/j.carbpol.2016.04.020.

Silva, L. P. da, Pereira, E., Prieto, M. A., Simal-Gandara, J., Pires, T. C. S. P., Alves, M. J., Calhelha, R., Barros, L., & Ferreira, I. C. F. R. (2019). Rubus ulmifolius schott as a novel source of food colorant: Extraction optimization of coloring pigments and incorporation in a bakery product. *Molecules (Basel, Switzerland)*, *24*, 2181. Available from https://doi.org/10.3390/molecules24112181.

Soleimanian, Y., Sanou, I., Turgeon, S. L., Canizares, D., & Khalloufi, S. (2022). Natural plant fibers obtained from agricultural residue used as an ingredient in food matrixes or packaging materials: A review. *Comprehensive Reviews in Food Science and Food Safety*, *21*, 371–415. Available from https://doi.org/10.1111/1541-4337.12875.

Stavropoulou, E., & Bezirtzoglou, E. (2019). Human microbiota in aging and infection: A review. *Critical Reviews in Food Science and Nutrition*, *59*, 537–545. Available from https://doi.org/10.1080/10408398.2017.1379469.

Subiria-Cueto, R., Coria-Oliveros, A. J., Wall-Medrano, A., Rodrigo-García, J., González-Aguilar, G. A., Martinez-Ruiz, N. del R., & Alvarez-Parrilla, E. (2021). Antioxidant dietary fiber-based bakery products: A new alternative for using plant-by-products. *Food Science and Technology*, *42*(February), ctaAR57520. Available from https://doi.org/10.1590/fst.57520.

Tome-Carneiro, J., Larrosa, M., Gonzalez-Sarrias, A., Tomas-Barberan, F. A., Garcia-Conesa, M. T., & Espin, J. C. (2013). Resveratrol and clinical trials: The crossroad from in vitro studies to human evidence. *Current Pharmaceutical Design*, *19*, 6064–6093.

Trautwein, E. A., Koppenol, W. P., de Jong, A., Hiemstra, H., Vermeer, M. A., Noakes, M., & Luscombe-Marsh, N. D. (2018). Plant sterols lower LDL-cholesterol and triglycerides in dyslipidemic individuals with or at risk of developing type 2 diabetes; a randomized, double-blind, placebo-controlled study. *Nutrition & Diabetes*, *8*, 1–13. Available from https://doi.org/10.1038/s41387-018-0039-8.

Ullah, R., & Khan, I. (2023). Biotechnological utilization of the marine environment for food, drugs, and energy. In M. D. Shah, J. Ransangan, & B. A. V. Maran (Eds.), *Marine biotechnology: Applications in food, drugs and energy* (edited by, pp. 23–46). Singapore: Springer Nature. Available from https://doi.org/10.1007/978-981-99-0624-6_2.

Vlaicu, P. A., Untea, A. E., Varzaru, I., Saracila, M., & Oancea, A. G. (2023). Designing nutrition for health—Incorporating dietary by-products into poultry feeds to create functional foods with insights into health benefits, risks, bioactive compounds, food component functionality and safety regulations. *Foods*, *12*, 4001. Available from https://doi.org/10.3390/foods12214001.

Vuksan, V., Jenkins, A. L., Rogovik, A. L., Fairgrieve, C. D., Jovanovski, E., & Leiter, L. A. (2011). Viscosity rather than quantity of dietary fibre predicts cholesterol-lowering effect in healthy individuals. *British Journal of Nutrition*, *106*, 1349–1352. Available from https://doi.org/10.1017/S0007114511001711.

Wezel, A., Herren, B. G., Kerr, R. B., Barrios, E., Gonçalves, A. L. R., & Sinclair, F. (2020). Agroecological principles and elements and their implications for transitioning to sustainable food systems. A review. *Agronomy for Sustainable Development*, *40*, 40. Available from https://doi.org/10.1007/s13593-020-00646-z.

Whitehead, A., Beck, E. J., Tosh, S., & Wolever, T. M. (2014). Cholesterol-lowering effects of oat β-glucan: A meta-analysis of randomized controlled trials. *The American Journal of Clinical Nutrition*, *100*, 1413–1421. Available from https://doi.org/10.3945/ajcn.114.086108.

Xiong, J., Wang, K., Yuan, C., Xing, R., Ni, J., Hu, G., Chen, F., & Wang, X. (2017). Luteolin protects mice from severe acute pancreatitis by exerting HO-1-mediated anti-inflammatory and antioxidant effects. *International Journal of Molecular Medicine*, *39*, 113–125. Available from https://doi.org/10.3892/ijmm.2016.2809.

Yegin, S., Kopec, A., Kitts, D. D., & Zawistowski, J. (2020). Chapter 24 - Dietary fiber: A functional food ingredient with physiological benefits. In H. G. Preuss, & D. Bagchi (Eds.), *Dietary sugar, salt and fat in human health* (edited by, pp. 531–555). Academic Press. Available from https://doi.org/10.1016/B978-0-12-816918-6.00024-X.

Yurko-Mauro, K., Alexander, D. D., & Van Elswyk, M. E. (2015). Docosahexaenoic acid and adult memory: A systematic review and meta-analysis. *PLoS One*, *10*, e0120391. Available from https://doi.org/10.1371/journal.pone.0120391.

Zawistowska-Rojek, A., Zaręba, T., Mrówka, A., & Tyski, S. (2016). Assessment of the microbiological status of probiotic products. *Polish Journal of Microbiology*, *65*, 97–104.

Zhang, S., Hu, H., Wang, L., Liu, F., & Pan, S. (2018). Preparation and prebiotic potential of pectin oligosaccharides obtained from citrus peel pectin. *Food Chemistry*, *244*(April), 232–237. Available from https://doi.org/10.1016/j.foodchem.2017.10.071.

Chapter 3

Functional foods for cardiovascular health: nurturing a strong heart

Rinku Sudarshan Agrawal[1] and Nilesh Prakash Nirmal[2]

[1]*MIT School of Food Technology, MIT Art, Design and Technology University, Pune, Maharashtra, India,* [2]*Institute of Nutrition, Mahidol University, Salaya, Nakhon Pathom, Thailand*

3.1 Introduction

The widespread occurrence of cardiovascular diseases (CVDs) stands as the foremost contributor to illness and death globally, placing a substantial strain on public health resources. CVDs encompass a group of disorders impacting both the heart and blood vessels, which encompass conditions such as coronary heart diseases. These diseases often result from atherosclerosis, the build-up of plaque in arteries, leading to reduced blood flow (Kiren et al., 2020). The human cardiovascular system, a complex network responsible for the circulation of blood, is susceptible to an array of maladies that compromise its functionality. Ranging from coronary artery disease and heart failure to stroke and peripheral vascular diseases, the array of cardiovascular disorders poses a significant challenge to public health. Therefore it is crucial to recognize both the factors that increase the risk and those that offer protection against CVDs in everyday life. As lifestyle factors play a pillar role in the development and control of CVDs, the exploration of functional foods as a therapeutic approach has garnered increasing attention.

Foods classified as functional foods have health benefits more than basic nourishment, that includes reducing high blood total cholesterol and low-density lipoprotein cholesterol. Functional foods are effective assets in preserving health and combating heart disease (Mpho & Shonisani, 2021). The involvement of functional foods in the treatment and prevention of CVDs signifies a fundamental change in preventive medicine. From the omega-3 fatty acids present in fatty fish to the polyphenols plentiful in fruits and vegetables, every functional food provides a distinct array of advantages for cardiovascular well-being. This chapter commences by discussing primary risk factors like high blood pressure and increased cholesterol levels. Furthermore, this chapter identifies the intersection of functional foods and cardiovascular well-being. Fruits, vegetables, seeds, whole grains, nuts, legumes, and fatty fish are among the highlighted foods, with a focus on their nutrient profiles and practical incorporation into a heart-healthy diet. The exploration extends to spices and herbs, showcasing the potential of ingredients such as turmeric, garlic, and cinnamon to contribute to cardiovascular wellness. Ultimately, this exploration of functional foods for cardiovascular health aims to empower individuals to make informed dietary choices, fostering a proactive approach to the prevention and treatment of CVDs.

3.2 Risk factors for cardiovascular health

CVDs are influenced by a myriad of risk factors, ranging from nonmodifiable genetic predispositions to modifiable lifestyle choices. Nonmodifiable risk factors for CVD are characteristics that cannot be altered, encompassing aspects such as age, ethnicity, and family medical history, whereas modifiable risk factors for CVD are those that can be decreased or managed through changes in behavior. Through implementing specific lifestyle adjustments, individuals can reduce their risk of developing CVD. The rise in CVD rates in developing countries can be attributed to shifts in the socioeconomic and cultural landscape, leading to changes in lifestyle among the population. Recognizing and comprehending these risk factors is essential for preventing, detecting early, and managing cardiovascular conditions effectively (Fig. 3.1).

Unleashing the Power of Functional Foods and Novel Bioactives. DOI: https://doi.org/10.1016/B978-0-443-28862-3.00003-0

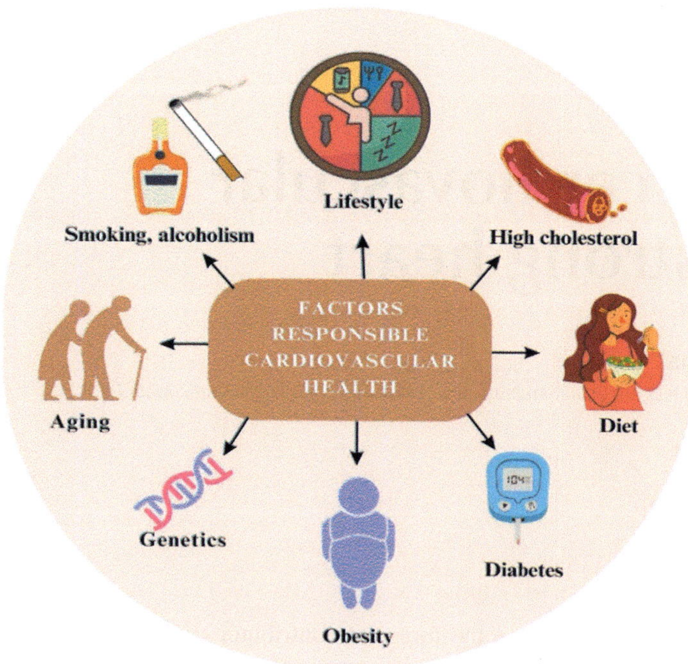

FIGURE 3.1 Factors responsible for cardiovascular diseases.

3.2.1 Nonmodifiable risk factors

1. **Age**: As individuals age, their likelihood of experiencing CVDs rises, with older individuals facing a heightened risk of developing such conditions. While aging itself is inevitable, adopting a generally healthy lifestyle is advised to lower the risk of developing heart and circulatory conditions.
2. **Gender**: Men typically have a greater susceptibility to CVDs, whereas for women, the risk escalates following menopause.
3. **Family history**: CVD has a genetic component, so having a family history of the condition is regarded as a risk factor. A family background of hypertension, high cholesterol, and type 2 diabetes can also elevate an individual's likelihood of developing CVD.

3.2.2 Modifiable risk factors

1. **Hypertension (high blood pressure):** Elevated blood pressure forces the heart to work harder, which increases the risk of stroke and heart disease.
2. **High cholesterol:** Elevated levels of LDL cholesterol and low levels of HDL cholesterol are factors that contribute to the development of atherosclerosis.
3. **Smoking:** Chemicals present in tobacco smoke harm blood vessels, decrease oxygen levels, and play a role in the progression of atherosclerosis.
4. **Diabetes:** People with diabetes face a heightened risk of CVDs.
5. **Obesity:** Having excess body weight, particularly abdominal obesity, is linked to a higher likelihood of heart disease and stroke.
6. **Physical inactivity:** Being physically inactive represents a significant risk factor that can be modified. A sedentary lifestyle can contribute to the development and progression of numerous cardiovascular conditions. Lack of regular exercise is directly linked to obesity, high blood pressure, etc.
7. **Unhealthy diet:** Consuming diets rich in saturated fats, trans fats, cholesterol, and salt, while low in fruits, vegetables, and whole grains contributes to cardiovascular risk.
8. **Excessive alcohol consumption:** Excessive and prolonged alcohol consumption can lead to elevated blood pressure, heart failure, and cardiomyopathy.
9. **Stress:** Persistent stress can lead to unhealthy lifestyle habits, like inadequate diet and physical inactivity, which can affect cardiovascular health.

3.3 Unlocking cardiovascular wellness through functional foods

Unlocking cardiovascular wellness through functional foods is a multifaceted approach that involves leveraging the nutritional properties of certain foods to promote heart health and prevent CVDs. Functional foods are defined as those providing supplementary health advantages beyond basic nutrition, typically because of the specific bioactive compounds they contain. Functional foods comprise physiologically active elements sourced from either plants or animals and are frequently promoted for their potential to mitigate the risk of heart disease, concentrating primarily on established risk factors such as blood cholesterol, diabetes, and hypertension. A diverse range of functional foods offers benefits in the prevention and treatment of CVDs. A dietary pattern abundant in functional foods like vegetables, legumes, whole grains, fruits, nuts, and olive oil, with moderate intake of fish and wine, and limited consumption of red and processed meat and whole-fat dairy products is widely acknowledged as a healthy dietary pattern. There is reliable evidence indicating that diet can positively influence major risk factors for CVD, such as dyslipidemia, diabetes mellitus, hypertension, and obesity, thereby reducing the incidence of CVD. From omega-3 fatty acid-packed fish and fiber-rich whole grains to antioxidant-laden fruits and vegetables, each category offers unique benefits, such as inflammation reduction and cholesterol regulation. Nuts, seeds, and legumes provide protein, fiber, and heart-healthy fats, while plant sterols and stanols, found naturally or fortified in select products, aid in cholesterol management. Incorporating heart-healthy herbs, spices, green tea, and dark chocolate exhibits protective effects against heart disease, attributed to their antiinflammatory and antioxidant properties. Embracing functional foods like olive oil as a source of healthy fats completes this dietary approach, fostering cardiovascular wellness alongside regular exercise and overall healthy lifestyle habits (Fig. 3.2).

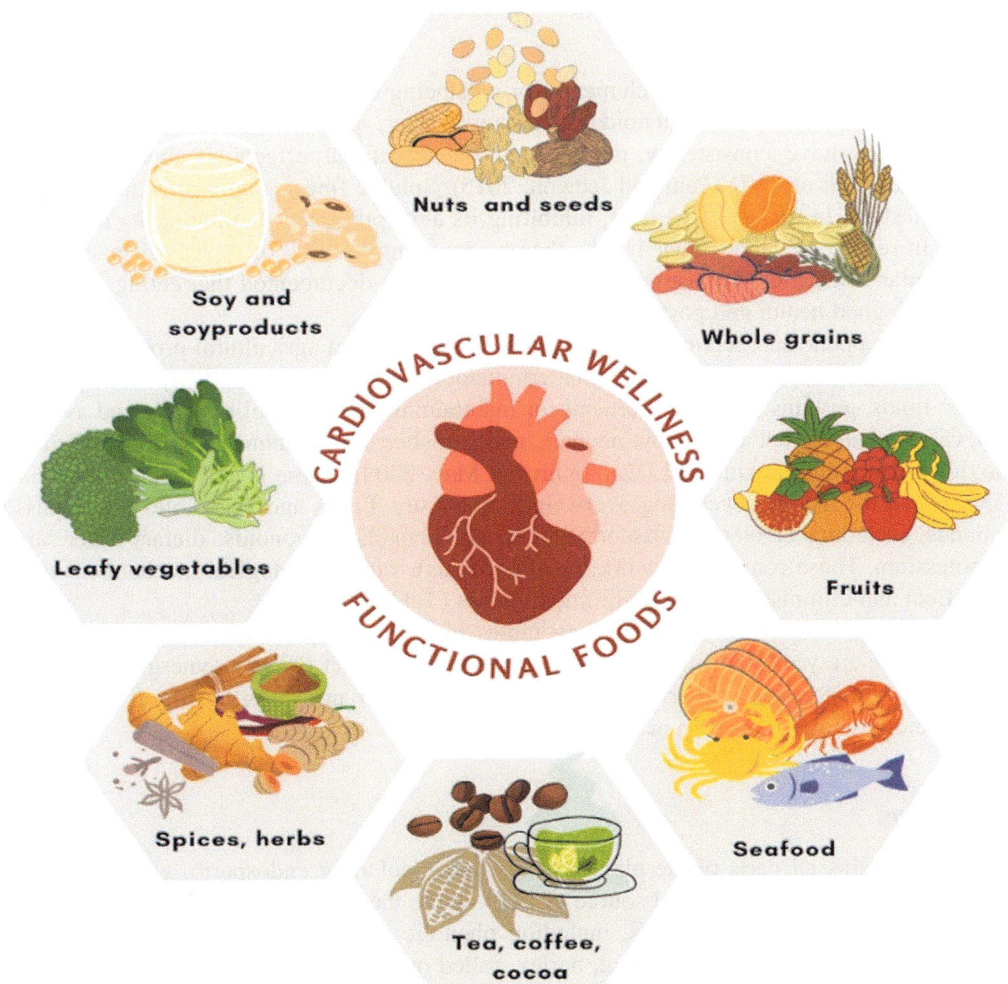

FIGURE 3.2 Cardiovascular wellness and respective functional foods.

TABLE 3.1 Cardio-Protective Mechanism by Fruits and Vegetables.

Fruits and Vegetables	Bioactive Compounds	Potential Mechanism	References
Apple	Polyphenols	Enhance vascular function, lower systolic blood pressure, and decrease cholesterol levels.	Bondonno et al. (2017)
Banana	Potassium	Maintains normal blood pressure and heart function	Kumar et al. (2012)
Dragon fruit	Antioxidants, phenol, tocotrienol	Vascular improvement	Luu et al. (2021)
Grapes	Polyphenols	Inhibition of LDL oxidation and exerting other favorable effects on cellular redox state, enhancing endothelial function, reducing blood pressure, inhibiting platelet aggregation, decreasing inflammation, and activating novel proteins.	Dohadwala and Vita (2009)
Berries	Anthocyanin	Increase in plasma or urinary antioxidant capacity, Reduction in LDL oxidation and lipid peroxidation, Reduction in plasma glucose or total cholesterol levels, and an increase in HDL cholesterol levels	Basu et al. (2010)
Tomato	Lycopene	To shield lipoproteins and vascular cells from oxidation	Willcox et al. (2003)

3.4 Fruits and vegetables

These are frequently recommended as crucial elements for enhancing cardiovascular health due to their abundance of nutrients such as vitamins, minerals, carotenoids, potassium, fiber, phytochemicals, and especially antioxidants. Numerous research studies have consistently documented the beneficial effects of diets abundant in fruits and vegetables on reducing the risk of CVD (Pem and Jeewon, 2015). Soluble fibers, such as pectin found in apples and citrus fruits, bind to cholesterol in the digestive tract, inhibiting its absorption and facilitating its removal from the body. Additionally, it aids in regulating blood sugar levels, thereby lowering the risk of type 2 diabetes, which represents a significant cardiovascular risk factor. Robust epidemiological evidence documented that eating diets abundant in fruits and vegetables promotes good health and postpones the onset of CVD.

Carotenoids such as lycopene and beta-carotene, found in deeply colored agricultural produce like carrots, tomatoes, and dark green vegetables, are dietary antioxidants that counteract free radicals in the body. This process helps prevent oxidative damage to lipids, proteins, and DNA, crucial for maintaining blood vessel integrity and averting atherosclerosis (Carol, 2009). Citrus, melons, red and yellow peppers, and strawberries are abundant sources of vitamin C. It acts as a powerful antioxidant and reduces oxidized LDL (Aguirre & May, 2008). There is an inverse correlation between fruit and vegetable intake and the risk of developing overweight or obesity. Fruits and vegetables encompass a multitude of bioactive compounds, including carotenoids, ascorbic acid, polyphenols, flavonoids, dietary fiber, and minerals like magnesium and potassium. These components work together through various biological mechanisms to foster an overall health-promoting effect and diminish the risk of chronic diseases (Table 3.1).

The cardioprotective mechanisms of fruits and vegetables involve multiple factors that collectively support heart health. Including a diverse array of colorful fruits and vegetables in the diet offers a synergistic blend of these cardioprotective mechanisms. A diverse and plant-rich diet, in conjunction with an overall healthy lifestyle, contributes to the prevention of CVDs and promotes long-term heart health.

3.5 Whole grains

A whole-grain kernel contains all parts of the plant's whole seed, including endosperm, germ, and bran in its natural form. The outer coating of the bran is a crucial source of fiber, while the inner germ contains essential nutrients such as vitamins, minerals, lignans, and phytochemicals, including phenolic acids, phytosterol compounds, and polyphenols. Whole-grain foods include brown rice, whole wheat, barley, rolled oats, and rye. Consuming whole grains is vital in the realm of functional foods as it has been associated with numerous health benefits owing to the presence of bioactive compounds that aid to prevent and control CVDs (Chung et al., 2022).

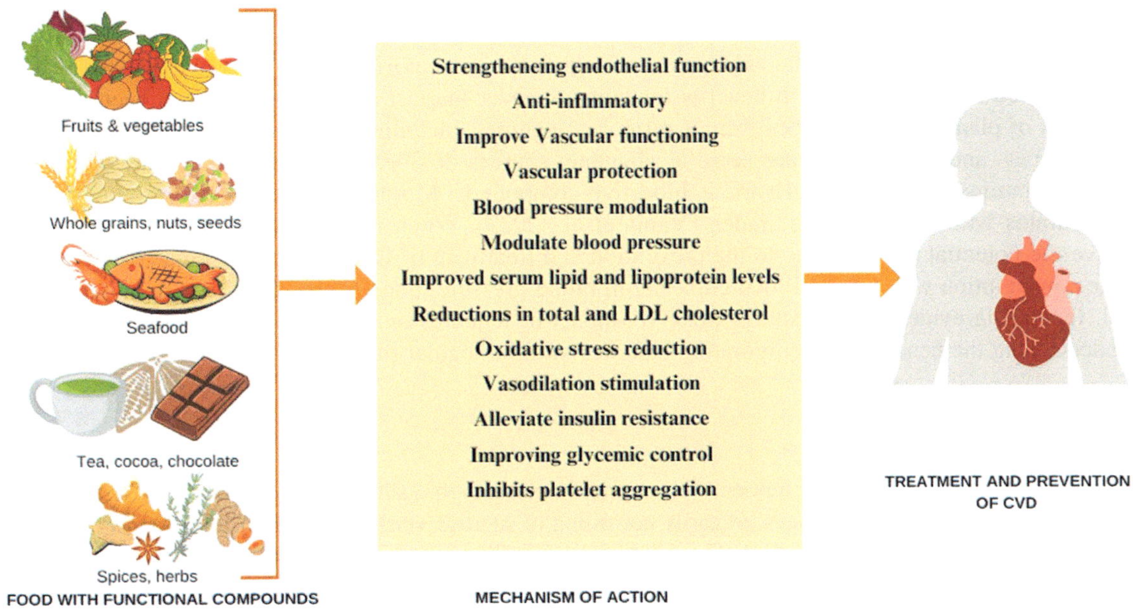

FIGURE 3.3 Mechanism of action of Foods to treat and prevent CVDs. *CVD*, Cardiovascular disease.

Whole grains, oats, and barley, which contain β-glucan fibers, play a significant role in reducing blood cholesterol, sustaining optimal blood pressure, and mitigating the risk of hypertension—a key contributor to CVD (Theuwissen and Mensink, 2007). Moreover, it helps in metabolic diseases such as decreased postprandial glucose and insulin (Biorklund et al., 2005). Regular consumption of whole grains has been shown to positively influence lipid profiles by lowering LDL cholesterol while preserving or increasing levels of beneficial HDL cholesterol. This balance is essential for preventing the build-up of arterial plaques and reducing the atherosclerosis risk. Numerous studies demonstrated the relation between whole-grain intake and a reduced CVD risk. Consuming whole grains in your diet has been suggested to lower the chances of developing type 2 diabetes, colorectal cancer, obesity, and CVD (Seal and Brownlee, 2015). The diverse range of nutrients and their multifaceted effects on risk factors make whole grains an essential component of a heart-friendly diet. As part of a balanced and varied diet, whole grains contribute significantly to the management of CVDs (Fig. 3.3).

3.6 Nuts and seeds

Nuts and seeds are integral components of heart-friendly diet. Nuts are botanically categorized as tree nuts and peanuts. Commonly consumed tree nuts comprise almonds, walnuts, hazelnuts, cashews, and pistachios. Tree nuts and peanuts share several nutritional similarities, although peanuts are classified botanically as legumes. These offer a diverse array of nutrients and bioactive components like macronutrients, fat-soluble bioactive components (monounsaturated and polyunsaturated fatty acids), vitamins, fiber, minerals, and phenolic compounds (flavonoids, stilbenes, lignans, phenolic acids) are believed to collectively contribute to their positive effects on cardiovascular health (Alasalvar et al., 2020). Being a powerhouse of these nutrients, nuts, and seeds play various roles in cardiovascular health, such as supporting overall heart function and promoting the repair of damaged tissues. Regular consumption of nuts, such as almonds, walnuts, and pistachios, has been linked to a reduced LDL level. Moreover, nuts and seeds are plentiful sources of omega-3 fatty acids, which have been linked to decreasing blood cholesterol levels and reducing the risk of coronary heart disease.

Flaxseeds are rich in alpha-linolenic acid (ALA), a plant-based omega-3 fatty acid, which is instrumental in their antiinflammatory and antiatherogenic qualities. This plays a vital role in lowering the risk of CVD (Delfin et al., 2010). The lignans present in flaxseeds serve as antioxidants, combating oxidative stress and inflammation, which are critical factors in the onset and advancement of cardiovascular conditions. The soluble fiber in flaxseeds aids in maintaining healthy blood pressure levels by enhancing arterial flexibility. It can also help to lower LDL by interfering with the absorption of dietary cholesterol (Mishra, 2016). Some seeds, like pumpkin seeds and sunflower seeds, contain plant sterols that can help lower LDL cholesterol levels. Plant sterols, which have a similar structure to cholesterol, compete with cholesterol absorption, consequently lowering its levels in the bloodstream. Additionally, chia seeds and sesame seeds play a role in reducing risk factors linked to CVD, including inflammation, high cholesterol, and hypertension.

3.7 Legumes

Recently, there has been increasing acknowledgment of legumes as an environmentally sustainable source of plant protein, which is linked to numerous health benefits for humans. Over the last few years, there has been a notable rise in the consumption of plant proteins sourced from a variety of legumes, including pea, mungbean, lupin, cowpea, soybean, jack bean, chickpea, and lentils. Legumes serve as abundant sources of fiber and essential minerals such as potassium, magnesium, B vitamins, iron, zinc, and various bioactive compounds. Moreover, legumes are low in saturated fat and offer carbohydrates with low glycaemic-index (Vania et al., 2023). When incorporated into a balanced, healthy diet, legumes have the potential to contribute to the prevention and treatment of CVD. Previous research has steadily associated legume consumption with reduced total cholesterol, blood pressure, obesity, and increased high-density lipoprotein cholesterol. Increasing evidence suggests the positive impact of legumes on cardiovascular health and cardiometabolic factors, underscoring the benefits of incorporating legumes into the regular diet (Bazzano et al., 2008).

3.8 Soy protein

Soybeans are globally esteemed for their nutrient-rich profile, boasting high-quality protein content (~40%), significant polyunsaturated fatty acids (18%), carbohydrates primarily consisting of sucrose, stachyose, and raffinose, as well as dietary fibers. Additionally, soybeans contain phytochemicals like phytosterols, isoflavones, and lecithins, along with polysaccharides, soluble fibers and saponins. These compounds may exert their effects either collectively or through independent mechanisms, which have been associated with various health benefits. Soybean has garnered significant attention as a heart-healthy food, particularly due to its beneficial effects on cholesterol levels and blood pressure. Extensive documentary evidence supports the notion that replacing animal protein with soy protein can lead to reductions in blood cholesterol levels and potentially offer other cardiovascular benefits. Soy protein has been extensively studied for its potential role in the treatment and prevention of CVD due to its beneficial effects on lipid profiles, blood pressure, endothelial function, and inflammation. Both the American Heart Association and the Food and Drug Administration recommend a daily intake of 25 g or more of soy protein containing phytoestrogens as part of a diet low in saturated fat and cholesterol. This dietary approach can potentially improve the lipid profile and lower the risk of heart disease (Rebholz et al., 2012). Dietary soy protein has extensively documented positive effects on plasma lipid and lipoprotein concentrations. These effects typically include reductions in LDL cholesterol of approximately 13%, reductions in plasma triglycerides of around 10%, and increases in HDL cholesterol. The extent of HDL cholesterol increase may vary among individuals, but on average, it is around 2%. Soy contains antioxidants like tocopherols and isoflavones, which help to reduce oxidative stress and protect against the damage caused by free radicals. Soy protein is commonly consumed in various traditional fermented and nonfermented soy foods, including miso, tofu, and tempeh, as well as in whole soybeans, soymilk, soy cheese, and soy yogurt. Incorporating soy protein into a balanced diet may represent a practical and sustainable approach to managing cardiovascular risk factors and reducing the chances of CVDs (Fig. 3.4).

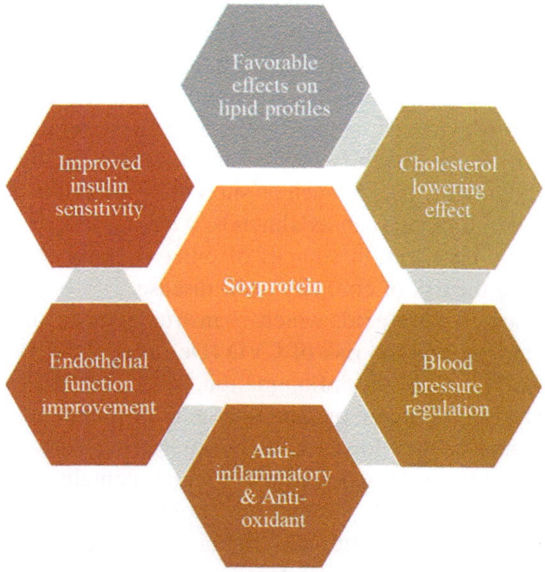

FIGURE 3.4 Soy protein action mechanism on CVD. *CVD*, Cardiovascular disease.

3.9 Fish

Fish is widely recognized as a vital source of functional food due to its rich nutritional profile. The nutrient content of fish differs greatly by species and in individual fish based on age, sex, season, and environment. The significance of fish in the context of CVD is primarily attributed to the presence of omega-3 fatty acids specifically polyunsaturated fats like eicosapentaenoic acid (EPA) and docosahexaenoic acid (DHA). Fatty fish species like salmon, tuna, herring, mackerel, and trout are abundant sources of omega-3 fatty acids, that have been extensively researched for their beneficial effects on heart health. Enhanced consumption of fish and fish oil supplements is recommended as it contributes to minimizing the incidence of CVDs and mitigating its risk (He et al., 2004). These fatty acids lower blood triglyceride levels, decrease inflammation, and improve arterial function. Moreover, they have been associated with a reduced incidence of arrhythmias and blood clot formation, resulting in overall cardiovascular health benefits.

Voluminous scientific studies have consistently concluded that omega-3 fatty acids have an important role in reducing the risk factors associated with CVDs. Fish oil supplements have a beneficial impact on blood pressure and lipid profile. Additionally, DHA and EPA have been shown to decrease the oxidative sensitivity of low-density lipoprotein in postmenopausal women, potentially aiding in the reduction of CVD risk (Lee and Wander, 2005). Dietary guidelines recommend consuming oily fish at least twice a week to prevent onset of CVD. Omega-3 fatty acids have the potential to prevent the formation of blood clots, thereby reducing the risk of thrombosis and associated cardiovascular symptoms. High-dose fish oil supplementation has demonstrated efficacy in reducing triglyceride levels in individuals with severe hypertriglyceridemia (Arnett et al., 2019).

3.10 Spices and herbs

Spices have been an integral part of Indian culture from the dawn of time and hold significant importance for both their culinary and medicinal virtues. Indian spices and their bioactive phytocompounds are well documented in the context of functional foods owing to their multifaceted role in health promotion and disease prevention. The components from spices and herbs have the potential to minimize or inhibit the risk for the development of degenerative diseases like obesity, diabetes, CVDs and cancer.

Spices like fenugreek, garlic, and onion are effective in humans with hyperlipidemic conditions. Garlic, a culinary and medicinal herb, contains bioactive compounds like allicin and sulfur compounds with cardiovascular benefits. Garlic consumption has been related to reduce cholesterol levels, blood pressure, and reduced risk of blood clot formation, contributing to cardiovascular health. Compounds from turmeric- curcumin, ginger-gingerol, black pepper- piperine, and other spices such as cinnamon, and coriander, have been found proactive and effective against CVD (Vasanthi and Parameswari, 2010). Curcumin, the active compound in turmeric, exhibits antioxidant and antiinflammatory properties that support cardiovascular health. Ashwagandha root extract improves cardiorespiratory endurance and enhances the quality of life in healthy athletic adults (Mohiuddin, 2019).

TABLE 3.2 Cardioprotective Mechanism of Some Indian Spices.

Spices and Herbs	Bioactive Compounds	Potential Mechanism	References
Garlic	Allicin	Reduces total cholesterol, and blood pressure, inhibits platelet aggregation, and increases antioxidant status	Vasanthi and Parameswari (2010)
Turmeric	Curcumin	Delay cellular senescence reduces oxidative stress, improves vascular endothelial function	Cox et al. (2022)
Red chili	Capsaicin	Reduces adipogenesis, alleviates insulin resistance, regulates glucose homeostasis	Sun et al. (2016)
Ginger	Gingerol. Zingerone	Lowers blood pressure, prevents obesity, and improves lipid profile, glycemic control, and vascular health	Cerdá et al. (2022)
Cinnamon	Cinnamaldehyde and cinnamic acid	Lowers blood glucose level, improves insulin sensitivity, antioxidant, anti–inflammatory effects	Das et al. (2022)
Mint	Flavonoids	Reduce cardiac depression, lipid peroxidation, antioxidant, hypo protective	Saddam et al. (2022)

Essential oils are natural organic compounds derived from different parts of aromatic plants. Research indicates that essential oils and their bioactive constituents possess a range of biological properties, including antioxidant and antiinflammatory activities. Essential oil improves lipid balance, reduces blood pressure, liver function, and inhibits diabetes development. Essential oils from medicinal plants such as *Allium sativum, Curcuma longa L., Foeniculum vulgare., Linum usitatissimum L., Mentha x villosa, Nigella sativa, and Rosa indica L.* have been found to exhibit cardioprotective action (Seol and Shin, 2018) (Table 3.2).

3.11 Coffee and tea

Coffee stands as one of the most widely consumed beverages globally and holds a significant place in the commercial food industry. Coffee, a complex beverage, contains a variety of bioactive compounds including caffeic acid, trigonelline, chlorogenic acids, diterpenes, and melanoidins. These compounds are known to exert potent effects on long-term human health (Bułdak et al., 2018). The chlorogenic acids and polyphenols are the significant prevalent forms of phenolic compounds present in coffee contributing to its antiinflammatory as well as antioxidant properties that help to mitigate oxidative stress and prevent the onset of atherosclerosis. The chlorogenic acids and caffeine have been linked to improved endothelial function and reduced inflammation. Furthermore, coffee consumption has been linked to reduced risks of developing conditions such as coronary heart disease, heart failure, and stroke (Dludla et al., 2023). However, it is essential to note that excessive coffee consumption or the addition of high-calorie ingredients like sugar and cream can negate these potential benefits and may even have adverse effects on cardiovascular health.

Tea ranks among the most widely consumed beverages globally and has been extensively researched for its potential health benefits, both in vitro and in vivo domain. Bioactive components in tea appear to have potential in the management of cardiovascular, metabolic, and neurodegenerative diseases. Tea leaves are rich in polyphenols, constituting approximately 30% of the dry substance, with flavonoids being the predominant type. The major class of flavonoids in tea are flavanols, consisting catechin, epicatechin (EC), epicatechin gallate (ECG), epigallocatechin (EGC) and epigallocatechin gallate (EGCG) (Kris-Etherton et al., 2002). In recent times, there has been significant interest in exploring the potential of tea consumption to lower the risk of CVD. EGCG is one of the most studied and bioactive compounds in tea, known for its potential health benefits, including its role in CVD prevention (Apranta Deka et al., 2011). The potential mechanism of benefit for tea against CVD is as follows:

1. **Antioxidant effects:** EGCG is indeed a potent antioxidant known for its ability to neutralize free radicals in the body. Free radicals have the potential to cause oxidative damage to cells, including those in the cardiovascular system, leading to inflammation and the development of CVD. By scavenging these free radicals, EGCG helps protect against oxidative stress and reduces the risk of cardiovascular damage.
2. **Antiinflammatory effects:** EGCG has been found to possess antiinflammatory potential that helps to reduce inflammation in the blood vessels and prevent the development of atherosclerosis and other inflammatory conditions associated with CVD.
3. **Lipid metabolism regulation:** EGCG has been suggested to play a role in regulating lipid metabolism by potentially reducing the absorption of dietary fats and cholesterol in the intestine, as well as enhancing their excretion from the body. By lowering levels of LDL cholesterol (the "bad" cholesterol) and triglycerides, EGCG helps to prevent the build-up of plaque in the arteries and reduces the risk of atherosclerosis and cardiovascular events.
4. **Blood Pressure Regulation**: EGCG has been shown to have a mild hypotensive (blood pressure-lowering) effect, which can help to reduce the risk of hypertension, a major risk factor for CVD. By promoting vasodilation and improving endothelial function, EGCG helps maintain healthy blood pressure levels.

3.12 Chocolate

Chocolate is indeed among the most popular foods globally and is gaining recognition for its potential benefits for cardiometabolic health. High cocoa and chocolate consumption have been closely linked with reduced CVD risk in several research studies. Dark chocolate has a distinctive bittersweet flavor due to its higher cocoa content and has been studied for its potential role in CVD prevention. Dark chocolate contains a variety of bioactives, like heobromine, catechins, procyanidins from cocoa, together with added sucrose and lipids. All of these can directly or indirectly affect the cardiovascular system via multiple mechanisms (Kerimi and Williamson, 2015). Several studies have demonstrated that moderate dark chocolate consumption helps to improve endothelial function, lipid profile and reduce blood lipid levels.

Dark chocolate possesses antioxidant properties due to flavanols and polyphenols that help in neutralization of free radicals and prevention of oxidative stress (Yang et al., 2024). Studies indicate that increasing your intake of dietary flavonoids is correlated with a reduced risk of coronary heart disease. Dark chocolate is rich in flavonoids, especially a type known as flavanols, which are linked to a decreased likelihood of heart disease.

3.13 Mushroom

Mushrooms are edible fungus and have been characterized due to its nutritional goodness. Mushrooms serve as exceptional sources of high-quality protein derived from agricultural and industrial byproducts. Additionally, they contain all nine essential amino acids that may help in reducing the risk of protein-energy malnutrition in humans. It is ideally preferred to formulate low-caloric functional foods due to its less fat content, high dietary fibers with low trans isomers of unsaturated fatty acids, and low concentration of sodium (Eva et al., 2010). Edible mushrooms are well-regarded as functional foods because of their diverse nutritional and bioactive compounds, which are known to positively impact cardiovascular health.

Several research studies documented the effect of mushroom intake on some metabolic markers (LDL, HDL, total cholesterol, fasting triacylglycerol, homocysteine, homeostatic function, blood pressure, oxidative and inflammatory damage), that may reduce the risk of CVDs. Mushrooms possess numerous bioactive flavonoids and more than 30 polyphenolic compounds, serving as potent antioxidants due to their remarkable ability to neutralize free radicals and function as reducing agents (Mwangi et al., 2022). Numerous research studies have established the beneficial health effects of consuming edible mushrooms in preventing or treating various chronic diseases. *Agaricus brasiliensis* polysaccharide includes glucose (78.38%), arabinose (10.46%), as well as mannose (8.51%), which was propitious to some CVDs and used to treat heart diseases as well as prevent cancer (Zhang et al., 2010). The low fat and high fiber content of mushrooms play a role in preventing hypertension and hypercholesterolemia, and they are also beneficial for weight control. Mushrooms are valuable sources of essential fatty acids, with a high proportion (52−87%) consisting of unsaturated fatty acids. Primarily, they provide linoleic acid, which is vital for health as it cannot be directly synthesized by the human body. Mushrooms are abundant in indigestible carbohydrates, which positions them as promising sources of innovative prebiotic components. The low glycemic index and high mannitol content of mushrooms are thought to offer benefits for individuals with diabetes (Das et al., 2021).

3.14 Bioactive dietary compounds with cardioprotective potentials

There are several bioactive dietary compounds having cardioprotective potential. These compounds are found in various foods and have been studied in-detail for their effects on cardiovascular health. Some of the key bioactive compounds are discussed below:

1. **Polyphenols**: These are plant-derived compounds associated with antioxidant and antiinflammatory properties. Flavonoids, such as quercetin and catechins, found abundantly in fruits, vegetables, red wine, and tea have been associated with reduced risk of CVD. Resveratrol, primarily found in grapes and red wine, has garnered attention for its potential cardioprotective effects, including antiinflammatory and vasodilatory properties.
2. **Omega-3 fatty acids:** Omega-3 fatty acids, notably EPA and DHA, are most essential fatty acids found in fatty fish, chia seeds, flaxseeds, and walnuts. Consumption of omega-3 fatty acids has been linked to reduced triglyceride levels, enhanced endothelial function, and decreased risk of arrhythmias and atherosclerosis, contributing to overall cardiovascular health.
3. **Dietary fiber:** Dietary fiber, prevalent in fruits, vegetables, whole grains, nuts, and seeds, exerts cardioprotective impact through various mechanisms. Soluble fiber aids in reducing cholesterol levels by binding to bile acids and facilitating their excretion, while insoluble fiber aids in weight management and regulation of blood sugar levels, reducing the risk of CVD.
4. **Phytosterols:** Phytosterols, plant-derived compounds structurally similar to cholesterol, are abundant in nuts, seeds, legumes, and whole grains. These compounds inhibit cholesterol absorption in the intestine, leading to reduced LDL cholesterol levels and mitigating the risk of atherosclerosis and cardiovascular events.
5. **Monounsaturated and polyunsaturated fats:** Healthy fats, including monounsaturated and polyunsaturated fats present in avocados, olive oil, nuts, and seeds, confer cardioprotective benefits. These fats improve lipid profiles, reduce inflammation, and lower the risk of CVD when substituted for saturated and trans fats in the diet.

6. **Green tea catechins:** Green tea catechins, particularly epigallocatechin gallate (EGCG), possess antioxidant and antiinflammatory properties that promote heart health. Green tea consumption has been linked to improved lipid metabolism, reduced oxidative stress, and enhanced endothelial function, offering protection against CVD.

These bioactive dietary compounds have a crucial role in preventing and managing CVD. Adding these bioactive compounds into a balanced diet can support heart health through antioxidant, antiinflammatory, lipid-modulating, and vasoprotective mechanisms. It's crucial to acknowledge that although these compounds have been linked to cardioprotective effects in research, individual responses may differ. Moreover, overall dietary habits and lifestyle choices significantly influence cardiovascular health.

3.15 Preventive measures for cardiovascular disease

Preventive measures for CVD focus on reducing risk factors and adopting a heart-healthy lifestyle. These preventive measures encompass a holistic approach that addresses lifestyle factors, risk factor management, and proactive health monitoring.

1. **Healthy diet:** Diet is an important part of the development and management of CVD, with certain bioactive compounds demonstrating cardioprotective properties. Promoting heart-healthy dietary habits involves adopting not only a balanced but also a nutrient-rich diet that includes a variety of fruits, vegetables, lean proteins, whole grains, and healthy fats. Reducing the intake of processed foods, sugars, and unhealthy fats while maintaining a calorie balance contributes to overall cardiovascular well-being. Dietary choices are integral to preventing and managing CVDs, making healthy eating habits a cornerstone of cardiovascular health promotion.
2. **Maintaining a healthy weight**: Being overweight or obese indeed constitutes significant risk factors for CVD. Body mass index (BMI) serves as a reliable predictor of CVD risk, especially at elevated levels. Having a BMI $>$ 25 is a risk factor for CVD (Stewart et al., 2017). The distribution of body fat also poses an additional risk, as abdominal obesity is an independent risk factor for coronary heart disease.
3. **Exercise**: Regular physical activity is another cornerstone of CVD prevention. Engaging in regular aerobic exercise and strength training aids in maintaining a healthy weight and also improves cardiovascular fitness, lowers blood pressure, and enhances overall well-being. Incorporating physical activity into daily routines can significantly reduce the risk of CVDs and contribute to a healthier lifestyle.
4. **SmokingCessation**: Smoking has long been recognized as a key risk factor for CVD. Quitting smoking not only reduces the risk of developing heart-related conditions but also improves overall health and quality of life (Piepoli et al., 2016).
5. **Limit alcohol consumption**: Limiting alcohol consumption is an important preventive measure for reducing the risk of developing CVDs. By limiting alcohol consumption, individuals can reduce their overall caloric intake, maintain a healthy weight, and lower their risk of developing obesity-related CVDs such as coronary artery disease and type 2 diabetes.
6. **Stress management**: Managing stress effectively is essential for heart health. Chronic stress contributes to the development of CVDs by elevating blood pressure, increasing inflammation, and promoting unhealthy coping behaviors such as overeating or smoking. Incorporating stress-reduction techniques such as mindfulness meditation, deep breathing exercises, or engaging in hobbies can help mitigate the detrimental effects of stress on cardiovascular health.
7. **Regular health checkups**: Regular health checkups play a pivotal role in CVD prevention by enabling early detection and management of risk factors. Routine screenings for blood pressure, cholesterol levels, blood glucose, and other relevant markers allow healthcare providers to identify individuals at risk and implement preventive interventions accordingly.
8. **Medication adherence:** Preventing CVDs requires a multifaceted approach that addresses modifiable risk factors through lifestyle modifications and appropriate medical interventions. By adopting a heart-healthy lifestyle and staying proactive in managing risk factors, individuals can significantly reduce their risk of developing CVDs and enjoy better heart health and overall well-being.

3.16 Future directions and concluding remarks

Functional foods with cardiovascular benefits showcase a vital role in preventive cardiology. The future of functional foods for CVD promises to be dynamic and multifaceted, with several key directions paving the way for innovative research and practical applications. The emphasis on personalized nutrition, driven by advancements in nutrigenomics and nutrigenetics is successively growing. Integration of digital health technologies, such as mobile applications and wearables, may offer new ways to monitor and enhance the impact of functional foods on cardiovascular outcomes. With progressive research in this field, the incorporation of functional foods into dietary guidelines holds promise for improving public health outcomes related to cardiovascular wellness. A holistic approach, combining a heart-healthy diet with regular physical activity and other healthy lifestyle choices, remains the cornerstone of CVD prevention.

References

Aguirre, R., & May, J. M. (2008). Inflammation in the vascular bed: Importance of vitamin C. *Pharmacology & Therapeutics*, *119*(1), 96–103. Available from https://doi.org/10.1016/j.pharmthera.2008.05.002.

Alasalvar, C., Salvado, J. S., & Ros, E. (2020). Bioactives and health benefits of nuts and dried fruits. *Food Chemistry*, *314*, 126192. Available from https://doi.org/10.1016/j.foodchem.2020.126192.

Apranta Deka, M. D., Joseph, A., & Vita, M. D. (2011). Tea and cardiovascular disease. *Pharmacological Research*, *64*(2), 136–145.

Arnett, D. K., Blumenthal, R. S., & Albert, M. A. (2019). ACC/AHA Guideline on the primary prevention of cardiovascular disease: a report of the American College of Cardiology/American Heart Association Task Force on Clinical Practice Guidelines. *Circulation*, *140*(11), e596–e646. Available from https://doi.org/10.1161/CIR.0000000000000678.

Basu, A., Rhone, M., & Lyons, T. J. (2010). Berries: Emerging impact on cardiovascular health. *Nutrition Reviews*, *68*(3), 168–177.

Bazzano, L., Tees, M. T., & Nguyen, C. H. (2008). Effect of non-soy legume consumption on cholesterol levels: A meta-analysis of randomized controlled trial. *Circulation*, *118*, S1122.

Biorklund, M., van Rees, A., Mensink, R. P., & Onning, G. (2005). Changes in serum lipids and postprandial glucose and insulin concentrations after consumption of beverages with beta-glucans from oats or barley: A randomised dose-controlled trial. *European Journal of Clinical Nutrition*, *59*, 1272–1281.

Bondonno N. P., Bondonno C.P., Ward N. C., Hodgson J. M., & Croft K. D. (2017). The cardiovascular health benefits of apples: Whole fruit vs. isolated compounds. *Trends in Food Science and Technology*, *69*(B), 243–256.

Bułdak, R. J., Hejmo, T., Osowski, M., Buldak, L., Kukla, M., Polaniak, R., & Birkner, E. (2018). The impact of coffee and its selected bioactive compounds on the development and progression of colorectal cancer in vivo and in vitro. *Molecules*, *23*, 3309. Available from https://doi.org/10.3390/molecules23123309.

Carol, J. (2009). Functional foods as modifiers of cardiovascular disease. *American Journal of Lifestyle Medicine*, *3*(1), 39S–43S.

Cerdá, B., Marhuenda, J., Arcusa, R., Villaño, D., Ballester, P., & Zafrilla, P. (2022). *Ginger in the prevention of cardiovascular diseases*. IntechOpen. Available from https://doi.org/10.5772/intechopen.103970.

Chung, S., Hwang, J.-T., & Park, S.-H. (2022). Physiological effects of bioactive compounds derived from whole grains on cardiovascular and metabolic diseases. *Applied Sciences*, *12*(2), 658.

Cox, F. F., Misiou, A., Vierkant, A., Ale-Agha, N., Grandoch, M., Haendeler, J., & Altschmied, J. (2022). Protective effects of curcumin in cardiovascular diseases—Impact on oxidative stress and mitochondria. *Cells*, *11*(3), 342. Available from https://doi.org/10.3390/cells11030342.

Das, A. K., Nanda, P. K., Dandapat, P., Bandyopadhyay, S., Gullón, P., Sivaraman, G. K., McClements, D. J., Gullón, B., & Lorenzo, J. M. (2021). Edible mushrooms as functional ingredients for development of healthier and more sustainable muscle foods: A flexitarian approach. *Molecules*, *26*(9), 2463. Available from https://doi.org/10.3390/molecules26092463, PMID: 33922630; PMCID: PMC8122938.

Das, G., Gonçalves, S., Basilio Heredia, J., Romano, A., Jiménez-Ortega, L. A., Gutiérrez-Grijalva, E. P., Shin, H. S., & Patra, J. K. (2022). Cardiovascular protective effect of cinnamon and its major bioactive constituents: An update. *Journal of Functional Foods*, *97*, 105045.

Delfin, R.-L., Bassett, C. M. C., McCullough, R., & Pierce, G. N. (2010). The cardiovascular effects of flaxseed and its omega-3 fatty acid, alpha-linolenic acid. *ogy*, *26*(9), 489–496.

Dludla, P. V., Cirilli, I., Marcheggiani, F., Silvestri, S., Orlando, P., Muvhulawa, N., Moetlediwa, M. T., Nkambule, B. B., Mazibuko-Mbeje, S. E., Hlengwa, N., Hanser, S., Ndwandwe, D., Marnewick, J. L., Basson, A. K., & Tiano, L. (2023). Potential benefits of coffee consumption on improving biomarkers of oxidative stress and inflammation in healthy individuals and those at increased risk of cardiovascular disease. *Molecules*, *28*(18), 6440.

Dohadwala, M. M., & Vita, J. A. (2009). Grapes and cardiovascular disease. *The Journal of Nutrition*, *139*(9), 1788S–1793SS.

Eva, G., Garcia-Lafuente, A., Lozano, M., Arrigo, M. D., Rostagno, M. A., Villares, A., & Alfredo Martínez, J. (2010). Edible mushrooms: Role in the prevention of cardiovascular diseases. *Fitoterapia*, *81*(7), 715–723.

He, K., Song, Y., Daviglus, M. L., Liu, K., Van Horn, L., Dyer, A. R., & Greenland, P. (2004). Accumulated evidence on fish consumption and coronary heart disease mortality a meta-analysis of cohort studies. *Circulation*, *109*(22), 2705–2711.

Kerimi, A., & Williamson, G. (2015). The cardiovascular benefits of dark chocolate. *Vascular Pharmacology*, *71*, 11–15. Available from https://doi.org/10.1016/j.vph.2015.05.011.

Kiren, M., Ajmal, I., Naz, T., Ahmad Fazili, A. B., Bai, X., & Song, Y. (2020). Bioactive functional foods for cardiovascular diseases. *American Journal of Biochemistry and Biotechnology*, *16*(3), 354–369.

Kris-Etherton, P. M., Hecker, K. D., Bonanome, A., Coval, S. M., Binkoski, A. E., & Hilpert, K. F. (2002). Bioactive compounds in foods: Their role in the prevention of cardiovascular disease and cancer. *The American Journal of Medicine*, *113*(Suppl 9B), 71S–88S.

Kumar, K. S., Bhowmik, D., Duraivel, S., & Umadevi, M. (2012). Traditional and medicinal uses of banana. *Journal of Pharmacognosy and Phytochemistry*, *1*(3), 51–63.

Lee, Y. S., & Wander, R. C. (2005). Reduced effect on apoptosis of 4-hydroxyhexenal and oxidized LDL enriched with n-3 fatty acids from postmenopausal women. *Journal of Nutritional Biochemistry, 16*(4), 213–221. Available from https://doi.org/10.1016/j.jnutbio.2004.09.006, www.elsevier.com/locate/jnutbio.

Luu, T. T. H., Le, T. L., Huynh, N., & Quintela-Alonso, P. (2021). Dragon fruit: A review of health benefits and nutrients and its sustainable development under climate changes in Vietnam. *Czech Journal of Food Sciences, 39*(2), 71–94. Available from https://doi.org/10.17221/139/2020-CJFS, https://www.agriculturejournals.cz/publicFiles/139_2020-CJFS.pdf.

Mishra, N. (2016). Effect of whole flaxseed and flaxseed oil in CVD patient. *Health sciences: An International Journal, 6*(1), 1–7.

Mohiuddin, A. K. (2019). Natural Foods and Indian herbs of cardiovascular interest. *Pharmacy & Pharmacology International Journal, 7*(2). Available from https://doi.org/10.15406/ppij.2019.07.00235.

Mpho, E. M., & Shonisani, E. R. (2021). Role of functional food in treating and preventing cardiovascular diseases. *Functional Foods - Phytochemicals and Health Promoting Potential*. Available from https://doi.org/10.5772/intechopen.96614.

Mwangi, R. W., Macharia, J. M., Wagara, I. N., & Bence, R. L. (2022). The antioxidant potential of different edible and medicinal mushrooms. *Biomedicine and Pharmacotherapy, 147*, 112621. Available from https://doi.org/10.1016/j.biopha.2022.112621.

Pem, D., & Jeewon, R. (2015). Fruit and vegetable intake: Benefits and progress of nutrition education interventions-narrative review article. *Journal of Public Health, 44*(10), 1309–1321. Available from http://www.ncbi.nlm.nih.gov/pmc/articles/PMC4644575/pdf/IJPH-44-1309.pdf.

Piepoli, M. F., Hoes, A. W., Agewall, S., Albus, C., Brotons, C., Catapano, A. L., Cooney, M. T., Corrà, U., Cosyns, B., Deaton, C., Graham, I., Hall, M. S., Hobbs, F. D. R., Løchen, M. L., Löllgen, H., Marques-Vidal, P., Perk, J., Prescott, E., Redon, J., ... Gale, C. (2016). European Guidelines on cardiovascular disease prevention in clinical practice. *European Heart Journal, 37*(29), 2315–2381. Available from https://doi.org/10.1093/eurheartj/ehw106, http://eurheartj.oxfordjournals.org/.

Rebholz, C. M., Friedman, E. E., Powers, L. J., Arroyave, W. D., He, J., & Kelly, T. N. (2012). Dietary protein intake and blood pressure: A meta-analysis of randomized controlled trials. *American Journal of Epidemiology, 176*, S27–S43.

Saddam, S., Ullah, F., Naeem, M., Younas, M., Ayaz, A., Ali, S., & Zaman, W. (2022). Mentha: Nutritional and health attributes to treat various ailments including cardiovascular diseases. *Molecules, 27*(19), 6728.

Seal, C. J., & Brownlee, I. A. (2015). Whole-grain foods and chronic disease: Evidence from epidemiological and intervention studies. *Proceedings of the Nutrition Society, 74*(3), 313–319.

Seol, G. H., & Shin, Y. K. (2018). *Essential oils and factors related to cardiovascular diseases*. IntechOpen. Available from https://doi.org/10.5772/intechopen.77278.

Stewart, J., Manmathan, G., & Wilkinson, P. (2017). Primary prevention of cardiovascular disease: A review of contemporary guidance and literature. *JRSM Cardiovasc Disease*; 6, 2048004016687211. https://doi.org/10.1177/2048004016687211. PMID: 28286646; PMCID: PMC5331469.

Sun, F., Xiong, S., & Zhu, Z. (2016). Dietary capsaicin protects cardiometabolic organs from dysfunction. *Nutrients, 8*(5), 174, 25.

Theuwissen, E., & Mensink, R. P. (2007). Simultaneous intake of β-glucan and plant stanol esters affects lipid metabolism in slightly hypercholesterolemic subjects. *Journal of Nutrition, 137*(3), 583–588. Available from https://doi.org/10.1093/jn/137.3.583, http://jn.nutrition.org/cgi/reprint/137/3/583.

Vania, M., Niforou, A., Kasdagli, M. I., Ververis, E., & Naska, A. (2023). Intake of legumes and cardiovascular disease: A systematic review and dose–response meta-analysis. *Nutrition, Metabolism, and Cardiovascular Diseases, 33*(1), 22–37.

Vasanthi, H. R., & Parameswari, R. P. (2010). Indian spices for healthy heart - An overview. *Current Cardiology Reviews, 6*(4), 274–279. Available from https://doi.org/10.2174/157340310793566172.

Willcox, J. K., Catignani, G. L., & Lazarus, S. (2003). Tomatoes and cardiovascular health. *Critical Reviews in Food Science and Nutrition, 43*(1), 1–18.

Yang, J., Zhou, J., Yang, J., Lou, H., Zhao, B., Chi, J., & Tang, W. (2024). Dark chocolate intake and cardiovascular diseases: a Mendelian randomization study. *Scientific Reports, 14*(1). Available from https://doi.org/10.1038/s41598-023-50351-6, https://www.nature.com/srep/.

Zhang, S., He, B., Ge, J., Zhai, C., Liu, X., & Liu, P. (2010). Characterization of chemical composition of Agaricus brasiliensis polysaccharides and its effect on myocardial SOD activity, MDA andcaspase-3 level in ischemia-reperfusion rats. *International Journal of Biological Macromolecules, 46*(3), 363–366.

Chapter 4

Digestive health: functional foods for a happy gut

Vaishnavi A. Pathak[1], Gitanjali S. Deokar[1], Sanjay J. Kshirsagar[1], Kapil S. Kulkarni[1], Yasmina Sultanbawa[2] and Nilesh Prakash Nirmal[3]

[1]MET's Institute of Pharmacy, Bhujbal Knowledge City, Adgaon, Nashik, Maharashtra, India, [2]Centre for Nutrition and Food Sciences, Queensland Alliance for Agriculture and Food Innovation (QAAFI), The University of Queensland Elkhorn Building (#1024), Indooroopilly, QLD, Australia, [3]Institute of Nutrition, Mahidol University, Salaya, Nakhon Pathom, Thailand

4.1 Introduction

Digestive health is a very important part of human being's health that consists of various physiological activities. To maintain a healthy body, it is important to have a healthy digestive system. The gastrointestinal (GI) tract also plays a vital role in the absorption of nutrients, transport of minerals, and regulation of metabolism (Isackson & Ashley, 2023). In recent years, many studies have been conducted on functional foods and have gained traction for their potential benefits in supporting GI health. These specialized foods offer enhanced health advantages beyond basic nourishment due to the presence of bioactive compounds like probiotics, prebiotics, dietary fibers, and phytochemicals (Nath et al., 2023). Extensive research explores how these components can influence gut microbe balance, optimize nutrient absorption, promote regular bowel movements, and reduce inflammation within the GI tract. Functional foods can be defined as basic, naturally occurring, processed foods that meet the body's nutritional needs and have the potential to improve the host's health in other ways as well. These benefits may include lowering disease rates by enhancing the immune system's ability to fight off infections from pathogens and diseases that alter the host's functioning (Damián et al., 2022). It is vital to comprehend the connection between diet, gut microorganisms, and digestive wellness. It assists in understanding the functional food ingredients, dietary approaches, and their interventions. This chapter aims to provide an overview of functional foods, their classification, and scientific evidence showing the role of functional foods in maintaining GI health. Our study is focused on potential mechanisms by which beneficial effects are exerted on digestive health by acknowledging the literature available.

4.1.1 Importance of digestive health for overall well-being

The optimum digestion process is essential to maintaining the human body's homeostasis. It can be affected by various important processes that are required for maintaining optimum health. Digestive health conducts various processes that involve digestion, absorption, metabolism, and excretion. Effective nutrition intake, balanced energy expenditure, and strong immunity are all dependent on a healthy digestive tract (Saha & Pathak, 2021). These progressions are essential for both health homeostasis and disease prevention. Nutritional deficits, stomach pain, reduced immunity, and long-term illnesses like metabolic disorders or inflammatory bowel diseases can all be brought on by digestive disorders (Corsello et al., 2020). Hence, putting intestinal health first is essential to attaining and maintaining health over the long term.

4.1.2 Significance of functional foods in promoting gut health

Ingestion of functional foods that improve GI health is very important. These meals provide extra benefits over basic nourishment. These support the gut flora homeostasis and regulate the optimum function of the GI process. For

Unleashing the Power of Functional Foods and Novel Bioactives. DOI: https://doi.org/10.1016/B978-0-443-28862-3.00004-2

instance, probiotics support the colonization of the gut flora. Prebiotics nourish and promote the formation of beneficial gut flora. Dietary fiber promotes normal digestion, increases feelings of fullness, and helps good gut flora proliferate. Numerous phytochemicals are present in fruits, vegetables, and whole grains that have been shown to have antiinflammatory properties and antioxidant properties, as well as supporting gut integrity and preventing various GI problems. Individuals can maintain the gut microbiome, improve digestive health, and lower their risk of GI illnesses by including functional foods in their normal diet (Banerjee et al., 2023). A variety of disorders can be treated and prevented with the use of functional dietary ingredients. Functional food ingredients that are biologically active can lower blood cholesterol and lessen the risk of several noncommunicable illnesses, including cancer, type II diabetes, cardiovascular disease, osteoporosis, and inflammation (Shaikh, 2022). Considering the consequence of functional foods in promoting gut health, emerging dietary strategies that aid digestive well-being by contributing to gut microbiome diversity are important to study.

4.2 The digestive process: an overview

The digestive system encompasses many different tissues and organs. The digestion process' main functions include the breakdown of food into simple molecules, absorption of nutrients, and excretion of waste. The process of digestion begins in the oral cavity where the breakdown of food takes place. The meal then passes into the stomach through the esophagus. Enzymes and gastric acids further break down the food into simple components (Patricia & Dhamoon, 2022). The small intestine then helps the body absorb nutrients. Waste material builds up concurrently as a stool in preparation for ultimate expulsion. Supporting organs such as the liver, pancreas, and gallbladder supply vital chemicals and enzymes throughout this process (Sensoy, 2021). Comprehending the intricate mechanisms of digestion is crucial for maintaining optimal digestive health and ensuring efficient nutrient assimilation.

4.2.1 Explanation of the gastrointestinal system

The digestive system comprises a complex network of organs, sometimes referred to as the GI tract. It helps to convert food into nutrients that can be absorbed. The seven major organs involved in the flow of digestion are the mouth, esophagus, stomach, small intestine, large intestine, rectum, and anus as shown in Fig. 4.1 (Derrickson & Tortora, 2019; Gastrointestinal Tract & Definition, 2019). It starts in the oral cavity and finishes in the anus. Let us understand a description of each organ of the digestive system concerning microbiomes.

4.2.1.1 Mouth

The mouth or oral cavity is the initial part of the digestive system, lined with mucus membranes. This area houses vital structures like the tongue, teeth, and salivary glands that play crucial roles. The tongue facilitates chewing and swallowing through its movements. Teeth mechanically break down food into smaller pieces for easier digestion. Salivary glands secrete saliva, which contains the enzyme amylase, initiating carbohydrate digestion (Tortora et al., 2021). The human oral cavity is home to a complex ecosystem of microorganisms, with an estimated 700 prokaryotic species identified to date. These species belong to 185 genera and 12 phyla, including *Firmicutes, Fusobacteria, Proteobacteria*, and *Bacteroidetes*, among others. This diverse microbiome encompasses bacteria, fungi, viruses, archaea, and protozoa, although most studies focus primarily on the bacterial components. Among Gram-positive bacteria, *cocci* genera include *Abiotrophia, Peptostreptococcus, Streptococcus*, and *Stomatococcus*, while Gram-positive rods encompass *Actinomyces, Bifidobacterium, Corynebacterium, Eubacterium, Lactobacillus, Propionibacterium, Pseudoramibacter, and Rothia*. On the Gram-negative side, the *cocci* genera feature *Moraxella, Neisseria, and Veillonella*. Gram-negative rods consist of *Campylobacter, Capnocytophaga, Desulfobacter, Desulfovibrio, Eikenella, Fusobacterium, Hemophilus, Leptotrichia, Prevotella, Selemonas, Simonsiella, Treponema*, and *Wolinella*. Additionally, certain bacteria contribute to saliva production and assist in breaking down carbohydrates during the chewing process, initiating digestion (Deo & Deshmukh, 2019). This extensive microbial diversity engages in a symbiotic relationship with the host, providing mutual benefits while inhibiting the growth of pathogenic species.

4.2.1.2 Esophagus

The esophagus is a muscular tube that connects the throat (pharynx) to the stomach. The pharynx, or throat, and the stomach are connected by the esophagus, a muscular tube. Its length is roughly 25 centimeters (10 in.). Food is moved from the mouth to the stomach by the esophagus through a series of synchronized muscle contractions called peristalsis

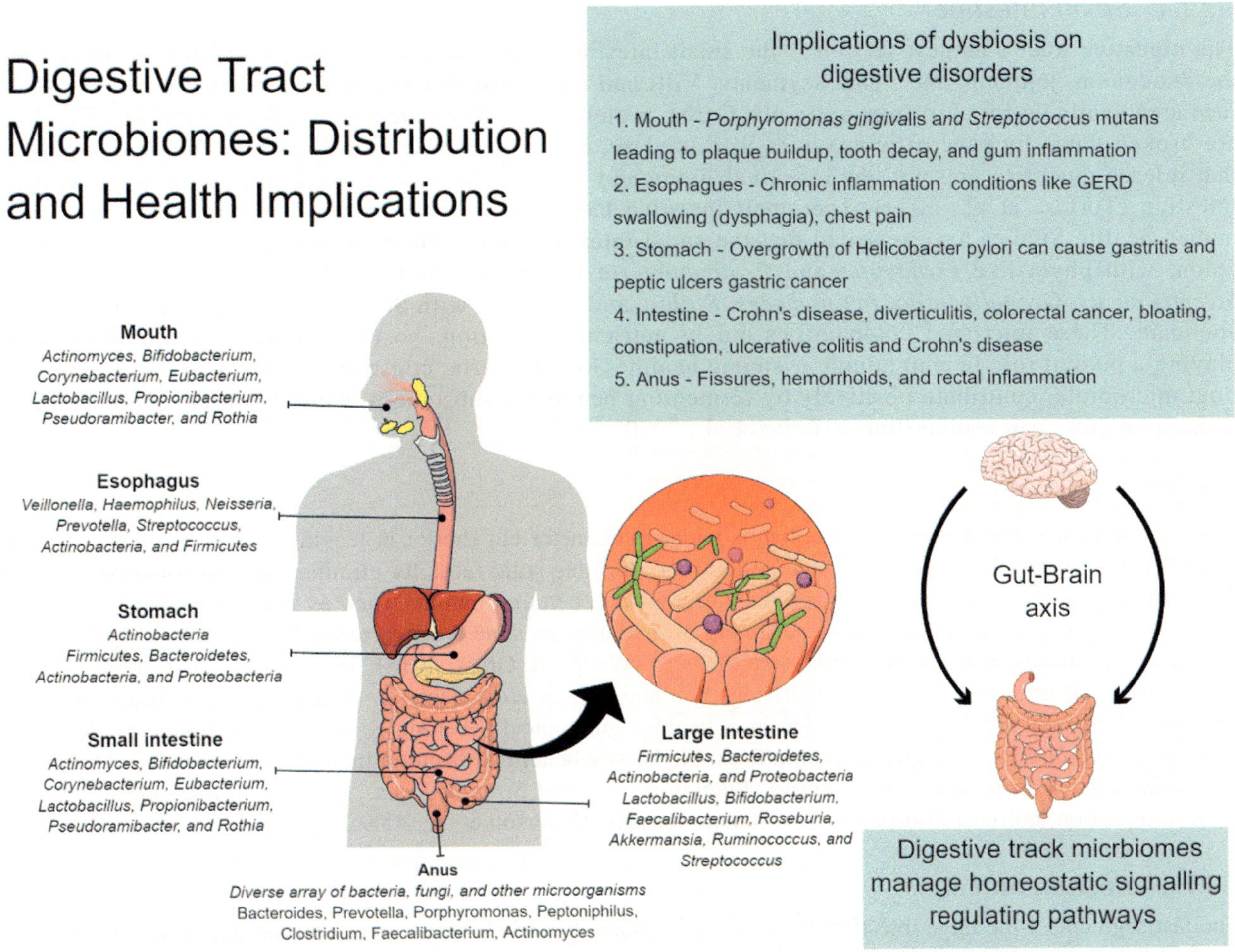

FIGURE 4.1 Digestive tract microbiomes, distribution, and health implication. *GERD*, Gastroesophageal reflux disease.

(Netter, 2019). The oral and native esophageal microbiomes are similar in composition, with a high relative abundance of the genera *Streptococcus* and the phylum *Firmicutes*. In a healthy esophagus, the most prevalent bacterial taxa are *Veillonella, Haemophilus, Neisseria, Prevotella, and Streptococcus*. Even in a normal esophagus, however, the makeup of bacteria might vary based on several circumstances (Park & Lee, 2020). The other six phyla are *Bacteroidetes* (20%), *Actinobacteria* (4%), *Proteobacteria* (2%), *Fusobacteria* (2%), *Firmicutes* (70%), and *TM7 (Saccharibacteria phylum)* (1%) (May & Abrams, 2018).

4.2.1.3 Stomach

The digestive system of the stomach is formed like a "J" shape. It generates digestive juices and acids that catalyze bodily chemical reactions. To enable food to move through to your small intestine, this mixture of digestive fluids and enzymes breaks it down. Hydrochloric acid and pepsin, the enzymes that break down proteins, are found in the gastric juice secreted by the stomach (17). To guard against harm from the acidic environment, mucous cells in the lining of the stomach secrete a coating of mucus. Considering gut microbiome in acidic environments, recent studies using culture-independent techniques, specifically 16 S rRNA sequencing, have revealed significant bacterial diversity in the human stomach. In individuals without major disruptions to their gastric microbiota—such as infection with *Helicobacter pylori* or the use of proton pump inhibitors (PPIs)—the bacterial population in the stomach and duodenum is markedly smaller than that of the lower GI tract, likely due to the lower pH in these upper GI organs. The primary bacterial phyla in the human stomach include *Firmicutes, Bacteroidetes, Actinobacteria, and Proteobacteria*. Unlike the lower GI tract and feces, where *Firmicutes* predominate followed by *Bacteroidetes*, the stomach and duodenum are primarily inhabited by *Firmicutes* and *Proteobacteria* (Ohno & Satoh-Takayama, 2020).

4.2.1.4 Small intestine

The digestive tract's longest section is the small intestine, which is around 6 m (20 ft) long. It is divided into the duodenum, jejunum, and ileum segments. Villi and microvilli that line the small intestine increase the surface area available for absorbing nutrients. Carbs, proteins, and lipids are easier to digest and absorb when they are broken down by pancreatic enzymes like amylase, esterase, lactase, and liver bile. Numerous goblet cells that release mucus to preserve the intestinal lining and aid in food passage are found in the walls of the small intestine (Tortora et al., 2021). The small intestine harbors a diverse array of microbial species crucial for human health. Studies have revealed that the small intestinal microbiome differs significantly from that of the colon, with phyla like *Firmicutes* and *Proteobacteria* being predominant. Commonly found species include *Streptococcus, Granulicatella, Actinomyces, Rothia*, and *Gemella*, with Streptococcus species being particularly abundant. These microbial communities aid in nutrient absorption, host metabolism, and immune function, playing a pivotal role in maintaining systemic health. Good bacteria, constituting 10%–20% of the small intestinal microbiota, contribute positively by fermenting beneficial substances, while the presence of bad bacteria, making up 20%, can lead to illness (Leite et al., 2020).

4.2.1.5 Large intestine

The large intestine, also known as the colon, is wider in diameter but shorter in length compared to the small intestine. It absorbs water and electrolytes from undigested food, forming solid feces for elimination. The colon contains bacteria that ferment undigested carbohydrates, producing gases and certain vitamins, such as vitamin K which shows gut protective activity (Lai et al., 2022). The inner lining of the large intestine is characterized by numerous crypts and glands, which secrete mucus to lubricate the passage of feces (Waugh & Grant, 2018). The human gut is home to a rich and diverse array of microbial species, comprising thousands of different bacteria, archaea, fungi, viruses, and protozoa. The most common and abundant species in a healthy gut typically belong to the phyla *Firmicutes, Bacteroidetes, Actinobacteria, and Proteobacteria*. Within these phyla, key beneficial bacteria include *Lactobacillus, Bifidobacterium, Faecalibacterium, Roseburia, Akkermansia, Ruminococcus, and Streptococcus*. These beneficial species play crucial roles in digestion, nutrient absorption, and immune function (Peterson et al., 2009).

4.2.1.6 Rectum and anus

The last segment of the large intestine, the rectum, is situated just before the anus. During defecation, it acts as a holding tank for the feces before they are released from the body. The rectal wall is made up of smooth muscle fibers and elastic tissue that allows it to expand and hold the feces (23). Anus is an orifice via which the body expels feces from the digestive tract. Sphincter muscles, such as the internal and external anal sphincters, which regulate feces transit, encircle it (Waugh & Grant, 2018). A study with 20 adolescent women as a sample shows the anus microbiome comprises a diverse array of bacteria, fungi, and other microorganisms. The genera Bacteroides (18.5% ± 11.6%) and Prevotella (42.2% ± 24.2%) dominated the anal microbiotas, with additional genera (*Porphyromonas, Peptoniphilus, Clostridium, Faecalibacterium*, and *Actinomyces*) (Smith et al., 2016). The microbiome processes operate harmoniously, and they support efficient digestion and nutrient absorption, thus contributing to energy production, immune response, and other essential functions. Assuring the effective breakdown of food and the extraction of nutrients necessary for sustaining health and vigor, each digestive system organ makes a distinct contribution to the processes of digestion, absorption, and evacuation.

4.2.2 Description of the digestion and absorption process

The breakdown of eaten food into absorbable nutrients and their subsequent reception into circulation is made possible by the intricate set of activities known as digestion and absorption, which take place within the GI tract (Patricia & Dhamoon, 2022). The digestive system's many organs and enzymes work together to coordinate mechanical, chemical, and biotransformative processes.

4.2.2.1 The digestion processes

The digestive process can be classified into two types: mechanical digestion and chemical digestion.

1. Mechanical digestion: To increase the surface area of food for enzymatic activity, food is physically broken down into smaller particles during mechanical digestion. It starts in the mouth, where food is broken down into a bolus

that may be taken by chewing and combining with saliva. Muscle spasms in the stomach combine the food with gastric secretions, churning it into a semiliquid termed chyme. Food is moved down the GI system by peristalsis, which is the regular contraction of the smooth muscle in the digestive tract. This movement helps in food absorption and digestion (Sensoy, 2021).

2. Chemical digestion: Chemical digestion also known as enzymatic digestion is the process by which complicated chemicals are broken down into simpler forms that the body can absorb (Introduction to the Digestive System, 2019). By dissolving starches into smaller sugars like maltose, the saliva produced by the mouth's salivary glands contains the enzyme amylase, which starts the breakdown of carbohydrates. Hydrochloric acid and pepsin, an enzyme that converts proteins into peptides, are secreted by the stomach's gastric glands. To facilitate simpler digestion of fats by pancreatic lipase in the small intestine, bile—which is generated by the liver and kept in the gallbladder—emulsifies fats. Pancreatic amylase, proteases, and lipases are among the digestive enzymes sent into the duodenum by the pancreas to aid in the further breakdown of carbohydrates, proteins, and lipids (Karpińska & Czauderna, 2022).
3. Microbial digestion: Gut microbiota, or microflora, play a key role in digestion by breaking down complex carbohydrates, fibers, and proteins that human enzymes cannot process. Through fermentation, these microbes produce short-chain fatty acids (SCFAs) like acetate, propionate, and butyrate, which support colon health and have antiinflammatory effects. They also help synthesize essential nutrients like vitamin K and certain B vitamins, aiding nutrient absorption (Liu et al., 2023). A balanced microbiota is crucial for optimal digestion and immune function, while imbalances can lead to digestive issues, emphasizing the need for a healthy diet and lifestyle to maintain gut health.

4.2.2.2 The absorption processes

Absorption chiefly arises in the small intestine where the maximum of nutrients are absorbed into the bloodstream. The small intestine is creased with finger-like projections called villi, and there is a rise in its surface area for nutrient absorption. Glucose, amino acids, fatty acids, vitamins, and minerals are the nutrients that are absorbed through the villi, and then they are transported into blood capillaries and lymphatic vessels (Chen et al., 2016). Water and electrolytes are also absorbed throughout the digestive tract, with the majority being absorbed in the small intestine and outstanding in the large intestine to form feces (Wang, Camilleri, et al., 2022). The absorption of nutrients in the small intestine involves various mechanisms, including active transport, passive diffusion, facilitated diffusion, and cotransport (symport and antiport). Here is a breakdown of each mechanism along with realistic examples of vitamins, macronutrients, and minerals as shown in Fig. 4.2.

4.2.2.2.1 Active transport

Active transport is a fundamental process within biological systems that enables the movement of ions, molecules, and other substances across cell membranes against their concentration gradient, from areas of lower concentration to areas of higher concentration (Chen & Lui, 2022). Active transport relies on cellular energy (usually ATP) to move substances against their concentration gradient. In the context of the gut microbiota, SCFAs like butyrate, produced by microbial fermentation, provide energy to colonocytes, thereby supporting active transport processes such as the sodium–potassium ATPase pump, which maintains ion gradients critical for nutrient absorption. ATP hydrolysis provides the necessary energy to drive the conformational changes in the carrier proteins, allowing them to transport molecules against their concentration gradients. For example, in humans, active transport mechanisms in the intestinal epithelium facilitate the absorption of glucose, amino acids, and minerals from the digestive tract into the bloodstream (Trommelen et al., 2021), as shown in Fig. 4.2.

4.2.2.2.2 Passive diffusion

Passive diffusion is a fundamental process by which substances move across cell membranes without the expenditure of energy, driven solely by the concentration gradient (Di & Kerns, 2016). In passive diffusion, molecules or ions move from regions of higher concentration to regions of lower concentration until equilibrium is reached. One example of passive diffusion is the movement of water through aquaporins. Lipid-soluble vitamins, including vitamins A, D, E, and K, have molecular structures that allow them to dissolve in and pass through the lipid bilayer of cell membranes (Reboul, 2023).

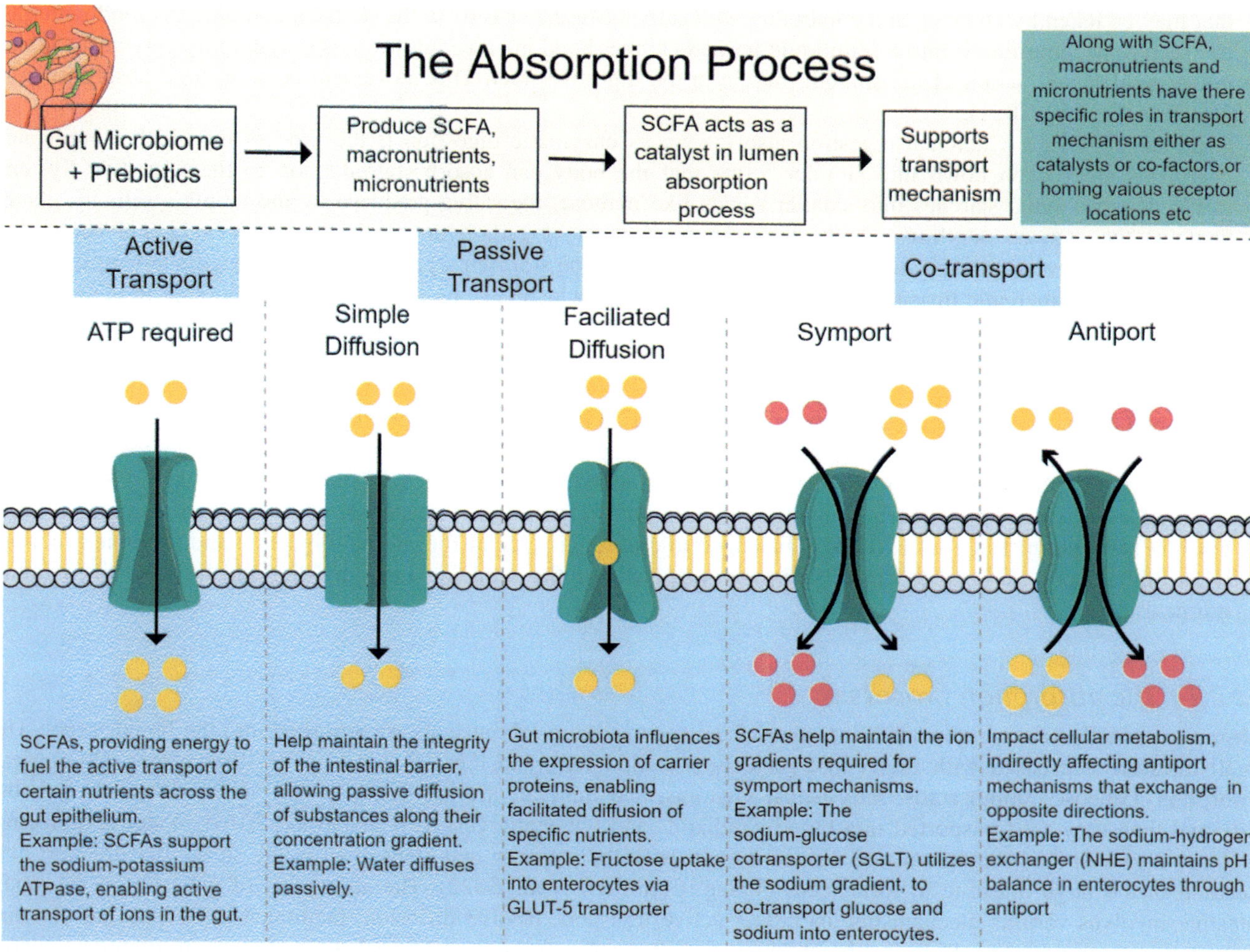

FIGURE 4.2 The absorption process (SCFA—short chain fatty acids, ATP—adenosine tri-phosphate, GLUT-5—glucose transporter 5, SGLT—sodium-glucose transporter, sodium hydrogen exchanger).

4.2.2.2.3 Facilitated diffusion

Facilitated diffusion is a pivotal mechanism by which substances are transported across cell membranes with the aid of carrier proteins, moving along their concentration gradient without the expenditure of cellular energy. This process allows for the selective and efficient transport of specific molecules that would otherwise face difficulty crossing the lipid bilayer unassisted as shown in Fig. 4.2. A compelling example of facilitated diffusion is the transportation of fructose into enterocytes, the absorptive cells of the small intestine (Martínez-Crespo et al., 2020). Gut microbiota influences the expression of carrier proteins, enabling facilitated diffusion of specific nutrients. For example, fructose uptake into enterocytes via GLUT-5 (glucose transporter-5) transporter is facilitated by carrier proteins, whose expression can be influenced by microbial activity (Ferraris et al., 2018).

4.2.2.2.4 Cotransport (symport and antiport) cotransport involves the simultaneous transport of two different substances across the cell membrane

- Symport: Two substances move in the same direction.
- Antiport: Two substances move in opposite directions.

Symport and antiport transport mechanisms are fundamental processes by which substances are transported across cell membranes in coordination with one another. These mechanisms play crucial roles in maintaining cellular homeostasis and facilitating the uptake of essential nutrients and ions (Cho et al., 2016; Satyanarayana, 2017). In symport, the gut microbiome produces SCFAs, which help maintain the ion gradients required for symport mechanisms. For example, the

TABLE 4.1 Fecal consistency, color, and microflora associated.

Sr. No.	Fecal consistency	Fecal colors	Normal or abnormal	Normal or disturbed microflora in abnormal feces	References
1.	Formed, soft	Brown	Normal	Coliforms, streptococci, and lactobacilli	van Houte and Gibbons (1966)
2.	Hard, lumpy	Dark brown	Abnormal	Reduced Bifidobacterium and Lactobacillus, increased Firmicutes and *Bacteroidetes*	Zhao and Yu (2016)
3.	Watery	Green	Abnormal	Increased *Escherichia coli, Clostridium difficile*, and other pathogenic bacteria	Allen et al. (2013)
4.	Loose, mushy	Yellow	Abnormal	Increased Clostridium, Bacteroides, or other dysbiotic species	Vandeputte et al. (2015)
5.	Soft with mucus	Pale	Abnormal	Reduced beneficial bacteria, and increased opportunistic pathogens like Enterobacteriaceae	Rustam et al. (2006)

sodium-glucose cotransporter (SGLT) utilizes the sodium gradient, influenced by SCFAs, to cotransport glucose and sodium into enterocytes. In antiport, the gut microbes impact cellular metabolism, indirectly affecting antiport mechanisms that exchange substances across the cell membrane in opposite directions. For example, the sodium-hydrogen exchanger (NHE) maintains pH balance in enterocytes through antiport, which may be affected by the metabolic activities of gut microbes (Nikolovska et al., 2022), as shown in Fig. 4.2.

4.2.2.3 Biotransformation (metabolism and elimination)

Once absorbed, nutrients are transported via the bloodstream to various cells and tissues throughout the body. Biotransformation is the process by which substances are chemically transformed in the body, often leading to changes in their biological activity and facilitating their elimination. This process typically involves enzymatic reactions, converting compounds into more water-soluble and easily excretable forms. In the context of metabolism and elimination, biotransformation occurs primarily in the liver (liver-gut axis), where enzymes like cytochrome P450 oxidize, reduce, or hydrolyze substances. The metabolites produced through biotransformation are then transported to the kidneys (kidney gut axis) or intestines for excretion via urine or feces, respectively. For example, amino acids are utilized for protein synthesis or converted into energy. Fatty acids are either oxidized for energy or stored as triglycerides in adipose tissue. Vitamins and minerals play essential roles as cofactors in enzymatic reactions, maintaining cellular functions, and supporting overall health (39). The kidney gut axis and liver gut axis play a major role in metabolism and elimination within the digestive system. These processes ensure the body receives vital nutrients for energy production, growth, repair, and various physiological functions while efficiently removing waste and toxins to maintain internal balance. As stool is expelled through the anus, it carries with it a snapshot of this complex microbiome, providing valuable insights into the health and composition of the gut's microbial community. By analyzing stool samples, scientists can identify which microbes are present and in what proportions, offering clues about the overall balance or imbalance of the gut microbiome. A common method used for this analysis is 16 S rRNA sequencing, which allows for the detection and classification of bacterial species in a sample. This technique can help identify potential deficiencies or excesses in the microbiome, guiding personalized approaches to restoring gut health and addressing digestive issues. Different fecal consistency can be associated with the presence of different microflora, as shown in Table 4.1.

4.3 Understanding what are poor dietary choices

Poor dietary choices refer to consuming foods and beverages that are high in unhealthy fats, sugars, refined carbohydrates, and processed ingredients while lacking essential nutrients such as vitamins, minerals, and dietary fiber. This starts causing a disturbance in homeostatic signaling and regulating digestive health. Therefore poor dietary choices could be defined as "food choices that interfere wrongly and create disturbance in homeostatic signaling regulating pathways in digestive health."

- Wrongly processed foods refer to food products that have undergone improper or nonoptimal manufacturing, handling, or storage practices, resulting in reduced quality, safety risks, or altered nutritional profiles. These processing errors can lead to contamination with harmful microorganisms, chemical residues, or the loss of essential nutrients. Common issues include:

- Contamination
- Wrong combination of ingredients
- Nutrient loss
- Chemical additives
- Improper packaging.

To avoid these issues, food manufacturers must adhere to strict safety and quality standards, ensuring that processing practices maintain the safety, nutritional integrity, and overall quality of the food.

- Highly processed foods: Processed foods, such as fast food, frozen meals, sugary snacks, and packaged foods, are often high in added sugars, unhealthy fats, and sodium. They typically lack essential nutrients, contain artificial additives, and can cause weight gain, which was proved in a clinical trial conducted on 20 weight-stable adults (Hall et al., 2019).
- Sugary beverages: Sugary drinks like soda, fruit juices with added sugars, sweetened teas, and energy drinks contribute excessive amounts of sugar to the diet without providing any nutritional benefits. Consuming these beverages regularly can lead to weight gain, insulin resistance, and an increased risk of chronic diseases like type 2 diabetes and cardiovascular disease (Yoshida & Simoes, 2018).
- Fried and fast foods: Foods that are deep-fried or prepared with unhealthy fats (e.g., trans fats and hydrogenated oils) contribute to inflammation, obesity, and heart disease. Fast food items like burgers, fries, fried chicken, and pizza are typically high in calories, unhealthy fats, and sodium while lacking essential nutrients (Mohammadbeigi et al., 2018).
- Low-fiber foods: Diets low in dietary fiber from fruits, vegetables, whole grains, and legumes can lead to constipation, irregular bowel movements, and an increased risk of digestive disorders like diverticulitis and colorectal cancer (Veettil et al., 2021).
- Excessive consumption of red and processed meats: Diets high in red and processed meats, such as bacon, sausage, hot dogs, and deli meats, are associated with an increased risk of heart disease, stroke, type 2 diabetes, and certain cancers. Processed meats contain harmful additives and preservatives like nitrates and nitrites, which may contribute to health problems (Di et al., 2023).

Layman lacks knowledge regarding gut microflora, homeostasis, and management as given above and is unaware of the "feed the feeder" concept.

4.3.1 Clinical evidence of effect of poor dietary choices on gut health

Clinical trials have demonstrated the adverse effects of poor dietary choices on gut health. For example, a 6-month randomized controlled trial involving 217 healthy young adults (aged 18–35, BMI <28 kg/m^2) (body mass index) investigated the effects of diets with varying fat content on gut microbiota, fecal metabolomics, and cardiometabolic risk factors. Participants were provided one of three isocaloric diets: lower fat (20% energy from fat), moderate-fat (30%), and higher fat (40%). The lower fat diet was linked to increased gut microbiota diversity and an abundance of beneficial bacteria like *Blautia* and *Faecalibacterium*, while the higher fat diet led to an increase in *Alistipes* and *Bacteroides*, with a decrease in *Faecalibacterium*. The higher fat diet elevated plasma proinflammatory factors. These findings suggest that choosing a high-fat diet may cause bad changes in gut microbiota (Wan, Wang, et al., 2019). For instance, Sidhu et al. investigated the impact of a short-term diet high in animal products and low in plant-based foods on the gut microbiota composition. The study found that participants consuming the animal-based diet exhibited a significant decrease in the abundance of beneficial bacteria such as *Bifidobacterium* and an increase in potentially harmful bacteria associated with inflammation and metabolic disorders (Sidhu et al., 2023). Modern lifestyles pose significant challenges to digestive health, with poor dietary choices being a primary concern. Diets high in processed foods, sugar, and unhealthy fats can disrupt the balance of beneficial bacteria in the gut, leading to dysbiosis and increased susceptibility to GI issues. For example, clinical studies have shown that diets rich in processed foods and low in fiber are associated with an increased risk of inflammatory bowel diseases like Crohn's disease and ulcerative colitis (Peters et al., 2022). A study involving 297 healthy young subjects investigated the effects of habitual animal fat consumption on gut microbiota, SCFAs, and bile acids (BAs). By using 16 S rRNA gene sequencing, researchers found that high animal fat intake was linked to reduced microbial diversity and lower concentrations of butyric acid and valeric acid, both important

SCFAs. The abundance of SCFA-producing bacteria like *Blautia, Eubacterium hallii*, and *Megamonas* was significantly reduced in the high animal-fat group compared to the low animal-fat group (Wan, Tong, et al., 2019).

Poor dietary choices not only lack essential nutrients but also contribute to severe health issues. To exemplify the impact of poor dietary choices on gut health, clinical trials and studies have demonstrated the detrimental effects of diets high in processed foods and low in fiber on gut microbiota composition and can lead to gut dysbiosis.

4.3.2 Gut dysbiosis

An imbalance in the gut microbial population that results in changes to both the quality and quantity of its activities is referred to as dysbiosis (Regunathan-Shenk et al., n.d.). Poor dietary choices can disrupt the delicate balance of the gut microbiota, leading to dysbiosis. Mechanistically, these dietary patterns promote the growth of pathogenic bacteria such as *Escherichia coli, Clostridium difficile*, and *Enterococcus faecalis* while suppressing beneficial microbes like *Bifidobacteria* and *Lactobacilli*, altering the composition and diversity of the gut microbiome (Ibragimova et al., 2021). Clinical trials have elucidated several mechanisms underlying this phenomenon. For instance, diets high in saturated fats and low in fiber have been associated with decreased abundance of beneficial bacteria such as *Bifidobacteria* and *Lactobacilli* and increased levels of potentially harmful bacteria like *Firmicutes* and *Proteobacteria* (Ibragimova et al., 2021). Moreover, excessive consumption of sugars and artificial sweeteners can disrupt the microbial balance by promoting the growth of sugar-loving bacteria, leading to microbial dysregulation and metabolic disturbances (Cronin et al., 2021).

Gut dysbiosis, often instigated by poor dietary choices, disrupts the intricate balance of the gut microbiota. The impact of gut dysbiosis on health affects various physiological systems beyond the GI tract. Dysbiosis-induced inflammation and intestinal permeability can contribute to systemic inflammation and immune dysfunction, increasing susceptibility to chronic inflammatory conditions such as inflammatory bowel disease (IBD), metabolic syndrome, and autoimmune disorders (Sadeghpour, 2024). Furthermore, dysbiosis-associated alterations in microbial metabolism can perturb host metabolism and energy homeostasis, predisposing individuals to obesity, type 2 diabetes, and cardiovascular disease (Al Bataineh et al., 2023) as shown in Fig. 4.3. Moreover, dysbiosis-induced disruption of the gut-brain axis can influence neurological function and mental health, contributing to conditions like depression, anxiety, and cognitive impairment (Kandpal et al., 2022) (Fig. 4.4).

4.3.3 Implications of dysbiosis on digestive disorders

Long-term consequences of digestive disorders can significantly increase the risk of developing severe complications that can arise from various digestive conditions, which may include:

Mouth: Dysbiosis in the oral microbiome can lead to various dental and periodontal diseases, such as cavities, gingivitis, and periodontitis. Harmful bacteria like *Porphyromonas gingivalis* and *Streptococcus mutans* can overpopulate, leading to plaque buildup, tooth decay, and gum inflammation (Santacroce et al., 2023). The imbalance in oral microbiota can also contribute to bad breath and affect the overall health of the mouth.

Esophagus: (Esophageal strictures) Chronic inflammation and irritation of the esophagus, often seen in conditions like GERD, can lead to the formation of scar tissue and narrowing of the esophageal lumen. Esophageal strictures can cause difficulty swallowing (dysphagia), chest pain, and recurrent food impactions, impairing the individual's ability to eat and leading to nutritional deficiencies (Desai & Moustarah, 2022).

Stomach: The stomach is a critical organ for digestion, where hydrochloric acid and enzymes break down food. Dysbiosis in the stomach, particularly due to the overgrowth of *H. pylori*, can cause gastritis and peptic ulcers. Chronic infection with *H. pylori* can lead to more severe conditions like gastric cancer. Other stomach issues related to dysbiosis may include reduced digestion efficiency and altered gastric acid production (Malfertheiner et al., 2023).

Intestinal: Conditions such as Crohn's disease, diverticulitis, and colorectal cancer can cause structural abnormalities, inflammation, or the formation of adhesions within the intestines, leading to partial or complete blockages. Intestinal obstructions result in severe abdominal pain, bloating, vomiting, and constipation, requiring prompt medical intervention to relieve the obstruction and prevent bowel perforation (Smith & Nehring, 2023). Colorectal cancer is observed in individuals with longstanding inflammatory bowel disease, particularly ulcerative colitis and Crohn's disease, who have an increased risk of developing colorectal cancer over time. Chronic inflammation of the intestinal lining predisposes to genetic mutations and dysplastic changes, which may progress to colorectal adenocarcinoma if left untreated. Regular screening and surveillance colonoscopies are essential for early detection and management of

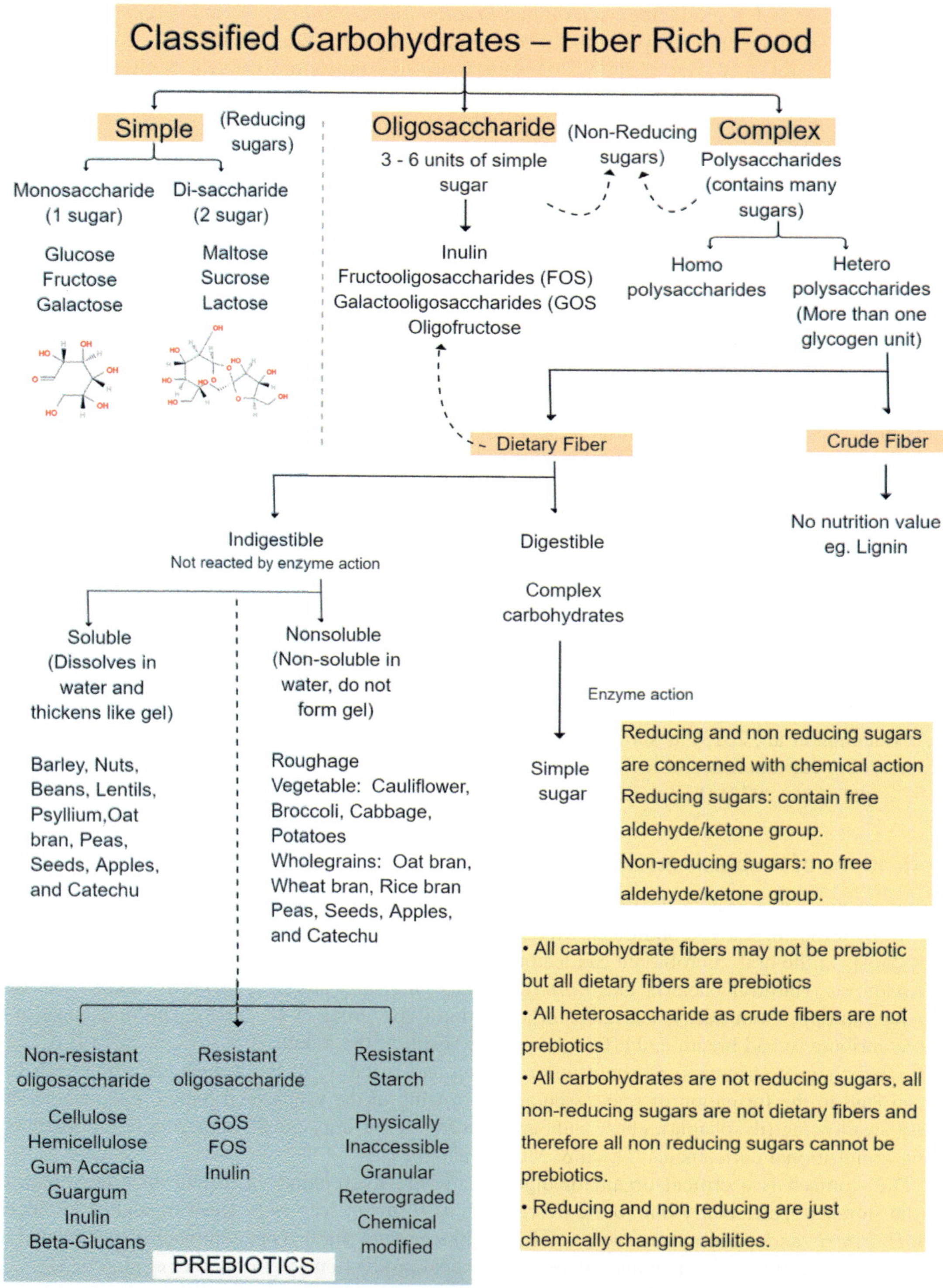

FIGURE 4.3 Classified carbohydrates–fiber-rich food (FOS, GOS). *FOS*, Fructooligosaccharides; *GOS*, galactooligosaccharides.

colorectal cancer in high-risk individuals (Nakanishi et al., n.d). Malabsorption syndromes: Malabsorption results in deficiencies of essential nutrients, vitamins, and minerals, leading to symptoms such as weight loss, fatigue, weakness, anemia, osteoporosis, and neurological complications (Hendifar et al., 2019).

Anus: Dysbiosis can affect the rectal and anal regions by causing inflammation and other GI disorders. Conditions like anal fissures, hemorrhoids, and rectal inflammation can be exacerbated by an imbalanced gut microbiota, leading

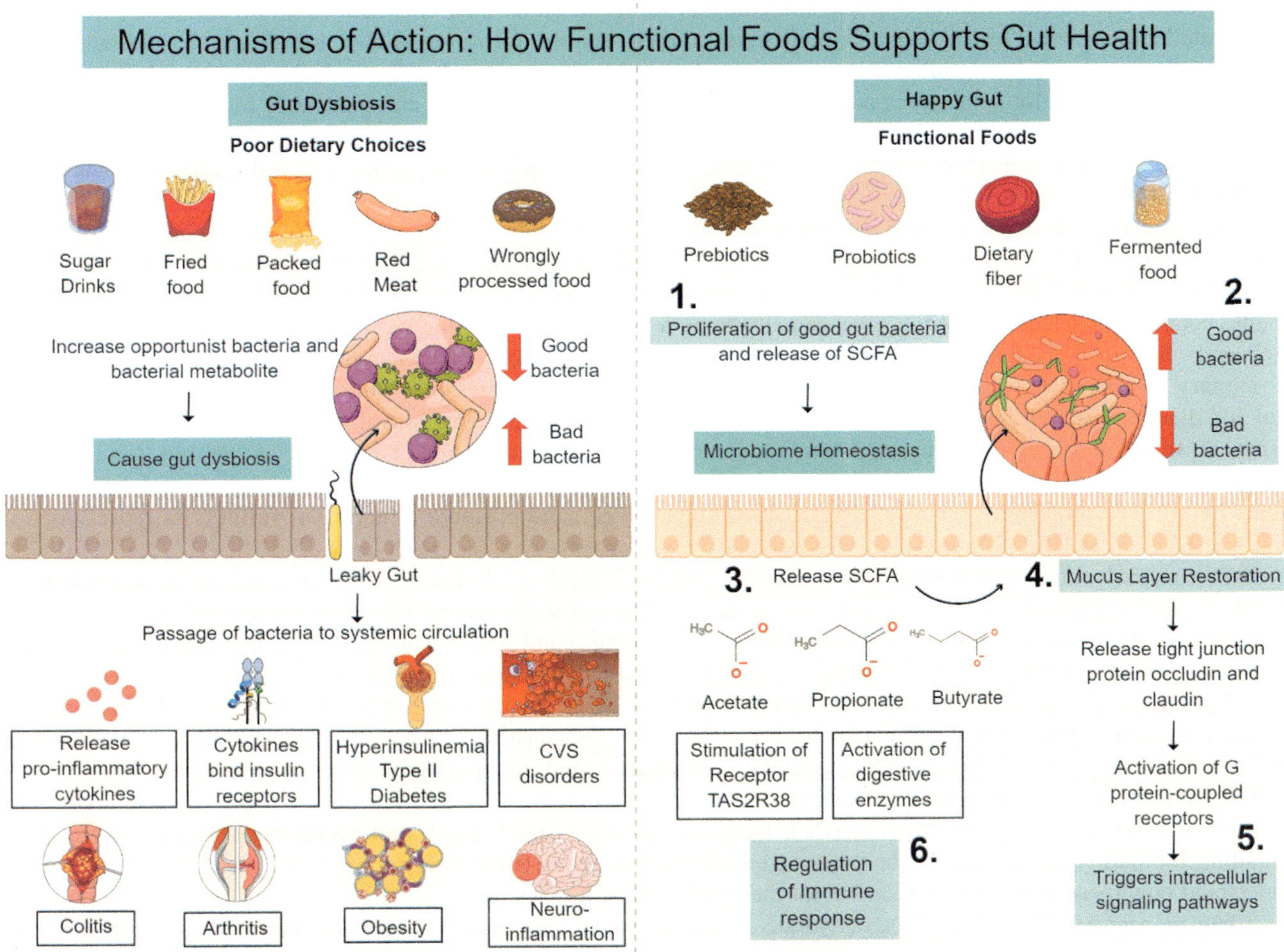

FIGURE 4.4 Mechanisms of action: how functional foods support gut health; CVS—cardiovascular disease, SCFA—short-chain fatty acid, TAS2R38—stands for taste 2 receptor member 38.

to discomfort and pain (Palumbo et al., 2023). The increased production of harmful metabolites and reduced production of beneficial ones, like SCFAs, can contribute to anal irritation and other issues.

In summary, dysbiosis can impact a wide range of digestive organs, leading to various complications and discomforts. Maintaining a healthy and balanced microbiome through a nutritious diet, probiotics, and prebiotics can help prevent or mitigate the adverse effects of dysbiosis on these organs.

4.4 Functional food for digestive health

Functional foods have grabbed attention for their potential to support digestive health and address GI issues effectively. Functional foods are defined as whole foods along with fortified, enriched, or enhanced foods that have a potentially beneficial effect on health when consumed as part of a varied diet regularly at effective levels. The functional foods focused on in this chapter are mainly concerned with the improvement of digestive health. These foods are specially formulated or naturally enriched with components, such as classified carbohydrates, fibers, probiotics, prebiotics, and digestive enzymes, which target specific aspects of digestive function. Incorporating these foods into a balanced diet can play a vital role in promoting GI health, alleviating digestive symptoms, and reducing the risk of long-term digestive complications (Granato et al., 2020).

4.4.1 Classified carbohydrates—fiber-rich food

Carbohydrates are essential macronutrients found in foods and play a crucial role in providing energy for the body's functions. They are composed of carbon, hydrogen, and oxygen atoms, with a general formula of $(CH_2O)n$.

Carbohydrates can be classified into simple and complex forms based on their chemical structure and how quickly they are digested and absorbed by the body. Carbohydrates in their simplest forms are known as monosaccharides and cannot be further broken down into smaller sugar molecules. Examples of monosaccharides include glucose, which is the primary source of energy for cells; fructose, commonly found in fruits and honey; and galactose, found in dairy products. Disaccharides, on the other hand, are composed of two monosaccharide units linked together. Common disaccharides include maltose (glucose + glucose), sucrose (glucose + fructose), and lactose (glucose + galactose) (Satyanarayana, 2017) as depicted in Fig. 4.3.

Complex carbohydrates, also known as polysaccharides, are made up of long chains of monosaccharide units. They can be further categorized into homopolysaccharides and heteropolysaccharides. Starch and glycogen are examples of homopolysaccharides, consisting of repeating glucose units as represented in Fig. 4.3. Starch is found in foods like grains, potatoes, and legumes, while glycogen serves as a storage form of glucose in animals. Heteropolysaccharides, such as dietary fibers, contain a variety of monosaccharides in their structure (Mohammed et al., 2021).

Dietary fibers are a type of complex carbohydrate that cannot be digested by human enzymes. They are important for digestive health and can be divided into soluble and insoluble fibers. Soluble fibers, such as pectins and gums, dissolve in water to form a gel-like substance in the digestive tract. Examples of soluble dietary fibers include barley, nuts, beans, lentils, psyllium, oat bran, peas, seeds, apples, carrots, cucumber, and beat. These fibers help lower cholesterol levels, stabilize blood sugar levels, and promote a feeling of fullness as represented in Fig. 4.3 (Chawla & Patil, 2010).

On the other hand, insoluble fibers, like cellulose and hemicellulose, do not dissolve in water and pass through the digestive system relatively intact. They add bulk to the stool and promote regular bowel movements. Examples of insoluble dietary fibers include roughage, whole grains, wheat bran, cauliflower, potatoes, nuts, and beans. These crude fibers and prebiotics help prevent constipation and maintain GI health (Stryer et al., 2019).

Indigestible or functional fibers can be further classified based on their structure and how they interact with the digestive system. These classifications include nonstarch oligosaccharides, resistant oligosaccharides, and resistant starch, as well as physically inaccessible, granular, retrograded, and chemically modified fibers. These fibers exert a prebiotic effect (Elleuch et al., 2011).

Research indicates that oligofructose (OF), lactulose, resistant starch (RS), and inulin meet each of the criteria, including promoting the growth of the advantageous bacterial genus Bifidobacterium (Weninger et al., 2023). Let us understand how these fibers are also known for their prebiotic properties.

It can be acknowledged that all carbohydrate fibers may not be prebiotic, but all dietary fibers are prebiotics. All heterosaccharides as crude fibers are not prebiotics. All carbohydrates are not reducing sugars, all nonreducing sugars are not dietary fibers, and therefore all nonreducing sugars cannot be prebiotics. Reducing and nonreducing are just chemically changing abilities. Reducing and nonreducing sugars are concerned with chemical action. Reducing sugars contain free aldehyde/ketone group. Nonreducing sugars: no free aldehyde/ketone group.

4.4.2 Prebiotics

4.4.2.1 Definition and types of prebiotics

Prebiotics are nondigestible dietary fibers that selectively stimulate the growth and activity of beneficial bacteria in the colon, thereby promoting GI health and overall well-being. These compounds serve as nourishment for probiotic bacteria, enhancing their colonization and activity within the gut microbiota. The definition of prebiotics has evolved, with the most widely accepted definition proposed by Gibson and Roberfroid in 1995, which defines prebiotics as "nondigestible food ingredients that beneficially affect the host by selectively stimulating the growth and/or activity of one or a limited number of bacteria in the colon, thus improving host health" (Davani-Davari et al., n.d). Prebiotics, classified based on their chemical structure and source, encompass a diverse array of nondigestible dietary fibers that selectively stimulate the growth and activity of beneficial bacteria in the colon, thereby promoting GI health and overall well-being. The detailed studies of prebiotics can be detailed as follows.

4.4.2.1.1 Inulin

Inulin is a naturally occurring polysaccharide composed of fructose molecules linked by β(2-1) glycosidic bonds. Sources of inulin include chicory root, Jerusalem artichokes, onions, and garlic. Inulin serves as a substrate for fermentation by beneficial gut bacteria, promoting the growth of *Bifidobacteria* and *Lactobacilli* (74).

4.4.2.1.2 Fructooligosaccharides

Fructooligosaccharides (FOS) are short-chain fructose polymers consisting of 2–9 fructose molecules linked by β(2-1) glycosidic bonds. FOS naturally occur in foods such as bananas, artichokes, wheat, and asparagus. FOS are resistant to digestion in the small intestine and selectively stimulate the growth of beneficial bacteria in the colon (75).

4.4.2.1.3 Galactooligosaccharides

Galactooligosaccharides (GOS) are oligosaccharides composed of galactose molecules linked by β(1-4) glycosidic bonds. Sources of GOS include legumes, beans, lentils, and certain dairy products. GOS serve as substrates for fermentation by colonic bacteria, promoting the growth of *Bifidobacteria* and other beneficial microbes (76).

4.4.2.1.4 Oligofructose

Oligofructose is a mixture of short-chain inulin and FOS. It is commonly derived from chicory root and is used as a prebiotic supplement and food ingredient. Oligofructose promotes the growth of beneficial bacteria in the gut and enhances GI health (77).

4.4.2.1.5 Resistant starches

Resistant starches are starch molecules that resist digestion in the small intestine and reach the colon intact. Sources of resistant starches include green bananas, legumes, whole grains, and cooked and cooled potatoes. Resistant starches serve as substrates for fermentation by colonic bacteria, contributing to the production of SCFAs and the growth of beneficial bacteria (78).

4.4.2.1.6 Other compounds

Other compounds with prebiotic properties may include polyphenols, such as flavonoids and phenolic acids, found in fruits, vegetables, and plant-based foods. Polyphenols can modulate the composition and activity of gut microbiota, exerting beneficial effects on GI health. Polyphenols are bioactive compounds found abundantly in various plant-based foods, including fruits, vegetables, legumes, nuts, seeds, and whole grains **(79)**. They encompass a diverse group of compounds, such as flavonoids, phenolic acids, lignans, and stilbenes.

- Flavonoids: Flavonoids are the most abundant and well-studied class of polyphenols. They include subclasses like flavonols, flavones, flavanones, flavan-3-ols (catechins), anthocyanins, and isoflavones. Flavonoids are known for their antioxidant, antiinflammatory, and antimicrobial properties. They can modulate the composition and activity of the gut microbiota by promoting the growth of beneficial bacteria like *Bifidobacteria* and *Lactobacilli* while inhibiting the proliferation of pathogenic microbes (80).
- Phenolic acids: Phenolic acids are another important group of polyphenols found in various plant foods. They include hydroxybenzoic acids (e.g., gallic acid) and hydroxycinnamic acids (e.g., caffeic acid and ferulic acid). Phenolic acids possess antioxidant and antiinflammatory properties and can exert prebiotic effects by selectively stimulating the growth of beneficial gut bacteria and enhancing microbial diversity in the gut ecosystem (81).

4.4.2.2 Role of prebiotics in nourishing beneficial gut bacteria

Prebiotics serve as essential components in promoting healthy gut homeostasis by nourishing beneficial gut bacteria through various mechanisms. They resist digestion in the upper GI tract, reaching the colon intact. There, they selectively ferment by beneficial gut bacteria, such as *Bifidobacteria* and *Lactobacilli*, which possess the necessary enzymes to break down these complex carbohydrates. This selective fermentation not only provides a source of nutrition specifically for these beneficial bacteria but also leads to the production of SCFAs (SCFAs), such as acetate, propionate, and butyrate. These SCFAs play vital roles in maintaining gut health, serving as an energy source for colonocytes, regulating inflammation, and promoting the growth of beneficial bacteria (Nogal et al., 2021). Additionally, prebiotics can interact with specific receptors on intestinal epithelial cells, such as G protein-coupled receptors (GPCRs), triggering signaling pathways that regulate various physiological processes, including immune responses and appetite regulation (Manzoor et al., 2022). Overall, incorporating prebiotic-rich foods into the diet supports a healthy gut microbiome and contributes to optimal digestive health.

4.4.2.3 Evidence-based health benefits associated with prebiotic consumption

Consuming prebiotics offers several health benefits, supported by scientific research and clinical studies. Some of the key health benefits associated with prebiotic consumption include:

Improved digestive health: Prebiotics promote the growth and activity of beneficial bacteria in the gut, such as *Bifidobacteria* and *Lactobacilli*, which contribute to digestive health. They help maintain a balanced gut microbiota, enhance intestinal barrier function, and regulate bowel movements, reducing the risk of GI disorders like irritable bowel syndrome (IBS), constipation, and diarrhea (Pham et al., 2021).

Enhanced nutrient absorption: Prebiotics stimulate the growth of beneficial gut bacteria, which, in turn, produce SCFAs (SCFAs) through fermentation. SCFAs, such as acetate, propionate, and butyrate, enhance nutrient absorption in the intestines, particularly of minerals like calcium and magnesium, as well as certain vitamins (Wang, Jiang, et al., 2023).

Support for immune function: The gut microbiota plays a crucial role in regulating immune responses and maintaining immune system balance. Prebiotics help promote the growth of beneficial bacteria that interact with immune cells in the gut-associated lymphoid tissue (GALT) (Bodera, 2008). This interaction helps modulate immune responses and reduce inflammation.

Reduced risk of chronic diseases: Prebiotics may contribute to a reduced risk of chronic diseases, including cardiovascular disease, obesity, and type 2 diabetes. By promoting healthy gut microbiota and improving metabolic parameters, such as lipid profiles and blood glucose levels, prebiotics help mitigate risk factors associated with these diseases (Mitchell et al., 2015, 2021).

Promotion of weight management: Prebiotics may aid in weight management and obesity prevention by promoting feelings of fullness and satiety, reducing energy intake, and modulating gut hormones involved in appetite regulation. Additionally, prebiotics can influence the metabolism of dietary fats and carbohydrates, potentially affecting energy balance and body composition (Ben Othman et al., 2023).

4.4.3 Probiotics

4.4.3.1 Definition and types of probiotics

Probiotics are live microorganisms that, when administered in adequate amounts, confer health benefits to the host (no date). These beneficial bacteria help maintain the balance of the gut microbiota and support various aspects of digestive and immune health. There are several types of probiotics commonly used, including strains of *Lactobacillus, Bifidobacterium, Streptococcus, and Saccharomyces. Lactobacillus and Bifidobacterium* genera are among the most extensively studied and widely used probiotics, known for their ability to survive the acidic environment of the stomach and colonize the intestines. *Streptococcus thermophilus* is another probiotic strain commonly found in dairy products. At the same time, *Saccharomyces boulardii* is a yeast probiotic known for its ability to support GI health and combat antibiotic-associated diarrhea (Kaźmierczak-Siedlecka et al., 2020). Each type of probiotic may offer unique health benefits, and the selection of specific strains depends on the desired therapeutic effects and individual health needs.

4.4.3.2 Mechanisms by which probiotics support gut health

Probiotics support gut health through a multifaceted set of mechanisms involving interactions with the intestinal epithelium, modulation of the gut microbiota, and regulation of immune responses. The stepwise mechanism by which probiotics exert their beneficial effects on gut health can be elucidated as follows.

4.4.3.2.1 Adhesion to intestinal epithelial cells

Probiotic bacteria possess surface structures such as pili, fimbriae, and adhesins that facilitate their adherence to the mucosal surface of the intestinal epithelium. These structures interact with host cell receptors, including mucin glycoproteins and epithelial cell surface proteins, promoting colonization and establishment within the gut (Gorreja & Walker, 2022).

4.4.3.2.2 Competitive exclusion of pathogens

Once adhered to the intestinal epithelium, probiotics compete with pathogenic microorganisms for nutrients and binding sites, preventing the adherence and colonization of pathogens. Probiotic strains such as *Lactobacillus* and

Bifidobacterium produce antimicrobial substances like bacteriocins, organic acids (e.g., lactic acid), and hydrogen peroxide, which inhibit the growth and proliferation of pathogenic bacteria (Haghshenas et al., 2023).

4.4.3.2.3 Reinforcement of intestinal barrier function

Probiotics enhance intestinal barrier function by stimulating the production of tight junction proteins (e.g., occludin and claudins) and mucin secretion by intestinal epithelial cells. These proteins help maintain the integrity of the intestinal epithelium, preventing the translocation of pathogens and harmful substances across the gut barrier (Camilleri, 2021).

4.4.3.2.4 Modulation of immune responses

Probiotics interact with immune cells within the gut-associated lymphoid tissue (GALT), including dendritic cells, macrophages, and T cells, through pattern recognition receptors (PRRs) such as Toll-like receptors (TLRs) and nucleotide-binding oligomerization domain (NOD)-like receptors. Activation of these receptors by probiotic-derived molecules, such as lipoteichoic acid and peptidoglycans, modulates immune signaling pathways, leading to the production of antiinflammatory cytokines (e.g., IL-10) and suppression of pro-inflammatory cytokines (e.g., TNF-alpha and IL-6) (Hemarajata & Versalovic, 2013).

4.4.3.2.5 Production of short-chain fatty acids

Probiotic bacteria ferment dietary fibers and undigested carbohydrates in the colon, resulting in the production of SCFAs such as acetate, propionate, and butyrate. SCFAs serve as an energy source for colonocytes, regulate intestinal pH, and promote the growth of beneficial bacteria, thereby contributing to gut homeostasis and health (Nagpal et al., 2018).

4.4.3.2.6 Enhancement of nutrient absorption

Probiotics aid in the digestion and absorption of nutrients by producing enzymes such as lactase, proteases, and lipases, which break down complex carbohydrates, proteins, and fats into absorbable forms. By improving nutrient bioavailability, probiotics support overall GI function and metabolic health (Barkhidarian et al., 2021).

4.4.3.3 Evidence of the benefits of probiotics in alleviating digestive issues

Evidence supporting the benefits of probiotics in alleviating digestive issues is substantial and spans various GI conditions. Clinical studies have demonstrated the efficacy of probiotics in managing symptoms associated with conditions such as irritable bowel syndrome (IBS), inflammatory bowel disease (IBD), diarrhea, constipation, and gastroenteritis (Jung et al., 2022). A study examined the impact of kefir, a fermented probiotic dairy product, on fecal microflora and symptoms in patients with inflammatory bowel disease (IBD). In this open-label trial, 45 IBD patients were divided into treatment and control groups. The treatment group received 400 mL/day of kefir for 4 weeks, and changes in stool *Lactobacillus* levels and symptoms like abdominal pain and bloating were monitored. Results showed that kefir increased fecal *Lactobacillus* counts significantly and reduced symptoms like bloating in Crohn's disease patients. Additionally, there were decreases in inflammatory markers like erythrocyte sedimentation rate and C-reactive protein, suggesting that kefir consumption could have beneficial effects on gut health and IBD-related symptoms in the short term (Yılmaz et al., 2019). Probiotics, particularly strains of *Lactobacillus* and *Bifidobacterium*, have been shown to restore microbial balance, improve gut barrier function, modulate immune responses, and reduce inflammation in the gut. For example, in individuals with IBS, probiotic supplementation has been associated with reductions in abdominal pain, bloating, and irregular bowel movements. A randomized, placebo-controlled trial studied the effects of dietary fibers and probiotics on functional constipation in 250 adults. Participants received polydextrose, psyllium husk, wheat bran + psyllium husk, or *Bifidobacterium animalis* + *Lacticaseibacillus rhamnosus*, with a maltodextrin placebo. Of the 242 who completed the 4-week study, all fiber/probiotic groups showed improved stool quality (Bristol stool scale score), while the placebo group did not. The fiber/probiotic interventions caused specific changes in gut microbiota, like increased Bifidobacterium in group A and Anaerostipes in groups B and C, linked to improved bowel movements (Lai et al., 2023). Similarly, in patients with ulcerative colitis and Crohn's disease, probiotics have been found to alleviate symptoms and reduce disease severity. Furthermore, probiotics are effective in preventing and treating antibiotic-associated diarrhea, traveler's diarrhea, and infectious gastroenteritis by promoting the growth of beneficial bacteria and inhibiting the proliferation of pathogens (Liao et al., 2021). Overall, the evidence supporting the use of probiotics in alleviating digestive issues underscores their potential as a safe and effective therapeutic intervention for GI health.

4.4.4 Fermented foods or postbiotics

4.4.4.1 Explanation of the fermentation process and its impact on gut health

Fermented foods play a crucial role in promoting gut microbiota balance by introducing beneficial bacteria into the GI tract and supporting the growth of diverse microbial communities. These foods undergo the fermentation process, which involves the action of beneficial bacteria and yeast that convert sugars and carbohydrates into organic acids, gases, and alcohol. It involves the breakdown of complex carbohydrates by beneficial bacteria in the colon, leading to the production of SCFAs (SCFAs) and other metabolites. This process occurs when indigestible carbohydrates, such as dietary fibers and prebiotics, reach the colon intact and serve as substrates for fermentation by gut microbiota. Beneficial bacteria, such as *Bifidobacteria* and *Lactobacilli*, possess the necessary enzymes to ferment these complex carbohydrates, converting them into SCFAs like acetate, propionate, and butyrate. As a result, fermented foods such as yogurt, kimchi, sauerkraut, kombucha, and miso are rich sources of probiotics, enzymes, and nutrients that contribute to the maintenance of a healthy gut microbiome (Dimidi et al., 2019).

4.4.4.2 Examples of fermented foods and their benefits

- Yogurt: Yogurt is made by fermenting milk with specific strains of bacteria, such as *Lactobacillus bulgaricus* and *S. thermophilus*. During fermentation, these bacteria produce lactic acid, which gives yogurt its characteristic tangy flavor and thick texture. Yogurt is rich in probiotics, which promote gut health by restoring microbial balance, improving digestion, and enhancing immune function. Regular consumption of yogurt has been associated with benefits such as improved lactose digestion, reduced risk of GI infections, and enhanced nutrient absorption (Mirjalili et al., 2023).
- Koshimbir/Kachumbar/Kosambari: Koshimbir or Kachumbar is a traditional Indian salad made with a mix of raw vegetables like cucumbers, tomatoes, onions, and carrots, seasoned with herbs and spices like coriander, mint, and lemon juice. This refreshing salad not only provides essential vitamins, minerals, and fiber but also serves as a source of prebiotics. The raw vegetables in Koshimbir contain dietary fiber, which acts as food for beneficial gut bacteria, promoting their growth and activity. Regular consumption of Koshimbir can help support a healthy gut microbiome, improve digestion, and enhance overall gut health (Srinivasan, 2010).
- Pickle: Pickles are preserved vegetables or fruits that undergo fermentation, resulting in a tangy and flavorful condiment. Traditional pickling methods involve fermenting vegetables or fruits in a brine solution containing salt and spices. During fermentation, beneficial bacteria, such as *Lactobacillus* species, produce lactic acid, which acts as a natural preservative and imparts a sour taste to the pickles. These beneficial bacteria also contribute to the probiotic content of pickles, promoting gut health by restoring microbial balance, improving digestion, and supporting immune function. Additionally, pickles are rich in antioxidants and may have antiinflammatory properties, further enhancing their health benefits (Behera et al., 2020).
- Paneer: Paneer is a type of fresh cheese commonly used in Indian cuisine. Made by curdling milk with an acidic agent like lemon juice or vinegar and then straining the curds, paneer is rich in protein, calcium, and probiotics. The fermentation process involved in paneer-making introduces beneficial bacteria, such as Lactobacillus acidophilus and Bifidobacterium bifidum, into the cheese. Including paneer in the diet can help promote gut health and overall well-being (Saleem et al., 2024).
- Kimchi: Kimchi is a traditional Korean dish made from fermented vegetables, typically cabbage or radishes, seasoned with spices, garlic, and chili peppers. The fermentation process gives kimchi its unique flavor profile and contributes to its probiotic content. Kimchi is rich in beneficial bacteria, such as *Lactobacillus plantarum and Lactobacillus kimchii*, which support gut health and may help reduce inflammation and boost immune function. Additionally, kimchi contains fiber, vitamins, and antioxidants, making it a nutritious addition to the diet (Jung et al., 2024).
- Sauerkraut: Sauerkraut is a fermented cabbage dish that originated in Eastern Europe. It is made by fermenting shredded cabbage with salt and allowing it to ferment for several weeks. During fermentation, lactic acid bacteria naturally present in the cabbage convert sugars into lactic acid, preserving the cabbage and giving sauerkraut its sour flavor. Sauerkraut is a good source of probiotics and fiber, which promote gut health, aid digestion, and support immune function. It is also rich in vitamins C and K, as well as antioxidants. Sauerkraut also acts as a source of natural yeast-containing food (Gaudioso et al., 2022).
- Kombucha: Kombucha is a fermented tea beverage made by fermenting sweetened tea with a symbiotic culture of bacteria and yeast (*SCOBY*). The fermentation process produces a tangy, slightly effervescent drink with a range of

potential health benefits. Kombucha contains probiotics, organic acids, and antioxidants, which may contribute to improved gut health, immune function, and detoxification (Pilipenko et al., 2022).

- Miso: Miso is a traditional Japanese seasoning made from fermented soybeans, salt, and koji (a type of fungus). It is commonly used to flavor soups, sauces, and marinades. Miso fermentation produces a rich, savory paste with a complex umami flavor. Miso is a source of probiotics, enzymes, and nutrients such as vitamins B and K. It may support gut health, aid digestion, and provide antioxidant and antiinflammatory benefits (Saeed et al., 2022).
- Various fermented foods are the natural source of yeast, for example, miso, sauerkraut, kombucha, and yogurt (Behera et al., 2020; Pilipenko et al., 2022; Saeed et al., 2022). Nowadays, people prefer bread, cakes, and biscuits as a source of yeast which comes under a poor dietary choice. However, we can rely beneficially on other natural foods for yeast rather than bread.

4.4.4.3 Role of fermented foods in gut microbiota balance

Regular consumption of fermented foods can help restore microbial balance, enhance gut barrier function, modulate immune responses, and promote overall gut health. By providing a source of beneficial bacteria and supporting the growth of diverse microbial communities, fermented foods contribute to the maintenance of gut microbiota balance. Moreover, SCFAs have been shown to enhance the absorption of minerals such as calcium and magnesium in the colon, contributing to overall nutrient absorption and bone health. They also help regulate intestinal motility and promote regular bowel movements, thereby preventing constipation and supporting digestive regularity (Dimidi et al., 2019).

4.5 Mechanisms of action: how functional foods support gut health

4.5.1 Modulation of gut microbiota composition

Functional foods contribute to the modulation of gut bacteria through mechanisms that both proliferate beneficial gut bacteria and reduce harmful ones.

4.5.1.1 Proliferation of good gut bacteria

Functional foods, particularly those containing probiotics and prebiotics, promote the proliferation of beneficial gut bacteria. Probiotics are live microorganisms that, when consumed in adequate amounts, confer health benefits on the host. These probiotics, such as *Lactobacillus* and *Bifidobacterium* species, colonize the GI tract and compete with pathogenic bacteria for nutrients and adhesion sites. Prebiotics, on the other hand, are nondigestible fibers that serve as food for beneficial gut bacteria. They pass undigested through the upper GI tract and reach the colon, where they are fermented by gut bacteria into SCFAs like acetate, propionate, and butyrate (Damián et al., 2022).

4.5.1.2 Reduction of bad gut bacteria

Functional foods also contribute to the reduction of harmful gut bacteria through various mechanisms. Some functional foods contain bioactive compounds like polyphenols, flavonoids, and essential oils with antimicrobial properties. These compounds inhibit the growth and virulence of pathogenic bacteria by disrupting their cell membranes, interfering with their metabolism, or inhibiting their adhesion to the gut epithelium. Additionally, certain functional foods contain substances like allicin in garlic and thymol in thyme, which exhibit broad-spectrum antimicrobial activity against pathogenic bacteria (Ried et al., 2020). Furthermore, the fermentation of prebiotic fibers into SCFAs creates an acidic environment in the colon, which is unfavorable for the growth of pathogenic bacteria. Moreover, functional foods containing probiotics produce antimicrobial substances like lactic acid and hydrogen peroxide, which inhibit the growth of pathogenic bacteria and contribute to a balanced gut microbiota as shown in Fig. 4.3 (Haghshenas et al., 2023).

4.5.2 Enhancement of digestive enzyme activities

Enhancement of digestive enzyme activities by functional foods involves complex mechanisms that facilitate the breakdown and absorption of nutrients in the GI tract.

4.5.2.1 Stimulation of receptors

Functional foods containing bioactive compounds, such as polyphenols and flavonoids, can interact with receptors on the surface of intestinal epithelial cells. One such receptor is the bitter taste receptor TAS2R38, which has been found to stimulate the secretion of digestive enzymes in response to bitter compounds. Activation of TAS2R38 triggers intracellular signaling pathways that lead to the release of digestive enzymes from pancreatic acinar cells and intestinal goblet cells (Choi et al., 2016).

4.5.2.2 Activation of digestive enzymes

Once released, digestive enzymes such as amylase, protease, lipase, and cellulase act on their respective substrates to break them down into absorbable components. For example, lipase facilitates the hydrolysis of dietary fats into fatty acids and glycerol, and cellulase breaks down cellulose into glucose molecules (Pirahanchi & Sharma, 2020).

4.5.2.3 Examples

- Ginger: Ginger contains bioactive compounds like gingerols and shogaols, which have been shown to stimulate the secretion of digestive enzymes such as amylase and lipase. These compounds activate receptors on intestinal epithelial cells, leading to increased enzyme production and enhanced digestion of carbohydrates and fats (Unuofin et al., 2021).
- Turmeric: Curcumin, the active compound in turmeric, has been found to stimulate the secretion of bile from the gallbladder, which contains BAs and bile salts that aid in the emulsification and digestion of dietary fats. Additionally, curcumin has been shown to enhance the activity of pancreatic lipase, the enzyme responsible for breaking down fats into absorbable components (Peterson et al., 2018).
- Papaya: Papaya contains the enzyme papain, which has proteolytic activity and aids in the digestion of proteins. Papain can help break down complex protein structures into smaller peptides and amino acids, facilitating their absorption in the small intestine (Sharma et al., n.d).

4.5.3 Promotion of intestinal barrier function

Promotion of intestinal barrier function by functional foods involves several mechanisms, including the production of SCFAs, interaction with specific receptors, and modulation of tight junction proteins.

4.5.3.1 Production of short-chain fatty acids

Prebiotics reach the colon intact, where they are fermented by gut bacteria into SCFAs, primarily acetate, propionate, and butyrate. These SCFAs play a crucial role in maintaining intestinal barrier function. Butyrate, in particular, is known for its ability to enhance the integrity of the intestinal epithelial barrier by promoting the expression of tight junction proteins, such as occludin and claudins, which regulate paracellular permeability (Sharma et al., n.d).

4.5.3.2 Interaction with receptors

SCFAs produced during the fermentation of prebiotics interact with specific receptors on intestinal epithelial cells, such as G protein-coupled receptors (GPCRs) like GPR41 and GPR43. Activation of these receptors by SCFAs triggers intracellular signaling pathways that regulate various physiological processes. For example, activation of GPR43 by SCFAs has been shown to increase the expression of mucin genes and antimicrobial peptides, enhancing mucosal barrier integrity and defense against pathogens (Liu et al., 2023).

4.5.3.3 Modulation of tight junction proteins

In addition to SCFAs, prebiotics like inulin and oat fibers can directly modulate the expression and assembly of tight junction proteins, which are essential for maintaining the integrity of the intestinal barrier. By promoting the expression of proteins like occludin, claudins, and zonulin, prebiotics strengthen the connections between adjacent epithelial cells, reducing paracellular permeability, and preventing the entry of harmful substances into the bloodstream (Sharma et al., n.d.).

4.5.3.4 Examples of prebiotics

Various examples of plant-based prebiotics include almonds, artichoke, barley, chia seeds, chicory, dandelion greens, flaxseeds, garlic, and oats (Kaur et al., 2021).

4.5.4 Support for immune function in the gut

Functional foods that support immune function in the gut exert their effects through various mechanisms, including interaction with specific receptors, modulation of signaling pathways, and enhancement of immune responses. Here is a detailed explanation, along with examples.

4.5.4.1 Interaction with receptors

Functional foods contain bioactive compounds that can interact with specific receptors on immune cells in the gut-associated lymphoid tissue (GALT). For example, certain polyphenols found in foods like berries, green tea, and cocoa can bind to receptors such as Toll-like receptors (TLRs) and aryl hydrocarbon receptors (AhR) on immune cells. Activation of these receptors triggers intracellular signaling pathways that regulate immune responses and inflammation (Wang, Qi, et al., 2022).

4.5.4.2 Modulation of signaling pathways

Bioactive compounds in functional foods can modulate various signaling pathways involved in immune function. For instance, polyphenols like epigallocatechin gallate (EGCG) found in green tea have been shown to inhibit nuclear factor kappa B (NF-κB) signaling, a key pathway involved in inflammation. By suppressing NF-κB activation, EGCG helps reduce the production of pro-inflammatory cytokines and enhance immune regulation in the gut (Mokra et al., 2023).

4.5.4.3 Enhancement of immune responses

Functional foods containing probiotics and prebiotics can enhance immune responses in the gut by promoting the growth of beneficial gut bacteria and modulating the activity of immune cells. Probiotics, such as strains of *Lactobacillus* and *Bifidobacterium*, interact with immune cells in the gut, including dendritic cells, macrophages, and T cells. These interactions stimulate the production of antimicrobial peptides, cytokines, and immunoglobulins, strengthening the immune defenses in the gut (Srivastava et al., 2021).

4.5.4.4 Examples of functional foods

- Fermented foods: Fermented foods like yogurt, kefir, and kimchi contain probiotics that support immune function in the gut. These probiotics interact with immune cells through receptors like TLRs, stimulating immune responses and enhancing gut barrier function (Averina et al., 2021).
- Polyphenol-rich foods: Foods rich in polyphenols, such as berries (200–300 mg), green tea (100 mg), and dark chocolate, contain bioactive compounds that modulate immune function (Pandey & Rizvi, 2009).
- Beta-glucans: Beta-glucans found in foods like mushrooms and oats are polysaccharides that have been shown to enhance immune function. Beta-glucans interact with immune cells through receptors like dectin-1, triggering immune responses and promoting the clearance of pathogens in the gut (Mata-Martínez et al., 2022).

4.6 International cuisine and digestive health

Functional foods, embedded within the culinary traditions of various regions worldwide, reflect a rich tapestry of ingredients, flavors, and cultural practices. Across continents, from America to Europe, Asia to Africa, and Australia, each region boasts a diverse array of functional foods that contribute to health and well-being.

4.6.1 Asian cuisine

In Asia, a continent celebrated for its vibrant culinary heritage, functional foods abound in a tapestry of flavors, textures, and colors. From Japan's renowned fermented soy products like miso and natto to China's diverse array of medicinal herbs and teas, Asian cuisine offers a wealth of functional ingredients known for their health-promoting properties. From India, ingredients like millet, pulses, turmeric, ginger, flaxseeds, chia seeds, fennel seeds, onion, garlic, spices, milk products, and tofu are staples in Asian diets, celebrated for their antiinflammatory, antioxidant, and digestive benefits. Asian cuisines employ various cooking techniques that promote gut health, including stir-frying, steaming, and boiling. Fermentation is a cornerstone of Asian culinary traditions, with foods like pickle, kachumbar, yogurt, lassi, miso, tempeh, soy sauce, and kimchi undergoing fermentation to enhance flavor and introduce probiotics. Traditional Asian diets emphasize fresh fruits and vegetables, whole grains, lean proteins, and fermented foods like kimchi, miso, and tempeh (Srinivasan, 2010). These foods are rich in probiotics, prebiotics, and digestive enzymes, which support gut health, improve digestion, and boost immunity. Spices and herbs used in Indian cooking, such as turmeric, ginger, pepper, dried onions, cinnamon, and garlic, have antiinflammatory and digestive properties, aiding in digestion and promoting overall well-being (Paswan et al., n.d.).

4.6.2 American cuisine

In America, the culinary landscape is as varied as its geography, with a focus on fresh, locally sourced ingredients and innovative culinary techniques. Functional foods in American cuisine include nutrient-dense staples like blueberries, kale, quinoa, and sweet potatoes, utilized for their antioxidant properties, fiber content, and nutritional benefits. Traditional Native American cooking methods include steaming, baking, and stewing foods like beans, corn, and squash. Slow-cooking techniques, such as simmering soups and stews, help break down tough fibers and enhance digestibility. American cuisine is diverse, reflecting the cultural influences of Native American, European, African, and Latin American traditions. The American diet often includes a variety of foods, ranging from processed convenience foods to fresh, locally sourced ingredients. Functional foods like beans, whole grains, fruits, and vegetables contribute to digestive health by providing dietary fiber, antioxidants, and essential nutrients (Sajid Arshad et al., 2021). However, the prevalence of processed foods high in sugar, salt, and unhealthy fats may contribute to digestive issues such as bloating, gas, and indigestion.

4.6.3 African cuisine

Africa's culinary traditions reflect functional foods deeply rooted in indigenous ingredients and traditional cooking methods. Staples like sorghum, millet, teff, and yams provide essential nutrients, dietary fiber, and energy, while regional specialties like moringa, baobab, and hibiscus offer unique medicinal and nutritional properties. African cooking techniques often involve slow-cooking methods like stewing and simmering, which help tenderize meats and enhance the digestibility of fibrous vegetables and grains. Grilling and roasting over open flames are common in African cuisine, imparting smoky flavors and caramelization to foods while preserving their nutritional integrity (Oktay & Sadıkoğlu, 2018).

African cuisine with staple foods like sorghum, millet, cassava, yams, and legumes forms the basis of many diets. These foods are high in dietary fiber, vitamins, and minerals, promoting digestive regularity and gut health. Traditional African dishes often feature lean meats, fish, and poultry, providing essential nutrients and proteins necessary for digestive function. However, factors like limited access to clean water and sanitation in certain regions may contribute to digestive diseases and infections (Fao, n.d).

4.6.4 Australian cuisine

Australia's culinary landscape reflects its diverse cultural influences and abundant natural resources, with functional foods ranging from native bush foods like finger lime and wattle seed to nutrient-rich staples like kangaroo meat and seafood. Indigenous ingredients like Kakadu plum, known for its high vitamin C content, and macadamia nuts, rich in healthy fats and antioxidants, are prized for their nutritional benefits and culinary versatility. Australian cuisine draws inspiration from indigenous Aboriginal traditions as well as influences from British, European, Asian, and Mediterranean cuisines. Traditional Australian foods include seafood, lean meats like kangaroo and emu, native fruits and vegetables, and grains like quinoa and barley. These foods are nutrient-dense and rich in fiber, supporting digestive health and overall well-being (Ma Rhea, 2016). Indigenous Australian cooking methods include baking foods in earth ovens, steaming in leaves, and roasting over open fires. Traditional bush tucker cooking involves slow-cooking meats like kangaroo and emu, which help tenderize tough cuts and improve digestibility.

4.6.5 Mediterranean cuisine

In Europe, olive oil, fresh fruits and vegetables, whole grains, and legumes, is renowned for its heart-healthy benefits and antiinflammatory properties. Scandinavian cuisine features nutrient-rich seafood, wild berries, and hearty grains, while Eastern European cuisine incorporates fermented foods like sauerkraut, kefir, and kvass, known for their probiotic benefits. European cuisine is characterized by its diversity, with culinary traditions ranging from Mediterranean to Nordic and Eastern European. Mediterranean diets, rich in olive oil, fruits, vegetables, whole grains, and fish, are

TABLE 4.2 Poor Dietary intervention and its impact on gut health.

Sr. no.	Continents	Poor dietary intervention	Impact on gut health	Clinical trial reference
1.	Asian	High intake of refined carbohydrates, fried foods, and spicy dishes. Use of MSG and excessive salt in cooking.	Disruption of gut microbiota balance leads to dysbiosis and increased susceptibility to digestive issues such as bloating and diarrhea	Therdtatha et al. (2022)
2.	American	High intake of processed foods, sugary beverages, and red meat. Lack of diversity in diet.	Increases the risk of gut dysbiosis, inflammation, and gastrointestinal disorders such as IBS and IBD. Sugary beverages cause a BP-lowering effect.	Statovci et al. (2017) and Wang, Liu, et al. (2023)
3.	African	High consumption of fried and oily foods, processed meats, and sugary snacks. Limited intake of fruits, vegetables, and fiber-rich foods	Contributes to gut inflammation, oxidative stress, and an increased risk of metabolic disorders and colon cancer	Abrahams et al. (2011) and Addae et al. (2024)
4.	Australian	Westernized diet with high intake of processed foods, fast food, and sugary drinks. Low intake of fiber and plant-based foods.	Impairs gut microbiota diversity and function, predisposing to gut dysbiosis, obesity, and chronic diseases	Machado et al. (2020)
5.	European	High consumption of refined grains, processed meats, and dairy products. Excessive alcohol consumption and low intake of fruits and vegetables.	Alters gut microbiota composition and reduces microbial diversity, leading to gut dysbiosis and increased risk of digestive disorders	Stefler et al. (2021)

associated with reduced risk of digestive disorders and chronic diseases. However, the consumption of processed meats, fried foods, and excessive alcohol in certain European cuisines may negatively impact digestive health and increase the risk of GI disorders (European Nowak, 2014).

4.6.6 Comparative analysis of the impact of international cuisines on gut microbiota

A comparative analysis of the impact of international cuisines on gut microbiota provides insights into how dietary patterns across different continents influence the composition and diversity of the gut microbial community. In American, Australian and European cuisines, there is a high consumption of processed foods, sugar, and unhealthy fats. It may contribute to imbalances in gut microbiota composition, promoting the growth of opportunistic pathogens and reducing microbial diversity. However, the inclusion of fiber-rich foods like beans, whole grains, and fruits and vegetables can support the growth of beneficial bacteria and improve gut health (Moles & Otaegui, 2020). Asian cuisines, such as Japanese, Chinese, Indian, and Korean, are rich in fermented foods, whole grains, vegetables, and seafood. Fermented foods like miso, kimchi, and tempeh are abundant in Asian diets, providing probiotics that enhance gut microbiota diversity and function. Traditional Asian diets are generally high in dietary fiber and plant-based foods, promoting the growth of beneficial bacteria like *Bifidobacteria and Lactobacilli* and supporting overall gut health as shown in Table 4.2. African cuisine varies widely across regions, with staple foods like sorghum, millet, yams, and legumes forming the basis of many diets. Understanding the interplay between diet and gut microbiota is crucial for promoting digestive health and overall well-being across diverse cultural and culinary traditions (Lerma-Aguilera et al., 2024).

4.7 Ayurveda and functional foods

4.7.1 Introduction to Ayurveda as a traditional system of medicine

Ayurveda, originating from ancient India, is a holistic system of medicine that has been practiced for thousands of years. It is founded on the principle of balance and harmony between the body, mind, and spirit to achieve optimal health and well-being. The word "Ayurveda" is derived from Sanskrit, with "Ayur" meaning life and "Veda" meaning knowledge or science, thus representing the science of life (Krishnamurty & Ayurveda, 2011).

Central to Ayurvedic philosophy is the belief that each individual is unique, with their constitution, or "prakriti," determined by a combination of three fundamental energies, or doshas: Vata (air and ether), Pitta (fire and water), and Kapha (earth and water). These doshas govern various physiological and psychological functions within the body and are influenced by factors such as diet, lifestyle, environment, and genetics (Kunja et al., 1963). Ayurveda aims to restore and maintain balance within the body and mind through personalized lifestyle practices, dietary modifications, herbal remedies, detoxification techniques, yoga, meditation, and other holistic therapies. It emphasizes prevention as the cornerstone of health, focusing on cultivating harmony with nature and living by natural rhythms and cycles.

4.7.2 Principles of Ayurveda for digestive health

Ayurveda offers a comprehensive approach to digestive health, focusing on maintaining balance and harmony within the GI system to support overall well-being. The principles of Ayurveda for digestive health are rooted in the understanding of digestion as a central pillar of health, influencing physical vitality, mental clarity, and emotional balance. Here are some key principles of Ayurveda for digestive health.

4.7.2.1 Maintaining agni (digestive fire)

According to Ayurveda, proper digestion depends on the strength of "agni," or digestive fire. Agni represents the transformative power within the body responsible for breaking down food, absorbing nutrients, and eliminating waste. To support healthy digestion, Ayurveda emphasizes the importance of kindling and maintaining balanced agni through mindful eating practices, appropriate food choices, and lifestyle habits (Chaukhambha Prakashana, 2008).

4.7.2.2 Eating according to dosha

Ayurveda recognizes that individuals have unique constitutional types or doshas—Vata, Pitta, and Kapha—each with distinct digestive tendencies. Understanding one's dosha can guide personalized dietary recommendations and lifestyle practices to optimize digestive health. For example, Vata types may benefit from warm, nourishing foods that calm and ground their airy nature, while Pitta types may thrive on cooling, soothing foods that pacify their fiery tendencies (Chaukhambha Prakashana, 2008).

4.7.2.3 Choosing digestive-friendly foods

Ayurveda emphasizes the importance of selecting foods that are easy to digest and compatible with one's constitution. Whole, unprocessed foods, cooked vegetables, grains, legumes, and herbal teas are generally favored for their nourishing and soothing qualities. Spices like ginger, cumin, coriander, and fennel are valued for their digestive benefits and ability to stimulate agni without aggravating the doshas (Chaukhambha Prakashana, 2009).

4.7.2.4 Mindful eating practices

Ayurveda emphasizes the significance of mindful eating practices to enhance digestion and promote overall wellness. This includes eating in a calm, relaxed environment, chewing food thoroughly to aid in digestion, and savoring the flavors and textures of each meal. Eating mindfully allows for greater awareness of hunger and satiety cues, fostering a deeper connection with food and the body's natural rhythms (Chaukhambha Prakashana, 2010).

4.7.2.5 Balancing aggravating factors

Ayurveda recognizes that certain factors can disrupt digestive balance and impair agni, leading to digestive discomfort and imbalances. These factors may include excessive consumption of processed foods, irregular eating habits, emotional stress, environmental toxins, and inadequate hydration. By minimizing these aggravating factors and adopting supportive lifestyle practices, individuals can cultivate optimal digestive health and vitality (Chaukhambha Prakashana, 2010).

4.7.2.6 Herbal support

Ayurveda employs a variety of herbs and botanical remedies known for their digestive benefits and ability to support overall GI function. Common digestive herbs include triphala, an herbal blend renowned for its gentle cleansing and detoxifying properties; licorice root, which soothes inflammation and supports mucous membrane health; and peppermint, valued for its carminative and antispasmodic effects (Chaukhambha Prakashana, 2009).

4.7.3 Ayurvedic functional foods and their role in promoting a happy gut

Ayurvedic functional foods represent a cornerstone of Ayurvedic medicine, a holistic healing system originating from ancient India. These foods are carefully selected as they are rooted in the principles of Ayurveda, which emphasizes balance and harmony between the body, mind, and spirit. Ayurvedic functional foods encompass a diverse array of ingredients, including herbs, spices, fruits, vegetables, grains, legumes, and medicinal plants. Each of these foods offers unique therapeutic properties and contributes to digestive health in its own way. For example, warming spices like ginger, turmeric, and cinnamon help kindle the digestive fire and reduce digestive sluggishness, while soothing herbs like fennel, coriander, and licorice root calm inflammation and support GI comfort as given in Bhavaprakasha by Bhavamishran (Banerjee et al., 2015).

Ayurvedic functional foods also include traditional formulations and herbal remedies that have been used for centuries to address digestive imbalances and promote gut health. Triphala, a classic Ayurvedic herbal blend consisting of three fruits (Amalaki, Bibhitaki, and Haritaki), is renowned for its gentle detoxifying and cleansing effects on the digestive tract, promoting regularity and optimal bowel function (Banerjee et al., 2015).

According to Ayurveda, a happy gut is intimately connected to emotional and mental health, and the consumption of wholesome, nourishing foods supports harmony and balance at all levels of being. By incorporating these foods into daily life, individuals can cultivate digestive resilience, enhance vitality, and experience a profound sense of well-being that emanates from within.

4.7.4 Examples of Ayurvedic herbs and spices beneficial for digestion

4.7.4.1 Shunthi (dry ginger)

It is a warming spice known for its digestive benefits in Ayurveda. It stimulates digestion, reduces bloating, and alleviates nausea. Ginger can be consumed fresh, as a tea, or as a spice in cooking (Chaukhambha Prakashana, 2009).

4.7.4.2 Haridra (turmeric)

Turmeric is renowned for its antiinflammatory and digestive properties. It helps relieve digestive discomfort, supports liver function, and aids in detoxification. Turmeric can be added to curries, teas, or taken as a supplement (Chaukhambha Prakashana, 2009).

4.7.4.3 Saunf (fennel seeds)

Fennel seeds are commonly used as a digestive aid in Ayurveda. They help alleviate gas, bloating, and indigestion. Fennel seeds can be chewed after meals or brewed into a tea (Chaukhambha Prakashana, 2009).

4.7.4.4 Dhanyaka (coriander seeds)

Coriander seeds aid digestion and help soothe GI inflammation. They possess carminative properties, reducing gas and bloating. Coriander seeds can be used in cooking or steeped into a tea (Chaukhambha Prakashana, 2009).

4.7.4.5 Yashtimadhu (licorice root)

Licorice root soothes and protects the GI tract. It helps reduce inflammation, support mucous membrane health, and alleviate acid reflux. Licorice root can be consumed as a tea or taken in supplement form (Chaukhambha Prakashana, 2009).

4.7.4.6 Yavan (ajwain seeds)

Ajwain seeds are known for their carminative and digestive properties. They help relieve flatulence, indigestion, and stomach cramps. Ajwain seeds can be chewed raw, added to cooking, or brewed into a tea (Chaukhambha Prakashana, 2009).

4.7.4.7 Jeeraka (cumin seeds)

Cumin seeds aid digestion, reduce bloating, and stimulate appetite. They help alleviate symptoms of indigestion, colic, and irritable bowel syndrome (IBS). Cumin seeds are commonly used in cooking or brewed into a tea (Chaukhambha Prakashana, 2009).

4.7.4.8 *Ela (cardamom)*

Cardamom supports digestion, relieves gas, and freshens breath. It has carminative properties and helps soothe GI discomfort. Cardamom can be added to beverages and desserts or used in cooking (Chaukhambha Prakashana, 2009).

4.7.4.9 *Hing (asafoetida)*

Asafoetida aids digestion, reduces flatulence, and relieves abdominal distension. It helps alleviate symptoms of irritable bowel syndrome (IBS) and supports gut health. Asafoetida is commonly used as a spice in cooking (Chaukhambha Prakashana, 2009).

4.7.4.10 *Triphala*

Triphala is a classic Ayurvedic formulation consisting of three fruits: Amalaki, Bibhitaki, and Haritaki. It supports healthy digestion, detoxification, and regular bowel movements. Triphala can be taken as a powder, capsule, or decoction for digestive support (Chaukhambha Prakashana, 2009).

These Ayurvedic herbs and spices offer an approach to promoting digestive health and overall well-being. Incorporating them into daily meals and routines can support optimal digestion and enhance vitality.

4.7.5 Ayurvedic dietary guidelines for optimal digestive health

Ayurveda offers comprehensive dietary guidelines for optimal digestive health. Here are the Ayurvedic dietary guidelines along with detailed explanations as given in Vedic verse *Bhavaprakasha*:

4.7.5.1 *Ahara Vidhi (guidelines for eating)*

4.7.5.1.1 Eat according to your dosha

Ayurveda recognizes three primary doshas: Vata, Pitta, and Kapha. Understanding your dosha can help tailor your diet to balance your unique constitution. Vata types benefit from warm, nourishing foods that calm and ground their airy nature. Pitta types thrive on cooling, soothing foods that pacify their fiery tendencies. Kapha types do well with light, warming foods that energize and invigorate their earthy nature (Guha, 2006).

4.7.5.1.2 Eat fresh, seasonal foods

Choose fresh, seasonal foods that are locally sourced whenever possible. Incorporate a variety of fruits, vegetables, grains, legumes, and herbs into your diet to ensure a diverse and balanced nutrient intake (Shastri & Bhavprakash, 1966).

4.7.5.1.3 Practice mindful eating

Cultivate awareness and mindfulness during meals. Sit down to eat in a calm, relaxed environment, free from distractions. Chew your food thoroughly and savor the flavors and textures of each bite. Mindful eating enhances digestion, promotes satiety, and fosters a deeper connection with food and the body (Shastri & Bhavprakash, 1966).

4.7.5.2 *Ahara Rasa (six tastes of food)*

Ayurveda categorizes foods into six tastes: sweet, sour, salty, pungent, bitter, and astringent. Each taste has specific effects on the doshas and digestion. Incorporate all six tastes into your meals to ensure balance and satisfaction. Aim for a variety of tastes in each meal to stimulate the palate and support optimal digestion (Shastri & Bhavprakash, 1966).

4.7.5.3 *Ahara Sambhava (food compatibility)*

Pay attention to food combinations to optimize digestion and prevent the formation of toxins (ama) in the body. Avoid incompatible food combinations, such as mixing dairy with sour fruits, as they can disrupt digestion and lead to digestive discomfort.

4.7.5.4 *Ahara Pramana (proper quantity of food)*

Practice moderation in food consumption to avoid overeating and digestive strain. Pay attention to your hunger and satiety cues, and eat until you feel comfortably satisfied, but not overly full. Avoid eating large meals late at night, as this can impair digestion and disrupt sleep.

4.7.5.5 *Ahara Kala (timing of meals)*

Establish regular meal times and adhere to a consistent eating schedule. Eating meals at the same time each day helps regulate digestion and metabolism. Avoid skipping meals or eating irregularly, as this can disturb digestive rhythms and lead to imbalances in the doshas (Shastri & Bhavprakash, 1966).

4.7.5.6 *Ahara Upayoga (food preparation and cooking methods)*

Opt for whole, minimally processed foods that are rich in nutrients and life force energy (prana). Fresh fruits, vegetables, whole grains, legumes, nuts, seeds, and healthy fats form the foundation of a nourishing Ayurvedic diet. Incorporate digestive spices and herbs into your cooking to enhance flavor and support digestion. Common digestive spices include ginger, turmeric, cumin, coriander, fennel, and cardamom. Use gentle cooking methods such as steaming, sautéing, boiling, and stewing to retain the nutritional integrity of foods while making them easier to digest (Shastri & Bhavprakash, 1966).

4.7.5.7 *Ahara Vidhana (eating habits)*

Approach meals with gratitude and appreciation for the nourishment they provide to your body, mind, and spirit. Create a peaceful and harmonious atmosphere during meals by avoiding stressful or distracting conversations. Enjoy the company of loved ones and engage in uplifting and nourishing conversations.

Ayurveda views food as not only nourishment for the body but also as a sacred source of healing and vitality when approached mindfully and with reverence.

4.7.6 Integration of Ayurvedic principles with modern functional food concepts

The integration of Ayurvedic principles with modern functional food concepts represents a harmonious approach to promoting health and well-being that combines ancient wisdom with contemporary science (Lakhotia, 2018). Here is how Ayurvedic principles can be integrated with modern functional food concepts.

4.7.6.1 *Personalized nutrition*

Ayurveda emphasizes personalized nutrition based on an individual's unique constitution, or dosha. Modern functional food concepts similarly recognize the importance of personalized nutrition, taking into account factors such as genetics, lifestyle, and health goals to tailor dietary recommendations to individual needs.

4.7.6.2 *Focus on whole foods*

Both Ayurveda and modern functional food concepts emphasize the importance of whole, minimally processed foods as the foundation of a healthy diet. Whole foods provide essential nutrients, antioxidants, and phytonutrients that support optimal health and vitality.

4.7.6.3 *Nutrient density and bioavailability*

Ayurvedic principles highlight the importance of nutrient density and bioavailability in food choices, focusing on foods that are rich in essential vitamins, minerals, and other micronutrients. Modern functional food concepts similarly prioritize nutrient-dense foods that provide maximum nutritional value per calorie.

4.7.6.4 *Emphasis on digestive health*

Ayurveda places great importance on digestive health, recognizing the gut as the cornerstone of overall well-being. Modern functional food concepts align with this perspective by emphasizing the importance of gut health and promoting foods that support digestive function, such as probiotics, prebiotics, and fiber-rich foods.

4.7.6.5 *Incorporation of adaptogens and herbs*

Ayurveda utilizes a variety of adaptogenic herbs and botanicals to support health and resilience in the face of stress and environmental challenges. Modern functional food concepts incorporate adaptogens and herbs into functional foods and beverages designed to promote energy, resilience, and mental clarity.

4.7.6.6 *Holistic approach to health*

Ayurveda takes a holistic approach to health and wellness, considering the interconnectedness of the body, mind, and spirit. Modern functional food concepts similarly embrace a holistic approach to health, recognizing the importance of addressing lifestyle factors, stress management, and emotional well-being in promoting overall vitality and resilience.

4.8 Evidence-based recommendations for optimal digestive health

4.8.1 Considerations for individuals with specific digestive conditions

Considerations for individuals with specific digestive conditions are crucial for managing symptoms, promoting healing, and optimizing overall well-being. Here are some tailored recommendations for common digestive conditions:

1. Irritable bowel syndrome (IBS):
   - Low-FODMAP diet: Some individuals with IBS find relief by following a low-FODMAP diet, which restricts certain fermentable carbohydrates that may trigger symptoms such as bloating, gas, and abdominal pain (Pedersen et al., 2017).
   - Fiber intake: Gradually increase fiber intake from soluble sources like oats, psyllium husk, and flaxseeds, as insoluble fiber can exacerbate symptoms in some cases.
   - Stress management: Stress and anxiety can worsen IBS symptoms. Techniques such as meditation, yoga, and deep breathing exercises can help manage stress levels and alleviate symptoms.
2. Inflammatory bowel disease (IBD) (Crohn's disease, ulcerative colitis):
   - Antiinflammatory diet: Focus on an antiinflammatory diet rich in fruits, vegetables, fatty fish, olive oil, nuts, seeds, and whole grains to help reduce inflammation and support healing (Lacerda et al., 2021). Seeds contain various bioactive components and foods that can be beneficial for gut microbiomes (Deokar et al., 2024).
   - Limit trigger foods: Identify and avoid trigger foods that exacerbate symptoms, such as spicy foods, caffeine, alcohol, dairy products, and high-fat foods.
   - Medication adherence: Follow prescribed medication regimens as directed by healthcare providers to help manage symptoms and prevent disease flares.
3. Celiac disease:
   - Gluten-free diet: Strictly adhere to a gluten-free diet, avoiding all sources of gluten, including wheat, barley, rye, and their derivatives. Choose naturally gluten-free grains such as quinoa, rice, millet, and corn (Nastro et al., 2022).
   - Label reading: Learn to read food labels carefully to identify hidden sources of gluten in processed foods, sauces, condiments, and medications.
   - Cross-contamination awareness: Be vigilant about preventing cross-contamination by using separate cooking utensils, cutting boards, and kitchen appliances for gluten-free foods.

Individuals with specific digestive conditions should work closely with healthcare providers, registered dietitians, or nutritionists to develop personalized dietary plans tailored to their unique needs and preferences. By implementing appropriate dietary modifications, managing stress levels, and adhering to medical recommendations, individuals can better manage their digestive conditions and improve their quality of life.

4.9 Conclusion

Functional foods, enriched with beneficial nutrients, prebiotics, probiotics, and phytochemicals, play a pivotal role in supporting optimal digestive health. From promoting a diverse gut microbiota to enhancing nutrient absorption and maintaining gut barrier integrity, functional foods offer a holistic approach to nurturing a healthy digestive system. Informed dietary choices are essential for maintaining a happy gut and fostering overall well-being. By prioritizing whole, nutrient-dense foods and incorporating functional foods into daily meals, individuals can nourish their bodies and support digestive health. Mindful eating practices, such as paying attention to hunger cues, savoring flavors, and practicing portion control, further enhance the digestive experience. As we navigate the complexities of modern life, we must prioritize our digestive well-being for optimal health and vitality. The addition of functional foods to the diet can help maintain a healthy gut microbiome and gut homeostasis signaling regulating pathways. In essence, may we remember that the path to vibrant health begins within, where the choices we make today shape the well-being of tomorrow. Let us cherish and honor our bodies and our temples of vitality and embark on a lifelong journey for digestive wellness and holistic harmony.

References

Abrahams, Z., McHiza, Z., & Steyn, N. P. (2011). Diet and mortality rates in Sub-Saharan Africa: Stages in the nutrition transition. *BMC Public Health*, *11*. Available from https://doi.org/10.1186/1471-2458-11-801.

Addae, H. Y., Apprey, C., & Kwarteng, A. (2024). Gut microbiome-targeted nutrition interventions and growth among children in low- and middle-income countries: A systematic review and meta-analysis. *Current Developments in Nutrition*, *8*(3), 102085. Available from https://doi.org/10.1016/j.cdnut.2024.102085.

Al Bataineh, M. T., Künstner, A., Dash, N. R., Alsafar, H. S., Ragab, M., Schmelter, F., Sina, C., Busch, H., & Ibrahim, S. M. (2023). Uncovering the relationship between gut microbial dysbiosis, metabolomics, and dietary intake in type 2 diabetes mellitus and in healthy volunteers: a multi-omics analysis. *Scientific Reports*, *13*(1). Available from https://doi.org/10.1038/s41598-023-45066-7, https://www.nature.com/srep/.

Allen, S. J., Wareham, K., Wang, D., Bradley, C., Hutchings, H., Harris, W., Dhar, A., Brown, H., Foden, A., Gravenor, M. B., & Mack, D. (2013). Lactobacilli and bifidobacteria in the prevention of antibiotic-associated diarrhoea and Clostridium difficile diarrhoea in older inpatients (PLACIDE): a randomised, double-blind, placebo-controlled, multicentre trial. *The Lancet*, *382*(9900), 1249–1257. Available from https://doi.org/10.1016/s0140-6736(13)61218-0.

Averina, O. V., Poluektova, E. U., Marsova, M. V., & Danilenko, V. N. (2021). Biomarkers and utility of the antioxidant potential of probiotic lactobacilli and bifidobacteria as representatives of the human gut microbiota. *Biomedicines*, *9*(10). Available from https://doi.org/10.3390/biomedicines9101340, https://www.mdpi.com/2227-9059/9/10/1340/pdf.

Banerjee, A., Somasundaram, I., Das, D., Jain Manoj, S., Banu, H., Mitta Suresh, P., Paul, S., Bisgin, A., Zhang, H., Sun, X.-F., Duttaroy, A. K., & Pathak, S. (2023). Functional foods: A promising strategy for restoring gut microbiota diversity impacted by SARS-CoV-2 variants. *Nutrients*, *15*(11), 2631. Available from https://doi.org/10.3390/nu15112631.

Banerjee, S., Debnath, P., & Debnath, P. K. (2015). Ayurnutrigenomics: Ayurveda-inspired personalized nutrition from inception to evidence. *Journal of Traditional and Complementary Medicine*, *5*(4), 228–233. Available from https://doi.org/10.1016/j.jtcme.2014.12.009, www.jtcm.org/.

Barkhidarian, B., Roldos, L., Iskandar, M. M., Saedisomeolia, A., & Kubow, S. (2021). Probiotic supplementation and micronutrient status in healthy subjects: A systematic review of clinical trials. *Nutrients*, *13*(9), 3001. Available from https://doi.org/10.3390/nu13093001.

Behera, S. S., El Sheikha, A. F., Hammami, R., & Kumar, A. (2020). Traditionally fermented pickles: How the microbial diversity associated with their nutritional and health benefits? *Journal of Functional Foods*, *70*, 103971. Available from https://doi.org/10.1016/j.jff.2020.103971.

Bodera, P. (2008). Influence of prebiotics on the human immune system (GALT). *Recent Patents on Inflammation and Allergy Drug Discovery*, *2*(2), 149–153. Available from https://doi.org/10.2174/187221308784543656, http://www.ingentaconnect.com/content/ben/iad/2008/00000002/00000002/art00010.

Camilleri, M. (2021). Human intestinal barrier: Effects of stressors, diet, prebiotics, and probiotics. *Clinical and Translational Gastroenterology*, *12*(1), e00308. Available from https://doi.org/10.14309/ctg.0000000000000308.

Chaukhambha Prakashana. (2008).

Chaukhambha Prakashana. (2009).

Chaukhambha Prakashana. (2010).

Chawla, R., & Patil, G. R. (2010). Soluble dietary fiber. *Comprehensive Reviews in Food Science and Food Safety*, *9*(2), 178–196. Available from https://doi.org/10.1111/j.1541-4337.2009.00099.x, http://onlinelibrary.wiley.com/doi/10.1111/j.1541-4337.2009.00099.x/pdf.

Chen, L., Tuo, B., & Dong, H. (2016). Regulation of intestinal glucose absorption by ion channels and transporters. *Nutrients*, *8*(1). Available from https://doi.org/10.3390/nu8010043, http://www.mdpi.com/2072-6643/8/1/43/pdf.

Chen, F. Lui, Active Physiology, Transport, PubMed. Treasure Island FL. 2022.

Cho, I., Jackson, M. R., & Swift, J. (2016). Roles of cross-membrane transport and signaling in the maintenance of cellular homeostasis. *Cellular and Molecular Bioengineering*, *9*(2), 234–246. Available from https://doi.org/10.1007/s12195-016-0439-6, http://www.springer.com/engineering/biomedical + eng/journal/12195.

Choi, J. H., Lee, J., Choi, I. J., Kim, Y. W., Ryu, K. W., & Kim, J. (2016). Genetic variation in the TAS2R38 bitter taste receptor and gastric cancer risk in Koreans. *Scientific Reports*, *6*. Available from https://doi.org/10.1038/srep26904, www.nature.com/srep/index.html.

Corsello, A., Pugliese, D., Gasbarrini, A., & Armuzzi, A. (2020). Diet and nutrients in gastrointestinal chronic diseases. *Nutrients*, *12*(9), 1–19. Available from https://doi.org/10.3390/nu12092693, https://www.mdpi.com/2072-6643/12/9/2693/pdf.

Cronin, P., Joyce, S. A., O'toole, P. W., & O'connor, E. M. (2021). Dietary fibre modulates the gut microbiota. *Nutrients*, *13*(5). Available from https://doi.org/10.3390/nu13051655, https://www.mdpi.com/2072-6643/13/5/1655/pdf.

Damián, M. R., Cortes-Perez, N. G., Quintana, E. T., Ortiz-Moreno, A., Noguez, C. G., Cruceño-Casarrubias, C. E., Pardo, M. E. S., & Bermúdez-Humarán, L. G. (2022). Functional foods, nutraceuticals and probiotics: A focus on human health. *Microorganisms*, *10*(5). Available from https://doi.org/10.3390/microorganisms10051065, https://www.mdpi.com/2076-2607/10/5/1065/pdf?version = 1653129062.

Davani-Davari, Negahdaripour, Karimzadeh, Seifan, Mohkam, Masoumi, et al., (n.d) Prebiotics: Definition, Types, Sources, Mechanisms, and Clinical Applications.

Deo, P. N., & Deshmukh, R. (2019). Oral microbiome: Unveiling the fundamentals. *Journal of Oral and Maxillofacial Pathology*, *23*(1), 122–128. Available from https://doi.org/10.4103/jomfp.JOMFP_304_18, http://www.jomfp.in/.

Deokar, G. S., Nirmal, N. P., & Kshirsagar, S. J. (2024). *Plant seeds: A potential bioresource for isolation of nutraceutical and bioactive compounds* (pp. 333–372). Springer Science and Business Media LLC. Available from https://doi.org/10.1007/978-1-0716-3601-5_14.

Derrickson, B. H., & Tortora, G. J. (2019). *Principles of Anatomy and Physiology*. Wiley, Wiley.

Desai, J. P., Moustarah, F. Stricture, Internet]. PubMed. Treasure Island. 2022.

Di, L., & Kerns, E. H. (2016). *Transporters* (pp. 113–140). Elsevier BV. Available from https://doi.org/10.1016/b978-0-12-801076-1.00009-5.

Di, Y., Ding, L., Gao, L., & Huang, H. (2023). Association of meat consumption with the risk of gastrointestinal cancers: a systematic review and meta-analysis. *BMC Cancer*, *23*(1). Available from https://doi.org/10.1186/s12885-023-11218-1.

Dimidi, E., Cox, S. R., Rossi, M., & Whelan, K. (2019). Fermented foods: Definitions and characteristics, impact on the gut microbiota and effects on gastrointestinal health and disease. *Nutrients*, *11*(8). Available from https://doi.org/10.3390/nu11081806, https://www.mdpi.com/2072-6643/11/8/1806/pdf.

Elleuch, M., Bedigian, D., Roiseux, O., Besbes, S., Blecker, C., & Attia, H. (2011). Dietary fibre and fibre-rich by-products of food processing: Characterisation, technological functionality and commercial applications: A review. *Food Chemistry*, *124*(2), 411–421. Available from https://doi.org/10.1016/j.foodchem.2010.06.077.

European Nowak, Z. (2014). Cuisine, Ethical Considerations. *Encyclopedia of Food and Agricultural Ethics*.

Fao, (n.d) Dimensions of need - Staple foods: What do people eat?.

Ferraris, R. P., Choe, J. Y., & Patel, C. R. (2018). Intestinal absorption of fructose. *Annual Review of Nutrition*, *38*, 41–67. Available from https://doi.org/10.1146/annurev-nutr-082117-051707, http://www.annualreviews.org/journal/nutr.

Gastrointestinal Tract | Definition, Organs, Diagram, & Facts Encyclopædia Britannica. (2019).

Gaudioso, G., Weil, T., Marzorati, G., Solovyev, P., Bontempo, L., Franciosi, E., Bertoldi, L., Pedrolli, C., Tuohy, K. M., & Fava, F. (2022). Microbial and metabolic characterization of organic artisanal sauerkraut fermentation and study of gut health-promoting properties of sauerkraut brine. *Frontiers in Microbiology*, *13*. Available from https://doi.org/10.3389/fmicb.2022.929738, https://www.frontiersin.org/journals/microbiology#.

Gorreja, F., & Walker, W. A. (2022). The potential role of adherence factors in probiotic function in the gastrointestinal tract of adults and pediatrics: a narrative review of experimental and human studies. *Gut Microbes*, *14*(1). Available from https://doi.org/10.1080/19490976.2022.2149214, http://www.tandfonline.com/toc/kgmi20/current.

Granato, D., Barba, F. J., Bursać Kovačević, D., Lorenzo, J. M., Cruz, A. G., & Putnik, P. (2020). Functional foods: Product development, technological trends, efficacy testing, and safety. *Annual Review of Food Science and Technology*, *11*, 93–118. Available from https://doi.org/10.1146/annurev-food-032519-051708, http://www.annualreviews.org/journal/food.

Guha, A. Ayurvedic Concept of Food and Nutrition. (2006).

Haghshenas, B., Kiani, A., Mansoori, S., Mohammadi-noori, E., & Nami, Y. (2023). Probiotic properties and antimicrobial evaluation of silymarin-enriched Lactobacillus bacteria isolated from traditional curd. *Scientific Reports*, *13*(1). Available from https://doi.org/10.1038/s41598-023-37350-3.

Hall, K. D., Ayuketah, A., Brychta, R., Cai, H., Cassimatis, T., Chen, K. Y., Chung, S. T., Costa, E., Courville, A., Darcey, V., Fletcher, L. A., Forde, C. G., Gharib, A. M., Guo, J., Howard, R., Joseph, P. V., McGehee, S., Ouwerkerk, R., Raisinger, K., . . . Zhou, M. (2019). Ultra-processed diets cause excess calorie intake and weight gain: An inpatient randomized controlled trial of ad libitum food intake. *Cell Metabolism*, *30*(1), 67. Available from https://doi.org/10.1016/j.cmet.2019.05.008, http://www.cellmetabolism.org/.

Hemarajata, P., & Versalovic, J. (2013). Effects of probiotics on gut microbiota: mechanisms of intestinal immunomodulation and neuromodulation. *Therapeutic Advances in Gastroenterology*, *6*(1), 39–51. Available from https://doi.org/10.1177/1756283x12459294.

Hendifar, A. E., Petzel, M. Q. B., Zimmers, T. A., Denlinger, C. S., Matrisian, L. M., Picozzi, V. J., Rahib, L., Hendifar, A., Tuli, R., Wolpin, B., Hidalgo, M., Ryan, D., Hingorani, S., Chiorean, E. G., Coveler, A., O'Reilly, E., Balachandran, V., Simeone, D., Lowy, A., . . . Simeone, D. (2019). *Pancreas Cancer-Associated Weight Loss. Oncologist*, *24*(5), 691–701. Available from https://doi.org/10.1634/theoncologist.2018-0266, http://theoncologist.alphamedpress.org.

van Houte, J., & Gibbons, R. J. (1966). Studies of the cultivable flora of normal human feces. *Antonie Van Leeuwenhoek*, *32*(1), 212–222. Available from https://doi.org/10.1007/BF02097463.

Ibragimova, S., Ramachandran, R., Ali, F. R., Lipovich, L., & Ho, S. B. (2021). Dietary patterns and associated microbiome changes that promote oncogenesis. *Frontiers in Cell and Developmental Biology*, *9*. Available from https://doi.org/10.3389/fcell.2021.725821, https://www.frontiersin.org/journals/cell-and-developmental-biology#.

Introduction to the Digestive System. cancer.gov. (2019).

Isackson, H., & Ashley, C. C. (2023). Secretory functions of the gastrointestinal tract. *Surgery (United Kingdom*, *41*(7), 397–404. Available from https://doi.org/10.1016/j.mpsur.2023.02.033, http://www.elsevier.com/wps/find/journaldescription.cws_home/709612/description#description.

Jung, H., Yun, Y.-R., Hong, S. W., & Shin, S. (2024). Association between kimchi consumption and obesity based on BMI and abdominal obesity in Korean adults: a cross-sectional analysis of the Health Examinees study. *BMJ Open*, *14*(2), e076650. Available from https://doi.org/10.1136/bmjopen-2023-076650.

Jung, S., Kim, K., & Youn, S.-M. (2022). Randomized, double-blind, placebo-controlled trial to evaluate the effects of multi-strain synbiotic in patients with functional diarrhea and high fecal calprotectin levels: A pilot study. *14*.

Kandpal, M., Indari, O., Baral, B., Jakhmola, S., Tiwari, D., Bhandari, V., Pandey, R. K., Bala, K., Sonawane, A., & Jha, H. C. (2022). Dysbiosis of gut microbiota from the perspective of the gut−brain axis: Role in the provocation of neurological disorders. *Metabolites*, *12*(11). Available from https://doi.org/10.3390/metabo12111064, http://www.mdpi.com/journal/metabolites.

Karpińska, M., & Czauderna. (2022). Pancreas—Its functions, disorders, and physiological impact on the mammals' organism. *Frontiers in Physiology*, *13*, 807632.

Kaur, A. P., Bhardwaj, S., Dhanjal, D. S., Nepovimova, E., Cruz-martins, N., Kuča, K., Chopra, C., Singh, R., Kumar, H., Şen, F., Kumar, V., Verma, R., & Kumar, D. (2021). Plant prebiotics and their role in the amelioration of diseases. *Biomolecules*, *11*(3), 1−28. Available from https://doi.org/10.3390/biom11030440, https://www.mdpi.com/2218-273X/11/3/440/pdf.

Kaźmierczak-Siedlecka, K., Ruszkowski, J., Fic, M., Folwarski, M., & Makarewicz, W. (2020). Saccharomyces boulardii CNCM I-745: A non-bacterial microorganism used as probiotic agent in supporting treatment of selected diseases. *Current Microbiology*, *77*(9), 1987−1996. Available from https://doi.org/10.1007/s00284-020-02053-9.

Krishnamurty, K. H. Ayurveda, Br Publishing Corporation. (2011).

Kunja, K. Bhishagratna, Sushruta, Varanasi, Chowkhamba Sanskrit Series Office. (1963).

Lacerda, J. F., Lagos, A. C., Carolino, E., Silva-Herdade, A. S., Silva, M., & Sousa Guerreiro, C. (2021). Functional food components, intestinal permeability and inflammatory markers in patients with inflammatory bowel disease. *Nutrients*, *13*(2), 642. Available from https://doi.org/10.3390/nu13020642.

Lai, H., Li, Y., He, Y., Chen, F., Mi, B., Li, J., Xie, J., Ma, G., Yang, J., Xu, K., Liao, X., Yin, Y., Liang, J., Kong, L., Wang, X., Li, Z., Shen, Y., Dang, S., Zhang, L., . . . Liu, X. (2023). Effects of dietary fibers or probiotics on functional constipation symptoms and roles of gut microbiota: a double-blinded randomized placebo trial. *Gut Microbes*, *15*(1). Available from https://doi.org/10.1080/19490976.2023.2197837.

Lai, Y., Masatoshi, H., Ma, Y., Guo, Y., & Zhang, B. (2022). Role of Vitamin K in Intestinal Health. *Frontiers in Immunology*, *12*. Available from https://doi.org/10.3389/fimmu.2021.791565.

Lakhotia, S. (2018). At the Anniversary General Meeting of the Indian National Science Academy held at the Physical research Laboratory. *Ahmedabad Proc Indian Natn Sci Acad*, *85*(4), 697−703.

Leite, G. G. S., Weitsman, S., Parodi, G., Celly, S., Sedighi, R., Sanchez, M., Morales, W., Villanueva-Millan, M. J., Barlow, G. M., Mathur, R., Lo, S. K., Jamil, L. H., Paski, S., Rezaie, A., & Pimentel, M. (2020). Mapping the segmental microbiomes in the human small bowel in comparison with stool: A REIMAGINE study. *Digestive Diseases and Sciences*, *65*(9), 2595−2604. Available from https://doi.org/10.1007/s10620-020-06173-x, www.wkap.nl/journalhome.htm/0163-2116.

Lerma-Aguilera, A. M., Pérez-Burillo, S., Navajas-Porras, B., León, E. D., Ruíz-Pérez, S., Pastoriza, S., Jiménez-Hernández, N., Cämmerer, B.-M., Rufián-Henares, J. Á., Gosalbes, M. J., & Francino, M. P. (2024). Effects of different foods and cooking methods on the gut microbiota: an in vitro approach. *Frontiers in Microbiology*, *14*. Available from https://doi.org/10.3389/fmicb.2023.1334623.

Liao, W., Chen, C., Wen, T., & Zhao, Q. (2021). Probiotics for the prevention of antibiotic-associated diarrhea in adults. *Journal of Clinical Gastroenterology*, *55*(6), 469−480. Available from https://doi.org/10.1097/mcg.0000000000001464.

Liu, X. F., Shao, J. H., Liao, Y. T., Wang, L. N., Jia, Y., Dong, P. J., Liu, Z. Z., He, D. D., Li, C., & Zhang, X. (2023). Regulation of short-chain fatty acids in the immune system. *Frontiers in Immunology*, *14*. Available from https://doi.org/10.3389/fimmu.2023.1186892, https://www.frontiersin.org/journals/immunology#.

Ma Rhea, Z. (2016). *Australian national cuisine: Beyond the frontiers of taste* (pp. 181−208). Springer Science and Business Media LLC. Available from https://doi.org/10.1007/978-981-10-1630-1_9.

Machado, P. P., Steele, E. M., Louzada, M. Ld. C., Levy, R. B., Rangan, A., Woods, J., Gill, T., Scrinis, G., & Monteiro, C. A. (2020). Ultra-processed food consumption drives excessive free sugar intake among all age groups in Australia. *European Journal of Nutrition*, *59*(6), 2783−2792. Available from https://doi.org/10.1007/s00394-019-02125-y, http://www.springerlink.com/content/1436-6207.

Malfertheiner, P., Camargo, M. C., El-Omar, E., Liou, J. M., Peek, R., Schulz, C., Smith, S. I., & Suerbaum, S. (2023). Helicobacter pylori infection. *Nature Reviews Disease Primers*, *9*(1). Available from https://doi.org/10.1038/s41572-023-00431-8, https://www.nature.com/nrdp/.

Manzoor, S., Wani, S. M., Ahmad Mir, S., & Rizwan, D. (2022). Role of probiotics and prebiotics in mitigation of different diseases. *Nutrition (Burbank, Los Angeles County, Calif.)*, *96*, 111602. Available from https://doi.org/10.1016/j.nut.2022.111602.

Martínez-Crespo, L., Sun-Wang, J. L., Sierra, A. F., Aragay, G., Errasti-Murugarren, E., Bartoccioni, P., Palacín, M., & Ballester, P. (2020). Facilitated diffusion of proline across membranes of liposomes and living cells by a Calix[4]pyrrole Cavitand. *Chem*, *6*(11), 3054−3070. Available from https://doi.org/10.1016/j.chempr.2020.08.018, http://www.cell.com/chem/home.

Mata-Martínez, P., Bergón-Gutiérrez, M., & del Fresno, C. (2022). Dectin-1 signaling update: New perspectives for trained immunity. *Frontiers in Immunology*, *13*. Available from https://doi.org/10.3389/fimmu.2022.812148, https://www.frontiersin.org/journals/immunology#.

May, M., & Abrams, J. A. (2018). Emerging insights into the esophageal microbiome. *Current Treatment Options in Gastroenterology*, *16*(1), 72−85. Available from https://doi.org/10.1007/s11938-018-0171-5.

Mirjalili, M., Salari Sharif, A., Sangouni, A. A., Emtiazi, H., & Mozaffari-Khosravi, H. (2023). Effect of probiotic yogurt consumption on glycemic control and lipid profile in patients with type 2 diabetes mellitus: A randomized controlled trial. *Clinical Nutrition ESPEN*, *54*, 144−149. Available from https://doi.org/10.1016/j.clnesp.2023.01.014.

Mitchell, C. M., Davy, B. M., Halliday, T. M., Hulver, M. W., Neilson, A. P., Ponder, M. A., & Davy, K. P. (2015). The effect of prebiotic supplementation with inulin on cardiometabolic health: Rationale, design, and methods of a controlled feeding efficacy trial in adults at risk of type 2 diabetes. *Contemporary Clinical Trials*, *45*, 328−337. Available from https://doi.org/10.1016/j.cct.2015.10.012, http://www.elsevier.com/wps/find/journaldescription.cws_home/704636/description#description.

Mitchell, C. M., Davy, B. M., Ponder, M. A., McMillan, R. P., Hughes, M. D., Hulver, M. W., Neilson, A. P., & Davy, K. P. (2021). Prebiotic inulin supplementation and peripheral insulin sensitivity in adults at elevated risk for type 2 diabetes: A pilot randomized controlled trial. *Nutrients, 13* (9). Available from https://doi.org/10.3390/nu13093235, https://www.mdpi.com/2072-6643/13/9/3235/pdf.

Mohammadbeigi, A., Asgarian, A., Moshir, E., Heidari, H., Afrashteh, S., Khazaei, S., & Ansari, H. (2018). Fast food consumption and overweight/obesity prevalence in students and its association with general and abdominal obesity. *Journal of Preventive Medicine and Hygiene*, *59*(3), E236. Available from https://doi.org/10.15167/2421-4248/jpmh2018.59.3.830, http://www.jpmh.org/index.php/jpmh/article/view/830/625.

Mohammed, A. S. A. Naveed, Jost N. Polysaccharides, Classification, Chemical Properties, and Future Perspective Applications in Fields of Pharmacology and Biological Medicine (A Review of Current Applications and Upcoming Potentialities). 29 (2021).

Mokra, D., Joskova, M., & Mokry, J. (2023). Therapeutic effects of green tea polyphenol (-)-epigallocatechin-3-gallate (EGCG) in relation to molecular pathways controlling inflammation, oxidative stress, and apoptosis. *International Journal of Molecular Sciences*, *24*(1). Available from https://doi.org/10.3390/ijms24010340, http://www.mdpi.com/journal/ijms.

Moles, L., & Otaegui, D. (2020). The impact of diet on microbiota evolution and human health. Is diet an adequate tool for microbiota modulation? *Nutrients*, *12*(6), 1654. Available from https://doi.org/10.3390/nu12061654.

Nagpal, R., Wang, S., Ahmadi, S., Hayes, J., Gagliano, J., Subashchandrabose, S., Kitzman, D. W., Becton, T., Read, R., & Yadav, H. (2018). Human-origin probiotic cocktail increases short-chain fatty acid production via modulation of mice and human gut microbiome. *Scientific Reports*, *8*(1). Available from https://doi.org/10.1038/s41598-018-30114-4.

Nakanishi, T. Shimizu, K. Kumagai, Takai, H. Marusawa, (n.d). Genetic Pathogenesis of Inflammation-Associated Cancers in Digestive Organs. Pathogens.

Nastro, F. F., Serra, M. R., Cenni, S., Pacella, D., Martinelli, M., Miele, E., Staiano, A., Tolone, C., Auricchio, R., & Strisciuglio, C. (2022). Prevalence of functional gastrointestinal disorders in children with celiac disease on different types of gluten-free diets. *World Journal of Gastroenterology, 28* (46), 6589–6598. Available from https://doi.org/10.3748/wjg.v28.i46.6589, https://www.wjgnet.com/1007-9327/full/v28/i46/6589.htm.

Nath, A., Vatai, G., & Bánvölgyi, S. (2023). Functional foods and bioactive compounds through environmentally benign emerging processes. *Processes*, *11*(4), 1182. Available from https://doi.org/10.3390/pr11041182.

Netter, F. H. (2019). *Atlas of Human Anatomy*. Elsevier.

Nikolovska, K., Seidler, U. E., & Stock, C. (2022). The role of plasma membrane sodium/hydrogen exchangers in gastrointestinal functions: Proliferation and differentiation, fluid/electrolyte transport and barrier integrity. *Frontiers in Physiology, 13*. Available from https://doi.org/10.3389/fphys.2022.899286, http://www.frontiersin.org/Physiology/archive/.

Nogal, A., Valdes, A. M., & Menni, C. (2021). The role of short-chain fatty acids in the interplay between gut microbiota and diet in cardio-metabolic health. *Gut Microbes*, *13*(1), 1–24. Available from https://doi.org/10.1080/19490976.2021.1897212, http://www.tandfonline.com/toc/kgmi20/current.

Ohno, H., & Satoh-Takayama, N. (2020). Stomach microbiota, Helicobacter pylori, and group 2 innate lymphoid cells. *Experimental and Molecular Medicine*, *52*(9), 1377–1382. Available from https://doi.org/10.1038/s12276-020-00485-8, https://www.nature.com/emm/.

Oktay, S., & Sadıkoğlu, S. (2018). The gastronomic cultures' impact on the African cuisine. *Journal of Ethnic Foods*, *5*(2), 140–146. Available from https://doi.org/10.1016/j.jef.2018.02.005, http://www.journals.elsevier.com/journal-of-ethnic-foods/.

Ben Othman, R., Ben Amor, N., Mahjoub, F., Berriche, O., El Ghali, C., Gamoudi, A., et al. (2023). A clinical trial about effects of prebiotic and probiotic supplementation on weight loss, psychological profile and metabolic parameters in obese subjects. *Endrocrine Diabetes Metabolism*, *6*(2).

Palumbo, V. D., Tutino, R., Messina, M., Santarelli, M., Nigro, C., Lo Secco, G., Piceni, C., Montanari, E., Barletta, G., Venturelli, P., Geraci, G., Bonventre, S., & Lo Monte, A. I. (2023). Altered gut microbic flora and haemorrhoids: Could they have a possible relationship? *Journal of Clinical Medicine*, *12*(6). Available from https://doi.org/10.3390/jcm12062198, https://www.mdpi.com/journal/jcm.

Pandey, K. B., & Rizvi, S. I. (2009). Plant polyphenols as dietary antioxidants in human health and disease. *Oxidative Medicine and Cellular Longevity*, *2*(5), 270–278. Available from https://doi.org/10.4161/oxim.2.5.9498, http://www.landesbioscience.com/journals/oximed/article/PandeyOMCL2-5.pdf.

Park, C. H., & Lee, S. K. (2020). Exploring esophageal microbiomes in esophageal diseases: A systematic review. *Journal of Neurogastroenterology and Motility*, *26*(2), 171–179. Available from https://doi.org/10.5056/jnm19240, http://www.jnmjournal.org/.

Paswan, V. S., Singh, C. S., Kukreja, G., Bunkar, D.S., Bhinchhar, B. K. Health Benefits and Functional and Medicinal Properties of Some Common Indian Spices.

Patricia, J. J., Dhamoon, A. S. Digestion. PubMed. Treasure Island. (2022).

Pedersen, N., Ankersen, D. V., Felding, M., Wachmann, H., Végh, Z., Molzen, L., Burisch, J., Andersen, J. R., & Munkholm, P. (2017). Low-FODMAP diet reduces irritable bowel symptoms in patients with inflammatory bowel disease. *World Journal of Gastroenterology*, *23*(18), 3356. Available from https://doi.org/10.3748/wjg.v23.i18.3356.

Peters, V., Bolte, L., Schuttert, E. M., Andreu-Sánchez, S., Dijkstra, G., Weersma, R. K., & Campmans-Kuijpers, M. J. E. (2022). Western and carnivorous dietary patterns are associated with greater likelihood of IBD development in a large prospective population-based cohort. *Journal of Crohn's and Colitis*, *16*(6), 931–939. Available from https://doi.org/10.1093/ecco-jcc/jjab219.

Peterson, C. T., Vaughn, A. R., Sharma, V., Chopra, D., Mills, P. J., Peterson, S. N., & Sivamani, R. K. (2018). Effects of turmeric and curcumin dietary supplementation on human gut microbiota: A double-blind, randomized, placebo-controlled pilot study. *Journal of Evidence-Based Integrative Medicine*, *23*. Available from https://doi.org/10.1177/2515690x18790725, 2515690X1879072.

Peterson, J., Garges, S., Giovanni, M., McInnes, P., Wang, L., Schloss, J. A., Bonazzi, V., McEwen, J. E., Wetterstrand, K. A., Deal, C., Baker, C. C., Di Francesco, V., Howcroft, T. K., Karp, R. W., Lunsford, R. D., Wellington, C. R., Belachew, T., Wright, M., Giblin, C., ... Guyer, M. (2009).

The NIH human microbiome project. *Genome Research, 19*(12), 2317–2323. Available from https://doi.org/10.1101/gr.096651.109, http://genome.cshlp.org/content/19/12/2317.full.pdf + html.

Pham, V. T., Calatayud, M., Rotsaert, C., Seifert, N., Richard, N., Van den Abbeele, P., Marzorati, M., & Steinert, R. E. (2021). Antioxidant vitamins and prebiotic FOS and XOS differentially shift microbiota composition and function and improve intestinal epithelial barrier in vitro. *Nutrients, 13*(4), 1125. Available from https://doi.org/10.3390/nu13041125.

Pilipenko, V. I., Isakov, V. A., Morozov, S. V., Vlasova, A. V., & Kochetkova, A. A. (2022). Efficacy of newly developed kombucha-based specialized food product for treatment of constipation-predominant irritable bowel syndrome. *Federation Voprosy Pitaniia, 91*(5), 95–104. Available from https://doi.org/10.33029/0042-8833-2022-91-5-95-104, https://www.voprosy-pitaniya.ru/ru/journals_diet/71.html?SSr = 390134afd807ffffffff27c__07e7010407270b-542c.

Pirahanchi, S. Sharma, Biochemistry, PubMed. Treasure Island. 2020.

Reboul, E. (2023). Proteins involved in fat-soluble vitamin and carotenoid transport across the intestinal cells: New insights from the past decade. *Progress in Lipid Research, 89*, 101208.

Regunathan-Shenk, R., Shah, N. B., Raj, D. S., Kopple, J. D., Massry, S. G., Kalantar-Zadeh, K., Fouque, D. Chapter 11 - The gut microbiome and the kidney. Academic Press, 147–161.

Ried, K., Travica, N., Dorairaj, R., & Sali, A. (2020). Herbal formula improves upper and lower gastrointestinal symptoms and gut health in Australian adults with digestive disorders. *Nutrition Research, 76*, 37–51. Available from https://doi.org/10.1016/j.nutres.2020.02.008, www.elsevier.com/locate/nutres.

Rustam, S., Noor-us-saba., Qayyum, M., Islam, B. U., & Qazilbash, A. A. (2006). Enterobacteriaceae: Etiological agents of diarrhea. *Journal of Medical Sciences, 6*(2), 149–154. Available from https://doi.org/10.3923/jms.2006.149.154.

Sadeghpour. (2024). Gut microbiota and autoimmune diseases: Mechanisms, treatment, challenges, and future recommendations. *Current Clinical Microbiology Reports.*

Saeed, F., Afzaal, M., Shah, Y. A., Khan, M. H., Hussain, M., Ikram, A., et al. (2022). A traditional nutritious & health-endorsing fermented product. *Food Science & Nutrition, 10.*

Saha, S. K., & Pathak, N. N. (2021). *Digestion, absorption and metabolism of nutrients* (pp. 219–246). Springer Science and Business Media LLC. Available from https://doi.org/10.1007/978-981-15-9125-9_14.

Sajid Arshad, M., Khalid, W., Shabir Ahmad, R., Kamran Khan, M., Haseeb Ahmad, M., Safdar, S., Kousar, S., Munir, H., Shabbir, U., Zafarullah, M., Nadeem, M., Asghar, Z., & Ansar Rasul Suleria, H. (2021). *Functional foods and human health: An overview.* IntechOpen. Available from https://doi.org/10.5772/intechopen.99000.

Saleem, G. N., Gu, R., Qu, H., Bahar Khaskheli, G., Rashid Rajput, I., Qasim, M., & Chen, X. (2024). Therapeutic potential of popular fermented dairy products and its benefits on human health. *Frontiers in Nutrition, 11.* Available from https://doi.org/10.3389/fnut.2024.1328620.

Santacroce, L., Passarelli, P. C., Azzolino, D., Bottalico, L., Charitos, I. A., Cazzolla, A. P., Colella, M., Topi, S., Godoy, F. G., & D'Addona, A. (2023). Oral microbiota in human health and disease: A perspective. *Experimental Biology and Medicine, 248*(15), 1288–1301. Available from https://doi.org/10.1177/15353702231187645.

Satyanarayana, U. Biochemistry - E-Book, Google Books. Elsevier Health Sciences, (2017).

Sensoy, I. (2021). A review on the food digestion in the digestive tract and the used in vitro models. *Current Research in Food Science, 4*, 308–319. Available from https://doi.org/10.1016/j.crfs.2021.04.004, https://www.journals.elsevier.com/current-research-in-food-science.

Shaikh, S. (2022). *Sources and health benefits of functional food components.* IntechOpen. Available from https://doi.org/10.5772/intechopen.104091.

Sharma, Sharma, Sharma, Kumar, M.D. Barbhai, J.M. Lorenzo, et al., (n.d) Carica papaya L. Leaves: Deciphering Its Antioxidant Bioactives, Biological Activities, Innovative Products, and Safety Aspects. Oxidative Medicine and Cellular Longevity.

Shastri, G. Bhavprakash In: Chikitsa Prakarana Verse. Sastu Sahitya Vardhaka Karyalaya. (1966).

Sidhu, S. R. K., Kok, C. W., Kunasegaran, T., & Ramadas, A. (2023). Effect of plant-based diets on gut microbiota: A systematic review of interventional studies. *Nutrients, 15*(6). Available from https://doi.org/10.3390/nu15061510, http://www.mdpi.com/journal/nutrients/.

Smith, B. C., Zolnik, C. P., Usyk, M., Chen, Z., Kaiser, K., Nucci-Sack, A., Peake, K., Diaz, A., Viswanathan, S., Strickler, H. D., Schlecht, N. F., & Burk, R. D. (2016). Distinct ecological niche of anal, oral, and cervical mucosal microbiomes in adolescent women. *Yale Journal of Biology and Medicine, 89*(3), 277–284. Available from https://www.ncbi.nlm.nih.gov/pmc/articles/PMC5045137/pdf/yjbm_89_3_277.pdf.

Smith, S.M. Nehring, Bowel Obstruction. Nih.gov. StatPearls Publishing. 2023.

Srinivasan, K. (2010). *Traditional Indian functional foods Functional Foods of the East* (pp. 61–84). India CRC Press. Available from https://www.taylorfrancis.com/books/e/9781420071931.

Srivastava, M., Chandra, A., Rahul, R., Nigam, J., Rajan, P., Parmar, D., Srivastava, R. N., & Gupta, V. (2021). Expression of antimicrobial peptides and cytokines in human omentum following abdominal surgery. *Cureus.* Available from https://doi.org/10.7759/cureus.17477.

Statovci, D., Aguilera, M., MacSharry, J., & Melgar, S. (2017). The impact of western diet and nutrients on the microbiota and immune response at mucosal interfaces. *Frontiers in Immunology, 8.* Available from https://doi.org/10.3389/fimmu.2017.00838, http://journal.frontiersin.org/article/10.3389/fimmu.2017.00838/full.

Stefler, D., Brett, D., Sarkadi-Nagy, E., Kopczynska, E., Detchev, S., Bati, A., Scrob, M., Koenker, D., Aleksov, B., Douarin, E., Simonova, G., Malyutina, S., Kubinova, R., Pajak, A., Ruiz, M., Peasey, A., Pikhart, H., & Bobak, M. (2021). Traditional Eastern European diet and mortality: Prospective evidence from the HAPIEE study. *European Journal of Nutrition, 60*(2), 1091–1100. Available from https://doi.org/10.1007/s00394-020-02319-9.

Stryer, L., Berg, J., Tymoczko, J., Gatto, G. Biochemistry, (2019).

Therdtatha, P., Shinoda, A., & Nakayama, J. (2022). Crisis of the Asian gut: Associations among diet, microbiota, and metabolic diseases. *Bioscience of Microbiota, Food and Health, 41*(3), 83–93. Available from https://doi.org/10.12938/bmfh.2021-085.

Tortora, G. J., Derrickson, B., Burkett, B., Peoples, G., Dye., Cooke, J., et al. (2021). *Principles of anatomy and physiology*. John Wiley & Sons.

Trommelen, J., Tomé, D., & van Loon, L. J. C. (2021). Gut amino acid absorption in humans: Concepts and relevance for postprandial metabolism. *Clinical Nutrition Open Science, 36*, 43–55. Available from https://doi.org/10.1016/j.nutos.2020.12.006, https://www.journals.elsevier.com/clinical-nutrition-open-science.

Unuofin, J. O., Masuku, N. P., Paimo, O. K., & Lebelo, S. L. (2021). Ginger from farmyard to town: Nutritional and pharmacological applications. *Frontiers in Pharmacology, 12*. Available from https://doi.org/10.3389/fphar.2021.779352, http://www.frontiersin.org/Pharmacology.

Vandeputte, D., Falony, G., Vieira-Silva, S., Tito, R. Y., Joossens, M., & Raes, J. (2015). Stool consistency is strongly associated with gut microbiota richness and composition, enterotypes and bacterial growth rates. *Gut, 65*(1), 57–62. Available from https://doi.org/10.1136/gutjnl-2015-309618.

Veettil, S. K., Wong, T. Y., Loo, Y. S., Playdon, M. C., Lai, N. M., Giovannucci, E. L., & Chaiyakunapruk, N. (2021). Role of diet in colorectal cancer incidence: Umbrella review of meta-analyses of prospective observational studies. *JAMA Network Open, 4*(2), E2037341. Available from https://doi.org/10.1001/jamanetworkopen.2020.37341, https://jamanetwork.com/journals/jamanetworkopen.

Wan, Y., Tong, W., Zhou, R., Li, J., Yuan, J., Wang, F., & Li, D. (2019). Habitual animal fat consumption in shaping gut microbiota and microbial metabolites. *Food & Function, 10*(12), 7973–7982. Available from https://doi.org/10.1039/c9fo01490j.

Wan, Y., Wang, F., Yuan, J., Li, J., Jiang, D., Zhang, J., Li, H., Wang, R., Tang, J., Huang, T., Zheng, J., Sinclair, A. J., Mann, J., & Li, D. (2019). Effects of dietary fat on gut microbiota and faecal metabolites, and their relationship with cardiometabolic risk factors: a 6-month randomised controlled-feeding trial. *Gut, 68*(8), 1417–1429. Available from https://doi.org/10.1136/gutjnl-2018-317609.

Wang, J., Jiang, M., Hu, Y., Lei, Y., Zhu, Y., Xiong, H., & He, C. (2023). Lactulose regulates gut microbiota dysbiosis and promotes short-chain fatty acids production in acute pancreatitis patients with intestinal dysfunction. *Biomedicine & Pharmacotherapy, 163*, 114769. Available from https://doi.org/10.1016/j.biopha.2023.114769.

Wang, W., Liu, Y., Li, Y., Luo, B., Lin, Z., Chen, K., & Liu, Y. (2023). Dietary patterns and cardiometabolic health: Clinical evidence and mechanism. *MedComm, 4*(1). Available from https://doi.org/10.1002/mco2.212, onlinelibrary.wiley.com/journal/26882663.

Wang, T. C., Camilleri, M., Lebwohl, B., Lok, A. S., Sandborn, W. J., Wang, K. K., & Wu, G. D. (2022). *Electrolyte secretion and absorption in the small intestine and colon. Yamada's Textbook of Gastroenterology* (pp. 283–312). Wiley. Available from https://doi.org/10.1002/9781119600206.ch16.

Wang, X., Qi, Y., & Zheng, H. (2022). Dietary polyphenol, gut microbiota, and health benefits. *Antioxidants, 11*(6), 1212. Available from https://doi.org/10.3390/antiox11061212.

Waugh, A., & Grant. (2018). *Ross & Wilson Anatomy and Physiology in Health and illness*. Elsevier.

Weninger, S. N., Herman, C., Meyer, R. K., Beauchemin, E. T., Kangath, A., Lane, A. I., Martinez, T. M., Hasneen, T., Jaramillo, S. A., Lindsey, J., Vedantam, G., Cai, H., Cope, E. K., Caporaso, J. G., & Duca, F. A. (2023). Oligofructose improves small intestinal lipid-sensing mechanisms via alterations to the small intestinal microbiota. *Microbiome, 11*(1). Available from https://doi.org/10.1186/s40168-023-01590-2, https://microbiomejournal.biomedcentral.com/.

Yoshida, Y., & Simoes, E. J. (2018). Sugar-sweetened beverage, obesity, and type 2 diabetes in children and adolescents: Policies, taxation, and programs. *Current Diabetes Reports, 18*(6). Available from https://doi.org/10.1007/s11892-018-1004-6, www.springer.com.

Yılmaz, İ., Enver Dolar, M., & Özpınar, H. (2019). Effect of administering kefir on the changes in fecal microbiota and symptoms of inflammatory bowel disease: A randomized controlled trial. *Turkish Journal of Gastroenterology, 30*(3), 242–253. Available from https://doi.org/10.5152/tjg.2018.18227, http://www.turkjgastroenterol.org/sayilar/313/buyuk/242-253.pdf.

Zhao, Y., & Yu, Y. B. (2016). Intestinal microbiota and chronic constipation. *SpringerPlus, 5*(1). Available from https://doi.org/10.1186/s40064-016-2821-1, http://www.springerplus.com/archive.

Chapter 5

Cognitive enhancement: fueling the brain with functional foods

Anandu Chandra Khanashyam[1], Bharathi Ramesh[2], M. Anjaly Shanker[3], Meetha James[4], Kartik Shah[5], Priyamvada Thorakkattu[6] and Nilesh Prakash Nirmal[7]

[1]*Department of Food Science and Nutrition, University of Minnesota, St Paul, MN, United States,* [2]*Icahn School of Medicine at Mount Sinai, New York, NY, United States,* [3]*Department of Agriculture and Environmental Sciences, National Institute of Food Technology Entrepreneurship and Management (NIFTEM), Sonepat, Haryana, India,* [4]*Kraft Heinz, Glenview, IL, United States,* [5]*Sargento Foods, Elkhart Lake, WI, 53020, United States,* [6]*Department of Animal Sciences and Industry, Food Science Institute, Kansas State University, Manhattan, KS, United States,* [7]*Institute of Nutrition, Mahidol University, Salaya, Nakhon Pathom, Thailand*

5.1 Introduction

The average life expectancy has increased dramatically in recent decades due to breakthroughs in healthcare and technology, which is evidence of societal progress (Kuhn et al., 2023). However, chronic diseases like diabetes, cancer, cardiovascular disease, and most significantly, neurodegenerative diseases, have also increased as a result of this demographic transition (Li et al., 2021). Age-related cognitive decline (ARCD) and brain aging are closely related biological processes that are major risk factors for neurodegeneration (Juan et al., 2019). The senior population is particularly concerned about ARCD since it can present in a variety of ways, including memory, executive functioning, attention, and processing speed reductions. To effectively maintain and improve cognitive health in older adults, it is imperative to comprehend the complex etiology of these cognitive losses.

It has been determined that oxidative stress plays a significant role in the pathophysiology of ARCD. Reactive oxygen species (ROS) generation and the brain's antioxidant defenses are out of balance, which leads to stress. While the activity of vital antioxidant enzymes like superoxide dismutase (SOD), catalase, glutathione, and glutathione peroxidase declines with age, especially in crucial cognitive regions like the hippocampus and cerebral cortex, the buildup of reactive iron with aging contributes to increased ROS generation (Rao & Balachandran, 2002). The brain's capacity to combat free radicals (FR) is weakened by this redox imbalance, which increases susceptibility to oxidative damage and neuroinflammatory processes. These mechanisms have the potential to cause neuronal malfunction or death, which will ultimately exacerbate cognitive decline and several neurodegenerative diseases. In light of these challenges, the concept of functional foods has emerged as a promising avenue for cognitive enhancement and neuroprotection. Functional foods are defined as foods that provide health benefits beyond basic nutrition. These foods are rich in omega-3 fatty acids, antioxidants, polyphenols, vitamins, and minerals, all of which play vital roles in maintaining brain health (Rao & Balachandran, 2002). The potential mechanisms through which functional foods exert their beneficial effects on the brain include modulating neuronal signaling pathways, reducing oxidative stress, and inhibiting neuroinflammatory processes. Omega-3 fatty acids, predominantly found in fish oils, are crucial components of neuronal membranes and have been shown to enhance synaptic plasticity and cognitive function (Su, 2010). Antioxidants help mitigate oxidative stress by neutralizing ROS, thus protecting neuronal integrity. Polyphenols, abundant in fruits, vegetables, and certain beverages like tea and red wine, exhibit potent antioxidant and antiinflammatory properties, further supporting cognitive health. Moreover, certain functional foods can influence gut microbiota composition, which is increasingly recognized for its role in the gut–brain axis, impacting brain function and behavior.

Emerging research provides compelling evidence for the cognitive benefits of functional foods. For instance, epidemiological studies have demonstrated that diets rich in fruits, vegetables, fish, and nuts are associated with a reduced risk of cognitive decline and neurodegenerative diseases (Dalile et al., 2022). Clinical trials have also shown that

Unleashing the Power of Functional Foods and Novel Bioactives. DOI: https://doi.org/10.1016/B978-0-443-28862-3.00005-4

supplementation with specific functional foods can improve memory, attention, and executive function in both healthy individuals and those with cognitive impairments. These findings underscore the potential of functional foods as a natural and accessible strategy for promoting brain health and mitigating the effects of aging on cognitive function. The purpose of this chapter is to delve into the intricate role of functional food in cognitive health and neuroprotection. Polyphenols, ubiquitous in various plant-based foods and beverages, have garnered significant attention for their potential to promote brain function and protect against neurodegenerative diseases. By exploring the mechanisms underlying their effects on cognitive health and neuroprotection, this chapter aims to shed light on the therapeutic potential of polyphenols in maintaining brain health across the lifespan.

5.2 Understanding cognitive function

Cognitive health encompasses processes like thinking, learning, and memory, along with motor functions such as movement control and balance, emotional interpretation and response, and tactile sensations (Puri et al., 2023). Optimal brain health allows individuals to recognize their abilities and adjust their cognitive, psychological, emotional, and behavioral responses to life events. Several factors influence brain health, including age-related changes, injuries, mood disorders, substance abuse, and diseases (Fig. 5.1). While some factors are immutable, many lifestyle factors, such as diet, physical activity, social engagement, cognitive activities, smoking, and alcohol consumption, can be modified to maintain or enhance cognitive function (Anstey et al., 2013). Brain imaging studies have revealed that the brain continues to develop throughout childhood and young adulthood, with different brain structures maturing at different rates. Good brain health is essential for individuals to effectively manage cognitive, psychological, emotional, and behavioral functions, which in turn helps them adapt and cope with life's various challenges (Fig. 5.2). Maintaining cognitive health involves more than just avoiding cognitive decline; it encompasses a holistic approach that includes understanding how different factors, including diet, affect brain function and development throughout life (Puri et al., 2023).

Early childhood nutrition is crucial as it impacts brain growth and function, often having lifelong implications. Protein and low-fat diets are known to be protective against cognitive decline. However, it is not just individual nutrients that matter; there is strong evidence supporting the "whole diet approach," which suggests that a balanced diet, rather than focusing on single nutrients, is more beneficial for cognitive health. Diets such as the Mediterranean, DASH, and MIND have been associated with a lower risk of cognitive decline and dementia (Puri et al., 2023). These diets emphasize the consumption of healthy foods, including vegetables, fruits, whole grains, nuts, and fish, while

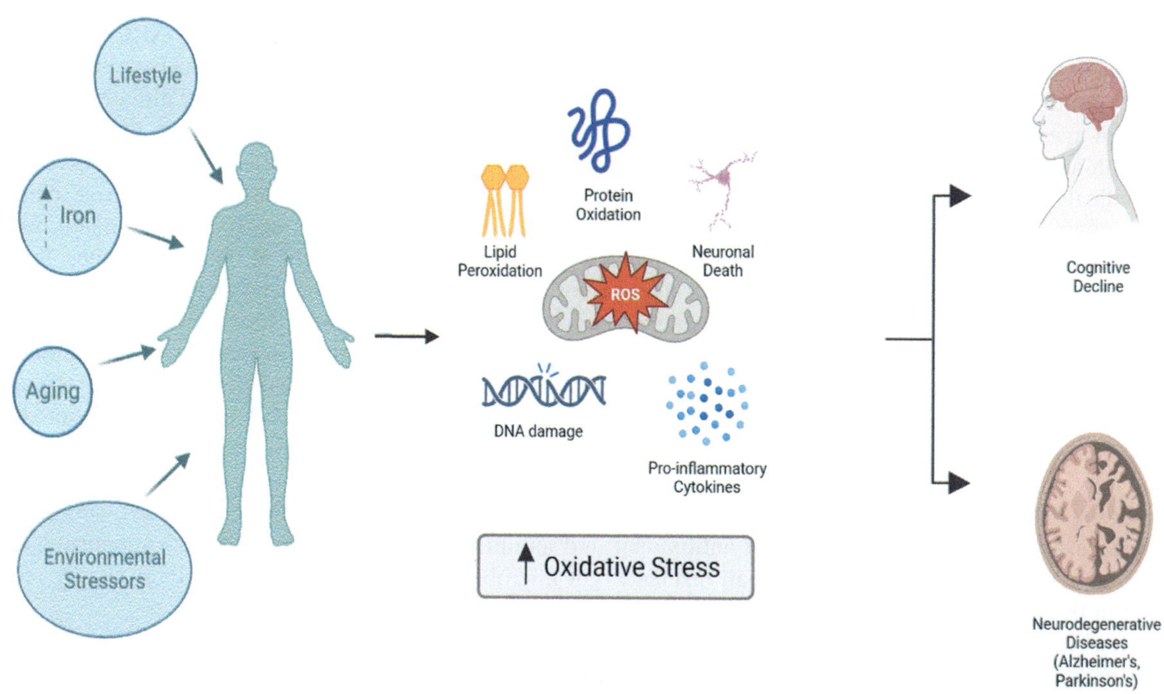

FIGURE 5.1 Factors affecting brain health.

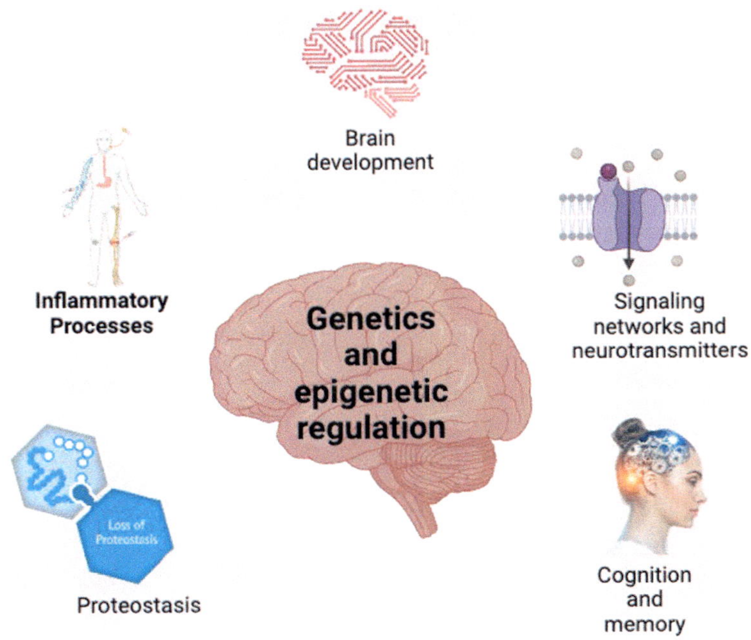

FIGURE 5.2 Genetic and epigenetic regulation of brain.

limiting the intake of red meat, sugar, and saturated fats. There is a growing body of evidence on the role of nutrition and lifestyle factors in cognitive development, function, and decline (Mintzer et al., 2019). A dietary approach that benefits cardiovascular health is likely effective against neurodegenerative disorders, highlighting the importance of a comprehensive, lifelong strategy for maintaining cognitive health (Dalile et al., 2022).

5.3 Functional foods and brain health: mechanisms and evidence

Functional foods, which are foods fortified with health-promoting ingredients, have garnered significant attention for their potential role in enhancing brain health. These foods are rich in bioactive compounds, such as omega-3 fatty acids, antioxidants, and polyphenols, which have been shown to positively influence cognitive function and neuroprotection (Fig. 5.3). Emerging evidence suggests that these compounds may modulate neuronal signaling pathways, reduce oxidative stress, and inhibit neuroinflammatory processes, thereby supporting brain health and mitigating the risk of neurodegenerative diseases. Consuming whole grains during childhood and adolescence appears to have varied effects on different cognitive domains. A longitudinal study found that diet scores related to whole grain intake did not correlate with cognitive outcomes at age 10 (Nyaradi et al., 2013). However, in adolescents, consuming 360 grams per day of a mixed-grain product over nine weeks helped mitigate the effects of induced mental fatigue on attention, vigilance, and response impulsivity (Chung et al., 2012). Higher consumption of fruits and vegetables is associated with a lower risk of cognitive impairment, according to a 2018 metaanalysis of observational studies (Mottaghi et al., 2018). However, there is conflicting evidence about the lifetime association between the consumption of fruits and vegetables and cognitive health. A systematic analysis conducted on children and adolescents showed that although poor snack consumption has a negative influence on executive function, eating a balanced diet, which includes fruits and vegetables, has a favorable effect (Cohen et al., 2016). Different cognitive domains may be affected differently by fruits and vegetables. A 13-year prospective cohort research in adults, for example, revealed a positive correlation between better verbal memory and the consumption of fruits and vegetables, particularly those high in vitamin C. Conversely, β-carotene-rich foods and vegetables had a negative correlation with executive function (Péneau et al., 2011). Nyaradi et al., (2013) reported that dairy intake at a young age was linked to better cognitive outcomes at age 10. Additionally, a 12-week high-dairy diet improved spatial working memory in overweight or obese adults (BMI ≥ 25) compared to a low-dairy diet (Crichton et al., 2012). Daily dairy consumption has also been positively associated with various cognitive functions

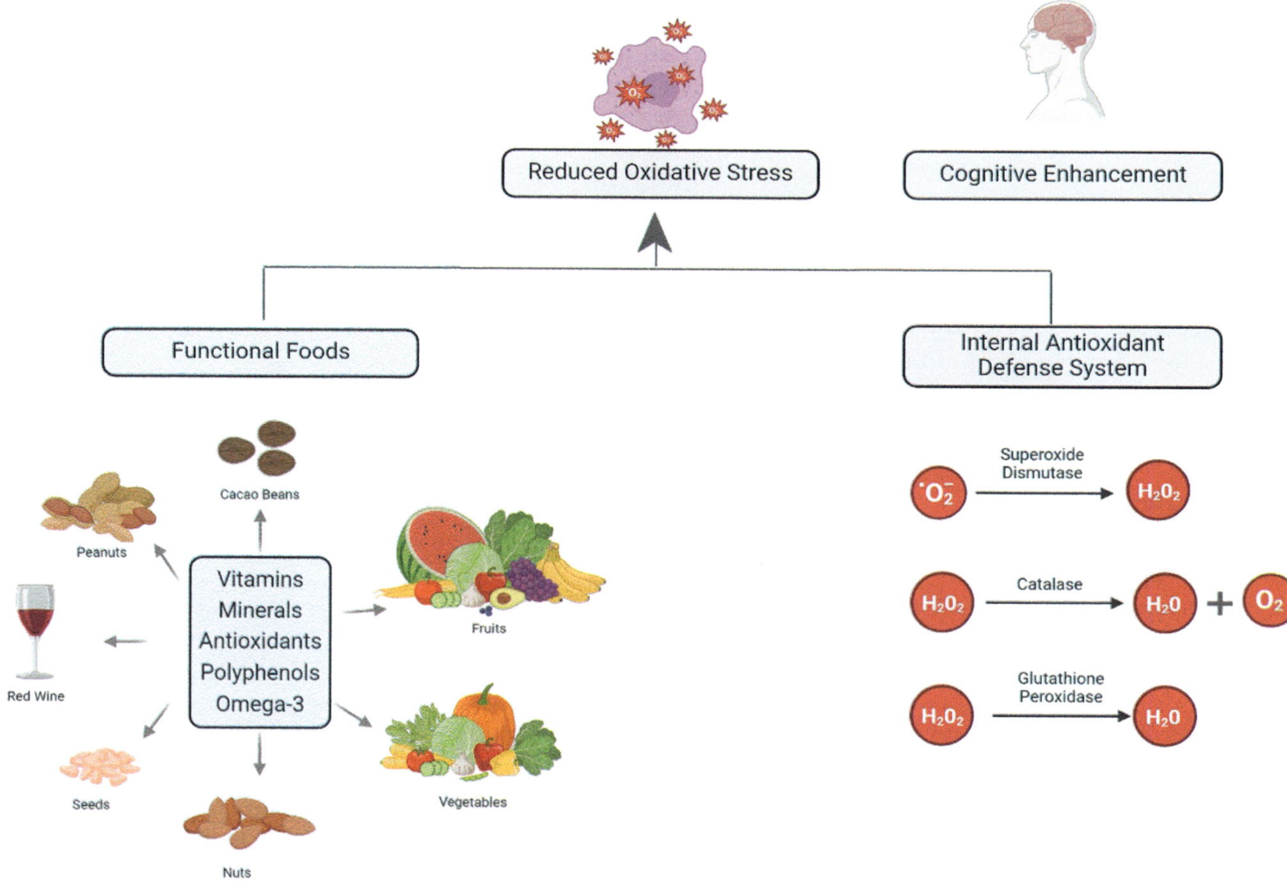

FIGURE 5.3 Impact of bioactive compounds and functional food in cognitive enhancement.

and better Mini-Mental State Examination (MMSE) scores compared to those who rarely consumed dairy. However, drinking more than one glass of milk daily between ages 45 and 64 was linked to a 10% decline in overall cognitive function and memory 20 years later (Petruski-Ivleva et al., 2017). The type and fat content of dairy products might influence this relationship, with potential differences between sexes. For instance, total dairy intake, particularly cheese, was positively correlated with faster information processing and overall cognitive performance, whereas high consumption of low-fat yogurt was linked to better memory recall in men, whereas whole-fat dairy products like ice cream and cream were associated with cognitive deficits (Crichton et al., 2012; Park & Fulgoni, 2013).

A systematic review conducted by Zhang, Hardie, et al. (2020) found no overall link between total meat consumption and cognitive function or cognitive disorders in adults. However, a submetaanalysis from the same review indicated a lower risk of cognitive disorders among those who consumed meat at least once a week. Furthermore, a large cohort study with nearly 500,000 participants found that an additional weekly serving of red meat was associated with reduced cognitive performance, such as lower fluid intelligence and memory (Zhang, Cade, et al., 2020). Some associations, including those related to reaction time, fluid intelligence, and prospective memory, were observed predominantly in men. Nevertheless, increased red meat consumption appeared to have a protective effect on visuospatial memory in both men and women. Numerous studies have demonstrated the long-term protective effects of fish consumption against cognitive decline in older adults. Eating at least four servings of fish per week can result in memory scores comparable to those of individuals who are four years younger (Samieri et al., 2018). Consuming one fish meal per week is linked to a 10% slower rate of cognitive decline, while two fish meals per week are associated with a 13% reduction in the rate of cognitive decline (Morris et al., 2005). In a Japanese cohort, higher fish consumption was inversely related to the onset of dementia, with an odds ratio of 0.84. This suggests that increasing fish intake to the highest quintile of consumption (over 85.7 g/day) could potentially prevent 5.6% of dementia cases globally, equivalent to 2.6 million cases (Tsurumaki et al., 2019). The relationship between fish consumption and cognitive function is complex. Fish provides beneficial nutrients, such as long-chain n-3 polyunsaturated fatty acids (PUFAs), but can also contain contaminants like mercury and dioxins. In one study, children who consumed a fish flour spread for 6 months exhibited better verbal learning and memory than those who had a placebo spread made of superfine rusk bread flour (Dalton et al., 2009). Additionally, when accounting for dietary compliance, children who ate an oily fish lunch three times a week for 16 weeks showed improved intelligence scores compared to those who ate a meat-based lunch (Øyen et al., 2018). A cross-sectional study found that while high seafood intake, particularly of large-mouth fish like tuna, raises mercury levels in the blood, it also increases levels of n-3 PUFAs. Up to three servings of large-mouth fish per week are associated with better cognition due to these n-3 PUFAs. However, high mercury levels (above 15 μg/L) can negate these benefits and worsen cognitive function. Khan et al. (2015) and Masley et al. (2012) found that children with low consumption of saturated fats showed improved cognitive flexibility. Conversely, higher intake of saturated fats and dietary cholesterol was linked to impaired working memory and cognitive control, especially during more challenging cognitive tasks. Some immediate effects of fat consumption have been noted in young adults aged 18 to 37. For instance, an acute dose of rapeseed oil (16 g; 10% ALA) improved attention and processing speed compared to a calorie-free placebo (Jones et al., 2012). In a randomized, placebo-controlled trial by Miller, Struyf, et al. (2018) consuming a milkshake with walnut oil (30 mL; 12% ALA) resulted in faster hippocampal-dependent learning compared to a milkshake with saturated fat (cream; 85 mL).

While the increase in average life expectancy is one of society's great achievements, it has also led to a rise in chronic diseases, including diabetes, cancer, cardiovascular diseases, and neurodegenerative diseases. Brain aging, a major risk factor for neurodegeneration, is a complex biological process linked with ARCD (Murman, 2015). ARCD involves declines in memory, executive function, attention, and processing speed, which are significant concerns for the elderly. The causes of these cognitive declines are multifactorial, with oxidative stress playing a crucial role in triggering neuroinflammation in neuronal cells (Devi & Satpati, 2016). In older adults, the shift toward a pro-oxidant redox state is primarily due to two factors: (1) increased production of ROS from greater reactive iron accumulation with aging (Jolitha et al., 2006), and (2) decreased activity of antioxidant enzymes such as SOD, catalase, glutathione, and glutathione peroxidase in critical brain areas like the hippocampus and cerebral cortex (Siqueira et al., 2005). This imbalance impairs the brain's ability to counteract FRs, increasing vulnerability to oxidative damage and leading to tissue harm and neuroinflammation. These neuroinflammatory processes can cause neuron dysfunction or death, ultimately contributing to cognitive decline (Pesce et al., 2018). One of the most well-known mechanisms of action of polyphenols is their antioxidant activity. Polyphenols act as potent scavengers of FRs and ROS, neutralizing their harmful effects and preventing oxidative damage to cells, lipids, proteins, and DNA. The antioxidant properties of polyphenols are attributed to their ability to donate hydrogen atoms or electrons to FRs, thereby stabilizing them and inhibiting chain reactions of lipid peroxidation and protein oxidation. Polyphenols also enhance the activity of endogenous antioxidant enzymes, such as SOD, catalase, and glutathione peroxidase, which further contribute to their antioxidant defenses (Akpoveso et al., 2023). Additionally, polyphenols chelate transition metal ions (e.g., iron and copper), which can catalyze the formation of ROS through Fenton and Haber–Weiss reactions, thereby preventing oxidative stress. In addition to their antioxidant properties, polyphenols exert potent antiinflammatory effects. Chronic inflammation is implicated in the pathogenesis of various chronic diseases, including cardiovascular disease, diabetes, cancer, and neurodegenerative disorders. Polyphenols modulate inflammatory pathways and reduce the production of pro-inflammatory cytokines and enzymes, such as tumor necrosis factor-alpha (TNF-α), interleukin-6 (IL-6), cyclooxygenase-2 (COX-2), and inducible nitric oxide synthase (iNOS) (Sobhani et al., 2021). Polyphenols inhibit the activation of nuclear factor-kappa B (NF-κB), a key transcription factor that regulates the expression of genes involved in inflammation and immune responses. By suppressing NF-κB activation, polyphenols attenuate the inflammatory cascade and mitigate tissue damage associated with chronic inflammation.

Fish oil, along with its primary omega-3 polyunsaturated fatty acids (n-3 PUFAs), such as eicosapentaenoic acid (EPA) and docosahexaenoic acid (DHA), has been shown to have beneficial effects in preventing atherosclerosis and cardiovascular diseases (Marckmann & Grønbæk, 1999). These fatty acids are integrated into cell membranes, where they exhibit strong antiinflammatory, antithrombotic, antiarrhythmic, and triacylglycerol-lowering properties. Additionally, growing evidence suggests that n-3 PUFAs have neuroprotective functions, which include enhancing learning and memory and slowing the progression of neurodegenerative diseases by decelerating cognitive decline (Su, 2010). However, the molecular mechanisms by which n-3 PUFAs exert these effects are diverse and not yet fully understood. It is believed that the modulation of membrane microorganization and the regulation of gene expression play significant roles in the functions of n-3 PUFAs. n-3 fatty acids enhance hippocampal function and learning memory by increasing CaMKII, CREB, and glutamate receptor expression, which promotes long-term potentiation (LTP) (Su, 2010). They also boost glutamate release and elevate phosphatidylethanolamine (PE) levels and synaptic/cytoskeletal protein expression, facilitating neurite outgrowth, synaptogenesis, dendritic spine density, and neurogenesis (Dyall et al., 2007; Puskás et al., 2003). These structural and molecular changes contribute to strengthened synaptic plasticity. Additionally, n-3 fatty acids offer antioxidative, antiinflammatory, and anti-apoptotic protection, counteract age-related changes, and help prevent Alzheimer's disease (AD), with DHA potentially acting through retinoid signaling (Boudrault et al., 2009). DHA functions as a ligand for retinoid X receptors (RXRs), which regulate genes involved in brain development, neuronal differentiation, LTP, neurite outgrowth, and neurogenesis (Urquiza et al., 2000). This signaling is crucial for neuron protection, inflammation modulation, neurotrophin regulation, and reducing AD pathology. During brain development, DHA synthesis and uptake support neuronal differentiation, neurite outgrowth, synaptogenesis, neurogenesis, and neuron protection. In the mature brain, DHA enhances synaptic protein expression and LTP, leading to increased dendritic spine formation, neurite outgrowth, synaptogenesis, c-Fos-positive neurons, BDNF secretion, and neurogenesis, thereby strengthening hippocampal synaptic plasticity, protecting neurons, preventing AD, and reversing age-related hippocampal changes (Cao et al., 2009; Su, 2010).

5.4 Dietary patterns and cognitive enhancement

The foundation of development and functional activity of the human brain revolves around the internal individual genotypic facet and certain external factors like social interactions, stress, nutrition, diseases, prenatal , and parental care. Among the external factors, the relationship between nutrition and mental or brain health is largely studied and recognized owing to the visible improvements that food is inflicting on cognitive function. This understanding is the basis of the concept of brain foods and encompasses the fact that nutrition has become an important aspect in the treatment of psychiatric disorders (Ansari et al., 2024). The nutrition component of human life is directly dependent on the day-to-day food intake and the type and constituents of diet included. To put it in another way, the development can be correlated to the type of diet of each individual, and the level of positives is totally dependent on the type of food products included in the diet. To understand that correlation, efforts have been made to explain in broader terms the relationship between the diet and the functional activity of the brain in the approaching portions of this subsection.

5.4.1 Mediterranean diet

The concept of the Mediterranean diet (MedDiet) was initially coined by Ancel Keys, who described it as featuring low levels of saturated fat and a high proportion of vegetable oils, based on dietary patterns observed in Greece and Southern Italy during the 1960s (Martínez-González & Sánchez-Villegas, 2004). It is characterized by a focus on the consumption of fruits, vegetables, whole grains, legumes, olive oil, and fish, along with a moderate intake of dairy, poultry, and eggs (Davis et al., 2015; Guasch-Ferré & Willett, 2021). Fresh fruit is consumed daily, and olive oil serves as the primary fat source. Moreover, low-to-moderate quantities of fish, seafood, poultry, and dairy products are included in the daily diet. A consistent, moderate consumption of wine is observed, alongside the intake of 0–4 eggs per week. The consumption of sweets, which contain sugar or honey, and red meat is limited and infrequent (Fu et al., 2022).

The Mediterranean diet has attracted considerable scientific attention for its potential benefits in enhancing cognitive health (Davis et al., 2015). Extensive research has explored the correlation between the Mediterranean diet and its impact on prolonging life expectancy, alongside reducing the mortality and morbidity rates associated with specific cancers and other diseases linked to nutrition. Nonetheless, the potential of MedDiet in the prevention or postponement of cognitive disorders, as well as its capability to enhance cognitive performance, remains understudied (Rosato et al., 2019; Schwingshackl et al., 2017). However, research shows that several mechanisms (as mentioned below) may underlie the Mediterranean diet's positive impact on cognitive health (Crichton et al., 2013; Gardener et al., 2012).

- **Antioxidant powerhouse:** This diet is rich in antioxidants, which combat FRs—molecules that damage brain cells and contribute to cognitive decline. Fruits, vegetables, and olive oil are particularly abundant in these protective compounds.
- **Essential omega-3 fatty acids:** The emphasis on fatty fish like salmon, tuna, and sardines provides a rich source of omega-3s, crucial for brain development and function, and potentially reducing the risk of neurodegenerative diseases.
- **Improved blood flow:** The Mediterranean diet may enhance blood flow to the brain, a vital factor for delivering oxygen and nutrients necessary for optimal cognitive function. This effect is likely due to the presence of healthy fats and moderate alcohol consumption (in some variations).

- **Reduced inflammation:** Chronic inflammation is linked to cognitive decline. The Mediterranean diet's focus on antiinflammatory foods like fruits, vegetables, and whole grains may contribute to a neuroprotective effect by mitigating inflammatory processes.
- **Gut microbiome influence:** Emerging research suggests that the gut microbiome plays a role in brain health. The Mediterranean diet, rich in fiber and prebiotics, may promote a beneficial gut microbiota composition, potentially impacting cognitive function through the gut–brain axis.

5.4.2 Dietary Approaches to Stop Hypertension diet

The Dietary Approaches to Stop Hypertension (DASH) diet is widely endorsed in international guidelines as a fundamental lifestyle intervention for managing blood pressure (Daskalopoulou et al., 2012; Kwan et al., 2013). This dietary pattern advocates for an increased intake of whole grains, fruits, vegetables, low-fat dairy products, lean meats, poultry, fish, nuts, and legumes. It is characterized by high levels of potassium, magnesium, calcium, and dietary fiber and recommends reducing the consumption of total fats, saturated fats, and cholesterol. Furthermore, it imposes a limitation on daily sodium intake to 2300 mg. The DASH diet is different from the MedDiet through several key nutritional aspects. The DASH diet advocates for a reduced intake of saturated fats and commercially prepared pastries and sweets, alongside a higher consumption of dairy products compared to the Mediterranean dietary pattern (Daniel et al., 2021; Tangney et al., 2014). Numerous epidemiological studies have explored the connection between adherence to the DASH diet and cognitive decline (Berendsen et al., 2017; Chen et al., 2019). Notably, a longitudinal study conducted in 2013 demonstrated a positive correlation between heightened adherence to the DASH diet and improved cognitive function, including enhancements in psychomotor speed, observed over 11 years within a cohort predominantly composed of elderly, non-Hispanic White individuals (Wengreen et al., 2013). A recent intervention called the MIND diet (Mediterranean-DASH Intervention for Neurodegenerative Delay diet) is gaining popularity to understand the effects of all these diets and their impact on slowing down cognitive decline. Recent scientific findings indicate that greater compliance with the Mediterranean, DASH, or MIND dietary patterns correlates with reduced cognitive decline and a diminished risk of AD, with the most significant correlations being noted for the MIND diet (van den Brink et al., 2019).

5.4.3 Plant-based diet and brain health

Positive impacts and correlations between diet patterns and brain health logically highlight the possibility of a plant-based diet owing to its nutritional, functional, and bioactive profile. Plant-based diets are generally distinguished by a higher intake of plant-based foods and low or no intake of animal foods (Williams & Patel, 2017). Compared to the restrictive nature of vegan and vegetarian diets, the former diet pattern allows flexibility, limiting and sometimes evading negative stimuli related to animal foods. In addition, plant-based diets confine the consumption of red meat, whole-fat cheese, stick margarine, sweets and pastries, and fried/fast foods which increase the incidence of saturated and trans-fat forms and arachidonic acid affecting cognitive function. Antioxidant and phytonutrient profiles of specific plant foods encompassed in a diet are found to be effective in reducing the oxidative burden on neuronal cells and inhibiting the deposition of β-amyloid plaques thereby protecting the brain and mental health (Gildawie et al., 2018). Reports show that the diet, including those high in palmitic acid, exhibits and aids in an increase in brain activation during execution of working tasks compared to high-oleic acid diets (Dumas et al., 2016). There is mounting evidence that supports the improvements of plant-based diets in the incidence and prevention of ARCD and in certain specific conditions like dementia related to mental health. The association of different plant-based diet patterns and components on brain health and cognitive function is given in detail in Table 5.1 Chen et al. (2017) conducted a detailed study on the effect of different diets (vegetable, meat, and traditional dietary patterns) on the cognitive function and brain health of a group of individuals. The vegetable diet involved in the study majorly included dark green leafy vegetables, tubers, and vegetables with oil characterized by a marginal amount of folates, flavonoids, vitamins, and carotenoids. This dietary pattern was found to be effective in reducing cognitive decline and dementia patterns in epidemiological studies. The author here also refers to the positive influences that the diet offers on cognitive improvement and in the prevention of neuronal damage in animal studies.

Compared to the former diet pattern, reported variance was reported in the case of the meat-based intake pattern posing a risk of verbal fluency decline in the elderly. The fat percentage in animal foods was reported to have a direct influence in increasing the incidence of dementia and is also related to worse executive function in individuals. In the case of traditional foods, including more fermented pickles and foods, a reported constructive pattern was observed in

TABLE 5.1 Importance of plant-based diet components in cognitive function and brain health.

Sl no.	Dietary patterns/ plant food components	Observations	References
1.	Japanese traditional diet	Fermented foods rich in isoflavones and different vitamin fractions showed protective and preventive effects in logical memory recall decline	Yoshinaga et al. (2012)
2.	Seven different diet patterns	Dietary patterns categorized with an intake of soybeans, vegetables, algae, milk, and other dairy products and a low intake of rice greatly influenced reduced risk of dementia	Ozawa et al. (2013)
3.	Vegetable dietary pattern, meat intake pattern and traditional intake pattern	Vegetable patterns prevented the logical memory decline and meat traditional intake patterns safeguarded the logical memory recall activity. Meat pattern of intake included a risk of decline in verbal fluency with some positive affirmations towards the attention decline.	Chen et al. (2017)
4.	Wheat-based diet and rice pork diet	A slower rate of decline in cognitive function was reported in the consumption of a wheat-based diet owing to the nutritional profile	Qin et al. (2015)
5.	Traditional diet	Vitamin fractions are known for a contributory role in nonverbal episodic memory and in preventing cognitive impairment	Kumar et al. (2012)
6.	Western dietary pattern and healthy vegetable-based diet	Western diet plans have increased the risk of cognitive impairment	Tsai (2015)
7.	Vegetables- fruit diet pattern and fish-meat diet pattern	The former was identified as influencing brain health with a reduced risk of cognitive impairment	Chan et al. (2013)

the case of logical memory recall activity. The author correlates the positive influence with the incidence of postbiotics like lactic acid bacteria in these fermented fractions which influences the overall functionality and body health. A similar pattern of constrictive development was reported that illustrates the effect of kimchi, a Korean traditional pickled cabbage rich in vitamin content, on brain activity and functionality (Kumar et al., 2012). High fractions of vitamin K are reported to have a contributory role in the consolidation of nonverbal episodic memory along with the influence of vitamin B_{12} in preventing cognitive impairment (Presse et al., 2013). Similarly, fruit juices and their inclusion in diet have been shown and reported to have a positive image in the case of cognitive functional development. For example, in a study involving the consumption of high flavanone content orange juice in the diet of individuals, it was observed to have a contributory role in global cognitive function in the cohort group (Kean et al., 2015). Analog patterns of increased or improved and preventative patterns of cognitive activity were stated in the case of these fruits, vegetables, and their juice fractions owing to the superior phenolic and flavonoid profiles of the former and latter fractions (Bookheimer et al., 2013; Miller, Hamilton, et al., 2018; Whyte et al., 2018).

5.5 Bioactive compounds and brain function

Neurodegenerative diseases represent a group of disorders characterized by progressive degeneration and dysfunction of neurons in the central nervous system (CNS). These diseases often result in gradual cognitive decline, motor impairment, and other neurological deficits, ultimately leading to significant disability and impairment of quality of life. Among the most common neurodegenerative diseases are AD and Parkinson's disease, each with distinct clinical features, underlying pathology, and disease mechanisms. AD is the most prevalent form of dementia, accounting for the majority of dementia cases worldwide (Breijyeh & Karaman, 2020). It is characterized by the accumulation of abnormal protein aggregates in the brain, including beta-amyloid plaques and tau tangles, which disrupt neuronal function and connectivity (Breijyeh & Karaman, 2020). AD typically presents with progressive memory loss, cognitive impairment, and behavioral changes, ultimately leading to profound dementia and loss of independent function. The exact cause of AD remains unknown, although genetic, environmental, and lifestyle factors are thought to contribute to disease development and progression. Currently, there is no cure for AD, and available treatments focus on managing symptoms and slowing disease progression. Parkinson's disease (PD) is a progressive movement disorder characterized by the loss of dopamine-producing neurons in the substantia nigra region of the brain (Khan et al., 2019). This loss of dopaminergic neurons leads to motor symptoms such as tremors, bradykinesia (slowness of movement), rigidity, and postural instability. PD is also associated with nonmotor symptoms, including cognitive impairment, autonomic dysfunction, and psychiatric disturbances. The underlying pathology of PD involves the accumulation of alpha-synuclein protein aggregates, known as Lewy bodies, within neurons. While the precise etiology of PD remains unclear, both genetic and environmental factors are believed to contribute to disease susceptibility. Treatment options for PD include dopamine replacement therapy, deep brain stimulation, and other symptomatic therapies aimed at improving motor function and quality of life. Despite the distinct features of each neurodegenerative disease, they share common underlying mechanisms of neuronal dysfunction and death, including oxidative stress, inflammation, mitochondrial dysfunction, and protein misfolding/aggregation. Understanding these shared mechanisms may provide insights into potential therapeutic strategies for treating neurodegenerative diseases. However, significant challenges remain in developing effective treatments that can halt or reverse the progressive neurodegeneration associated with these devastating disorders. Ongoing research efforts are focused on elucidating the pathophysiology of neurodegenerative diseases and identifying novel dietary therapeutic targets to address these conditions.

Polyphenols are a broad class of naturally occurring compounds found in various plant-based foods and beverages. They are characterized by the presence of multiple phenolic (aromatic) rings and are known for their diverse biological activities, including antioxidant, antiinflammatory, and antimicrobial properties (Tijjani et al., 2020). Polyphenols are widely distributed in the plant kingdom and can be found in fruits, vegetables, whole grains, nuts, seeds, legumes, herbs, spices, tea, coffee, cocoa, and wine (Mustafa et al., 2020). The chemical structure of polyphenols is characterized by the presence of one or more phenolic (aromatic) rings with one or more hydroxyl (−OH) groups attached (Vuolo et al., 2019). These phenolic rings can be linked together by different types of chemical bonds, leading to the formation of various subclasses of polyphenols. Major subclasses include flavonoids (e.g., flavonols, flavones, flavanones, flavanols, and anthocyanins), phenolic acids (e.g., hydroxybenzoic and hydroxycinnamic acids), stilbenes (e.g., resveratrol), and lignans (Vuolo et al., 2019). Flavonoids are the most studied subclass of polyphenols and are further classified based on their chemical structure and the degree of oxidation of the central pyran ring (Mutha et al., 2021). They are abundant in fruits, vegetables, tea, and wine and contribute to the vibrant colors of plant-based foods. Phenolic acids, on the other hand, are divided into hydroxybenzoic acids and hydroxycinnamic acids, depending on the number and position of hydroxyl groups on the benzene ring (Vuolo et al., 2019). They are found in a wide range of plant foods, including fruits, vegetables, grains, and beverages like tea and coffee. Table 5.2 summarizes the types of polyphenols and their dietary sources.

Polyphenols are renowned for their diverse array of health benefits. As potent antioxidants, polyphenols play a crucial role in combating oxidative stress and protecting the body against various chronic diseases (Rudrapal et al., 2022). Their importance in human health extends beyond their antioxidant properties, encompassing antiinflammatory, cardioprotective, neuroprotective, and anticancer effects (Rudrapal et al., 2022). By mitigating oxidative stress, polyphenols help maintain cellular integrity and function, which is essential for overall health and longevity. Polyphenols also possess potent antiinflammatory properties, modulating inflammatory pathways and reducing the production of proinflammatory cytokines and enzymes (Sobhani et al., 2021). Furthermore, polyphenols exert cardioprotective effects by improving vascular function, lowering blood pressure, reducing LDL cholesterol oxidation, and inhibiting platelet aggregation (Iqbal et al., 2023). In addition to cardiovascular benefits, polyphenols have emerged as promising agents for promoting brain health and cognitive function. Epidemiological and preclinical studies suggest that polyphenol-rich diets are associated with improved cognitive performance and a reduced risk of ARCD and neurodegenerative diseases such as Alzheimer's and Parkinson's disease (Potì et al., 2019). Polyphenols exert neuroprotective effects through multiple mechanisms, including antioxidant and antiinflammatory actions, modulation of neuronal signaling pathways, and promotion of synaptic plasticity and neurogenesis.

In a review evaluating 28 studies, a combination of cross-sectional and cohort studies, and 55 trials, it was shown that certain polyphenols, when taken in a single dose, offer acute benefits, particularly enhancing attention function and working memory (Yang et al., 2021). These polyphenols notably affect memory and executive function, possibly by improving cerebral blood flow and hippocampal connectivity, while reducing oxidative stress and neuroinflammation. These mechanisms are closely tied to cognitive processes involved in memory and frontal executive function. In a study by Karimipour et al. (2019), a rat model was used to investigate quercetin's capacity to induce neurogenesis. Three groups of rats were randomly assigned to control Alzheimer's (AD) and saline, and AD and quercetin. Rats in the AD and quercetin group received 40 mg/kg/day of quercetin orally for one month following the administration of amyloid-beta. The results showed that while quercetin treatment improved retention and learning, amyloid-beta had a

TABLE 5.2 List of polyphenols and food sources.

Type	Subtypes	Food sources
Flavonoids	Flavonols (quercetin, kaempferol, myricetin)	Apples, onions, berries, citrus fruits, kale, spinach, broccoli, cranberries, red grapes, tea
	Flavones (apigenin, luteolin)	Parsley, celery, chamomile tea, celery, thyme, green peppers
	Flavanones (hesperetin, naringenin)	Citrus fruits, grapefruits, tomatoes, cocoa
	Flavanols (catechin, epicatechin, epigallocatechin gallate)	Tea, apples, cocoa, berries, green tea
	Anthocyanins (cyanidin, delphinidin, pelargonidin)	Berries, cherries, red cabbage, grapes, strawberries, raspberries, red apples
Phenolic acids	Hydroxybenzoic acids (gallic acid, protocatechuic acid)	Grapes, tea, green tea, berries, grains
	Hydroxycinnamic acids (caffeic acid, ferulic acid, sinapic acid)	Coffee, apples, pears, mustard seeds, kale, cauliflower
Stilbenes	Resveratrol	Red wine, grapes, peanuts
Lignans	Secoisolariciresinol, enterolactone	Flaxseeds, sesame seeds, whole grains
Others	Curcumin	Turmeric
	Ellagic acid	Berries, nuts, and pomegranates
	Isoflavones (genistein, daidzein)	Soybeans

detrimental effect on both. In the hippocampus, quercetin increases neural stem/progenitor cell multiplication and drives their growth. Additionally, it increased neurogenesis in adults, possibly by upregulating neurogenesis-related genes such as BDNF, NGF, CREB, and EGR-1. The consumption of green tea by humans can lead to the presence of epigallocatechin gallate (EGCG), a polyphenol, in the brain at low levels, which may encourage the growth of neurites, thereby potentially preventing cognitive decline (Pervin et al., 2019). Additionally, EGCG and its metabolites that reach the brain can help reduce oxidative damage, as evidenced by decreased lipid peroxidation levels in studies on senescence-accelerated mice. These metabolites also exhibit antioxidant properties. However, the composition of intestinal microbiota varies among individuals, affecting the production and absorption rates of these metabolites (Pervin et al., 2019). Despite this, there is currently no research on the in vivo neuroprotective effects of microbial ring-fission metabolites of EGCG. Epidemiological evidence suggests that consuming green tea may help suppress cognitive decline. A study by Carrillo et al. (2019) investigated the impact of polyphenols, particularly flavonoids, on cognitive functions, emphasizing their role in modulating proteins like CREB and BDNF, cerebral blood flow, and memory. Polyphenols were found to exert neuroprotective and antioxidant effects, influencing signaling pathways crucial for cognitive health, particularly in the hippocampus, a key region for memory and learning. Flavonoids were found to enhance synaptic plasticity and cognitive capacities by increasing cerebral blood flow, while lifestyle factors like diet, physical activity, alcohol, and caffeine intake also affected cognitive performance. Furthermore, polyphenols, notably from sources like green tea and cocoa, demonstrated protective effects on cognition and memory, reducing biomarkers of stress and inflammation and enhancing neural growth and connectivity, especially in older individuals and those with neurodegenerative diseases. Bensalem et al. (2019) examined the impact of a polyphenol-rich grape and blueberry extract (PEGB) on memory in older, healthy adults between the ages of 60 and 70 in a double-blind, randomized, and placebo-controlled trial. A total of 215 participants were randomly assigned to receive 600 mg/day of PEGB or a placebo for 6 months. The main outcome measure was the CANTAB Paired Associate Learning (PAL) exam, which evaluates episodic memory and visuospatial learning. PEGB supplementation significantly increased verbal episodic memory (VRM) free recall, even though no discernible effect of PEGB was seen on PAL across the board in the cohort. After placing individuals into quartiles according to their initial PAL scores, a subset known as decliners with advanced cognitive decline responded favorably to PEGB, improving in both PAL and VRM-delayed recognition.

5.6 Challenges and future directions

Dietary interventions, particularly those incorporating polyphenols, hold immense promise in promoting cognitive health and potentially mitigating cognitive decline associated with aging and neurodegenerative diseases. As research continues to uncover the complex interplay between dietary factors, polyphenols, and cognitive function, several key avenues for future investigation and therapeutic applications are emerging. Precision medicine principles can be applied to dietary interventions targeting cognitive health, considering individual variability in genetic makeup, lifestyle factors, and cognitive resilience. Advances in omics technologies enable the identification of molecular signatures and biomarkers associated with dietary responsiveness, cognitive function, and brain health. By stratifying individuals based on their dietary profiles and cognitive phenotypes, precision dietary interventions aim to optimize cognitive outcomes and reduce the risk of cognitive decline across diverse populations. Polyphenols, abundant in various plant-based foods and beverages, have garnered significant attention for their potential neuroprotective properties. Polyphenols exert antioxidant, antiinflammatory, and antiamyloidogenic effects, which may help mitigate oxidative stress, neuroinflammation, and the accumulation of amyloid-beta plaques and neurofibrillary tangles—hallmarks of neurodegenerative diseases such as AD. Moreover, polyphenols can enhance synaptic plasticity, neurogenesis, and neuronal survival, supporting overall brain health and cognitive function. Personalized nutrition approaches, tailored to individual dietary preferences, metabolic profiles, and cognitive health status, offer opportunities for optimizing polyphenol intake and cognitive outcomes. Nutrigenomic approaches enable the identification of genetic variants and biomarkers associated with polyphenol metabolism, cognitive function, and neurodegenerative risk. By integrating personalized dietary recommendations, supplementation strategies, and lifestyle modifications, personalized polyphenol interventions aim to support cognitive resilience, delay cognitive decline, and improve quality of life in aging populations. In conclusion, the future of dietary interventions, particularly those incorporating polyphenols, holds tremendous potential for promoting cognitive health and resilience against neurodegenerative diseases. By leveraging precision medicine principles, neuroprotective mechanisms of polyphenols, epigenetic regulation, brain-targeted delivery strategies, and personalized nutrition approaches, dietary interventions may advance cognitive health promotion and disease prevention strategies. Continued interdisciplinary collaboration and translational efforts are essential to realize the full potential of dietary interventions in supporting cognitive function and improving brain health across the lifespan.

References

Akpoveso, O. O. P., Ubah, E. E., & Obasanmi, G. (2023). Antioxidant phytochemicals as potential therapy for diabetic complications. MDPI, Jamaica. *Antioxidants*, *12*(1). Available from https://doi.org/10.3390/antiox12010123, www.mdpi.com/journal/antioxidants.

Ansari, A. H., Singh, D., & Singh, S. (2024). *Effect of plant-based diets on the brain. Nutraceutical fruits and foods for neurodegenerative disorders* (pp. 249–260). Elsevier.

Anstey, K. J., Cherbuin, N., & Herath, P. M. (2013). Development of a new method for assessing global risk of Alzheimer's disease for use in population health approaches to prevention. Springer Science and Business Media, LLC, Australia. *Prevention Science*, *14*(4), 411–421. Available from https://doi.org/10.1007/s11121-012-0313-2, www.springer.com/journal/11121.

Bensalem, J., Dudonné, S., Etchamendy, N., Pellay, H., Amadieu, C., Gaudout, D., Dubreuil, S., Paradis, M.-E., Pomerleau, S., Capuron, L., Hudon, C., Layé, S., Desjardins, Y., & Pallet, V. (2019). Polyphenols From grape and blueberry improve episodic memory in healthy elderly with lower level of memory performance: A bicentric double-blind, randomized, placebo-controlled clinical study. *The Journals of Gerontology: Series A*, *74* (7), 996–1007. Available from https://doi.org/10.1093/gerona/gly166.

Berendsen, A. M., van de Rest, O., Feskens, E. J. M., de Groot, L. C. P. G. M., Kang, J. H., Grodstein, F., & Grodstein, F. (2017). The dietary approaches to stop hypertension diet, cognitive function, and cognitive decline in American Older Women. *Journal of the American Medical Directors Association*, *18*(5), 427–432. Available from https://doi.org/10.1016/j.jamda.2016.11.026.

Bookheimer, S. Y., Renner, B. A., Ekstrom, A., Li, Z., Henning, S. M., Brown, J. A., Jones, M., Moody, T., & Small, G. W. (2013). Pomegranate juice augments memory and fMRI activity in middle-aged and older adults with mild memory complaints. *Evidence-based Complementary and Alternative Medicine*, *2013*, 946298. Available from https://doi.org/10.1155/2013/946298.

Boudrault, C., Bazinet, R. P., & Ma, D. W. L. (2009). Experimental models and mechanisms underlying the protective effects of n-3 polyunsaturated fatty acids in Alzheimer's disease. *Journal of Nutritional Biochemistry*, *20*(1), 1–10. Available from https://doi.org/10.1016/j.jnutbio.2008.05.016.

Breijyeh, Z., & Karaman, R. (2020). Comprehensive review on Alzheimer's disease: Causes and treatment. *Molecules*, *25*(24), 5789. Available from https://doi.org/10.3390/molecules25245789.

Cao, D., Kevala, K., Kim, J., Moon, H. S., Jun, S. B., Lovinger, D., & Kim, H. Y. (2009). Docosahexaenoic acid promotes hippocampal neuronal development and synaptic function. *Journal of Neurochemistry*, *111*(2), 510–521. Available from https://doi.org/10.1111/j.1471-4159.2009.06335.x.

Carrillo, J. Á., Zafrilla, M. P., & Marhuenda, J. (2019). Cognitive function and consumption of fruit and vegetable polyphenols in a young population: Is there a relationship? *Foods*, *8*(10), 507. Available from https://doi.org/10.3390/foods8100507.

Chan, R., Chan, D., & Woo, J. (2013). A cross sectional study to examine the association between dietary patterns and cognitive impairment in older Chinese people in Hong Kong. *The Journal of nutrition, health and aging*, *17*(9), 757–765. Available from https://doi.org/10.1007/s12603-013-0348-5.

Chen, X., Maguire, B., Brodaty, H., & O'Leary, F. (2019). Dietary patterns and cognitive health in older adults: A systematic review. *Journal of Alzheimer's Disease*, *67*(2), 583–619.

Chen, Y. C., Jung, C. C., Chen, J. H., Chiou, J. M., Chen, T. F., Chen, Y. F., Tang, S. C., Yeh, S. J., & Lee, M. S. (2017). Association of dietary patterns with global and domain-specific cognitive decline in Chinese elderly. *Journal of the American Geriatrics Society*, *65*(6), 1159–1167. Available from https://doi.org/10.1111/jgs.14741, http://www.blackwellpublishing.com/journal.asp?ref = 0002-8614&site = 1.

Chung, Y. C., Park, C. H., Kwon, H. K., Park, Y. M., Kim, Y. S., Doo, J. K., Shin, D. H., Jung, E. S., Oh, M. R., & Chae, S. W. (2012). Improved cognitive performance following supplementation with a mixed-grain diet in high school students: A randomized controlled trial. *Nutrition*, *28*(2), 165–172. Available from https://doi.org/10.1016/j.nut.2011.05.017.

Cohen, J. F. W., Gorski, M. T., Gruber, S. A., Kurdziel, L. B. F., & Rimm, E. B. (2016). The effect of healthy dietary consumption on executive cognitive functioning in children and adolescents: A systematic review. *British Journal of Nutrition*, *116*(6), 989–1000. Available from https://doi.org/10.1017/s0007114516002877.

Crichton, G. E., Murphy, K. J., Howe, P. R. C., Buckley, J. D., & Bryan, J. (2012). Dairy consumption and working memory performance in overweight and obese adults. *Appetite*, *59*(1), 34–40. Available from https://doi.org/10.1016/j.appet.2012.03.019, http://www.elsevier.com/inca/publications/store/6/2/2/7/8/5/index.htt.

Crichton, G. E., Bryan, J., Hodgson, J. M., & Murphy, K. J. (2013). Mediterranean diet adherence and self-reported psychological functioning in an Australian sample. *Appetite*, *70*, 53–59. Available from https://doi.org/10.1016/j.appet.2013.06.088.

Dalile, B., Kim, C., Challinor, A., Geurts, L., Gibney, E. R., Galdos, M. V., Fata., Mathers, J. C., & Vauzour, D. (2022). The EAT–Lancet reference diet and cognitive function across the life course. *The Lancet Planetary Health*, *6*(9), e749–e759.

Dalton, A., Wolmarans, P., Witthuhn, R. C., van Stuijvenberg, M. E., Swanevelder, S. A., & Smuts, C. M. (2009). A randomised control trial in schoolchildren showed improvement in cognitive function after consuming a bread spread, containing fish flour from a marine source. *Prostaglandins, Leukotrienes, and Essential Fatty Acids*, *80*(2-3), 143–149. Available from https://doi.org/10.1016/j.plefa.2008.12.006.

Daniel, G. D., Chen, H., Bertoni, A. G., Rapp, S. R., Fitzpatrick, A. L., Luchsinger, J. A., Wood, A. C., Hughes, T. M., Burke, G. L., & Hayden, K. M. (2021). DASH diet adherence and cognitive function: Multi-ethnic study of atherosclerosis. *Clinical Nutrition ESPEN*, *46*, 223–231. Available from https://doi.org/10.1016/j.clnesp.2021.10.004, http://www.journals.elsevier.com/clinical-nutrition-espen.

Daskalopoulou, S. S., Khan, N. A., Quinn, R. R., Ruzicka, M., McKay, D. W., Hackam, D. G., Rabkin, S. W., Rabi, D. M., Gilbert, R. E., Padwal, R. S., Dawes, M., Touyz, R. M., Campbell, T. S., Cloutier, L., Grover, S., Honos, G., Herman, R. J., Schiffrin, E. L., Bolli, P., … Tobe, S. W. (2012). The 2012 Canadian hypertension education program recommendations for the management of hypertension: blood pressure measurement, diagnosis, assessment of risk, and therapy. *Canadian Journal of Cardiology*, *28*(3), 270–287. Available from https://doi.org/10.1016/j.cjca.2012.02.018.

Davis, C., Bryan, J., Hodgson, J., & Murphy, K. (2015). Definition of the Mediterranean diet; A literature review. *Nutrients*, *7*(11), 9139–9153. Available from https://doi.org/10.3390/nu7115459.

Devi, S. A., & Satpati, A. (2016). *Oxidative stress and the brain: An insight into cognitive aging. Topics in biomedical gerontology* (pp. 123–140). India: Springer Singapore. Available from https://doi.org/10.1007/978-981-10-2155-8, https://doi.org/10.1007/978-981-10-2155-8_8.

Dumas, J. A., Bunn, J. Y., Nickerson, J., Crain, K. I., Ebenstein, D. B., Tarleton, E. K., Makarewicz, J., Poynter, M. E., & Kien, C. L. (2016). Dietary saturated fat and monounsaturated fat have reversible effects on brain function and the secretion of pro-inflammatory cytokines in young women. *Metabolism: Clinical and Experimental*, *65*(10), 1582–1588. Available from https://doi.org/10.1016/j.metabol.2016.08.003, http://www.elsevier.com/inca/publications/store/6/2/3/3/1/9/index.htt.

Dyall, S. C., Michael, G. J., Whelpton, R., Scott, A. G., & Michael-Titus, A. T. (2007). Dietary enrichment with omega-3 polyunsaturated fatty acids reverses age-related decreases in the GluR2 and NR2B glutamate receptor subunits in rat forebrain. *Neurobiology of Aging*, *28*(3), 424–439. Available from https://doi.org/10.1016/j.neurobiolaging.2006.01.002.

Fu, J., Tan, L. J., Lee, J. E., & Shin, S. (2022). Association between the mediterranean diet and cognitive health among healthy adults: A systematic review and meta-analysis. *Frontiers in Nutrition*, *9*, 946361. Available from https://doi.org/10.3389/fnut.2022.946361, journal.frontiersin.org/journal/nutrition.

Gardener, S., Gu, Y., Rainey-Smith, S. R., Keogh, J. B., Clifton, P. M., Mathieson, S. L., Taddei, K., Mondal, A., Ward, V. K., Scarmeas, N., Barnes, M., Ellis, K. A., Head, R., Masters, C. L., Ames, D., Macaulay, S. L., Rowe, C. C., Szoeke, C., & Martins, R. N. (2012). Adherence to a Mediterranean diet and Alzheimer's disease risk in an Australian population. *Translational Psychiatry*, *2*(10), e164. Available from https://doi.org/10.1038/tp.2012.91.

Gildawie, K. R., Galli, R. L., Shukitt-Hale, B., & Carey, A. N. (2018). Protective effects of foods containing flavonoids on age-related cognitive decline. *Current Nutrition Reports*, *7*, 39–48. Available from https://doi.org/10.1007/s13668-018-0227-0, http://www.springer.com/new + %26 + forthcoming + titles + %28default%29/journal/13668?changeHeader.

Guasch-Ferré, M., & Willett, W. C. (2021). The Mediterranean diet and health: A comprehensive overview. *Journal of Internal Medicine*, *290*(3), 549–566. Available from https://doi.org/10.1111/joim.13333.

Iqbal, I., Wilairatana, P., Saqib, F., Nasir, B., Wahid, M., Latif, M. F., Iqbal, A., Naz, R., & Mubarak, M. S. (2023). Plant polyphenols and their potential benefits on cardiovascular health: A review. *Molecules*, *28*(17), 6403. Available from https://doi.org/10.3390/molecules28176403, http://www.mdpi.com/journal/molecules.

Jolitha, A. B., Subramanyam, M. V. V., & Asha Devi, S. (2006). Modification by vitamin E and exercise of oxidative stress in regions of aging rat brain: Studies on superoxide dismutase isoenzymes and protein oxidation status. *Experimental Gerontology*, *41*(8), 753–763. Available from https://doi.org/10.1016/j.exger.2006.04.007.

Jones, E. K., Sünram-Lea, S. I., & Wesnes, K. A. (2012). Acute ingestion of different macronutrients differentially enhances aspects of memory and attention in healthy young adults. *Biological Psychology*, *89*(2), 477–486. Available from https://doi.org/10.1016/j.biopsycho.2011.12.017.

Juan, S. M., & Adlard, P. A. (2019). Ageing and cognition. *Subcellular Biochemistry*, *91*(2019), 107–122. Available from https://doi.org/10.1007/978-981-13-3681-2_5, http://www.springer.com/series/6515.

Karimipour, M., Rahbarghazi, R., Tayefi, H., Shimia, M., Ghanadian, M., Mahmoudi, J., & Bagheri, H. S. (2019). Quercetin promotes learning and memory performance concomitantly with neural stem/progenitor cell proliferation and neurogenesis in the adult rat dentate gyrus. *International Journal of Developmental Neuroscience*, *74*, 18–26. Available from https://doi.org/10.1016/j.ijdevneu.2019.02.005, www.elsevier.com/locate/ijdevneu.

Kean, R. J., Lamport, D. J., Dodd, G. F., Freeman, J. E., Williams, C. M., Ellis, J. A., Butler, L. T., & Spencer, J. P. E. (2015). Chronic consumption of flavanone-rich orange juice is associated with cognitive benefits: An 8-wk, randomized, double-blind, placebo-controlled trial in healthy older adults. *American Journal of Clinical Nutrition*, *101*(3), 506–514. Available from https://doi.org/10.3945/ajcn.114.088518, http://ajcn.nutrition.org/content/101/3/506.full.pdf + html.

Khan, A. U., Akram, M., Daniyal, M., & Zainab, R. (2019). Awareness and current knowledge of Parkinson's disease: a neurodegenerative disorder. *International Journal of Neuroscience*, *129*(1), 55–93. Available from https://doi.org/10.1080/00207454.2018.1486837, http://www.tandfonline.com/loi/ines20.

Khan, N. A., Raine, L. B., Drollette, E. S., Scudder, M. R., & Hillman, C. H. (2015). The relation of saturated fats and dietary cholesterol to childhood cognitive flexibility. *Appetite*, *93*, 51–56. Available from https://doi.org/10.1016/j.appet.2015.04.012, http://www.elsevier.com/inca/publications/store/6/2/2/7/8/5/index.htt.

Kuhn, M., Minniti, A., Prettner, K., & Venturini, F. (2023). Medical innovation, life expectancy, and economic growth. *SSRN Electronic Journal*. Available from https://doi.org/10.2139/ssrn.4491818.

Kumar, M., Ghosh, M., & Ganguli, A. (2012). Mitogenic response and probiotic characteristics of lactic acid bacteria isolated from indigenously pickled vegetables and fermented beverages. *World Journal of Microbiology and Biotechnology*, *28*(2), 703–711. Available from https://doi.org/10.1007/s11274-011-0866-4.

Kwan, M. W. M., Wong, M. C. S., Wang, H. H. X., Liu, K. Q. L., Lee, C. L. S., Yan, B. P. Y., Yu, C. M., & Griffiths, S. M. (2013). Compliance with the dietary approaches to stop hypertension (DASH) diet: A systematic review. *PLoS ONE*, *8*(10), e78412. Available from https://doi.org/10.1371/journal.pone.0078412, http://www.plosone.org/article/fetchObject.action?uri = info:doi/10.1371/journal.pone.0078412&representation = PDF.

Li, Z., Zhang, Z., Ren, Y., Wang, Y., Fang, J., Yue, H., Ma, S., & Guan, F. (2021). Aging and age-related diseases: from mechanisms to therapeutic strategies. *Biogerontology*, *22*(2), 165–187. Available from https://doi.org/10.1007/s10522-021-09910-5.

Marckmann, P., & Grønbæk, M. (1999). Fish consumption and coronary heart disease mortality. A systematic review of prospective cohort studies. *European Journal of Clinical Nutrition*, *53*(8), 585–590. Available from https://doi.org/10.1038/sj.ejcn.1600832.

Martínez-González, M. Á., & Sánchez-Villegas, A. (2004). The emerging role of Mediterranean diets in cardiovascular epidemiology: monounsaturated fats, olive oil, red wine or the whole pattern? *European Journal of Epidemiology*, *19*(1), 9–13.

Masley, S. C., Masley, L. V., & Gualtieri, C. T. (2012). Effect of mercury levels and seafood intake on cognitive function in middle-aged adults. *Integrative Medicine*, *11*(3), 32–39.

Miller, H. C., Struyf, D., Baptist, P., Dalile, B., Van Oudenhove, L., & Van Diest, I. (2018). A mind cleared by walnut oil: The effects of polyunsaturated and saturated fat on extinction learning. *Appetite*, *126*, 147–155. Available from https://doi.org/10.1016/j.appet.2018.04.004, http://www.elsevier.com/inca/publications/store/6/2/2/7/8/5/index.htt.

Miller, M. G., Hamilton, D. A., Joseph, J. A., & Shukitt-Hale, B. (2018). Dietary blueberry improves cognition among older adults in a randomized, double-blind, placebo-controlled trial. *European Journal of Nutrition*, *57*, 1169–1180.

Mintzer, J., Donovan, K. A., Kindy, A. Z., Lock, S. L., Chura, L. R., & Barracca, N. (2019). Lifestyle choices and brain health. *Frontiers in Medicine*, *6*. Available from https://doi.org/10.3389/fmed.2019.00204.

Morris, M. C., Evans, D. A., Tangney, C. C., Bienias, J. L., & Wilson, R. S. (2005). Fish consumption and cognitive decline with age in a large community study. *Archives of Neurology*, *62*(12), 1849–1853. Available from https://doi.org/10.1001/archneur.62.12.noc50161, http://archneur.ama-assn.org/cgi/reprint/62/12/1849, United States.

Mottaghi, T., Amirabdollahian, F., & Haghighatdoost, F. (2018). Fruit and vegetable intake and cognitive impairment: a systematic review and meta-analysis of observational studies. *European Journal of Clinical Nutrition*, *72*(10), 1336–1344. Available from https://doi.org/10.1038/s41430-017-0005-x.

Murman, D. L. (2015). The impact of age on cognition. *Seminars in hearing*, *36*(3), 111–121. Available from https://doi.org/10.1055/s-0035-1555115, http://www.thieme-connect.com/ejournals/toc/sih.

Mustafa, S. K., Oyouni, A. A. W. A., Aljohani, M. M. H., & Ayaz Ahmad, M. (2020). Polyphenols more than an antioxidant: Role and scope. *Journal of Pure and Applied Microbiology, Saudi Arabia Journal of Pure and Applied Microbiology*, *14*(1), 47–61. Available from https://doi.org/10.22207/JPAM.14.1.08, https://microbiologyjournal.org/polyphenols-more-than-an-antioxidant-role-and-scope/.

Mutha, R. E., Tatiya, A. U., & Surana, S. J. (2021). Flavonoids as natural phenolic compounds and their role in therapeutics: An overview. *Future Journal of Pharmaceutical Sciences*, *7*(1). Available from https://doi.org/10.1186/s43094-020-00161-8.

Nyaradi, A., Li, J., Hickling, S., Whitehouse, A. J. O., Foster, J. K., & Oddy, W. H. (2013). Diet in the early years of life influences cognitive outcomes at 10 years: A prospective cohort study. *Acta Paediatrica, International Journal of Paediatrics*, *102*(12), 1165–1173. Available from https://doi.org/10.1111/apa.12363.

Øyen, J., Kvestad, I., Midtbø, L. K., Graff, I. E., Hysing, M., Stormark, K. M., Markhus, M. W., Baste, V., Frøyland, L., & Koletzko, B. (2018). Fatty fish intake and cognitive function: FINS-KIDS, a randomized controlled trial in preschool children. *BMC medicine*, *16*, 1–15. Available from https://doi.org/10.1186/s12916-018-1020-z, http://www.biomedcentral.com/bmcmed/.

Ozawa, M., Ninomiya, T., Ohara, T., Doi, Y., Uchida, K., Shirota, T., Yonemoto, K., Kitazono, T., & Kiyohara, Y. (2013). Dietary patterns and risk of dementia in an elderly Japanese population: The Hisayama Study. *The American Journal of Clinical Nutrition*, *97*(5), 1076–1082. Available from https://doi.org/10.3945/ajcn.112.045575.

Park, K. M., & Fulgoni, V. L. (2013). The association between dairy product consumption and cognitive function in the National Health and Nutrition Examination Survey. *British Journal of Nutrition*, *109*(6), 1135–1142. Available from https://doi.org/10.1017/S0007114512002905.

Péneau, S., Galan, P., Jeandel, C., Ferry, M., Andreeva, V., Hercberg, S., Kesse-Guyot, E., Vogt, L., Escande, M., Sérot, J. M., Vasseur, E., Debray, M., Hussonnois, C., Iehl-Robert, M., Le Sommer, M., Boge, T., Rajaonarivo, J., Jouseau, J., Frison, M., … Cézard, O. (2011). Fruit and vegetable intake and cognitive function in the SU. VI. MAX 2 prospective study. *The American Journal of Clinical Nutrition*, *94*(5), 1295–1303.

Pervin, M., Unno, K., Takagaki, A., Isemura, M., & Nakamura, Y. (2019). Function of green tea catechins in the brain: Epigallocatechin gallate and its metabolites. *International Journal of Molecular Sciences*, *20*(15), 3630. Available from https://doi.org/10.3390/ijms20153630.

Pesce, M., Tatangelo, R., La Fratta, I., Rizzuto, A., Campagna, G., Turli, C., Ferrone, A., Franceschelli, S., Speranza, L., Patruno, A., Ballerini, P., De Lutiis, M. A., Felaco, M., & Grilli, A. (2018). Aging-related oxidative stress: Positive effect of memory training. *Neuroscience*, *370*, 246–255. Available from https://doi.org/10.1016/j.neuroscience.2017.09.046.

Petruski-Ivleva, N., Kucharska-Newton, A., Palta, P., Couper, D., Meyer, K., Graff, M., Haring, B., Sharrett, R., & Heiss, G. (2017). Milk intake at midlife and cognitive decline over 20 years. The Atherosclerosis Risk in Communities (ARIC) Study. *Nutrients*, *9*(10), 1134. Available from https://doi.org/10.3390/nu9101134.

Potì, F., Santi, D., Spaggiari, G., Zimetti, F., & Zanotti, I. (2019). Polyphenol health effects on cardiovascular and neurodegenerative disorders: A review and meta-analysis. *International Journal of Molecular Sciences*, *20*(2), 351. Available from https://doi.org/10.3390/ijms20020351.

Presse, N., Belleville, S., Gaudreau, P., Greenwood, C. E., Kergoat, M. J., Morais, J. A., Payette, H., Shatenstein, B., & Ferland, G. (2013). Vitamin K status and cognitive function in healthy older adults. *Neurobiology of Aging*, *34*(12), 2777–2783. Available from https://doi.org/10.1016/j.neurobiolaging.2013.05.031.

Puri, S., Shaheen, M., & Grover, B. (2023). Nutrition and cognitive health: A life course approach. *Frontiers in Public Health*, *11*, 1023907. Available from https://doi.org/10.3389/fpubh.2023.1023907.

Puskás, L. G., Kitajka, K., Nyakas, C., Barcelo-Coblijn, G., & Farkas, T. (2003). Short-term administration of omega 3 fatty acids from fish oil results in increased transthyretin transcription in old rat hippocampus. *Proceedings of the National Academy of Sciences*, *100*(4), 1580–1585. Available from https://doi.org/10.1073/pnas.0337683100.

Qin, B., Adair, L. S., Plassman, B. L., Batis, C., Edwards, L. J., Popkin, B. M., & Mendez, M. A. (2015). Dietary patterns and cognitive decline among Chinese older adults. *Epidemiology*, *26*(5), 758–768. Available from https://doi.org/10.1097/EDE.0000000000000338, http://journals.lww.com/epidem/pages/default.aspx.

Rao, A. V., & Balachandran, B. (2002). Role of oxidative stress and antioxidants in neurodegenerative diseases. *Nutritional Neuroscience*, *5*(5), 291–309. Available from https://doi.org/10.1080/1028415021000033767.

Rosato, V., Temple, N. J., La Vecchia, C., Castellan, G., Tavani, A., & Guercio, V. (2019). Mediterranean diet and cardiovascular disease: A systematic review and meta-analysis of observational studies. *European Journal of Nutrition*, *58*(1), 173–191. Available from https://doi.org/10.1007/s00394-017-1582-0, http://www.springerlink.com/content/1436-6207.

Rudrapal, M., Khairnar, S. J., Khan, J., Dukhyil, A. B., Ansari, M. A., Alomary, M. N., Alshabrmi, F. M., Palai, S., Deb, P. K., & Devi, R. (2022). Dietary polyphenols and their role in oxidative stress-induced human diseases: Insights into protective effects, antioxidant potentials and mechanism(s) of action. *Frontiers in Pharmacology*, *13*. Available from https://doi.org/10.3389/fphar.2022.806470, http://www.frontiersin.org/Pharmacology.

Samieri, C., Morris, M. C., Bennett, D. A., Berr, C., Amouyel, P., Dartigues, J. F., Tzourio, C., Chasman, D. I., & Grodstein, F. (2018). Fish intake, genetic predisposition to Alzheimer disease, and decline in global cognition and memory in 5 cohorts of older persons. *American Journal of Epidemiology*, *187*(5), 933–940. Available from https://doi.org/10.1093/aje/kwx330, http://aje.oxfordjournals.org/.

Schwingshackl, L., Schwedhelm, C., Galbete, C., & Hoffmann, G. (2017). Adherence to Mediterranean diet and risk of cancer: An updated systematic review and meta-analysis. *Nutrients*, *9*(10), 1063. Available from https://doi.org/10.3390/nu9101063.

Siqueira, I. R., Fochesatto, C., De Andrade, A., Santos, M., Hagen, M., Bello-Klein, A., & Netto, C. A. (2005). Total antioxidant capacity is impaired in different structures from aged rat brain. *International Journal of Developmental Neuroscience*, *23*(8), 663–671. Available from https://doi.org/10.1016/j.ijdevneu.2005.03.001.

Sobhani, M., Farzaei, M. H., Kiani, S., & Khodarahmi, R. (2021). Immunomodulatory; anti-inflammatory/antioxidant effects of polyphenols: A comparative review on the parental compounds and their metabolites. *Food Reviews International*, *37*(8), 759–811. Available from https://doi.org/10.1080/87559129.2020.1717523, www.tandf.co.uk/journals/titles/87559129.asp.

Su, H. M. (2010). Mechanisms of n-3 fatty acid-mediated development and maintenance of learning memory performance. *Journal of Nutritional Biochemistry*, *21*(5), 364–373. Available from https://doi.org/10.1016/j.jnutbio.2009.11.003.

Tangney, C. C., Li, H., Wang, Y., Barnes, L., Schneider, J. A., Bennett, D. A., & Morris, M. C. (2014). Relation of DASH- and Mediterranean-like dietary patterns to cognitive decline in older persons. *Neurology*, *83*(16), 1410–1416. Available from https://doi.org/10.1212/WNL.0000000000000884.

Tijjani, H., Zangoma, M. H., Mohammed, Z. S., Obidola, S. M., Egbuna, C., & Abdulai, S. I. (2020). *Polyphenols: Classifications, biosynthesis and bioactivities* (pp. 389–414). Springer Science and Business Media LLC. Available from https://doi.org/10.1007/978-3-030-42319-3_19.

Tsai, H. J. (2015). Dietary patterns and cognitive decline in Taiwanese aged 65 years and older. *International Journal of Geriatric Psychiatry*, *30*(5), 523–530. Available from https://doi.org/10.1002/gps.4176, http://onlinelibrary.wiley.com/journal/10.1002/(ISSN)1099-1166.

Tsurumaki, N., Zhang, S., Tomata, Y., Abe, S., Sugawara, Y., Matsuyama, S., & Tsuji, I. (2019). Fish consumption and risk of incident dementia in elderly Japanese: The Ohsaki cohort 2006 study. *British Journal of Nutrition*, *122*(10), 1182–1191. Available from https://doi.org/10.1017/s0007114519002265.

Urquiza, A. M. D., Liu, S., Sjoberg, M., Zetterstrom, R. H., Griffiths, W., Sjovall, J., & Perlmann, T. (2000). Docosahexaenoic acid, a ligand for the retinoid X receptor in mouse brain. *Science*, *290*(5499), 2140–2144.

van den Brink, A. C., Brouwer-Brolsma, E. M., Berendsen, A. A. M., & van de Rest, O. (2019). The Mediterranean, Dietary Approaches to Stop Hypertension (DASH), and Mediterranean-DASH Intervention for Neurodegenerative Delay (MIND) Diets Are Associated with Less Cognitive Decline and a Lower Risk of Alzheimer's Disease-A Review. *Advances in Nutrition*, *10*(6), 1040–1065. Available from https://doi.org/10.1093/advances/nmz054.

Vuolo, M. M., Lima, V. S., & Junior, M. R. M. (2019). *Phenolic Compounds. Bioactive Compounds: Health Benefits and Potential Applications* (2019, pp. 33–50). Brazil: Elsevier. Available from https://www.sciencedirect.com/book/9780128147740, https://doi.org/10.1016/B978-0-12-814774-0.00002-5.

Wengreen, H., Munger, R. G., Cutler, A., Quach, A., Bowles, A., Corcoran, C., Tschanz, J. A. T., Norton, M. C., & Welsh-Bohmer, K. A. (2013). Prospective study of Dietary Approaches to Stop Hypertension-and Mediterranean-style dietary patterns and age-related cognitive change: The Cache County Study on Memory, Health and Aging. *American Journal of Clinical Nutrition*, *98*(5), 1263–1271. Available from https://doi.org/10.3945/ajcn.112.051276, http://ajcn.nutrition.org/content/98/5/1263.full.pdf + html, United States.

Whyte, A. R., Cheng, N., Fromentin, E., & Williams, C. M. (2018). A randomized, double-blinded, placebo-controlled study to compare the safety and efficacy of low dose enhanced wild blueberry powder and wild blueberry extract (Thinkblue™) in maintenance of episodic and working memory in older adults. *Nutrients*, *10*(6). (2018), Available from:. Available from https://doi.org/10.3390/nu10060660, http://www.mdpi.com/2072-6643/10/6/660/pdf.

Williams, K. A., & Patel, H. (2017). Healthy plant-based diet: What does it really mean? *Journal of the American College of Cardiology*, *70*(4), 423–425. Available from https://doi.org/10.1016/j.jacc.2017.06.006, www.elsevier.com/locate/jacc.

Yang, W., Cui, K., Li, X., Zhao, J., Zeng, Z., Song, R., Qi, X., & Xu, W. (2021). Effect of polyphenols on cognitive function: Evidence from population-based studies and clinical trials. *The Journal of nutrition, health and aging*, *25*(10), 1190–1204. Available from https://doi.org/10.1007/s12603-021-1685-4.

Yoshinaga, M., Toda, N., Tamura, Y., Terakado, S., Ueno, M., Otsuka, K., Numabe, A., Kawabata, Y., & Uehara, Y. (2012). Japanese traditional miso soup attenuates salt-induced hypertension and its organ damage in Dahl salt-sensitive rats. *Nutrition*, *28*(9), 924–931. Available from https://doi.org/10.1016/j.nut.2011.09.010.

Zhang, H., Hardie, L., Bawajeeh, A. O., & Cade, J. (2020). Meat consumption, cognitive function and disorders: a systematic review with narrative synthesis and meta-analysis. *Nutrients*, *12*(5), 1528.

Zhang, H., Cade, J., & Hadie, L. (2020). Consumption of red meat is negatively associated with cognitive function: a cross-sectional analysis of UK Biobank. *Current Developments in Nutrition*, *4*, nzaa061_138.

Chapter 6

Weight management: functional foods for a balanced body

Zahra Emam-Djomeh[1], Salma Samieitousi[1], Sara Gashtasbi[1], Homa Behmadi[2], Elham Azarpazhooh[3] and Hosahalli S. Ramaswamy[4]

[1]*Functional Food Research Core (FFRC), Transfer Phenomena Laboratory (TPL), College of Agriculture & Natural Resources, University of Tehran, Karaj Campus, Tehran, Iran,* [2]*Agricultural Engineering Research Institute, Agricultural Research, Education and Extension Organization (AREEO), Karaj, Iran,* [3]*Agricultural Engineering Research Department, Khorasan Razavi Agricultural and Natural Resources Research and Education Center, AREEO, Mashhad, Iran,* [4]*Department of Food Science, Macdonald Campus, McGill University, Ste Anne de Bellevue, QC, Canada*

6.1 Introduction

Underdeveloped and developed nations have been confronting health challenges and chronic diseases such as obesity. In recent decades, obesity has become a prevalent universal epidemic due to various reasons such as genetic predisposition, environmental factors, inappropriate lifestyles, like eating habits, unbalanced diet, high intake of processed food, and inadequate physical activity (Tsoi *et al.*, n.d.). As stated by WHO, in 2016, 1.9 billion adults aged 18 and above were classified as overweight, and through them, more than 650 million adults were classified as obese (Ruiz *et al.*, 2020). The adverse effects of obesity include the expansion of type 2 diabetes mellitus, hypertension, dyslipidemia, metabolic syndrome, asthma, and cardiovascular diseases (Tsoi *et al.*, n.d.).

Triacylglycerol plays a vital role in providing energy. Disrupting equality between the intake of calories and energy consumption leads to the accumulation of excess fatty tissue and obesity. Obesity is described as a rise in the amount and magnitude of fat cells, identified by their improvement from fibroblastic preadipocytes (Haththotuwa et al., 2016; Ruiz *et al.*, 2020). Adipose tissue (AT) is a significant energy storage and endocrine organ. The AT generates adipokines like adiponectin and leptin and pro-inflammatory factors such as TNF-α and IL-6. To sustain energy regulation. Under normal circumstances, when the body receives immoderate energy, it increases the size and number of ATs that need more oxygen and nutrients for the entire tissue. In the condition of obesity, fatty tissue undergoes changes such as decreased angiogenesis, increased hypoxia, and heightened immune cell levels, which induce low-grade inflammation. Obesity causes a reduction of antiinflammatories such as adiponectin and an increase in promoting adipocytokines and interleukins such as IL-6 (interleukin-6), TNF-α tumor necrosis factor-alpha), and leptin. Production of these inflammatory adipocytokines participates in systemic inflammation, insulin resistance, and various metabolic disorders associated with obesity (Blüher, 2016; Otelea *et al.*, 2019).

A rise in quantity and considerable adipocytes is associated with inflammation, ROS generation, and changing the concentration of the substances involved in inflammation. Oxidative stress is described as a condition owning to the inequality between the intracellular oxidation and reduction systems. The disbalance causes infusing cellular stress responses which in turn stimulate cytotoxicity and promote cell death, the occurrence of metabolic disease, and the development of obesity (Zuo *et al.*, 2019).

ROS generation occurs in adipocytes due to fatty acid oxidation in both mitochondria and peroxisomes, conceivably leading to a rise in oxidative stress under obesity.

Increasing reactive oxygen species (ROS) levels may diminish mitochondrial function, hindering the respiratory process. Consecutively, it could decrease adipocyte energy expenditure while enhancing energy storage in AT. Diets rich in lipids contribute to the production of ROS by disturbing oxygen metabolism, resulting in a remarkable decrease in antioxidant enzymes like superoxide dismutase, catalase, and glutathione peroxidase. Consequently, this could give rise to obesity-related comorbidities (Nono Nankam *et al.*, 2021).

Unleashing the Power of Functional Foods and Novel Bioactives. DOI: https://doi.org/10.1016/B978-0-443-28862-3.00006-6

More effective procedures to control weight management and prevent obesity include increasing energy expenditure and intake of low-calorie foods while restricting high-calorie foods. Choosing an adequate diet, such as the Mediterranean diet coincident with increasing physical exertion, could contribute to a more beneficial strategy (Rolls, 2014; Torres-Fuentes *et al.*, 2015). Dramatic rates of morbidity and mortality have caused people to realize the correlation between their dietary choices and the incidence of disease. Improved health and well-being drew people's attention and interest to the benefits and consumption of functional food. Functional foods, referred to as nutraceuticals, are interpreted as food ingredients consisting of bioactive compounds such as polyphenols, prebiotic polysaccharides, and essential fatty acids, positively impacting consumer health. These bioactive compounds, which can be phytochemicals taken as supplements or have medicinal value when consumed as whole foods, have been conducive to the increasing popularity of functional foods. These foods are looked after for their potential to prevent various diseases, promote growth, and boost host metabolic activity (Scientific Opinion on establishing Food-Based Dietary Guidelines, 2010).

6.2 Overweight and obesity

Obesity becomes terrifyingly an international health danger when the body mass index rises with Class I BMI (moderate risk), Class II BMI (high risk), and Class III BMI > 40 (very high risk) of mortality. This widespread noncommunicable health issue impacts 1.1 billion adults globally, with 312 million classified as obese, highlighting the urgent need for impactful interventions (Baboota *et al.*, 2013). Within the last decade, several industrialized nations have witnessed a concerning growth in obesity rates, with the general population experiencing a doubling or even tripling of prevalence. This is a disturbing trend that is not a phenomena limited to North America but rather a global fact driven by the widespread "Western lifestyle" characterized by consumption of high-fat, high-refined carbohydrate food stuffs and predominantly sedentary activities. The complex interaction of genetic, metabolic, behavioral, and environmental factors contributes to overweight and obesity. The rapid growth of obesity implies that the epidemic is primarily driven by behavioral and environmental influences rather than inherent biological changes. This surge is attributed to an increase in energy consumption, a decrease in energy expenditure, or a combination of both, resulting in a positive energy balance and a significant rise in weight across societies (Green et al., 2020; Stein & Colditz, 2004).

6.2.1 Adipose tissue

AT boundlessly extends during overweightness as it is a vital part of the body that is actively dispersed all through the body which regulates various processes in the body. Moreover, it affects the overall metabolism of the body level through adipocytokines. Changes within the primary adipokines have numerous obesity-related metabolic issues, such as type 2 diabetes, metabolic disorders, and cardiovascular illnesses (Heinonen *et al.*, 2020). It comprises various cells found in the empty spaces between other cells. The cells interplaying to determine AT homeostasis are adipocytes, adipose stem cells, fibroblast, endothelial, nerve, and immune cells (Schulz & Tseng, 2013).

Two significant sorts of AT are white and brown in mammals. The biggest part of body fat is located around important organs and arteries in the place inside the belly and under the skin is white AT (WAT) in which extra power in the shape of triglycerides is kept by gathering extra fats and sugar from the blood, and it guards other body parts from an unhealthy increase of triglycerides. Moreover, elevated WAT gathering, especially in visceral depots, is a major determinant of the relative risk of cardiometabolic disorders, hypertension, and cardiovascular disease (Lee et al., 2013; Piché et al., 2020). If depot capacity is disrupted, fats can leak into other parts of the body, such as organs and blood vessels. This can cause mild inflammation and problems with insulin and metabolism. Interestingly, both not having enough fat tissue in lipodystrophies and having too much unhealthy fat tissue in obesity can cause the same problems, like accumulating fat in the liver and resistance to insulin (Heinonen *et al.*, 2020). It is confirmed that individuals with higher visceral AT and storage of TG in tissues other than AT have an increased prevalence of cardiometabolic disorders; however, similarly obese people with lower visceral AT have moderately more subcutaneous AT (SAT). So, using only BMI to measure obesity does not accurately show the real risk of cardiovascular disease (Hall *et al.*, 2015; Piché et al., 2020).

Unlike WAT, brown adipose tissue (BAT) makes up only about 4.3% of all AT in grown-up humans. In animals like mammals, there are two different types of brown fat cells. The first type, classical brown adipocytes or cBAT, develops before birth. The second type, called beige or brite AT (having blended characteristics of both white and brown fat cells), develops after birth in white fat cells or skeletal muscle. This second type can also be called recruitable BAT (Giralt & Villarroya, 2013; Schulz & Tseng, 2013). It has a unique brown color because it contains a lot of iron and cytochrome in its mitochondria and blood vessels. In newborn children and little children, cBAT is fully evolved, and the reason is hypothermia may occur because they have more surface area compared to their size. This means that it is really important for them to work properly to keep a normal body temperature. The BAT is a special place in the body that generates heat by a protein called UCP1 (also called thermogenin). This protein uncouples the respiratory chain to produce heat, and the mitochondria in BAT can break down fat. So, the BAT can help "burn" fat (Giralt & Villarroya, 2013). Brown fat cells can do this because they have a lot of mitochondria that have UCP1, which is responsible for separating the process of making energy from the process of making ATP. The balance of electrons and protons in the mitochondria changes, which causes energy to be lost as heat. There are two types of brown fat cells, one with a high ability to generate heat and the other with a low ability to generate heat dependent on the UCP1 expression, mitochondrial substance, and population of brown adipocytes (Giralt & Villarroya, 2013). Furthermore, cold exposure causes a decrease in the amount of glucose taken up by brown fat and a decrease in blood flow in people who are overweight or have type 2 diabetes (Carpentier *et al.*, 2018). The amount of BAT in grown-up humans is very small, although people are still discussing its importance and how it contributes to our energy usage (Carpentier *et al.*, 2018). It can be found in various parts of the body, including the neck, shoulder, armpit, back, chest, and abdomen. BAT has properties that can help with obesity and diabetes. It also has health benefits for the heart and overall wellness in people (Becher *et al.*, 2021). BTA action is contrarily related to the body mass index, and impaired BAT activity is subscribed to obesity (Wijers et al., 2010). In comparison to the single-chamber white adipocytes having big triglyceride droplets, brown adipocytes have small, multilocular lipid droplets leading to a high proportion of lipid oxidation. WAT plays a vital part in keeping up energy hemostasias assisted by endocrine communication where the vitality capacity is located; meanwhile, BAT wastes energy to deliver heat (Chen et al., 2017).

6.3 Functional food

Persistent health conditions, such as heart disease, cancer, diabetes, and obesity, are significant public health issues. These conditions are generally a consequence of consuming excessive dietary highs in fat, refined sugar, salt, and cholesterol. The increasing rates of chronic disease in the elderly community and adverse pharmaceutics effects have led to high demand for the development of nutritionally enriched foods and healthy products that promote well-being and are confirmed to be safe. The intake of foods containing functional elements such as vitamins, probiotics, minerals, fiber, and antioxidants can lower the probability of disease. Functional food can be assorted into four groups, including conventional food, modified foods, foods for particular dietary necessities, and therapeutic foods (Kamerow, 2004; Sun-Waterhouse, 2011).

Functional foods originated in Japan during the 1980s. They are classified as processed food with compounds that perform specific bodily activities. This term was introduced as part of the Japanese Ministry of Health & Welfare's initiative to enhance the health of the aging Japanese society and moderate healthcare expenses. Functional foods are commonly referred to as healthy food products; nevertheless, there is no global explanation. In Japan, foods categorized as "functional foods" are termed Foods for Specified Health Use (FOSHU). Their ability to influence the structure and function of the human body by regulating certain medical conditions has been recognized (Ohama et al., 2006).

Health Canada characterizes a "functional food" as a sort of food that is similar to routine foods and generally consumed in part of a regular diet and has proven physiological benefits beyond providing essential nutritional functions like alleviating the danger of chronic diseases, as stated on the Health Canada website (http://hc-sc.gc.ca).

The American Dietetic Association explains "functional foods" as enriched, whole, fortified, or enhanced foods that create functional benefits, well-being, and essential nutrients. Foods are described as available when, in addition to their crucial nutritional effects, they demonstrate potential beneficial effects on specific functions within the human body, eventually contributing to developed physical well-being and a reduced risk of developing chronic diseases (Hasler et al., 2004).

Scientists claim that functional food, as a regular diet, can positively influence health, which divides from prepared meals to fortified foods and beverages. Healthy ingredients like fiber, omega-3, antioxidants, and probiotics have been utilized in a wide range of food products such as oil products, pastry and dairy goods, and beverages (Hasler et al., 2004; Konstantinidi & Koutelidakis, 2019).

In 2009 according to PricewaterhouseCoopers, the functional foods market displayed annual growth rates ranging from 8.5% to 20%. The functional foods market has a bright future. In 2021 the global functional food market was valued at USD 280.7 billion and is forecast to increase by a compound annual growth rate of 8.5% between 2022 and 2030 (source https://www.grandviewresearch.com/).

Functional foods include compounds that do not usually exist in food and are not essential as macro- or micronutrients; however, they have been used due to beneficial effects. Natural bioactive compounds, such as polyphenols, dietary lipids, dietary fiber, and probiotics, can alleviate obesity and its associated complications (Kamerow, 2004).

6.3.1 Function of phytochemicals on obesity

Lately, chemical antioxidants produced by natural plants named phytochemicals attract researchers' attention because of their therapeutic feature in hindering and curing diseases such as obesity and metabolic disorders. Among the phytochemicals, polyphenols get more attention. Polyphenols are various bioactive compounds that naturally distribute in plants as secondary metabolites. These compounds are defined as molecules with aromatic rings and hydroxyl groups. Plentiful polyphenols have been detected in legumes, fruits, vegetables, and other plant origins, which are classified into phenolic acids, flavonoids, lignans, and stilbenes (Mechanisms, 2021).

Consuming dietary polyphenols has demonstrated diverse, profitable biological effects, such as antiinflammatory, particularly antioxidant activity that can potentially safeguard cells from oxidative stress by neutralizing ROS and reconstructing cell functions (Heim et al., 2002). Furthermore, polyphenols provide other characteristics like bonding metals such as Fe^{2+} and Cu^{2+} and suppressing enzymes taking part in producing ROS, such as phosphate oxidase, nicotinamide adenine dinucleotide, or xanthine oxidase. In addition, dietary polyphenols can significantly affect obesity patients by replacing electrophile responsive elements located on promoter sites with intrinsic antioxidant enzymes' gene expression, thereby increasing the activity of internal antioxidant enzymes such as superoxide dismutase, catalase, and glutathione peroxidase.(Bräunlich *et al.*, 2013).

Several in vivo and animal scientific research studies have indicated polyphenolic compounds' impact and considered them a viable method to prevent obesity. They explore the antiobesity effects of polyphenols on animal cell cultures (3T3-L1) for adipogenesis in high-fat diet-induced obese animals, which indicates that dietary polyphenols might hinder preadipocyte differentiation into adipocytes (Moghe *et al.*, 2012). They can induce apoptosis in adipocytes, reduce fat absorption in the gut, decrease glucose uptake by skeletal muscles, inhibit lipid biosynthesis, their prothermogenic properties, and stimulate catabolism in AT, liver, and other organs positioning them as potential antiobesity metabolites (Fernández-Sánchez *et al.*, 2011).

Despite this, in recent years, researchers have concentrated on and investigated the function of polyphenols in clinical trials and human experiments.

Curcumin is a lipophilic polyphenol that forms the more significant portion of Curcuma longa.

Curcumin has various medical properties, such as antiinflammation, antiangiogenesis, and antioxidation, in different parts of the body, including fatty tissue (Aggarwal, 2010). There is considerable outcome about the profitable efficiency of curcumin, which can trigger β-oxidation, inhibit fatty acid synthesis, decline fat accumulation, and moderate unlashing of pro-inflammatory mediators, for instance, IL-6, TNFα, and IL-1β. Furthermore, it restrains the Janus Kinase enzyme (JAK), which participates in developing obesity (Bradford, 2013). An investigation conducted on 84 obese patients shows the consumption of two 40 mg curcumin capsules/day for three months causes a reduction in serum inflammatory markers such as IL-6, high-sensitive C-reactive protein, and TNFα (Jazayeri-Tehrani *et al.*, 2019). Similar results were achieved in the clinical trial carried out on 60 youthful girls who were on a diet to lose mild weight; the intake of curcumin (500 mg/day) for 10 weeks led to a considerable reduction in hs-CRP and IL-6 compared to those who received a placebo supplement (Saraf-Bank *et al.*, 2019).

The maximum daily usage advised by WHO and the Food and Agriculture Organization is 1 mg/kg body weight; however, few studies report that the adverse side effects of daily consumption of curcumin, such as liver toxicity and higher doses of curcumin, can induce gastrointestinal upset, inflamed skin, and chest tightness (Zhao *et al.*, 2017).

6.3.1.1 *Dietary lipids for weight control*

There has been remarkable buyer intrigue within the health-promoting part of determined foods and specifically, active food components, particularly about utilizing fatty acids as a functional food. The alteration of dietary fat type displays a way for weight control. In many industrialized societies, dietary lipids make up more than 35% of the daily caloric intake. Therefore because of its weight management effects, it would definitely be beneficial to incorporate dietary lipid ingredients (Donahoo *et al.*, 2008; Kaur et al., 2014).

Even though we have two groups of ω-3 and ω-6 polyunsaturated fatty acids, they have different functionalities as dietary omega-3 polyunsaturated fatty acids (PUFAs). Main types for human well-being are α-linolenic acid (ALA, C18:3n-3), eicosapentaenoic acid (EPA, C20:5n-3), and docosahexaenoic acid (DHA, C22:6n-3) from the n-3 family with an 18-carbon-chain backbone and three double bonds, which can alleviate inflammation in AT. On the other hand, omega-6 PUFAs linoleic acid (LA, C18:2n-6), dihomo-γ-linolenic acid (DGLA, 20:3n-6), and arachidonic acid (AA, C20:4n-6) are in the group of omega-6 PUFAs, known for their pro-inflammatory properties, which exhibit a different impact on obesity (Di Pasquale, 2009; Pagotto *et al.*, 2006).

Fatty acid is essentially a long aliphatic chain, with a carboxyl on one end and a methyl at a different terminal. The class of fatty acids is actually classified into three main classes based on the degree of saturation, and they include the saturated fatty acids (SFA), monounsaturated fatty acids (MUFAs), and polyunsaturated fatty acid (PUFA) (Albracht-Schulte *et al.*, 2018). Saturated fatty acids (SFAs) consist of a carbon chain without any double bonds, monounsaturated fatty acids (MUFAs) contain one double bond, and polyunsaturated fatty acids (PUFAs) are characterized by carbon chains containing two or more double bonds. These structural differences across the classes can result in particular physiological impacts. For instance, SFAs have been related to the onset of metabolic dysfunction, whereas MUFAs and PUFAs show advantageous impacts on the digestion system. The primary way to title each composition is by checking from the end tail and looking for the first position of the double bond which is omega-3 (Jeromson *et al.*, 2015).

Omega-6 and omega-3 fatty acids ingested in the form of triglycerides of different food origins get digested within the small intestine with the potential of absorption and transportation with the bloodstream, following the digestion, and afterward get integrated in various tissues, inclusive those in the brain, retina, and others. During digestion, multiple things may happen to dietary fatty acids; much like the process of β-oxidation, these serve to provide energy in the form of ATP, including the conversion into cellular lipids, encompassing triglycerides, cholesterol esters, and phospholipids, through the process of esterification and other important longer chain, more unsaturated compounds through active desaturation and elongation reactions, primarily occurring in the liver but to a lesser extent in other tissues (Kaur et al., 2014).

The only source from which humans can obtain linoleic acid (LA) and alpha-linolenic acid (ALA) is dietary consumption; however, due to modern eating habits, elevated levels of linoleic acid (LA) in comparison to alpha-linolenic acid (ALA) are present in dietary intake. This trend is driven by the competition of LA and ALA with certain enzymes that support elongation and desaturation, which leads to the inhibition of the development of ALA, preferably with the metabolic substance for the Δ6 desaturase, into eicosapentaenoic acid (EPA) and docosahexaenoic acid (DHA), as well as the increased synthesis of arachidonic acid (AA) through small amounts of arachidonic acid (AA), which are paramount to functions like reproduction, and highest levels of AA are considered problematic in the initiation or development of certain chronic health matters (Calder, 2013; Haley & Freeman, 2018). The reason that it has great significance to know more and follow the process of changing ALA into EPA and DHA is that it has been addressed in the science area if ALA which can be defined as a diverse combination of fatty acids applies its health advantages only post its metabolism to the active forms eicosapentaenoic acid (EPA) and docosahexaenoic acid (DHA) as the most bioactive of the ω-3 species; however, docosapentaenoic acid (DPA, 22:5), which acts as an intermediary between EPA and DHA, might also possess beneficial health attributes, or demonstrate distinctive impacts in living organisms (Burdge, 2004). Nevertheless, while we discuss the advantageous effects of omega-3, it is crucial to acknowledge that omega-6 also exerts notable impacts on the human body, given its inability to be synthesized internally but it will undergo further metabolization through the phases of elongation and desaturation. Δ6 desaturases and Δ5 desaturases correspondingly are capable of metabolizing the ALA, although arachidonic acid (AA 22:4n-6) is converted from LA. Research indicates that adding stearidonic acid (18:3n-3) through supplementation may enhance the conversion efficiency to DHA, highlighting that Δ6 desaturase is a crucial factor limiting this process (Jeromson *et al.*, 2015; Nording *et al.*, 2013).

The overall setpoint of different appetitive or pro-nutritional behaviors and the development of pleasure involve regulation within the body, affecting processes such as lipogenesis, adipogenesis, glucose metabolism, and lipoprotein metabolism. The endocannabinoid system (ECS) plays a pivotal role in these peripheral regulatory functions (Di Marzo, 2008; Rossi *et al.*, 2018). The human body has a built-in messaging system called the endocannabinoid system (ECS). It is made up of specific receptors, CB1 and CB2, along with natural messengers (endocannabinoids) and enzymes that create and break down these messengers. It is like a natural communication network within our body (Schulz *et al.*, 2021). Both omega-3 and omega-6 fatty acids play a role in producing lipid messengers like endocannabinoids. These two components are pretty crucial in things like managing how much we eat, sensing energy levels, dealing with food-related issues, taking care of reproduction matters, handling inflammation, responding to stress, and even dealing with the big C (cancer)—among other important stuff. This intricate interaction can be compared to an endogenous management network organizing a range of physiological tasks inside the body (Pagotto *et al.*, 2006). The essential metabolic functions for n-3 and n-6 PUFAs are in the transmission of signals, which often require the PUFAs to be released from the membrane by phospholipases. Excepting this, PUFAs favor the β-oxidation process and increase membrane fluidity that plays an immense role in regulation of genes either directly or indirectly by its derived secondary messenger molecules such as the lipid mediators octadecadienoids (C18), eicosanoids (C20), and docosanoids (C22) found in the cytoplasm (Bentsen, 2017).

6.3.1.2 Gut microbiota and obesity

More than a thousand unique bacterial strains comprise the complex gut microbiota ecosystem, consisting of *Bacteroides*, *Proteus*, *Firmicutes*, *Fusobacteria*, *Actinomycetes*, and *Verrucomicrobia* (Structure, function and diversity of the healthy human microbiome, 2012). A combination of items such as dietary factors, sex, and genetics impacts the diversity and structure of the host microbiome, and diet is recognized as the most influential factor among them. Healthy gut microbiota participates in human well-being by generating numerous active substances like short-chain fatty acid vitamins and maintaining body and energy (Lloyd-Price et al., 2016).

To sustain metabolic hemostasis, the microbiome responds to physiological signals like food intake, energy demand, and stress, among many others. Modern researchers consider the gut microbiome because of its effects on human health regulation. Gut microbiome has the potential to ferment the indigestible carbohydrates like dietary fibers and produce short-chain fatty acids (Canfora *et al.*, 2019). The significant number of microbial cells in our gut is a crucial metabolic center that boosts physiological balance and homeostasis as well as supports immune function through a symbiotic association with the host. The human microbiome affects the digestive system and acts as a moderator to connect the gut, enteric nervous system (ENS), and the brain. The disturbance of the gut microbiome correlates with various metabolic, gastrointestinal, and cognitive pathologies, enhancing appetite and resulting in obesity (Canfora *et al.*, 2019).

Gut microbiota can affect adiposity by modulating fat storage, energy absorption, chronic inflammation, and central appetite.

Many microbial researchers demonstrate the obese microbiome and identify the particular strain that participates in improving obesity. Based on some research, lean phenotypes are related to an increasing ratio of Bacteroidetes: Firmicutes; however, this ratio is altered in obese mice. The gut microbiota of obese mice indicates a decline in the Bacteroidetes community and an increase in Firmicutes (Indiani *et al.*, 2018). A study on Ukrainian people demonstrates that the ratio of Firmicutes/Bacteroidetes grows with increasing BMI (Koliada *et al.*, 2017). Nevertheless, some researchers are against these results. Based on the US Public Gastrointestinal Programme database, an investigation was conducted to examine gut microbiotas of 1655 normal and 898 overweight subjects. They figured out that the ratio of Firmicutes/Bacteroidetes is comparatively low in obese adults (Wei & Wen-wei, 2020).

On the other hand, some studies related fatness with particular bacteria, such as the family Christensenellaceae, consisting of the genera Bifidobacteria, *Methanobacteriales*, *Lactobacillus*, and *Akkermansia* (Waters & Ley, 2019).

Early research determines the impact of a new class of bacteria. The family Christensenellaceae was figured out to be related to weight loss and hurt the BMI host (Waters & Ley, 2019). Based on investigations, *Akkermansia muciniphila* is found to be crucial bacteria which positively correlated with weight loss. Intake supplements, including *A. muciniphila*, can progress metabolic factors such as insulin sensitivity and reduce body weight, fat mass, and hip circumference in obese patients (Depommier *et al.*, 2019). Similarly, *Bifidobacterium* and *Lactobacillus* are conventional probiotics that participate in making human intestinal microecology balanced. Among them, *Limosilactobacillus reuteri* and *Lactobacillus gasseri* are considerably related to obesity (Crovesy *et al.*, 2017). Some studies show Bifidobacterium resistance through animal trials. Based on results from animal models with diet-induced obesity, the intake of Bifidobacterium demonstrates varied effects reliant on bacterial strain. This evidence infers that the microorganisms connected with obesity are specific to particular species even though bacteria with the same genes can show opposition effects, which can be associated with the convoluted metabolic mechanism of obesity (Yin *et al.*, 2010). As mentioned, the abundance of Firmicutes/Bacteroidetes is determined to be a characteristic of obesity. This rise of Firmicutes in obesity is intimately related to markers for brown adipocytes in subcutaneous AT; nevertheless, this correlation is not observed in visceral fatty tissue (Moreno-Navarrete *et al.*, 2018). Probiotics positively correlate with visceral obesity. The rising Akkermansia community in mice with a high-fat/high-sugar diet causes a reduction in body weight and visceral obesity (Anhê *et al.*, 2015).

The combination of probiotics, including *Lactobacillus paracasei*, *Pediococcus pentosaceus*, *Lactobacillus acidophilus*, *Lacticaseibacillus rhamnosus*, *Bifidobacterium lactis*, and *Bifidobacterium breve*, considerably decreased BMI and intrahepatic fat fraction in nonalcoholic fatty liver patients following a 12-week administration (Ahn *et al.*, 2018). Tavella et al. indicate that declining visceral AT in the gut microbiota of older people is related to the significant numbers of Porphyromonadaceae, Rikenellaceae, and Christensenellaceae (Tavella *et al.*, 2021). Moreover, bacterial diversity is an essential factor in host health and is related to obesity. Many investigations indicate the correlation between gut microbiota diversity and adiposity, which is the wealthiest gut microbiota relevance with decreased obesity in patients (Denou *et al.*, 2016). Rigorous statistical analysis shows a notable relation between bacterial diversity and "microbiota-related diseases" in only about one-third of the cases, and bacterial diversity seems closely related to the occurrence and evolution of diseases. Obesity may be related to dysbiosis in the bacteria ecosystem (Ma et al., 2019).

6.4 Obesity mechanisms induced by the gut microbiota

Some investigations indicate that obese mice utilize more proteins and carbohydrates genetically through the gut microbiota to supply energy. Previous studies found that animal trials on mice without differences in weight or diet show an increase of total body fat in germ-free mice colonized by the "obese microbiota" compared to the mice colonized by lean microbiota. This proposes that the gut microbiota of obesity has the potential to enhance the absorption of energy from food, which is a consequence of accumulating excessive energy and raising weight gain (Turnbaugh *et al.*, 2006).

Digesting nondigestible carbohydrates is one of the core functions of gut microbiota that converts them to short-chain fatty acid (SCFA). SCFA, including propionate, acetate, and butyrate, is an essential factor for moderating dominant energy homeostasis (Cani *et al.*, 2019). Acetate generates profitable substances such as peptide YY, glucagon-like peptide-1, and other intestinal hormones, which can decrease lipolysis and proinflammatory cytokine as well as grow energy expenditure and lipid oxidation. Propionate facilitates mice's intestinal lipolysis and energy homeostasis via the AMPK/LSD1 pathway (Wang *et al.*, 2019). Butyrate is the primary energy fountain for the colon, and intestinal epithelial cells receive a large proportion of it through butyrate oxidation. The enhancement of butyrate-producing bacteria in the gut microbiota raises the production of butyrate, thereby promoting lipid metabolism through the butyrate-SESN2/CRTC2 pathway; in contrast, a high abundance of butyrate can alter the metabolite effects (Miyamoto, 2006). Based on recent research, a significant number of fecal SCFAs have an adverse efficacy on gut permeability, obesity, and metabolic disorder markers. It seems that SCFA has dual effects, whereas they can safeguard the host from obesity. On the other hand, immoderate SCFA supplies more energy for the host, subsequently improving obesity (Teixeira *et al.*, 2013).

6.4.1 Central appetite

The function of gut microbiota goes beyond gastrointestinal; it uses different procedures like endocrine, immune, and neural pathways to connect the brain and gut (Cryan *et al.*, 2019). The gut microbiota can affect food consumption by moderating brain function in different ways, like participating in generating serotonin, which has an essential pattern in modulating gastrointestinal ability. Moreover, the lactate generated by Lactobacillus and Bifidobacterium is important in lengthening satisfaction after a meal (Silberbauer *et al.*, 2000).

The gut microbiota balances and develops gut hormones such as GLP-1, pancreatic polypeptide, and peptide YY from enteroendocrine cells. These hormones have various effects; for instance, peptide YY and pancreatic polypeptide cause anorexia; similarly, GLP-1 reduces food consumption, diminishes glucan levels, and slows gastric emptying (Salehi & Purnell, 2019). Also, some research studies indicate that the levels of peptide YY and GLP-1 are notable plunges in overweight patients. Studies found that gut microbiota and their by-products intensify the feelings of fullness in the digestive system (Federico *et al.*, 2016).

6.4.2 Fat storage

Based on the research done, they figured out the relevance between gut microbiota and fat storage. Fredrik Backed et al. relieve the result of their investigation, and the integration of adult germ-free mice with ordinary microbiota gathered from the distal intestine resulted in an escalation in body fat to 60% and insulin resistance in 14 days. The gut microbiota is involved in processing carbohydrates and raising glucose absorption in the intestines, enhancing glucose content, and increasing two expression transcriptions, ChREBP and SREBP-1, which play a role in fat synthesis in the liver. Intestinal epithelial cells secrete fasting-induced adipocyte factor (Fiaf), suppressing lipoprotein lipase and enhancing energy accumulation. LPL promotes the transfer of triglycerides to the stream, eventually absorbed by fat cells (Bäckhed *et al.*, 2004). Huizhen Li et al. published antiobesity effects of a mixture of lactobacilli (*Lactobacillus plantarum* KLDS1.0386 and *L. plantarum* KLDS1.0344) through the in vivo trial; they decreased body weight gain and body fat rate. The mixture of lactobacilli was investigated on C57BL/6 J mice for eight weeks. The research outcome shows results in the development of blood lipid levels, liver function, and ease of liver oxidative stress. Besides that, they suppress lipid storage in the liver and moderate lipid metabolism in AT (Li *et al.*, 2020). Zhijing Liu et al. elevate the effect of *L. paracasei* 24 (LP24) on HFD-induced obese mice. The consequence exhibits that the consumption of LP24 decreases the body weight in HDF mice and develops blood lipid levels, reducing inflammatory response to liver oxidative stress. And, it moderates the fat metabolism. More LP24 modulates the diversity of gut microbiota, declines the ratio of Firmicutes/Bacteroidetes, and raises plenty of *Akkermansia references.*

Furthermore, Aronsson et al. indicate *that L. paracasei* can diminish lipid storage in obese mice by moderating and expressing Angiopoietin-like protein 4 (ANGPTL4) as a main role that participates in fat storage (Aronsson *et al.*, 2010).

6.4.3 Inflammation

Low-grade inflammation indicates metabolic diseases such as obesity and type 2 diabetes. This metabolic disorder results from the conversion of microbiota composition and metabolites. As a result of relocating from the gut, it affects other parts of the body, such as the liver and fatty tissue, which participate in metabolic inflammation (Tilg *et al.*, 2020). Bacterial lipopolysaccharide is a factor that triggers inflammation. Based on studies, a diet rich in fat causes alternation in gut microbiota and an increase in adiposity and inflammation. These changes following the elevation of gram-negative bacterial product, LPS (lipopolysaccharide), and the subcutaneous injection of LPS for four weeks in mice caused increased markers of inflammation, liver triglyceride, and AT weight compared with HFD mice (Cani *et al.*, 2007).

Linking LPS to their receptors CD14 TLR4 on immune cells can set off the transcription factors, NF-κB, AP-1, and interferon regulatory factors, which initiate a proinflammatory cascade within the gut (Janssen & Kersten, 2017). Based on the studies conducted by Robert Caesar on mice administrated with lard and fish oil, the mice provided with lard reduced insulin sensitivity and increased white adipose tissue inflammation through the activation of Toll-like receptor (TLR), as well as the escalation of the TLR4 bond LPS was observed in mice fed lard (Caesar *et al.*, 2015). HFD proliferates both the plasma and fecal endotoxin due to increasing the *Firmicutes to Bacteroidetes* ratio, infusing growth of Enterobacteriaceae, and generating endotoxin.

Chao Kang et al. assess the effect of administrating supplements containing Capsaicin (CAP) on HFD mice. The result exhibits that capsaicin causes an amplify in butyrate-producing Ruminococcaceae and Lachnospiraceae while reducing the community of the (LPS)-producing family S24_7 through decreasing chronic low-grade information and restrain of cannabinoid receptor type 1 collaborating in avoiding HFD-induced gut barrier dysfunction. The endocannabinoid system is a central modulator of fat formation in the gut and fat cells, and its activation can enhance the desire to eat. Treatment with (CB1) antagonist reduces gut permeability and body weight (Kang *et al.*, 2017).

6.5 The role of pre and probiotics on obesity and metabolic syndrome

Pre and probiotics have been known for their health benefits and positive effects on gastrointestinal health from the past to the present. Probiotics are live bacterial cells delivered to the host through fermented food products or capsules. At the same time, prebiotics are components that are fermented by gut microbes and increase their growth. FAO/WHO characterizes probiotics as a live microorganism that provides health benefits to the host when intake is sufficient. Lately, they have identified profound effects in moderating the host metabolic process of weight gain and obesity. Also mixing with prebiotic fibers can enhance the growth and their activities. This combinatorial approach, called synbiotics, may have a useful impact on enhancing the beneficial effects of probiotics further. It is crucial to recognize that not all probiotics are alike, and their effects on the host vary greatly depending on the specific strain and dosage (Sanders & Marco, 2010).

Clinical trial on the use of probiotics to treat obesity:

Lactobacillus and Bifidobacterium are the most studied probiotic strains in humans and animals. In further research conducted on various strains, 85% of probiotic supplements led to decreased body weight or fat mass compared to placebo-treated control (Ejtahed *et al.*, 2019).

Some particular strains of Lactobacillus and Bifidobacterium such as *L. rhamnosus*, *L. plantarum*, *L. gasseri*, *L. casei*, B. infantis, and B. longum, have constant antiobesogenic properties through human and animals studies (Ejtahed *et al.*, 2019).

Animal investigation demonstrates that probiotic treatment positively affects prevention and obesity treatment. Lee et al. show that administering the conjugated linoleic acid (CLA) produced by *L. rhamnosus* for 8 weeks significantly decreased body weight and white AT without changing energy consumption. In addition, administering the

Lactobacillus curvatus HY7601 and *L. plantarum* KY1032 to mice indicates diminished body weight, leptin, fat storage, liver toxicity biomarkers, and total cholesterol (Lee *et al.*, 2006).

Ultimately, hamsters administered with microencapsulated Lactobacillus fermentum ATCC 11976, which produces feruloyl esterase, led to enhanced lipid profiles by reducing the amount of hepatic free cholesterol, phospholipids, triglycerides, and esterified cholesterol phospholipids. Moreover, treated animals experienced decreased serum levels of total cholesterol, uric acid, triglycerides, and insulin resistance (Bhathena *et al.*, 2013).

Additionally, clinical trials in humans demonstrate the beneficial effects of probiotic supplements on body weight and metabolic markers. The research was conducted on children supplemented with mixed probiotics, including Streptococcus thermophilus DSM24731, *L. paracasei* DSM24733, and L. delbrueckii subsp. Bulgaricus DSM24724, *L. acidophilus* DSM24735, *L. plantarum* DSM24730, B. longum DSM24736, *B. breve* DSM24732, and B. infantis DSM24737 for 4 months, reducing BMI raising the GLP-1 compared to control (Alisi *et al.*, 2014). Furthermore, the clinical trial of intaking fermented milk consisting of *L. gasseri* SBT2055 for 12 weeks makes a critical deduction of visceral fat, subcutaneous fat, and body weight compared to the control experience (Kadooka *et al.*, 2013).

In similar research, intake of synbiotics containing Lactobacillus casei, *L. acidophilus*, and Bifidobacterium bifidum plus inulin notably plunge the plasma triglycerides, body weight, and total cholesterol in a group of overweight and obese adult subjects (Hadi *et al.*, 2019).

Furthermore, 10 weeks of consumption of nutritious yogurt enriched with *B. lactis* Bb-12 and inulin by obese subjects led to a reduction of triglyceride level, waist circumference, and body fat percentage in comparison to those who consumed plain yogurt (Mohammadi-Sartang *et al.*, 2018).

6.6 Dietary fiber and its effect on obesity

Raising the intake of natural products and dietary fiber as suggested by the World Health Organization may be a way of changing lifestyle that can help reduce the risk of communicable diseases (NCDs), and it is because of intricate physiological processes associated with obesity. Dietary fiber (DF) is a term applied to intricate constituents of apparent chemical, physical, and other properties; both natural and modified products show substantial variance in physical and chemical properties, which are not hydrolyzed by human digestive enzymes in the small intestine and potentially have physiological effects. Furthermore, their beneficial impacts on health are distinguished based on their characteristics, for example, solubility, fermentability, water absorption, binding ability, viscosity, and bulking ability (Müller et al., 2018; Poutanen *et al.*, 2018). Enhancing glycemic index, reducing lipid levels, and showing prebiotic effects are some of the principal roles that it plays which have a crucial role in lowering the risk of weight gain. Moreover, it can ameliorate individual energy balance by modifying food structure and digestive processes as well as appetitive cues in humans (Khan *et al.*, 2018).

β-Glucan, psyllium, pectin, guar gum, arabinoxylans, and inulin are strongly associated with few benefits toward human organisms, such as cholesterol diminishment, gastric emptying decrease, small intestine transit time decrease, prebiotic effect, and fecal bulk impact that are examples of soluble dietary fibers (SDF); however, insoluble dietary fibers (iIDF) such as cellulose, hemicellulose, chitosan, and lignin are examples that have positive effect due to their properties such as water insolubility, low fermentability, and stool bulk forming (Surampudi *et al.*, 2016).

This therapeutic approach is gaining popularity as it manipulates the gut microbiomes which are mainly influenced by diet for preventing obesity (Baboota *et al.*, 2013).

Because the gut microbiota is known as a center stage in human well-being, prebiotic fibers are the wise choice for consumers as they are considered for their functional properties that cause an increase of intestinal microbes via fermentation into short fatty acids that could increase satiety (Hill *et al.*, 2014). Although prebiotic fibers support the growth of Bifidobacterium and Lactobacillus, they provide bactericidal activity for *Clostridium perfringens* and *Escherichia coli* whose growth is decreased by an acidic medium regulated by these components (Kaur & Gupta, 2002). Compared to digestible polysaccharides, the indigestibility of fiber leads to longer transit times in the intestinal lumen and a greater feeling of satiety. One of its other functions is to prolong the time between meals by evoking and enhancing chewing when satiety through presumed cephalic and peripheral effects. As a result of the fermentation of dietary fibers by gut bacteria in the large intestine, the initiation of glucose-dependent insulinotropic peptide (GIP) is presently being linked with gastrointestinal satiety peptide hormones such as glucagon-like peptide (GLP-1) and peptide YY (PYY) or dietary fiber (Lim & Poppitt, 2019). Fermented products from dietary fiber, which are known as short-chain fatty acids (SCFAs), are another feasible mechanism to help in body weight control. Proximal small intestinal digestion and nutrient absorption occur in the human stomach. These complex glycans can be degraded by saccharolytic microorganisms, which can then supply the host with a variety of metabolites. These include SCFAs, which are essential for controlling food and energy intake and are also a fantastic source of energy (Morrison & Preston, 2016). SCFs

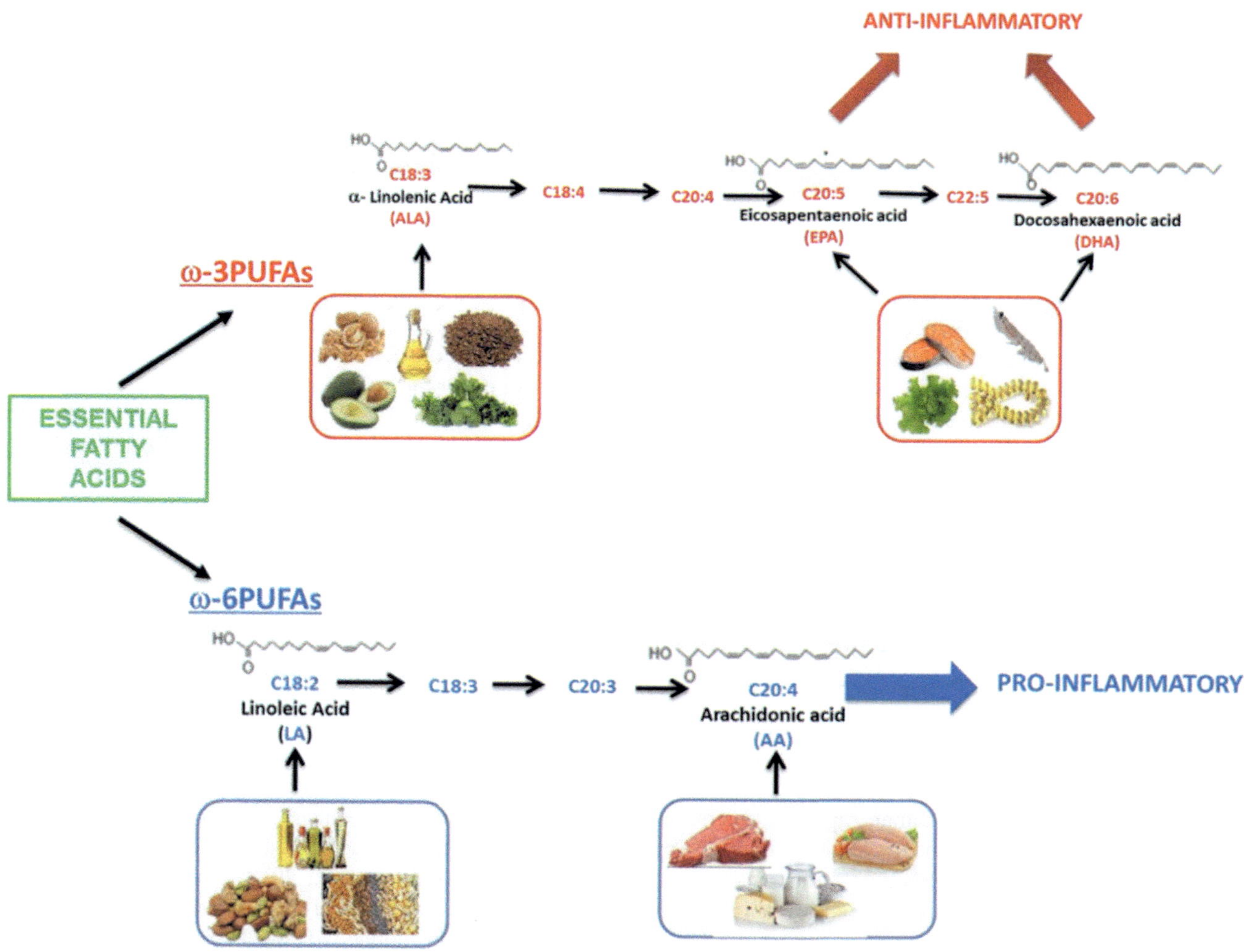

FIGURE 6.1 Essential fatty acids and dietry fiber sources. *AA*, arachidonic acid; *ALA*, α-linolenic acid; *DHA*, docosahexaenoic acid; *EPA*, eicosapentaenoic acid; *LA*, linoleic acid; *PUFA*, polyunsaturated fatty acid.

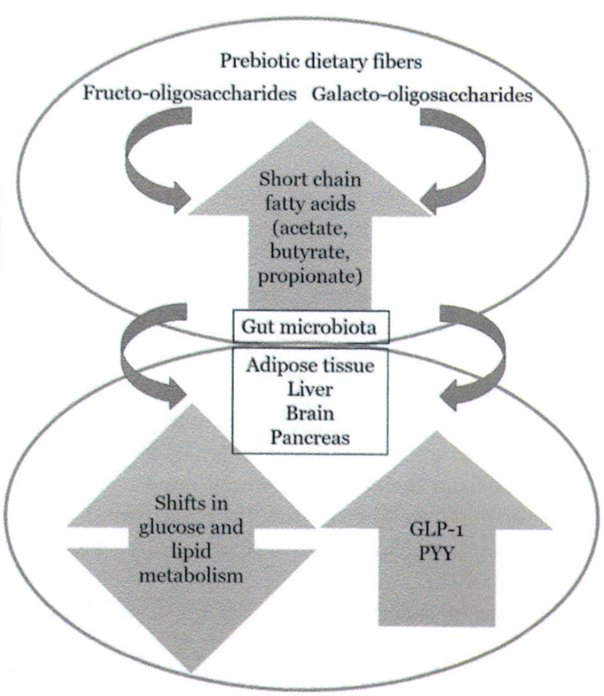

FIGURE 6.2 Effect of Dietry Fibers and Fermentation on the glucose and lipid metabolism.

TABLE 6.1 Effect of different polyphenols on weight management.

Polyphenol	Participant	Dosage and intervention period	Result	Reference
Curcumin	Randomized placebo-controlled double-blind 152 overweight/obese adults randomized placebo-controlled double-blind 118 patients with type 2 diabetes Randomized placebo-controlled double-blind 59 patients with metabolic syndrome randomized, double-blind, placebo crossover trial randomized, double-blind, placebo-controlled trial 84 overweight/obese patients with NAFLD	Received 160 mg curcumin/day alone or with fish oil (2000 mg docosahexaenoic acid + 400 mg eicosapentaenoic acid per day) for 16 weeks Received 1000 mg curcumin with 1000 mg piperine for 12 weeks Administrate 1000 mg/day of curcumin for eight weeks Receive 1000 mg curcumin /day for four weeks Receive 40 mg Nano-curcumin capsules per day for three months.	Consume fish oils regularly, but not curcumin affects cardiovascular biomarkers and cerebrovascular function Decrease serum levels of leptin TNF-α and leptin: adiponectin ratio while increasing serum adiponectin levels Decrease TNF-a, IL-6, TGF-b and MCP-1 levels Decrease IL-1β, IL-4, VEGF Decrease QUICKI↑, HDL↑, LDL-C↓, WC↓, ALT↓, AST↓, TC↓, HbA1c↓, TG↓, FBG↓, TNF-α↓, HOMA-IR↓, IL-6↓, hs-CRP↓, and NAFLD severity↓	Diet (2017), Ganjali *et al.* (2014), Jazayeri-Tehrani *et al.* (2019), Kuszewski *et al.* (2020), Panahi *et al.* (2016)
Quercetin	Randomized, double-blind, placebo-controlled trial 102 overweight and obese Korean patients	Receive onion peel extract including 100 mg quercetin for 12 weeks.	↓ Body fat and weight ↓ Blood glucose ↓ Leptin ↑Resting energy expenditure and respiratory quotient	Lee *et al.* (2016)
Resveratrol	Randomized, double-blind, placebo-controlled trial 25 overweight and obese humans randomized, double-blind, placebo-controlled trial 25 obese adults with metabolic syndrome randomized, double-blind, placebo-controlled trial 41 overweight/obese adult	Receive a combination of 80 mg epigallocatechin-gallate/day And 282 mg resveratrol for 12 weeks Combination of exercise program, 250 mg resveratrol with a diet for three months Receive 150 mg resveratrol daily for six months	↓Apoptosis ↓Pathways contributing to adipogenesis ↓Oxidative stress ↓Expression of pathways related to energy metabolism ↑HDL ↓ Total cholesterol, albumin, urea, creatinine, and VLDL No effect on insulin sensitivity ↓HbA1c	Batista-Jorge *et al.* (2020), De Ligt *et al.* (2020), Most *et al.* (2018)

(*Continued*)

TABLE 6.1 (Continued)

Polyphenol	Participant	Dosage and intervention period	Result	Reference
Epigallocatechin	Randomized, double-blind, placebo-controlled trial 115 women with central obesity single-blind, placebo-controlled parallel, clinical trial 84 obese patients randomized, double-blind, placebo-controlled trial 60 healthy Japanese males and females	Received green tea extract with 856.8 mg EGCG/day for 12 weeks Receive a cup of green tea daily for 8 and 12 weeks Combination of 178 mg α-glucosyl hesperidin and 146 mg EGCG for 12 weeks	↓BMI ↓Waist circumference ↓Total cholesterol and LDL ↑Adiponectin ↓BMI ↓BW ↓Waist circumference Prevent weight gain ↓BMI ↓LDL/HDL ratio ↓ Body fat percentage ↓ TG	Chen *et al.* (2015), Nabi *et al.* (2018), Yoshitomi *et al.* (2021)

TABLE 6.2 Impact of different prebiotics on weight management.

Study	Prebiotic-dose-duration	Source of prebiotic	Subject	Impacts
Hiel *et al.* (2020)	Native inulin-16 g/d-3 months maltodextrin-16 g/d- 3 months	Chicory root, Cosucra, Belgium Cargill, Belgium	A randomized, single-blinded, multicentric, placebo-controlled trial- 150 obese patients	Prebiotics and placebo reduced energy intake and influenced external food intake, making it lower and restrained food intake higher
Ghavami *et al.* (2019)	High performance inulin- 10 g/day- 8 weeks-	Sensus, Borchwef 3, 4704 RG Roosendaal the Netherlands	A randomized, double-blind, placebo-controlled trial -46 patients with type 2 diabetes	Significant decreases in WC, HC, BMI and energy intake in the high satiety inulin group. Additionally, overall satiety levels were remarkably high in the same group.
Chambers *et al.* (2019)	Inulin and inulin-propionate ester (IPE)-20 g/d- 42 days		A randomized, double-blind, placebo-controlled, parallel design- 18 adults	In the inulin-control group an increase in IHCL was observed and not in the IPE group and mice, diet-induced body weight loss was shown which greatly reduced the insulin level rates of hepatic DNL
Alptekin et al. (2022)	Beta-glucan and inulin- 6 g/day- 5 weeks		Three-group, parallel, single-blinded randomized controlled intervention study of -24 females	Participants in the inulin group saw the highest reduction in body fat percentage, while the beta-glucan group showed improvements in weight and waist circumference
Kao *et al.* (2018)	Fructooligosaccharide and Resistant maltodextrin- 0.97 and 1.94 g/kg body weight- 8 weeks		Eight weight classes of four each-32 Sprague–Dawley male rats (6 weeks old)	Reducing total body fat, feed intake and C. perfringens counts and increasing total bifidobacteria counts and total short-chain fatty acids in stool
Mistry *et al.* (2020)	GOS -with or without β-GOS (7% w/w)-15 weeks		Two groups of ad libitum with control and GOS-supplemented diets- Male C57BL/6OlaHsd mice (9 weeks of age)	The Beta-GOS diet reduces weight gain, fat absorption, insulin resistance and improves the lipid profile.
Hul (2020)	FOS or SCF- 8 weeks		Different groups: control diet, high-fat diet, a high-fat diet supplemented with FOS, and a high-fat diet supplemented with soluble corn fiber- Nine-week-old male C57BL/6 J mice	Both prebiotic fibers had similar effects on body weight and inflammation, and SCF affected energy excretion while FOS did not
Merino-Aguilar *et al.* (2014)	FOS Fraction (FOS)-12 weeks	Psacalium decompositum "Matarique" (medical plant)	Two groups and the second group divided into 3 groups- 24 male Wistar rats (12 weeks)	Significant reductions in weight, cholesterol, triglycerides, and inflammatory markers in rats fed by FOS fraction
Li et al. (2019)	TF and FOS- 250 mg/kg body weight -8 weeks		Five experimental groups of male Kunming mice (weighing 18–22 g)	FOS and TF reduce the influence of HS on cholesterol levels; Their combination also has a positive effect on HDL and LDL.

DNL, De novo lipogenesis; *FOS*, fructooligosaccharides; *GOS*, galactooligosaccharides; *IHCL*, intrahepatocellular lipid; *SCF*, soluble corn fiber; *TF*, Tea flavonoids.

and their receptors have been found to play a key role in mediating the interactions between diet, gut microbiota, and host physiology. These interactions occur through the control of endocrine responses, leukocyte development, enzyme function and activity, and transcription factors. Two GPRs specific or SCFAs are commonly expressed on intestinal enteroendocrine cells, adipocytes, and immune cells. These are FFAR2/GPR43 and the free fatty acid receptor (FFAR) 3/G protein-coupled receptor (GPR) 41. The stimulation of the secretion of the intestinal hormone PYY, which is part of a signaling cascade that produces a feeling of satiety and, as a result, a reduced food intake, is directly influenced by GPR41 activation on enteroendocrine cells. Nevertheless, GPR43 signaling has been suggested to contribute to host insulin sensitivity through stimulated GLP-1 release (Samuel *et al.*, 2008; Tolhurst *et al.*, 2012). Another possible technique of antiobesity property in probiotics is the combined effect with the probiotic bacteria, which leads to an alteration in the activity of the center of appetite, activation of thermogenesis in brown fat, and intensification of lipolysis in white AT and CLA (trans-10, cis-12 conjugated linoleic acid) production during fermentation (Lee *et al.*, 1996). In regard to texture-enhancing features, the integration of dietary fibers into commercial food products as fat and sugar replacers without devaluation of their taste and texture and its unique property directly comes from their gelling properties which give rise to bulk and viscosity (Guimarães *et al.*, 2020).

6.7 Conclusion

Obesity is indeed a global health concern that can lessen the quality of life due to the participation in preventing diseases such as cardiovascular diseases, type 2 diabetes, and some cancers. Functional foods can influence preventing and treating obesity by influencing gut microbiota, energy intake through modulating appetite and satiety, and energy expenditure by modulating thermogenesis and adipogenesis. Dietary lipids account for a significant portion of daily caloric intake in many societies in which the consumption of dietary lipid compounds with antiobesity properties can affect weight management such as conjugated linoleic acid, omega-6 and omega-3 fatty acid, as well as fiber, polyphenols, and probiotics. Moreover, polyphenols like curcumin, quercetin, and resveratrol can decrease inflammation biomarkers, weight, and body fat, hemoglobin-A1c, and improve lipid profile.

6.8 Future perspective

As far as the prediction of the food system is concerned, it is vital to look in a joined manner at today's structure of the alimentary process in which environment, people, and well-being-related boundaries and infrastructure must be taken into account (Godfray *et al.*, 2010). The history of functional food products and the physiological changes that may happen upon their consumption are simultaneously must studied. Moreover, studying the intricate system is an alternative to bioactive compounds which helps in better understanding in future investigations. Furthermore, bioaccessibility is the main indicator most often; however, it has limited data. Meanwhile, recognizing its method and the desired concentration of it during digestion and targeted organs would be more effectual and helpful in the field of food design. Despite the oral coconsumption of (de Vries *et al.*, 2018) food and drugs by sick people, not enough information is revealed about the interaction between them. The opposite relation of drugs and food with the potential of bioactive components available could guide in regard to the alteration of drug dosage. Another possible way to have proper food production in the following years is waste usage as it is known as an advantageous way that has the dual purpose of reducing trash as well as producing functional products (Alongi & Anese, 2021) (Figs. 6.1 and 6.2, Tables 6.1 and 6.2).

References

Aggarwal, B. B. (2010). Targeting lammation-induced obesity and metabolic diseases by curcumin and other nutraceuticals. *Annual Review of Nutrition, 30*, 173–199. Available from https://doi.org/10.1146/annurev.nutr.012809.104755.

Ahn, S. B., Jun, D. W., Kang, B., Lim, J. H., Lim, S. (2018., Placebo-controlled Study of a Multispecies Probiotic Mixture in Nonalcoholic Fatty Liver Disease. 1–9, Available from https://doi.org/10.1038/s41598-019-42059-32018.

Albracht-Schulte, K., Kalupahana, N. S., Ramalingam, L., Wang, S., Rahman, S. M., Robert-McComb, J., & Moustaid-Moussa, N. (2018). Omega-3 fatty acids in obesity and metabolic syndrome: A mechanistic update. *Journal of Nutritional Biochemistry, 58*, 1–16. Available from https://doi.org/10.1016/j.jnutbio.2018.02.012, www.elsevier.com/locate/jnutbio.

Alisi, A., Bedogni, G., Baviera, G., Giorgio, V., Porro, E., Paris, C., Giammaria, P., Reali, L., Anania, F., & Nobili, V. (2014). Randomised clinical trial: the beneficial effects of VSL #3 in obese children with non-alcoholic steatohepatitis. *Alimentary Pharmacology & Therapeutics, 39*(11), 1276–1285. Available from https://doi.org/10.1111/apt.12758.

Alongi, M., & Anese, M. (2021). Re-thinking functional food development through a holistic approach. *Journal of Functional Foods, 81*104466. Available from https://doi.org/10.1016/j.jff.2021.104466.

Alptekin, İ. M., Çakiroğlu, F. P., & Örmeci, N. (2022). Effects of β-glucan and inulin consumption on postprandial appetite, energy intake and food consumption in healthy females: A randomized controlled trial. *Nutrition and Health*, *28*(3), 433–442. Available from https://doi.org/10.1177/02601060211023256, https://journals.sagepub.com/home/NAH.

Anhê, F. F., Roy, D., Pilon, G., Dudonné, S., Matamoros, S., Varin, T. V., Garofalo, C., Moine, Q., Desjardins, Y., Levy, E., & Marette, A. (2015). A polyphenol-rich cranberry extract protects from diet-induced obesity, insulin resistance and intestinal inflammation in association with increased *Akkermansia* spp. population in the gut microbiota of mice. *Gut*, *64*(6), 872–883. Available from https://doi.org/10.1136/gutjnl-2014-307142, http://gut.bmj.com/content/64/6/872.full.pdf + html.

Aronsson, L., Huang, Y., Parini, P., Korach-André, M., Håkansson, J., Gustafsson, J. A., Pettersson, S., Arulampalam, V., & Rafter, J. (2010). Decreased fat storage by Lactobacillus paracasei is associated with increased levels of angiopoietin-like 4 protein (ANGPTL4). *PLoS One*, *5*(9), 1–7. Available from https://doi.org/10.1371/journal.pone.0013087Sweden, http://www.plosone.org/article/fetchObjectAttachment.action?uri = info%3Adoi%2F10.1371%2Fjournal.pone.0013087&representation = PDF.

Baboota, R. K., Bishnoi, M., Ambalam, P., Kondepudi, K. K., Sarma, S. M., Boparai, R. K., & Podili, K. (2013). Functional food ingredients for the management of obesity and associated co-morbidities - A review. *Journal of Functional Foods*, *5*(3), 997–1012. Available from https://doi.org/10.1016/j.jff.2013.04.014.

Bäckhed, F., Ding, H., Wang, T., Hooper, L. V., G, Y. K., Nagy, A., Semenkovich, C. F., & Gordon, J. I. (2004). The gut microbiota as an environmental factor that regulates fat storage. *Proceedings of the National Academy of Sciences of the United States of America*, *101*(44), 15718–15723. Available from https://doi.org/10.1073/pnas.0407076101.

Batista-Jorge, G. C., Barcala-Jorge, A. S., Silveira, M. F., Lelis, D. F., Andrade, J. M. O., de Paula, A. M. B., Guimarães, A. L. S., & Santos, S. H. S. (2020). Oral resveratrol supplementation improves Metabolic Syndrome features in obese patients submitted to a lifestyle-changing program. *Life Sciences*, *256*117962. Available from https://doi.org/10.1016/j.lfs.2020.117962.

Becher, T., Palanisamy, S., Kramer, D. J., Eljalby, M., Marx, S. J., Wibmer, A. G., Butler, S. D., Jiang, C. S., Vaughan, R., Schöder, H., Mark, A., & Cohen, P. (2021). Brown adipose tissue is associated with cardiometabolic health. *Nature Medicine*, *27*(1), 58–65. Available from https://doi.org/10.1038/s41591-020-1126-7.

Bentsen, H. (2017). Dietary polyunsaturated fatty acids, brain function and mental health. *Microbial Ecology in Health and Disease*, *28*(sup1), 1281916. Available from https://doi.org/10.1080/16512235.2017.1281916.

Bhathena, J., Martoni, C., Kulamarva, A., Tomaro-Duchesneau, C., Malhotra, M., Paul, A., Urbanska, A. M., & Prakash, S. (2013). Oral probiotic microcapsule formulation ameliorates non-alcoholic fatty liver disease in bio F1B golden syrian hamsters. *PLoS One*, *8*(3). Available from https://doi.org/10.1371/journal.pone.0058394Canada, http://www.plosone.org/article/fetchObjectAttachment.action?uri = info%3Adoi%2F10.1371%2Fjournal.pone.0058394&representation = PDF.

Blüher, M. (2016). Adipose tissue inflammation: A cause or consequence of obesity-related insulin resistance? *Clinical Science*, *130*(18), 1603–1614. Available from https://doi.org/10.1042/CS20160005, http://www.clinsci.org/content/ppclinsci/130/18/1603.full.pdf.

Bradford, P. G. (2013). Curcumin and obesity. *Biofactors (Oxford, England)*, *39*(1), 78–87. Available from https://doi.org/10.1002/biof.1074.

Bräunlich, M., Slimestad, R., Wangensteen, H., Brede, C., Malterud, K., & Barsett, H. (2013). Extracts, anthocyanins and procyanidins from aronia melanocarpa as radical scavengers and enzyme inhibitors. *Nutrients*, *5*(3), 663–678. Available from https://doi.org/10.3390/nu5030663.

Burdge, G. (2004). α-Linolenic acid metabolism in men and women: Nutritional and biological implications. *Current Opinion in Clinical Nutrition and Metabolic Care*, *7*(2), 137–144. Available from https://doi.org/10.1097/00075197-200403000-00006.

Caesar, R., Tremaroli, V., Kovatcheva-Datchary, P., Cani, P. D., & Bäckhed, F. (2015). Crosstalk between gut microbiota and dietary lipids aggravates WAT inflammation through TLR signaling. *Cell Metabolism*, *22*(4), 658–668. Available from https://doi.org/10.1016/j.cmet.2015.07.026, http://www.cellmetabolism.org/.

Calder, P. C. (2013). Omega-3 polyunsaturated fatty acids and inflammatory processes: Nutrition or pharmacology? *British Journal of Clinical Pharmacology*, *75*(3), 645–662. Available from https://doi.org/10.1111/j.1365-2125.2012.04374.x.

Canfora, E. E., Meex, R. C. R., Venema, K., & Blaak, E. E. (2019). Gut microbial metabolites in obesity, NAFLD and T2DM. *Nature Reviews Endocrinology*, *15*(5), 261–273. Available from https://doi.org/10.1038/s41574-019-0156-z, http://www.nature.com/nrendo/index.html.

Cani, P. D., Amar, J., Iglesias, M. A., Poggi, M., Knauf, C., Bastelica, D., Neyrinck, A. M., Fava, F., Tuohy, K. M., Chabo, C., Waget, A., Delmée, E., Cousin, B., Sulpice, T., Chamontin, B., Ferrières, J., Tanti, J. F., Gibson, G. R., Casteilla, L., … Burcelin, R. (2007). Metabolic endotoxemia initiates obesity and insulin resistance. *Diabetes*, *56*(7), 1761–1772. Available from https://doi.org/10.2337/db06-1491France, http://diabetes.diabetesjournals.org/cgi/reprint/56/7/1761.

Cani, P. D., Van Hul, M., Lefort, C., Depommier, C., Rastelli, M., & Everard, A. (2019). Microbial regulation of organismal energy homeostasis. *Nature Metabolism*, *1*(1), 34–46. Available from https://doi.org/10.1038/s42255-018-0017-4, https://www.nature.com/natmetab/.

Carpentier, A. C., Blondin, D. P., Virtanen, K. A., Richard, D., Haman, F., & Turcotte, É. E. (2018). Brown adipose tissue energy metabolism in humans. *Frontiers in Endocrinology*, *9*. Available from https://doi.org/10.3389/fendo.2018.00447, https://www.frontiersin.org/articles/10.3389/fendo.2018.00447/full.

Chambers, E. S., Byrne, C. S., Rugyendo, A., Morrison, D. J., Preston, T., Tedford, C., Bell, J. D., Thomas, L., Akbar, A. N., Riddell, N. E., Sharma, R., Thursz, M. R., Manousou, P., & Frost, G. (2019). The effects of dietary supplementation with inulin and inulin-propionate ester on hepatic steatosis in adults with non-alcoholic fatty liver disease. *Diabetes, Obesity and Metabolism*, *21*(2), 372–376. Available from https://doi.org/10.1111/dom.13500.

Chen, I., Liu, C., Chiu, J., & Hsu, C. (2015). Therapeutic effect of high-dose green tea extract on weight reduction: A randomized, double-blind, placebo-controlled clinical trial. *Clinical Nutrition (Edinburgh, Scotland)*, 1–8. Available from https://doi.org/10.1016/j.clnu.2015.05.0032015.

Chen, Y., Pan, R., & Pfeifer, A. (2017). Regulation of brown and beige fat by microRNAs. *Pharmacology and Therapeutics, 170*, 1–7. Available from https://doi.org/10.1016/j.pharmthera.2016.10.004, www.elsevier.com/locate/pharmthera.

Crovesy, L., Ostrowski, M., Ferreira, D. M. T. P., Rosado, E. L., & Soares-Mota, M. (2017). Effect of *Lactobacillus* on body weight and body fat in overweight subjects: A systematic review of randomized controlled clinical trials. *International Journal of Obesity, 41*(11), 1607–1614. Available from https://doi.org/10.1038/ijo.2017.161, http://www.nature.com/ijo/index.html.

Cryan, J. F., O'riordan, K. J., Cowan, C. S. M., Sandhu, K. V., Bastiaanssen, T. F. S., Boehme, M., Codagnone, M. G., Cussotto, S., Fulling, C., Golubeva, A. V., Guzzetta, K. E., Jaggar, M., Long-Smith, C. M., Lyte, J. M., Martin, J. A., Molinero-Perez, A., Moloney, G., Morelli, E., Morillas, E., ... Dinan, T. G. (2019). The microbiota-gut-brain axis. *Physiological Reviews, 99*(4), 1877–2013. Available from https://doi.org/10.1152/physrev.00018.2018, https://www.physiology.org/doi/pdf/10.1152/physrev.00018.2018.

De Ligt, M., Bergman, M., Fuentes, R. M., Essers, H., Moonen-Kornips, E., Havekes, B., Schrauwen-Hinderling, V. B., & Schrauwen, P. (2020). No effect of resveratrol supplementation after 6 months on insulin sensitivity in overweight adults: A randomized trial. *American Journal of Clinical Nutrition, 112*(4), 1029–1038. Available from https://doi.org/10.1093/ajcn/nqaa125, http://www.ajcn.org/contents-by-date.2005.shtml.

de Vries, H., Axelos, M. A. V., Sarni-Manchado, P., & O'Donohue, M. (2018). Meeting new challenges in food science technology: The development of complex systems approach for food and biobased research. *Innovative Food Science and Emerging Technologies, 46*, 1–6. Available from https://doi.org/10.1016/j.ifset.2018.04.004, http://www.elsevier.com/locate/ifset.

Denou, E., Marcinko, K., Surette, M. G., Steinberg, G. R., & Schertzer, J. D. (2016). High-intensity exercise training increases the diversity and metabolic capacity of the mouse distal gut microbiota during diet-induced obesity. *American Journal of Physiology - Endocrinology and Metabolism, 310*(11), E982. Available from https://doi.org/10.1152/ajpendo.00537.2015, http://ajpendo.physiology.org/content/ajpendo/310/11/E982.full.pdf.

Depommier, C., Everard, A., Druart, C., Plovier, H., Van Hul, M., Vieira-Silva, S., Falony, G., Raes, J., Maiter, D., Delzenne, N. M., de Barsy, M., Loumaye, A., Hermans, M. P., Thissen, J. P., de Vos, W. M., & Cani, P. D. (2019). Supplementation with Akkermansia muciniphila in overweight and obese human volunteers: a proof-of-concept exploratory study. *Nature Medicine, 25*(7), 1096–1103. Available from https://doi.org/10.1038/s41591-019-0495-2, http://www.nature.com/nm/index.html.

Di Marzo, V. (2008). The endocannabinoid system in obesity and type 2 diabetes. *Diabetologia, 51*(8), 1356–1367. Available from https://doi.org/10.1007/s00125-008-1048-2.

Di Pasquale, M. G. (2009). The essentials of essential fatty acids. *Journal of Dietary Supplements, 6*(2), 143–161. Available from https://doi.org/10.1080/19390210902861841, http://www.tandfonline.com/loi/ijds20.

Diet H., crossm Gut Microbiota Mediates the Protective Effects of Dietary Capsaicin against Chronic Low-Grade Inflammation and Associated Obesity Induced by. (2017), 2017.

Donahoo, W., Wyatt, H. R., Kriehn, J., Stuht, J., Dong, F., Hosokawa, P., Grunwald, G. K., Johnson, S. L., Peters, J. C., & Hill, J. O. (2008). Dietary fat increases energy intake across the range of typical consumption in the United States. *Obesity, 16*(1), 64–69. Available from https://doi.org/10.1038/oby.2007.31.

Ejtahed, H. S., Angoorani, P., Soroush, A. R., Atlasi, R., Hasani-Ranjbar, S., Mortazavian, A. M., & Larijani, B. (2019). Probiotics supplementation for the obesity management; A systematic review of animal studies and clinical trials. *Journal of Functional Foods, 52*, 228–242. Available from https://doi.org/10.1016/j.jff.2018.10.039, http://www.elsevier.com/wps/find/journaldescription.cws_home/717426/description#description.

Federico, A., Dallio, M., Tolone, S., Gravina, A. G., Patrone, V., Romano, M., Tuccillo, C., Mozzillo, A. L., Amoroso, V., Misso, G., Morelli, L., Docimo, L., & Loguercio, C. (2016). Gastrointestinal hormones, intestinal microbiota and metabolic homeostasis in obese patients: Effect of bariatric surgery. *In Vivo (Athens, Greece), 30*(3), 321–330. Available from http://iv.iiarjournals.org/.

Fernández-Sánchez, A., Madrigal-Santillán, E., Bautista, M., Esquivel-Soto, J., Morales-González, A., Esquivel-Chirino, C., Durante-Montiel, I., Sánchez-Rivera, G., Valadez-Vega, C., & Morales-González, J. A. (2011). Inflammation, oxidative stress, and obesity. *International Journal of Molecular Sciences, 12*(5), 3117–3132. Available from https://doi.org/10.3390/ijms12053117Mexico, http://www.mdpi.com/1422-0067/12/5/3117/pdf.

Ganjali, S., Sahebkar, A., Mahdipour, E., Jamialahmadi, K., Torabi, S., Akhlaghi, S., Ferns, G., Parizadeh, S. M. R., & Ghayour-Mobarhan, M. (2014). Investigation of the effects of curcumin on serum cytokines in obese individuals: A randomized controlled trial. *The Scientific World Journal, 2014*. Available from https://doi.org/10.1155/2014/898361.

Ghavami, A., Roshanravan, N., Nattagh-Eshtivani, E., Sharifi, S., Arzhang, P., Sani, M. A., Dinarvand, M. H., Shokri, A., & Ostadrahimi, A. (2019). The effect of high performance inulin on appetite, energy intake and anthropometric indices in patient with type 2 diabetes. *Progress in Nutrition, 21*, 121–126. Available from https://doi.org/10.23751/pn.v21i2-S.6824, https://www.mattioli1885journals.com/index.php/progressinnutrition/article/view/6824/7670.

Giralt, M., & Villarroya, F. (2013). White, brown, beige/brite: Different adipose cells for different functions? *Endocrinology, 154*(9), 2992–3000. Available from https://doi.org/10.1210/en.2013-1403Spain, http://endo.endojournals.org/content/154/9/2992.full.pdf + html.

Godfray, H. C. J., Beddington, J. R., Crute, I. R., Haddad, L., Lawrence, D., Muir, J. F., Pretty, J., Robinson, S., Thomas, S. M., & Toulmin, C. (2010). Food security: The challenge of feeding 9 billion people. *Science (New York, N.Y.), 327*(5967), 812–818. Available from https://doi.org/10.1126/science.1185383.

Green, M., Arora, K., & Prakash, S. (2020). Microbial medicine: Prebiotic and probiotic functional foods to target obesity and metabolic syndrome. *International Journal of Molecular Sciences, 21*(8). Available from https://doi.org/10.3390/ijms21082890, https://www.mdpi.com/1422-0067/21/8/2890/pdf.

Guimarães, J. T., Balthazar, C. F., Silva, R., Rocha, R. S., Graça, J. S., Esmerino, E. A., Silva, M. C., Sant'Ana, A. S., Duarte, M. C. K. H., Freitas, M. Q., & Cruz, A. G. (2020). Impact of probiotics and prebiotics on food texture. *Current Opinion in Food Science, 33*, 38–44. Available from https://doi.org/10.1016/j.cofs.2019.12.002, http://www.journals.elsevier.com/current-opinion-in-food-science/.

Hadi, A., Sepandi, M., Marx, W., Moradi, S., & Parastouei, K. (2019). Clinical and psychological responses to synbiotic supplementation in obese or overweight adults: A randomized clinical trial. *Complementary Therapies in Medicine, 47*102216. Available from https://doi.org/10.1016/j.ctim.2019.102216.

Haley, W. E., & Freeman. (2018). *Physiology & Behavior, 176*, 139–148. Available from https://doi.org/10.1097/MCO.0000000000000254. Desaturase2018.

Hall, J. E., Do Carmo, J. M., Da Silva, A. A., Wang, Z., & Hall, M. E. (2015). Obesity-Induced hypertension: Interaction of neurohumoral and renal mechanisms. *Circulation Research, 116*(6), 991–1006. Available from https://doi.org/10.1161/CIRCRESAHA.116.305697, https://www.ovid.com/product-details.454.html.

Hasler, C. M., Bloch, A. S., & Thomson, C. A. (2004). Position of the American dietetic association: Functional foods. *Journal of the American Dietetic Association, 104*(5), 814–826. Available from https://doi.org/10.1016/j.jada.2004.03.015.

Haththotuwa R.N., C.N. Wijeyaratne, U. Senarath, (2016), 2016.

Heim, K. E., Tagliaferro, A. R., & Bobilya, D. J. (2002). Flavonoid antioxidants: Chemistry, metabolism and structure-activity relationships. *Journal of Nutritional Biochemistry, 13*(10), 572–584. Available from https://doi.org/10.1016/S0955-2863(02)00208-5.

Heinonen, S., Jokinen, R., Rissanen, A., & Pietiläinen, K. H. (2020). White adipose tissue mitochondrial metabolism in health and in obesity. *Obesity Reviews, 21*(2). Available from https://doi.org/10.1111/obr.12958, http://onlinelibrary.wiley.com/journal/10.1111/(ISSN)1467-789X.

Hiel, S., Gianfrancesco, M. A., Rodriguez, J., Portheault, D., Leyrolle, Q., Bindels, L. B., Gomes da Silveira Cauduro, C., Mulders, M. D. G. H., Zamariola, G., Azzi, A. S., Kalala, G., Pachikian, B. D., Amadieu, C., Neyrinck, A. M., Loumaye, A., Cani, P. D., Lanthier, N., Trefois, P., Klein, O., ... Delzenne, N. M. (2020). Link between gut microbiota and health outcomes in inulin -treated obese patients: Lessons from the Food4Gut multicenter randomized placebo-controlled trial. *Clinical Nutrition, 39*(12), 3618–3628. Available from https://doi.org/10.1016/j.clnu.2020.04.005, http://www.elsevier-international.com/journals/clnu/.

Hill, C., Guarner, F., Reid, G., Gibson, G. R., Merenstein, D. J., Pot, B., Morelli, L., Canani, R. B., Flint, H. J., Salminen, S., Calder, P. C., & Sanders, M. E. (2014). Expert consensus document: The international scientific association for probiotics and prebiotics consensus statement on the scope and appropriate use of the term probiotic. *Nature Reviews Gastroenterology and Hepatology, 11*(8), 506–514. Available from https://doi.org/10.1038/nrgastro.2014.66, http://www.nature.com/nrgastro/index.html.

Indiani, C. M. D. S. P., Rizzardi, K. F., Castelo, P. M., Ferraz, L. F. C., Darrieux, M., & Parisotto, T. M. (2018). Childhood Obesity and Firmicutes/Bacteroidetes Ratio in the Gut Microbiota: A Systematic Review. *Childhood Obesity, 14*(8), 501–509. Available from https://doi.org/10.1089/chi.2018.0040, www.liebertonline.com/obe.

Janssen, A. W. F., & Kersten, S. (2017). Potential mediators linking gut bacteria to metabolic health: a critical view. *Journal of Physiology, 595*(2), 477–487. Available from https://doi.org/10.1113/JP272476, http://www.wiley.com/bw/editors.asp?ref = 0022-3751&site = 1.

Jazayeri-Tehrani, S. A., Rezayat, S. M., Mansouri, S., Qorbani, M., Alavian, S. M., Daneshi-Maskooni, M., & Hosseinzadeh-Attar, M. J. (2019). Nano-curcumin improves glucose indices, lipids, inflammation, and Nesfatin in overweight and obese patients with non-alcoholic fatty liver disease (NAFLD): A double-blind randomized placebo-controlled clinical trial. *Nutrition and Metabolism, 16*(1). Available from https://doi.org/10.1186/s12986-019-0331-1, http://www.nutritionandmetabolism.com/home/.

Jeromson, S., Gallagher, I. J., Galloway, S. D. R., & Hamilton, D. L. (2015). Omega-3 fatty acids and skeletal muscle health. *Marine Drugs, 13*(11), 6977–7004. Available from https://doi.org/10.3390/md13116977, http://www.mdpi.com/1660-3397/13/11/6977/pdf.

Kadooka, Y., Sato, M., Ogawa, A., Miyoshi, M., Uenishi, H., Ogawa, H., Ikuyama, K., Kagoshima, M., & Tsuchida, T. (2013). Effect of Lactobacillus gasseri SBT2055 in fermented milk on abdominal adiposity in adults in a randomised controlled trial. *The British Journal of Nutrition, 110*(9), 1696–1703. Available from https://doi.org/10.1017/S0007114513001037.

Kamerow, D. (2004). Food, functional food. *BMJ (Clinical Research ed.), 328*(7440), E277. Available from https://doi.org/10.1136/bmj.328.7440.E277.

Kang, C., Wang, B., Kaliannan, K., Wang, X., Lang, H., Hui, S., Huang, L., Zhang, Y., Zhou, M., Chen, M., & Mi, M. (2017). Gut microbiota mediates the protective effects of dietary capsaicin against chronic low-grade inflammation and associated obesity induced by high-fat diet. *mBio, 8*(3). Available from https://doi.org/10.1128/mBio.00470-17, http://mbio.asm.org/content/8/3/e00470-17.full.pdf.

Kao, W. M., Chang, C. R., Chang, T. J., Li, S. Y., Chen, W. J., & Chau, C. F. (2018). Inclusion of fructooligosaccharide and resistant maltodextrin in high fat diets promotes simultaneous improvements on body fat reduction and fecal parameters. *Molecules (Basel, Switzerland), 23*(9). Available from https://doi.org/10.3390/molecules23092169, http://www.mdpi.com/1420-3049/23/9/2169/pdf.

Kaur, N., & Gupta, A. K. (2002). Applications of inulin and oligofructose in health and nutrition. *Journal of Biosciences, 27*(7), 703–714. Available from https://doi.org/10.1007/BF02708379, http://www.ias.ac.in/jbiosci/.

Kaur, N., Chugh, V., & Gupta, A. K. (2014). Essential fatty acids as functional components of foods- a review. *Journal of Food Science and Technology, 51*(10), 2289–2303. Available from https://doi.org/10.1007/s13197-012-0677-0, http://www.springerlink.com/content/121580/.

Khan, K., Jovanovski, E., Ho, H. V. T., Marques, A. C. R., Zurbau, A., Mejia, S. B., Sievenpiper, J. L., & Vuksan, V. (2018). The effect of viscous soluble fiber on blood pressure: A systematic review and meta-analysis of randomized controlled trials. *Nutrition, Metabolism and Cardiovascular Diseases, 28*(1), 3–13. Available from https://doi.org/10.1016/j.numecd.2017.09.007.

Koliada, A., Syzenko, G., Moseiko, V., Budovska, L., Puchkov, K., Perederiy, V., Gavalko, Y., Dorofeyev, A., Romanenko, M., Tkach, S., Sineok, L., Lushchak, O., & Vaiserman, A. (2017). Association between body mass index and Firmicutes/Bacteroidetes ratio in an adult Ukrainian population. *BMC Microbiology, 17*(1). Available from https://doi.org/10.1186/s12866-017-1027-1, http://www.biomedcentral.com/bmcmicrobiol/.

Konstantinidi, M., & Koutelidakis, A. E. (2019). Functional foods and bioactive compounds: A review of its possible role on weight management and obesity's metabolic consequences. *Medicines, 6*(3), 94. Available from https://doi.org/10.3390/medicines6030094.

Kuszewski, J. C., Wong, R. H. X., Wood, L. G., & Howe, P. R. C. (2020). Effects of fish oil and curcumin supplementation on cerebrovascular function in older adults: A randomized controlled trial. *Nutrition, Metabolism and Cardiovascular Diseases*, *30*(4), 625–633. Available from https://doi.org/10.1016/j.numecd.2019.12.010, http://www.elsevier.com/wps/find/journaldescription.cws_home/704955/description#description.

Hul M.V., Keywords: dietary fibers, metabolism, obesity, gut microbiota 1. (2020), 2020.

Lee, H. Y., Park, J. H., Seok, S. H., Baek, M. W., Kim, D. J., Lee, K. E., Paek, K. S., Lee, Y., & Park, J. H. (2006). Human originated bacteria, *Lactobacillus rhamnosus* PL60, produce conjugated linoleic acid and show anti-obesity effects in diet-induced obese mice. *Biochimica et Biophysica Acta - Molecular and Cell Biology of Lipids*, *1761*(7), 736–744. Available from https://doi.org/10.1016/j.bbalip.2006.05.007.

Lee, J.-S., Cha, Y.-J., Lee, K.-H., & Yim, J.-E. (2016). Onion peel extract reduces the percentage of body fat in overweight and obese subjects: a 12-week, randomized, double-blind, placebo-controlled study. *Nutrition Research and Practice*, *10*(2), 175. Available from https://doi.org/10.4162/nrp.2016.10.2.175.

Lee, K.-U., Park, J. Y., Kim, C. H., Hong, S. K., Suh, K. I., Park, K. S., & Park, S. W. (1996). Effect of decreasing plasma free fatty acids by acipimox on hepatic glucose metabolism in normal rats. *Metabolism: Clinical and Experimental*, *45*(11), 1408–1414. Available from https://doi.org/10.1016/s0026-0495(96)90123-7.

Lee, M. J., Wu, Y., & Fried, S. K. (2013). Adipose tissue heterogeneity: Implication of depot differences in adipose tissue for obesity complications. *Molecular Aspects of Medicine*, *34*(1), 1–11. Available from https://doi.org/10.1016/j.mam.2012.10.001.

Li, H., Liu, F., Lu, J., Shi, J., Guan, J., Yan, F., Li, B., & Huo, G. (2020). Probiotic mixture of Lactobacillus plantarum strains improves lipid metabolism and gut microbiota structure in high fat diet-fed mice. *Frontiers in Microbiology*, *11*. Available from https://doi.org/10.3389/fmicb.2020.00512, https://www.frontiersin.org/journals/microbiology#.

Li, W., Zhang, K., & Zhao, Q. (2019). Fructooligosaccharide enhanced absorption and anti-dyslipidemia capacity of tea flavonoids in high sucrose-fed mice. *International Journal of Food Sciences and Nutrition*, *70*(3), 311–322. Available from https://doi.org/10.1080/09637486.2018.1511688, http://www.tandfonline.com/loi/iijf20.

Lim, J. J., & Poppitt, S. D. (2019). How satiating are the 'satiety' peptides: A problem of pharmacology versus physiology in the development of novel foods for regulation of food intake. *Nutrients*, *11*(7). Available from https://doi.org/10.3390/nu11071517, https://www.mdpi.com/2072-6643/11/7/1517/pdf.

Lloyd-Price, J., Abu-Ali, G., & Huttenhower, C. (2016). The healthy human microbiome. *Genome Medicine*, *8*(1). Available from https://doi.org/10.1186/s13073-016-0307-y, http://www.genomemedicine.com/.

Ma, Z., Li, L., & Gotelli, N. J. (2019). Diversity-disease relationships and shared species analyses for human microbiome-associated diseases. *ISME Journal*, *13*(8), 1911–1919. Available from https://doi.org/10.1038/s41396-019-0395-y, http://www.nature.com/ismej/marketing/aims_scope.html.

Mechanisms M., Antioxidant and Anti-Inflammatory Potential of Polyphenols. (2021), 2021.

Merino-Aguilar, H., Arrieta-Baez, D., Jiménez-Estrada, M., Magos-Guerrero, G., Hernández-Bautista, R. J., Susunaga-Notario, Ad. C., Almanza-Pérez, J. C., Blancas-Flores, G., Román-Ramos, R., & Alarcón-Aguilar, F. J. (2014). Effect of fructooligosaccharides fraction from Psacalium decompositum on inflammation and dyslipidemia in rats with fructose-induced obesity. *Nutrients*, *6*(2), 591–604. Available from https://doi.org/10.3390/nu6020591, http://www.mdpi.com/2072-6643/6/2/591/pdf.

Mistry, R. H., Liu, F., Borewicz, K., Lohuis, M. A. M., Smidt, H., Verkade, H. J., & Tietge, U. J. F. (2020). Long-term β-galacto-oligosaccharides supplementation decreases the development of obesity and insulin resistance in mice fed a western-type diet. *Molecular Nutrition & Food Research*, *64*(12). Available from https://doi.org/10.1002/mnfr.201900922.

Miyamoto, A. (2006). Author copy only 331. *The Journal of Endocrinology*, 2006.

Moghe, S. S., Juma, S., Imrhan, V., & Vijayagopal, P. (2012). Effect of blueberry polyphenols on 3T3-F442A preadipocyte differentiation. *Journal of Medicinal Food*, *15*(5), 448–452. Available from https://doi.org/10.1089/jmf.2011.0234.

Mohammadi-Sartang, M., Bellissimo, N., Totosy de Zepetnek, J. O., Brett, N. R., Mazloomi, S. M., Fararouie, M., Bedeltavana, A., Famouri, M., & Mazloom, Z. (2018). The effect of daily fortified yogurt consumption on weight loss in adults with metabolic syndrome: A 10-week randomized controlled trial. *Nutrition, Metabolism and Cardiovascular Diseases*, *28*(6), 565–574. Available from https://doi.org/10.1016/j.numecd.2018.03.001.

Moreno-Navarrete, J. M., Serino, M., Blasco-Baque, V., Azalbert, V., Barton, R. H., Cardellini, M., Latorre, J., Ortega, F., Sabater-Masdeu, M., Burcelin, R., Dumas, M. E., Ricart, W., Federici, M., & Fernández-Real, J. M. (2018). Gut microbiota interacts with markers of adipose tissue browning, insulin action and plasma acetate in morbid obesity. *Molecular Nutrition and Food Research*, *62*(3). Available from https://doi.org/10.1002/mnfr.201700721, www.mnf-journal.de.

Morrison, D. J., & Preston, T. (2016). Formation of short chain fatty acids by the gut microbiota and their impact on human metabolism. *Gut Microbes*, *7*(3), 189–200. Available from https://doi.org/10.1080/19490976.2015.1134082, http://www.tandfonline.com/toc/kgmi20/current.

Most, J., Warnke, I., Boekschoten, M. V., Jocken, J. W. E., de Groot, P., Friedel, A., Bendik, I., Goossens, G. H., & Blaak, E. E. (2018). The effects of polyphenol supplementation on adipose tissue morphology and gene expression in overweight and obese humans. *Adipocyte*, *7*(3), 190–196. Available from https://doi.org/10.1080/21623945.2018.1469942, http://www.tandfonline.com/loi/kadi20.

Müller, M., Canfora, E. E., & Blaak, E. E. (2018). Gastrointestinal transit time, glucose homeostasis and metabolic health: Modulation by dietary fibers. *Nutrients*, *10*(3). Available from https://doi.org/10.3390/nu10030275, http://www.mdpi.com/2072-6643/10/3/275/pdf.

Nabi, B. N., Sedighinejad, A., Haghighi, M., Farzi, F., Rimaz, S., Atrkarroushan, Z., & Biazar, G. (2018). The anti-obesity effects of green tea: A controlled, randomized, clinical trial. *Iranian Red Crescent Medical Journal*, *20*(1). Available from https://doi.org/10.5812/ircmj.55950, http://cdn.neoscriber.org/cdn/serve/3144b/5ab316297831c7d2d07e2980de4436b0b04a3d6e/ircmj-20-01-55950.pdf.

Nono Nankam, P. A., Nguelefack, T. B., Goedecke, J. H., & Blüher, M. (2021). Contribution of adipose tissue oxidative stress to obesity-associated diabetes risk and ethnic differences: Focus on women of African ancestry. *Antioxidants*, *10*(4). Available from https://doi.org/10.3390/antiox10040622, https://www.mdpi.com/2076-3921/10/4/622/pdf.

Nording, M. L., Yang, J., Georgi, K., Hegedus Karbowski, C., German, J. B., Weiss, R. H., Hogg, R. J., Trygg, J., Hammock, B. D., & Zivkovic, A. M. (2013). Individual variation in lipidomic profiles of healthy subjects in response to omega-3 fatty acids. *PLoS One*, *8*(10). Available from https://doi.org/10.1371/journal.pone.0076575Sweden, http://www.plosone.org/article/fetchObject.action;jsessionid = CE05B6C445 9C88F3D428AAAB8DE97123?uri = info%3Adoi%2F10.1371%2Fjournal.pone.0076575&representation = PDF.

Ohama, H., Ikeda, H., & Moriyama, H. (2006). Health foods and foods with health claims in Japan. *Toxicology*, *221*(1), 95–111. Available from https://doi.org/10.1016/j.tox.2006.01.015, www.elsevier.com/locate/toxicol.

Otelea, M. R., Streinu-Cercel, A., Baicus, C., & Nitescu, M. (2019). The adipokine profile and the cardiometabolic risk in non-obese young adults. *Balkan Medical Journal*, *36*(3), 155–161. Available from https://doi.org/10.4274/balkanmedj.galenos.2018.2018.0789, http://balkanmedicaljournal.org/pdf.php?&id = 2062.

Pagotto, U., Marsicano, G., Cota, D., Lutz, B., & Pasquali, R. (2006). The emerging role of the endocannabinoid system in endocrine regulation and energy balance. *Endocrine Reviews*, *27*(1), 73–100. Available from https://doi.org/10.1210/er.2005-0009Italy, http://edrv.endojournals.org/cgi/reprint/27/1/73.

Panahi, Y., Hosseini, M. S., Khalili, N., Naimi, E., Simental-Mendía, L. E., Majeed, M., & Sahebkar, A. (2016). Effects of curcumin on serum cytokine concentrations in subjects with metabolic syndrome: A post-hoc analysis of a randomized controlled trial. *Biomedicine and Pharmacotherapy*, *82*, 578–582. Available from https://doi.org/10.1016/j.biopha.2016.05.037, www.elsevier.com/locate/biomedpharm.

Piché, M. E., Tchernof, A., & Després, J. P. (2020). Obesity phenotypes, diabetes, and cardiovascular diseases. *Circulation Research*, *126*(11), 1477–1500. Available from https://doi.org/10.1161/CIRCRESAHA.120.316101, https://www.ovid.com/product-details.454.html.

Poutanen, K. S., Fiszman, S., Marsaux, C. F. M., Pentikäinen, S. P., Steinert, R. E., & Mela, D. J. (2018). Recommendations for characterization and reporting of dietary fibers in nutrition research. *American Journal of Clinical Nutrition*, *108*(3), 437–444. Available from https://doi.org/10.1093/ajcn/nqy095, http://www.ajcn.org/contents-by-date.2005.shtml.

Rolls, B. J. (2014). What is the role of portion control in weight management. *International Journal of Obesity*, *38*(1), S1–S8. Available from https://doi.org/10.1038/ijo.2014.82, http://www.nature.com/ijo/index.html.

Rossi, F., Punzo, F., Umano, G. R., Argenziano, M., & Miraglia Del Giudice, E. (2018). Role of cannabinoids in obesity. *International Journal of Molecular Sciences*, *19*(9). Available from https://doi.org/10.3390/ijms19092690, http://www.mdpi.com/1422-0067/19/9/2690/pdf.

Ruiz, L. D., Zuelch, M. L., Dimitratos, S. M., & Scherr, R. E. (2020). Adolescent obesity: Diet quality, psychosocial health, and cardiometabolic risk factors. *Nutrients*, *12*(1). Available from https://doi.org/10.3390/nu12010043, https://www.mdpi.com/2072-6643/12/1/43/pdf.

Salehi, M., & Purnell, J. Q. (2019). The role of glucagon-like peptide-1 in energy homeostasis. *Metabolic Syndrome and Related Disorders*, *17*(4), 183–191. Available from https://doi.org/10.1089/met.2018.0088, www.liebertonline.com/met/.

Samuel, B. S., Shaito, A., Motoike, T., Rey, F. E., Backhed, F., Manchester, J. K., Hammer, R. E., Williams, S. C., Crowley, J., Yanagisawa, M., & Gordon, J. I. (2008). Effects of the gut microbiota on host adiposity are modulated by the short-chain fatty-acid binding G protein-coupled receptor, Gpr41. *Proceedings of the National Academy of Sciences of the United States of America*, *105*(43), 16767–16772. Available from https://doi.org/10.1073/pnas.0808567105, http://www.pnas.org/content/105/43/16767.full.pdf.

Sanders, M. E., & Marco, M. L. (2010). Food formats for effective delivery of probiotics. *Annual Review of Food Science and Technology*, *1*(1), 65–85. Available from https://doi.org/10.1146/annurev.food.080708.100743.

Saraf-Bank, S., Ahmadi, A., Paknahad, Z., Maracy, M., & Nourian, M. (2019). Effects of curcumin supplementation on markers of inflammation and oxidative stress among healthy overweight and obese girl adolescents: A randomized placebo-controlled clinical trial. *Phytotherapy Research*, *33*(8), 2015–2022. Available from https://doi.org/10.1002/ptr.6370.

Schulz, P., Hryhorowicz, S., Rychter, A. M., Zawada, A., Słomski, R., Dobrowolska, A., & Krela-Kaźmierczak, I. (2021). What role does the endocannabinoid system play in the pathogenesis of obesity? *Nutrients*, *13*(2), 1–24. Available from https://doi.org/10.3390/nu13020373, https://www.mdpi.com/2072-6643/13/2/373/pdf.

Schulz, T. J., & Tseng, Y. H. (2013). Brown adipose tissue: Development, metabolism and beyond. *Biochemical Journal*, *453*(2), 167–178. Available from https://doi.org/10.1042/BJ20130457, http://www.biochemj.org/bj/453/0167/4530167.pdf.

Scientific Opinion on establishing Food-Based Dietary Guidelines. EFSA Journal. 8 (3) (2010), doi: 10.2903/j.efsa.2010.1460.

Silberbauer, C. J., Surina-Baumgartner, D. M., Arnold, M., & Langhans, W. (2000). Prandial lactate infusion inhibits spontaneous feeding in rats. *American Journal of Physiology - Regulatory Integrative and Comparative Physiology*, *278*(3), R646. Available from https://doi.org/10.1152/ajpregu.2000.278.3.r646, ajpregu.physiology.org.

Stein, C. J., & Colditz, G. A. (2004). The epidemic of obesity. *Journal of Clinical Endocrinology and Metabolism*, *89*(6), 2522–2525. Available from https://doi.org/10.1210/jc.2004-0288.

Structure, function and diversity of the healthy human microbiome. Nature. 486 (7402) (2012), 207–214, doi: 10.1038/nature11234.

Sun-Waterhouse, D. (2011). The development of fruit-based functional foods targeting the health and wellness market: A review. *International Journal of Food Science and Technology*, *46*(5), 899–920. Available from https://doi.org/10.1111/j.1365-2621.2010.02499.x.

Surampudi, P., Enkhmaa, B., Anuurad, E., & Berglund, L. (2016). Lipid lowering with soluble dietary fiber. *Current Atherosclerosis Reports*, *18*(12). Available from https://doi.org/10.1007/s11883-016-0624-z.

Tavella, T., Rampelli, S., Guidarelli, G., Bazzocchi, A., Gasperini, C., Pujos-Guillot, E., Comte, B., Barone, M., Biagi, E., Candela, M., Nicoletti, C., Kadi, F., Battista, G., Salvioli, S., O'Toole, P. W., Franceschi, C., Brigidi, P., Turroni, S., & Santoro, A. (2021). Elevated gut microbiome abundance of Christensenellaceae, Porphyromonadaceae and Rikenellaceae is associated with reduced visceral adipose tissue and healthier metabolic profile in Italian elderly. *Gut Microbes*, *13*(1), 1–19. Available from https://doi.org/10.1080/19490976.2021.1880221, http://www.tandfonline.com/toc/kgmi20/current.

Teixeira, T. F. S., Grześkowiak, Ł., Franceschini, S. C. C., Bressan, J., Ferreira, C. L. L. F., & Peluzio, M. C. G. (2013). Higher level of faecal SCFA in women correlates with metabolic syndrome risk factors. *British Journal of Nutrition*, *109*(5), 914–919. Available from https://doi.org/10.1017/S0007114512002723.

Tilg, H., Zmora, N., Adolph, T. E., & Elinav, E. (2020). The intestinal microbiota fuelling metabolic inflammation. *Nature Reviews. Immunology*, *20* (1), 40–54. Available from https://doi.org/10.1038/s41577-019-0198-4, http://www.nature.com/nri/index.html.

Tolhurst, G., Heffron, H., Lam, Y. S., Parker, H. E., Habib, A. M., Diakogiannaki, E., Cameron, J., Grosse, J., Reimann, F., & Gribble, F. M. (2012). Short-chain fatty acids stimulate glucagon-like peptide-1 secretion via the G-protein-coupled receptor FFAR2. *Diabetes*, *61*(2), 364–371. Available from https://doi.org/10.2337/db11-1019, http://diabetes.diabetesjournals.org/content/61/2/364.full.pdf + html.

Torres-Fuentes, C., Schellekens, H., Dinan, T. G., & Cryan, J. F. (2015). A natural solution for obesity: Bioactives for the prevention and treatment of weight gain. A review. *Nutritional Neuroscience*, *18*(2), 49–65. Available from https://doi.org/10.1179/1476830513Y.0000000099, http://www.maneyonline.com/doi/pdfplus/10.1179/1476830513Y.0000000099.

Tsoi M.F., H.L. Li, Q. Feng, C.L. Cheung, T.T. Cheung, B.M.Y. Cheung, Prevalence of Childhood Obesity in the United States in 1999-2018: A 20-Year Analysis. Obes. Facts. 15. Available from https://doi.org/10.1159/000524261.n.d

Turnbaugh, P. J., Ley, R. E., Mahowald, M. A., Magrini, V., Mardis, E. R., & Gordon, J. I. (2006). An obesity-associated gut microbiome with increased capacity for energy harvest. *Nature*, *444*(7122), 1027–1031. Available from https://doi.org/10.1038/nature05414.

Wang, D., Liu, C. D., Tian, M. L., Tan, C. Q., Shu, G., Jiang, Q. Y., Zhang, L., & Yin, Y. L. (2019). Propionate promotes intestinal lipolysis and metabolic benefits via AMPK/LSD1 pathway in mice. *Journal of Endocrinology*, *243*(3), 187–197. Available from https://doi.org/10.1530/JOE-19-0188, https://joe.bioscientifica.com/view/journals/joe/243/3/JOE-19-0188.xml.

Waters, J. L., & Ley, R. E. (2019). The human gut bacteria Christensenellaceae are widespread, heritable, and associated with health. *BMC Biology*, *17*(1). Available from https://doi.org/10.1186/s12915-019-0699-4, http://www.biomedcentral.com/bmcbiol/.

Wei C., L.U. Wen-wei, 肥胖人群肠道菌群特征分析及机器学习模型 Characteristics of gut microbiota of obese people and machine learning model. 47 (2020), 4328–4337, doi: 10.13344/j.microbiol.china.2000982020.

Wijers, S. L. J., Saris, W. H. M., & Lichtenbelt, W. D. V. M. (2010). Cold-induced adaptive thermogenesis in lean and obese. *Obesity*, *18*(6), 1092–1099. Available from https://doi.org/10.1038/oby.2010.74, http://onlinelibrary.wiley.com/journal/10.1002/(ISSN)1930-739X.

Yin, Y. N., Yu, Q. F., Fu, N., Liu, X. W., & Lu, F. G. (2010). Effects of four Bifidobacteria on obesity in high-fat diet induced rats. *World Journal of Gastroenterology*, *16*(27), 3394–3401. Available from https://doi.org/10.3748/wjg.v16.i27.3394, http://www.wjgnet.com/1007-9327/16/3394.pdf.

Yoshitomi, R., Yamamoto, M., Kumazoe, M., Fujimura, Y., Yonekura, M., Shimamoto, Y., Nakasone, A., Kondo, S., Hattori, H., Haseda, A., Nishihira, J., & Tachibana, H. (2021). The combined effect of green tea and α-glucosyl hesperidin in preventing obesity: A randomized placebo-controlled clinical trial. *Scientific Reports*, *11*(1). Available from https://doi.org/10.1038/s41598-021-98612-6, www.nature.com/srep/index.html.

Zhao, Y., Chen, B., Shen, J., Wan, L., Zhu, Y., Yi, T., & Xiao, Z. (2017). The beneficial effects of quercetin, curcumin, and resveratrol in obesity. *Oxidative Medicine and Cellular Longevity*, *2017*. Available from https://doi.org/10.1155/2017/1459497, http://www.hindawi.com/journals/oximed/.

Zuo, L., Prather, E. R., Stetskiv, M., Garrison, D. E., Meade, J. R., Peace, T. I., & Zhou, T. (2019). Inflammaging and oxidative stress in human diseases: From molecular mechanisms to novel treatments. *International Journal of Molecular Sciences*, *20*(18). Available from https://doi.org/10.3390/ijms20184472, https://www.mdpi.com/1422-0067/20/18/4472/pdf.

Chapter 7

Metabolic health: unleashing the potential of bioactive compounds

Prabina Bhattarai[1], Merina Dahal[2], Kiran Tiwari[3] and Nilesh Prakash Nirmal[4]

[1]Department of Health and Human Development, Montana State University, Bozeman, MT, United States, [2]College of Health Solutions, Downtown Phoenix Campus, Arizona State University, Tempe, AZ, United States, [3]School of business and hospitality, Food and Nutrition Management, Algonquin College, Ottawa, ON, Canada, [4]Institute of Nutrition, Mahidol University, Salaya, Nakhon Pathom, Thailand

7.1 Introduction

Metabolic health is typically defined as a healthy metabolic state with ideal blood sugar, blood pressure, lipid profile, and waist circumference level, where imbalances in these factors are the major contributors to chronic diseases such as heart disease, hypertension, and diabetes. The prevalence of metabolic syndrome has significantly increased in the USA, reaching 37.6% in 2011−12, 41.8% in 2017−18 and even higher in the rest of the world (An et al., 2023). Recent reports suggested that there has been an increasing mortality rate related to type 2 diabetes and obesity over the past 20 years, while some downward trends of mortality attributed to HTN and HLD were observed. Metabolic diseases that contribute to a large part of premature deaths worldwide have been projected to cost more than US $5000 for the health system worldwide (Chew et al., 2023). An individual with certain predisposed factors has a higher risk of developing these diseases. Although there is no such defined single cause for these diseases, some personal characteristics, like family history, genetic makeup, sex, and age, which cannot be changed, are the plausible causes of such diseases. However, dietary factors, which can be modulated by individuals, account equally for the development of metabolic syndrome. Researchers and scientists have identified a potent correlation between the transition of people's lifestyles to sedentary and unhealthy diet consumption and the changing metabolic health of individuals.

Inflammation is one of the vital changes that are elevated in the pathophysiology of metabolic syndrome and associated complications. For instance, in the initiation of diabetes, the increased expressions of inflammatory markers (interleukin-6 [IL-6], IL-1β, and tumor necrosis factor-α [TNF-α]) are observed. The activated inflammatory markers majorly contribute to the initiation and development of the complications associated with diseases (Vasim et al., 2022). Thus targeting the different signaling pathways of inflammation effectively minimizes the complications associated with such diseases. Evidence-based studies, both in vivo and in vitro, illustrate the health-promoting properties of several functional foods enriched with bioactive compounds and phytochemicals. Bioactive compounds, such as curcumin, have a regulatory role in metabolic health by regulating gene expression, inhibiting oxidation and inflammation signaling pathways, neutralizing free radicals, and suppressing certain receptors responsible for metabolic syndrome (Jabczyk et al., 2021). Therefore this chapter discusses the potential role of bioactive compounds in promoting metabolic health to serve the following goals: to prevent and/or reduce further damage to organs and to prevent the development of metabolic disorders in unaffected individuals.

7.2 Overview of metabolic diseases

7.2.1 Obesity/overweight

The changing lifestyle and food habits have turned obesity into a global epidemic. Obesity, particularly visceral obesity, is the initiation of metabolic syndrome and associated complications. Evidence-based studies have shown that central obesity is the major cause of metabolic syndrome, with the symptoms of insulin resistance, hypertension, diabetes, dyslipidemia, and cardiovascular diseases. Visceral obesity is responsible for alterations in adipokines and free fatty acids

Unleashing the Power of Functional Foods and Novel Bioactives. DOI: https://doi.org/10.1016/B978-0-443-28862-3.00007-8

and the onset of insulin resistance. In individuals with obesity, white adipose tissue (WAT) is a lipid storage organ that is crucial in the development of obesity-associated complications (Longo et al., 2019).

Adipocytes secrete adipokines and cytokines, including leptin and adiponectin, which affect inflammation and metabolism along with lipid storage. Leptin is a satiety hormone that also has a proinflammatory function and acts oppositely to the function of adiponectin. Adipokines (retinol-binding protein-4 and resistin), on the other hand, are responsible for decreasing insulin sensitivity (Klop et al., 2013). Effective storage of lipids prevents the accumulation and deposition of ectopic lipid on organs like the liver, heart, and muscle, preventing lipotoxicity, and is associated with various metabolic functions. Adipocyte precursors, adipocytes, and several immune cells, including macrophages, T cells, B cells, and dendritic cells, are present in WAT. Specifically, immune cells in WAT maintain and retain the integrity of adipocytes, metabolic processes, and sensitivity to hormones. Adipose tissue macrophages become polarized into proinflammatory macrophages during obesity and release multiple proinflammatory cytokines, like TNF, and activate the NF-κB signaling pathway, which eventually can disrupt insulin signaling and accelerate the development of insulin resistance. The most significant proinflammatory cytokines reported to disrupt insulin signaling are IL-1β and TNF; in the case of IL-1β, this is accomplished by targeting insulin receptor substrate-1 (Hildebrandt et al., 2023).

7.2.2 Insulin resistance and diabetes

Insulin resistance is the condition of an impaired body response to insulin, resulting in an elevation of the blood sugar level, and is the key to diabetes. Reduction of insulin-stimulated muscle glycogen synthesis results in insulin resistance, which is primarily due to reduced insulin-stimulated glucose transport (GLUT 4) function. This is specifically due to the accumulation of intracellular lipid metabolites such as diacylglycerol and fatty acyl CoAs in skeletal muscle and hepatocytes (Petersen & Shulman, 2006). Insulin resistance in individuals is well associated with obesity and its resultant inflammation. In insulin resistance, glucose regulation functions like plasma glucose uptake, glycogen synthesis, lipolysis, and suppression of hepatic glucose production are limited (Lee et al., 2022). This, in turn, results in inflammatory reactions and their related damages.

The onset of obesity triggers proinflammatory cytokine release by adipocytes that is driven by activated B cells (NF-kB) and the production of immune cells (Shoelson et al., 2003). This causes adipose tissue macrophage accumulation, which in turn triggers the formation of more proinflammatory cytokines, like TNFα and IL-6. These cytokines serve as feed-forward mechanisms that lead to chronic inflammation, adipose tissue dysfunction, decreased insulin sensitivity, and IR (Shimobayashi et al., 2018; Williamson & Sheedy, 2020). Insulin receptor substrate-1 (IRS-1) can be inhibited by TNFα-signaling, which lessens its capacity to promote downstream insulin signaling. Such an activated inflammatory pathway is also evident in the liver and muscle (Jiang et al., 2014).

The excessive supply of glucose in obese and insulin-resistant individuals leads to further production of reactive oxygen species (ROS) via endoplasmic reticulum stress, which eventually reduces the potential of β-cells to secrete insulin and further fosters oxidative stress and inflammation (Keane et al., 2015). The immune system is activated in type 2 diabetes due to endothelial dysfunction and immune cell attacks by neutrophils and macrophages. These immune cells damage the endothelium's integrity and increase ROS production. Several factors contribute to the production of ROS, oxidative stress in endothelial tissue, inflammation aggravation, cellular adhesion molecule expression, and malfunction of vascular endothelial tissue. Furthermore, ROS exacerbated pathophysiological conditions and insulin resistance in type 2 diabetic individuals by elevating growth factors and proinflammatory cytokines (An et al., 2023).

7.2.3 Dyslipidemia

Dyslipidemia, a chronic metabolic disorder, is diagnosed with elevated levels of low-density lipoprotein (LDL), total cholesterol, triglycerides, and/or a reduced high-density lipoprotein (HDL) level. Dyslipidemia can result in progressive cardiovascular disease if left untreated (Ji et al., 2019). During obesity, the lipolysis of triglycerides and lipoproteins is hindered due to a decrease in the expression of mRNA for lipoprotein lipase in adipose tissue, decreased lipoprotein lipase in muscle, and the onset of competitive lipolysis between chylomicrons and VLDL. Lipoprotein lipase attached to IDL and VLDL promotes triglyceride depletion. The production of small, dense LDL is eventually caused by the exchange of triglycerides from these residues for cholesterol esters from HDL by cholesteryl ester transfer protein (CETP) and the coordinated action of hepatic lipase. In hypertriglyceridemia, the mechanism of action of CETP causes the cholesterol-ester of LDL to decrease, while the triglyceride in LDL increases. Hepatic lipase hydrolyzes the elevated triglyceride content in LDL, resulting in the production of small, dense LDL particles (Klop et al., 2013). Individuals with dyslipidemia are often diagnosed with other metabolic syndrome-associated disorders, as modifications in LDL promote the activation of the endocannabinoid system.

7.2.4 Atherosclerosis and coronary artery diseases

Atherosclerosis is the primary risk factor for coronary artery diseases and CVD, the world's largest cause of death. The onset of atherosclerosis is due to endothelium activation, which sets off a series of processes that result in the accumulation of lipids, fibrous components, and calcification. These processes ultimately cause artery narrowing and the activation of inflammatory pathways. Initiation of atherosclerosis is signaled by the dysfunction of the endothelial system along with LDL retention and its modification in the intima (Hermida & Balligand, 2013). Despite other atherogenic factors, modified LDLs stimulate endothelial cells, which leads to the recruitment of monocytes in the intima. Also, modified LDLs are attracted by VSCM and differentiated monocytes, which facilitate foam cell development. Simultaneously, a number of inflammation signaling pathways are activated that facilitate fatty streak formation. This results in the inability of endothelial cells to maintain homeostasis; thus vessel walls are susceptible to vasoconstriction, lipid infiltration, leukocyte adhesion, oxidative stress, and platelet activation. Throughout the process, nitric oxide plays a key role in reducing platelet aggregation, inflammation, tissue oxidation, thrombogenic factor activation, and cell proliferation (Jebari-Benslaiman et al., 2022). However, different mediators activated by oxidative stress restrain the activity of eNOS and restrict the function of NO, as oxidative stress is known to promote proatherogenic cytokines, such as interleukins IL-1 and IL-6 and TNF-α synthesis, and chemokines like MCP-1 via heat-shock proteins-mediated NF-kB activation (Yu et al., 2015). Through a series of processes, this results in fibrous plaque development, where the necrotic core and the fibrous cap constitute the hallmarks of advanced atherosclerosis.

7.2.5 Hypertension

The condition of elevated blood pressure is characterized as hypertension, which is a progressive condition that can result in other complications (CKD and CVD). Inhibiting the enzyme that converts angiotensin I to angiotensin II, known as the angiotensin-converting enzyme (ACE), has been used in the treatment of hypertension and associated inflammation (Ji et al., 2005). Hypertensive patients often show endothelium-derived NO system defect due to abnormal endothelium-dependent vasodilatation (Rahman et al., 2021). Lack of exercise, heredity, and being overweight are all associated with high blood pressure, and over 40% of patients with hypertension have been identified with hypercholesterolemia (Behl et al., 2020). Apart from genetics, increased vascular aging and lifestyle might be considered the cause of hypertension-induced vascular diseases.

Elevated wall tension-related cellular stretch driven on by increased pressure causes NADPH oxidases to be induced and upregulated, which in turn increases the formation of ROS in the mitochondria. This leads to oxidative stress in endothelial cells and VSMCs. ROS in vascular cells activates a transcription factor called NRF_2, which causes the expression of several genes related to antioxidants. The severity of hypertension-induced oxidative stress and cellular damage is considered to result from dysfunction of NRF_2-mediated free radical detoxification pathways in the vasculature. Upon aging, cell-autonomous and nonautonomous mechanisms that have been causally linked to NRF_2 malfunction include age-related IGF1 insufficiency and dysregulation of microRNAs like miR-144. Due to this, the vasculature's cellular resistance to oxidative stress is compromised, and the antiinflammatory effect of NRF_2 is hindered by blocking NF-κB, which in turn promotes angiogenesis (Ungvari et al., 2021).

Sound metabolic health can be maintained by the adoption of prevention measures for these diseases, which begin with obesity, and a series of complications can be experienced. The extension of complications is mainly due to oxidative stress and alteration in the antiinflammatory pathway and its signaling factors.

7.3 Bioactive compounds promoting metabolic health

Bioactive compounds are natural compounds present in a wide variety of plants, animals, and marine sources (Pai et al., 2022). Compounds can be broadly classified into polyphenols, terpenoids, phytosterols, vitamins, bioactive peptides, polysaccharides, dietary fibers, capsaicinoids, and alkaloids that exhibit health-promoting functions. Most often, these bioactive compounds are extracted from plants, except for bioactive peptides, which are usually obtained from the hydrolysis of proteins in both plants and animals. These compounds play a dynamic role in regulating a wide array of metabolic pathways and neutralizing the free radicles that are formed during the metabolism process (Fig. 7.1).

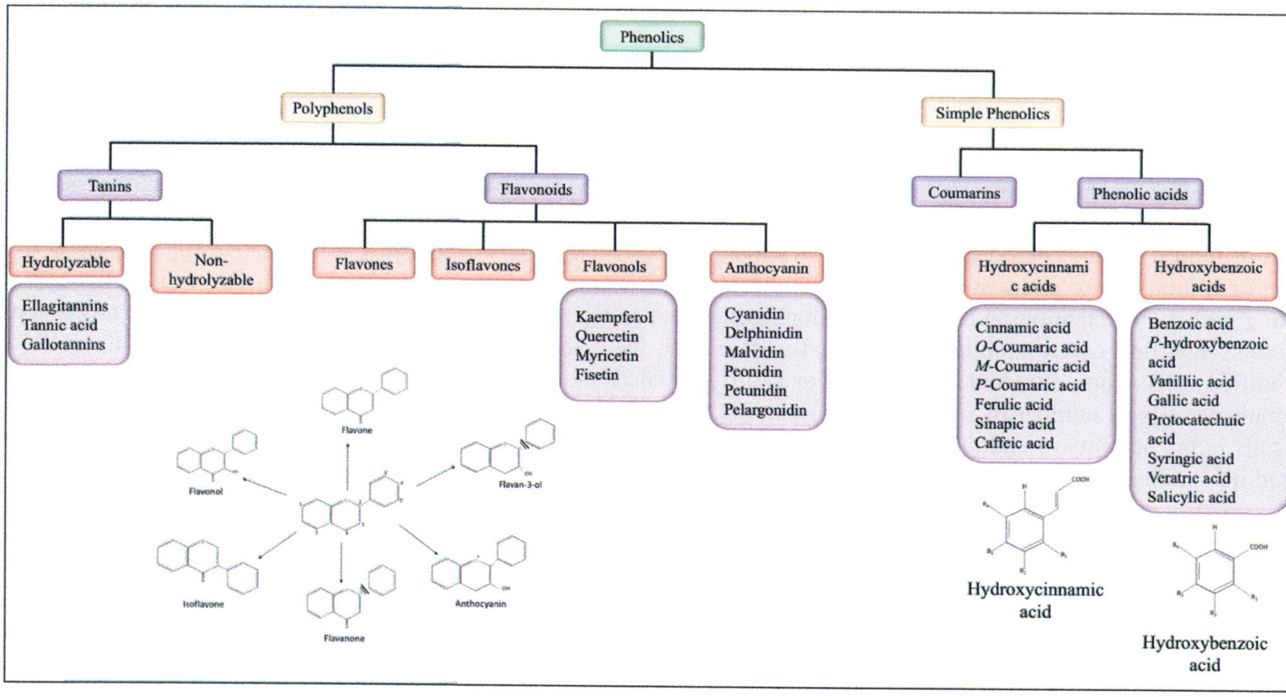

FIGURE 7.1 Polyphenols and its types with basic structures.

7.3.1 Polyphenols

Phenolics are a heterogeneous group of compounds of plant secondary metabolites synthesized during metabolism. These compounds are broadly classified into polyphenols and simple phenols, with subgroups of tannin and flavonoids for polyphenols and coumarins and phenolic acid for simple phenols. Phenols have at least one aromatic ring. One or more hydroxyl groups, which can be either aromatic or aliphatic, are attached to these aromatic rings. Flavonoids, also known as glycosides, are heterocyclic compounds with two aromatic rings connected by oxygen. These groups of phenols are further divided into five different types (flavones, isoflavones, flavonols, flavan-3-ols, and anthocyanins). Tannins are nonflavonoids with two subgroups, that is, hydrolyzable and nonhydrolyzable. Phenolic acids, on the other hand, are categorized as hydroxycinnamic acid and hydroxybenzoic acid (Goleniowski et al., 2013). The primary component of dietary polyphenols, including ferulic acid, caffeic acid, tartaric acid, and others, is hydroxycinnamic acid. Conversely, the dietary contributions of hydroxybenzoic acid are negligible, as it is mostly found in small amounts, where gallic and ellagic acids are the most studied hydroxybenzoic acids (Shahwan et al., 2022). Some other groups of polyphenols are stilbene (resveratrol is the most studied stilbene), coumarin, and lignans (Oluwole et al., 2022). The functional properties of these phenolics are phenolic hydroxyls, and the antioxidant capacity is directly dependent on the position and number of hydroxyls. Besides, carboxylic acid and methoxy groups also contribute to the antioxidant properties of phenolic compounds (Chen et al., 2020).

A phenolic molecule exhibits antioxidant activity via the hydrogen atom transfer mechanism, transition metal chelation, sequential proton loss electron transfer, or single-electron transfer via proton transfer (Zeb, 2020). Each of these compounds exhibits a distinct physiological function in humans, with a predominant bioactivity in free radical scavenging and inflammatory cytokine binding. These compounds exhibit substantial protective properties against neurological diseases, diabetes, tumor growth, proliferation, and metastasis. Except for flavonoids, other free phenolic acids, including cinnamic acid and benzoic acid, have excellent solubility in water as well as high bioavailability. These phenols can be absorbed directly in the GI tract; however, flavonoids are not directly absorbed in the GI, and only a limited amount of flavonoids are diffused passively in the bloodstream through the intestinal wall (Chen et al., 2020).

7.3.2 Terpenes and terpenoids

Terpenoids and terpenes are a group of compounds with a carbon backbone and are found especially in the essential oils of plants. Structurally, terpenes consist of a carbon backbone of 2-methylbuta-1,3-diene (isoprene units) and can rearrange into cyclic structures (Hyldgaard et al., 2012). This structural variation in terpenes is mostly caused by the number of isoprene units. Based on this, there are six groups of compounds: monoterpenes (C10), sesquiterpenes (C15), diterpenes (C20), triterpenes (C30), tetraterpenes (C40), and hemiterpenes (one unit of isoprene at C5) (Masyita et al., 2022). Some examples of terpenes are tiglic, angelic, isovaleric, and so on.

Terpenoids, on the other hand, are metabolites derived from terpenes and contain oxygen and several cyclic groups in them. Terpenoids are the form of terpenes and have certain additional functional groups like alcohols, carboxylic acids, and esters. Terpenoids are classified into several groups, including phenols, epoxides, alcohols, aldehydes, esters, and ethers. Carvacrol, geraniol, citronellal, piperitone, linalool, thymol, and menthol are some examples of terpenoids. Numerous biological activities are conferred by these bioactive compounds, including antibacterial, antioxidant, anticancer, and antiallergic (Banwo et al., 2021; Masyita et al., 2022). Terpenoids are either semivolatile or nonvolatile, in contrast to terpenes, which are known for being volatile. Terpenes and terpenoids can be found in a variety of foods, such as lemons, lavender, oranges, pepper, green tea, basil, bay leaves, parsley, pine, cannabis, and hops (Banwo et al., 2021).

Likewise, there are certain compounds classified as phenylpropanoids, which contain a six-carbon aromatic phenol group that is attached to the three-carbon propene tail of cinnamic acid. These compounds are often oxygenated in the third, fourth, or fifth position and have a carbon–carbon double bond. Anethole, eugenol, isoeugenol, cinnamaldehyde, myristicin, vanillin, and safrole are some examples of phenylpropanoids. These compounds have certain biological properties, such as myristicin, which has antiproliferative and antiinflammatory effects, and safrole, which shows analgesic, antibacterial, and antidiabetic effects (Masyita et al., 2022).

7.3.3 Phytosterols

Phytosterols are phytosteroids that include plant stanols and sterols and have similar structural and biological functions to cholesterol. Phytosterols belong to the triterpene family, which differs from cholesterol in one aspect as it possesses an extra side chain (Feng et al., 2020). Structurally, phytosterols have a long, flexible side chain at the C-17 carbon atom in the tetracyclic cyclopenta[α]phenanthrene ring. Compared to cholesterol, phytosterols are relatively more hydrophobic due to their side chain, which is made up of nine or ten carbons (Nattagh-Eshtivani et al., 2022). So far, over 250 distinct phytosterols have been identified, with the most prevalent forms being campesterol, stigmasterol, and β-sitosterol. In plant tissues, free and conjugated sterols are the most common forms of phytosterol, where the conjugated forms are classified as steryl glycosides, steryl esters, and acylated steryl glycosides. These compounds are found in the cell membranes of plants and are responsible for regulating cell membrane permeability and fluidity. They are found in almost all plant-based food sources. Campesterol (24α-methylcholesterol), stigmasterol (Δ22, 24α-ethylcholesterol), and sitosterol (24α-ethylcholesterol) are the three most common phytosterols that are available in our diet (Feng et al., 2020). Numerous investigations have documented the protective properties of phytosterols against a number of chronic diseases, including diabetes and cardiovascular disease.

7.3.4 Capsaicinoids and capsinoid compounds

Capsaicinoids, a group of molecules, are acid amides with branched-chain fatty acids (C9–C11) and vanillylamide acids. These compounds are present in plants of the genus Capsicum and impart a pungent sensation to the plant. Capsaicinoids have more than 10 structures, and capsaicin and dihydrocapsaicin are the most abundant among others. These compounds have excellent pharmacological properties. Compound capsaicin acts on the sensory receptor and sensory neurons by influencing the release of neuropeptides (calcitonin gene-related peptide and substance P) and transient receptor potential vanilloid subtype 1 (TRPV1), resulting in different neurophysical functions (Suntrup-Krueger et al., 2021; Whiting et al., 2012). Apart from this, it also has different metabolic health-promoting functions.

7.3.5 Alkaloids

Alkaloids are a class of diverse low-molecular-weight molecules with heterocyclic structures containing nitrogen. The heterocyclic structures, including piperidine and isoquinoline, give alkaloids distinct flavors and potent biological functions. Alkaloids are usually derived from amino acids found in plants, animals, and microbes. The structure and bioactivity of alkaloids are largely dependent on the techniques used for their extraction and purification. Indole, tropane, pyrrolidine, quinolone, izidine, and isoquinolone are the six main groups of alkaloids (Banwo et al., 2021). Indole is predominantly found in jasmine and orange blossom; quinolone is found in Howard and *Calendula officinalis* L.; and tropane is found in plant families of erythroxylaceae (cocaine, erythroxylum coca, etc.), *solanaceae*, and *convolvulaceae* (Thawabteh et al., 2019; Smolinske et al., 2007). Essential bioactive alkaloids called isoquinolones are found in herbal medicinal plants like the opium poppy, *Citrus aurantium*, *Papaver somniferum* L., and *Pausinystalia yohimbe* which is used to synthesize the analgesic morphine (Banwo et al., 2021). These alkaloids have diverse functions as stimulants, antiinflammatory agents, sports performance enhancers, and so on.

7.3.6 Vitamins

Vitamins are organic molecules having bioactive properties that are involved in several biochemical and metabolic pathways in the human body, including the regulation of gene expression, the control of enzymatic and chemical reactions, carbohydrates, and protein metabolism. Additionally, certain vitamins have antioxidant properties that combat the detrimental effects of free radicals. The most common sources of these vitamins include different plant and animal derivatives. These vitamins can be broadly divided into two groups: hydrophilic (vitamins B-complex and C) and hydrophobic (vitamins A, E, D, and K). Lipophilic vitamins are polypentadiene compounds with thick rings or long hydrocarbon chains that contain ring structures and long aliphatic hydrocarbons. These lipophilic vitamins are necessary for physiological functions such as promoting healthy bone development, combating free radicals, and so on (An et al., 2023). All water-soluble vitamins, however, serve as cofactors for enzymes, possibly improving energy metabolism. Vitamin A includes vitamers retinol, retinal, retinoic acid, and carotenoids, where carotenoids show excellent free radical inhibition properties. Likewise, two forms of vitamin D, cholecalciferol (vitamin D3) and ergocalciferol (vitamin D2), have been proven to have significant biological benefits for humans, which facilitate intestinal absorption, maintain homeostasis of calcium, and aid in parathyroid hormone's normal activity. It is also expressed in white blood cell activation (T and B cells and monocytes). Likewise, vitamin E, a strong antioxidant, is classified as a tocopherol, and tocotrienols have protective activity against DNA oxidation, LDL, and fatty acids, as well as modulating the immune system.

The B-complex vitamins are water-soluble vitamins that include thiamine (B1), riboflavin (B2), niacin (B3), choline (B4), pantothenic acid (B5), pyridoxine (B6), biotin (B8), folate (B9), and cobalamin (B12). B vitamins are primarily involved in metabolism, immune system activation, digestion, and cell repair. Vitamin B is essential for tissues since it acts as a cofactor for enzymes involved in several metabolic pathways. Vitamin C, also known as ascorbic acid, is also a water-soluble vitamin present in different vegetables and fruits. Vitamin C particularly acts as an antioxidant, protecting from oxidative damage and also participating in nonoxidative stress function.

7.3.7 Bioactive peptides

The short peptide chains, comprising two to twenty amino acids and a molar mass lower than 60 kD, are the key characteristic of the bioactive peptides. They are synthesized during the food processing process by the proteolytic clipping of proteins from animal, plant, and/or microbiological sources by both endogenous and exogenous enzymes (Toldrá et al., 2018). The functional potency of these peptides is determined by sequence, affinity after proteolysis, protein source, and N- and C-terminal amino acids (Koirala et al., 2023). The specific amino acids found in the peptide sequence that have excellent radical scavenger properties—phenylalanine, histidine, cysteine, lysine, methionine, proline, isoleucine, tyrosine, threonine, tryptophan, alanine, and leucine—have been associated with the antioxidant and antiinflammatory activity of peptides (Fan et al., 2022).

Plant protein and milk protein-derived peptides have promising metabolic health benefits, such as antioxidative, antiinflammatory, appetite-regulating, antidiabetic, antihypertensive, and antihypercholesterolemic. These peptides have the potential to treat metabolic syndrome because of their effects on various physiological systems, which include the immunological, endocrine, circulatory, and cardiovascular systems (Fan et al., 2022; Koirala et al., 2023). The biological activities of bioactive peptides are achieved via the modulation of several signaling pathways and molecular mechanisms, such as sterol regulatory element binding protein 1, CCAAT/enhancer-binding protein-α, and peroxisome proliferator-activated-γ in obesity; ACE inhibition in hypertension; Kelch-like ECH-associated protein 1/nuclear factor erythroid 2-related factor 2/antioxidant response element *in oxidative stress*; and AMP-activated protein kinase and insulin receptor substrate-1/phosphatidylinositol 3-kinase/protein kinase B in diabetes (Qiao et al., 2021). In diabetes, these bioactive peptides are essential for regulating cholecystokinin, a hormone that stimulates the release of pancreatic enzymes, glucose absorption, insulin signaling, adipocyte differentiation, and even insulin hormone mimicking (Samtiya et al., 2022).

7.3.8 Bioactive polysaccharides

Polysaccharides are macromolecules that consist of repeating units called monosaccharides, ranging from 20 to 10,000. Polysaccharides can be categorized as xyloglucan, glucan, arabinoxylan, glucomannan, and pectin based on their chemical composition. Based on dietary sources, it is also often classified as animal-, plant-, and microbe-derived polysaccharides. (Shi et al., 2023). Xanthan gum, guar gum, inulin, arabinogalactan, glucomannan, carrageenan, xylan, araboxylan, fucoidan, and glucan are a few of the extensively researched bioactive polysaccharides. Marine plants and animals are abundant sources of bioactive polysaccharides, which are present either in sulfated or nonsulfated forms. The monosaccharides in the polysaccharides are linked to each other by glycosidic linkage. The repeating units are of the same monosaccharide; they are defined as homopolysaccharides, while units with different monosaccharides are heteropolysaccharides (Hentati et al., 2020). The biological activity of these polysaccharides is significantly dependent on its source and repeating units.

7.3.9 Role of functional components in metabolic health

Bioactive compounds typically have strong antiinflammatory and antioxidative properties. Free radicals are neutralized by bioactive compounds in a number of ways, such as by chelating metal ions, giving protons and/or electrons, inhibiting lipid peroxidation, and boosting the body's natural antioxidant defense mechanism (Wen et al., 2020). In vivo, the regulation of antioxidant pathways (Keap1-Nrf2-ARE, NF-κB, mitogen-activated protein kinase, and many more) is signaled by ROS, and bioactive compounds can regulate these signaling pathways (Lv et al., 2022). The potential mechanism of bioactive compounds for the prevention of metabolic diseases (Fig. 7.2) has been elaborated on in the following section, along with examples of the recently identified bioactivity of functional compounds (Table 7.1).

7.3.10 Obesity/overweight

7.3.10.1 Flavonoids

Different studies have shown that flavonoids reduce the size of adipose tissues, stimulate beta-oxidation, and reduce adipogenesis and lipogenesis by decreasing the expression of LPL, SREBP1c, and PPAR-γ (Shirakura et al., 2011).

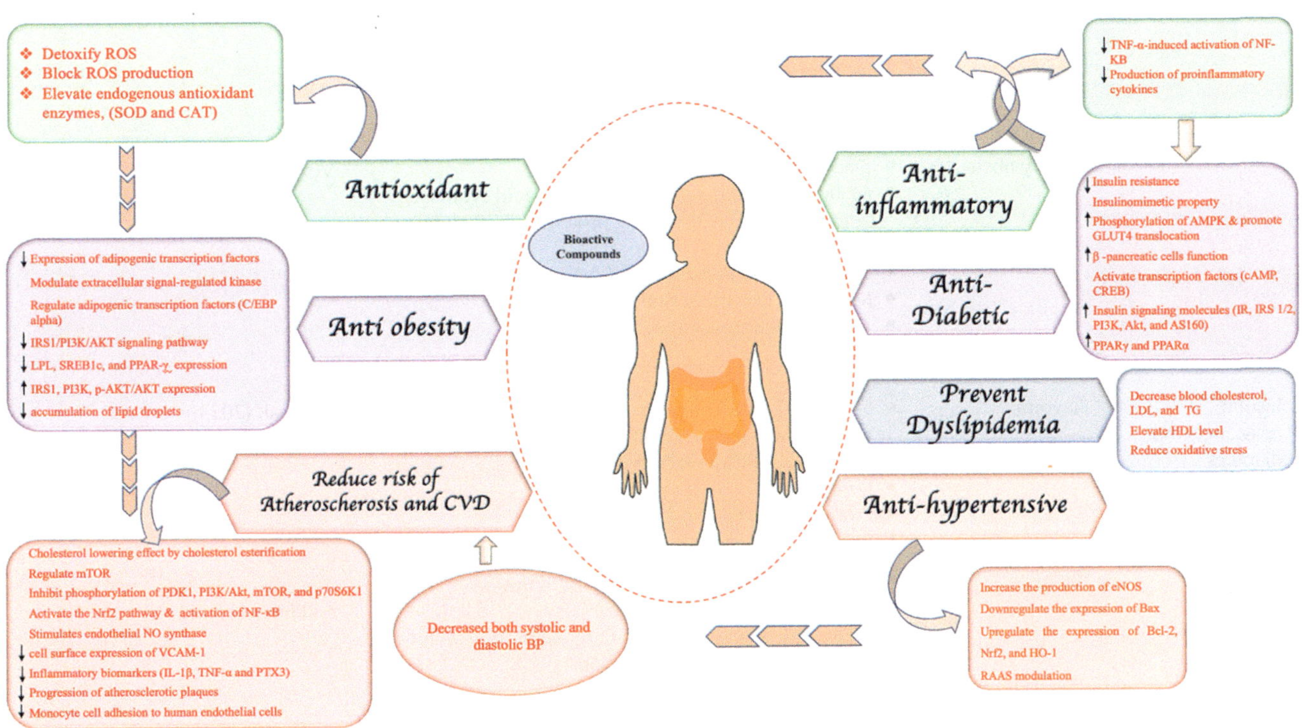

FIGURE 7.2 Different role of bioactive compounds in maintenanc of metabolic diseases.

TABLE 7.1 Recent updates in the promising role of phytonutrient in metabolic diseases prevention and treatment.

Metabolic Condition	Bioactive Compounds	Metabolism Health Promoting Mechanism	References
Obesity and overweight	Carotenoids	• Downregulate gene expression of adipocytes • Downregulate adipocyte differentiation • Regulate C/EBP alpha and PPAR-γ	Inoue et al. (2012) and Shirakura et al. (2011)
	Flavonoids	• Increase the expression of PPAR-alpha • Decrease the expression of LPL, SREBP-1c, and PPAR-γ • Induces apoptosis of mature adipocytes	Kim et al. (2017)
	Vitamins	• Vitamin D enhances adipocyte differentiation and lipid accumulation • Retinoic acid inhibits C/EBP-dependent gene transcription and PPAR-γ	Cordeiro et al. (2022)
	Capsaicinoids	• Agonist of TRP channels, activate UCP1 • Increase RMR, thermogenesis • Fat oxidation	Irandoost et al. (2021)
	Alkaloids	• Inhibit CD-36 and PPAR-gamma • Promote PPAR-alpha, adiponectin • Promote beta oxidation • Modulate firmicutes to the bacteroides ratio • Upregulate the expression of IRS1, PI3K, p-AKT/AKT • Downregulate the expression of SREBP-1c	He et al. (2022) and Liu et al. (2023)
	Bioactive polysaccharides	• Suppress upregulation of ACC1, FAS, PPAR-γ, SCD1, SREBP-1c, and C/EBP alpha • Modulates gut microbiota • Increase SCFA production • Stimulate GLP-1 • Activate brown fat tissue	Yu et al. (2022)
	Bioactive peptides	• Reduce the mRNA expression of FAS, --Increase fat excretion • Increase the release of cholecystokinin, gastrin • Inhibit C/EBPs • Decrease the expression of PPAR-γ • Activate Wnt/β-catenin pathway	
	Dietary fibers	• Decreased fat absorption • Modulate resistin, adiponectin, fatty acid synthase, adipocyte fatty acid binding protein, C/EBP alpha, PPAR-γ • Downregulate PI3K/Akt, ERK pathway • Modulate foxo transcription factor • Activate Wnt/Beta-catenin	Vezza et al. (2020)
	Polyphenols	• Decrease G3P, inhibit PPAR-γ	
Insulin resistance and diabetes	Flavonoids	• Stimulate glucose uptake in adipocytes and myocytes via the PI3K/Akt pathway • Increase AMPK phosphorylation • Improve oxidative stress • Promote GLUT4 translocation • Inhibit NF-kb cascade	An et al. (2023)
	Vitamins	• Vitamin D improve the sensitivity of insulin receptors to insulin • Vitamin D Binds to vitamin-D receptor in beta-cells, helping release insulin secretion	Asbaghi et al. (2019) and Rafiq and Jeppesen (2021)

(Continued)

TABLE 7.1 (Continued)

Metabolic Condition	Bioactive Compounds	Metabolism Health Promoting Mechanism	References
	Carotenoids	• Upregulate SHBG • Upregulate GLUT3, GLUT4, and IRS-1	Li et al. (2022)
	Capsaicinoids	• Modulates CAMKK2, AMPK, • Activate transcription factors such as CREB • Stimulate GLUT4	Ferdowsi et al. (2023)
	Alkaloids	• Activate AMPK pathway, • Activate protein kinase • Decrease the activity of the alpha-glucosidase enzyme • Reduce free radical • Improve the functioning of beta pancreatic cells • Downregulate PPAR-γ and upregulate PPAR- alpha	El-Nashar et al. (2021), Gjorgieva Ackova et al. (2023), and Zafar et al. (2016)
	Bioactive polysaccharides	• Increase IR, IRS-2, Akt and GLUT4 expression level. • Reduce beta cell dysfunction, elevate beta cell mass • Activate PI3/Akt and MAPK/ERK pathways	Ganesan and Xu (2019)
	Bioactive peptides	• Upregulate Akt phosphorylation, ERK½ phosphorylation • Increase phosphorylation of IRS-1 stimulating GLUT4 • Suppress appetite by controlling hormones such as CCK, GLP-1, and peptide YY	Jahandideh and Wu (2022)
	Dietary fibers	• Decrease gut glucose absorption. • Enhance IR, IRS-1, PI3K, Akt and AS160, GLUT4 • Suppress inflammation	Prasad et al. (2022)
	Polyphenols	• Inhibit intestinal glucose transport	
Hyperlipidemia	Polyphenols	• Inhibit plasma CETP activity • Reduce systemic cholesterol production by promoting fecal bile acid excretion • Inhibit the intestinal expression of NPC1L1, elevate hepatic LDLR • Activate JNK and SREBP2 pathway • Inhibit Apo-b, HMGR and the activity of ACAT	Sun et al. (2021)
	Flavonoids	• Suppress inflammation, oxidative stress • Inhibit VCAM-1 and ICAM • Regulate cellular cholesterol efflux, and hepatic paraoxonase-1 expression	Zeka et al. (2017)
	Capsaicinoids	• Increase thermogenic genes such as UCP-2, BMP8b, SIRT-1, PGC-1 alpha, PRDM-16 and trpv1 • Inhibit PPAR-γ and C/EBP alpha • Inhibit the expression of leptin • Induce upregulation of adiponectin	Baskaran et al. (2017)
	Alkaloids	• Increase LDL-receptor • Inhibit ERK and PCSK9 • Promote cholesterol excretion • Inhibit enterocyte cholesterol uptake • Regulate bile acid synthesis by increasing hepatic expression of mitochondrial sterol 27- hydroxylase, 7 alpha-hydroxylase • Inhibit HMG-CoA • Upregulate CPT-1 alpha gene	Wang and Zidichouski (2018)

(Continued)

TABLE 7.1 (Continued)

Metabolic Condition	Bioactive Compounds	Metabolism Health Promoting Mechanism	References
	Bioactive polysaccharides	• Upregulate AMPK-alpha • Downregulate acetyl CoA carboxylase, SREBP-1c, and β-hydroxy-β-methylglutaryl coenzyme A • Increase viscosity of intestinal lumen affecting the diffusion of micelles to the intestinal epithelium • Sequester bile salts • Promote SCFA production interfering with cholesterol biosynthesis	Silva et al. (2021)
	Bioactive peptides	• Upregulate the expression of ABCG5 and ABCG8, FGF15/19 • Downregulate those of CYP7A1 and CYP8B • Inhibit FAS, HMG-CoA reductase • Downregulate PPAR-γ, SREBP-1 • Upregulate LXR-alpha • Decrease apoB and increase apoA1 levels	Ma et al. (2023)
	Dietary fibers	• Reduce cholesterol absorption • Reduces cholesterol esterification by affecting the expression of ACAT2, MTP • Inhibit LDLR and LRP1 • Regulate HMG-CoA reductase • Promote LXR-alpha expression	Li et al. (2022)
	Vitamins	• Decrease the production of angiotensin-II • Decrease oxidative stress • Prevents proliferation of pathological fibrous and fatty atheroma • Pantothenic acid- a part of CoA, promotes fat oxidation • Vitamin E prevent oxidative damage of lipids and endothelial cells • Vitamin K regulates clotting and calcium deposition in blood vessel	Surdu et al. (2021) and Tang et al. (2021)

Additionally, it decreases the expression of adipogenic transcription factors and induces the apoptosis of mature adipocytes through the modulation of the extracellular signal-regulated kinase. In accordance with these mechanisms, a study by Solverson et al. (2018) showed that participants consuming 600 g/day of blackberries (1500 mg/day flavonoids) for seven days lowered respiration quotient and increased fat oxidation in overweight and obese people. Yousefi et al. (2021) showed that supplementing grape seed extract (300 mg/day) for 12 weeks significantly decreased the visceral adiposity index compared with the baseline in overweight and obese individuals. During 40% VO2max exercise and in the recovery period, a single dose (600 mg) of licorice flavonoid oil showed a decrease in respiratory exchange ratio, indicating improved fat oxidation with the supplementation (Mori et al., 2015).

7.3.10.2 Nonflavonoids polyphenols

Polyphenols are known to exert antilipogenic effects by inhibiting glycerol 3-phosphate. This leads to inhibiting the conversion of dihydroxyacetone phosphate to glycerol three phosphates, which serves as a backbone for triglyceride synthesis. Besides, polyphenols inhibit PPAR gamma which leads to the downregulation of gene expression relating to preadipocyte differentiation to mature adipocytes and encoding enzymes involved in fatty acid uptake, synthesis, and storage. Saraf-Bank et al. (2019) showed that consuming curcumin tablet supplementation for ten weeks significantly reduced BMI, waist circumference, and hip circumference in obese and overweight individuals. Quercetin supplementation (150 mg/day) for eight weeks in healthy male subjects with apo-E genotype led to a significant decrease in waist circumference and body mass index (Pfeuffer et al., 2013).

7.3.10.3 Carotenoids

Carotenoids are known to restrict adipogenesis and hypertrophy of adipocytes. They downregulate gene expression in adipocytes, inhibit adipocyte differentiation, and have antiadipogenic effects via regulating adipogenic transcription factors, such as C/EBP alpha and PPAR-gamma (Mounien et al., 2019). Supplementation of 20 mg/day of lutein in obese individuals for ten weeks showed a decrease in the percentage of body fat and significantly preserved fat-free mass during calorie restriction (Azzini et al., 2017). Similarly, supplementing high lycopene + low lutein for eight weeks showed significantly decreased waist circumference in obese Japanese individuals (Takagi et al., 2020).

7.3.10.4 Vitamins

Vitamins are known to have a synergistic effect on fat synthesis. Vitamin B, specifically vitamins B_1 and B_6, is required to synthesize fat from carbohydrates and proteins. Likewise, Vitamin D enhances adipocyte differentiation and lipid accumulation (Cordeiro et al., 2022), while retinoic acid increases brown adipocyte activity, brown fat production, and energy expenditure (Novin et al., 2018). Also, retinoic acid blocks adipocyte differentiation and inhibits adipogenesis, inhibiting C/EBP-dependent gene transcription and PPAR gamma activity. A dietary clinical trial with the supplementation of 1800 IU/day of vitamin D for 12 months after the bariatric surgery led to a significant decrease in visceral adiposity index compared to the 800 IU/day (Cordeiro et al., 2022). Another study, which used a four-week supplementation of a moderate deficit calorie diet, showed that the supplementation of branched chain amino acids (BCAA) (6 g/day) with 40 mg/day of vitamin B_6 led to a significant decrease in the waist-to-hip ratio, left leg, and right leg (Novin et al., 2018).

7.3.10.5 Phytosterols

Phytosterols-induced reduction in body weight is hypothesized to be associated with decreased fat absorption following the consumption of phytosterols. Besides saringosterol, a steroid isolated from edible brown algae showed antiobesity properties by modulating the expression of several adipogenic genes, such as resistin, adiponectin, fatty acid synthase, and adipocyte fatty acid binding protein, and suppressing adipocyte differentiation, possibly by impacting C/EPB alpha and PPAR gamma. Besides fucosterol has shown a reduction in the accumulation of lipid droplets, downregulation of PI3K/Akt and ERK pathway, and modulating the foxo transcription factor. Fucosterol regulates adipogenic differentiation by activating the Wnt/Beta-catenin signaling pathways and its other major components (Vezza et al., 2020). However, a randomized controlled trial where NAFLD subjects were supplemented with either 3.3 g/day phytosterol, 450 mg EPA + 1500 mg DHA/day, 3 g/day phytosterol, and 450 mg EPA + 1500 mg DHA/day for 12 weeks did not show a significant change in BMI compared to the baseline (Song et al., 2020). On the other hand, a 12-month supplementation of two sachets of Dioscorea extracts containing 12 mg/dose of phytosterol reduced the BMI (Hsu et al., 2017). Likewise, a significant reduction in waist circumference was shown with the supplementation of phytosterol in people with metabolic syndrome compared to the placebo group (Palmeiro-Silva et al., 2020).

7.3.10.6 Capsaicinoids

Studies indicate that capsaicinoids increase RMR, thermogenesis, and fat oxidation. Capsaicinoids/Capsinoids act as agonists of TRP channels and activate the sympathetic nervous system, which in turn triggers uncoupling protein 1 (UCP1) as a thermogenic gene (TRP-SNS-UCP1 pathway). In accordance with this mechanism, a systematic review of RCT concluded that the supplementation of capsaicin significantly decreases BMI, waist circumference, and body weight. The study showed that supplementing healthy overweight subjects with capsifen (4 mg capsaicinoids/day) for 28 days decreased 2.1% of body weight, 4% of waist-to-hip ratio, and 2.2% of BMI compared to placebo (An et al., 2023). Another study, however, showed no effect of Kochujang (32 g/day) supplementation for 12 weeks on overweight/obese subjects and showed no effect on body composition (Cha et al., 2013).

7.3.10.7 Alkaloids

Alkaloids such as Sangzhi-A inhibited CD36 and mRNA expression of PPAR gamma while promoting mRNA expression of PPAR alpha and adiponectin secretion, suggesting that Sangzhi-A may decrease hepatic lipid accumulation and steatosis by inhibiting de novo lipogenesis and fatty acid uptake while promoting β-oxidation. The same study indicated a decrease in body weight in Sangzhi-A -treated mice compared to the control group. Moreover, a change in the gut microbiota composition was seen after treatment with Sangzhi-A, which involves modulating the ratio of firmicutes to the Bacteroides ratio, where firmicutes have strong energy utilization efficiency. In contrast, Bacteroides have low nutrient absorption efficiency. Jatrorrhizine exerted an antiobesity effect through the IRS1/PI3K/AKT signaling pathway (upregulate IRS1, PI3K, p-AKT/AKT expression; downregulates SREBP-1c expression). However, a randomized controlled trial with 16 weeks of supplementation of Sangzhi-A showed no effect on body weight and BMI compared to the placebo (Qu et al., 2022).

7.3.10.8 Bioactive polysaccharides

The possible mechanism of bioactive polysaccharides supplementation alleviating hepatic triglyceride production and accumulation is through upregulating lipolysis-degrading enzymes, boosting fatty acid β-oxidation, and inhibiting lipogenic enzyme production in the liver. Lycium barbarum polysaccharide supplementation has shown suppression of ACC1, FAS, PPAR-γ, SCD1, SREBP-1c, and C/ebpα expression in adipose tissues of high-fat diet-fed mice. SREBP-1c can mediate the expression of fatty acid synthesis genes and activate lipogenic transcription factors such as ACC1, FAS, and SCD1, which subsequently induces lipogenesis and the accumulation of lipids. Besides, it modulates the gut microbiota, which regulates energy homeostasis. Polysaccharides also increase short-chain fatty acid production, stimulating glucagon-like peptide-1 production and activating brown fat tissue, leading to sustained satiety and fat oxidation enhancement. However, supplementation with 10 g inulin plus 10 g resistant maltodextrin or 20 g of placebo with a 500 kcal/day energy-restricted diet showed no significant differences in weight loss or body composition between the groups (Hess et al., 2020). But 4.5 g polyGlycopleX as soft gels, 5 g as granules, or 5 g rice flour control supplementation for 12 weeks showed a reduction in body weight (−1.4 kg) and BMI reduction (−0.5) (Onakpoya & Heneghan, 2015).

7.3.10.9 Bioactive peptides

Soybean peptides have been used extensively in food items for their body fat-decreasing properties. Isolates from soy protein reduce the mRNA expression of fatty acid synthase in adipose tissue in Wistar rats, while soy isolate hydrolysate decreases fat accumulation by increasing fat excretion in rats (Aoyama et al., 2000). Protease and pepsin-prepared egg white hydrolysates reduced total body fat in rats (Garcés-Rimón et al., 2016). Zhang and Beynen reported that whey protein increased the release of cholecystokinin, also known as the appetite-suppressing hormone (Zhang & Beynen, 1993). Antiappetizing peptides from milk suppress appetite and thus prevent weight gain and obesity. Some marine peptides also release gastrin and cholecystokinin and/or stimulate their release, resulting in appetite control (Cudennec et al., 2008). Peptides from boiled tuna inhibited CCAAT/enhancer-binding proteins (C/EBPs). These peptides, including peptides GlyProLeu and IleTyr, decrease the expression of PPAR-γ, which causes activation of the Wnt/β-catenin pathway, inhibiting preadipocytes differentiation into fat globule cells (Kim et al., 2015).

7.3.11 Insulin resistance and diabetes

7.3.11.1 Flavonoids

Flavanol extracted from grape seeds has shown an insulino-mimetic property by stimulating glucose uptake in adipocytes and myocytes via the PI3K/Akt pathway (Pinent et al., 2004). EGCG increased the phosphorylation of AMPK and improved oxidative stress, promoting GLUT4 translocation (An et al., 2023). Additionally, EGCG inhibited TNF-α-induced activation of nuclear factor kappa-light-chain-enhancer of activated B cells (NF-kb) signaling cascade, which decreased insulin resistance; quercetin improved insulin signaling, leading to the restoration of AS160 phosphorylation and GLUT4 translocation (An et al., 2023). A similar effect was shown in type 2 diabetes patients, where 500 mg rutin supplementation for three months led to decreased fasting blood glucose, insulin, HbA1c, and HOMA-IR in the rutin group compared with the placebo group (Bazyar et al., 2023).

7.3.11.2 Nonflavonoids polyphenols

In healthy participants, either water or cacao polyphenol-rich chocolate plus water was given 15 min before a 50 g oral glucose tolerance test. The incremental plasma glucose for the polyphenol group was significantly lower, while the incremental serum insulin and plasma GLP-1 AUC did not differ significantly between groups (Kawakami et al., 2021). Similarly, a study on postmenopausal women showed that after consuming 600 mg apple polyphenol + 600 mg blackcurrant anthocyanins-rich diet with a starch and sucrose meal, there was a significant reduction in insulin, C-peptide, and gastric inhibitory polypeptide concentrations relative to control (Castro-Acosta et al., 2017). The mechanism is assumed to be related to inhibition of intestinal glucose transport.

7.3.11.3 Carotenoids

Beta-carotene is known to improve insulin sensitivity by promoting the expression of sex hormone-binding globulin, which upregulates GLUT3, GLUT4, and IRS-1 and enhances glucose consumption in insulin-resistant cells (Li et al., 2022). The effect of daily supplementation of mixed carotenoids containing a mixture of zeaxanthin, lycopene, astaxanthin, and γ-tocopherol or placebo was observed in obese children. The study showed a decrease in HOMAIR at three weeks and six months compared to placebo (Canas et al., 2017). In another study, patients under methadone maintenance treatment received either 15 mg/day of crocin or placebo two times/day for eight weeks, where crocin administration resulted in a significant reduction in fasting glucose, insulin levels, insulin resistance, and a significant increase in insulin sensitivity compared with the placebo (Ghaderi et al., 2019).

7.3.11.4 Vitamins

Vitamin D is an epigenetic factor affecting the transcription level of genes involved in insulin sensitivity, like insulin receptor substrate (IRS). Vitamin D improves the sensitivity of insulin receptors to insulin and glucose transport and promotes the conversion of proinsulin to insulin (Rafiq & Jeppesen, 2021). Besides, vitamin D binds to VDR in β-cells, helping to release insulin secretion; also, binding to VDR regulates calcium flux, which strongly regulates calcium (Asbaghi et al., 2019; Rafiq & Jeppesen, 2021). However, in overweight/obese individuals, vitamin D3 4000 IU was supplemented for 24 months which showed no significant changes in HOMAIR between the two groups (Mesinovic et al., 2023). Likewise, in adults with prediabetes and vitamin D deficiency, the supplementation of vitamin D3 for six months showed no significant difference between fasting glucose or 2 h-OGTT postprandial glucose in the two groups. However, the HOMA-IR score was significantly lower in the vitamin D group (Niroomand et al., 2019). In another study, a single dose of 300,000 IU cholecalciferol followed by 1400 IU cholecalciferol + 500 mg of calcium daily for 150 days led to 13% lower fasting serum insulin concentrations than the placebo-treated group and 19% lower HOMA-IR (Holt et al., 2024).

7.3.11.5 Alkaloid

The antidiabetic effect of alkaloids was mediated by activating the AMP pathway, activating protein kinase, which leads to the translocation of GLUT4 (El-Nashar et al., 2021). Additionally, these alkaloids decrease the activity of the α-glucosidase enzyme, reducing glucose absorption in the body (Zafar et al., 2016). The antioxidant effect of alkaloids also reduces free radicals, improving the functioning of beta-pancreatic cells and upregulating the PPAR-γ and PPAR-α (Gjorgieva Ackova et al., 2023). In accordance with that, supplementation of Berberine phytosome (2 tablets/day, 550 mg/tablet) for 90 days in overweight and obese individuals showed a significance decrease in plasma glucose and insulin compared to the placebo group (Rondanelli et al., 2023). Likewise, a placebo-controlled study showed that berberine supplementation on overweight/obese patients with type 2 diabetes mellitus (T2DM) for six months decreased HOMAIR, blood glucose, and insulin compared to the baseline (Guarino et al., 2017).

7.3.11.6 Capsaicinoids

Capsaicin improves glucose metabolism by elevating insulin sensitivity, reducing inflammatory factors, increasing fatty acid oxidation, and stimulating insulin secretion from pancreatic β cells.

Moreover, it modulates calcium/calmodulin-dependent protein kinase 2 (CaMKK2) and AMP-activated protein kinase (AMPK) pathway, activating transcription factors such as CREB eventually, stimulating glucose uptake and GLUT4 translocation to the cell membrane (Ferdowsi et al., 2023). However, a study on low (2 mg/day) and high (4 mg/day) capsimax or placebo for 12 weeks did not affect the insulin response and sensitivity after an OGTT (Urbina et al., 2017). On the other hand, when pregnant women with GDM were supplemented with 5 mg/day of capsaicin for four weeks, there was a decrease in 2-h postprandial insulin concentrations, HOMAIR (Yuan et al., 2016). Similarly, supplementing meals containing chili (5 · 82 mg total capsaicinoids) showed a smaller decrease in insulin AUC and glucose AUC postprandially (Kroff et al., 2017).

7.3.11.7 Phytosterol and dietary fiber

B-sitosterol is known to lower blood glucose by decreasing gut glucose absorption or increasing the glycogenic and glycolytic pathways with a corresponding reduction in the gluconeogenesis and glycogenolysis pathways. Phytosterol enhances insulin signaling molecules, such as IR, IRS 1/2, PI3K, Akt, and AS160, which promotes GLUT4 synthesis and glucose absorption and suppresses inflammatory events, affecting insulin signaling and sensitivity (Prasad et al., 2022).

For example, when pregnant women suffering from GDM were given margarine spread with phytosterols daily for 16 weeks, they showed a significant reduction in fasting plasma glucose, serum insulin levels, the quantitative insulin check index, HOMAIR, and β-cell function (Li & Xing, 2016). Likewise, 8 weeks of dietary fiber supplementation showed markedly improved postprandial blood glucose levels and reduced incidence of impaired glucose tolerance compared to the control group (Zhang et al., 2021). Likewise, the 5.6 g of RPG (R + PolyGly) dietary fiber consumption in 12 healthy subjects showed improved satiety, increased GLP-1 after a high glucose meal, and reduced postprandial blood glucose but increased serum insulin and insulin AUC (Wu et al., 2023).

7.3.11.8 Bioactive polysaccharide

Bioactive polysaccharides stimulate the insulin-signaling pathway and increase IRS-2, Akt, and GLUT4 expression levels, stimulating glycogen synthesis. Polysaccharides have also shown reduced beta cell dysfunction, elevated beta cell mass, and enhanced glucose uptake by activating the PI3K/Akt and MAPK−ERK pathways (Ganesan & Xu, 2019). For example, supplementation of 8 g and 16 g of galactomannan derivative significantly improved 2-h postprandial glucose levels compared to the baseline in type 2 diabetes mellitus (Trask et al., 2014). In another study, in healthy adults, there was a 33% reduction in postprandial glucose iAUC in the fiber-rich muffin group (11.6 TDF fiber), while only an 8% decrease was seen in the control group (0.9 g). Likewise, a decrease in serum iAUC was seen in the fiber muffin group compared to the control muffin top (Stewart & Zimmer, 2018). In a study, 100 g standard noodles (polysaccharide), with 75 g carbohydrates, increased incretin in type 2 diabetes patients (Deng et al., 2015).

7.3.11.9 Bioactive peptides

Egg white hydrolysate has shown insulin effects on the upregulation of Akt phosphorylation (insulin sensitizing) and increased ERK1/2 phosphorylation to a level similar to that of insulin (insulin-mimetic). Treatment of insulin-resistant muscle cells with egg white hydrolysate reversed insulin resistance through increased phosphorylation of IRS-1 (at tyrosine residue) and Akt as well as decreased IRS-1 serine residue phosphorylation, which stimulates GLUT4 abundance on the muscle cell membrane and by recovering TMF-induced impaired glucose uptake. Similarly, whey protein hydrolysate showed enhanced GLUT-4 translocation and glycogen synthesis. Some peptides suppress appetite by controlling hormones, such as CCK, GLP-1, and peptide YY, inhibiting food intake, gastric emptying, and energy homeostasis, eventually improving insulin sensitivity (Jahandideh & Wu, 2022).

7.3.12 Cholesterol and lipid disorders

7.3.12.1 Flavonoids

Flavonoids exert antiatherogenic effects by lowering lipids, suppressing inflammation and oxidative stress, and inhibiting adhesion molecules such as VCAM-1 and ICAM. The mechanism is likely due to a decrease in the production of vascular oxygen through directly scavenging oxygen and preventing the gene expressions associated with increased oxygen production. Besides, flavonoids regulate cellular cholesterol efflux from macrophages, hepatic paraoxonase-1 expression, and their antiatherogenic activity (Zeka et al., 2017). For example—12 weeks of supplementation of high-dose freeze-dried strawberries (50 g/day) decreased serum total and LDL-cholesterol compared to the control group with a similar fiber content (Basu et al., 2014). Another study on older subjects showed that consuming flavonoid-rich beverages once/day for up to 12 weeks improved glycemia, triglyceridemia, HDL, LDL, and oxidative stress markers (Munguia et al., 2019). Another study with the supplementation of 500 mg rutin showed significantly lower LDL, cholesterol, and fasting blood glucose in type 2 diabetes while HDL increased compared with the placebo group (Bazyar et al., 2023).

7.3.12.2 Nonflavonoid polyphenols

Anthocyanins have shown inhibition of the plasma CETP activity, reduced cholesterol absorption, and mediate bile acid metabolism, improving total cholesterol. Cyanidin-3-o-β-glucoside and curcumin inhibit systemic cholesterol production by promoting fecal bile acid excretion and inhibiting the intestinal expression of NPC1L1, respectively. Curcumin also elevates the expression of hepatic LDLR, activating the JNK signaling pathway and SREBP2 processing, followed by upregulation of LDLR. Also, decreased secretion of apob, inhibition of the expression of HMG-CoA-reductase, and the activity of ACAT were seen with the treatment with genistein (Sun et al., 2021). In an RCT on overweight and obese individuals, it was shown that consuming 450 mL of polyphenol cranberry extract beverage for eight weeks led to a significant reduction of fasting CRP, serum insulin, and increased HDL cholesterol compared to placebo (Chew et al., 2019). In another study of postmenopausal women, 400 mg EGCG or 800 mg EGCG supplemented for two months led to significantly decreased LDL-C in both groups and a significantly different LDL-C in EGCG group compared to placebo. Glucose and insulin decreased in EGCG groups but increased in the placebo (Wu et al., 2012). Similarly, another study where 19.2 mg resveratrol +136 mg polyphenols were supplemented daily for 8 weeks led to significant decrement in LDL-C, TG, IL-6, and Sirt1, and increment in p-AMPK expression indicates improved lipid metabolism (Kitada et al., 2020).

7.3.12.3 Carotenoids

Carotenoids are associated with reducing oxidative stress and ROS as they have higher electron transfer capacity. This leads to an increase in the bioavailability of NO, improving endothelium-dependent vasodilation and preventing the oxidation of protein lipids, DNA, and mitochondrial damage. In addition, carotenoids reduce expression of ICAM-1 and interaction between monocytes and endothelial cells, improving the CVD. Besides, carotenoids are involved in reducing levels of inflammation and downregulate COX-2, impairing PGE2, and reducing the progression of CVD (do Nascimento et al., 2020; Mozos et al., 2018). Beta-carotene fortified symbiotic was supplemented for 6 weeks, which led to a detectable decrease in insulin, HOMA-IR, triglycerides, VLDL-cholesterol, and total cholesterol/HDL ratio compared to the beta-carotene deficient diet. Moreover, beta-carotene fortified foods led to increased plasma NO and glutathione, all of which indicate improved cardiovascular and lipid metabolism (Asemi et al., 2016). Another study where 5 g/day of chlorella was supplemented for 4-week led to a remarkable decrease in total cholesterol, VLDL, TG, lutein/zeaxanthin, and alpha-carotene compared to the control group, which is possibly due to inhibition of the absorption of dietary and endogenous lipids in the intestine (Ryu et al., 2014). A 20 mg/day of lutein was supplemented for ten weeks, which led to a decrease in TC, LDL-C, and visceral fat. A statistical difference between the placebo and lutein group was observed for total cholesterol (Hajizadeh-Sharafabad et al., 2021).

7.3.12.4 Vitamins

Vitamin D promotes cardiovascular health by reducing antiinflammatory markers that impact activation of endothelial adhesion and vascular tone. It also decreased the production of angiotensin II, which decreases oxidative stress and inhibits cellular senescence, preventing the proliferation of pathological fibrous and fatty atheroma and atherogenesis (Surdu et al., 2021). Pantothenic acid promotes fat oxidation as a component of CoA required for converting fatty acids to their acyl-CoA derivatives. Vitamin B7 regulates the synthesis of fatty acid. Vitamin E improves cardiovascular health through its antioxidative properties, preventing oxidative damage of lipids and endothelial cells and preventing the initiation of atherosclerosis. Lastly, vitamin K regulates lipid metabolism and cardiovascular health by playing a role in clotting function and regulating calcium deposition in blood vessels (Fidanza & Audisio, 1982). However, a RCT showed that supplementation of 400 IU/day for 48 weeks in the diabetic population did not show any changes in CVD risk, lipid profile, or CRP. However, in patients not on cholesterol medication, vitamin D supplementation reduced TG compared to placebo (Angellotti et al., 2019). In participants with a history of vascular disease, 100 mcg, vitamin K2 was supplemented for 6 months, which led to a decrease in desphospho-uncarboxylated Matrix Gla compared to the placebo group but no changes in endothelial functions were seen (Fulton et al., 2016).

7.3.12.5 Alkaloid

Treatment with berberine (BBR) has shown an increase in LDL-receptor expression by stabilizing LDL-receptor mRNA through activation of the ERK pathway and the proprotein convertase subtilisin/kexin type 9 (PCSK9)-LDL-receptor pathway. PCSK9 pathway diverts LDL receptors toward lysosomal degradation, which is suppressed by BBR, consequently improving the concentration of circulating LDL-C by promoting cholesterol excretion from the liver into bile. Besides, BBR has shown a decreased enterocyte cholesterol uptake by interfering with intraluminal cholesterol micellization and decreased gene and protein expression of acyl-coenzyme A cholesterol acyltransferase-2 in vivo in the small intestine of rats. BBR also increases hepatic expression of mitochondrial sterol 27-hydroxylase, 7 alpha-hydroxylase expression regulating bile acids synthesis. Besides, it inhibits the expression of HMG-CoA, upregulating the CPT-1 alpha gene, preventing the formation of in vivo cholesterol synthesis, and promoting fat oxidation (Wang & Zidichouski, 2018). In accordance with these mechanisms, a RCT showed that supplementation of 1100 mg/day of berberine in participants with impaired fasting blood glucose for two months led to decreased glycemia, total cholesterol, total cholesterol/HDL, TG, insulin, Apob/Apoa, VAT, and fat mass compared to the placebo group (Rondanelli et al., 2023). In another study, patients were randomized to receive nutraceutical-combined pill containing BBR (500 mg) for 12 months, which led to significant reduction in total cholesterol, compared to placebo, but no changes in HDL-C were seen (Marazzi et al., 2011).

7.3.12.6 Capsaicinoids

Capsaicinoids (CAP) increase the expression of the thermogenic genes such as UCP-2, BMP 8b, SIRT-1, PGC-1 alpha, PRDM-16, and TRPV1 involved in BAT thermogenesis, promoting the burning of stored fat. Besides, CAP inhibits adipogenic transcription factors such as PPAR gamma and C/EBP-alpha, preventing preadipocyte differentiation into mature adipocytes (Baskaran et al., 2017). CAP also inhibits the expression of leptin and induces adiponectin upregulation, which consequently regulates appetite, promotes antiinflammation, and improves insulin sensitivity. Adiponectin also inhibits maturation of 3T3-L1 preadipocytes into adipocytes, reducing overall lipid storage. Dietary capsaicin stimulates glucagon-like peptide-1 (GLP-1) and supports the growth of the "antiobesity bacterium," Akkermansia muciniphila, by increasing mucin production (Szallasi, 2022). In accordance with these mechanisms, gestational diabetic women were randomly given 5 mg/day capsaicin for four weeks, which led to a decrease in postprandial glucose, insulin, HOMA-IR, fasting total cholesterol, and triglycerides compared to the placebo group, while serum Apob increased in the capsaicin group (Yuan et al., 2016). In another study, capsaicin was supplemented for three months, which led to an increase in fasting serum HDL-C, while TG, CRP, and phospholipid transfer protein activity decreased compared with the control group (Qin et al., 2017). In healthy participants, either 2 mg/day of CAP and 4 mg/day of CAP or placebo was supplemented for 12 weeks, which led to decreased kilocalorie consumption in the four mg group. There was a significant increase in fasting serum insulin and a decrease in HDL cholesterol in response to CAP which is not a favorable change but did not affect insulin response to administered OGTT and/or other indices of insulin sensitivity (Urbina et al., 2017).

7.3.12.7 Phytosterol and dietary fiber

Cholesterol and phytosterols have similar chemical structures and metabolic mechanisms. Phytosterols compete with cholesterol in micelles in the intestinal lumen and brush border membrane (BBM), thereby reducing cholesterol absorption. Besides, PS affects the expression of ACAT2 and MTP, reducing cholesterol esterification and the amount of cholesterol entering the chylomicron. Cholesterol in the chylomicron remnants enters the liver through the action of LDLR and LRP1, which is inhibited by phytosterol. Besides, phytosterol regulates HMG-CoA-R, preventing the de novo synthesis of cholesterol. Cholesterol is converted to bile acids in the liver by CYP7A1 and LXR-α which is an upstream regulatory gene of CYP7A1. Phytosterol can promote LXR-α expression, but the regulatory role for CYP7A1 is controversial. Likewise, phytosterol can decrease hepatic VLDL production to reduce circulating LDL-C levels (Li et al., 2022). However, in a study where participants were given either 1.5 g/day of phytosterols or two g/day of sunflower oil for 8 weeks, there was no difference between groups on LDL-C, TC, HDL-C, insulin, TG, systolic blood pressure, and diastolic blood pressure (Tavares et al., 2021). In hyperlipidemic patients, either a placebo or 3.4 g phytosterol ester-enriched soymilk powder was given for 6 months which showed decrement in total cholesterol, non-HDL, and LDL in the phytosterol group compared to the placebo group. No changes were seen in TG, HDL-C, apoe3, and apoe4 carriers (Dong et al., 2016). In another study of normo-cholesterolaemic participants, 2 g /day of phytosterols was given for 3 weeks, which led to a decrease in LDL cholesterol compared to baseline in the phytosterol group, but no changes in other lipid parameters were seen (Chau et al., 2020).

7.3.12.8 Bioactive polysaccharide

Polysaccharides improve plasma and liver lipid metabolism and accelerate cecum total bile acid, short-chain fatty acid, and lipid metabolism, which is mostly by upregulating AMPK α and downregulating the expression of acetyl-coenzyme A carboxylase, sterol regulatory element-binding protein 1c, and β-hydroxy-β-methylglutaryl coenzyme A. In a mice study, polysaccharide supplementation significantly reduced high-fat–induced fat accumulation in the liver and downregulated the gene relating to fat synthesis. Besides, polysaccharides affect the viscosity of intestinal lumen content, which affects the diffusion of dietary mixed micelles loaded with cholesterol to the intestinal epithelium membrane, limiting cholesterol availability. Also, polysaccharides sequester bile salts, lowering the amount of bile salts in the solution and reducing the emulsification power toward cholesterol, leading to its precipitation and excretion in the feces. Also, polysaccharide promotes SCFA production which interferes with cholesterol biosynthesis and converts primary into secondary BS, which is relevant for cholesterol emulsification (Silva et al., 2021). In accordance with this, 2 g/day of SXRG84 supplementation for 6 weeks in overweight and obese people, showed a significant reduction in non-HDL, atherogenic index, while CRP was reduced with the 4 g/day doses (Roach et al., 2022). In another study, polyglycoplex (PGX) was supplemented for 12 months in overweight and obese individuals, which showed that insulin and total cholesterol were significantly lowered in the PGX group compared to the placebo at 3 and 6 months. Serum glucose was lower at 3 months, and HDL was increased compared to control at 12 months (Pal et al., 2017). In another study, polysaccharide (750 mg/day) was given for 90 days in the unstable angina group leading to slightly increased SOD levels, decreased MDA, circulating endothelial cell (CEC), and endothelial progenitor cell (EPC) counts (Sargowo et al., 2018).

7.3.12.9 *Bioactive peptides*

Bioactive peptides from soybean hydrolysates promoted cholesterol excretion by upregulating the expressions of ABCG5 and ABCG8 in small intestinal cells and inhibiting hepatobiliary acid synthesis by upregulating the expression of FGF15/19 and downregulating CYP7A1 and CYP8B1. Peptides extracted from chickpeas are shown to inhibit the activities of FAS and HMG-CoA reductase (HMGR) and downregulate the expressions of pparγ and SREBP-1. At the same time, peptides upregulated the expression of LXR-alpha. Similarly, rice bran protein hydrolysate restricts the recycling of bile salts to the liver via direct excretion and exhibits inhibition of cholesterol entry into micelles. Walnut meal peptides are associated with increased Apo-B and reduced Apo-A1 levels, along with improved gene expression changes of LCAT, CYP7A1, HMGR, and FAS (Ma et al., 2023). In healthy adults, a single dose (20 g) of fish protein hydrolysate (FPH), whey protein hydrolysates (WHP), or placebo (PLA) was given, and flow-mediated dilatation before and at 30, 60, and 120 min after supplementation. There was a significant increase of endothelium-dependent dilation at 30 min after WPH but not after FPH as compared to PLA. There was a significantly greater total antioxidant capacity (TAC) in FPH than in the WPH supplement (Oliveira et al., 2020). In another study, 1 g lupin protein hydrolysate was given for 28 days, which showed decreased LDL-C/HDL and total cholesterol (Cruz-Chamorro et al., 2021).

7.3.13 Atherosclerosis

Evidence-based studies have proven the protective effect of aforementioned bioactive compounds against atherosclerosis progression and CVD. Bioactive compounds are involved in the regulation of several modulating pathways, which are responsible for treating atherosclerosis. Polyphenols are useful in reducing mTOR signaling. Targeting the mammalian target of rapamycin (mTOR) is the therapeutic approach for CVD, and bioactive compounds are actively involved in the regulation of mTOR. Bioactive phenols promote deptor/mTOR interaction to inhibit mTORC1 activation; inhibit phosphorylation of PDK1, PI3K/Akt, mTOR, and p70S6 (K1); activate phosphorylation of AMPK and AMPK-dependent inhibition of the mTOR pathway; reduce the expression of mTOR signaling proteins; activate the mTORC2-Rictor survival pathway; and inhibit p300 histone acetyltransferase-dependent acetylation of GATA4 (Sanches-Silva et al., 2020; Ziółkiewicz et al., 2023).

Polyphenols participate in stimulation of endothelial NO synthase, modulate several mechanisms (blocking ROS production, detoxifying ROS, insulin sensitivity, DNA repair), decrease cell surface expression of VCAM-1, and improve microvascular endothelial reactivity. Also, it is involved in association with inflammatory biomarkers (TNF-α, IL-1β, and PTX3) reduction, mitigates atherosclerosis pathophysiology, reduces the progression of atherosclerotic plaques, inflammatory cell infiltration, and the activity of NF-$\kappa\beta$ (Behl et al., 2020). The main mechanisms by which polyphenols inhibit atherosclerosis are reducing circulating cholesterol and adhering to LDL particles. Also, it enhances antioxidant activity by increasing glutathione and preventing DNA from oxidative damage. Studies revealed that introducing phenolic extracts to a diet lowers plasma levels of the cell adhesion molecules P-selectin and β-thromboglobulin (Ahmadi et al., 2022). For instance, curcumin has proven effective in improving plasma catalase, NO, and myeloperoxidase. Additionally, in cases of atherosclerosis and CVD, certain compounds, such as EGCG and curcumin, activate the Nrf2 pathway and reduce the activation of NF-κB (Sanches-Silva et al., 2020). High-dose catechin supplementation also increased levels of NO, reduced monocyte chemoattractant protein-1, CD40, and plasma asymmetric dimethylarginine (Bahramsoltani et al., 2019).

Phenolic acids, such as caffeic acid, ellagic acid, and vanillic acid, show excellent antioxidative, antiinflammatory, and cadioprodective properties. In streptozotocin-induced diabetic rats, ellagic and caffeic acids show cardioprotective benefits. These acids lessen oxidative stress and dyslipidemia, boost insulin production, and enhance glycemic control. Ellagic acid has antilipid peroxidation properties and can manage plasma lipid profiles (Oluwole et al., 2022). Another phenolic compound, lignans, is also involved in the active reduction of CVD as it prevents vascular inflammation and endothelial dysfunction, which are key to CVD (Rodríguez-García et al., 2019). The production of lipid peroxides and oxygen-free radicals by platelet adhesion to the vascular endothelium can inhibit the endothelial production of nitrous oxide and prostacyclin. Flavonoids, such as kaempferol, quercetin, and myricetin, are found to maintain the levels of prostacyclin and nitric oxide in the endothelium (Oluwole et al., 2022). Resveratrol, one of the stilbenes, has the potential to decrease the adherence of monocyte cells to human endothelial cells by lowering proinflammatory mediators such as M-CSF, IL-6, and MCP-1 in addition to ICAM-1, VCAM-1, and E-selectin (Bahramsoltani et al., 2019; Calabriso et al., 2016). This suggests that phenolic extract supplements are vital in minimizing the risk of atherosclerosis and CVD via modulation of several pathways, free radical scavenging, and inflammation reduction.

Alkaloids have the potential to overcome some of the features of atherosclerosis development, including limiting the accumulation of oxidatively modified LDL, which causes oxidative stress, accumulates ROS, and induces endothelial cell dysfunction. Sangzhi alkaloid, a novel alkaloid obtained from mulberry branches, has shown potent inhibition of vascular inflammation and protection against atherosclerosis by modulating the polarization of M1/M2 macrophages and reducing macrophage infiltration. The proinflammatory mediator C-X-C motif chemokine ligand (CXCL)-10, which is mostly released by M1 macrophages, was inhibited by Sangzhi alkaloid. This decrease in CXCL-10 prevented the inflammatory amplification effect, decreased the recruitment of new macrophages, and enhanced endothelial cell function (Peng et al., 2024). Likewise, two alkaloids, epi-aszonalenin A and aszonalenin, from fungus suppressed VEGF protein expression, ox-LDL-induced LOX-1, inflammatory factors (IL-1β, IL-6, and TNF-α), and MAPK and PI3K/AKT pathways phosphorylation. Aszonalenin inhibited platelet-derived growth factor, VEGF receptor, intercellular adhesion molecule-1, and vascular cell adhesion molecule-1. Furthermore, by inhibiting apoptosis and inflammation via the cleaved caspase-3, Bax/Bcl-2, and NF-κB pathways, it prevented ox-LDL-induced atherosclerosis (Li et al., 2022).

Different vitamins are responsible for the prevention of CVD by preventing plaque formation, as these vitamins act as antioxidant reservoirs and reduce ROS and inflammatory markers (Ziegler et al., 2020). Vitamins C and E delay the development of common carotid atherosclerosis, and vitamin K hydroquinone acts as a cofactor and regulates the γ-carboxylase enzyme within the endoplasmic reticulum. Similarly, vitamin D has a considerable effect on cells associated with atherosclerosis, which includes VSMCs, ECs, and immune cells (monocytes, lymphocytes, macrophages, and so on) (Danziger et al., 2016; Khan et al., 2020).

Damage to the atherosclerotic endothelium led to a decrease in endothelial NO synthase, a compromised release of NO, and an increase in ROS production in the arterial wall. Different bioactive peptides can be effective in treating these conditions. An in vivo study on animals revealed that kefir peptides prevent hyperlipidemia in obese rats by inhibiting the lipogenesis pathway via the enzyme fatty acid synthase reduction, boosting the protein p-ACC, and stimulating the lipid oxidation pathway through elevating the expression of PPAR-α, CPT1, and p-AMPK. Kefir peptides suppressed the lesion macrophage, which successfully reduced the production of TNF-α and IL-1β. Kefir peptides inhibit endothelial cell activation as well as THP-1 monocyte adhesion and migration (Tung et al., 2020). Bioactive peptides reduce endothelial permeability, inflammatory response, and atherogenic indicators while increasing overall antioxidant activity. Significant contribution of bioactive peptides in the reduction of inflammation, oxidative stress, and hyperlipidemia—all important aspects of atherosclerosis (He et al., 2022; Santos-Sánchez et al., 2022). This suggests that unleashing novel bioactive peptides with antiatherosclerosis and cardioprotective properties can help treat CVD.

Furthermore, atherosclerotic plaque can be efficiently stabilized by moderate autophagic activation, which inhibits inflammatory reactions by controlling macrophages; thereby, autophagy could serve as an effective way to reduce atherosclerosis and stabilize atherosclerotic plaque. Due to their distinct antiinflammatory, antithrombotic, and lipid-lowering properties, sulfated polysaccharides have emerged as a key active ingredient in the stabilization of atherosclerotic plaque. Within plaque, sulfated polysaccharides are responsible for downregulating the expression of LC3B and CD68 while upregulating the expression of P62, which indicates an enhancement of autophagy flux (Xiong et al., 2020) (Fig. 7.3).

7.3.14 Hypertension

The enzyme (ACE) responsible for the conversion of angiotensin I to angiotensin II is key in the development of inflammation associated with hypertension (Ji et al., 2005). The figure below shows the role of bioactive compounds in the treatment of hypertension. The ACE inhibition properties of the phenolics are evident. Phenolics such as anthocyanins possess an endothelium-dependent vasorelaxant action, which is responsible for lowering the blood pressure. As mentioned earlier, phenolics inhibit different signaling pathways of inflammatory cytokines. In rats treated with Nω-nitro-L-arginine methyl ester, vanillic acid demonstrated a reduction in hypertension by increasing the production of eNOS and decreasing cardiac markers such as lactate dehydrogenase and creatine kinase (Li et al., 2019). The tannins

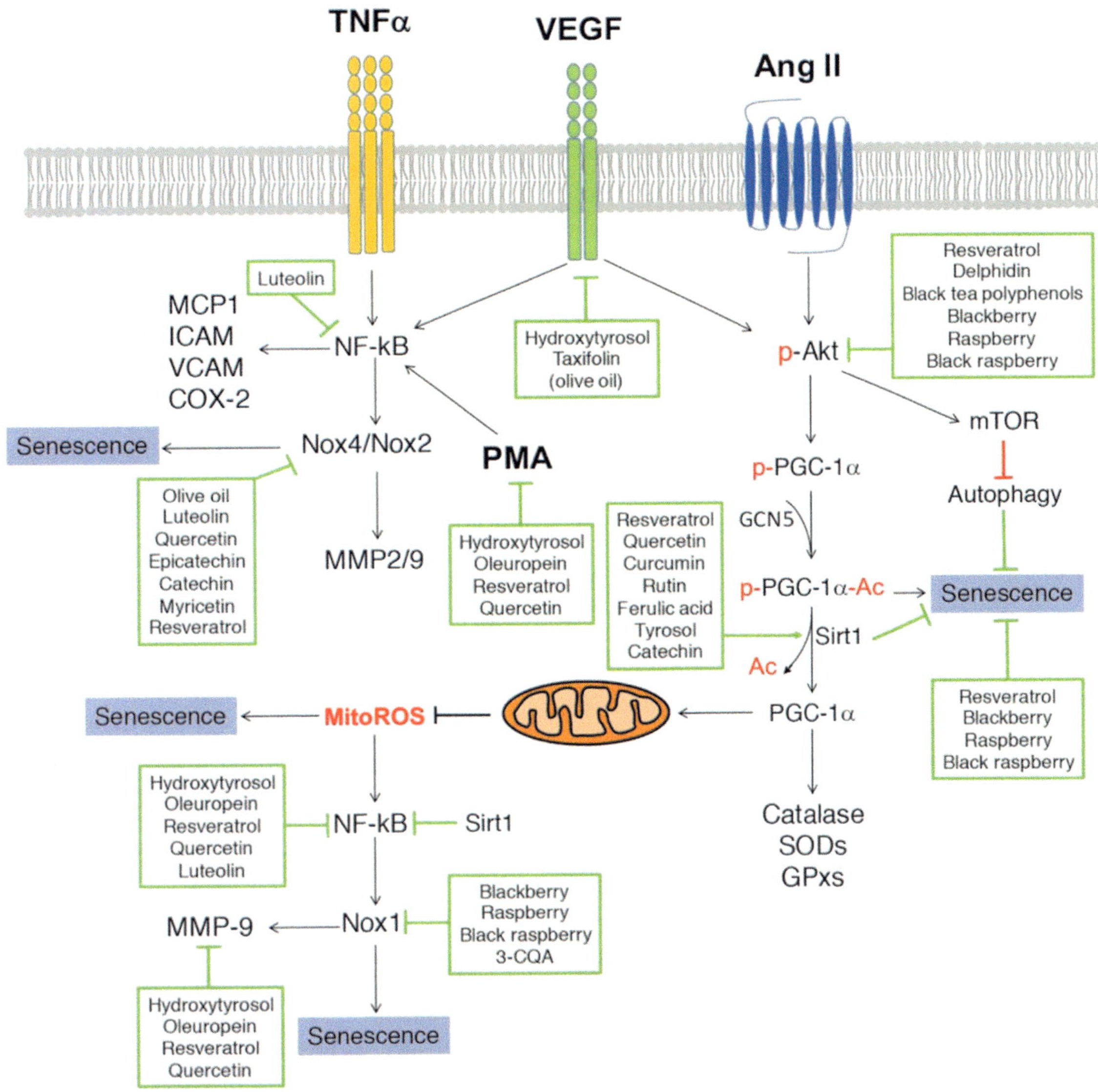

FIGURE 7.3 Modulation of oxidative stress-induced pathways, including Ang II, VEGF, and TNFα (Serino & Salazar, 2019). *Reproduced from Serino, A., & Salazar, G. (2019). Protective role of polyphenols against vascular inflammation, aging and cardiovascular disease.* Nutrients, 11*(1)*, *53, https://doi.org/10.3390/nu11010053. This article is an open access article distributed under the terms and conditions of the Creative Commons Attribution (CC BY) license.*

contribute to oxidation resistance and antiinflammatory effects by decreasing the expression of Bax in pulmonary artery endothelial cells and increasing the expression of Bcl-2, Nrf2, and HO-1. It also prevented H_2O_2-induced pulmonary artery endothelial cell death and ROS generation (Aimaier et al., 2023). Hypertensive patients often show endothelium-derived NO system defects due to abnormal endothelium-dependent vasodilatation (Rahman et al., 2021).

Several studies have reported antihypertensive mechanism of phenolics as direct vasodilation, suppression of NLRP3 inflammasome activation, and amelioration of endothelial dysfunction (Theofilis et al., 2021). In a double-blind randomized controlled trial, prehypertensive patients' blood pressure was decreased after consuming a phenolic-rich extract derived from grape seed and skins (330 mg), green tea (100 mg), resveratrol (60 mg), and a combination of quercetin, ginkgo biloba, and bilberry (60 mg) for 28 days (Biesinger et al., 2016). Catechins and other polyphenols are abundant in tea, particularly Camellia sinensis tea. For eight days of consumption of black tea, hypertensive individuals experienced a reduction in blood pressure (Grassi et al., 2016). This result can be explained by the phytochemical ability to inhibit NADPH oxidase activity and lower the concentration of ROS within the arteries (de Brito Alves et al., 2023) (Fig. 7.4).

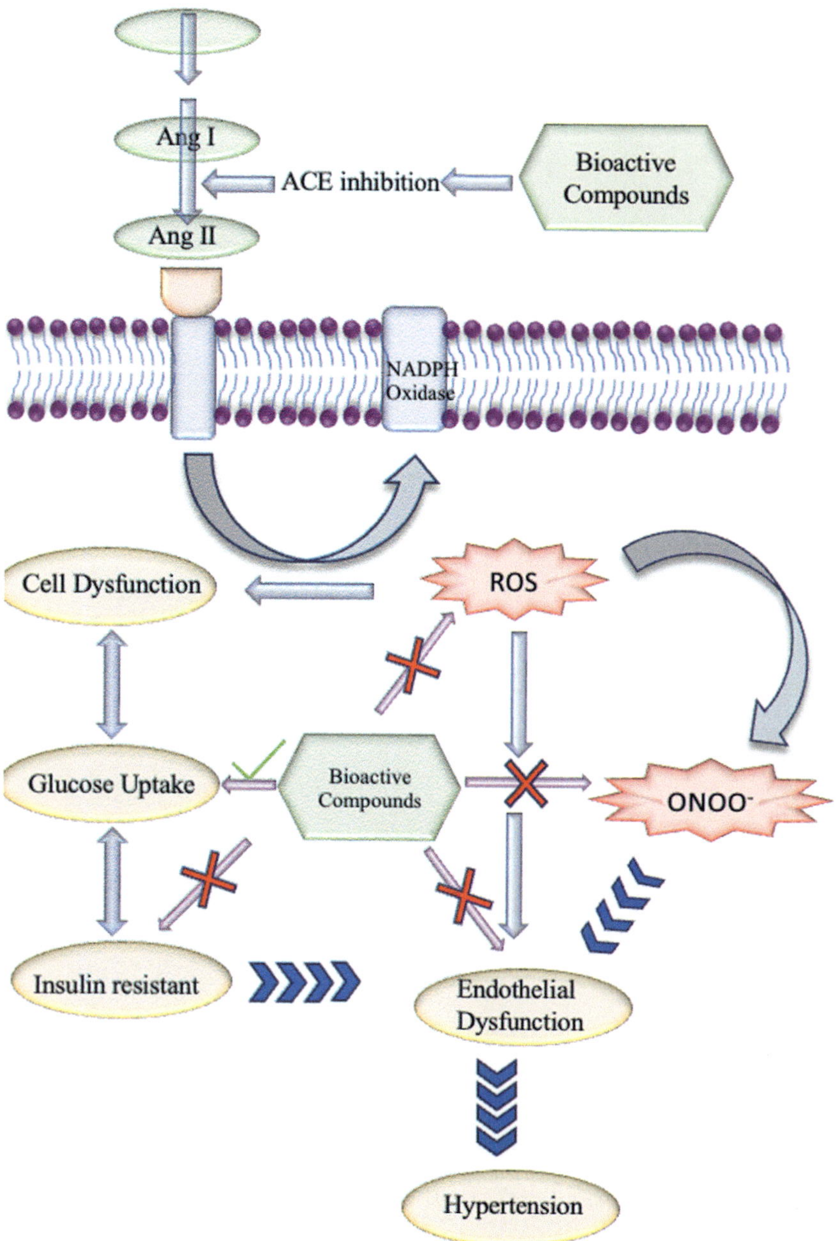

FIGURE 7.4 Preventive mechanism of bioactive compounds against hypertension.

Similarly, capsaicin administration in animals demonstrated a decrease in systolic blood pressure starting in the fourth month of regular administration of capsaicin (15 mg/kg) in rats (Yang et al., 2010). Xanthophylls, oxygenated carotenoids, supplementation with a paprika xanthophyll capsule at a dose of 0.9 mg xanthophyll for three months resulted in a reduction in both systolic and diastolic blood pressure; however, the effect was not significant (Kakutani et al., 2018). Even though the antihypertensive properties of capsaicin are controversial, a metaanalysis recently carried out by Amini et al. (2021) has shown an association between capsaicin ingestion and hypertension management. There have been reports of the involvement of several mechanisms for hypertension reduction, which include stimulating diuresis and natriuresis, releasing vasodilator neuropeptides through transient receptor potential vanilloid 1 activation, L-type $Ca2+$ channel inhibition in muscle cells, and ACE inhibitory activity (Amini et al., 2021). Beside these, the highest ACE inhibitory activity is shown by novel peptides like IPP, VPP, and VLPVPQK that are extracted from simulated gastrointestinal digestion of milk casein. These peptides also exhibit antihypertensive effects through proinflammatory cytokine expression, RAAS modulation, increased endothelial nitric oxide and monocyte activity, and/or decreased oxidative stress in vascular smooth muscle and endothelial dysfunction (Koirala et al., 2023).

7.4 Conclusion

In the last decades, there have been a number of intensive studies conducted to explore the potential health benefits of bioactive active compounds with a promising role in preventing and/or reducing the complications linked with impaired metabolic health. With the aim of enhancing the metabolic health of individuals, bioactive compounds have proven to have an effect on the downregulation mechanism of inflammation mediators and free radicles responsible for oxidative damage. Traditional medicinal therapy relying on the utilization of bioactive compounds and phytoextracts is now an effective approach to healing different metabolisms and endocrine diseases. The several in vitro and in vivo studies reported offer a strong foundation for considering medical assertions and the multiorgan-protecting functions of bioactive compounds in humans. Recent advancements in technology have further aided to illustrate the potential mechanism of bioactive compounds in promoting the metabolic health of individuals. The approaches of combined therapy, where medicine and bioactive compounds can be used in the treatment of metabolic syndrome and associated complications, have opened up novel insights in medicine and pharmaceutics to promote the metabolic health of people. Thus the promising results outlined show promising prospects for further utilizing bioactive compounds in medical science, yet this requires large sample randomized controlled trials. Unless there is sufficient exploration of bioactive compounds in a human model with a larger population, unleashing the proven effects of bioactive compounds will still be confined to lab research.

References

Ahmadi, A., Jamialahmadi, T., & Sahebkar, A. (2022). Polyphenols and atherosclerosis: A critical review of clinical effects on LDL oxidation. *Pharmacological Research*, *184*, 106414. Available from https://doi.org/10.1016/j.phrs.2022.106414.

Aimaier, S., Tao, Y., Lei, F., Yupeng, Z., Wenhui, S., Aikemu, A., & Maimaitiyiming, D. (2023). Protective effects of the Terminalia bellirica tannin-induced Nrf2/HO-1 signaling pathway in rats with high-altitude pulmonary hypertension. *BMC Complementary Medicine and Therapies*, *23*(1). Available from https://doi.org/10.1186/s12906-023-03981-2.

Amini, M. R., Sheikhhossein, F., Bazshahi, E., Hajiaqaei, M., Shafie, A., Shahinfar, H., Azizi, N., Eghbaljoo Gharehgheshlaghi, H., Naghshi, S., Fathipour, R. B., & Shab-Bidar, S. (2021). The effects of capsinoids and fermented red pepper paste supplementation on blood pressure: A systematic review and meta-analysis of randomized controlled trials. *Clinical Nutrition*, *40*(4), 1767–1775. Available from https://doi.org/10.1016/j.clnu.2020.10.018, http://www.elsevier-international.com/journals/clnu/.

An, Y., Xu, Bt, Wan, Sr, Ma, Xm, Long, Y., Xu, Y., & Jiang, Zz (2023). The role of oxidative stress in diabetes mellitus-induced vascular endothelial dysfunction. *Cardiovascular Diabetology*, *22*(1). Available from https://doi.org/10.1186/s12933-023-01965-7, https://cardiab.biomedcentral.com/.

Angellotti, E., D'Alessio, D., Dawson-Hughes, B., Chu, Y., Nelson, J., Hu, P., Cohen, R. M., & Pittas, A. G. (2019). Effect of vitamin D supplementation on cardiovascular risk in type 2 diabetes. *Clinical Nutrition*, *38*(5), 2449–2453. Available from https://doi.org/10.1016/j.clnu.2018.10.003, http://www.elsevier-international.com/journals/clnu/.

Aoyama, T., Fukui, K., Takamatsu, K., Hashimoto, Y., & Yamamoto, T. (2000). Soy protein isolate and its hydrolysate reduce body fat of dietary obese rats and genetically obese mice (yellow KK). *Nutrition (Burbank, Los Angeles County, Calif.)*, *16*(5), 349–354. Available from https://doi.org/10.1016/s0899-9007(00)00230-6.

Asbaghi, O., Khosroshahi, M. Z., Kashkooli, S., & Abbasnezhad, A. (2019). Effect of Calcium-vitamin D co-supplementation on insulin, insulin sensitivity, and glycemia: a systematic review and meta-analysis of randomized clinical trials. *Hormone and Metabolic Research*, *51*(5), 288–295. Available from https://doi.org/10.1055/a-0887-0205, http://www.thieme-connect.com/ejournals/toc/hmr.

Asemi, Z., Alizadeh, S. A., Ahmad, K., Goli, M., & Esmaillzadeh, A. (2016). Effects of beta-carotene fortified synbiotic food on metabolic control of patients with type 2 diabetes mellitus: A double-blind randomized cross-over controlled clinical trial. *Clinical Nutrition*, *35*(4), 819–825. Available from https://doi.org/10.1016/j.clnu.2015.07.009, http://www.elsevier-international.com/journals/clnu/.

Azzini, E., Venneria, E., Ciarapica, D., Foddai, M. S., Intorre, F., Zaccaria, M., Maiani, F., Palomba, L., Barnaba, L., Tubili, C., Maiani, G., & Polito, A. (2017). Effect of red orange juice consumption on body composition and nutritional status in overweight/obese female: A pilot study. *Oxidative Medicine and Cellular Longevity*, *2017*, 1–9. Available from https://doi.org/10.1155/2017/1672567.

Bahramsoltani, R., Ebrahimi, F., Farzaei, M. H., Baratpourmoghaddam, A., Ahmadi, P., Rostamiasrabadi, P., Rasouli Amirabadi, A. H., & Rahimi, R. (2019). Dietary polyphenols for atherosclerosis: A comprehensive review and future perspectives. *Critical Reviews in Food Science and Nutrition*, *59*(1), 114–132. Available from https://doi.org/10.1080/10408398.2017.1360244, https://www.tandfonline.com/loi/bfsn20.

Banwo, K., Olojede, A. O., Adesulu-Dahunsi, A. T., Verma, D. K., Thakur, M., Tripathy, S., Singh, S., Patel, A. R., Gupta, A. K., Aguilar, C. N., & Utama, G. L. (2021). Functional importance of bioactive compounds of foods with Potential Health Benefits: A review on recent trends. *Food Bioscience*, *43*. Available from https://doi.org/10.1016/j.fbio.2021.101320, http://www.journals.elsevier.com/food-bioscience/.

Baskaran, P., Krishnan, V., Fettel, K., Gao, P., Zhu, Z., Ren, J., & Thyagarajan, B. (2017). TRPV1 activation counters diet-induced obesity through sirtuin-1 activation and PRDM-16 deacetylation in brown adipose tissue. *International Journal of Obesity*, *41*(5), 739–749. Available from https://doi.org/10.1038/ijo.2017.16.

Basu, A., Betts, N. M., Nguyen, A., Newman, E. D., Fu, D., & Lyons, T. J. (2014). Freeze-dried strawberries lower serum cholesterol and lipid peroxidation in adults with abdominal adiposity and elevated serum lipids. American Society for Nutrition, United States. *Journal of Nutrition*, *144*(6), 830–837. Available from https://doi.org/10.3945/jn.113.188169, http://jn.nutrition.org/content/144/6/830.full.pdf.

Bazyar, H., Moradi, L., Zaman, F., & Javid, A. Z. (2023). The effects of rutin flavonoid supplement on glycemic status, lipid profile, atherogenic index of plasma, brain-derived neurotrophic factor (BDNF), some serum inflammatory, and oxidative stress factors in patients with type 2 diabetes mellitus: A double-blind, placebo-controlled trial. *Phytotherapy Research, 37*(1), 271–284. Available from https://doi.org/10.1002/ptr.7611.

Behl, T., Bungau, S., Kumar, K., Zengin, G., Khan, F., Kumar, A., Kaur, R., Venkatachalam, T., Tit, D. M., Vesa, C. M., Barsan, G., & Mosteanu, D. E. (2020). Pleotropic effects of polyphenols in cardiovascular system. *Biomedicine and Pharmacotherapy, 130*. Available from https://doi.org/10.1016/j.biopha.2020.110714, https://www.journals.elsevier.com/biomedicine-and-pharmacotherapy.

Biesinger, S., Michaels, H. A., Quadros, A. S., Qian, Y., Rabovsky, A. B., Badger, R. S., & Jalili, T. (2016). A combination of isolated phytochemicals and botanical extracts lowers diastolic blood pressure in a randomized controlled trial of hypertensive subjects. *European Journal of Clinical Nutrition, 70*(1), 10–16. Available from https://doi.org/10.1038/ejcn.2015.88.

de Brito Alves, J. L., Alves Brasil, J. M., Maia, L. A., M.d.C. Lima, K. B., Sampaio, E. L., & de Souza. (2023). Phenolic compounds in hypertension: Targeting gut-brain interactions and endothelial dysfunction. *Journal of Functional Foods, 104*. Available from https://doi.org/10.1016/j.jff.2023.105531, http://www.elsevier.com/wps/find/journaldescription.cws_home/717426/description#description.

Calabriso, N., Massaro, M., Scoditti, E., Pellegrino, M., Ingrosso, I., Giovinazzo, G., & Carluccio, M. (2016). Red grape skin polyphenols blunt matrix metalloproteinase-2 and -9 activity and expression in cell models of vascular inflammation: Protective role in degenerative and inflammatory diseases. *Molecules (Basel, Switzerland), 21*(9), 1147. Available from https://doi.org/10.3390/molecules21091147.

Canas, J. A., Lochrie, A., McGowan, A. G., Hossain, J., Schettino, C., & Balagopal, P. B. (2017). Effects of mixed carotenoids on adipokines and abdominal adiposity in children: A pilot study. *Journal of Clinical Endocrinology and Metabolism, 102*(6), 1983–1990. Available from https://doi.org/10.1210/jc.2017-00185, https://oup.silverchair-cdn.com/oup/backfile/Content_public/Journal/jcem/102/6/10.1210_jc.2017-00185/2/jc.2017-00185.pdf.

Castro-Acosta, M. L., Stone, S. G., Mok, J. E., Mhajan, R. K., Fu, C. I., Lenihan-Geels, G. N., Corpe, C. P., & Hall, W. L. (2017). Apple and blackcurrant polyphenol-rich drinks decrease postprandial glucose, insulin and incretin response to a high-carbohydrate meal in healthy men and women. *Journal of Nutritional Biochemistry, 49*, 53–62. Available from https://doi.org/10.1016/j.jnutbio.2017.07.013, www.elsevier.com/locate/jnutbio.

Cha, Y. S., Kim, S. R., Yang, J. A., Back, H. I., Kim, M. G., Jung, S. J., Song, W. O., & Chae, S. W. (2013). Kochujang, fermented soybean-based red pepper paste, decreases visceral fat and improves blood lipid profiles in overweight adults. *Nutrition and Metabolism, 10*(1). Available from https://doi.org/10.1186/1743-7075-10-24, http://www.nutritionandmetabolism.com/home/.

Chau, Y. P., Cheng, Y. C., Sing, C. W., Tsoi, M. F., Cheng, V. K. F., Lee, G. K. Y., Cheung, C. L., & Cheung, B. M. Y. (2020). The lipid-lowering effect of once-daily soya drink fortified with phytosterols in normocholesterolaemic Chinese: a double-blind randomized controlled trial. *European Journal of Nutrition, 59*(6), 2739–2746. Available from https://doi.org/10.1007/s00394-019-02119-w, http://www.springerlink.com/content/1436-6207.

Chen, J., Yang, J., Ma, L., Li, J., Shahzad, N., & Kim, C. K. (2020). Structure-antioxidant activity relationship of methoxy, phenolic hydroxyl, and carboxylic acid groups of phenolic acids. *Scientific Reports, 10*(1). Available from https://doi.org/10.1038/s41598-020-59451-z, www.nature.com/srep/index.html.

Chew, B., Mathison, B., Kimble, L., McKay, D., Kaspar, K., Khoo, C., Chen, C. Y. O., & Blumberg, J. (2019). Chronic consumption of a low calorie, high polyphenol cranberry beverage attenuates inflammation and improves glucoregulation and HDL cholesterol in healthy overweight humans: A randomized controlled trial. *European Journal of Nutrition, 58*(3), 1223–1235. Available from https://doi.org/10.1007/s00394-018-1643-z, http://www.springerlink.com/content/1436-6207.

Chew, N. W. S., Ng, C. H., Tan, D. J. H., Kong, G., Lin, C., Chin, Y. H., Lim, W. H., Huang, D. Q., Quek, J., Fu, C. E., Xiao, J., Syn, N., Foo, R., Khoo, C. M., Wang, J. W., Dimitriadis, G. K., Young, D. Y., Siddiqui, M. S., Lam, C. S. P., Wang, Y., Figtree, G. A., Chan, M. Y., Cummings, D. E., Noureddin, M., Wong, V. W. S., Ma, R. C. W., Mantzoros, C. S., Sanyal, A., & Muthiah, M. D. (2023). The global burden of metabolic disease: Data from 2000 to 2019. *Cell Metabolism, 35*(3), 414. Available from https://doi.org/10.1016/j.cmet.2023.02.003, http://www.cellmetabolism.org/.

Cordeiro, A., Pereira, S. E., Saboya, C. J., & Ramalho, A. (2022). Vitamin D Supplementation and Its Relationship with Loss of Visceral Adiposity. *Obesity Surgery, 32*(10), 3419–3425. Available from https://doi.org/10.1007/s11695-022-06239-x, http://www.obesitysurgery.comhttps://link.springer.com/journal/11695.

Cruz-Chamorro, I., Álvarez-Sánchez, N., Álvarez-Ríos, A. I., Santos-Sánchez, G., Pedroche, J., Millán, F., Carrera Sánchez, C., Fernández-Pachón, M. S., Millán-Linares, M. C., Martínez-López, A., Lardone, P. J., Bejarano, I., Guerrero, J. M., & Carrillo-Vico, A. (2021). Safety and efficacy of a beverage containing lupine protein hydrolysates on the immune, oxidative and lipid status in healthy subjects: An intervention study (the Lupine-1 Trial). *Molecular Nutrition and Food Research, 65*(14). Available from https://doi.org/10.1002/mnfr.202100139, http://onlinelibrary.wiley.com/journal/10.1002/(ISSN)1613-4133.

Cudennec, B., Ravallec-Plé, R., Courois, E., & Fouchereau-Peron, M. (2008). Peptides from fish and crustacean by-products hydrolysates stimulate cholecystokinin release in STC-1 cells. *Food Chemistry, 111*(4), 970–975. Available from https://doi.org/10.1016/j.foodchem.2008.05.016.

Danziger, J., Young, R. L., Shea, M. K., Tracy, R. P., Ix, J. H., Jenny, N. S., & Mukamal, K. J. (2016). Vitamin K-dependent protein activity and incident ischemic cardiovascular disease: The multi-ethnic study of atherosclerosis. *Arteriosclerosis, Thrombosis, and Vascular Biology, 36*(5), 1037–1042. Available from https://doi.org/10.1161/ATVBAHA.116.307273, http://atvb.ahajournals.org/.

Deng, Y., Zhang, Y., Zheng, S., Hong, J., Wang, C., Liu, T., Sun, Z., Gu, W., Gu, Y., Shi, J., Yao, S., Wang, W., & Ning, G. (2015). Postprandial glucose, insulin and incretin responses to different carbohydrate tolerance tests. *Journal of Diabetes, 7*(6), 820–829. Available from https://doi.org/10.1111/1753-0407.12245.

Dong, S., Zhang, R., Ji, Y. C., Hao, J. Y., Ma, W. W., Chen, X. D., Xiao, R., & Yu, H. L. (2016). Soy milk powder supplemented with phytosterol esters reduced serum cholesterol level in hypercholesterolemia independently of lipoprotein E genotype: a random clinical placebo-controlled trial. *Nutrition Research, 36*(8), 879–884. Available from https://doi.org/10.1016/j.nutres.2016.05.006, www.elsevier.com/locate/nutres.

El-Nashar, H. A. S., Mostafa, N. M., El-Shazly, M., & Eldahshan, O. A. (2021). The role of plant-derived compounds in managing diabetes mellitus: A review of literature from 2014 to 2019. *Current Medicinal Chemistry, 28*(23), 4694–4730. Available from https://doi.org/10.2174/0929867328999201123194510, https://www.eurekaselect.com/node/188269.

Fan, H., Liu, H., Zhang, Y., Zhang, S., Liu, T., & Wang, D. (2022). Review on plant-derived bioactive peptides: biological activities, mechanism of action and utilizations in food development. *Journal of Future Foods, 2*(2), 143–159. Available from https://doi.org/10.1016/j.jfutfo.2022.03.003.

Feng, S., Belwal, T., Li, L., Limwachiranon, J., Liu, X., & Luo, Z. (2020). Phytosterols and their derivatives: Potential health-promoting uses against lipid metabolism and associated diseases, mechanism, and safety issues. *Comprehensive Reviews in Food Science and Food Safety, 19*(4), 1243–1267. Available from https://doi.org/10.1111/1541-4337.12560, http://onlinelibrary.wiley.com/journal/10.1111/(ISSN)1541-4337.

Ferdowsi, P. V., Ahuja, K. D. K., Beckett, J. M., & Myers, S. (2023). Capsaicin and zinc signalling pathways as promising targets for managing insulin resistance and type 2 diabetes. *Molecules (Basel, Switzerland), 28*(6). Available from https://doi.org/10.3390/molecules28062861, http://www.mdpi.com/journal/molecules.

Fidanza, A., & Audisio, M. (1982). Vitamins and lipid metabolism. *Acta Vitaminologica et Enzymologica, 4*(1-2), 105–114.

Fulton, R. L., McMurdo, M. E. T., Hill, A., Abboud, R. J., Arnold, G. P., Struthers, A. D., Khan, F., Vermeer, C., Knapen, M. H. J., Drummen, N. E. A., & Witham, M. D. (2016). Effect of vitamin K on vascular health and physical function in older people with vascular disease—a randomised controlled trial. *The Journal of nutrition, health and aging, 20*(3), 325–333. Available from https://doi.org/10.1007/s12603-015-0619-4.

Ganesan., & Xu. (2019). Anti-diabetic effects and mechanisms of dietary polysaccharides. *Molecules (Basel, Switzerland), 24*(14), 2556. Available from https://doi.org/10.3390/molecules24142556.

Garcés-Rimón, M., López-Expósito, I., López-Fandiño, R., & Miguel, M. (2016). Egg white hydrolysates with in vitro biological multiactivities to control complications associated with the metabolic syndrome. *European Food Research and Technology, 242*(1), 61–69. Available from https://doi.org/10.1007/s00217-015-2518-7.

Ghaderi, A., Rasouli-Azad, M., Vahed, N., Banafshe, H. R., Soleimani, A., Omidi, A., Ghoreishi, F. S., & Asemi, Z. (2019). Clinical and metabolic responses to crocin in patients under methadone maintenance treatment: A randomized clinical trial. *Phytotherapy Research, 33*(10), 2714–2725. Available from https://doi.org/10.1002/ptr.6445, http://onlinelibrary.wiley.com/journal/10.1002/(ISSN)1099-1573.

Gjorgieva Ackova, D., Maksimova, V., Smilkov, K., Buttari, B., Arese, M., & Saso, L. (2023). Alkaloids as natural NRF2 inhibitors: Chemoprevention and cytotoxic action in cancer. *Pharmaceuticals, 16*(6), 850. Available from https://doi.org/10.3390/ph16060850.

Goleniowski, M., Bonfill, M., Cusido, R., & Palazón, J. (2013). *Phenolic acids. Natural Products: Phytochemistry, Botany and Metabolism of Alkaloids, Phenolics and Terpenes* (pp. 1951–1973). Springer Berlin Heidelberg. Available from http://doi.org/10.1007/978-3-642-22144_64.

Grassi, D., Draijer, R., Schalkwijk, C., Desideri, G., D'Angeli, A., Francavilla, S., Mulder, T., & Ferri, C. (2016). Black tea increases circulating endothelial progenitor cells and improves flow mediated dilatation counteracting deleterious effects from a fat load in hypertensive patients: A randomized controlled study. *Nutrients, 8*(11), 727. Available from https://doi.org/10.3390/nu8110727.

Guarino, G., Strollo, F., Carbone, L., Della Corte, T., Letizia, M., Marino, G., & Gentile, S. (2017). Bioimpedance analysis, metabolic effects and safety of the association berberis aristataisilybum marianum: A 52-week double-blind, placebo-controlled study in obese patients with type 2 diabetes. *Journal of Biological Regulators and Homeostatic Agents, 31*(2), 495–502. Available from http://www.biolifesas.org/contentsJBRHA.htm.

Hajizadeh-Sharafabad, F., Tarighat-Esfanjani, A., Ghoreishi, Z., & Sarreshtedari, M. (2021). Lutein supplementation combined with a low-calorie diet in middle-aged obese individuals: effects on anthropometric indices, body composition and metabolic parameters. *British Journal of Nutrition, 126*(7), 1028–1039. Available from https://doi.org/10.1017/s0007114520004997.

He, H., Deng, J., Yang, M., An, L., Ye, X., & Li, X. (2022). Jatrorrhizine from Rhizoma Coptidis exerts an anti-obesity effect in db/db mice. *Journal of Ethnopharmacology, 298*, 115529. Available from https://doi.org/10.1016/j.jep.2022.115529.

Hentati, F., Tounsi, L., Djomdi, D., Pierre, G., Delattre, C., Ursu, A. V., Fendri, I., Abdelkafi, S., & Michaud, P. (2020). Bioactive polysaccharides from seaweeds. *Molecules (Basel, Switzerland), 25*(14). Available from https://doi.org/10.3390/molecules25143152, https://www.mdpi.com/1420-3049/25/14/3152/pdf.

Hermida, N., & Balligand, J.-L. (2013). Low-density lipoprotein-cholesterol-induced endothelial dysfunction and oxidative stress: The role of statins. *Antioxidants & Redox Signaling, 20*(8), 1216–1237. Available from https://doi.org/10.1089/ars.2013.5537.

Hess, A. L., Benítez-Páez, A., Blædel, T., Larsen, L. H., Iglesias, J. R., Madera, C., Sanz, Y., & Larsen, T. M. (2020). The effect of inulin and resistant maltodextrin on weight loss during energy restriction: a randomised, placebo-controlled, double-blinded intervention. *European Journal of Nutrition, 59*(6), 2507–2524. Available from https://doi.org/10.1007/s00394-019-02099-x, http://www.springerlink.com/content/1436-6207.

Hildebrandt, X., Ibrahim, M., & Peltzer, N. (2023). Cell death and inflammation during obesity: "Know my methods, WAT(son). *Cell Death & Differentiation, 30*(2), 279–292. Available from https://doi.org/10.1038/s41418-022-01062-4.

Holt, R., Jorsal, M. J., Yahyavi, S. K., Qin, S., Juul, A., Jørgensen, N., & Blomberg Jensen, M. (2024). High-dose cholecalciferol supplementation to obese infertile men is sufficient to reach adequate vitamin D status. *British Journal of Nutrition, 131*(4), 642–647. Available from https://doi.org/10.1017/s0007114523002222.

Hsu, C. C., Kuo, H. C., & Huang, K. E. (2017). The Effects of Phytosterols Extracted from Diascorea alata on the Antioxidant Activity, Plasma Lipids, and Hematological Profiles in Taiwanese Menopausal Women. *Nutrients, 9*(12). Available from https://doi.org/10.3390/nu9121320.

Hyldgaard, M., Mygind, T., & Meyer, R. L. (2012). Essential oils in food preservation: mode of action, synergies, and interactions with food matrix components. *Frontiers in microbiology*, *3*, 20029.

Inoue, M., Tanabe, H., Matsumoto, A., Takagi, M., Umegaki, K., Amagaya, S., & Takahashi, J. (2012). Astaxanthin functions differently as a selective peroxisome proliferator-activated receptor γ modulator in adipocytes and macrophages. *Biochemical Pharmacology*, *84*(5), 692–700. Available from https://doi.org/10.1016/j.bcp.2012.05.021.

Irandoost, P., Lotfi Yagin, N., Namazi, N., Keshtkar, A., Farsi, F., Mesri Alamdari, N., & Vafa, M. (2021). The effect of Capsaicinoids or Capsinoids in red pepper on thermogenesis in healthy adults: A systematic review and meta-analysis. *Phytotherapy Research*, *35*(3), 1358–1377. Available from https://doi.org/10.1002/ptr.6897.

Jabczyk, M., Nowak, J., Hudzik, B., & Zubelewicz-Szkodzińska, B. (2021). Curcumin in Metabolic Health and Disease. *Nutrients*, *13*(12), 4440. Available from https://doi.org/10.3390/nu13124440.

Jahandideh, F., & Wu, J. (2022). A review on mechanisms of action of bioactive peptides against glucose intolerance and insulin resistance. *Food Science and Human Wellness*, *11*(6), 1441–1454. Available from https://doi.org/10.1016/j.fshw.2022.06.001.

Jebari-Benslaiman, S., Galicia-García, U., Larrea-Sebal, A., Olaetxea, J. R., Alloza, I., Vandenbroeck, K., Benito-Vicente, A., & Martín, C. (2022). Pathophysiology of Atherosclerosis. *International Journal of Molecular Sciences*, *23*(6), 3346. Available from https://doi.org/10.3390/ijms23063346.

Ji, X., Shi, S., Liu, B., Shan, M., Tang, D., Zhang, W., Zhang, Y., Zhang, L., Zhang, H., Lu, C., & Wang, Y. (2019). Bioactive compounds from herbal medicines to manage dyslipidemia. *Biomedicine & Pharmacotherapy*, *118*, 109338. Available from https://doi.org/10.1016/j.biopha.2019.109338.

Ji, Z., Huang, C., Liang, C., Chen, B., Chen, S., & Sun, W. (2005). Protective effects of blocking renin-angiotensin system on the progression of renal injury in glomerulosclerosis. *Cellular & Molecular Immunology*, *2*(2), 150–154.

Jiang, Y., Biswas, S. K., Steinle, J. J., Steinle, J. J., & Steinle, J. J. (2014). Serine 307 on insulin receptor substrate 1 is required for SOCS3 and TNF-α signaling in the rMC-1 cell line. *Molecular Vision, United States Molecular Vision*, *20*, 1463–1470. Available from http://www.molvis.org/molvis/v20/1463/mv-v20-1463.pdf.

Kakutani, R., Hokari, S., Nishino, A., Ichihara, T., Sugimoto, K., Takaha, T., Kuriki, T., & Maoka, T. (2018). Effect of Oral Paprika Xanthophyll Intake on Abdominal Fat in Healthy Overweight Humans: A Randomized, Double-blind, Placebo-controlled Study. *Journal of Oleo Science*, *67*(9), 1149–1162. Available from https://doi.org/10.5650/jos.ess18076.

Kawakami, Y., Watanabe, Y., Mazuka, M., Yagi, N., Sawazaki, A., Koganei, M., Natsume, M., Kuriki, K., Morimoto, T., Asai, T., & Arai, H. (2021). Effect of cacao polyphenol-rich chocolate on postprandial glycemia, insulin, and incretin secretion in healthy participants. *Nutrition (Burbank, Los Angeles County, Calif.)*, *85*, 111128. Available from https://doi.org/10.1016/j.nut.2020.111128.

Keane, K. N., Cruzat, V. F., Carlessi, R., De Bittencourt, P. I. H., & Newsholme, P. (2015). Molecular Events Linking Oxidative Stress and Inflammation to Insulin Resistance and β-Cell Dysfunction. *Oxidative Medicine and Cellular Longevity*, *2015*. Available from https://doi.org/10.1155/2015/181643, http://www.hindawi.com/journals/oximed/.

Khan, S. A., Bhattacharjee, S., Ghani, M. O. A., Walden, R., & Chen, Q. M. (2020). Vitamin c for cardiac protection during percutaneous coronary intervention: A systematic review of randomized controlled trials. *Nutrients*, *12*(8), 1–21. Available from https://doi.org/10.3390/nu12082199, https://www.mdpi.com/2072-6643/12/8/2199/pdf.

Kim, Y. J., Choi, M. S., Woo, J. T., Jeong, M. J., Kim, S. R., & Jung, U. J. (2017). Long-term dietary supplementation with low-dose nobiletin ameliorates hepatic steatosis, insulin resistance, and inflammation without altering fat mass in diet-induced obesity. *Molecular Nutrition and Food Research*, *61*(8). Available from https://doi.org/10.1002/mnfr.201600889, www.mnf-journal.de.

Kim, Y. M., Kim, I. H., Choi, J. W., Lee, M. K., & Nam, T. J. (2015). The anti-obesity effects of a tuna peptide on 3T3-L1 adipocytes are mediated by the inhibition of the expression of lipogenic and adipogenic genes and by the activation of the Wnt/β-catenin signaling pathway. *International Journal of Molecular Medicine*, *36*(2), 327–334. Available from https://doi.org/10.3892/ijmm.2015.2231, http://www.spandidos-publications.com/ijmm/36/2/327/download.

Kitada, M., Ogura, Y., Monno, I., & Koya, D. (2020). Supplementation with red wine extract increases insulin sensitivity and peripheral blood mononuclear Sirt1 expression in nondiabetic humans. *Nutrients*, *12*(10), 3108. Available from https://doi.org/10.3390/nu12103108.

Klop, B., Elte, J. W., & Cabezas, M. C. (2013). Dyslipidemia in obesity: Mechanisms and potential targets. *Nutrients*, *5*(4), 1218–1240. Available from https://doi.org/10.3390/nu5041218.

Koirala, P., Dahal, M., Rai, S., Dhakal, M., Nirmal, N. P., Maqsood, S., Al-Asmari, F., & Buranasompob, A. (2023). Dairy milk protein–derived bioactive peptides: Avengers against metabolic syndrome. *Current Nutrition Reports*, *12*(2), 308–326. Available from https://doi.org/10.1007/s13668-023-00472-1, https://www.springer.com/journal/13668.

Kroff, J., Hume, D. J., Pienaar, P., Tucker, R., Lambert, E. V., & Rae, D. E. (2017). The metabolic effects of a commercially available chicken peri-peri (African bird's eye chilli) meal in overweight individuals. *British Journal of Nutrition*, *117*(5), 635–644. Available from https://doi.org/10.1017/S0007114515003104, http://journals.cambridge.org/BJN.

Lee, S. H., Park, S. Y., & Choi, C. S. (2022). Insulin resistance: From mechanisms to therapeutic strategies. *Diabetes Metab J*, *46*(1), 15–37. Available from https://doi.org/10.4093/dmj.2021.0280.

Li, B., He, X., Lei, S. S., Zhou, F. C., Zhang, N. Y., Chen, Y. H., Wang, Y. Z., Su, J., Yu, J. J., Li, L. Z., Zheng, X., Luo, R., Kołodyńska, D., Xiong, S., Lv, G. Y., & Chen, S. H. (2019). Hypertensive rats treated chronically with N(ω)-Nitro-L-arginine methyl ester (L-NAME) induced disorder of hepatic fatty acid metabolism and intestinal pathophysiology. *Front Pharmacol*, *10*, 1677. Available from https://doi.org/10.3389/fphar.2019.01677.

Li, Q., & Xing, B. (2016). A phytosterol-enriched spread improves lipid profile and insulin resistance of women with gestational diabetes mellitus: A randomized, placebo-controlled double-blind clinical trial. *Diabetes Technology & Therapeutics*, *18*(8), 499–504. Available from https://doi.org/10.1089/dia.2016.0103.

Li, X., Xin, Y., Mo, Y., Marozik, P., He, T., & Guo, H. (2022). The bioavailability and biological activities of phytosterols as modulators of cholesterol metabolism. *Molecules (Basel, Switzerland)*, *27*(2), 523. Available from https://doi.org/10.3390/molecules27020523.

Liu, D., Ye, J., Yan, Y., Chen, Y., Wang, H., Wang, M., Feng, Y., Li, R., Xu, X., Jiang, Y., Lian, C., Yang, Y., Meng, Y., Liu, Y., & Jiang, W. (2023). Ramulus mori (Sangzhi) alkaloids regulates gut microbiota disorder and its metabolism profiles in obese mice induced by a high-fat diet. *Frontiers in Pharmacology*, *14*. Available from https://doi.org/10.3389/fphar.2023.1166635.

Longo, M., Zatterale, F., Naderi, J., Parrillo, L., Formisano, P., Raciti, G. A., Beguinot, F., & Miele, C. (2019). Adipose tissue dysfunction as determinant of obesity-associated metabolic complications. *International Journal of Molecular Sciences*, *20*(9). Available from https://doi.org/10.3390/ijms20092358, https://www.mdpi.com/1422-0067/20/9/2358/pdf.

Lv, R., Dong, Y., Bao, Z., Zhang, S., Lin, S., & Sun, N. (2022). Advances in the activity evaluation and cellular regulation pathways of food-derived antioxidant peptides. *Trends in Food Science & Technology*, *122*, 171–186. Available from https://doi.org/10.1016/j.tifs.2022.02.026.

Ma, W., Li, N., Lin, L., Wen, J., Zhao, C., & Wang, F. (2023). Research progress in lipid metabolic regulation of bioactive peptides. *Food Production, Processing and Nutrition*, *5*(1). Available from https://doi.org/10.1186/s43014-022-00123-y.

Marazzi, G., Cacciotti, L., Pelliccia, F., Iaia, L., Volterrani, M., Caminiti, G., Sposato, B., Massaro, R., Grieco, F., & Rosano, G. (2011). Long-term effects of nutraceuticals (berberine, red yeast rice, policosanol) in elderly hypercholesterolemic patients. *Advances in Therapy*, *28*(12), 1105–1113. Available from https://doi.org/10.1007/s12325-011-0082-5.

Masyita, A., Mustika Sari, R., Dwi Astuti, A., Yasir, B., Rahma Rumata, N., Emran, T. B., Nainu, F., & Simal-Gandara, J. (2022). Terpenes and terpenoids as main bioactive compounds of essential oils, their roles in human health and potential application as natural food preservatives. *Food Chemistry: X*, *13*, 100217. Available from https://doi.org/10.1016/j.fochx.2022.100217.

Mesinovic, J., Rodriguez, A. J., Cervo, M. M., Gandham, A., Xu, C. L. H., Glavas, C., de Courten, B., Zengin, A., Ebeling, P. R., & Scott, D. (2023). Vitamin D supplementation and exercise for improving physical function, body composition and metabolic health in overweight or obese older adults with vitamin D deficiency: a pilot randomized, double-blind, placebo-controlled trial. *European Journal of Nutrition*, *62*(2), 951–964. Available from https://doi.org/10.1007/s00394-022-03038-z, https://www.springer.com/journal/394.

Wu, A. H., Spicer, D., Stanczyk, F. Z., Tseng, C. C., Yang, C. S., & Pike, M. C. (2012). Effect of 2-month controlled green tea intervention on lipoprotein cholesterol, glucose, and hormone levels in healthy postmenopausal women. *Cancer Prevention Research*, *5*(3), 393–402. Available from https://doi.org/10.1158/1940-6207.CAPR-11-0407, http://cancerpreventionresearch.aacrjournals.org/content/5/3/393.full.pdf + html.

Mori, N., Nakanishi, S., Shiomi, S., Kiyokawa, S., Kakimoto, S., Nakagawa, K., Hosoe, K., Minami, K., & Nadamoto, T. (2015). Enhancement of Fat Oxidation by Licorice Flavonoid Oil in Healthy Humans during Light Exercise. *Journal of Nutritional Science and Vitaminology*, *61*(5), 406–416. Available from https://doi.org/10.3177/jnsv.61.406.

Mounien, L., Tourniaire, F., & Landrier, J. F. (2019). Anti-obesity effect of carotenoids: Direct impact on adipose tissue and adipose tissue-driven indirect effects. *Nutrients*, *11*(7). Available from https://doi.org/10.3390/nu11071562.

Mozos, I., Stoian, D., Caraba, A., Malainer, C., Horbańczuk, J. O., & Atanasov, A. G. (2018). Lycopene and Vascular Health. *Frontiers in Pharmacology*, *9*(MAY). Available from https://doi.org/10.3389/fphar.2018.00521.

Munguia, L., Rubio-Gayosso, I., Ramirez-Sanchez, I., Ortiz, A., Hidalgo, I., Gonzalez, C., Meaney, E., Villarreal, F., Najera, N., Ceballos, G., & Newman, A. (2019). High flavonoid cocoa supplement ameliorates plasma oxidative stress and inflammation levels while improving mobility and quality of life in older subjects: A double-blind randomized clinical trial. *The Journals of Gerontology: Series A*, *74*(10), 1620–1627. Available from https://doi.org/10.1093/gerona/glz107.

do Nascimento, T. C., Cazarin, C. B. B., Maróstica, M. R., Mercadante, A. Z., Jacob-Lopes, E., & Zepka, L. Q. (2020). Microalgae carotenoids intake: Influence on cholesterol levels, lipid peroxidation and antioxidant enzymes. *Food Research International*, *128*. Available from https://doi.org/10.1016/j.foodres.2019.108770, www.elsevier.com/inca/publications/store/4/2/2/9/7/0.

Nattagh-Eshtivani, E., Barghchi, H., Pahlavani, N., Barati, M., Amiri, Y., Fadel, A., Khosravi, M., Talebi, S., Arzhang, P., Ziaei, R., & Ghavami, A. (2022). Biological and pharmacological effects and nutritional impact of phytosterols: A comprehensive review. *Phytotherapy Research*, *36*(1), 299–322. Available from https://doi.org/10.1002/ptr.7312.

Niroomand, M., Fotouhi, A., Irannejad, N., & Hosseinpanah, F. (2019). Does high-dose vitamin D supplementation impact insulin resistance and risk of development of diabetes in patients with pre-diabetes? A double-blind randomized clinical trial. *Diabetes Research and Clinical Practice*, *148*, 1–9. Available from https://doi.org/10.1016/j.diabres.2018.12.008.

Novin, Z. S., Ghavamzadeh, S., & Mehdizadeh, A. (2018). The weight loss effects of branched chain amino acids and vitamin B6: A randomized controlled trial on obese and overweight women. *International Journal for Vitamin and Nutrition Research. Internationale Zeitschrift fur Vitamin- und Ernahrungsforschung. Journal International de Vitaminologie et de Nutrition*, *88*(1-2), 80–89. Available from https://doi.org/10.1024/0300-9831/a000511.

Oliveira, G. Vd, Volino-Souza, M., Cordeiro, E. M., Conte-Junior, C. A., & Alvares, T. S. (2020). Effects of fish protein hydrolysate ingestion on endothelial function compared to whey protein hydrolysate in humans. Taylor and Francis Ltd, Brazil. *International Journal of Food Sciences and Nutrition*, *71*(2), 242–248. Available from https://doi.org/10.1080/09637486.2019.1635090, http://www.tandfonline.com/loi/iijf20.

Oluwole, O., Fernando, W. M. A. D. B., Lumanlan, J., Ademuyiwa, O., & Jayasena, V. (2022). Role of phenolic acid, tannins, stilbenes, lignans and flavonoids in human health – A review. *International Journal of Food Science & Technology*, *57*(10), 6326–6335. Available from https://doi.org/10.1111/ijfs.15936.

Onakpoya, I. J., & Heneghan, C. J. (2015). Effect of the novel functional fibre, polyglycoplex (PGX), on body weight and metabolic parameters: A systematic review of randomized clinical trials. *Clinical Nutrition, 34*(6), 1109–1114. Available from https://doi.org/10.1016/j.clnu.2015.01.004, http://www.elsevier-international.com/journals/clnu/.

Pai, S., Hebbar, A., & Selvaraj, S. (2022). A critical look at challenges and future scopes of bioactive compounds and their incorporations in the food, energy, and pharmaceutical sector. *Environmental Science and Pollution Research, 29*(24), 35518–35541. Available from https://doi.org/10.1007/s11356-022-19423-4.

Pal, S., Ho, S., Gahler, R. J., & Wood, S. (2017). Effect on insulin, glucose and lipids in overweight/obese australian adults of 12 months consumption of two different fibre supplements in a randomised trial. *Nutrients, 9*(2). Available from https://doi.org/10.3390/nu9020091, http://www.mdpi.com/2072-6643/9/2/91/pdf.

Palmeiro-Silva, Y. K., Aravena, R. I., Ossio, L., & Fluxa, J. P. (2020). Effects of daily consumption of an aqueous dispersion of free-phytosterols nanoparticles on individuals with metabolic syndrome: A randomised, double-blind, placebo-controlled clinical trial. *Nutrients, 12*(8), 1–18. Available from https://doi.org/10.3390/nu12082392, https://www.mdpi.com/2072-6643/12/8/2392/pdf.

Peng, D., Zhuge, F., Wang, M., Zhang, B., Zhuang, Z., Zhou, R., Zhang, Y., Li, J., Yu, Z., & Shi, J. (2024). Morus alba L. (Sangzhi) alkaloids mitigate atherosclerosis by regulating M1/M2 macrophage polarization. *Phytomedicine: International Journal of Phytotherapy and Phytopharmacology, 128*, 155526. Available from https://doi.org/10.1016/j.phymed.2024.155526.

Petersen, K. F., & Shulman, G. I. (2006). Etiology of insulin resistance. *American Journal of Medicine, 119*(5), S10. Available from https://doi.org/10.1016/j.amjmed.2006.01.009, www.elsevier.com/locate/amjmed.

Pfeuffer, M., Auinger, A., Bley, U., Kraus-Stojanowic, I., Laue, C., Winkler, P., Rüfer, C. E., Frank, J., Bösch-Saadatmandi, C., Rimbach, G., & Schrezenmeir, J. (2013). Effect of quercetin on traits of the metabolic syndrome, endothelial function and inflammation in men with different APOE isoforms. *Nutrition, Metabolism and Cardiovascular Diseases, 23*(5), 403–409. Available from https://doi.org/10.1016/j.numecd.2011.08.010.

Pinent, M., Blay, M., Bladé, M. C., Salvadó, M. J., & Arola, L. (2004). A. Ardévol, Grape seed-derived procyanidins have an antihyperglycemic effect in streptozotocin-induced diabetic rats and insulinomimetic activity in insulin-sensitive cell lines. *Endocrinology, 145*(11), 4985–4990. Available from https://doi.org/10.1210/en.2004-0764.

Prasad, M., Jayaraman, S., Eladl, M. A., El-Sherbiny, M., Abdelrahman, M. A. E., Veeraraghavan, V. P., Vengadassalapathy, S., Umapathy, V. R., Jaffer Hussain, S. F., Krishnamoorthy, K., Sekar, D., Palanisamy, C. P., Mohan, S. K., & Rajagopal, P. (2022). A comprehensive review on therapeutic perspectives of phytosterols in insulin resistance: A mechanistic approach. *Molecules (Basel, Switzerland), 27*(5). Available from https://doi.org/10.3390/molecules27051595, https://www.mdpi.com/1420-3049/27/5/1595/pdf.

Qiao, Q., Chen, L., Li, X., Lu, X., Xu, Q., & Deng, W. (2021). Roles of dietary bioactive peptides in redox balance and metabolic disorders. *Oxidative Medicine and Cellular Longevity, 2021*, 1–27. Available from https://doi.org/10.1155/2021/5582245.

Qin, Y., Ran, L., Wang, J., Yu, L., Lang, H. D., Wang, X. L., Mi, M. T., & Zhu, J. D. (2017). Capsaicin supplementation improved risk factors of coronary heart disease in individuals with low HDL-C levels. *Nutrients, 9*(9). Available from https://doi.org/10.3390/nu9091037, http://www.mdpi.com/2072-6643/9/9/1037/pdf.

Qu, L., Liang, Xc, Tian, Gq, Zhang, Gl, Wu, Ql, Huang, Xm, Cui, Yz, Liu, Yl, Shen, Zf, Ma, Gq, Lu, H., Li, Y., Jiang, H., Yang, Xy, Zhang, Gd, & Yang, Ch (2022). Efficacy and safety of mulberry twig alkaloids tablet for treatment of type 2 diabetes: A randomized, double-blind, placebo-controlled multicenter clinical study. *Chinese Journal of Integrative Medicine, 28*(4), 304–311. Available from https://doi.org/10.1007/s11655-021-2885-9, http://www.springerlink.com/content/1993-0402.

Rafiq, S., & Jeppesen, P. B. (2021). Vitamin d deficiency is inversely associated with homeostatic model assessment of insulin resistance. *Nutrients, 13*(12). Available from https://doi.org/10.3390/nu13124358, https://www.mdpi.com/2072-6643/13/12/4358/pdf.

Rahman, M. M., Rahaman, M. S., Islam, M. R., Rahman, F., Mithi, F. M., Alqahtani, T., Almikhlafi, M. A., Alghamdi, S. Q., Alruwaili, A. S., & Hossain, M. S. (2021). Role of phenolic compounds in human disease: current knowledge and future prospects. *Molecules (Basel, Switzerland), 27*(1), 233.

Roach, L. A., Meyer, B. J., Fitton, J. H., & Winberg, P. (2022). Improved plasma lipids, anti-inflammatory activity, and microbiome shifts in overweight participants: Two clinical studies on oral supplementation with algal sulfated polysaccharide. *Marine Drugs, 20*(8). Available from https://doi.org/10.3390/md20080500, http://www.mdpi.com/journal/marinedrugs.

Rodríguez-García, C., Sánchez-Quesada, C., Toledo, E., Delgado-Rodríguez, M., & Gaforio, J. J. (2019). Naturally lignan-rich foods: A dietary tool for health promotion? *Molecules (Basel, Switzerland), 24*(5). Available from https://doi.org/10.3390/molecules24050917, https://www.mdpi.com/1420-3049/24/5/917/pdf.

Rondanelli, M., Gasparri, C., Petrangolini, G., Allegrini, P., Avenoso, D., Fazia, T., Bernardinelli, L., Peroni, G., Patelli, Z., Mansueto, F., Tartara, A., Cavioni, A., & Riva, A. (2023). Berberine phospholipid exerts a positive effect on the glycemic profile of overweight subjects with impaired fasting blood glucose (IFG): A randomized double-blind placebo-controlled clinical trial. *European Review for Medical and Pharmacological Sciences, 27*(14), 6718–6727. Available from https://doi.org/10.26355/eurrev_202307_33142.

Ryu, N. H., Lim, Y., Park, J. E., Kim, J., Kim, J. Y., Kwon, S. W., & Kwon, O. (2014). Impact of daily Chlorella consumption on serum lipid and carotenoid profiles in mildly hypercholesterolemic adults: A double-blinded, randomized, placebo-controlled study. *Nutrition Journal, 13*(1). Available from https://doi.org/10.1186/1475-2891-13-57, http://www.nutritionj.com/home/.

Samtiya, M., Samtiya, S., Badgujar, P. C., Puniya, A. K., Dhewa, T., & Aluko, R. E. (2022). Health-promoting and therapeutic attributes of milk-derived bioactive peptides. *Nutrients, 14*(15). Available from https://doi.org/10.3390/nu14153001, http://www.mdpi.com/journal/nutrients/.

Sanches-Silva, A., Testai, L., Nabavi, S. F., Battino, M., Pandima Devi, K., Tejada, S., Sureda, A., Xu, S., Yousefi, B., Majidinia, M., Russo, G. L., Efferth, T., Nabavi, S. M., & Farzaei, M. H. (2020). Therapeutic potential of polyphenols in cardiovascular diseases: Regulation of mTOR signaling pathway. *Pharmacological Research*, *152*. Available from https://doi.org/10.1016/j.phrs.2019.104626, http://www.elsevier.com/inca/publications/store/6/2/2/9/3/1/index.htt.

Santos-Sánchez, G., Cruz-Chamorro, I., Álvarez-Ríos, A. I., Álvarez-Sánchez, N., Rodríguez-Ortiz, B., Álvarez-López, A. I., Fernández-Pachón, M.-S., Pedroche, J., Millán, F., Millán-Linares, M. d C., Lardone, P. J., Bejarano, I., & Carrillo-Vico, A. (2022). Bioactive peptides from lupin (*Lupinus angustifolius*) prevent the early stages of atherosclerosis in western diet-fed ApoE−/− mice. *Journal of Agricultural and Food Chemistry*, *70*(27), 8243−8253. Available from https://doi.org/10.1021/acs.jafc.2c00809.

Saraf-Bank, S., Ahmadi, A., Paknahad, Z., Maracy, M., & Nourian, M. (2019). Effects of curcumin on cardiovascular risk factors in obese and overweight adolescent girls: a randomized clinical trial. *Sao Paulo Medical Journal*, *137*(5), 414−422. Available from https://doi.org/10.1590/1516-3180.2018.0454120419.

Sargowo, D., Ovianti, N., Susilowati, E., Ubaidillah, N., Widya Nugraha, A., Vitriyaturrida, K., Siwi Proboretno, M., Failasufi, F., Ramadhan, H., Wulandari, Y., Waranugraha, D., & Hayuning Putri. (2018). The role of polysaccharide peptide of Ganoderma lucidum as a potent antioxidant against atherosclerosis in high risk and stable angina patients. *Indian Heart Journal*, *70*(5), 608−614. Available from https://doi.org/10.1016/j.ihj.2017.12.007.

Serino, A., & Salazar, G. (2019). Protective role of polyphenols against vascular inflammation, aging and cardiovascular disease. *Nutrients*, *11*(1), 53. Available from https://doi.org/10.3390/nu11010053.

Shahwan, M., Alhumaydhi, F., Ashraf, G. M., Hasan, P. M. Z., & Shamsi, A. (2022). Role of polyphenols in combating Type 2 Diabetes and insulin resistance. *International Journal of Biological Macromolecules*, *206*, 567−579. Available from https://doi.org/10.1016/j.ijbiomac.2022.03.004, www.elsevier.com/locate/ijbiomac.

Shi, R., Dan, B., & Lü, L. (2023). Bioactive effects advances of natural polysaccharides. *Journal of Future Foods*, *3*(3), 234−239. Available from https://doi.org/10.1016/j.jfutfo.2023.02.005.

Shimobayashi, M., Albert, V., Woelnerhanssen, B., Frei, I. C., Weissenberger, D., Meyer-Gerspach, A. C., Clement, N., Moes, S., Colombi, M., Meier, J. A., Swierczynska, M. M., Jenö, P., Beglinger, C., Peterli, R., & Hall, M. N. (2018). Insulin resistance causes inflammation in adipose tissue. *Journal of Clinical Investigation*, *128*(4), 1538−1550. Available from https://doi.org/10.1172/JCI96139, https://www.jci.org/articles/view/96139/pdf.

SHIRAKURA, Y., TAKAYANAGI, K., MUKAI, K., TANABE, H., & INOUE, M. (2011). β-cryptoxanthin suppresses the adipogenesis of 3T3-L1 cells via RAR activation. *Journal of Nutritional Science and Vitaminology*, *57*(6), 426−431. Available from https://doi.org/10.3177/jnsv.57.426.

Shoelson, S. E., Lee, J., & Yuan, M. (2003). Inflammation and the IKKβ/IκB/NF-κB axis in obesity-and diet-induced insulin resistance. *International Journal of Obesity*, *27*(3), S49−S52.

Silva, I. M. V., Machado, F., Moreno, M. J., Nunes, C., Coimbra, M. A., & Coreta-Gomes, F. (2021). Polysaccharide structures and their hypocholesterolemic potential. *Molecules (Basel, Switzerland)*, *26*(15). Available from https://doi.org/10.3390/molecules26154559, https://www.mdpi.com/1420-3049/26/15/4559/pdf.

Smolinske, S. C., Daubert, G. P., & Spoerke, D. G. (2007). Chapter 24 - Poisonous plants. In M. W. Shannon, S. W. Borron, & M. J. Burns (Eds.), *Haddad and Winchester's clinical management of poisoning and drug overdose (Fourth Edition)* (pp. 473−506). W.B. Saunders. Available from https://doi.org/10.1016/B978-0-7216-0693-4.50029-3.

Solverson, P. M., Rumpler, W. V., Leger, J. L., Redan, B. W., Ferruzzi, M. G., Baer, D. J., Castonguay, T. W., & Novotny, J. A. (2018). Blackberry feeding increases fat oxidation and improves insulin sensitivity in overweight and obese males. *Nutrients*, *10*(8). Available from https://doi.org/10.3390/nu10081048, http://www.mdpi.com/2072-6643/10/8/1048/pdf.

Song, L., Zhao, X. G., Ouyang, P. L., Guan, Q., Yang, L., Peng, F., Du, H., Yin, F., Yan, W., Yu, W. J., & Yan, H. (2020). Combined effect of n-3 fatty acids and phytosterol esters on alleviating hepatic steatosis in non-alcoholic fatty liver disease subjects: A double-blind placebo-controlled clinical trial. *British Journal of Nutrition*, *123*(10), 1148−1158. Available from https://doi.org/10.1017/S0007114520000495, http://journals.cambridge.org/BJN.

Stewart, M. L., & Zimmer, J. P. (2018). Postprandial glucose and insulin response to a high-fiber muffin top containing resistant starch type 4 in healthy adults: A double-blind, randomized, controlled trial. *Nutrition (Burbank, Los Angeles County, Calif.)*, *53*, 59−63. Available from https://doi.org/10.1016/j.nut.2018.01.002, www.elsevier.com/locate/nut.

Sun, P., Zhao, L., Zhang, N., Zhou, J., Zhang, L., Wu, W., Ji, B., & Zhou, F. (2021). Bioactivity of dietary polyphenols: The role in LDL-C lowering. *Foods*, *10*(11), 2666. Available from https://doi.org/10.3390/foods10112666.

Suntrup-Krueger, S., Muhle, P., Kampe, I., Egidi, P., Ruck, T., Lenze, F., Jungheim, M., Gminski, R., Labeit, B., Claus, I., Warnecke, T., Gross, J., & Dziewas, R. (2021). Effect of capsaicinoids on neurophysiological, biochemical, and mechanical parameters of swallowing function. *Neurotherapeutics: the Journal of the American Society for Experimental NeuroTherapeutics*, *18*(2), 1360−1370. Available from https://doi.org/10.1007/s13311-020-00996-2.

Surdu, A. M., Pînzariu, O., Ciobanu, D. M., Negru, A. G., Căinap, S. S., Lazea, C., Iacob, D., Săraci, G., Tirinescu, D., Borda, I. M., & Cismaru, G. (2021). Vitamin D and its role in the lipid metabolism and the development of atherosclerosis. *Biomedicines*, *9*(2), 1−16. Available from https://doi.org/10.3390/biomedicines9020172, https://www.mdpi.com/2227-9059/9/2/172.

Szallasi, A. (2022). Dietary capsaicin: A spicy way to improve cardio-metabolic health? *Biomolecules*, *12*(12), 1783. Available from https://doi.org/10.3390/biom12121783.

Takagi, T., Hayashi, R., Nakai, Y., Okada, S., Miyashita, R., Yamada, M., Mihara, Y., Mizushima, K., Morita, M., Uchiyama, K., Naito, Y., & Itoh, Y. (2020). Dietary intake of carotenoid-rich vegetables reduces visceral adiposity in obese Japanese men—A randomized, double-blind trial. *Nutrients*, *12*(8), 2342. Available from https://doi.org/10.3390/nu12082342.

Tang, J., Feng, Y., Zhang, B., Wu, Y., Guo, Z., Liang, S., Zhou, Z., Xie, M., & Hou, S. (2021). Severe pantothenic acid deficiency induces alterations in the intestinal mucosal proteome of starter Pekin ducks. *BMC Genomics*, *22*(1). Available from https://doi.org/10.1186/s12864-021-07820-x.

Tavares, A. K. M. M., Ribas, S. A., Paravidino, V. B., Sgambato, M. R., Rodrigues, Rd. R. M., da Rocha, C. M. M., Sichieri, R., & Cunha, D. B. (2021). Effect of phytosterol capsule supplementation associated with the National Cholesterol Education Program Step 2 diet on low-density lipoprotein in children and adolescents with dyslipidemia: A double-blind crossover trial. *Nutrition*, *82*. Available from https://doi.org/10.1016/j.nut.2020.111051, www.elsevier.com/locate/nut.

Thawabteh, A., Juma, S., Bader, M., Karaman, D., Scrano, L., Bufo, S., & Karaman, R. (2019). The biological activity of natural alkaloids against herbivores, cancerous cells and pathogens. *Toxins*, *11*(11), 656. Available from https://doi.org/10.3390/toxins11110656.

Theofilis, P., Sagris, M., Oikonomou, E., Antonopoulos, A. S., Siasos, G., Tsioufis, C., & Tousoulis, D. (2021). Inflammatory mechanisms contributing to endothelial dysfunction. *Biomedicines*, *9*(7). Available from https://doi.org/10.3390/biomedicines9070781, https://www.mdpi.com/2227-9059/9/7/781/pdf.

Toldrá, F., Reig, M., Aristoy, M. C., & Mora, L. (2018). Generation of bioactive peptides during food processing. *Food Chemistry*, *267*, 395–404. Available from https://doi.org/10.1016/j.foodchem.2017.06.119, www.elsevier.com/locate/foodchem.

Trask, L. E., Chaidarun, S. S., Platt, D., & Parkin, C. G. (2014). Treatment with novel galactomannan derivative reduces 2-hour postprandial glucose excursions in individuals with type 2 diabetes treated with oral medications and/or insulin. *Journal of Diabetes Science and Technology*, *8*(5), 1018–1022. Available from https://doi.org/10.1177/1932296814538939, http://dst.sagepub.com/content/by/year.

Tung, M. C., Lan, Y. W., Li, H. H., Chen, H. L., Chen, S. Y., Chen, Y. H., Lin, C. C., Tu, M. Y., & Chen, C. M. (2020). Kefir peptides alleviate high-fat diet-induced atherosclerosis by attenuating macrophage accumulation and oxidative stress in ApoE knockout mice. *Scientific Reports*, *10* (1). Available from https://doi.org/10.1038/s41598-020-65782-8, www.nature.com/srep/index.html.

Ungvari, Z., Toth, P., Tarantini, S., Prodan, C. I., Sorond, F., Merkely, B., & Csiszar, A. (2021). Hypertension-induced cognitive impairment: from pathophysiology to public health. Nature Research, United States. *Nature Reviews Nephrology*, *17*(10), 639–654. Available from https://doi.org/10.1038/s41581-021-00430-6, http://www.nature.com/nrneph/archive/index.html.

Urbina, S. L., Roberts, M. D., Kephart, W. C., Villa, K. B., Santos, E. N., Olivencia, A. M., Bennett, H. M., Lara, M. D., Foster, C. A., Purpura, M., Jäger, R., Taylor, L. W., & Wilborn, C. D. (2017). Effects of twelve weeks of capsaicinoid supplementation on body composition, appetite and self-reported caloric intake in overweight individuals. *Appetite*, *113*, 264–273. Available from https://doi.org/10.1016/j.appet.2017.02.025, http://www.elsevier.com/inca/publications/store/6/2/2/7/8/5/index.htt.

Vasim, I., Majeed, C. N., & DeBoer, M. D. (2022). Intermittent fasting and metabolic health. *Nutrients*, *14*(3), 631.

Vezza, T., Canet, F., Marañón, A. M. de, Bañuls, C., Rocha, M., & Víctor, V. M. (2020). Phytosterols: Nutritional health players in the management of obesity and its related disorders. *Antioxidants*, *9*(12), 1–20. Available from https://doi.org/10.3390/antiox9121266, https://www.mdpi.com/2076-3921/9/12/1266.

Wang, Y., & Zidichouski, J. A. (2018). Update on the benefits and mechanisms of action of the bioactive vegetal alkaloid berberine on lipid metabolism and homeostasis. *Cholesterol*, *2018*. Available from https://doi.org/10.1155/2018/7173920, http://www.hindawi.com/journals/chol/.

Wen, C., Zhang, J., Zhang, H., Duan, Y., & Ma, H. (2020). Plant protein-derived antioxidant peptides: Isolation, identification, mechanism of action and application in food systems: A review. *Trends in Food Science & Technology*, *105*, 308–322. Available from https://doi.org/10.1016/j.tifs.2020.09.019.

Whiting, S., Derbyshire, E., & Tiwari, B. K. (2012). Capsaicinoids and capsinoids. A potential role for weight management? A systematic review of the evidence. *Appetite*, *59*(2), 341–348. Available from https://doi.org/10.1016/j.appet.2012.05.015.

Williamson, G., & Sheedy, K. (2020). Effects of polyphenols on insulin resistance. *Nutrients*, *12*(10), 3135. Available from https://doi.org/10.3390/nu12103135.

Wu, S., Jia, W., He, H., Yin, J., Xu, H., He, C., Zhang, Q., Peng, Y., & Cheng, R. (2023). A new dietary fiber can enhance satiety and reduce postprandial blood glucose in healthy adults: A randomized cross-over trial. *Nutrients*, *15*(21), 4569. Available from https://doi.org/10.3390/nu15214569.

Xiong, Q., Hu, Y., Ye, X., Song, Z., Yuan, J., Xiong, B., Jing, Y., Shi, Y., Xu, T., Wu, J., Zhang, Q., Liang, J., & Zhou, L. (2020). Extraction, purification and characterization of sulphated polysaccharide from Bellamya quadrata and its stabilization roles on atherosclerotic plaque. *International Journal of Biological Macromolecules*, *152*, 314–326. Available from https://doi.org/10.1016/j.ijbiomac.2020.02.243.

Yang, D., Luo, Z., Ma, S., Wong, W. T., Ma, L., Zhong, J., He, H., Zhao, Z., Cao, T., Yan, Z., Liu, D., Arendshorst, W. J., Huang, Y., Tepel, M., & Zhu, Z. (2010). Activation of TRPV1 by dietary capsaicin improves endothelium-dependent vasorelaxation and prevents hypertension. Cell Press, China. *Cell Metabolism*, *12*(2), 130–141. Available from https://doi.org/10.1016/j.cmet.2010.05.015, http://www.cellmetabolism.org/.

Yousefi, R., Parandoosh, M., Khorsandi, H., Hosseinzadeh, N., Madani Tonekaboni, M., Saidpour, A., Babaei, H., & Ghorbani, A. (2021). Grape seed extract supplementation along with a restricted-calorie diet improves cardiovascular risk factors in obese or overweight adult individuals: A randomized, placebo-controlled trial. *Phytotherapy Research*, *35*(2), 987–995. Available from https://doi.org/10.1002/ptr.6859.

Yu, W., Zeng, D., Xiong, Y., Shan, S., Yang, X., Zhao, H., & Lu, W. (2022). Health benefits of functional plant polysaccharides in metabolic syndrome: An overview. *Journal of Functional Foods*, *95*. Available from https://doi.org/10.1016/j.jff.2022.105154, http://www.elsevier.com/wps/find/journaldescription.cws_home/717426/description#description.

Yu, X.-H., Zheng, X.-L., & Tang, C.-K. (2015). Chapter One - Nuclear factor-κB activation as a pathological mechanism of lipid metabolism and atherosclerosis. In G. S. Makowski (Ed.), *Advances in Clinical Chemistry* (Vol. 70, pp. 1–30). Elsevier. Available from https://doi.org/10.1016/bs.acc.2015.03.004.

Yuan, L. J., Qin, Y., Wang, L., Zeng, Y., Chang, H., Wang, J., Wang, B., Wan, J., Chen, S. H., Zhang, Q. Y., Zhu, J. D., Zhou, Y., & Mi, M. T. (2016). Capsaicin-containing chili improved postprandial hyperglycemia, hyperinsulinemia, and fasting lipid disorders in women with gestational diabetes mellitus and lowered the incidence of large-for-gestational-age newborns. *Clinical Nutrition*, *35*(2), 388–393. Available from https://doi.org/10.1016/j.clnu.2015.02.011, http://www.elsevier-international.com/journals/clnu/.

Zafar, M., Khan, H., Rauf, A., Khan, A., & Lodhi, M. A. (2016). In silico study of alkaloids as α-glucosidase inhibitors: Hope for the discovery of effective lead compounds. *Frontiers in Endocrinology*, *7*. Available from https://doi.org/10.3389/fendo.2016.00153, http://journal.frontiersin.org/article/10.3389/fendo.2016.00153/full.

Zeb, A. (2020). Concept, mechanism, and applications of phenolic antioxidants in foods. *Journal of Food Biochemistry*, *44*(9). Available from https://doi.org/10.1111/jfbc.13394.

Zeka, K., Ruparelia, K., Arroo, R., Budriesi, R., & Micucci, M. (2017). Flavonoids and their metabolites: Prevention in cardiovascular diseases and diabetes. *Diseases*, *5*(3), 19. Available from https://doi.org/10.3390/diseases5030019.

Zhang, X., & Beynen, A. C. (1993). Lowering effect of dietary milk-whey protein v. casein on plasma and liver cholesterol concentrations in rats. *British Journal of Nutrition*, *70*(1), 139–146. Available from https://doi.org/10.1079/BJN19930111.

Zhang, Z., Li, J., Hu, T., Xu, C., Xie, N., & Chen, D. (2021). Interventional effect of dietary fiber on blood glucose and pregnancy outcomes in patients with gestational diabetes mellitus. *Zhejiang Da Xue xue Bao. Yi xue Ban = Journal of Zhejiang University. Medical Sciences*, *50*(3), 305–312. Available from https://doi.org/10.3724/zdxbyxb-2021-0115.

Ziegler, M., Wallert, M., Lorkowski, S., & Peter, K. (2020). Cardiovascular and metabolic protection by vitamin E: A matter of treatment strategy? *Antioxidants*, *9*(10), 935. Available from https://doi.org/10.3390/antiox9100935.

Ziółkiewicz, A., Kasprzak-Drozd, K., Rusinek, R., Markut-Miotła, E., & Oniszczuk, A. (2023). The influence of polyphenols on atherosclerosis development. *International Journal of Molecular Sciences*, *24*(8), 7146. Available from https://doi.org/10.3390/ijms24087146.

Chapter 8

Sports nutrition: boosting performance with functional foods

Prabina Bhattarai[1], Kritee Niroula[2] and Nilesh Prakash Nirmal[3]

[1]Department of Health and Human Development, Montana State University, Bozeman, MT, United States, [2]School of Nutrition and Food Sciences, Louisiana State University, Baton Rouge, LA, United States, [3]Institute of Nutrition, Mahidol University, Salaya, Nakhon Pathom, Thailand

8.1 Introduction

Nutrition has an essential role in determining the performance of an athlete, and it is referred to as "invisible training" (Saura et al., 2019). The key to utmost athletic performance depends on the diet that provides energy for training, nutrients for body maintenance, and tissue repair and regulation of body metabolism. Intense training and performance cause oxidative cell damage and inflammation by producing free radicals or reactive oxygen species (ROS). Exercise-induced inflammation, muscle damage, and pain altogether contribute to decreased body movement and limit daily training in addition to affecting daily performance. Several foods containing antioxidants such as phenols, flavonoids, and vitamins E and C are known to combat free radicals induced during exercise, which subsequently impact the downstream oxidative and inflammatory pathways (Nikolaidis et al., 2012). Free radicals are converted into nonradicals which reduces their reactivity and therefore prevents the conversion to the reactive components that are responsible for cellular damage (Powers et al., 2014).

Several nutrients aid in accelerating the recovery process, shielding muscles and tissues from the damage caused by rigorous exercise, and eventually improving the performance of athletes. To optimize athletic performance and ensure the best possible health and wellness for athletes, biofunctional nutrients can be administered as appropriate through prudent sports nutritional therapy (Liu et al., 2023). An appropriate and well-balanced diet that satisfies their elevated needs for vitamins, minerals, and functional compounds, along with an ample quantity of water, offers a safe and wholesome substitute that can enhance optimal athletic performance. An adequate and balanced diet should be consumed particularly during periods of high physical activity to ensure that energy and macronutrient requirements are met for maintaining body weight, replenishing glycogen stores, providing enough protein to build and repair tissues, and providing essential fatty acids and fat-soluble vitamins (Gammone et al., 2014).

Exercise increases the number of antagonistic mediators such as proinflammatory cytokines, like tumor necrosis factor-alpha (TNFα), interleukin-1β (IL-1β), and IL-8 (Liu et al., 2023). Therefore nutrient supplements can be targeted to minimize the adverse effects of exercise by regulating the various signaling pathways associated with inflammation and oxidative stress. In the last decades, plant-based nutrients such as phytosterol, phenolic acids, and flavonoids have garnered researchers' interest in the utilization of these functional phytoextracts in the field of sports nutrition. These nutrients provide positive metabolic benefits by controlling gene expression, blocking oxidative and inflammatory signaling pathways, quenching free radicals, and inhibiting specific receptors associated with stress and inflammation. Thus this chapter explored the potential role of bioactive compounds in promoting athletes' health and additional organ damage as well as the development of certain illnesses.

8.2 Importance of bioactive nutrients

8.2.1 Functional fat

Fat, especially omega-3 polyunsaturated fatty acids (PUFA), derived primarily from fish, seafood, nuts, and seeds, is essential for humans due to its several health-promoting benefits. There are three major types of omega-3 fatty acids:

Unleashing the Power of Functional Foods and Novel Bioactives. DOI: https://doi.org/10.1016/B978-0-443-28862-3.00008-X

eicosapentaenoic acid (EPA) and docosahexaenoic acid (DHA), which are derived from animals, mainly fish ($\sim$300 mg/g oil); alpha-linolenic acid (ALA), which is derived from plant sources, mainly chia seed ($\sim$0.6 g/g oil). During exercise, particularly eccentric exercise, the muscle undergoes stress, which may lead to exercise-induced muscle damage. In such cases, the body responds to inflammation by releasing muscle-specific creatine kinase and releasing mediators such as interleukin-1 receptor antagonists, interleukin (IL)-6, IL-10, and acute-phase proteins (Baird et al., 2012; Kyriakidou et al., 2021). Supplementation of omega-3 has proven to be an effective way to reduce inflammation in the muscles and enhance functional recovery after intense exercise. Omega-3 PUFAs are mostly stored in cell membranes, which, upon activation by injury, are released to the cytosol, eventually leading to antiinflammatory pathways by producing antiinflammatory eicosanoids and inhibiting the formation of inflammatory eicosanoids. Omega-3 is linked with muscle inflammation as it helps to downregulate proinflammatory cytokines, like IL-6 and TNF-α, and decreases the production of ROS, which eventually reduces inflammation (Jannas-Vela et al., 2023). Ingestion of n-3 PUFA improves different physiological parameters, which are associated with improved performance and regulated oxygen utilization (Calder, 2017). n-3 PUFAs supplementation inhibits inflammation by inhibiting the cyclooxygenase-2 (COX-2) (Cui et al., 2022). Also, n-3 PUFAs inhibit inflammation by inhibiting the production of proinflammatory cytokines, as well as by lowering the production of ROS and arachidonic acid (Papadopoulou et al., 2022). Besides, the role of n-3 fatty acids on mitochondrial biogenesis is also important for improving the performance of athletes. Greater mitochondrial density enables the ability to optimize adenosine triphosphate (ATP) production, which increases endurance power and improves training adaptation in athletes. Research employing EPA supplementation on mitochondrial biogenesis has found increased expression of genes involved in mitochondrial biogenesis in overweight individuals (Laiglesia et al., 2016).

Apart from omega-3, isomers of conjugated linoleic acid (trans10 and cis 12) enhanced the exercise endurance of mice and promoted the formation of oxidative muscle fiber type of gastrocnemius muscle. t10, c12-conjugated linoleic acid isomer increased TLR4 signaling expression in skeletal muscle and C2C12 myotubes. More importantly, the knockdown of TLR4 eliminated the t10, c12-conjugated linoleic acid isomer-induced enhancement of exercise endurance in mice and elevation of oxidative muscle fiber type in C2C12 myotubes and gastrocnemius muscle (Duan et al., 2021). Conjugated linoleic acid supplementation improves energy metabolism by promoting significant changes in lipid metabolic pathways and body composition (Tavakoli-Rouzbehani et al., 2021).

8.2.2 Biofunctional carbohydrates

Carbohydrates are the predominant source of energy for human metabolism. As a substrate, it is utilized with either anaerobic glycolysis during short, high-intensity exercise or oxidative phosphorylation during aerobic exercise. Muscle glycogen is preferentially utilized as the source of carbohydrates during high-intensity exercise (Mul et al., 2015). The transportation of glucose is dependent on insulin activity and is transported to tissues via glucose transporters (GLUT) present in the cell membrane. Apart from the direct glucose source and stored glycogen, the liver converts various sources such as amino acids, glycerol, and lactate, into glucose through the gluconeogenesis pathway. There are other functional bioactive carbohydrates such as oligosaccharides, lactulose, and fucans, which are reported to have significant impacts on athlete's performance by improving the storage and utilization of energy (Cui et al., 2022).

8.2.3 Bioactive protein/peptide

About one-third of the protein in skeletal muscle is composed of branched-chain amino acids (BCAAs), which include leucine, valine, and isoleucine. BCAAs contribute to the formation of β-hydroxyl group, β-methylbutyrate, and α-ketoisohexanoic acid, which enhance muscular growth and decrease body fat. Consumption of BCAAs before an aerobic activity has been associated with decreased fatigue, delayed glycogen utilization, and lowered protein degradation (Cui et al., 2022).

Short peptides are superior to amino acids when it comes to faster transit, lower energy consumption, and less carrier saturation. They are easier for tissues and organs to absorb and can compensate for amino acid–based nutritional requirements. Through pinocytosis, peptides mainly enter intestinal epithelial cells via the M-cell route. Through the processes of endocytosis and exocytosis, M cells can absorb intact peptides and then transfer them to intestinal epithelial cells. Moreover, peptides may enter intestinal epithelial cells by the paracellular pathway, which does not require energy and is reliant on variations in concentration and electrochemical potential between the two sides of the intestinal epithelial cells (Wu et al., 2019). Currently, the exploration of the bioactive peptides from different sources has highlighted their potential antiinflammatory, antioxidant, and healing potential. Peptides isolated from the hydrolysis of plant peptides, dairy products, and marine sources have shown potent biofunctional activity (Gammone et al., 2014; Koirala et al., 2023; Nirmal et al., 2024). As a result, these peptides can be introduced into functional foods or utilized as nutraceuticals to help prevent diseases and tissue/cell damage; as such, they are excellent supplements for athletes.

8.2.4 Vitamins

Vitamins are fundamental to various metabolic pathways related to exercise, tissue growth, and general metabolic health. They have a wide range of functions, including red blood cell formation, energy metabolism, and antioxidative properties; thus they are vital bioactive components necessary for athletes to improve exercise-related performance. In athletes, the increase in demand for vitamins is mainly due to decreased absorption from the GI tract, increased utilization by exercise-related stress and maintenance of musculoskeletal mass. Vitamins A, C, and E are some highly needed vitamins for athletes as they are utilized in the quenching of free radicals produced during exercise. Vitamin E supplementation has shown improvement in muscle recovery after exercise-induced membrane disruptions, which are common in muscle contraction and relaxation and are susceptible to ROS attacks. Vitamin E supplementation has been shown to repair damaged cell membranes (Khor et al., 2014).

Likewise, vitamin D is involved in signaling different anabolic and catabolic pathways in skeletal muscle health (Latham et al., 2021). It is involved in increasing osteocalcin, fibroblast growth factor 23, osteoglycin, insulin-like growth factor 1, and vascular endothelial growth factor. The rates of protein synthesis and its degradation are essential to maintaining the balance of skeletal muscle health. Most often, the lysosomal system, the ATP-ubiquitin-dependent system, and the cytosolic calcium-activated system are described as proteolytic pathways in muscle mass maintenance. Vitamin D is found to be involved in the ATP-ubiquitin-dependent system, where its deficiency leads to an increase in the expression of the E2-ubiquitin conjugating enzyme, 2 muscle-specific E3 ligases, and ubiquitin conjugates. Also, muscle atrophy is mostly dependent on Atrogin-1 and Muscle RING finger 1 (MuRF1), which are in charge of intracellular proteolysis, and vitamin D deficiency has been found to increase Atrogin-1 and MuRF1 twofold (Bhat et al., 2013). Moreover, vitamin D deficiency is linked with ROS generation, vitamin D receptor (VDR) ablation, and mitochondrial dysfunction, eventually resulting in muscle atrophy (Dzik & Kaczor, 2019). B-complexes have an immunomodulating effect through different pathways, as shown in Fig. 8.1. Vitamin B_1 interacts with immune cells to release intercellular adhesion molecules and also functions as an antioxidant, preventing oxidative damage; B_2 supports the production of interferons (IFN), IL-17, and macrophage phagocytosis; B_3 reduces inflammatory factors (IL-6, TNF-alpha), eventually reducing oxidative stress, and also aids in limiting lipid deposition. The self-explanatory figure next shows the involvement of several B-complex vitamins in immunomodulatory effects in an individual.

8.2.5 Phyto extracts

Phytoextracts are most importantly involved in antioxidative, antiinflammatory activity, and associated pathways. Studies indicate that aerobic endurance exercise is more complex than anaerobic exercise, and there is convincing evidence that both chronic and moderate physical training increase endogenous antioxidant capacity. A study evaluating various cycling intensities indicated that moderate-intensity exercise appears to have beneficial benefits, even though continuous exercise increases ROS formation at higher exercise intensities (Maryama Awang Daud & Ahmedy, 2022). The phospholipase A_2 and NADPH oxidases in the sarcoplasm produce ROS by cleaving membrane phospholipids and releasing arachidonic acid, a substrate that activates ROS-producing enzyme systems. In such conditions, antioxidant compounds can act in two different ways: one as RONS sequestrants and another as nuclear factor erythroid 2—related factor 2 (Nrf-2) activators. According to reports, reactive oxygen and nitrogen species scavengers reduced the development of antioxidant endogenous enzymes such as glutathione peroxidase (GPX) and mitochondrial superoxide dismutase by preventing the transitory rise of free radicals (Li et al., 2022). Polyphenols function as xenobiotics, inducing the hermetic cellular response and endogenous antioxidant synthesis (including glutathione reductase, superoxide dismutase, catalase, glutathione transferase, and glutathione peroxidase). This process can further improve the antioxidant status of the human body, including that of athletes (Ali Redha et al., 2024). The antioxidant ability of phenolic acids, such as anthocyanins, is dependent on the number and location of phenolic hydroxyls and the donation of a hydrogen atom from the phenolic hydroxyl group of anthocyanins (reference). On the other hand, compounds such as flavonoids and resveratrol act as Nrf-2 activators. Through the upregulation of the Nrf2 cellular stress signaling system, flavonoids aid in the recovery from exercise-induced muscle injury (Carey et al., 2021). The process by which polyphenols trigger signaling pathways is linked to cellular stress, which in turn mobilizes Nrf2 and activates the nuclear antioxidant

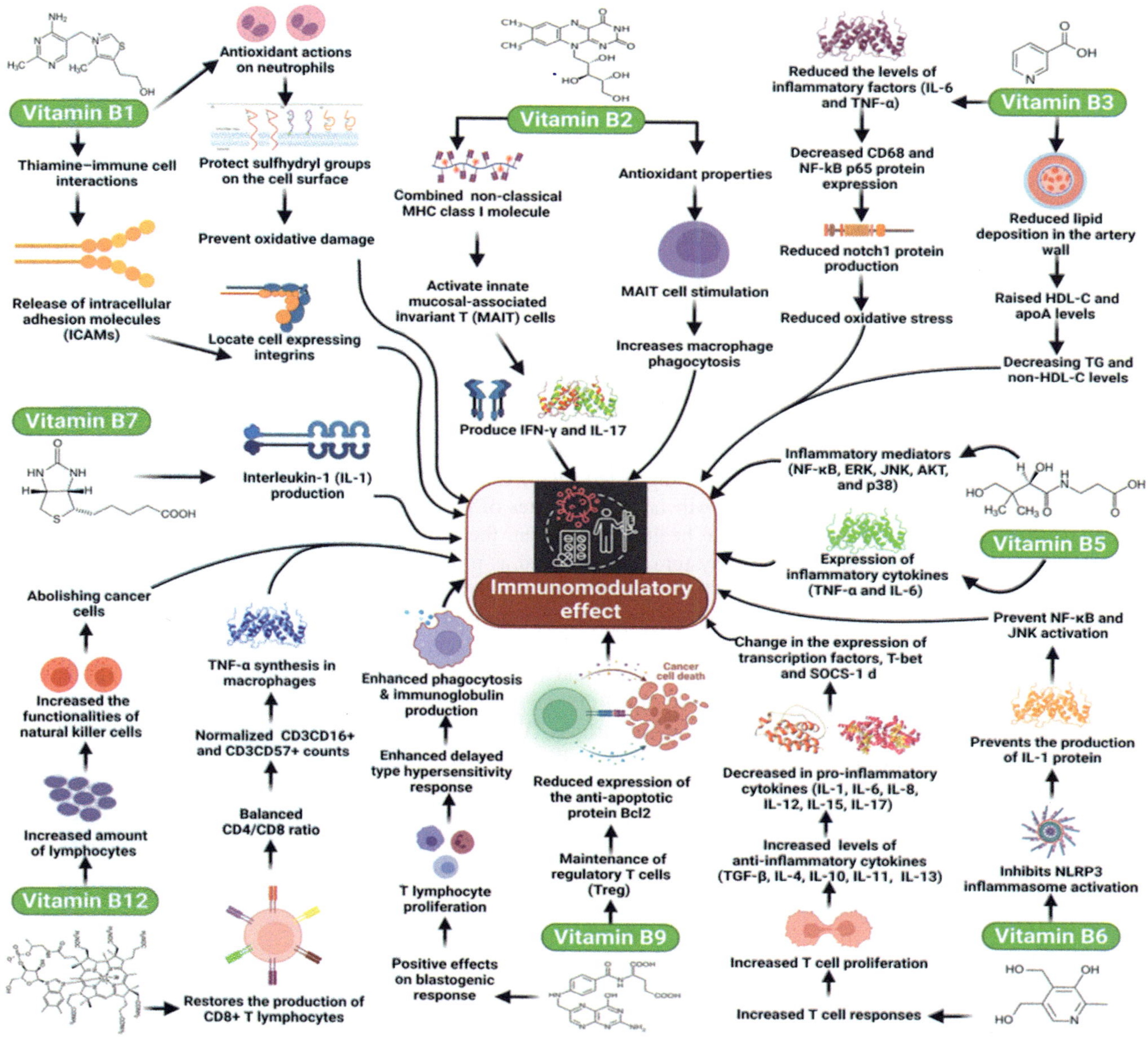

FIGURE 8.1 Immune-boosting functions of B-complex vitamins outsourced from Mitra et al. (2022) which is an open-access article distributed under the terms and conditions of the creative commons attribution (CC BY) license.

response element (ARE). The ARE's activation stimulates the synthesis of antioxidants and Phase II enzymes, including glutathione (Fig. 8.1) (Ali Redha et al., 2024).

Apart from this, the phytoextracts alleviate inflammation, which is most common among athletes. Athletes must overcome significant physical and psychological stress during extremely taxing exercises during everyday physical endeavors. Thus for better performance, it is demanding physical fitness by overcoming these issues. Many sportsmen have inflammation and musculoskeletal issues despite having a higher pain threshold. The most common sports injuries are to the lower extremities, where they mostly manifest as ligament rips and deformities, occasionally as fractures. Additionally, there is an immunological response to stress: In the event of intense exercise, there is a higher risk of infections and transient immunosuppression. The supplementation of bioactive compounds aids in reducing inflammation and compromised immune systems. It has been discovered that compounds such as fucoxanthin can effectively increase the thermogenic potential of brown adipose tissue and the expression of the uncoupling protein (UCP) 1 gene in white adipose tissue, functioning as a regulator of energy expenditure and lipid metabolism in adipose tissues. Also, fucoxanthin is a potent antioxidant that strengthens the immune system and shields cells from oxidative damage (Jeon et al., 2010).

TABLE 8.1 Biofunctional Proteins, Peptides, and Oligosaccharides With a Potent Role in Enhancing Athletics Health.

Protein/ Biofunctional Carbohydrates	Mechanism	Role in Sport Nutrition	References
Collagen	A framework that makes up the skeleton	Muscle tissue regeneration	Cui et al. (2022)
lentinan	Act as an enhancer and immune activator	Enhancing immune function	
Phycocyanin	Increase the activity of lymphocytes and enhance human immunity	Improve immunity	
L-carnitine	Promotes oxidation and decomposition of fatty acids into mitochondria	Weight control	
Creatine	Stored in the muscle as extra ATP production during training	Improve endurance	
Chondroitin:	Promote cartilage regeneration, inhibit cartilage-destroying enzyme activity and synthesis and supplement synovial fluid	Body recovery	
Oligosaccharides	The body's energy supply and strengthen the body's endurance.	Increasing energy storage and utilization	
Konjac	Changes the fluidity of cell membranes and increases the rate of fat oxidation	Wellness	
Glucosamine Chitosan monomer	Prevent collagen degradation and enhance collagen synthesis	Collagen synthesis and recovery	Momomura et al. (2013) and Yoshimura et al. (2009)

At the site of tissue damage, an enzyme called COX-2 is produced, causing prostaglandin E2, an anabolic molecule that increases pain and inflammation. In addition to COX, additional molecules that can disrupt the processes involved in the regulation of gene expression, including nuclear factor kappa B (NF-κB), should also be considered possible anti-inflammatory compounds. In this regard, it has recently been demonstrated that marine natural bioactives contain not only antioxidant agents but also steroids and a variety of molecular entities that may be able to target cyclooxygenase-1 (COX-1), cyclooxygenase-2 (COX-2), and the NF-κB pathway. This can help to block pain and inflammation while occasionally avoiding the need for medication in athletes (Gammone et al., 2014). Table 8.1 highlights the recent findings for the potential application of several bioactive compounds as antioxidative and antiinflammatory molecules to overcome oxidative stress, inflammation, and immunosuppression in athletes to maintain overall well-being.

8.3 Sports activity and nutrition

8.3.1 Enhancing muscle strength

There are a variety of underlying factors contributing to an athlete's performance. Muscular strength is a modifiable factor directly correlated to the athlete's performance. Muscular strength can be modified through the synergistic effects of nutrition and resistance training. Muscular strength is associated with enhanced performance, improved power output, resistance to fatigue, and body injuries. Stronger muscles lead to increased force production of the muscles, leading to faster muscular contraction due to active recruitment of the motor units, subsequently increasing the speed of movement and helping athletes reach their full potential. Certain bioactive compounds are effective in enhancing the muscle strength of individuals.

8.3.1.1 Peptides

Strength training is mostly related to protein consumption, and the role of bioactive peptides in building muscle has recently garnered research interest in sports nutrition. Bioactive peptides are known to have random interactions with receptors or endogenous proteins, such as the mammalian target of rapamycin (mTOR), glucose transporter type 4

(GLUT-4), or glycogen synthase, which stimulates muscular protein synthesis (König et al., 2021). For example, one randomized controlled trial study showed that ingesting whole eggs or egg whites for 12 weeks along with resistance training increased knee extension and handgrip strength (Bagheri et al., 2021). There was an absolute change in the group who ate whole eggs, indicated by a more significant increase in quadriceps strength, handgrip strength for the left hand, and handgrip strength for the right hand. The impact study of 6 months of egg white protein supplementation on muscle strength in old age found increased muscular strength (handgrip strength) compared to the placebo group (isocaloric maltodextrin) (Ullevig et al., 2022).

8.3.1.2 Omega-3

The beneficial effect of omega-3 fatty acids is increased muscular strength by enhancing the rates of muscle protein synthesis by increasing the enhancement of anabolic mTOR Ser2448 and p70S6K1 Thr389 phosphorylation in skeletal muscle, supporting gains in skeletal muscle mass and size over time (Gingras et al., 2007). Six months of n-3 PUFA supplementation in older adults showed a significant increase in handgrip strength and 1-RM muscle strength and tended to increase average isokinetic power compared to the corn oil (Kunz et al., 2022). Compared with the control group, six months of supplementation with krill oil in older adults increased knee extensor maximal torque and grip strength, respectively (Alkhedhairi et al., 2022). A comparison of supplementation of 3 g omega-3 and corn pill placebo per day in older adults engaging in a 12-week resistance exercise program showed an increase in isometric knee-extensor strength and leg press strength improved only in the omega-3 group (Dalle et al., 2021). However, no improvements in strength were observed in competitive male and female soccer players who supplemented their diet with omega-3 fatty acids over 4-week training period, indicating that consumption of omega-3 fatty acids may enhance muscle strength in older adults, but not in healthy young population (Gravina et al., 2017).

8.3.1.3 Dietary nitrate

The efficacy of using dietary nitrate food products to enhance muscular strength is equivocal, which is partly attributed to choosing different outcomes to measure muscle strength. Beetroot juice supplementation has been shown to reduce the phosphocreatine cost of force production and improve the local perfusion and contractility of low-oxygenated type II (fast twitch) muscle fibers, indicating improved maximal strength (Fulford et al., 2013). For instance, a randomized crossover clinical trial on older subjects showed a significant reduction of handgrip strength declination observed 30 min after exercise with 100 g of beetroot-based gel compared to placebo (Oliveira et al., 2017). Healthy older adults showed increased maximal knee extensor power with the consumption of nitrate-rich beetroot juice compared to nitrate beetroot juice (Coggan et al., 2020). Likewise, young recreationally active males with the supplementation of 6 days of 140 mL/day nitrate-rich (BR) and nitrate-depleted (PLA; 0.37 mg/day) beetroot juice showed significantly higher isokinetic knee flexion power following BR compared with PLA ingestion at $60° \cdot s^{-1}$, but not at $120° \cdot s^{-1}$, $180° \cdot s^{-1}$, and $300° \cdot s^{-1}$ (Nyakayiru et al., 2017). No significant improvements were found in isometric strength and isokinetic knee extension power between treatments, indicating no improvement in maximal strength in healthy, active males (Jonvik et al., 2021).

8.3.1.4 Catechins

Catechins, which belong to the flavonoid group, are the main secondary metabolites of tea. Animal studies have indicated that catechins significantly attenuate the loss of muscle fiber cross-sectional area and hindlimb plantaris muscle mass, along with increasing satellite cell proliferation and differentiation in skeletal muscles and increasing the expression of anabolic factors, simultaneously reducing protein degradation through the ubiquitin-proteasome pathway (Alway et al., 2015). The combination of epicatechin (1 mg/kgbw) and resistance training led to a detectable increase in muscle strength (leg press and chest press) compared to the placebo group. In another study, there were no changes in muscular strength (knee extension strength and grip strength) with either exercise and tea catechin supplementation (540 mg/day), exercise, tea catechin supplementation (540 mg/day), or health education (Mafi et al., 2019). A 24-week randomized controlled trial (RCT) in older adults with sarcopenia allocated to resistance exercise (RE), RE with essential amino acids (EAA) supplementation (RE + 3 g EAA), or RE with 3 g EAA and 540 mg of tea catechins supplementation (RE + 3 g EAA + 540 mg tea catechins—TCC) groups showed a significant increase in skeletal muscle mass in the RE + EAA + TCC group than in the RE group (Cardoso et al., 2013).

8.3.1.5 Quercetin

Quercetin, a bioactive flavonol compound, has shown potent antiinflammatory and antioxidant potential, which has been hypothesized to prevent free radical-induced disruption of muscle fibers. Moreover, quercetin has been shown to affect Ca^{2+} release from the sarcoplasmic reticulum (SR), increasing myofibrils' sensitivity and positively affecting muscle strength (Lee et al., 2002). Also, the quercetin blocking effect on the adenosine receptors may influence motor unit recruitment capacity, which in turn can also affect isometric strength. A 14-day crossover study on 16 young men showed that 1000 mg/day supplementation of quercetin significantly increased the isometric strength compared to baseline (Bazzucchi et al., 2019). A double-blind RCT crossover study showed on young men that the consumption of 1 g/day of quercetin 3 hours before a resistance training session enhanced the torque–velocity curve of knee extensors and lowered MVIC reduction (Ferreira et al., 2022).

8.3.1.6 Caffeine

Caffeine improves muscular strength by sensitizing calcium channels and increasing the release of calcium ions from the SR. With more calcium ions available, there is a greater potential for muscle fibers to contract with greater force, allowing for more efficient muscle contractions and improving muscular strength. A crossover, randomized, double-blind, placebo-controlled study showed that consuming 8 mg · kg/bw of caffeine significantly improves the muscular strength measured with bench press and squat compared to placebo on muscle strength in recreationally resistance-trained participants (Ferreira et al., 2022). However, the supplementation of 3 or 6 mg/kg BM of caffeine or placebo on strength-trained females using hormonal contraception showed no improvement in muscular strength measured with 1 RM test (Jones et al., 2021). Other studies showed improved bench press 1RM (repetition maximum) and bench press RTF (repetition to failure) with 4 mg · /kg caffeine ingestion compared to placebo in resistance-trained females during the early follicular phase (Norum et al., 2020).

8.3.2 Improving endurance

Improved endurance is crucial for any athlete as it ensures the ability of athletes to perform prolonged tests, better recovery, less fatigue, and handle larger training volume. Improved endurance is associated with improved aerobic capacity, which relates to the body's ability to take in, transport, and utilize oxygen during sustained physical activity. VO2 max is the indicator of aerobic capacity, and with increased VO2 max, it indicates greater aerobic capacity, meaning the ability to sustain longer physical activities without fatigue. Therefore much research has been done to study functional foods that may improve endurance in athletes and other populations.

8.3.2.1 Peptides

Human studies have indicated an increase in endurance performance in response to bioactive peptide consumption, even though the mechanism is unclear. It is assumed that the significant increase in fat-free mass and strength may enhance muscle work efficiency and increase fat oxidation, which saves carbohydrate stores, positively impacting performance. The possible explanations could be increased glycogen uptake and storage in muscle muscles, as indicated in vitro studies and rats (Morifuji et al., 2010). Also, increased glycogen synthase and increased translocation of GLUT-4 transporters into the cell membrane lead to increased glucose uptake and utilization, producing energy for exercise performance. Peptides from whey hydrolysates showed improved endothelial function by suppressing the angiotensin-converting enzyme (ACE), which improves oxygen consumption (König et al., 2021). A 1-hour time trial showed that the collagen peptides group (15 g) had a significantly higher increase in running distance and increased ventilatory lactate threshold compared to the control group in the time trial (Jerger et al., 2023). Another study conducted in recreationally active men showed that after 12 weeks of 15 g creatinine phosphate (CP) supplementation, there was a higher increase in running distance and increase in velocity at lactate and anaerobic threshold. The 12 weeks of supplementation of collagen peptides (15 g/day) in young men showed significantly increased fat-free mass compared to the placebo (Oertzen-Hagemann et al., 2019). However, no differences were observed with fiber cross-sectional area (fCSA) of type II muscle fibers between groups (Jendricke et al., 2020; Kirmse et al., 2019).

8.3.2.2 Omega-3

Omega-3 fatty acids are considered a potential nutritional supplement to improve endurance performance in sports personnel; however, there is a lack of consensus, partly due to a lack of data and mostly because the studies were conducted on nonprofessionals. The available evidence suggests that EPA stimulates mitochondrial biogenesis in obese participants, which improves endurance regulated via the PGC-1a pathway. EPA/DHA also increases RBC's deformability, increasing muscle oxygen delivery (Thielecke & Blannin, 2020b). Besides, EPA upregulates specific genes involved in beta-oxidation, such as carnitine PMT-II. A placebo-controlled randomized control trial conducted on amateur male long-distance runners with omega-3 fatty acid capsules (omega group, 2234 mg of EPA and 916 mg of DHA daily) or medium-chain triglycerides capsules as placebo (medium-chain triglyceride [MCT] group, 4000 mg of MCT daily) during 12 weeks of endurance training showed a detectable increase in VO2 max in the omega group only (Tomczyk et al., 2023). Another 8-week intervention with EPA (600 mg) and DHA (260 mg) showed no improvement in oxygen saturation in muscle tissue (StO2), an index of muscle oxygen availability with the supplementation in healthy subjects (Morishima et al., 2020). In contrast, a 4-week supplementation of n-3 FA showed improvement in Yo-Yo test distance with training in the n-3 FA group only with a mean difference of 203 (66-340) m for n-3 FA and 62 (-94-217) m for placebo (Gravina et al., 2017).

8.3.2.3 Dietary nitrate

Dietary nitrate is popular in sports nutrition for its ergogenic properties; however, the exact mechanism underlying it has not yet been established in humans. Dietary nitrate is converted to NO inside the body, which is a vasodilator. Vasodilator modulates skeletal muscle function through its role in blood flow regulation, contractility, glucose and calcium homeostasis, and mitochondrial biogenesis, eventually leading to improved glucose transport and muscle uptake during exercise (Hord et al., 2009). Mitochondrial biogenesis leads to increased mitochondrial protein, oxygen consumption, and muscle contraction through calcium leakage from the SR. A human intervention trial has shown that seven days of beetroot supplementation (BR) with 12.4 mmol NO_3^- per day on a 10-km cycling time trial (TT) performance in 12 well-trained cyclists in normoxia and normobaric hypoxia revealed improved TT performance with BR supplementation ($\sim$1.6%), improved VO2 and VE (Rokkedal-Lausch et al., 2019). Another study showed that long-term nitrate supplementation (14 days) showed a significant decrease in time to completion and increased average power and speed in the 8 km cycling time trial compared to single preexercise dosing (Jo et al., 2019). Another study tested the effects of NO3 – rich beetroot juice (BJ) on performance in a 30-second Wingate cycle test. It was shown that compared to placebo, supplementation with BJ increased peak power output (Wpeak) and lowered the time to reach Wpeak during the Wingate test (Jodra et al., 2020).

8.3.2.4 Catechins

Catechins may impact VO2 max through their antioxidant properties, as ROS bioactivity/oxidative stress can modulate responsiveness to beta-adrenergic receptor stimulation by the sympathoadrenal system in sedentary individuals. Green tea catechins affect SIRT1, which increases the activity of PGC-1a, consequently improving mitochondrial function (Afzalpour et al., 2017). Catechins also increase endothelial NO synthesis and vasodilation, which improves the perfusion of oxygen to the active muscles and endurance performance. Catechins/green tea extract also increases fat oxidation at rest and/or during exercise, which is related to improved endurance as well (Nobari et al., 2021). The effect of catechins on nonathlete male subjects was studied, where participants received test beverages with or without tea catechins (570 mg) daily for eight weeks, along with a training program twice a week. A significant increase in ventilatory threshold during exercise and a higher recovery rate of oxygenated myoglobin and hemoglobin levels were observed after graded cycle exercise in the catechins group compared to the placebo group (Ota et al., 2016). Another trial done on physically active men with the supplementation of 500 mg of polyphenols showed increased mean duration of the maximal endurance test and delayed reach to the maximal perceived exertion with polyphenols (Deley et al., 2017). Consuming dark chocolate (20 g) for 3 months increased VO2 max and maximum work achieved in sedentary subjects. The same study showed a significant increase in protein levels for LKB1, AMPK, and peroxisome proliferator-activated receptor-gamma coactivator-1 alpha (PGC1α) and in their active forms (phosphorylated AMPK and LKB1), as well as in citrate synthase activity, which implicated the mechanism as well (Taub et al., 2016). Decaffeinated green tea extract (dGTE) consumption for four weeks in 24 recreationally active males showed improvement in performance distance covered and 50-min performance trials, which was after cycling for 1 h at 50% (Roberts et al., 2015).

8.3.2.5 Quercetin

Cell culture studies have indicated that quercetin activates the AMPK and MAPK signaling pathways, both of which are upstream of PGC-1a activation. As indicated before, an increase in SIRT1 deacetylase activity with quercetin and with phosphorylation of liver kinase B1 (LKB1) leads to PGC-1α activation (Nieman et al., 2010). Quercetin also increases whole-body insulin-stimulated glucose uptake and attenuates exercise-induced oxygen stress, and proinflammation (Tsao et al., 2022). However, there are mixed findings. On trained cyclists, there was no effect of 2 weeks of quercetin supplementation on postexercise (14 h) muscle messenger RNA expression for peroxisome proliferator-activated receptor F coactivator, citrate synthase, or cytochrome (Nieman et al., 2009). Two weeks of quercetin supplementation on untrained young adults showed increased skeletal muscle messenger RNA for sirtuin 1, PPAR-gamma 1, cytochrome C oxidase, citrate synthase, and muscle mitochondrial DNA compared to placebo (Nieman et al., 2010). Another randomized controlled trial on 58 healthy, moderately trained men and women showed no changes in the quercetin group's VO2 peak and physical performance (Bigelman et al., 2010; Scholten et al., 2015).

8.3.2.6 *Caffeine*

There is well-established evidence that caffeine acts as an adenosine A1 and A2A receptor antagonist, which blocks the adenosine receptors, affecting the release of norepinephrine, dopamine, acetylcholine, and serotonin, reducing pain and perceived exertion during exercise, and delaying fatigue. Moreover, it is known to preserve muscle glycogen by better distributing fatty acids in the bloodstream and increasing the release of calcium ions by enhancing muscle fibers' contraction power (Ferreira et al., 2022; Martins et al., 2020). A 6 mg/kg body weight supplementation of caffeine 60-minute pretrial in 26 triathletes resulted in a 3.7% reduction in swing time and a 1.3% reduction in time to completion (Potgieter et al., 2018). Another study investigated the effect of Turkish coffee and decaffeinated Turkish coffee, which showed significantly higher energy levels at 30 minutes for Turkish coffee compared to the decaffeinated coffee group during the 5 km run. Moreover, upper body reaction performance and respiratory exchange ratio (RER) were greater for Turkish coffee; however, no significant differences were observed in the 5 km run time (Church et al., 2015). Trained male cyclists were randomly given Red Bull (9.4 mL/kg body mass [BM] containing 3 mg/kg BM caffeine), anhydrous caffeine (3 mg/kg BM in capsule form), or a placebo 1.5 hours before starting a time trial (1 h cycling at 75% peak power output). Caffeine consumption improved performance by 120 s after caffeine compared with placebo (Quinlivan et al., 2015).

8.3.3 Body recovery and preventing injuries

While muscular strength and endurance are crucial, prioritizing recovery is equally essential for athletes. Any imbalance between exercise stress and recovery over extended periods can affect an athlete's performance, which can have long-term debilitating consequences in the form of overtraining. The recovery process may take several minutes to several days, where an altered biological system, including the metabolome, is restored to its original state. There are two stages of metabolic recovery: a fast stage where oxygen, ATP, and phosphocreatine are replenished, and a subsequent slow stage in which the adaptations of innate metabolism are restored. Glucosamine, a chitosan monomer, exerts a chondroprotective action by preventing collagen degradation and enhancing collagen synthesis. Strenuous training and exercise increase the risk of articular cartilage degeneration resulting in osteoarthritis and joint disorder (Isao Nagaoka & Masafumi Yoshimura, 2019). Among groups of soccer players and bicycle racers, the administration of glucosamine helped maintain collagen synthesis (Momomura et al., 2013; Yoshimura et al., 2009).

8.3.3.1 *Peptides*

The use of bioactive peptides as a nutrition strategy for athletes is recommended for muscle recovery, repair, and growth as it stimulates muscle protein synthesis compared to exercise alone. For example, whey protein supplementation accelerates satellite cell proliferation during recovery from eccentric exercise (Farup et al., 2014). Physically active males were given either β-hydroxy-β methylbutyrate free acid (HMB-FA) or placebo groups 30 minutes before performing an acute plyometric exercise protocol. At 1 h postexercise, greater increases in oxidative stress markers were observed in the placebo group compared to the HMB-FA group, and the WBC level (leukocyte response) was greater for the placebo group in comparison to the HMB-FA group at postexercise (Arazi et al., 2019). This indirectly indicates that HMB-FA decreases oxidative stress markers and leukocyte responses postexercise. Oral glucose tolerance tests (oral-GTT) were performed preexercise (cycled to exhaustion at 70% VO2 peak) and after 1, 3, and 6 days of creatine (20 g/day) and placebo supplementation along with a high carbohydrate diet. Creatine supplementation increased muscle total-Cr, free-Cr, and phosphocreatine (PCr) content above placebo following 1, 3, and 6 days of supplementation. Creatine supplementation also increased muscle glycogen content noticeably above placebo after one day of supplementation, which was sustained after that (Roberts et al., 2016). Another study was done on the supplementation of 0.3 g/kg of creatine or placebo before and during recovery (48 h) from 6 sets of 8 repetitions of eccentric exercise. No group differences in fatigue index were observed (Boychuk et al., 2016). Peres et al. (2023) studied the supplementation of 50 g of maltodextrin and four tablets of 700 mg whey protein (hydrolyzed) enriched with 175 mg of glutamine dipeptide (MGln) or four tablets of 700 mg maltodextrin plus 50 g maltodextrin d30 minutes after a progressive incremental test on an ergometer. MGln decreased plasma lactate dehydrogenase (LDH) and creatine kinase activities, indicating protection from muscle damage. No change in plasma cytokine and C-reactive protein levels was detected across the study periods (Peres et al., 2023). In another study, participants were given a placebo or an L-carnitine tartrate group for five weeks, where compared to a placebo, L-carnitine tartrate supplementation was able to improve perceived recovery and soreness and lower serum creatine kinase (Stefan et al., 2021).

L-carnitine, derived from amino acid, has a significant role in energy metabolism and postexercise recovery among athletes. Carnitine has a fundamental role in the β oxidation of fatty acids. Intense exercise leads to severe depletion of L-carnitine in the muscles. Its supplementation even for a couple of weeks improves glucose and ammonia levels in the plasma (Broad et al., 2008). Likewise, glutamine, one of the most abundant amino acids, is the precursor for the synthesis of nucleotides. Continuous exercise reduces plasma glutamine levels and results in impaired immune function. Therefore supplementation of glutamine reduces the incidence of sickness (Castell, 2002). Evidence-based outcomes also claim that the supplementation of L-glutamine postexercise enhances muscle recovery. It reduces muscle soreness which might be associated with reduced muscle damage (Legault et al., 2015).

8.3.3.2 Omega-3

Omega-3 fatty acids, once consumed, are incorporated in the phospholipids of the membrane, which promote muscle recovery by stimulating muscle protein synthesis by activating the mTORC1-p70S6k1 pathway and also by promoting antiinflammatory action, which heals muscle damage (Witard & Davis, 2021). Healthy males were supplemented with four weeks of 3 g/day n-3 supplementation or placebo, following which a 60 min downhill running test at 65% VO2 max, -10% gradient was performed. Muscle soreness was significantly lower in the n-3 versus placebo group at 24 h post-EIMD, and IL-6 was increased in placebo but not in n-3 following EIMD. EIMD altered maximal voluntary isometric contraction (MVIC), CK, and TNF-α but did not differ between groups (Jakeman et al., 2017). Thirty healthy women (22.2 years) received either omega-3 rich fish oil (3.2 g/day) or placebo (olive oil) at dinner—after doing the 10 sets of 10 unilateral eccentric contractions in a knee extension chair, as well as at lunch for the three subsequent days or placebo. During the 3 days after exercise, participants experienced greater muscle soreness and decreased muscular strength; however, no difference between groups was found. Another study also showed that 5 g/ day of fish oil for four weeks did not decrease the cumulative creative kinase response, inflammation, muscle soreness, or muscle function following eccentric exercise (Mackay et al., 2023).

8.3.3.3 Dietary nitrate

The rates of oxygen availability and mitochondrial efficiency are crucial for body recovery after exercise. Dietary nitrates enhance oxygen availability by improving blood flow, optimizing local perfusion, and improving mitochondrial efficiency by reducing the expression of mitochondrial membrane proteins such as adenine nucleotide translocase and uncoupling protein 3 (Nair et al., 2011). Mitochondrial efficiency means the efficient conversion of ADP to ATP subsequently preserving the muscle glycogen and phosphocreatine. NO also promotes better recovery through its antiinflammatory properties, which prevent prolonged inflammation states after exercise, restoring the metabolic state to its natural equilibrium (Jädert et al., 2014). A single-blinded trial was done on healthy adults where participants were given 12.5 mmol of nitrate per day through beetroot juice before ascent or a nonnitrate calorie-matched control. There was no decline in fitness scores compared to baseline in the BRJ group, but no change in heart rate recovery speed was observed (Marshall et al., 2021).

A 9-week supplementation of 3 g/day of citrulline plus 2.1 g/day of beetroot juice (300 mg/day of nitrates (NO_3-)) led to significant differences in the distance covered in the cooper test, cortisol, and testosterone/cortisol. There were no differences in urea, creatinine, aspartate aminotransferase (AST), alanine transaminase (ALT), gamma-glutamyl transferase (GGT), LDH, and CK between groups, namely, placebo, BR group, citrulline (CIT) group, and BR + CIT group (Burgos et al., 2022). Another study showed that the ingestion of beetroot extract (600 mg in a capsule before exercise) accelerates the recovery of systolic blood pressure (SBP) following physical effort and improves HR recovery to baseline resting levels (beetroot protocol: change in ~62% vs. placebo protocol: change in ~80%) and intensifies the return of vagal HR control during recovery after exercise (Benjamim et al., 2021).

8.3.3.4 Catechins

Not many studies have been done on understanding catechins' mechanisms to improve body recovery and prevent injuries. An in vitro study indicated that catechin might prevent cellular injury by regulating miR-92a and c-Jun N-terminal kinase signaling pathways (Fang et al., 2018). Besides, catechins possess antiinflammatory and antioxidative properties, which potentially combat free radicals and prevent the oxidative stress chronic inflammatory phase in athletes. After 15 days of supplementation (500 mg/day) with green tea extract on nontrained participants, there was a reduction in muscle damage. However, no changes in muscle soreness, plasma oxidative damage marker, and antioxidant status were observed (da Silva et al., 2018). After 13 weeks of supplementation, a high dose of polyphenolic (PB) (2000 mg/day) reduced whole-body and hamstring soreness compared to the placebo. All groups had increased serum cortisol and creatine kinase (CK), but cortisol and CK returned to preexercise levels after supplementation in 96 hours (Herrlinger et al., 2015).

8.3.3.5 Quercetin

Quercetin supports body recovery after exercise as an antioxidant and antiinflammatory agent. Quercetin induces copper and ferrous through catechol in its composition which activates antioxidant capacity preventing lipid peroxidation and inflammation (Yang et al., 2020). Besides, it assists the glutathione pathway in regulating the increase in glutathione synthesis, which catalyzes the degradation of hydrogen peroxide to water molecules. Free radicals activate transcription factors to produce proinflammatory cytokines, which can be neutralized by quercetin and lead to a decrease in inflammatory markers. Moreover, it has shown antiinflammatory actions on endothelial and monocyte/macrophage systems (Lotito & Frei, 2006). The activity of COX-2 and inducible nitric oxide synthase (iNOS) was inhibited by Q by suppressing activator protein-1 (AP-1), NF-κB, and signal transducer and activator of transcription 1 (STAT-1) signaling in cytokine- or LPS-induced human umbilical vein endothelial cells (HUVECs) and macrophages (Hämäläinen et al., 2007). These properties of quercetin in the inflammation process assist in repairing long-term adaptive responses (Cerqueira et al., 2019). The 30 days supplementation of quercetin (500 mg) led to a decrement in the malondialdehyde levels of the quercetin group compared to baseline while increasing the levels of antioxidant enzymes superoxide dismutases (SOD), catalase (CAT), and glutathione (GSH) (Demirci, 2017). The supplementation of 1 g/day of quercetin or placebo for 14 days led to a more marked increase in insulin-like growth factor 1 (IGF-I) levels, and notably, the insulin-like growth factor 2 (IGF-II) peak was found earlier, compared to placebo. Quercetin significantly reduced plasma markers of cell damage CK, lactate dehydrogenase (LDH), and the interleukin-6 level during the recovery period following exercise-induced muscle damage compared to placebo (Sgrò et al., 2021). Another study showed that a quercetin supplementation of 1000 mg/day for seven days led to significantly decreased glucose-induced insulin response, increased antioxidant capacity, SO, and mitigated malondialdehyde (MDA) levels during the recovery period of 3 hours after 70% VO2 max cycling. Lower IL-6 responses and creatine kinase were found at two hours in quercetin treatment, but no significant differences in glucose, respiratory exchange ratio (RER), TNF-alpha, myoglobin, and hs-CRP were found between treatments (Tsao et al., 2022).

8.3.3.6 Caffeine

In vitro and in vivo studies have shown that coffee components caffeic acid and caffeine have a positive effect in stimulating glucose receptor translocation, phosphorylation, and activation of calcium/calmodulin (CaM)-dependent protein kinases (CaMK), phosphorylation, and activation of AMPK, and phosphorylation and inactivation of acetyl-CoA carboxylase (ACC) in muscle cells. Cafestol and caffeic acid stimulate insulin secretion from the beta cells positively. There is also a positive effect of exercise, contraction, and depression of glycogen on AMPK phosphorylation and activation in muscle cells (Lawler & Cialdella-Kam, 2020; Loureiro et al., 2018). Endurance-trained participants did an exhaustive cycle ergometer, followed by a cycling protocol the next morning. After the second cycling protocol, participants were randomized to receive either a test beverage (coffee + milk) or a control (milk) and a breakfast meal. The consumption of the test beverage resulted in greater muscle glycogen recovery and greater glucose and insulin total area under the curve compared with the control (Loureiro et al., 2021). In another study, after completing a 164 km endurance cycling event, subjects ingested 3 mg/kg body mass of caffeine or placebo pills immediately after the ride and for the next four mornings and three afternoons. With caffeine ingestion, there was a greater perceived lower extremity functionality (LEF) in the afternoon on the first-day postride, and a test group had lower overall ratings of perceived muscle soreness (RPMS) in the afternoon compared to the placebo (Caldwell et al., 2017). Healthy individuals were supplemented with caffeine (400 mg) or placebo pills, followed by a maximal treadmill test to exhaustion. Interestingly, heart rate (HR), mean arterial pressure (MAP), and diastolic blood pressure (DBP) remained elevated with caffeine during recovery. There was an increase in the natural log transformation of the low-to-high frequency ratio (LnLF/LnHF) of heart rate variability and corrected QT interval compared to the baseline (Bunsawat et al., 2015). The effect of caffeine congestion with carbohydrate (CHO) during recovery from exhaustive exercise in trained subjects showed higher glycogen accumulation in the caffeine + CHO group compared to the CHO group. Phosphorylation of CaMKThr286 was higher in the caffeine + CHO than in the CHO only group after 4 h. CaMKII activity has been shown to affect insulin sensitivity and glucose uptake in myocytes and modulate kinases and phosphatases involved in insulin signaling (Pedersen et al., 2008).

8.3.4 Boosting immunity and well-being

Immune health and well-being of individuals, either the general population or athletes, are important for being protective against diseases and overall physiological performance. The bioactive compounds have immunomodulating and immunity-boosting properties. ROS produced during physical activity are thought to activate PGC1-α and MAPK, two biochemical pathways essential for both muscle growth and aerobic capacity. Oxidative stress and elevated ROS levels may damage tissues and cells and induce inflammation (Clemente-Suárez et al., 2023). The biofunctional compounds promote immunological health and general well-being by protecting from oxidative stress, inflammation, and/or activation of several immunoregulatory pathways. Most often, B vitamins are involved in immunomodulation (Fig. 8.1). However, bioactive extracts are also found to participate in the immunomodulating effect, inflammation reduction, and prevention of oxidative stress. Table 8.1 and Fig. 8.1 illustrate the different mechanisms by which bioactive extracts maintain immunological health in individuals. Fruit and vegetable extracts high in polyphenols are used to reduce the physiological stress brought on by exercise and can act as ibuprofen alternatives (Nieman et al., 2013).

Curcumin, an active ingredient of turmeric, is found to have antiinflammatory properties. Researchers, in a study of mice models, reported supplementation of 5000 ppm for 6 months suppressed the incidence of inflammation and oxidative damage in the brain. They concluded both high and low doses of curcumin lowered the proinflammatory cytokine IL-1 by 57%–61.8%, thus reducing inflammation (Giselle et al., 2001). Curcumin for a supplementation period of 12 days improved cognitive function and decreased lipid peroxidation in the brain tissue of rats (Belviranlı et al., 2013). Lycopene is a naturally occurring antioxidant found in tomatoes. Creatine phosphokinase (CPK) and lactate dehydrogenase (LDH) are known as the biomarkers of exercise-induced muscle damage. Administration of tomato juice to a group of athletes for 2 months, having increased levels of CPK and LDH at baseline, led to a significant decrease in their levels probably due to its antioxidant properties. The levels of C-reactive protein were also significantly lowered (Tsitsimpikou et al., 2013). Researchers claim that capsaicin has multiple metabolic effects that potentially influence performance during intense exercise. High-intensity exercise induces an inflammatory response which at elevated levels can be detrimental to the body. Capsaicin can reduce respiratory quotient and shift the energy breakdown from carbohydrates to fats during endurance training. Based on animal model research, it is found to reduce the inflammatory response in response to intense exercise (Opheim & Rankin, 2012). The supplementation of capsaicin is involved in the modulation of the transient receptor potential vanilloid 1 (TRPV1) channel. The activation increases the release of calcium in the SR, increasing fatty acid oxidation and sparing glycogen, which reduces body fatigue and increases performance (Haramizu et al., 2006).

Resveratrol, a naturally occurring polyphenol, improved systemic metabolic rate and altered substrate utilization in mice models. Researchers claimed resveratrol may help reduce fatigue and exercise intolerance (Sung et al., 2017). It counteracts oxidative stress and inflammation in response to exercise. Supplementation of 120 mg resveratrol and 225 mg quercetin for the first 6 days and 240 mg resveratrol and 450 mg quercetin on day 7 before exercise significantly reduced the exercise-induced lipid peroxidation (McAnulty et al., 2013). Supplementation of 500 mg resveratrol with 10 mg piperine for 4 weeks with submaximal endurance training among healthy adults enhanced mitochondrial capacity (Polley et al., 2016). Further, more research is needed to explore the effects of resveratrol supplementation on athletes and sports performance.

Vitamins C and E: Supplementations of vitamins C and E have been found to have a role in reducing muscle damage markers during aerobic exercises. A 4-week double-blinded clinical trial among 64 female athletes with the supplementation of either vitamin C, E, or both vitamin E reported a decrease in creatine kinase and lactate dehydrogenase, concluding that the supplementation of these vitamins decreases oxidative stress markers (Taghiyar et al., 2013). Researchers studying the effect of vitamin E (800 IU) supplementation on muscular and oxidative damage induced by eccentric exercise concluded that vitamin E supplementation is an important factor of defense against oxidative stress and muscle damage in humans. On analyzing the blood samples, there were decreased muscle soreness, lactose dehydrogenase activity, lipid peroxidation, protein carbonylation, tumor necrosis factor-α (TNF-α), and interleukin-10 (IL-10) levels after 14 days of supplementation when compared to placebo (Silva et al.,

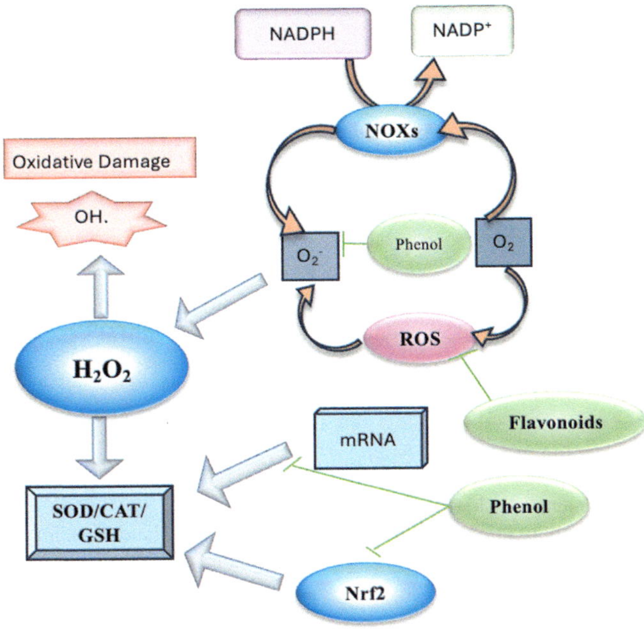

FIGURE 8.2 Activation of antioxidant cascade by phenolic compounds.

2010). There is also evidence of vitamin E having protective effects against cellular velum and other fatty cellular parts by gifting electrons to free radicals which helps to reduce muscle damage. Vitamin D is necessary for optimal bone health reducing the risk of stress fracture, body inflammation, illnesses, and impaired muscle function. It upregulates the gene expression of broad-spectrum antimicrobial peptides which have been known to be important for innate immunity (Larson-Meyer & Willis, 2010). In a group of college athletes, low vitamin D was found to be associated with an increased incidence of the common cold, influenza, and gastroenteritis (Halliday et al., 2011). Its deficiency has been known to decrease skeletal muscle function and increase recovery time from training. Supplementation of 5000 IU vitamin D_3 per day for 8 weeks among 30 athletes increased their serum vitamin D concentrations and also improved their performance in terms of sprint times and vertical jump (Close et al., 2013).

Omega-3 fatty acids, especially DHA and EPA, have been found to have beneficial effects on athletic performance through improved endurance and delayed onset of muscle soreness. They also enhance recovery and immune modulation (Thielecke & Blannin, 2020a). Research conducted among 20 professional rugby players given a supplement containing 551 mg EPA and 551 mg DHA twice daily during 5 weeks of preseason training reported beneficial effects on fatigue, and body muscle soreness was lower on day 35 (Black et al., 2018). Omega-3 fatty acids are also proven to have beneficial effects on cardiovascular function. Supplementation of 6 gm/day of DHA among Australian football players for 5 weeks of training concluded decreased triglycerides and diastolic blood pressure (Buckley et al., 2009) Fig. 8.2.

8.4 Future perspectives and conclusion

Sports have become more competitive in recent years, and researchers are looking for the best way to optimize the performance of athletes by increasing their strength, endurance power, immunity power, and recovery. Exercise-induced inflammation, muscle damage, and pain are frequently associated with athletes' lives, making sports nutrition a crucial field to work in. Several nutrients improve strength and endurance and accelerate the body's recovery process, preventing the tissues and muscles from the deleterious effects of intense training and ultimately causing a direct impact on the athlete's performance. Moreover, the consumption of bioactive compounds boosts immunity and promotes the well-being of athletes, preventing them from falling ill and missing important sports events. However, the impact of several bioactive compounds is not consistently evident across all research findings. Therefore specific research needs to be done based on age, sex, exercise intensity, duration, timing, and mode of ingestion. Besides, the synergistic effects of nutrients and bioactive compounds need to be studied extensively. It has become evident that single nutrients from different food sources provide different health benefits, likely because of the interaction between nutrients, which provides synergistic benefits. Lastly, the nutrients mentioned above can be utilized appropriately through an evidence-based sports nutrition approach to maximize athletic performance and ensure optimal health and wellness of athletes (Table 8.2).

TABLE 8.2 Mechanism of Bioactive Compounds in the Health of Athletes.

Bioactive Compound	Mechanism	Role in the Health of Athletes	References
Quercetin	Affect Ca^{2+} release from the SR, increasing myofibrils' sensitivity. Quercetin activates the AMPK and MAPK signaling pathways Quercetin induces copper and ferrous iron through catechol	Increases muscle strength and endurance capacity. Improves antiinflammatory capacity	Lee et al. (2002)
Catechins	Reduces protein degradation through the ubiquitin-proteasome pathway Affects silent mating type information regulation 2 homolog 1 (SIRT1), which increases the activity of the peroxisome proliferator-activated receptor-gamma coactivator (PGC-1a) Regulates miR-92a and JNK signaling pathways	Increases muscular strength Improves the mitochondrial function Prevent cellular injury	Afzalpour et al. (2017), Alway et al. (2015)
Caffeine	Sensitize calcium channels and increase the release of calcium ions from the SR Stimulate glucose receptor translocation, phosphorylation, and activation of CaMK, phosphorylation, activation of AMPK, and phosphorylation and inactivation of ACC in muscle cells Acts as an adenosine A1 and A2A receptor antagonist, which blocks the adenosine receptors, affecting the release of norepinephrine, dopamine, acetylcholine, and serotonin	Efficient muscle contractions and improving muscular strength Improve endurance delay pain and fatigue	Ferreira et al. (2022), Lawler and Cialdella-Kam (2020), Loureiro et al. (2018)
Peptides	Interactions with receptors or endogenous proteins, such as the mammalian target of rapamycin (mTOR), glucose transporter type 4 (GLUT-4), or glycogen synthase A significant increase in fat-free mass and strength may enhance muscle work efficiency and increase fat oxidation Increased glycogen synthase and increased translocation of GLUT-4 transporters into the cell membrane	Stimulate muscular protein synthesis. Increased muscular strength Positively impacting performance Increased glucose uptake and utilization, producing energy for exercise performance	König et al. (2021)
Omega-3	Increases the enhancement of anabolic mTOR Ser2448 and p70S6K1 Thr389 phosphorylation in skeletal muscle	Increased muscular strength	Gingras et al. (2007)
Nitrate	Reduce the phosphocreatine cost of force production and improve the local perfusion and contractility of low-oxygenated type II (fast twitch) muscle fibers Converts to NO inside the body working as a vasodilator	Improves maximal strength, improves mitochondrial biogenesis, improves blood flow	Fulford et al. (2013) and Nyakayiru et al. (2017)

AMPK, AMP-activated protein kinase; *JNK*, Jun N-terminal kinase; *MAPK*, mitogen-activated protein kinase; *SR*, sarcoplasmic reticulum.

References

Afzalpour, M. E., Ghasemi, E., & Zarban, A. (2017). Effects of 10 weeks of high intensity interval training and green tea supplementation on serum levels of Sirtuin-1 and peroxisome proliferator-activated receptor gamma co-activator 1-alpha in overweight women. *Science & Sports*, *32*(2), 82–90. Available from https://doi.org/10.1016/j.scispo.2016.09.004.

Ali Redha, A., Anusha Siddiqui, S., Zare, R., Spadaccini, D., Guazzotti, S., Feng, X., Bahmid, N. A., Wu, Y. S., Ozeer, F. Z., & Aluko, R. E. (2024). Blackcurrants: A nutrient-rich source for the development of functional foods for improved athletic performance. *Food Reviews International*, *40*(1), 135–157. Available from https://doi.org/10.1080/87559129.2022.2162076, www.tandf.co.uk/journals/titles/87559129.asp.

Alkhedhairi, S. A., Aba Alkhayl, F. F., Ismail, A. D., Rozendaal, A., German, M., MacLean, B., Johnston, L., Miller, A. A., Hunter, A. M., Macgregor, L. J., Combet, E., Quinn, T. J., & Gray, S. R. (2022). The effect of krill oil supplementation on skeletal muscle function and size in older adults: A randomised controlled trial. *Clinical Nutrition*, *41*(6), 1228–1235. Available from https://doi.org/10.1016/j.clnu.2022.04.007, http://www.elsevier-international.com/journals/clnu/.

Alway, S. E., Bennett, B. T., Wilson, J. C., Sperringer, J., Mohamed, J. S., Edens, N. K., & Pereira, S. L. (2015). Green tea extract attenuates muscle loss and improves muscle function during disuse, but fails to improve muscle recovery following unloading in aged rats. *Journal of Applied Physiology*, *118*(3), 319–330. Available from https://doi.org/10.1152/japplphysiol.00674.2014, http://jap.physiology.org/content/118/3/319.full-text.pdf + html.

Arazi, H., Hosseini, Z., Asadi, A., Ramirez-Campillo, R., & Suzuki, K. (2019). β-Hydroxy-β-methylbutyrate free acid attenuates oxidative stress induced by a single bout of plyometric exercise. *Frontiers in Physiology*, *10*. Available from https://doi.org/10.3389/fphys.2019.00776.

Bagheri, R., Hooshmand Moghadam, B., Ashtary-Larky, D., Forbes, S. C., Candow, D. G., Galpin, A. J., Eskandari, M., Kreider, R. B., & Wong, A. (2021). Whole egg vs. egg white ingestion during 12 weeks of resistance training in trained young males: A randomized controlled trial. *Journal of Strength and Conditioning Research*, *35*(2), 411–419. Available from https://doi.org/10.1519/JSC.0000000000003922, http://journals.lww.com/nsca-jscr.

Baird, M. F., Graham, S. M., Baker, J. S., & Bickerstaff, G. F. (2012). Creatine-kinase-and exercise-related muscle damage implications for muscle performance and recovery. *Journal of Nutrition and Metabolism*, *2012*.

Bazzucchi, I., Patrizio, F., & Ceci, R. (2019). Guglielmo Duranti, Paolo Sgrò, Stefania Sabatini, Luigi Di Luigi, Massimo Sacchetti, Francesco Felici, The Effects of Quercetin Supplementation on Eccentric Exercise-Induced Muscle Damage. *Nutrients.*, *11*(1), 205. Available from https://doi.org/10.3390/nu11010205.

Belviranlı, M., Okudan, N., Esra Nurullahoğlu Atalık, K., & Öz, M. (2013). Curcumin improves spatial memory and decreases oxidative damage in aged female rats. *Biogerontology*, *14*(2), 187–196. Available from https://doi.org/10.1007/s10522-013-9422-y.

Benjamim, C. J. R., Francisco, F. W., de Figueirêdo, M. Í. L. S., Benjamim, C. J. R., Cavalcante, T. C. F., da Silva, A. A. M., Monteiro, L. R. L., Santana, M. D. R., Garner, D. M., & Valenti, V. E. (2021). Beetroot (*Beta vulgaris* L.) extract acutely improves heart rate variability recovery following strength exercise: A randomized, double-blind, placebo-controlled crossover trial-pilot study. *Journal of the American College of Nutrition*, *40*(4), 307–316. Available from https://doi.org/10.1080/07315724.2020.1774441, http://www.tandfonline.com/toc/uacn20/current.

Bhat, M., Kalam, R., Qadri, S. S. Y. H., Madabushi, S., & Ismail, A. (2013). Vitamin D deficiency-induced muscle wasting occurs through the ubiquitin proteasome pathway and is partially corrected by calcium in male rats. *Endocrinology*, *154*(11), 4018–4029. Available from https://doi.org/10.1210/en.2013-1369.

Bigelman, K. A., Fan, E. H., Chapman, D. P., Freese, E. C., Trilk, J. L., & Cureton, K. J. (2010). Effects of six weeks of quercetin supplementation on physical performance in ROTC cadets. *Military Medicine*, *175*(10), 791–798. Available from https://doi.org/10.7205/MILMED-D-09-00088, http://docserver.ingentaconnect.com/deliver/connect/amsus/00264075/v175n10/s31.pdf?expires = 1286976020&id = 59090946&titleid = 10681&accname = Elsevier + Science&checksum = 95D7622E5602791754E3BBCA066BFF4B.

Black, K. E., Witard, O. C., Baker, D., Healey, P., Lewis, V., Tavares, F., Christensen, S., Pease, T., & Smith, B. (2018). Adding omega-3 fatty acids to a protein-based supplement during pre-season training results in reduced muscle soreness and the better maintenance of explosive power in professional Rugby Union players. *European Journal of Sport Science*, *18*(10), 1357–1367. Available from https://doi.org/10.1080/17461391.2018.1491626, http://www.tandf.co.uk/journals/journal.asp?issn = 1746-1391&linktype = 1.

Boychuk, K. E., Lanovaz, J. L., Krentz, J. R., Lishchynsky, J. T., Candow, D. G., & Farthing, J. P. (2016). Creatine supplementation does not alter neuromuscular recovery after eccentric exercise. *Muscle and Nerve*, *54*(3), 487–495. Available from https://doi.org/10.1002/mus.25091, http://onlinelibrary.wiley.com/journal/10.1002/(ISSN)1097-4598.

Broad, E. M., Maughan, R. J., & Galloway, S. D. R. (2008). Carbohydrate, protein, and fat metabolism during exercise after oral carnitine supplementation in humans. *International Journal of Sport Nutrition and Exercise Metabolism*, *18*(6), 567–584. Available from https://doi.org/10.1123/ijsnem.18.6.567, http://www.humankinetics.com/eJournalMedia/pdfs/16427.pdf.

Buckley, J. D., Burgess, S., Murphy, K. J., & Howe, P. R. C. (2009). DHA-rich fish oil lowers heart rate during submaximal exercise in elite Australian Rules footballers. *Journal of Science and Medicine in Sport*, *12*(4), 503–507. Available from https://doi.org/10.1016/j.jsams.2008.01.011, http://www.elsevier.com/wps/find/journaldescription.cws_home/707423/description#description.

Bunsawat, K., White, D. W., Kappus, R. M., & Baynard, T. (2015). Caffeine delays autonomic recovery following acute exercise. *European Journal of Preventive Cardiology*, *22*(11), 1473–1479. Available from https://doi.org/10.1177/2047487314554867, https://academic.oup.com/eurjpc.

Burgos, J., Viribay, A., Calleja-González, J., Fernández-Lázaro, D., Olasagasti-Ibargoien, J., Seco-Calvo, J., & Mielgo-Ayuso, J. (2022). Long-term combined effects of citrulline and nitrate-rich beetroot extract supplementation on recovery status in trained male triathletes: A randomized, double-blind, placebo-controlled trial. *Biology*, *11*(1), 75. Available from https://doi.org/10.3390/biology11010075.

Calder, P. C. (2017). Omega-3 fatty acids and inflammatory processes: From molecules to man. *Biochemical Society Transactions*, *45*(5), 1105–1115. Available from https://doi.org/10.1042/BST20160474, http://www.biochemsoctrans.org/content/45/5/1105.full-text.pdf.

Caldwell, A. R., Tucker, M. A., Butts, C. L., McDermott, B. P., Vingren, J. L., Kunces, L. J., Lee, E. C., Munoz, C. X., Williamson, K. H., Armstrong, L. E., & Ganio, M. S. (2017). Effect of caffeine on perceived soreness and functionality following an endurance cycling event.

Journal of Strength and Conditioning Research, *31*(3), 638–643. Available from https://doi.org/10.1519/JSC.0000000000001608, http://journals.lww.com/nsca-jscr.

Cardoso, G. A., Salgado, J. M., Cesar, M. D. C., & Donado-Pestana, C. M. (2013). The effects of green tea consumption and resistance training on body composition and resting metabolic rate in overweight or obese women. *Journal of Medicinal Food*, *16*(2), 120–127. Available from https://doi.org/10.1089/jmf.2012.0062.

Carey, C. C., Lucey, A., & Doyle, L. (2021). Flavonoid containing polyphenol consumption and recovery from exercise-induced muscle damage: A systematic review and meta-analysis. *Sports Medicine*, *51*(6), 1293–1316. Available from https://doi.org/10.1007/s40279-021-01440-x, http://rd.springer.com/journal/40279.

Castell, L. M. (2002). Can glutamine modify the apparent immunodepression observed after prolonged, exhaustive exercise? *Nutrition (Burbank, Los Angeles County, Calif.)*, *18*(5), 371–375. Available from https://doi.org/10.1016/S0899-9007(02)00754-2, 08999007.

Cerqueira, É., Marinho, D. A., Neiva, H. P., & Lourenço, O. (2019). Inflammatory effects of high and moderate intensity exercise—A systematic review. *Front Physiol*, *10*, 1550. Available from https://doi.org/10.3389/fphys.2019.01550.

Church, D. D., Hoffman, J. R., LaMonica, M. B., Riffe, J. J., Hoffman, M. W., Baker, K. M., Varanoske, A. N., Wells, A. J., Fukuda, D. H., & Stout, J. R. (2015). The effect of an acute ingestion of Turkish coffee on reaction time and time trial performance. *Journal of the International Society of Sports Nutrition*, *12*(1). Available from https://doi.org/10.1186/s12970-015-0098-3, http://www.jissn.com/.

Clemente-Suárez, V. J., Bustamante-Sanchez, Á., Mielgo-Ayuso, J., Martínez-Guardado, I., Martín-Rodríguez, A., & Tornero-Aguilera, J. F. (2023). Antioxidants and sports performance. *Nutrients*, *15*(10). Available from https://doi.org/10.3390/nu15102371, http://www.mdpi.com/journal/nutrients/.

Close, G. L., Russell, J., Cobley, J. N., Owens, D. J., Wilson, G., Gregson, W., Fraser, W. D., & Morton, J. P. (2013). Assessment of vitamin D concentration in non-supplemented professional athletes and healthy adults during the winter months in the UK: implications for skeletal muscle function. *Journal of Sports Sciences*, *31*(4), 344–353. Available from https://doi.org/10.1080/02640414.2012.733822.

Coggan, A. R., Hoffman, R. L., Gray, D. A., Moorthi, R. N., Thomas, D. P., Leibowitz, J. L., Thies, D., & Peterson, L. R. (2020). A single dose of dietary nitrate increases maximal knee extensor angular velocity and power in healthy older men and women. *Journals of Gerontology - Series A Biological Sciences and Medical Sciences*, *75*(6), 1154–1160. Available from https://doi.org/10.1093/GERONA/GLZ156, http://biomedgerontology.oxfordjournals.org/.

Cui, P., Li, M., Yu, M., Liu, Y., Ding, Y., Liu, W., & Liu, J. (2022). Advances in sports food: Sports nutrition, food manufacture, opportunities and challenges. *Food Research International*, *157*, 111258. Available from https://doi.org/10.1016/j.foodres.2022.111258.

da Silva, W., Machado, Á. S., Souza, M. A., Mello-Carpes, P. B., & Carpes, F. P. (2018). Effect of green tea extract supplementation on exercise-induced delayed onset muscle soreness and muscular damage. *Physiology and Behavior*, *194*, 77–82. Available from https://doi.org/10.1016/j.physbeh.2018.05.006, www.elsevier.com/locate/physbeh.

Dalle, S., Van Roie, E., Hiroux, C., Vanmunster, M., Coudyzer, W., Suhr, F., Bogaerts, S., Van Thienen, R., Koppo, K., & Le Couteur, D. (2021). Omega-3 supplementation improves isometric strength but not muscle anabolic and catabolic signaling in response to resistance exercise in healthy older adults. *The Journals of Gerontology: Series A*, *76*(3), 406–414. Available from https://doi.org/10.1093/gerona/glaa309.

Deley, G., Guillemet, D., Allaert, F. A., & Babault, N. (2017). An acute dose of specific grape and apple polyphenols improves endurance performance: A randomized, crossover, double-blind versus placebo controlled study. *Nutrients.*, *9*(8). Available from https://doi.org/10.3390/nu9080917, http://www.mdpi.com/2072-6643/9/8/917/pdf.

Demirci, N. (2017). Protective effect of prolonged quercetin supplement on oxidative stress and antioxidant enzyme activities in boxers. *Studies on Ethno-Medicine*, *11*(2), 168–173. Available from https://doi.org/10.1080/09735070.2017.1305225.

Duan, C., Yin, C., Ma, Z., Li, F., Zhang, F., Yang, Q., Lin, M., Feng, S., Zhu, C., Wang, L., Zhu, X., Gao, P., Jiang, Q., Shu, G., & Wang, S. (2021). trans 10, cis 12, but Not cis 9, trans 11 conjugated linoleic acid isomer enhances exercise endurance by increasing oxidative skeletal muscle fiber type via Toll-like receptor 4 signaling in mice. *Journal of Agricultural and Food Chemistry*, *69*(51), 15636–15648. Available from https://doi.org/10.1021/acs.jafc.1c06280.

Dzik, K. P., & Kaczor, J. J. (2019). Mechanisms of vitamin D on skeletal muscle function: oxidative stress, energy metabolism and anabolic state. *European Journal of Applied Physiology*, *119*(4), 825–839. Available from https://doi.org/10.1007/s00421-019-04104-x, link.springer.de/link/service/journals/00421/index.htm.

Fang, J. F., Dai, J. H., Ni, M., Cai, Z. Y., & Liao, Y. F. (2018). Catechin protects rat cardiomyocytes from hypoxia-induced injury by regulating microRNA-92a. *Int J Clin Exp Pathol*, *11*(7), 3257–3266.

Farup, J., Rahbek, S. K., Knudsen, I. S., De Paoli, F., Mackey, A. L., & Vissing, K. (2014). Whey protein supplementation accelerates satellite cell proliferation during recovery from eccentric exercise. *Amino Acids*, *46*(11), 2503–2516. Available from https://doi.org/10.1007/s00726-014-1810-3, link.springer.de/link/service/journals/00726/index.htm.

Ferreira, L. H. B., Forbes, S. C., Barros, M. P., Smolarek, A. C., Enes, A., Lancha-Junior, A. H., Martins, G. L., & Souza-Junior, T. P. (2022). High doses of caffeine increase muscle strength and calcium release in the plasma of recreationally trained men. *Nutrients*, *14*(22). Available from https://doi.org/10.3390/nu14224921, http://www.mdpi.com/journal/nutrients/.

Fulford, J., Winyard, P. G., Vanhatalo, A., Bailey, S. J., Blackwell, J. R., & Jones, A. M. (2013). Influence of dietary nitrate supplementation on human skeletal muscle metabolism and force production during maximum voluntary contractions. *Pflugers Archiv European Journal of Physiology*, *465*(4), 517–528. Available from https://doi.org/10.1007/s00424-013-1220-5.

Gammone, M. A., Gemello, E., Riccioni, G., & D'Orazio, N. (2014). Marine bioactives and potential application in sports. *Marine Drugs*, *12*(5), 2357–2382. Available from https://doi.org/10.3390/md12052357, http://www.mdpi.com/1660-3397/12/5/2357/pdf.

Gingras, A. A., White, P. J., Chouinard, P. Y., Julien, P., Davis, T. A., Dombrowski, L., Couture, Y., Dubreuil, P., Myre, A., Bergeron, K., Marette, A., & Thivierge, M. C. (2007). Long-chain omega-3 fatty acids regulate bovine whole-body protein metabolism by promoting muscle insulin signalling to the Akt-mTOR-S6K1 pathway and insulin sensitivity. *Journal of Physiology*, *579*(1), 269–284. Available from https://doi.org/10.1113/jphysiol.2006.121079, http://onlinelibrary.wiley.com/journal/10.1111/(ISSN)1469-7793.

Giselle, P. L., Teresa, C., Fusheng, Y., Walter, B., Sally, A. F., & Greg, M. C. (2001). The curry spice curcumin reduces oxidative damage and amyloid pathology in an Alzheimer transgenic mouse. *The Journal of Neuroscience*, *21*. Available from https://doi.org/10.1523/JNEUROSCI.21-21-08370.20012001.

Gravina, L., Brown, F. F., Alexander, L., Dick, J., Bell, G., Witard, O. C., & Galloway, S. D. R. (2017). N-3 fatty acid supplementation during 4 weeks of training leads to improved anaerobic endurance capacity, but not maximal strength, speed, or power in soccer players. *International Journal of Sport Nutrition and Exercise Metabolism*, *27*(4), 305–313. Available from https://doi.org/10.1123/ijsnem.2016-0325, http://journals.humankinetics.com/doi/pdf/10.1123/ijsnem.2016-0325.

Halliday, T. M., Peterson, N. J., Thomas, J. J., Kleppinger, K., Hollis, B. W., & Larson-Meyer, D. E. (2011). Vitamin D status relative to diet, Lifestyle, Injury, and Illness in College Athletes. *Medicine and Science in Sports and Exercise*, *43*(2), 335–343. Available from https://doi.org/10.1249/MSS.0b013e3181eb9d4d.

Hämäläinen, M., Nieminen, R., Vuorela, P., Heinonen, M., & Moilanen, E. (2007). Anti-inflammatory effects of flavonoids: Genistein, kaempferol, quercetin, and daidzein inhibit STAT-1 and NF- κ B activations, whereas flavone, isorhamnetin, naringenin, and pelargonidin inhibit only NF- κ B activation along with their inhibitory effect on iNOS expression and NO production in activated macrophages. *Mediators of Inflammation*, *2007*, 1–10. Available from https://doi.org/10.1155/2007/45673.

Haramizu, S., Mizunoya, W., Masuda, Y., Ohnuki, K., Watanabe, T., Yazawa, S., & Fushiki, T. (2006). Capsiate, a nonpungent capsaicin analog, increases endurance swimming capacity of mice by stimulation of vanilloid receptors. *Bioscience, Biotechnology, and Biochemistry*, *70*(4), 774–781. Available from https://doi.org/10.1271/bbb.70.774, http://www.jstage.jst.go.jp/article/bbb/70/4/774/_pdf, Japan.

Herrlinger, K. A., Chirouzes, D. M., & Ceddia, M. A. (2015). Supplementation with a polyphenolic blend improves post-exercise strength recovery and muscle soreness. *Food and Nutrition Research* (59). Available from https://doi.org/10.3402/fnr.v59.30034, http://www.foodandnutritionresearch.net/index.php/fnr/article/view/30034/44200.

Hord, N. G., Tang, Y., & Bryan, N. S. (2009). Food sources of nitrates and nitrites: The physiologic context for potential health benefits. *American Journal of Clinical Nutrition*, *90*(1), 1–10. Available from https://doi.org/10.3945/ajcn.2008.27131, http://www.ajcn.org/cgi/reprint/90/1/1, United States.

Isao Nagaoka, A. T., & Masafumi Yoshimura, C. (2019). Action of glucosamine, a chitosan monomer, on the joint health of athletes. *International Journal of Biological Macromolecules*, *132*, 795–800. Available from https://doi.org/10.1016/j.ijbiomac.2019.03.234.

Jädert, C., Phillipson, M., Holm, L., Lundberg, J. O., & Borniquel, S. (2014). Preventive and therapeutic effects of nitrite supplementation in experimental inflammatory bowel disease. *Redox Biology*, *2*(1), 73–81. Available from https://doi.org/10.1016/j.redox.2013.12.012, http://www.journals.elsevier.com/redox-biology.

Jakeman, J. R., Lambrick, D. M., Wooley, B., Babraj, J. A., & Faulkner, J. A. (2017). Effect of an acute dose of omega-3 fish oil following exercise-induced muscle damage. *European Journal of Applied Physiology*, *117*(3), 575–582. Available from https://doi.org/10.1007/s00421-017-3543-y.

Jannas-Vela, S., Espinosa, A., Candia, A. A., Flores-Opazo, M., Peñailillo, L., & Valenzuela, R. (2023). The role of omega-3 polyunsaturated fatty acids and their lipid mediators on skeletal muscle regeneration: A narrative review. *Nutrients.*, *15*(4), 871. Available from https://doi.org/10.3390/nu15040871.

Jendricke, P., Kohl, J., Centner, C., Gollhofer, A., & König, D. (2020). Influence of specific collagen peptides and concurrent training on cardiometabolic parameters and performance indices in women: A randomized controlled trial. *Frontiers in Nutrition*, *7*. Available from https://doi.org/10.3389/fnut.2020.580918.

Jeon, S. M., Kim, H. J., Woo, M. N., Lee, M. K., Chul Shin, Y., Bok Park, Y., & Choi, M. S. (2010). Fucoxanthin-rich seaweed extract suppresses body weight gain and improves lipid metabolism in high-fat-fed C57BL/6J mice. *Biotechnology Journal*, *5*(9), 961–969. Available from https://doi.org/10.1002/biot.201000215, http://onlinelibrary.wiley.com/doi/10.1002/biot.201000215/pdf, South Korea.

Jerger, S., Jendricke, P., Centner, C., Bischof, K., Kohl, J., Keller, S., Gollhofer, A., & König, D. (2023). Effects of specific bioactive collagen peptides in combination with concurrent training on running performance and indicators of endurance capacity in men: A randomized controlled trial. *Sports Medicine - Open*, *9*(1). Available from https://doi.org/10.1186/s40798-023-00654-9.

Jo, E., Fischer, M., Auslander, A. T., Beigarten, A., Daggy, B., Hansen, K., Kessler, L., Osmond, A., Wang, H., & Wes, R. (2019). The effects of multi-day vs. Single pre-exercise nitrate supplement dosing on simulated cycling time trial performance and skeletal muscle oxygenation. *Journal of Strength and Conditioning Research*, *33*(1), 217–224. Available from https://doi.org/10.1519/JSC.0000000000001958, http://journals.lww.com/nsca-jscr.

Jodra, P., Domínguez, R., Sánchez-Oliver, A. J., Veiga-Herreros, P., & Bailey, S. J. (2020). Effect of beetroot juice supplementation on mood, perceived exertion, and performance during a 30-second wingate test. *International Journal of Sports Physiology and Performance*, *15*(2), 243–248. Available from https://doi.org/10.1123/ijspp.2019-0149, https://journals.humankinetics.com/view/journals/ijspp/15/2/article-p243.xml.

Jones, L., Johnstone, I., Day, C., Le Marquer, S., & Hulton, A. T. (2021). The dose-effects of caffeine on lower body maximal strength, muscular endurance, and rating of perceived exertion in strength-trained females. *Nutrients.*, *13*(10). Available from https://doi.org/10.3390/nu13103342, https://www.mdpi.com/2072-6643/13/10/3342/pdf.

Jonvik, K. L., Hoogervorst, D., Peelen, H. B., de Niet, M., Verdijk, L. B., van Loon, L. J. C., & van Dijk, J.-W. (2021). The impact of beetroot juice supplementation on muscular endurance, maximal strength and countermovement jump performance. *European Journal of Sport Science*, *21*(6), 871–878. Available from https://doi.org/10.1080/17461391.2020.1788649.

Khor, S. C., Abdul Karim, N., Wan Ngah, W. Z., Mohd Yusof, Y. A., & Makpol, S. (2014). Vitamin e in sarcopenia: Current evidences on its role in prevention and treatment. *Oxidative Medicine and Cellular Longevity, 2014*. Available from https://doi.org/10.1155/2014/914853, http://www.hindawi.com/journals/oximed/.

Kirmse, M., Oertzen-Hagemann, V., de Marées, M., Bloch, W., & Platen, P. (2019). Prolonged collagen peptide supplementation and resistance exercise training affects body composition in recreationally active men. *Nutrients., 11*(5). Available from https://doi.org/10.3390/nu11051154, https://www.mdpi.com/2072-6643/11/5/1154/pdf.

Koirala, P., Dahal, M., Rai, S., Dhakal, M., Nirmal, N. P., Maqsood, S., Al-Asmari, F., & Buranasompob, A. (2023). Dairy milk protein−derived bioactive peptides: Avengers against metabolic syndrome. *Current Nutrition Reports, 12*(2), 308−326. Available from https://doi.org/10.1007/s13668-023-00472-1, https://www.springer.com/journal/13668.

König, D., Kohl, J., Jerger, S., & Centner, C. (2021). Potential relevance of bioactive peptides in sports nutrition. *Nutrients., 13*(11), 3997. Available from https://doi.org/10.3390/nu13113997.

Kunz, H. E., Michie, K. L., Gries, K. J., Zhang, X., Ryan, Z. C., & Lanza, I. R. (2022). A randomized trial of the effects of dietary n3-PUFAs on skeletal muscle function and acute exercise response in healthy older adults. *Nutrients, 14*(17). Available from https://doi.org/10.3390/nu14173537, http://www.mdpi.com/journal/nutrients/.

Kyriakidou, Y., Wood, C., Ferrier, C., Dolci, A., & Elliott, B. (2021). The effect of Omega-3 polyunsaturated fatty acid supplementation on exercise-induced muscle damage. *Journal of the International Society of Sports Nutrition, 18*(1). Available from https://doi.org/10.1186/s12970-020-00405-1.

Laiglesia, L. M., Lorente-Cebrián, S., Prieto-Hontoria, P. L., Fernández-Galilea, M., Ribeiro, S. M. R., Sáinz, N., Martínez, J. A., & Moreno-Aliaga, M. J. (2016). Eicosapentaenoic acid promotes mitochondrial biogenesis and beige-like features in subcutaneous adipocytes from overweight subjects. *The Journal of Nutritional Biochemistry, 37*, 76−82. Available from https://doi.org/10.1016/j.jnutbio.2016.07.019.

Larson-Meyer, D. E., & Willis, K. S. (2010). Vitamin D and athletes. *Current Sports Medicine Reports, 9*(4), 220−226. Available from https://doi.org/10.1249/JSR.0b013e3181e7dd45.

Latham, C. M., Brightwell, C. R., Keeble, A. R., Munson, B. D., Thomas, N. T., Zagzoog, A. M., Fry, C. S., & Fry, J. L. (2021). Vitamin D promotes skeletal muscle regeneration and mitochondrial health. *Frontiers in Physiology, 12*. Available from https://doi.org/10.3389/fphys.2021.660498, http://www.frontiersin.org/Physiology/archive/.

Lawler, T. P., & Cialdella-Kam, L. (2020). Non-carbohydrate dietary factors and their influence on post-exercise glycogen storage: A review. *Current Nutrition Reports, 9*(4), 394−404. Available from https://doi.org/10.1007/s13668-020-00335-z, http://www.springer.com/new + %26 + forthcoming + titles + %28default%29/journal/13668?changeHeader.

Lee, E. H., Meissner, G., & Kim, D. H. (2002). Effects of quercetin on single Ca2 + release channel behavior of skeletal muscle. *Biophysical Journal, 82*(3), 1266−1277. Available from https://doi.org/10.1016/S0006-3495(02)75483-0, http://www.sciencedirect.com/science/journal/00063495.

Legault, Z., Bagnall, N., & Kimmerly, D. S. (2015). The influence of oral L-glutamine supplementation on muscle strength recovery and soreness following unilateral knee extension eccentric exercise. *International Journal of Sport Nutrition and Exercise Metabolism, 25*(5), 417−426. Available from https://doi.org/10.1123/ijsnem.2014-0209, http://journals.humankinetics.com/AcuCustom/Sitename/Documents/DocumentItem/01%20Legault%20IJSNEM_2014_0209_417_426.pdf.

Li, S., Fasipe, B., & Laher, I. (2022). Potential harms of supplementation with high doses of antioxidants in athletes. *Journal of Exercise Science & Fitness, 20*(4), 269−275. Available from https://doi.org/10.1016/j.jesf.2022.06.001.

Liu, Y., Shen, X., Sha, M., Feng, Z., & Liu, Y. (2023). Natural bioactive flavonoids as promising agents in alleviating exercise-induced fatigue. *Food Bioscience, 51*, 102360. Available from https://doi.org/10.1016/j.fbio.2023.102360.

Lotito, S. B., & Frei, B. (2006). Dietary flavonoids attenuate tumor necrosis factor α-induced adhesion molecule expression in human aortic endothelial cells: Structure-function relationships and activity after first pass metabolism. *Journal of Biological Chemistry, 281*(48), 37102−37110. Available from https://doi.org/10.1074/jbc.M606804200United, http://www.jbc.org/cgi/reprint/281/48/37102.

Loureiro, L. M. R., Neto, Ed. S., Molina, G. E., Amato, A. A., Arruda, S. F., Reis, C. E. G., & Da Costa, T. H. M. (2021). Coffee increases post-exercise muscle glycogen recovery in endurance athletes: A randomized clinical trial. *Nutrients., 13*(10). Available from https://doi.org/10.3390/nu13103335, https://www.mdpi.com/2072-6643/13/10/3335/pdf.

Loureiro, L. M. R., Reis, C. E. G., & Da Costa, T. H. M. (2018). Effects of coffee components on muscle glycogen recovery: A systematic review. *International Journal of Sport Nutrition and Exercise Metabolism, 28*(3), 284−293. Available from https://doi.org/10.1123/ijsnem.2017-0342, https://journals.humankinetics.com/doi/pdf/10.1123/ijsnem.2017-0342.

Mackay, J., Bowles, E., Macgregor, L. J., Prokopidis, K., Campbell, C., Barber, E., Galloway, S. D. R., & Witard, O. C. (2023). Fish oil supplementation fails to modulate indices of muscle damage and muscle repair during acute recovery from eccentric exercise in trained young males. *European Journal of Sport Science, 23*(8), 1666−1676. Available from https://doi.org/10.1080/17461391.2023.2199282, http://www.tandf.co.uk/journals/journal.asp?issn = 1746-1391&linktype = 1.

Mafi, F., Biglari, S., Ghardashi Afousi, A., & Ali Gaeini, A. (2019). Improvement in skeletal muscle strength and plasma levels of follistatin and myostatin induced by an 8-week resistance training and epicatechin supplementation in sarcopenic older adults. *Journal of Aging and Physical Activity, 27*(3), 384−391. Available from https://doi.org/10.1123/japa.2017-0389.

Marshall, A. R., Rimmer, J. E., Shah, N., Bye, K., Kipps, C., Woods, D. R., O'Hara, J., Boos, C. J., & Barlow, M. (2021). Marching to the Beet: The effect of dietary nitrate supplementation on high altitude exercise performance and adaptation during a military trekking expedition. *Nitric Oxide - Biology and Chemistry, 113-114*, 70−77. Available from https://doi.org/10.1016/j.niox.2021.05.002, http://www.elsevier.com/inca/publications/store/6/2/2/9/2/6/index.htt.

Martins, G. L., Guilherme, J. P. L. F., Ferreira, L. H. B., Souza-Junior, T. P. de, & Lancha, A. H. (2020). Caffeine and exercise performance: Possible Directions for definitive findings. *Frontiers in Sports and Active Living*, *2*. Available from https://doi.org/10.3389/fspor.2020.574854.

Maryama Awang Daud, D., & Ahmedy, F. (2022). Dayang Marshitah Pg Baharuddin, Zainul Amiruddin Zakaria, Oxidative Stress and Antioxidant Enzymes Activity after Cycling at Different Intensity and Duration. *Applied Sciences*, *12*(18), 9161. Available from https://doi.org/10.3390/app12189161.

McAnulty, L. S., Miller, L. E., Hosick, P. A., Utter, A. C., Quindry, J. C., & McAnulty, S. R. (2013). Effect of resveratrol and quercetin supplementation on redox status and inflammation after exercise. Applied Physiology. *Nutrition and Metabolism*, *38*(7), 760–765. Available from https://doi.org/10.1139/apnm-2012-0455.

Mitra, S., Paul, S., Roy, S., Sutradhar, H., Emran, T. B., Nainu, F., Khandaker, M. U., Almalki, M., Wilairatana, P., & Mubarak, M. S. (2022). Exploring the immune-boosting functions of vitamins and minerals as nutritional food bioactive compounds: A comprehensive review. *Molecules (Basel, Switzerland)*, *27*(2). Available from https://doi.org/10.3390/molecules27020555, https://www.mdpi.com/1420-3049/27/2/555/pdf.

Momomura, R. E. I., Naito, K. I. Y. O. H. I. T. O., Igarashi, M. A. M. O. R. U., Watari, T. A. I. J. I., Terakado, A. T. S. U. H. I. K. O., Oike, S. H. I. N. J. I., Sakamoto, K. O. J. I., Nagaoka, I. S. A. O., & Kaneko, K. A. Z. U. O. (2013). Evaluation of the effect of glucosamine administration on biomarkers of cartilage and bone metabolism in bicycle racers. *Molecular Medicine Reports*, *7*(3), 742–746. Available from https://doi.org/10.3892/mmr.2013.1289.

Morifuji, M., Kanda, A., Koga, J., Kawanaka, K., & Higuchi, M. (2010). Post-exercise carbohydrate plus whey protein hydrolysates supplementation increases skeletal muscle glycogen level in rats. *Amino Acids*, *38*(4), 1109–1115. Available from https://doi.org/10.1007/s00726-009-0321-0.

Morishima, T., Tsuchiya, Y., Ueda, H., & Ochi, E. (2020). Muscular endurance and muscle metabolic responses to 8 weeks of omega-3 polyunsaturated fatty acids supplementation. *Physiological Reports*, *8*(16). Available from https://doi.org/10.14814/phy2.14546.

Mul, J. D., Stanford, K. I., Hirshman, M. F., Goodyear, L. J. (2015). Exercise and Regulation of Carbohydrate Metabolism. *Progress in Molecular Biology and Translational Science*, *135*, 17–37. Available from https://doi.org/10.1016/bs.pmbts.2015.07.020, http://www.elsevier.com/books/book-series/progress-in-molecular-biology-and-translational-science#. Elsevier B.V. United States.

Nair, K. S., Irving, B. A., & Lanza, I. R. (2011). Can dietary nitrates enhance the efficiency of mitochondria? *Cell Metabolism*, *13*(2), 117–118. Available from https://doi.org/10.1016/j.cmet.2011.01.013, http://www.cellmetabolism.org/.

Nieman, D. C., Gillitt, N. D., Knab, A. M., Shanely, R. A., Pappan, K. L., Jin, F., & Lila, M. A. (2013). Influence of a polyphenol-enriched protein powder on exercise-induced inflammation and oxidative stress in athletes: A randomized trial using a metabolomics approach. *PLoS One*, *8*(8). Available from https://doi.org/10.1371/journal.pone.0072215, http://www.plosone.org/article/fetchObjectAttachment.action;jsessionid = D3145D5A9DA440B78145B2EEFECBAAD8?uri = info%3Adoi%2F10.1371%2Fjournal.pone.0072215&representation = PDF, United States.

Nieman, D. C., Henson, D. A., Maxwell, K. R., Williams, A. S., Mcanulty, S. R., Jin, F., Shanely, R. A., & Lines, T. C. (2009). Effects of quercetin and egcg on mitochondrial biogenesis and immunity. *Medicine and Science in Sports and Exercise*, *41*(7), 1467–1475. Available from https://doi.org/10.1249/MSS.0b013e318199491f.

Nieman, D. C., Williams, A. S., Shanely, R. A., Jin, F., McAnulty, S. R., Triplett, N. T., Austin, M. D., & Henson, D. A. (2010). Quercetin's influence on exercise performance and muscle mitochondrial biogenesis. *Medicine and Science in Sports and Exercise*, *42*(2), 338–345. Available from https://doi.org/10.1249/MSS.0b013e3181b18fa3.

Nikolaidis, M. G., Kerksick, C. M., Lamprecht, M., & McAnulty, S. R. (2012). Does vitamin C and e supplementation impair the favorable adaptations of regular exercise? *Oxidative Medicine and Cellular Longevity*. Available from https://doi.org/10.1155/2012/707941.

Nirmal, N., Khanashyam, A. C., Shah, K., Awasti, N., Sajith Babu, K., Ucak, İ., Afreen, M., Hassoun, A., & Tuanthong, A. (2024). Plant protein-derived peptides: Frontiers in sustainable food system and applications. *Frontiers in Sustainable Food Systems*, *8*. Available from https://doi.org/10.3389/fsufs.2024.1292297, www.frontiersin.org/journals/sustainable-food-systems#.

Nobari, H., Saedmocheshi, S., Chung, L. H., Suzuki, K., Maynar-Mariño, M., & Pérez-Gómez, J. (2021). An overview on how exercise with green tea consumption can prevent the production of reactive oxygen species and improve sports performance. *International Journal of Environmental Research and Public Health*, *19*(1). Available from https://doi.org/10.3390/ijerph19010218.

Norum, M., Risvang, L. C., Bjørnsen, T., Dimitriou, L., Rønning, P. O., Bjørgen, M., & Raastad, T. (2020). Caffeine increases strength and power performance in resistance-trained females during early follicular phase. *Scandinavian Journal of Medicine and Science in Sports*, *30*(11), 2116–2129. Available from https://doi.org/10.1111/sms.13776, http://onlinelibrary.wiley.com/journal/10.1111/(ISSN)1600-0838.

Nyakayiru, J., Jonvik, K. L., Trommelen, J., Pinckaers, P. J. M., Senden, J. M., van Loon, L. J. C., & Verdijk, L. B. (2017). Beetroot juice supplementation improves high-intensity intermittent type exercise performance in trained soccer players. *Nutrients*, *9*(3). Available from https://doi.org/10.3390/nu9030314, http://www.mdpi.com/2072-6643/9/3/314/pdf.

Oertzen-Hagemann, V., Kirmse, M., Eggers, B., Pfeiffer, K., Marcus, K., Marées, M. de, & Platen, P. (2019). Effects of 12 weeks of hypertrophy resistance exercise training combined with collagen peptide supplementation on the skeletal muscle proteome in recreationally active men. *Nutrients*, *11*(5), 1072. Available from https://doi.org/10.3390/nu11051072.

Oliveira, G. V. de, Morgado, M., Conte-Junior, C. A., Alvares, T. S., & Sandbakk, Ø. (2017). Acute effect of dietary nitrate on forearm muscle oxygenation, blood volume and strength in older adults: A randomized clinical trial. *PLoS One*, *12*(11), e0188893. Available from https://doi.org/10.1371/journal.pone.0188893.

Opheim, M. N., & Rankin, J. W. (2012). Effect of capsaicin supplementation on repeated sprinting performance. *Journal of Strength and Conditioning Research*, *26*(2), 319–326. Available from https://doi.org/10.1519/JSC.0b013e3182429ae5.

Ota, N., Soga, S., & Shimotoyodome, A. (2016). Daily consumption of tea catechins improves aerobic capacity in healthy male adults: A randomized double-blind, placebo-controlled, crossover trial. *Bioscience, Biotechnology, and Biochemistry*, *80*(12), 2412–2417. Available from https://doi.org/10.1080/09168451.2016.1224638.

Papadopoulou, S. K., Mantzorou, M., Kondyli-Sarika, F., Alexandropoulou, I., Papathanasiou, J., Voulgaridou, G., & Nikolaidis, P. T. (2022). The key role of nutritional elements on sport rehabilitation and the effects of nutrients intake. *Sports, 10*(6). Available from https://doi.org/10.3390/sports10060084, https://www.mdpi.com/2075-4663/10/6/84/pdf?version = 1653554203.

Pedersen, D. J., Lessard, S. J., Coffey, V. G., Churchley, E. G., Wootton, A. M., Ng, T., Watt, M. J., & Hawley, J. A. (2008). High rates of muscle glycogen resynthesis after exhaustive exercise when carbohydrate is coingested with caffeine. *Journal of Applied Physiology, 105*(1), 7–13. Available from https://doi.org/10.1152/japplphysiol.01121.2007, http://jap.physiology.org/cgi/reprint/105/1/7, Australia.

Peres, F. P., Levada-Pires, A. C., Vieira, M., Hatanaka, E., Cury-Boaventura, M. F., Folador, A., Gorjão, R., Hirabara, S. M., Santos-Silva, P. R., Deuster, P. A., Curi, R., & Pithon-Curi, T. C. (2023). Hydrolyzed whey protein enriched with glutamine dipeptide attenuates skeletal muscle damage and improves physical exhaustion test performance in triathletes. *Frontiers in Sports and Active Living, 4*. Available from https://doi.org/10.3389/fspor.2022.1011240, www.frontiersin.org/journals/sports-and-active-living.

Polley, K. R., Jenkins, N., O'Connor, P., & McCully, K. (2016). Influence of exercise training with resveratrol supplementation on skeletal muscle mitochondrial capacity. *Applied Physiology, Nutrition, and Metabolism, 41*(1), 26–32. Available from https://doi.org/10.1139/apnm-2015-0370.

Potgieter, S., Wright, H. H., & Smith, C. (2018). Caffeine improves triathlon performance: A field study in males and females. *International Journal of Sport Nutrition and Exercise Metabolism, 28*(3), 228–237. Available from https://doi.org/10.1123/ijsnem.2017-0165, https://journals.humankinetics.com/doi/pdf/10.1123/ijsnem.2017-0165.

Powers, S. K., Sollanek, K. J., & Wiggs, M. P. (2014). Endurance exercise and antioxidant supplementation: Sense or nonsense? *Part 1. Sport Sci Exch, 27*(137), 1–4, 2014.

Quinlivan, A., Irwin, C., Grant, G. D., Anoopkumar-Dukie, S., Skinner, T., Leveritt, M., & Desbrow, B. (2015). The effects of red bull energy drink compared with caffeine on cycling time-trial performance. *International Journal of Sports Physiology and Performance, 10*(7), 897–901. Available from https://doi.org/10.1123/ijspp.2014-0481, http://journals.humankinetics.com/AcuCustom/Sitename/Documents/DocumentItem/13_Quinlivan_IJSPP_2014-0481_987-901.pdf.

Roberts, J. D., Roberts, M. G., Tarpey, M. D., Weekes, J. C., & Thomas, C. H. (2015). The effect of a decaffeinated green tea extract formula on fat oxidation, body composition and exercise performance. *Journal of the International Society of Sports Nutrition, 12*, 1–9.

Roberts, P. A., Fox, J., Peirce, N., Jones, S. W., Casey, A., & Greenhaff, P. L. (2016). Creatine ingestion augments dietary carbohydrate mediated muscle glycogen supercompensation during the initial 24 h of recovery following prolonged exhaustive exercise in humans. *Amino Acids, 48*, 1831–1842.

Rokkedal-Lausch, T., Franch, J., Poulsen, M. K., Thomsen, L. P., Weitzberg, E., Kamavuako, E. N., Karbing, D. S., & Larsen, R. G. (2019). Chronic high-dose beetroot juice supplementation improves time trial performance of well-trained cyclists in normoxia and hypoxia. *Nitric Oxide - Biology and Chemistry, 85*, 44–52. Available from https://doi.org/10.1016/j.niox.2019.01.011, http://www.elsevier.com/inca/publications/store/6/2/2/9/2/6/index.htt.

Saura, R. A., Rentero, M. P. Z., Hernandez, J. M. (2019). Sports Nutrition and Performance - Our Challenges Now and Forthcoming Time Intechopen Limited. (2019), 2019.

Scholten, S., Sergeev, I., Birger, C., & Song, Q. (2015). Effects of vitamin D and quercetin, alone and in combination, on cardiorespiratory fitness and muscle function in physically active male adults. *Open Access Journal of Sports Medicine*, 229. Available from https://doi.org/10.2147/OAJSM.S83159.

Sgrò, P., Ceci, R., Lista, M., Patrizio, F., Sabatini, S., Felici, F., Sacchetti, M., Bazzucchi, I., Duranti, G., & Di Luigi, L. (2021). Quercetin modulates IGF-I and IGF-II levels after eccentric exercise-induced muscle-damage: A placebo-controlled study. *Frontiers in Endocrinology, 12*. Available from https://doi.org/10.3389/fendo.2021.745959.

Silva, L. A., Pinho, C. A., Silveira, P. C. L., Tuon, T., De Souza, C. T., Dal-Pizzol, F., & Pinho, R. A. (2010). Vitamin e supplementation decreases muscular and oxidative damage but not inflammatory response induced by eccentric contraction. *Journal of Physiological Sciences, 60*(1), 51–57. Available from https://doi.org/10.1007/s12576-009-0065-3.

Stefan, M., Sharp, M., Gheith, R., Lowery, R., Ottinger, C., Wilson, J., Durkee, S., & Bellamine, A. (2021). L-Carnitine tartrate supplementation for 5 weeks improves exercise recovery in men and women: A randomized, double-blind, placebo-controlled trial. *Nutrients, 13*(10), 3432. Available from https://doi.org/10.3390/nu13103432.

Sung, M. M., Byrne, N. J., Robertson, I. M., Kim, T. T., Samokhvalov, V., Levasseur, J., Soltys, C. L., Fung, D., Tyreman, N., Denou, E., Jones, K. E., Seubert, J. M., Schertzer, J. D., & Dyck, J. R. B. (2017). Resveratrol improves exercise performance and skeletal muscle oxidative capacity in heart failure. *American Journal of Physiology - Heart and Circulatory Physiology, 312*(4), H842. Available from https://doi.org/10.1152/ajpheart.00455.2016, http://ajpheart.physiology.org/content/312/4/H842.full.pdf.

Taghiyar, M., Darvishi, L., Askari, G., Feizi, A., Hariri, M., Mashhadi, N. S., & Ghiasvand, R. (2013). The effect of vitamin C and e supplementation on muscle damage and oxidative stress in female athletes: A clinical trial. *International Journal of Preventive Medicine, 2013*, 16–23.

Taub, P. R., Ramirez-Sanchez, I., Patel, M., Higginbotham, E., Moreno-Ulloa, A., Román-Pintos, L. M., Phillips, P., Perkins, G., Ceballos, G., & Villarreal, F. (2016). Beneficial effects of dark chocolate on exercise capacity in sedentary subjects: Underlying mechanisms. *A double blind, randomized, placebo controlled trial. Food and Function, 7*(9), 3686–3693. Available from https://doi.org/10.1039/c6fo00611f, http://www.rsc.org/Publishing/Journals/FO/about.asp.

Tavakoli-Rouzbehani, O., Rezaei, A., Safaei, E., Iranshani, A., & Amirpour, M. (2021). The potential effect of conjugated linoleic acid on endurance exercise: A mechanistic review. Austin. *Sports Medicine (Auckland, N.Z.), 6*(1), 2021.

Thielecke, F., & Blannin, A. (2020a). Omega-3 fatty acids for sport performance—Are they equally beneficial for athletes and amateurs? A narrative review. *Nutrients, 12*(12). Available from https://doi.org/10.3390/nu12123712.

Thielecke, F., & Blannin, A. (2020b). Omega-3 fatty acids for sport performance—Are they equally beneficial for athletes and amateurs? A narrative review. *Nutrients*, *12*(12), 3712. Available from https://www.mdpi.com/2072-6643/12/12/3712.

Tomczyk, M., Jost, Z., Chroboczek, M., Urbański, R., Calder, P. C., Fisk, H. L., Sprengel, M., & Antosiewicz, J. (2023). Effects of 12 wk of omega-3 fatty acid supplementation in long-distance runners. *Medicine and Science in Sports and Exercise*, *55*(2), 216–224. Available from https://doi.org/10.1249/MSS.0000000000003038, https://journals.lww.com/acsm-msse/Pages/issuelist.aspx.

Tsao, J. P., Bernard, J. R., Hsu, H. C., Hsu, C. L., Liao, S. F., & Cheng, I. S. (2022). Short-term oral quercetin supplementation improves post-exercise insulin sensitivity, antioxidant capacity and enhances subsequent cycling time to exhaustion in healthy adults: A pilot study. *Frontiers in Nutrition*, *9*. Available from https://doi.org/10.3389/fnut.2022.875319, journal.frontiersin.org/journal/nutrition.

Tsitsimpikou, C., Kioukia-Fougia, N., Tsarouhas, K., Stamatopoulos, P., Rentoukas, E., Koudounakos, A., Papalexis, P., Liesivuori, J., & Jamurtas, A. (2013). Administration of tomato juice ameliorates lactate dehydrogenase and creatinine kinase responses to anaerobic training. *Food and Chemical Toxicology*, *61*, 9–13. Available from https://doi.org/10.1016/j.fct.2012.12.023.

Ullevig, S. L., Zuniga, K., Austin Lobitz, C., Santoyo, A., & Yin, Z. (2022). Egg protein supplementation improved upper body muscle strength and protein intake in community-dwelling older adult females who attended congregate meal sites or adult learning centers: A pilot randomized controlled trial. *Nutrition and Health*, *28*(4), 611–620. Available from https://doi.org/10.1177/02601060211051592, https://journals.sagepub.com/home/NAH.

Witard, O. C., & Davis, J.-K. (2021). Omega-3 fatty acids for training adaptation and exercise recovery: A muscle-centric perspective in athletes. *SSE*, *29*(211), 1–6, 2021.

Wu, W., He, L., Liang, Y., Yue, L., Peng, W., Jin, G., & Ma, M. (2019). Preparation process optimization of pig bone collagen peptide-calcium chelate using response surface methodology and its structural characterization and stability analysis. *Food Chemistry*, *284*, 80–89. Available from https://doi.org/10.1016/j.foodchem.2019.01.103.

Yang, D., Wang, T., Long, M., Li, P., & Quiles, J. L. (2020). Quercetin: Its main pharmacological activity and potential application in clinical medicine. *Oxidative Medicine and Cellular Longevity*, *2020*, 1–13. Available from https://doi.org/10.1155/2020/8825387.

Yoshimura, M., Sakamoto, K., Tsuruta, A., Yamamoto, T., Ishida, K., Yamaguchi, H., & Nagaoka, I. (2009). Evaluation of the effect of glucosamine administration on biomarkers for cartilage and bone metabolism in soccer players. *International Journal of Molecular Medicine*, *24*(4), 487–494. Available from https://doi.org/10.3892/ijmm_00000257, http://www.spandidos-publications.com/serveFile/ijmm_24_4_487_PDF.pdf?type = article&article_id = ijmm_24_4_487&item = PDF, Japan.

Chapter 9

Functional foods and aging and antiaging: a recipe for longevity

Sarra Akermi[1], Ashwani Sharma[2], Abira Dey[3], Moufida Chaari[1], Khaoula Elhadef[1], Altaf Choudhary[4], Subrata Sinha[5], Lotfi Mellouli[1] and Slim Smaoui[6]

[1]*Laboratory of Microbial Biotechnology, Enzymatic and Biomolecules, Center of Biotechnology of Sfax (CBS), University of Sfax, Sfax, Tunisia,* [2]*Insight Biosolutions, Biopole Rennes, Rennes, France,* [3]*Moldoc Biotech Private, SINE Limited Business Center, IIT Bombay, Mumbai, Maharashtra, India,* [4]*Pharma Department, Dr APJ Abdul Kalam Technical University, AKTU CDRI RD, Lucknow, Uttar Pradesh, India,* [5]*Department of Computational Sciences, Brainware University, Kolkata, West Bengal, India,* [6]*Laboratory of Microbial, Enzymes Biotechnology and Biomolecules (LMEBB), Centre of Biotechnology of Sfax (CBS), University of Sfax, Sfax, Tunisia*

9.1 Introduction

In the quest for a healthier and longer life, the intricate interplay between nutrition and aging has become a focal point of scientific inquiry. The aging process, a complex and multifaceted phenomenon, involves a myriad of biological, genetic, and environmental factors. As individuals age, they experience physiological and metabolic changes that can contribute to the development of chronic diseases and a decline in overall well-being (Fraile et al., 2022). In recent years, researchers and health professionals have increasingly turned their attention to the role of functional foods in mitigating the effects of aging and promoting longevity (Miyazawa et al., 2022). Many scientific studies reported the richness of functional foods in bioactive compounds which have several biological properties, including antioxidant, antiinflammatory, antimicrobial, anticancer, immunomodulatory, and neuroprotective effects, and were suggested as promising alternatives in food preservation, flavoring, coloring as well as enhancing food products' nutritional values (Akermi et al., 2024; Chaari et al., 2023; Elhadef et al., 2024). Other research discussed the existence of an interesting relationship between diet, aging, and lifestyle and how superfood could affect our biological metabolism, health, and lifespan.

Aging is a natural and inevitable biological process that involves the decay of an organism's structure and function. Aging is associated with declines in cellular function and the disruption of molecular functions in tissues, leading to a significant increase in the risks of various diseases. These include neurodegenerative processes associated with neuronal diseases, cardiovascular dysfunctions, metabolic disorders, musculoskeletal damage, and wear and tear diseases, as well as a decline in the immune system (Guo et al., 2022). The buildup of molecular mistakes affecting the functions of adult stem cells happens due to a combination of genetic and epigenetic interactions. This process is influenced by both hereditary and environmental factors, as well as random, unpredictable elements (Pagiatakis et al., 2021). Apart from molecular and genetic factors, diet, lifestyle, and exposure to oxidative stress also contribute significantly. Cellular damage, accumulated over time, leads to a decline in the function of various organs and systems, ultimately manifesting as the aging phenotype. Free radicals, generated as byproducts of metabolism, can damage cellular structures and DNA, leading to the accumulation of errors and mutations. Additionally, chronic low-grade inflammation, often referred to as "inflamm-aging," plays a pivotal role in the aging process and the development of age-related diseases (Asejeje & Ogunro, 2023) (Figure 1.1).

9.2 Understanding the role of functional foods in aging prevention

Functional foods, defined as foods that provide health benefits beyond basic nutrition, have gained prominence in the realm of aging research. These foods often enriched with bioactive compounds, vitamins, and minerals are designed to enhance overall well-being and mitigate the impact of aging on the body (Temple, 2022). A growing body of evidence

Unleashing the Power of Functional Foods and Novel Bioactives. DOI: https://doi.org/10.1016/B978-0-443-28862-3.00009-1

suggests that incorporating functional foods into the diet can positively influence various physiological processes, offering a promising approach to healthy aging.

Antioxidants, found abundantly in fruits, vegetables, and certain spices, are among the key bioactive compounds present in functional foods (Temple, 2022). The incorporation of regularly consumed nutritious foods is essential. Examples of such healthy foods with functional properties include beetroot (Tan & Hamid, 2021), peanuts (Toomer, 2020), sweet potato (Amagloh et al., 2021), pomegranate juice (Fahmy et al., 2020), and strawberries (Villamil-Galindo et al., 2021) (Fig. 9.1, Table 9.1). These foods have the potential to improve health and act as preventive measures against diseases due to their rich content of phytochemicals and micronutrients. These compounds play a crucial role in neutralizing free radicals, thereby reducing oxidative stress and mitigating cellular damage. Polyphenols, such as resveratrol in red wine and catechins in green tea, have garnered attention for their potential antiaging properties, demonstrated in numerous preclinical and clinical studies. Moreover, functional foods rich in omega-3 fatty acids, such as fatty fish and flaxseeds, have been linked to improved cognitive function, cardiovascular health, and a reduced risk of age-related diseases. The antiinflammatory properties of these essential fatty acids contribute to their potential in modulating the aging process and promoting healthy aging.

A diverse and well-balanced diet is essential for promoting overall health and well-being. The table highlights a variety of foods categorized into different types, each offering unique nutritional benefits. Fruits such as berries, kiwis, pears, peaches, apples, oranges, and bananas provide a rich source of vitamins, minerals, and antioxidants. Vegetables like broccoli, cauliflower, kale, spinach, and zucchini contribute essential nutrients and fiber. Nuts, including almonds, cashews, pistachios, macadamia nuts, and Brazil nuts, offer healthy fats, protein, and micronutrients. Seeds such as chia seeds, flaxseeds, hemp seeds, and pumpkin seeds provide additional sources of healthy fats, fiber, and omega-3 fatty acids. Legumes like black beans, chickpeas, navy beans, and lentils are excellent plant-based protein sources. Whole grains, including oats, barley, buckwheat, brown rice, and couscous, offer complex carbohydrates and fiber. Finally, herbs and spices like turmeric, cinnamon, ginger, and cayenne not only enhance flavor but also contribute antiinflammatory and antioxidant properties. Incorporating a diverse array of these foods into one's diet ensures a well-rounded nutritional profile, supporting overall health and longevity.

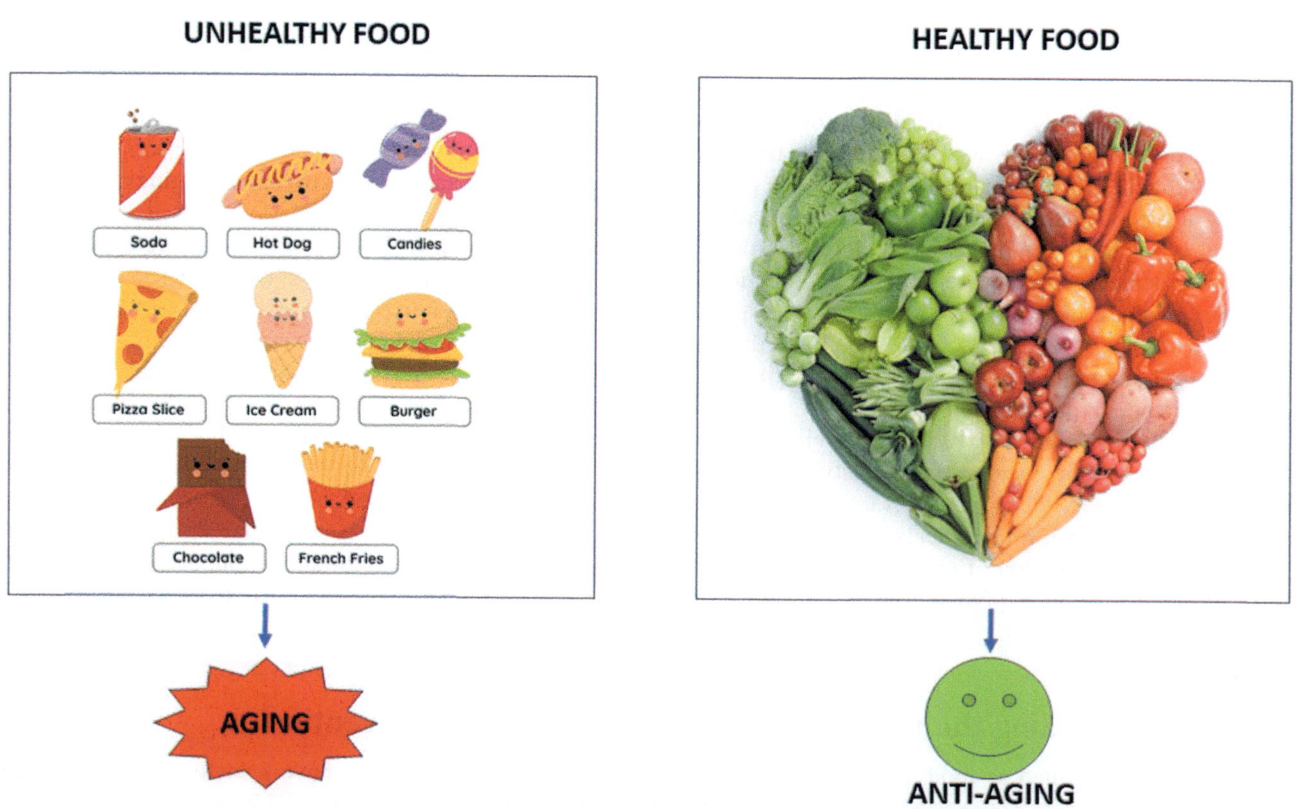

FIGURE 9.1 Different classifications of foods, healthy and unhealthy foods, which are responsible for aging or antiaging effects.

TABLE 9.1 List of Conventional Functional Food With Antiaging Effect.

Foods	Types
Fruits	Berries, kiwi, pears, peaches, apples, oranges, bananas
Vegetables	Broccoli, cauliflower, kale, spinach, zucchini
Nuts	Almonds, cashews, pistachios, macadamia nuts, Brazil nuts
Seeds	Chia seeds, flaxseeds, hemp seeds, pumpkin seeds
Legumes	Black beans, chickpeas, navy beans, lentils
Whole grains	Oats, barley, buckwheat, brown rice, couscous
Herbs and spices	Turmeric, cinnamon, ginger, cayenne

9.3 List of Nutrients from food and their effect on Biomarker genes in the Body

Vitamins and biomarkers play critical roles in maintaining optimal health and preventing deficiencies. Vitamin A is essential for vision, immune function, and skin health, with sources like carrots, sweet potatoes, spinach, kale, liver, and dairy products. It is associated with the retinol-binding protein (RBP). Vitamin D facilitates calcium absorption for bone health and supports immune system modulation, with sources including sun exposure, fatty fish, egg yolks, and fortified dairy products. Biomarkers like D-25-hydroxylase and 25-hydroxyvitamin D-1-hydroxylase are associated with vitamin D. Vitamin B9, crucial for DNA synthesis and red blood cell formation, is found in leafy greens, legumes, nuts, and fortified cereals. Its biomarker is dihydrofolate reductase (DHFR). Vitamin B12, vital for nerve function and DNA synthesis, is primarily present in animal products, and its associated biomarker is haptocorrin. Iodine, a key thyroid hormone component, is sourced from iodized salt, seaweed, fish, dairy, and certain fruits and vegetables. Biomarkers include urine iodine concentration (UIC), thyroid-stimulating hormone (TSH), thyroglobulin (Tg), T4 and T3, and goiter. Iron, crucial for oxygen transport and immune function, is found in red meat, poultry, fish, beans, lentils, and fortified cereals. Biomarkers like BMP6, BMPR, DMT1, FPN, HJV, RBC, SIRPα, SMAD, and TSAT are associated with iron. Zinc, vital for immune function and DNA synthesis, is sourced from meat, dairy, nuts, and seeds, with a biomarker linked to nonalcoholic fatty liver disease (NAFLD). Polyphenols, antioxidants with health benefits, are found in fruits, vegetables, tea, coffee, red wine, and dark chocolate. Biomarkers include polyphenol excretion (TPE), urinary polyphenols (TUP), and total dietary polyphenols (TDP). Carotenoids, precursors to vitamin A, are in colorful fruits and vegetables, with biomarkers like skin carotenoid status (SCS) and plasma carotenoids. Understanding these nutrients and their associated biomarkers is essential for crafting a balanced and health-promoting diet (Table 9.2).

9.4 Bioactive compounds—longevity recipes

In the quest for a longer and healthier life, scientists and researchers have turned their attention to the intricate world of bioactive compounds found in various foods. These compounds, often referred to as "longevity recipes," have been studied extensively for their potential to influence the aging process and promote overall well-being. The goal of longevity recipes is to create a balanced and nutritious eating plan that may contribute to overall health, support antiaging processes, and potentially extend the quality and duration of life. These recipes often draw inspiration from traditional diets, scientific research on longevity-promoting foods, and a holistic approach to nutrition and lifestyle. As our understanding of the molecular mechanisms behind aging deepens, the role of bioactive compounds in modulating these processes becomes increasingly significant.

Bioactive compounds are naturally occurring chemicals found in plants, animals, and microorganisms that exert specific physiological effects on the human body. They are not nutrients in the traditional sense, as the body does not require them for basic survival, but their presence in our diet has been linked to various health benefits (Pham et al., 2019). The aging process is a complex phenomenon influenced by various factors, and researchers have increasingly turned their attention to bioactive compounds found in natural sources for their potential role in promoting healthy aging. Notable bioactive compounds, such as polyphenols, flavonoids, and carotenoids, have garnered significant

TABLE 9.2 List of Important Nutrients Available In Functional Food and Used In Anti-aging Remedies And Regulation Of The Human Body.

Nutrients	Food Surces	Biomarker Genes
Vitamin A (Cheng et al., 2021; Huang et al., 2022)	Function: Essential for vision, immune function, and skin health. It also plays a role in cell differentiation and reproduction. Sources: Found in foods like carrots, sweet potatoes, spinach, kale, liver, and dairy products.	RBP
Vitamin D (Jeenduang et al., 2020)	Function: Facilitates calcium absorption for bone health and supports immune system modulation. Sources: Sun exposure, fatty fish (salmon, mackerel), egg yolks, and fortified dairy products.	D-25-hydroxylase, 25-hydroxyvitamin D-1-hydroxylase
Vitamin B9 Folate (Rotstein et al., 2022)	Function: Crucial for DNA synthesis, cell division, and the formation of red blood cells. Particularly important during pregnancy. Sources: Leafy green vegetables (spinach, kale), legumes (beans, lentils), nuts, and fortified cereals.	DHFR
Vitamin B12 (Kornerup et al., 2019)	Function: Vitamin B12 is essential for nerve function and DNA synthesis. Sources: Vitamin B12 is primarily present in animal products like meat, fish, and dairy.	Haptocorrin
Iodine Biomarker (Liu et al., 2022; Neven et al., 2021)	Function: Key component of thyroid hormones, regulating metabolism, and supporting thyroid function. Sources: Iodized salt, seaweed, fish, dairy products, and some fruits and vegetables.	UIC, TSH, Tg, T4 and T3, and goiter
Iron Biomarker (Masini et al., 2022)	Function: Essential for oxygen transport in the blood, energy production, and immune function. Sources: Red meat, poultry, fish, beans, lentils, and fortified cereals.	BMP6; BMPR; DMT1; Fe; FPN; HJV; RBC; SIRPα; SMAD; TSAT
Zinc Biomarker (Vogel-González et al., 2021)	Function: Important for immune function, wound healing, and DNA synthesis. Sources: Meat, dairy products, nuts, and seeds.	NAFLD
Biomarker of Polyphenol (Murphy et al., 2018)	Function: Antioxidants with potential health benefits, including antiinflammatory and cardiovascular protective effects. Sources: Fruits, vegetables, tea, coffee, red wine, and dark chocolate.	TPE, TUP, and TDP
Biomarker of Carotenoid (Page et al., 2021)	Function: Precursors to vitamin A, with antioxidant properties that support eye health and immune function. Sources: Colorful fruits and vegetables like carrots, tomatoes, peppers, and leafy greens.	SCS and plasma carotenoids

BMP6, Bone morphogenetic protein 6; *BMPR*, bone morphogenetic protein receptor; *DHFR*, Dihydrofolate reductase; *DMT1*, divalent metal transporter 1; *Fe*, iron/ferrum; *FPN*, ferroportin; *HJV*, hemojuvelin; *NAFLD*, nonalcoholic fatty liver disease; *RBC*, red blood cell; *RBP*, Retinol-binding protein; *SCS*, skin carotenoid status; *SIRPα*, signal regulatory protein alpha; *SMAD*, small-body-size mothers against decapentaplegic homolog 1; *TPE*, polyphenol excretion, *TUP*, urinary polyphenols, *TDP*, total dietary polyphenols; *TSAT*, percentage transferrin saturation; *UIC*, urine iodine concentration, *TSH*, thyroid-stimulating hormone, *Tg*, thyroglobulin

interest due to their antioxidant and anti-inflammatory properties. While they are abundant in fruits, vegetables, nuts, seeds, and whole grains, their concentrations can vary widely among different foods (Michalak et al., 2021).

Researchers emphasize the correlation between a well-balanced diet and the overall condition of the human body, encompassing both the appearance and functionality of the skin. The presence of essential nutrients in one's daily dietary intake plays a crucial role in supporting the biological processes occurring in both youthful and aging skin. Given the skin's high proliferative potential as a tissue, ensuring an ample supply of proteins, carbohydrates, and fats, vital for cellular regeneration, becomes imperative. Growing evidence indicates that maintaining a balanced diet significantly impacts the aging process of the skin. Incorporating functional antiaging elements into the diet involves substances that participate in the synthesis and metabolism of skin components, such as protein peptides and essential fatty acids.

Bioactive compounds exhibit potential as supplements for mature skincare, particularly due to their ability to safeguard the skin from harmful UV-induced effects. This protection is attributed to their antimutagenic, antioxidant, and free radical scavenging properties (Michalak, 2022).

Chronic inflammation is associated with a range of age-related diseases, including arthritis, cardiovascular disease, and neurodegenerative disorders. Bioactive compounds like flavonoids have been shown to possess anti-inflammatory effects, potentially mitigating the inflammatory processes that contribute to age-related diseases (Al-Khayri et al., 2022). Furthermore, some bioactive compounds have demonstrated the ability to influence cellular signaling pathways involved in aging and longevity. Resveratrol, found in red wine and grapes, is a well-known example. Studies have suggested that resveratrol may activate sirtuins, a family of proteins associated with longevity and cellular health. While the exact mechanisms are still under investigation, these findings highlight the intricate ways in which bioactive compounds may interact with cellular processes to promote longevity. Green et al. (2022) and Kim et al. (2019) explored the potential protective effects of grape peel extract (GPE) and resveratrol against the development of skin wrinkles induced by ultraviolet (UV) exposure. Administering either 2 g GPE or 2 mg resveratrol per kg body weight to mice orally showed a reduction in UVB-induced epidermal thickening. The thickness was decreased by approximately 63% and 55% with GPE and resveratrol consumption before UVB exposure, respectively, compared to the condition treated only with UVB. Additionally, both GPE and resveratrol demonstrated a modest protective impact on UVB-induced wrinkle formation in the skin. The introduction of GPE or resveratrol led to the activation of Nrf2-dependent antioxidant enzymes, including heme oxygenase-1 (HO-1), in both the liver and skin. Moreover, the substances inhibited metalloproteinases. This suggests a high likelihood that the extract or resveratrol mitigated UVB-induced photoaging by activating the Nrf2/HO-1 signaling pathway (Kim et al., 2019). Indications propose that individuals may experience advantages from plant phenolics acquired either through dietary intake or through skin application, as they possess the capacity to alleviate symptoms and hinder the onset of diverse skin disorders. With their natural source and minimal toxicity, phenolic compounds emerge as a promising resource for addressing the origins and consequences of skin aging, various skin diseases, as well as skin injuries such as wounds and burns. Additionally, polyphenols serve a protective role, aiding in the prevention or mitigation of the progression of specific skin issues, ranging from common concerns like wrinkles and acne to more severe, potentially life-threatening conditions like cancer (Liu et al., 2023).

For centuries, people in tropical regions have traditionally utilized virgin coconut oil (VCO) as a moisturizer. Clinical studies have affirmed its efficacy in improving skin disorder symptoms through moisturization and soothing effects. Despite this, the precise in vitro mechanisms of VCO and its skin benefits remain unclear. In in vitro studies on Reconstructed Human Epidermis (RHE) and NIH3T3 cells, VCO demonstrated nonirritating qualities and nonphototoxicity. The research also unveiled VCO's antiinflammatory activity, evidenced by the suppression of inflammatory markers and the fortification of skin barrier function. This study represents the initial documentation of VCO's in vitro antiinflammatory and skin-protective advantages. In summary, these results advocate for the integration of VCO into skincare formulations (Varma et al., 2019). Omega-3 fatty acids, prevalent in fish oil, demonstrate cardiovascular benefits and may contribute to maintaining cognitive health (Mora et al., 2022). Moreover, bioactive compounds like quercetin, found in apples and onions, and epigallocatechin gallate (EGCG) in green tea are being investigated for their potential to modulate cellular processes that impact aging, including cellular senescence and autophagy.

While the intriguing potential benefits of bioactive compounds on longevity warrant attention, it is crucial to approach this subject with a well-rounded perspective. The field of nutritional science is intricate, and individual responses to bioactive compounds can differ based on factors like genetics, diet, and overall health. A significant obstacle in researching the effects of bioactive compounds lies in the complexity of the human diet. Foods consist of a combination of diverse bioactive compounds, and their interactions can significantly impact their overall effects on health. Researchers face methodological challenges when attempting to isolate the effects of a specific compound within the context of a varied diet. Furthermore, the bioavailability of these compounds, determining how effectively the body absorbs and utilizes them, can vary. Factors such as food processing, cooking methods, and individual differences in metabolism play a role in influencing the bioavailability of bioactive compounds, thereby affecting their potential health benefits (Martirosyan et al., 2022).

Venturing into the realm of bioactive compounds offers a compelling avenue toward achieving healthier and extended lives. The intricate correlation between these compounds and the aging process accentuates the complexity inherent in human biology. While the potential benefits are promising, it is vital to approach this subject with a nuanced understanding of the challenges and considerations entailed in translating scientific discoveries into practical guidance. With the expansion of our knowledge, the integration of bioactive compounds into dietary strategies emerges as a comprehensive approach to nurturing longevity and overall well-being. Navigating the dynamic landscape of longevity research transcends the reliance on a single miraculous solution; instead, it involves thoughtful decision-making, embracing a diverse array of nutrient-rich foods, and adopting a holistic approach to well-being. The amalgamation of bioactive compounds drawn from diverse sources, combined with lifestyle factors and a sprinkle of culinary wisdom, establishes a roadmap for longevity that extends beyond the dining table, delving into the intricate choreography of life itself.

9.4.1 Impact of bioactive compounds on aging oxidative stress

Aging is a complex biological process characterized by a gradual decline in physiological functions and an increased susceptibility to diseases. One of the key factors contributing to aging is oxidative stress, which results from an imbalance between the production of reactive oxygen species and the body's ability to detoxify them. Oxidative stress can lead to cellular damage, inflammation, and, ultimately, the aging of tissues and organs (Luo et al., 2020). In recent years, there has been growing interest in the potential role of bioactive compounds in mitigating the impact of oxidative stress on aging. These compounds are recognized for their antioxidant properties, meaning that they can neutralize reactive oxygen species and protect cells from oxidative damage.

The impact of bioactive compounds on aging and oxidative stress is attributed to their ability to modulate various cellular and molecular pathways. One primary mechanism involves the scavenging of reactive oxygen species. Bioactive compounds act as antioxidants by donating electrons to reactive oxygen species, neutralizing their harmful effects on cellular components such as proteins, lipids, and DNA. This scavenging activity helps maintain cellular homeostasis and reduces the risk of oxidative damage. Furthermore, bioactive compounds can activate cellular defense mechanisms. They upregulate the expression of antioxidant enzymes, such as superoxide dismutase (SOD), catalase, and glutathione peroxidase, which enhance the cell's capacity to neutralize reactive oxygen species. Additionally, these compounds may influence signaling pathways associated with inflammation, apoptosis, and cell survival, providing further protection against oxidative stress-induced damage (López-Otín et al., 2023).

Cellular senescence is a state in which cells lose their ability to divide and contribute to tissue repair. It is a hallmark of aging and is closely linked to oxidative stress. Bioactive compounds have shown promise in mitigating cellular senescence by modulating key molecular pathways. Yao et al. (2022) and Zhou et al. (2021) discussed the protective effects of Astragalus polysaccharide (APS) against hydrogen peroxide-induced hepatocyte senescence. APS demonstrated strong protection in cell lines and aged mice, reducing oxidative stress, apoptosis, and pyroptosis while maintaining mitochondrial homeostasis. The mechanism involved AMP-activated protein kinase (AMPK) activation, inhibition of the mammalian target of rapamycin (mTOR), and promotion of mitophagy. However, the protective effect was weakened in the presence of chloroquine, suggesting a role for autophagy in APS's benefits. Overall, APS showed promise in alleviating hepatocyte senescence both in vitro and in vivo. Corina et al. (2019) and Diwan and Sharma (2022) explored the impact of vitamin E intake on cellular aging biomarkers in individuals with cardiovascular disease. Analyzing data from 1002 participants, researchers found that those with insufficient vitamin E intake had shorter leukocyte telomere length (LTL), a marker of cellular aging. Adequate vitamin E intake is correlated with longer LTL. Additionally, positive associations were observed between LTL and olive oil as well as fish consumption, highlighting the potential role of diet in modulating the aging process and emphasizing the importance of sufficient antioxidant intake (Corina Baba, 2020).

Mitochondria, the powerhouse of the cell, are particularly susceptible to oxidative damage due to their role in energy production and the generation of reactive oxygen species. Mitochondrial functioning is crucial for high-energy-demand organs like the heart and brain. In cardiovascular diseases, mitochondrial dysfunction leads to reactive oxygen species overproduction, reducing mitochondrial membrane potential and activating signaling proteins that induce apoptosis. Aging exacerbates oxidative stress, a key factor in cardiovascular issues, diminishing antioxidant response and increasing reactive oxygen species production. This process influenced by mitochondrial dysfunction and DNA damage results in extensive cellular damage and reduced life expectancy (Kowalska et al., 2020). Bioactive compounds have been demonstrated to protect mitochondrial function and maintain cellular energy balance. Flavonoids, such as quercetin, kaempferol, and epicatechin, protect cells from mitochondria-mediated cell death and may mitigate diseases linked to oxidative stress. A study screening five major subclasses of flavonoids found that these compounds inhibit H_2O_2 production by mitochondria from rat brain and heart. Quercetin, kaempferol, and epicatechin are potent inhibitors, with quercetin and kaempferol also affecting complex I activity. These findings suggest that flavonoids, by targeting mitochondria, contribute to their reported preventive effects against oxidative stress and mitochondrial dysfunction-related diseases (Hajam et al., 2022). Resveratrol exhibits effects aligned with the activation of AMP-activated protein kinase (AMPK), SIRT1, and PPARγ coactivator 1α (PGC-1α), crucial in regulating lipid and glucose balance and managing oxidative stress. In a study on type 2 diabetes, resveratrol demonstrated protective effects on the kidneys, potentially preventing diabetic nephropathy in mice. The mechanism involves phosphorylation of AMPK and activation of SIRT1-PGC-1α signaling, which may safeguard against lipotoxicity-induced apoptosis and oxidative stress in the kidney (Pyo et al., 2020).

Chronic inflammation is closely linked to oxidative stress and contributes significantly to the aging process. Bioactive compounds with antiinflammatory properties may exert their antiaging effects by modulating inflammatory pathways and reducing oxidative stress. Omega-3 fatty acids, specifically polyunsaturated fatty acids of the n-3 series, play a crucial role in blood coagulation and resolving inflammatory processes. Their antiinflammatory effects involve various mechanisms, including changes in cell membrane lipid composition, inhibition of NF-κB signaling that activates proinflammatory mediators, activation of the antiinflammatory transcription factor peroxisome proliferator-activated receptor delta, and binding to the G-protein coupled receptor, which suppresses macrophage-mediated tissue inflammation (Stromsnes et al., 2021).

The aging process often involves cognitive decline and an increased risk of neurodegenerative disorders such as Alzheimer's disease. Bioactive compounds have been investigated for their neuroprotective effects, which may be attributed, in part, to their ability to reduce oxidative stress in the brain. Polyphenols, including those in green tea and berries, have shown promise in protecting neurons from oxidative damage and preserving cognitive function. Resveratrol, in addition to its effects on mitochondrial function, has been studied for its potential in preventing age-related cognitive decline and reducing the risk of neurodegenerative diseases (Kim et al., 2019).

The research exploring the impact of bioactive compounds on aging through the reduction of oxidative stress is a rapidly evolving field. Polyphenols, flavonoids, carotenoids, and other antioxidants have demonstrated their ability to counteract oxidative stress, modulate inflammatory pathways, preserve mitochondrial function, and exert neuroprotective effects. As our understanding of the intricate mechanisms involved in aging continues to expand, incorporating a diverse range of bioactive compounds into dietary patterns holds great potential for enhancing overall health and longevity. While the existing research provides valuable insights, ongoing studies are needed to delve deeper into the specific mechanisms by which bioactive compounds exert their antiaging effects. Moreover, exploring the synergistic interactions between different compounds and understanding their optimal dosage and bioavailability will be crucial for developing personalized strategies to promote healthy aging. Ultimately, the integration of bioactive compounds into preventive and therapeutic approaches may pave the way for a healthier and more vibrant aging process.

9.4.2 Polyphenols for antiaging benefits

Polyphenols, a diverse group of natural compounds found in plants, are gaining prominence as promising antiaging nutraceuticals due to their ability to counteract cellular senescence—the process of irreversible cell cycle arrest associated with aging. These compounds, abundantly present in foods such as fruits, vegetables, tea, and red wine, exhibit a range of biological activities that contribute to their antisenescence effects (Fig. 9.2). One key mechanism through which polyphenols exert their antiaging properties is by acting as potent antioxidants. Polyphenols, including resveratrol, quercetin, and catechins, scavenge free radicals and reduce oxidative stress, which is a major contributor to cellular damage and senescence (Rudrapal et al., 2022). By mitigating oxidative stress, polyphenols help preserve cellular integrity and function. Moreover, polyphenols are known to activate longevity-associated pathways within cells. Resveratrol, for example, activates sirtuins, a family of proteins linked to cellular maintenance and stress response (Di Lorenzo et al., 2021). Other polyphenols, such as quercetin, modulate signaling pathways like AMP-activated protein kinase (AMPK), which regulates cellular energy metabolism and has implications for longevity (Meccariello and D'Angelo, 2021).

Research suggests that regular consumption of polyphenol-rich foods or supplements may contribute to the prevention or delay of age-related conditions and promote overall health and well-being. However, it is crucial to note that the efficacy and optimal dosages of polyphenols for antiaging benefits may vary, and further investigation is needed to establish specific recommendations. Nevertheless, the growing body of evidence supports the potential of polyphenols as antisenescence nutraceuticals, offering a natural and holistic approach to promoting healthy aging.

9.4.2.1 Saponins

Saponins, a class of natural compounds widely distributed in plants, have garnered interest for their potential as antiaging agents. These amphipathic glycosides, found in various plant sources such as ginseng, soybeans, and quinoa, exhibit diverse biological activities, including antioxidant, antiinflammatory, and immunomodulatory effects, which contribute to their antiaging properties (Timilsena et al., 2023). One key mechanism through which saponins exert antiaging

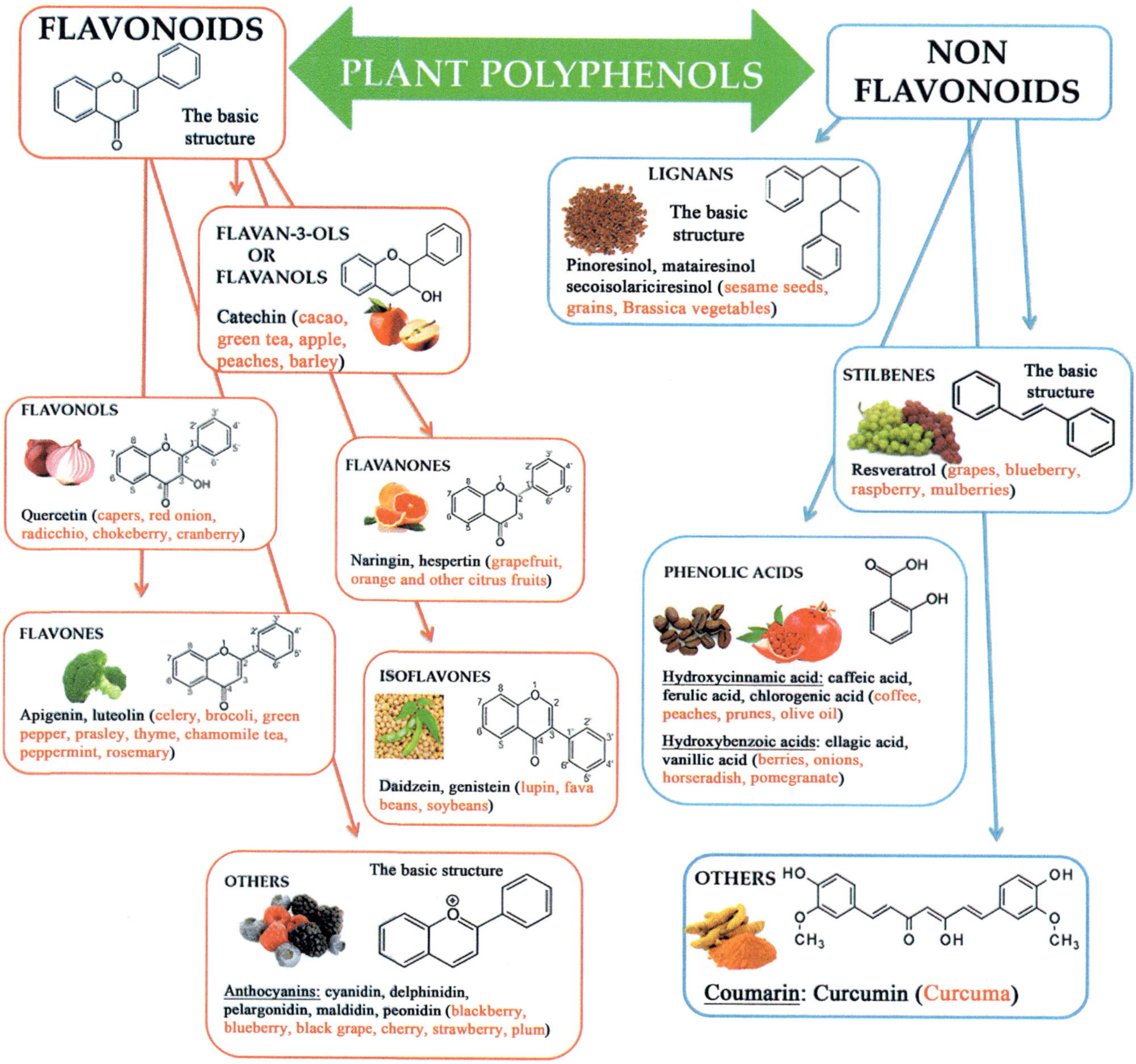

FIGURE 9.2 List of polyphenols for antiaging benefits.

effects is their ability to combat oxidative stress. Oxidative stress, resulting from an imbalance between free radicals and antioxidants in the body, is a major contributor to cellular damage and aging. Saponins, acting as potent antioxidants, scavenge free radicals, reducing oxidative damage and preserving cellular integrity. Additionally, saponins have been shown to have antiinflammatory properties. Chronic inflammation is associated with various age-related conditions, and by mitigating inflammatory responses, saponins may contribute to overall health and longevity. Furthermore, some studies suggest that saponins may enhance collagen synthesis and promote skin health. Collagen is a crucial protein that provides structure and elasticity to the skin. As we age, collagen production tends to decline, leading to wrinkles and sagging skin. Saponins may help address this by supporting collagen synthesis, thereby contributing to antiaging effects on the skin. While research on the antiaging potential of saponins is ongoing, the existing evidence highlights their multifaceted mechanisms of action. Incorporating saponin-rich foods or supplements into a balanced diet may offer a natural approach to supporting healthy aging. However, it is important to note that more comprehensive studies are needed to establish specific recommendations for saponin intake and understand their antiaging benefits (Rai et al., 2021).

9.4.2.2 *Curcumin*

Curcumin, the active compound found in turmeric, has gained attention for its potential antiaging properties. Turmeric, a yellow spice commonly used in traditional medicine, has been associated with various health benefits, and curcumin is considered its primary bioactive component. The antiaging effects of curcumin are attributed to its diverse biological activities, including antioxidant, antiinflammatory, and anticarcinogenic properties (Sharifi-Rad et al., 2020). One of the key mechanisms through which curcumin may exert its antiaging effects is by combating oxidative stress. Oxidative stress, resulting from an imbalance between free radicals and antioxidants, contributes to cellular damage and aging. Curcumin acts as a potent antioxidant, scavenging free radicals and reducing oxidative damage, which helps preserve cellular integrity (Wolf et al., 2022). Additionally, curcumin has been shown to have antiinflammatory effects. Chronic inflammation is implicated in various age-related diseases, and by modulating inflammatory pathways, curcumin may contribute to overall health and longevity. Moreover, curcumin has been studied for its potential in promoting cognitive health and neuroprotection. It may enhance brain function by crossing the blood-brain barrier and exerting antiinflammatory and antioxidant effects in the central nervous system. Cognitive decline is a common aspect of aging, and curcumin's neuroprotective properties are of interest in the context of antiaging interventions (Shen et al., 2023). While research on curcumin as an antiaging compound is promising, it is important to note that its bioavailability is a challenge, and efforts to enhance its absorption are ongoing. Incorporating turmeric into the diet or considering curcumin supplements may offer potential antiaging benefits, but more rigorous clinical studies are needed to establish specific recommendations and better understand the full range of its effects on aging and age-related conditions.

9.4.2.3 *Stilbenes*

Stilbenes, a group of natural compounds characterized by a common stilbene backbone structure, have gained attention for their potential antiaging properties. One of the most well-known stilbenes is resveratrol, which is found in certain fruits (such as grapes), red wine, and peanuts. Stilbenes exhibit various biological activities, including antioxidant, antiinflammatory, and anticarcinogenic effects, contributing to their potential as antiaging compounds. One of the primary mechanisms through which stilbenes, particularly resveratrol, may exert antiaging effects is by activating sirtuins (Benabbes et al., 2023). Sirtuins are a class of proteins involved in cellular regulation, metabolism, and stress response. Resveratrol has been shown to activate sirtuins, particularly SIRT1, which plays a crucial role in cellular homeostasis, DNA repair, and longevity. Activation of sirtuins by stilbenes may enhance cellular resilience and promote healthy aging. Stilbenes also demonstrate antioxidant properties, helping to neutralize free radicals and reduce oxidative stress. Oxidative stress is a major contributor to cellular damage and aging, and the antioxidant effects of stilbenes may help protect cells from this damage. Furthermore, stilbenes, including resveratrol, have been studied for their potential to promote cardiovascular health. They may have protective effects on the cardiovascular system by improving blood vessel function, reducing inflammation, and lowering oxidative stress. Cardiovascular health is closely linked to the aging process, and interventions that support heart health may contribute to overall longevity (Koo et al., 2022). While stilbenes show promise as antiaging compounds, it is essential to note that the research is ongoing, and the optimal dosage and long-term effects are still areas of investigation. Including stilbene-rich foods, such as grapes and red wine, in the diet or considering stilbene supplements may offer potential benefits, but more comprehensive clinical studies are needed to establish specific recommendations for antiaging interventions.

9.4.2.4 *Anthocyanins*

Anthocyanins, a group of naturally occurring pigments responsible for the red, purple, and blue colors in many fruits and vegetables, have been studied for their potential antiaging properties. These compounds are abundant in berries (such as blueberries, strawberries, and blackberries), cherries, red grapes, and other colorful fruits (Wang et al., 2022). Anthocyanins possess a range of bioactive properties that contribute to their potential benefits in counteracting the aging process. One significant mechanism through which anthocyanins may exert antiaging effects is their antioxidant activity. Anthocyanins act as free radical scavengers, neutralizing reactive oxygen species (ROS) and reducing oxidative stress. Oxidative stress is a key factor in cellular damage and the aging process, and by mitigating this stress, anthocyanins contribute to cellular protection and longevity. Anthocyanins also display antiinflammatory properties. Chronic inflammation is linked to various age-related diseases, and the antiinflammatory effects of anthocyanins may help mitigate inflammation, supporting overall health and potentially slowing down the aging process. Moreover, anthocyanins have been investigated for their potential role in promoting cardiovascular health. They may enhance blood vessel function, reduce blood pressure, and have positive effects on lipid metabolism (Mostafa et al., 2023). Cardiovascular health is crucial for longevity, and interventions that support heart health can contribute to overall antiaging benefits. Studies have suggested that anthocyanins may also have positive effects on cognitive function. These compounds may protect against age-related cognitive decline by influencing neuronal signaling, reducing oxidative stress in the brain, and promoting neuroplasticity. While the research on anthocyanins and antiaging is promising, it is important to note that more comprehensive clinical studies are needed to establish specific recommendations regarding dosage and long-term effects. Including a variety of anthocyanin-rich foods in the diet, such as berries and colorful fruits, may offer potential antiaging benefits as part of a holistic approach to maintaining health and longevity.

9.4.2.5 Apigenin

Apigenin, a natural flavonoid present in various fruits, vegetables, and herbs, has been investigated for its potential antiaging properties. Flavonoids are known for their antioxidant and antiinflammatory effects, and apigenin is no exception. Several studies suggest that apigenin may contribute to cellular protection and longevity through various mechanisms. One key aspect of apigenin's potential antiaging effects is its antioxidant activity. By scavenging free radicals and reducing oxidative stress, apigenin helps protect cells from damage (Yoon et al., 2023). Oxidative stress is a major contributor to the aging process, and antioxidants play a crucial role in maintaining cellular health. Apigenin also exhibits antiinflammatory properties, which can be beneficial in combating chronic inflammation associated with aging. Chronic inflammation is linked to various age-related diseases, and by modulating inflammatory pathways, apigenin may contribute to overall health and potentially slow down the aging process. Moreover, apigenin has been studied for its potential impact on cellular senescence, a process in which cells lose their ability to divide and function properly. Some research suggests that apigenin may influence pathways related to cellular senescence and promote a more youthful cellular environment. Additionally, apigenin has been investigated for its effects on skin health. It may have benefits for skin aging by promoting collagen synthesis, inhibiting enzymes that degrade collagen, and protecting against UV-induced damage (Woo et al., 2020). While the research on apigenin and antiaging is promising, it is important to note that more comprehensive clinical studies are needed to establish specific recommendations regarding dosage and long-term effects. Including apigenin-rich foods in the diet, such as parsley, celery, and chamomile tea, may offer potential antiaging benefits as part of a well-rounded approach to maintaining health and longevity. As always, it is advisable to consult with a healthcare professional before incorporating new supplements or making significant changes to one's diet.

9.5 Challenges and opportunities in functional foods for aging

The variability in individual responses to functional foods due to genetic and environmental factors poses another challenge. Personalized nutrition, tailoring dietary recommendations based on an individual's unique genetic makeup and health status, may offer a solution to enhance the effectiveness of functional foods in promoting healthy aging. Furthermore, the integration of functional foods into dietary patterns and cultural preferences is essential for long-term adherence. Developing innovative food products that are both nutritious and palatable, along with effective public health campaigns, can encourage widespread adoption of functional foods as a part of a healthy aging strategy.

- **Need for robust scientific evidence:**
  Due to a lack of sufficient scientific evidence for the efficacy of functional foods in promoting healthy aging. However, this can be solved by conducting well-designed clinical trials to establish the effectiveness of specific functional foods in mitigating the effects of aging.
- **Bioavailability and optimal dosage:**
  There is uncertainty regarding the bioavailability and optimal dosage of bioactive compounds in functional foods, which can be further investigated to ensure the bioavailability and optimal dosage of bioactive compounds in real-world scenarios.
- **Variability in individual responses:**
  Due to varied individual responses to functional foods influenced by genetic and environmental factors, we need to implement personalized nutrition strategies, tailoring dietary recommendations based on an individual's unique genetic makeup and health status.
- **Integration into dietary patterns:**
  It is very difficult to integrate functional foods into diverse dietary patterns and cultural preferences; however, the solution could be to emphasize the development of innovative, nutritious, and palatable food products that align with cultural preferences for long-term adherence.

- **Effective public health campaigns:**

There is limited awareness and adoption of functional foods in the broader population, which can be solved by implementing effective public health campaigns to educate and encourage the widespread adoption of functional foods as a crucial component of a healthy aging strategy.

9.6 Conclusion

In conclusion, the intricate relationship between functional foods and aging presents a compelling avenue for research and intervention in the pursuit of longevity and well-being. The aging process, influenced by a myriad of factors, can be modulated through dietary choices, with functional foods emerging as key players in this endeavor. Antioxidants, antiinflammatory compounds, and bioactive molecules found in these foods have demonstrated the potential to mitigate cellular damage, modulate senescence, and promote gut health. As we unravel the complex mechanisms of aging, it becomes increasingly clear that a holistic approach, encompassing both genetic and environmental factors, is necessary for effective intervention. Functional foods offer a practical and accessible means to incorporate health-promoting compounds into everyday diets, potentially influencing the trajectory of aging and contributing to a longer, healthier life. As we embark on this journey into the realm of functional foods and aging, ongoing research and collaboration between scientists, healthcare professionals, and the food industry, as well as public awareness and education, will be crucial. By combining scientific rigor with practical solutions, we can unlock the full potential of functional foods as a recipe for longevity and pave the way for a healthier, more vibrant aging population.

References

Akermi, S., Smaoui, S., Chaari, M., Elhadef, K., Gentile, R., Hait, M., Roymahapatra, G., & Mellouli, L. (2024). Combined in vitro/in silico approaches, molecular dynamics simulations and safety assessment of the multifunctional properties of thymol and carvacrol: A comparative insight. *Chemistry & Biodiversity*. Available from https://doi.org/10.1002/cbdv.202301575.

Al-Khayri, J. M., Sahana, G. R., Nagella, P., Joseph, B. V., Alessa, F. M., & Al-Mssallem, M. Q. (2022). Flavonoids as potential anti-inflammatory molecules: A review. *Molecules (Basel, Switzerland)*, *27*. Available from https://doi.org/10.3390/molecules27092901.

Amagloh, F. C., Yada, B., Tumuhimbise, G. A., Amagloh, F. K., & Kaaya, A. N. (2021). The potential of sweetpotato as a functional food in sub-saharan africa and its implications for health: A review. *Molecules (Basel, Switzerland)*, *26*. Available from https://doi.org/10.3390/molecules26102971.

Asejeje, F. O., & Ogunro, O. B. (2023). Deciphering the mechanisms, biochemistry, physiology, and social habits in the process of aging Aging process: Deciphering the mechanisms, biochemistry, physiology, and social habits. *Archives of Gerontology and Geriatrics Plus*. Available from https://doi.org/10.1016/j.aggp.2023.100003.

Benabbes, R., Ouahhoud, S., Moueqqit, M., Addi, M., Hano, C., Delporte, C., Nacoulma, A. P., & Megalizzi, V. (2023). The major stilbene compound accumulated in the roots of a resistant variety of *Phoenix dactylifera* L. activates proteasome for a path in anti-aging strategy. *Cells*, *12*. Available from https://doi.org/10.3390/cells12010071.

Chaari, M., Elhadef, K., Akermi, S., Hlima, H. B., Fourati, M., Mtibaa, A. C., Ennouri, M., DÁmore, T., Ali, D. S., Mellouli, L., Khaneghah, A. M., & Smaoui, S. (2023). Potentials of beetroot (Beta vulgaris L.) peel extract for quality enhancement of refrigerated beef meat. *Quality Assurance and Safety of Crops and Foods*, *15*, 99–115. Available from https://doi.org/10.15586/qas.v15i4.1376.

Cheng, J., Balbuena, E., Miller, B., & Eroglu, A. (2021). The role of β-carotene in colonic inflammation and intestinal barrier integrity. *Frontiers in Nutrition*, *8*. Available from https://doi.org/10.3389/fnut.2021.723480.

Corina, A., Rangel-Zúñiga, O. A., Jiménez-Lucena, R., Alcalá-Díaz, J. F., Quintana-Navarro, G., Yubero-Serrano, E. M., López-Moreno, J., Delgado-Lista, J., Tinahones, F., Ordovás, J. M., López-Miranda, J., & Pérez-Martínez, P. (2019). Low intake of vitamin E accelerates cellular aging in patients with established cardiovascular disease: The CORDIOPREV study. *The Journals of Gerontology: Series A*, *74*, 770–777. Available from https://doi.org/10.1093/gerona/gly195.

Corina Baba, A. (2020). The relationship between nutrients and biological aging. *Relación entre los nutrientes y el grado de envejecimiento biológico*.

Diwan, B., & Sharma, R. (2022). Nutritional components as mitigators of cellular senescence in organismal aging: a comprehensive review. *Food Science and Biotechnology*, *31*, 1089–1109. Available from https://doi.org/10.1007/s10068-022-01114-y.

Elhadef, K., Chaari, M., Akermi, S., Ennouri, K., Ben Hlima, H., Fourati, M., Chakchouk Mtibaa, A., Ennouri, M., Sarkar, T., Shariati, M. A., Gökşen, G., Pateiro, M., Mellouli, L., Lorenzo, J. M., & Smaoui, S. (2024). Gelatin-sodium alginate packaging film with date pits extract: An eco-friendly packaging for extending raw minced beef shelf life. *Meat Science*, *207*. Available from https://doi.org/10.1016/j.meatsci.2023.109371.

Fahmy, H., Hegazi, N., El-Shamy, S., & Farag, M. A. (2020). Pomegranate juice as a functional food: A comprehensive review of its polyphenols, therapeutic merits, and recent patents. *Food and Function*, *11*, 5768–5781. Available from https://doi.org/10.1039/d0fo01251c.

Fraile, M., Eiro, N., Costa, L. A., Martín, A., & Vizoso, F. J. (2022). Aging and mesenchymal stem cells: Basic concepts, challenges and strategies. *Biology*, *11*. Available from https://doi.org/10.3390/biology11111678.

Green, C. L., Lamming, D. W., & Fontana, L. (2022). Molecular mechanisms of dietary restriction promoting health and longevity. *Nature Reviews. Molecular Cell Biology*, *23*, 56–73. Available from https://doi.org/10.1038/s41580-021-00411-4.

Guo, J., Huang, X., Dou, L., Yan, M., Shen, T., Tang, W., & Li, J. (2022). Aging and aging-related diseases: from molecular mechanisms to interventions and treatments. *Signal Transduction and Targeted Therapy*, *7*. Available from https://doi.org/10.1038/s41392-022-01251-0.

Hajam, Y. A., Rani, R., Ganie, S. Y., Sheikh, T. A., Javaid, D., Qadri, S. S., Pramodh, S., Alsulimani, A., Alkhanani, M. F., Harakeh, S., Hussain, A., Haque, S., & Reshi, M. S. (2022). Oxidative stress in human pathology and aging: Molecular mechanisms and perspectives. *Cells*, *11*. Available from https://doi.org/10.3390/cells11030552.

Huang, Q., Wang, X., Bu, X., Song, Y., You, J., Zhang, C., Qin, C., Qin, J., & Chen, L. (2022). Dietary vitamin A affects growth performance, immunity, antioxidant capacity, and lipid metabolism of juvenile Chinese mitten crab Eriocheir sinensis. *Aquaculture (Amsterdam, Netherlands)*, *548*. Available from https://doi.org/10.1016/j.aquaculture.2021.737556.

Jeenduang, N., Plyduang, T., & Horpet, D. (2020). Association of 25-hydroxyvitamin D levels and metabolic syndrome in Thai postmenopausal women. *Diabetes & Metabolic Syndrome: Clinical Research & Reviews*, *14*, 1585–1590. Available from https://doi.org/10.1016/j.dsx.2020.08.018.

Kim, J., Oh, J., Averilla, J. N., Kim, H. J., Kim, J. S., & Kim, J. S. (2019). Grape peel extract and resveratrol inhibit wrinkle formation in mice model through activation of Nrf2/HO-1 signaling pathway. *Journal of Food Science*, *84*, 1600–1608. Available from https://doi.org/10.1111/1750-3841.14643.

Koo, H. B., Hwang, H. S., Han, J. Y., Cheong, E. J., Kwon, Y. S., & Choi, Y. E. (2022). Enhanced production of pinosylvin stilbene with aging of Pinus strobus callus and nematicidal activity of callus extracts against pinewood nematodes. *Scientific Reports*, *12*. Available from https://doi.org/10.1038/s41598-022-04843-6.

Kornerup, L. S., Hvas, C. L., Abild, C. B., Richelsen, B., & Nexo, E. (2019). Early changes in vitamin B12 uptake and biomarker status following Roux-en-Y gastric bypass and sleeve gastrectomy. *Clinical Nutrition*, *38*, 906–911. Available from https://doi.org/10.1016/j.clnu.2018.02.007.

Kowalska, M., Piekut, T., Prendecki, M., Sodel, A., Kozubski, W., & Dorszewska, J. (2020). Mitochondrial and nuclear DNA oxidative damage in physiological and pathological aging. *DNA and Cell Biology*, *39*, 1410–1420. Available from https://doi.org/10.1089/dna.2019.5347.

Liu, H. M., Cheng, M. Y., Xun, M. H., Zhao, Z. W., Zhang, Y., Tang, W., Cheng, J., Ni, J., & Wang, W. (2023). Possible mechanisms of oxidative stress-induced skin cellular senescence, inflammation, and cancer and the therapeutic potential of plant polyphenols. *International Journal of Molecular Sciences*, *24*. Available from https://doi.org/10.3390/ijms24043755.

Liu, S., Sharp, A., Villanueva, E., & Ma, Z. F. (2022). Breast milk iodine concentration (BMIC) as a biomarker of iodine status in lactating women and children <2 years of age: A systematic review. *Nutrients.*, *14*. Available from https://doi.org/10.3390/nu14091691.

Di Lorenzo, C., Colombo, F., Biella, S., Stockley, C., & Restani, P. (2021). Polyphenols and human health: The role of bioavailability. *Nutrients*, *13*. Available from https://doi.org/10.3390/nu13010273.

Luo, J., Mills, K., le Cessie, S., Noordam, R., & van Heemst, D. (2020). Ageing, age-related diseases and oxidative stress: What to do next? *Ageing Research Reviews*, *57*. Available from https://doi.org/10.1016/j.arr.2019.100982.

López-Otín, C., Blasco, M. A., Partridge, L., Serrano, M., & Kroemer, G. (2023). Hallmarks of aging: An expanding universe. *Cell*, *186*, 243–278. Available from https://doi.org/10.1016/j.cell.2022.11.001.

Martirosyan, D., Lampert, T., & Lee, M. (2022). A comprehensive review on the role of food bioactive compounds in functional food science. *Functional Food Science*, *2*, 64. Available from https://doi.org/10.31989/ffs.v2i3.906.

Masini, G., Graham, F. J., Pellicori, P., Cleland, J. G. F., Cuthbert, J. J., Kazmi, S., Inciardi, R. M., & Clark, A. L. (2022). Criteria for iron deficiency in patients with heart failure. *Journal of the American College of Cardiology*, *79*, 341–351. Available from https://doi.org/10.1016/j.jacc.2021.11.039.

Meccariello, R., & D'Angelo, S. (2021). Impact of polyphenolic-food on longevity: An elixir of life. An overview. *Antioxidants*, *10*. Available from https://doi.org/10.3390/antiox10040507.

Michalak, M. (2022). Plant-derived antioxidants: Significance in skin health and the ageing process. *International Journal of Molecular Sciences*, *23*. Available from https://doi.org/10.3390/ijms23020585.

Michalak, M., Pierzak, M., Kręcisz, B., & Suliga, E. (2021). Bioactive compounds for skin health: A review. *Nutrients*, *13*. Available from https://doi.org/10.3390/nu13010203.

Miyazawa, T., Abe, C., Burdeos, G. C., Matsumoto, A., & Toda, M. (2022). Food antioxidants and aging: Theory, current evidence and perspectives. *Nutraceuticals*, *2*, 181–204. Available from https://doi.org/10.3390/nutraceuticals2030014.

Mora, I., Arola, L., Caimari, A., Escoté, X., & Puiggròs, F. (2022). Structured long-chain omega-3 fatty acids for improvement of cognitive function during aging. *International Journal of Molecular Sciences*, *23*. Available from https://doi.org/10.3390/ijms23073472.

Mostafa, H., Meroño, T., Miñarro, A., Sánchez-Pla, A., Lanuza, F., Zamora-Ros, R., Rostgaard-Hansen, A. L., Estanyol-Torres, N., Cubedo-Culleré, M., Tjønneland, A., Landberg, R., Halkjær, J., & Andres-Lacueva, C. (2023). Dietary sources of anthocyanins and their association with metabolome biomarkers and cardiometabolic risk factors in an observational study. *Nutrients*, *15*. Available from https://doi.org/10.3390/nu15051208.

Murphy, N., Achaintre, D., Zamora-Ros, R., Jenab, M., Boutron-Ruault, M. C., Carbonnel, F., Savoye, I., Kaaks, R., Kühn, T., Boeing, H., Aleksandrova, K., Tjønneland, A., Kyrø, C., Overvad, K., Quirós, J. R., Sánchez, M. J., Altzibar, J. M., María Huerta, J., Barricarte, A., ... Scalbert, A. (2018). A prospective evaluation of plasma polyphenol levels and colon cancer risk. *International Journal of Cancer*, *143*, 1620–1631. Available from https://doi.org/10.1002/ijc.31563.

Neven, K. Y., Cox, B., Cosemans, C., Gyselaers, W., Penders, J., Plusquin, M., Roels, H. A., Vrijens, K., Ruttens, A., & Nawrot, T. S. (2021). Lower iodine storage in the placenta is associated with gestational diabetes mellitus. *BMC Medicine*, *19*. Available from https://doi.org/10.1186/s12916-021-01919-4.

Page, M. J., McKenzie, J. E., Bossuyt, P. M., Boutron, I., Hoffmann, T. C., Mulrow, C. D., Shamseer, L., Tetzlaff, J. M., Akl, E. A., Brennan, S. E., Chou, R., Glanville, J., Grimshaw, J. M., Hróbjartsson, A., Lalu, M. M., Li, T., Loder, E. W., Mayo-Wilson, E., McDonald, S., ... Moher, D.

(2021). The PRISMA 2020 statement: An updated guideline for reporting systematic reviews. *International Journal of Surgery*, *88*. Available from https://doi.org/10.1016/j.ijsu.2021.105906.

Pagiatakis, C., Musolino, E., Gornati, R., Bernardini, G., & Papait, R. (2021). Epigenetics of aging and disease: a brief overview. *Aging Clinical and Experimental Research*, *33*, 737–745. Available from https://doi.org/10.1007/s40520-019-01430-0.

Pham, J. V., Yilma, M. A., Feliz, A., Majid, M. T., Maffetone, N., Walker, J. R., Kim, E., Cho, H. J., Reynolds, J. M., Song, M. C., Park, S. R., & Yoon, Y. J. (2019). A review of the microbial production of bioactive natural products and biologics. *Frontiers in Microbiology*, *10*. Available from https://doi.org/10.3389/fmicb.2019.01404.

Pyo, I. S., Yun, S., Yoon, Y. E., Choi, J. W., & Lee, S. J. (2020). Mechanisms of aging and the preventive effects of resveratrol on age-related diseases. *Molecules (Basel, Switzerland)*, *25*. Available from https://doi.org/10.3390/molecules25204649.

Rai, S., Acharya-Siwakoti, E., Kafle, A., Devkota, H. P., & Bhattarai, A. (2021). Plant-derived saponins: A review of their surfactant properties and applications. *Sci*, *3*. Available from https://doi.org/10.3390/sci3040044.

Rotstein, A., Kodesh, A., Goldberg, Y., Reichenberg, A., & Levine, S. Z. (2022). Serum folate deficiency and the risks of dementia and all-cause mortality: A national study of old age. *Evidence Based Mental Health*, *25*, 63–68. Available from https://doi.org/10.1136/ebmental-2021-300309.

Rudrapal, M., Khairnar, S. J., Khan, J., Dukhyil, A. B., Ansari, M. A., Alomary, M. N., Alshabrmi, F. M., Palai, S., Deb, P. K., & Devi, R. (2022). Dietary polyphenols and their role in oxidative stress-induced human diseases: Insights into protective effects, antioxidant potentials and mechanism(s) of action. *Frontiers in Pharmacology*, *13*. Available from https://doi.org/10.3389/fphar.2022.806470.

Sharifi-Rad, J., Rayess, Y. E., Rizk, A. A., Sadaka, C., Zgheib, R., Zam, W., Sestito, S., Rapposelli, S., Neffe-Skocińska, K., Zielińska, D., Salehi, B., Setzer, W. N., Dosoky, N. S., Taheri, Y., El Beyrouthy, M., Martorell, M., Ostrander, E. A., Suleria, H. A. R., Cho, W. C., . . . Martins, N. (2020). Turmeric and its major compound curcumin on health: Bioactive effects and safety profiles for food, pharmaceutical, biotechnological and medicinal applications. *Frontiers in Pharmacology*, *11*. Available from https://doi.org/10.3389/fphar.2020.01021.

Shen, R., Yang, X., & Lin, D. (2023). PH sensitive double-layered emulsions stabilized by bacterial cellulose nanofibers/soy protein isolate/chitosan complex enhanced the bioaccessibility of curcumin: In vitro study. *Food Chemistry*, *402*134262. Available from https://doi.org/10.1016/j.foodchem.2022.134262.

Stromsnes, K., Correas, A. G., Lehmann, J., Gambini, J., & Olaso-Gonzalez, G. (2021). Anti-inflammatory properties of diet: Role in healthy aging. *Biomedicines*, *9*. Available from https://doi.org/10.3390/biomedicines9080922.

Tan, M. L., & Hamid, S. B. S. (2021). Beetroot as a potential functional food for cancer chemoprevention, a narrative review. *Journal of Cancer Prevention*, *26*, 1–17. Available from https://doi.org/10.15430/jcp.2021.26.1.1.

Temple, N. J. (2022). A rational definition for functional foods: A perspective. *Frontiers in Nutrition*, *9*. Available from https://doi.org/10.3389/fnut.2022.957516.

Timilsena, Y. P., Phosanam, A., & Stockmann, R. (2023). Perspectives on saponins: Food functionality and applications. *International Journal of Molecular Sciences*, *24*, 13538. Available from https://doi.org/10.3390/ijms241713538.

Toomer, O. T. (2020). A comprehensive review of the value-added uses of peanut (Arachis hypogaea) skins and by-products. *Critical Reviews in Food Science and Nutrition*, *60*, 341–350. Available from https://doi.org/10.1080/10408398.2018.1538101.

Varma, S. R., Sivaprakasam, T. O., Arumugam, I., Dilip, N., Raghuraman, M., Pavan, K. B., Rafiq, M., & Paramesh, R. (2019). In vitro anti-inflammatory and skin protective properties of Virgin coconut oil. *Journal of Traditional and Complementary Medicine*, *9*, 5–14. Available from https://doi.org/10.1016/j.jtcme.2017.06.012.

Villamil-Galindo, E., Van de Velde, F., & Piagentini, A. M. (2021). Strawberry agro-industrial by-products as a source of bioactive compounds: Effect of cultivar on the phenolic profile and the antioxidant capacity. *Bioresour Bioprocess*, *8*, 61. Available from https://doi.org/10.1186/s40643-021-00416-z.

Vogel-González, M., Talló-Parra, M., Herrera-Fernández, V., Pérez-Vilaró, G., Chillón, M., Nogués, X., Gómez-Zorrilla, S., López-Montesinos, I., Arnau-Barrés, I., Sorli-Redó, M. L., Horcajada, J. P., García-Giralt, N., Pascual, J., Díez, J., Vicente, R., & Güerri-Fernández, R. (2021). Low zinc levels at admission associates with poor clinical outcomes in SARS-CoV-2 infection. *Nutrients*, *13*. Available from https://doi.org/10.3390/nu13020562.

Wang, B., Tang, X., Mao, B., Zhang, Q., Tian, F., Zhao, J., Cui, S., & Chen, W. (2022). Anti-aging effects and mechanisms of anthocyanins and their intestinal microflora metabolites. *Critical Reviews in Food Science and Nutrition*, 1–17. Available from https://doi.org/10.1080/10408398.2022.2123444.

Wolf, C. P. J. G., Rachow, T., Ernst, T., Hochhaus, A., Zomorodbakhsch, B., Foller, S., Rengsberger, M., Hartmann, M., & Hübner, J. (2022). Interactions in cancer treatment considering cancer therapy, concomitant medications, food, herbal medicine and other supplements. *Journal of Cancer Research and Clinical Oncology*, *148*, 461–473. Available from https://doi.org/10.1007/s00432-021-03625-3.

Woo, J. S., Choo, G. S., Yoo, E. S., Kim, S. H., Lee, J. H., Han, S. H., Kim, H. J., Jung, S. H., Park, Y. S., Kim, B. S., Kim, S. K., Park, B. K., Cho, S. D., Nam, J. S., Choi, C. S., Che, J. H., & Jung, J. Y. (2020). Apigenin induces apoptosis by regulating Akt and MAPK pathways in human melanoma cell A375SM. *Molecular Medicine Reports*, *22*, 4877–4889. Available from https://doi.org/10.3892/mmr.2020.11572.

Yao, T., Chen, J. M., Shen, L. E., Yu, Y. S., Tang, Z. H., Zang, G. Q., Zhang, Y., & Chen, X. H. (2022). Astragalus polysaccharide alleviated hepatocyte senescence via autophagy pathway. *Kaohsiung Journal of Medical Sciences*, *38*, 457–468. Available from https://doi.org/10.1002/kjm2.12495.

Yoon, J. H., Kim, M.-Y., & Cho, J. Y. (2023). Apigenin: A therapeutic agent for treatment of skin inflammatory diseases and cancer. *International Journal of Molecular Sciences*, *24*, 1498. Available from https://doi.org/10.3390/ijms24021498.

Zhou, D. D., Luo, M., Huang, S. Y., Saimaiti, A., Shang, A., Gan, R. Y., & Li, H. B. (2021). Effects and es. *Oxidative Medicine and Cellular Longevity*, *2021*. Available from https://doi.org/10.1155/2021/9932218.

Chapter 10

The role of functional foods in inflammation management

Ruchira Nandasiri[1,2,3], Anuruddika Hewage[1,4], Chamali Kodikara[1,4,5] and N. A. Michael Eskin[1]

[1]*Department of Food and Human Nutritional Sciences, University of Manitoba, Winnipeg, MB, Canada,* [2]*Division of Neurodegenerative Disorders (DND), St. Boniface Hospital Albrechtsen Research Centre, Winnipeg, MB, Canada,* [3]*Canadian Centre for Agri-Food Research in Health and Medicine (CCARM), St. Boniface Hospital Albrechtsen Research Centre, Winnipeg, MB, Canada,* [4]*Richardson Centre for Food Technology and Research, Winnipeg, MB, Canada,* [5]*Agriculture Agri-Food Canada, Morden Research and Development Centre, Morden, MB, Canada*

10.1 Introduction

10.1.1 Functional foods

The term functional food was first coined in 1993 in an article in Nature News magazine titled "Japan explores the boundary between food and medicine" (Swinbanks & O'Brien, 1993). Japan was the first country to develop specific regulations for the approval of functional foods, defining them as the food products that provide additional health benefits beyond their normal nutritional contributions (Roberfroid, 2002). In addition to their nutritional benefits functional foods are excellent sources of nutraceuticals, medical foods, probiotics, and designer foods (Chhikara et al., 2021). Even though the term functional food was introduced in 1993, the application of functional ingredients began in the early 1900s. Food scientists/nutritionists recommended fortification of the salt with iodine to prevent the occurrence of goiters. However, this fortification strategy was also very effective in improving the overall health of the public at the same time. Functional foods also provide health benefits, including protecting against noncommunicable diseases such as type 2 diabetes, cardiovascular diseases, cancer, and hypertension. However, these functional foods might not provide health benefits to all the members of the population (Chhikara et al., 2021).

Over the years the market demand for functional foods has increased. According to the statistics published by Grand View Research, Inc., the global market for functional foods is expected to reach over 275 billion USD by 2025, primarily in North America, Europe, and Japan, considering the type of functional foods available. European countries primarily produce dairy and cereal functional products, whereas Japan and North American countries produce more functional drinks, cereal products, and confectionery products (Vicentini et al., 2016). The increasing demand for the functional foods is associated with many other factors, including age, gender, income level, education, and availability of the products. Improving customer awareness could create more opportunities and further growth of functional foods.

Over the years functional foods have been defined in many different ways. Yet, a more concise definition was provided by the Functional Food Centre (FFC) defining them as "natural or processed foods that contain known or unknown biologically active compounds; which, in defined, effective, and nontoxic amounts, provide a clinically proven and documented health benefit for the prevention, management, or treatment of chronic disease" (Martirosyan & Singh, 2015). Functional foods can be classified as first-generation (supplements), second-generation (whole), and third-generation (novel) foods. Also, these could be categorized as conventional foods, modified foods, and functional food ingredients (Chhikara et al., 2021). In general, most of the food items we consume every day include fruits, vegetables, cereals, legumes, oilseeds, herbs, and spices all contain bioactive compounds and may be defined as functional foods (Wani et al., 2022). In addition, fortified foods, including cereals (with vitamin B complex), enriched milk (with vitamin D), or enhanced foods, including eggs (with DHA), and probiotics (dairy products), can all be considered functional foods (Ellis, 2022).

Unleashing the Power of Functional Foods and Novel Bioactives. DOI: https://doi.org/10.1016/B978-0-443-28862-3.00010-8

10.1.2 Inflammation

Inflammation is part of the complex biological response by the vascular tissues to harmful stimuli, such as damaged cells, pathogens, or irritants. Inflammation is a protective mechanism by the organism to remove injurious stimuli and initiate a healing process (Stankov, 2012). In an acute inflammatory process, there are various ways that the physical signs and symptoms of inflammation can be observed and felt (Szade et al., 2015). The following sequence of events that occurs in a specific type of tissue is designed to get rid of a pathogen (an agent causing disease) or repair some form of trauma, usually in a characteristic pattern. Essentially, an inflammatory response is a defense mechanism that protects an organism from infection and helps to heal any damage caused by the infection and other forms of irritation (Stankov, 2012). Two types of inflammation can be distinguished, acute and chronic, with each having its own characteristic pattern of response (Blázquez-Prieto et al., 2018). These symptoms and the severity of the inflammatory response depend upon the cause of the inflammation, the affected tissue, and the degree of damage. An acute inflammation is the body's immediate response to injury to defend itself against an invading bacteria, virus, or fungi and to get rid of the cause of the injury and the necrotic cells and tissues damaged from the original insult (Nailwal & Chan, 2019). Necrosis is the premature death of cells in living tissue usually caused by factors such as trauma, infection, toxins, and, most importantly, inflammation.

The cardinal signs of acute inflammation are redness, heat, pain, and swelling. An alteration to the tissue function can also be considered a fifth sign as loss of function can be from severe pain or destruction of the tissue so that it cannot perform its function (Immler et al., 2018). It is now generally accepted that there is a sixth sign of acute inflammation which is an alteration of the leukocyte blood count. During acute inflammation, various proinflammatory mediators are released in response to the injurious stimuli. These mediators can have different effects. Some dilate the blood vessels, increasing blood flow to the affected area (this is responsible for the redness and heat felt in the inflamed site and its neighboring areas). Others facilitate the movement of leukocytes to the site of injury and activation at the affected area. The mediators and leukocytes brought to the site can remove the cause of the inflammation and necrotic cells and tissues (Schebb et al., 2022). This is done via phagocytosis which involves engulfing and destroying cells and particles. Once this is done, the acute inflammatory process will terminate with the mediators being broken down and the leukocytes dying off and being removed from the site by the lymphatics (Blázquez-Prieto et al., 2018). Finally, the affected tissue can be repaired if the inflammation and the damage are mild so that the affected tissue can return to its normal structure and function. Alternatively, if the causative agent is removed quickly and there is little or no tissue damage, the normal structure and function can also be restored. However, if the damage is beyond repair, the tissue will be replaced with scar tissue.

This histopathology of acute inflammation can last from a few minutes to several days, is characterized by exudation of fluid and plasma proteins (edema), emigration of leukocytes particularly neutrophils, and is marked by a rapid resolution of signs and a restoration of normal structure and function (Feng et al., 2024). Chronic inflammation is a prolonged, smoldering form of the acute process that can last for several weeks to even years. In cases where an injurious agent persists or repeat episodes of acute inflammation and chronic inflammation can develop without becoming acute (Blázquez-Prieto et al., 2018). An immediate tell-tale sign of chronic inflammation within a couple of days is the infiltration of mononuclear cells, macrophages, and lymphocytes. Chronic inflammation is a complex immune response in emerging host cells and modified tissue of persistent injurious stimuli (Nazmi et al., 2019). It can be divided into chronic active and chronic persistent inflammation determined by the type of immune response and injurious agent.

Inflammation can be classified as a complex biological response of body tissues in response to harmful stimuli, such as pathogens, damaged cells, or irritants. It is actually a protective mechanism by the organism to remove the injurious stimuli and initiate the healing process. Inflammation can be acute or chronic. Acute inflammation is usually rapid onset and of short duration, usually lasting from a few minutes to several days. It is characterized by five cardinal signs: an acute inflammatory process.

10.2 Importance of recognizing signs and symptoms

An acute-phase response is a systemic response to inflammation, infection, trauma, or other tissue damage and is marked by specific changes in the plasma concentration of acute-phase proteins (positive or negative) and is usually accompanied by alterations in circulating cells (leukocytes) and platelets (Viola et al., 2019). It is now recognized that this response is largely regulated at the level of gene transcription by nuclear factor κB and other related transcription factors that are activated by receptor-mediated cell signaling, cytokines, and other proinflammatory stimuli (Pendurthi et al., 1997). This opened the way to new approaches for stratifying patient status and predicting prognosis from molecular profiles of gene expression in the context of different disease processes.

Recognition of signs and symptoms of inflammation required an active catalyst by the introduction of quantitative measurements of plasma proteins as indicators of increased vascular permeability at about the time when the first Hageman factor-dependent protease was discovered and named coagulation factor XII (Pendurthi et al., 1997). The recognition that biological processes, including inflammation and host defense, are regulated by proteolytic cascades and that activated cell-derived proteases have a direct role in proinflammatory and antimicrobial pathways has stimulated interest in understanding the balance between activation and control of these complex cascade systems.

10.2.1 Types of inflammation

Chronic inflammation is a prolonged and dysregulated process occurring in the tissue that can last for several months or years (Moyse et al., 2022). It often involves simultaneous active inflammation, ongoing tissue destruction, and attempts at repair. The predominant cells involved in chronic inflammation are the monocytes/macrophages and lymphocytes, whereas the predominant cells in acute inflammation are the neutrophils. There are many causes of chronic inflammation, but the most common is persistent injury or irritation to tissue, such as in the case of autoimmune reactions against self-antigens in conditions such as rheumatoid arthritis, systemic sclerosis, systemic lupus, and immune reactions against persistent foreign antigens, resulting in the against of chronic inflammation and granuloma formation as seen in some fungal and mycobacterial infections (Zatterale et al., 2020). Other causes of chronic inflammation include chronic ischemia and tissue necrosis, and also some acute conditions if the causative agent is not fully removed. An example of this is acute appendicitis, which can develop into a chronic state if the inflamed appendix is not removed.

10.2.2 Causes of inflammation

The two main types of inflammation described in the medical literature are acute and chronic (Blázquez-Prieto et al., 2018). Both involve a complex series of events in the body that are mediated by a variety of chemical substances produced by cells as a result of injury or infection. Acute inflammation usually involves a short-lived process that promotes healing and recovery. Under acute inflammation, the blood vessels at the site of injury constrict and then dilate (vasodilation), which results in an increased blood flow to the area. This causes the redness and heat typical of inflammation and is the process that can lead to swelling from the buildup of fluid in the damaged tissue. The increased flow of blood to the area also results in the movement of plasma and leukocytes (white blood cells) out of the blood and into the damaged tissue, where they initiate the removal of any foreign agents or damaged cells by phagocytosis. Following this, the plasma and cells are removed by the lymphatic system. This causes the swelling to decrease and is an indication that the inflammatory process is coming to an end, as the damaged tissue returning to normal or, in the case of more severe damage, tissue regeneration or reparative processes occurs with the formation of scar tissue (Feng et al., 2024).

There are many causes of inflammation, and the anatomic structure of the inflamed tissue can differ greatly by various types of reactions (Boehncke, 2018). The causes of inflammation can be classified as either extrinsic or intrinsic. Extrinsic causes include those causing inflammation by physical agents or those causing inflammation by living agents. Inflammation from physical agents can be caused by trauma, frostbite, burns, X-rays, and various forms of environmental pollution (Stankov, 2012). The most significant inflammatory problems today are caused by living agents, resulting in infections. The most important problem is the identification of the specific factor or factors responsible for the virulence of various bacteria and viruses, with future studies of microbial genetics likely to provide the best answers (Ernandes & Kagan, 2021). The virulence of such living agents is further related to the production of chronic inflammation and granuloma, which is an area that is neither well understood nor well defined. Bacteria utilize various agents such as toxins and enzymes, and it is clear that the host's response to bacteria plays a large part in determining its efficacy, with the specific mechanisms involved often being more confusing than those involved in any other type of inflammation. Charring, which is the coagulation of tissue protein by strong dry heat, is an outstanding example of localized thermal injury, but the mechanism in which less severe heat or cold causes inflammation is not clearly understood (Antunes & Kassiotis, 2010). Lastly, there are different reactions to foreign bodies that are usually involved in very chronic forms of inflammation. This occurs when the foreign body retards the activity of macrophages, so that granuloma is induced to quarantine the foreign material. This explains why inflammation often cannot be resolved when the agent causing it is no longer present.

10.2.3 Mechanisms of inflammation

Inflammation from cellular and molecular stimuli sets into motion detectable harmful stimuli. The process leads to the recognition of pathogens, damaged cells, or irritants by pattern recognition receptors (PRRs) expressed on immune cells (Hall & Agrawal, 2016). This recognition triggers a complex cascade of events, culminating in the activation of transcription factors such as nuclear factor-kappa B (NF-κB) and the subsequent expression of proinflammatory genes. The release of cytokines, chemokines, and inflammatory mediators orchestrates the recruitment and activation of immune cells to the site of injury or infection, amplifying the inflammatory response and facilitating tissue repair (Pendurthi et al., 1997).

The initiation of inflammation results in the recognition of harmful stimuli by pattern recognition receptors (PRRs), which are expressed in various immune cells, including macrophages, dendritic cells, and epithelial cells (Pendurthi et al., 1997). PRRs encompass a diverse array of receptors such as Toll-like receptors (TLRs), NOD-like receptors (NLRs), and RIG-I-like receptors (RLRs), each specialized in detecting specific molecular patterns associated with pathogens (pathogen-associated molecular patterns, PAMPs) or cellular damage (damage-associated molecular patterns, DAMPs). Upon binding to their cognate ligands, PRRs trigger downstream signaling cascades, initiating the inflammatory response (Hall & Agrawal, 2016).

PRRs consist of a diverse array of receptors, each containing unique recognition capabilities tailored to detect specific molecular patterns characteristic of infectious agents or tissue injury. Among the prominent classes of PRRs are TLRs, NLRs, and RLRs, each specialized in recognizing distinct classes of molecular patterns. TLRs, localized on the cell surface or within endosomal compartments, excel in sensing PAMPs, including bacterial lipopolysaccharides, viral nucleic acids, and fungal cell wall components (Hall & Agrawal, 2016).

Upon encountering their cognate ligands, PRRs undergo conformational changes, triggering downstream signaling cascades that culminate in the activation of transcription factors and induction of inflammatory gene expression. PAMP recognition by TLRs typically elicits MyD88-dependent or TRIF-dependent signaling pathways, leading to the activation of NF-κB and interferon regulatory factors (IRFs), which drive the expression of proinflammatory cytokines, type I interferons, and antimicrobial effectors (Hall & Agrawal, 2016; Hung & Suzuki, 2017) Similarly, the engagement of NLRs or RLRs by DAMPs triggers the assembly of multiprotein complexes known as inflammasomes or MAVS signaling platforms, respectively, initiating caspase activation and cytokine maturation, thereby amplifying the inflammatory response (Hall & Agrawal, 2016).

Proinflammatory cytokines, such as tumor necrosis factor-alpha (TNF-α) and interleukin-1 beta (IL-1β), are rapidly synthesized and released, promoting vasodilation, increased vascular permeability, and recruitment of immune cells to the site of infection or injury (Babaeijandaghi et al., 2022). Furthermore, the activation of PRR signaling pathways primes immune cells for enhanced antimicrobial activity and antigen presentation, facilitating pathogen clearance and initiation of adaptive immune responses (Park et al., 2017).

10.2.4 Activation of transcription factors

Activation of PRRs initiates intracellular signaling cascades that converge on key transcription factors, most significantly the NF-κB and activator protein-1 (AP-1). NF-κB serves as a master regulator of inflammation, controlling the expression of a wide array of proinflammatory genes involved in cytokine production, cell adhesion molecules, and antimicrobial peptides (Pendurthi et al., 1997). Its activation involves the degradation of inhibitory proteins (IκBs), liberating NF-κB to translocate into the nucleus and induce gene transcription. Similarly, AP-1 activation contributes to the transcriptional regulation of inflammatory mediators, further amplifying the inflammatory response.

10.2.5 Nuclear factor-kappa B (NF-κB): master regulator of inflammation

NF-κB emerges as the first step of inflammation, exerting multifaceted control over the transcriptional factor of immune and inflammatory genes. In its inactive state, NF-κB resides in the cytoplasm bound to inhibitory proteins known as IκBs, maintaining quiescence and preventing aberrant activation. Upon stimulation by inflammatory cues, such as PAMPs or DAMPs, the canonical NF-κB pathway is triggered. This pathway involves the phosphorylation and subsequent degradation of IκBs by the IκB kinase (IKK) complex, liberating NF-κB to translocate into the nucleus. Within the nucleus, NF-κB forms transcriptional complexes with other cofactors, binding to specific DNA sequences known as κB sites and driving the expression of a diverse array of proinflammatory genes. These include cytokines (e.g., TNF-α, IL-1β, IL-6), cell adhesion molecules (e.g., ICAM-1, VCAM-1), and antimicrobial peptides (e.g., defensins), orchestrating an inflammatory milieu conducive to pathogen clearance and tissue repair (Babaeijandaghi et al., 2022; Park et al., 2017).

10.3 AP-1: amplifier of inflammatory response

In parallel to NF-κB, the activator protein-1 (AP-1) serves as another critical transcription factor implicated in the transcriptional regulation of inflammatory mediators (Jiang et al., 2023). The AP-1 complex comprises members of the Jun (c-Jun, JunB, JunD) and Fos (c-Fos, FosB, Fra-1, Fra-2) families, which dimerize and bind to specific DNA elements known as AP-1 sites within the promoters of target genes. Activation of AP-1 signaling is mediated by diverse upstream kinases and growth factor receptors, culminating in the phosphorylation and activation of AP-1 components (Fu et al., 2018). Once activated, AP-1 complexes modulate the expression of genes involved in inflammation, proliferation, and apoptosis, thereby amplifying the inflammatory response and promoting tissue remodeling. AP-1 collaborates with NF-κB to synergistically regulate the expression of overlapping sets of inflammatory genes, reinforcing the inflammatory cascade and fine-tuning the immune response (Fain, 2010).

By controlling the expression of genes encoding cytokines, chemokines, adhesion molecules, and antimicrobial effectors, NF-κB and AP-1 foster an inflammatory milieu conducive to host defense and tissue repair (Kany et al., 2019). Moreover, cross-talk between NF-κB and AP-1 pathways amplifies and diversifies the transcriptional response, ensuring robust and coordinated regulation of inflammatory gene expression (Frejo & Lopez-Escamez, 2022). Cytokines such as tumor necrosis factor-alpha (TNF-α), interleukin-1 (IL-1), and interleukin-6 (IL-6) exert pleiotropic effects on various cell types, promoting inflammation, fever, and acute-phase protein synthesis (Padoan et al., 2019). Chemokines, on the other hand, guide the migration of immune cells, facilitating their recruitment to the site of inflammation. Additionally, lipid mediators such as prostaglandins and leukotrienes contribute to the vascular changes associated with inflammation, including vasodilation and increased vascular permeability (Bartekova et al., 2018).

10.3.1 Cytokines

Cytokines are a class of small proteins secreted by immune cells, exerting pleiotropic effects on various cell types involved in inflammation and immune responses (Bartekova et al., 2018). Among the key proinflammatory cytokines are tumor necrosis factor-alpha (TNF-α), interleukin-1 (IL-1), and interleukin-6 (IL-6), which play pivotal roles in amplifying and sustaining the inflammatory cascade. TNF-α, produced primarily by activated macrophages and T cells, stimulates endothelial cells to upregulate adhesion molecules, promoting leukocyte recruitment and extravasation into inflamed tissues (Sato et al., 2018). IL-1, produced by a variety of immune cells, induces fever, enhances vascular permeability, and promotes the synthesis of acute-phase proteins, amplifying the systemic inflammatory response. IL-6, produced by immune cells and stromal cells, contributes to the acute-phase response, stimulates B cell activation and antibody production, and modulates hematopoiesis, thereby orchestrating a broad range of inflammatory and immune functions (Song et al., 2016).

10.3.2 Chemokines

Chemokines represent a family of small chemotactic cytokines that guide the migration and trafficking of immune cells within the body (Alberto et al., 2019; Ehteshamfar et al., 2020). Through interactions with specific chemokine receptors expressed on immune cells, chemokines direct the recruitment of leukocytes to sites of inflammation in a precise and coordinated manner. For instance, chemokines such as CCL2 (also known as MCP-1) and CXCL8 (also known as IL-8) promote the recruitment of monocytes and neutrophils, respectively, to inflamed tissues, facilitating their extravasation from the bloodstream and subsequent infiltration into the site of injury or infection (Tilg & Moschen, 2006). Additionally, chemokines play key roles in shaping the composition and dynamics of immune cell populations within inflamed tissues, thereby modulating the intensity and duration of the inflammatory response (Suzuki, 2019).

10.3.3 Lipid mediators

Lipid mediators, including prostaglandins and leukotrienes, represent another class of inflammatory signaling molecules derived from arachidonic acid metabolism (Fu et al., 2018). Prostaglandins, synthesized by cyclooxygenase (COX) enzymes, exert diverse effects on inflammation, vasodilation, and pain perception. Prostaglandin E2 (PGE2), for instance, promotes vasodilation and vascular permeability, facilitating the recruitment of immune cells to sites of inflammation, while prostaglandin D2 (PGD2) modulates allergic responses and inflammation in various tissues. Leukotrienes, synthesized by 5-lipoxygenase (5-LOX) enzymes, play critical roles in allergic reactions and asthma, mediating bronchoconstriction, vascular permeability, and leukocyte recruitment to inflamed airways (Bretscher et al., 2015). Additionally, lipid mediators exhibit crosstalk with cytokine signaling pathways, amplifying and modulating the inflammatory response in a context-dependent manner.

The release of inflammatory mediators initiates the recruitment and activation of immune cells, such as neutrophils, macrophages, and lymphocytes, to the site of injury or infection (Garg et al., 2017). Neutrophils are among the first responders, swiftly migrating to the site of inflammation guided by chemotactic signals. Once recruited, they phagocytose pathogens and release antimicrobial molecules to aid in pathogen clearance. Macrophages play a dual role in inflammation, serving as phagocytes and antigen-presenting cells, while also producing a plethora of inflammatory mediators. Lymphocytes, including T cells and B cells, contribute to the adaptive immune response, further amplifying and modulating the inflammatory cascade (Luo et al., 2022).

10.4 Neutrophil recruitment and function

Neutrophils, the most abundant type of white blood cells in circulation, serve as frontline defenders, rapidly recruited to the sites of inflammation in response to chemotactic signals (Garg et al., 2017). Chemokines such as CXCL8 (IL-8) guide neutrophil migration from the bloodstream to the site of injury or infection, where they extravasate through the endothelial lining of blood vessels and infiltrate the affected tissue. Once at the site of inflammation, neutrophils employ an arsenal of antimicrobial strategies, including phagocytosis, degranulation, and release of reactive oxygen species (ROS) and antimicrobial peptides (Blázquez-Prieto et al., 2018). By engulfing and destroying invading pathogens, neutrophils play a critical role in the initial stages of host defense, limiting the spread of infection and facilitating tissue sterilization.

10.4.1 Macrophage recruitment and plasticity

Macrophages, versatile immune cells derived from circulating monocytes, play a multifaceted role in inflammation, serving as phagocytes, antigen-presenting cells, and mediators of tissue repair (Pahler et al., 2008). Upon recruitment to the sites of inflammation, macrophages undergo phenotypic polarization, adopting distinct activation states dictated by the local microenvironment. Classically activated (M1) macrophages, stimulated by microbial products or proinflammatory cytokines such as interferon-gamma (IFN-γ), exhibit potent antimicrobial and proinflammatory properties, promoting pathogen clearance and orchestrating tissue remodeling (Rigamonti et al., 2014). Alternatively, activated (M2) macrophages, induced by antiinflammatory cytokines such as interleukin-4 (IL-4) and interleukin-13 (IL-13), participate in tissue repair, extracellular matrix deposition, and resolution of inflammation. Through their plasticity and functional diversity, macrophages contribute to the dynamic regulation of inflammation and tissue homeostasis (Rigamonti et al., 2014).

10.4.2 Lymphocyte involvement in adaptive immune response

Lymphocytes, including T cells and B cells, are key players in the adaptive immune response, further amplifying and modulating the inflammatory cascade initiated by innate immune cells. T cells, including CD4 + helper T cells and CD8 + cytotoxic T cells, recognize antigenic peptides presented by antigen-presenting cells such as dendritic cells and macrophages, thereby initiating specific immune responses tailored to the invading pathogen (Alberto et al., 2019). Helper T cells secrete cytokines that modulate the activity of other immune cells, augmenting inflammation and facilitating pathogen clearance. Cytotoxic T cells, on the other hand, directly target and eliminate infected or aberrant cells, contributing to host defense and immune surveillance. B cells, upon activation by antigens and helper T cells, differentiate into plasma cells, which produce antibodies capable of neutralizing pathogens and promoting their clearance by other immune cells (Abdel Hammed et al., 2022). Through their coordinated efforts, lymphocytes bolster the immune response, providing long-lasting protection against recurrent infections and fostering immune memory.

10.4.3 Facilitation of tissue repair

Besides its role in host defense, inflammation plays a crucial role in tissue repair and regeneration. Inflammatory mediators promote angiogenesis, fibroblast proliferation, and extracellular matrix deposition, facilitating the restoration of tissue integrity following injury (Gómez-Ambrosi, 2023). Moreover, macrophages transition from a proinflammatory (M1) phenotype to an antiinflammatory (M2) phenotype, promoting tissue modeling and resolution of inflammation (Fain, 2010).

Angiogenesis, the process of new blood vessel formation, represents a critical step in tissue repair, ensuring adequate oxygen and nutrient supply to regenerating tissues. Inflammatory mediators, including vascular endothelial growth factor (VEGF) and fibroblast growth factor (FGF), serve as potent inducers of angiogenesis, stimulating endothelial cell proliferation, migration, and vessel sprouting (Pendurthi et al., 1997; Szade et al., 2015). By promoting neovascularization, these inflammatory signals facilitate the delivery of oxygen and nutrients to injured tissues, accelerating the healing process and supporting tissue regeneration.

10.4.4 Stimulation of fibroblast proliferation and extracellular matrix deposition

Fibroblasts are specialized cells responsible for synthesizing extracellular matrix components such as collagen, elastin, and fibronectin, which play a central role in tissue repair and remodeling (Jasso et al., 2022). Inflammatory mediators, including transforming growth factor-beta (TGF-β) and platelet-derived growth factor (PDGF), stimulate fibroblast proliferation and activation, promoting the synthesis and deposition of extracellular matrix proteins at the site of injury. This process, known as fibroplasia, reinforces tissue structure, enhances tensile strength, and provides a scaffold for cell migration and tissue regeneration (Kang et al., 2019).

10.4.5 Transition of macrophages to an antiinflammatory phenotype

Macrophages, dynamic immune cells with plasticity, undergo phenotypic switching in response to microenvironmental cues, transitioning from a proinflammatory (M1) phenotype to an antiinflammatory (M2) phenotype during the resolution phase of inflammation. M1 macrophages, activated by proinflammatory stimuli, contribute to tissue sterilization, phagocytosis of debris, and secretion of inflammatory mediators (Viola et al., 2019). Conversely, M2 macrophages, induced by antiinflammatory cytokines such as interleukin-10 (IL-10) and interleukin-4 (IL-4), promote tissue repair, resolution of inflammation, and remodeling of extracellular matrix. M2 macrophages facilitate the clearance of apoptotic cells, secrete growth factors that stimulate tissue regeneration, and orchestrate the transition from inflammatory to reparative phase, thereby restoring tissue homeostasis and functionality (Rigamonti et al., 2014; Viola et al., 2019).

10.4.6 Implications of inflammation in health and disease

While acute inflammation serves as a vital defense mechanism against infections and injuries, chronic inflammation poses a significant risk factor for the development of various chronic diseases (Moyse et al., 2022). Previous research found that the chronic inflammation in the pathogenesis of a spectrum of disorders, including cardiovascular diseases, metabolic syndrome, autoimmune conditions, neurodegenerative disorders, and cancer. Persistent activation of inflammatory pathways induces tissue damage, promotes oxidative stress, fosters insulin resistance, and fuels genomic instability, thereby contributing to disease progression and exacerbation of symptoms (Bartekova et al., 2018).

10.4.7 Cardiovascular diseases

Chronic low-grade inflammation emerges as a key player in the pathogenesis of cardiovascular diseases, including atherosclerosis, myocardial infarction, and stroke (Boehncke, 2018). Persistent activation of inflammatory pathways within the vascular wall promotes endothelial dysfunction, leukocyte recruitment, and foam cell formation, fostering the initiation and progression of atherosclerotic plaques. Moreover, inflammatory mediators contribute to plaque destabilization, increasing the risk of rupture and subsequent thrombotic events. Additionally, systemic inflammation promotes vascular remodeling, hypertension, and myocardial fibrosis, further exacerbating cardiovascular pathology (Feijóo-Bandín et al., 2020). Chronic low-grade inflammation emerges as a pivotal contributor to the pathogenesis of cardiovascular diseases, with a series of conditions such as atherosclerosis, myocardial infarction, and stroke (Boehncke, 2018).

10.4.8 Metabolic syndrome and diabetes

Chronic inflammation disrupts insulin signaling pathways, leading to insulin resistance and impaired glucose homeostasis. Adipose tissue serves as a reservoir of proinflammatory cytokines, with adipocytes and infiltrating immune cells releasing a milieu of inflammatory mediators. This adipose tissue inflammation contributes to systemic insulin resistance, dyslipidemia, and endothelial dysfunction, amplifying the risk of cardiovascular complications in individuals with diabetes (Dandona et al., 2005; Reinehr & Roth, 2018). Chronic inflammation effects insulin signaling pathways, undermining the ability of cells to respond to insulin and regulating glucose uptake and utilization. Inflammatory cytokines such as tumor necrosis factor-alpha (TNF-α) and interleukin-6 (IL-6) interfere with insulin receptor signaling cascades, promoting serine phosphorylation of insulin receptor substrate proteins and inhibiting downstream activation of phosphatidylinositol 3-kinase (PI3K) and Akt pathways (Huerta-Delgado et al., 2020). This disruption of insulin signaling pathways leads to insulin resistance, characterized by impaired glucose uptake in skeletal muscle and adipose tissue, as well as increased hepatic glucose production, contributing to hyperglycemia and metabolic dysregulation (Onalan et al., 2022). Adipose tissue serves as a dynamic endocrine organ, secreting adipokines and inflammatory mediators that regulate energy metabolism and systemic inflammation. In obesity, adipose tissue undergoes extensive remodeling, characterized by hypertrophy of adipocytes, infiltration of immune cells, and dysregulation of adipokine secretion (Zatterale et al., 2020). Adipocytes themselves secrete proinflammatory cytokines such as TNF-α, IL-6, and monocyte chemoattractant protein-1 (MCP-1), while infiltrating immune cells, particularly macrophages, contribute to the production of additional inflammatory mediators. This adipose tissue inflammation creates a proinflammatory milieu that exacerbates insulin resistance, impairs adipocyte function, and promotes lipolysis, leading to elevated circulating free fatty acids and dyslipidemia (Onalan et al., 2022). The systemic consequences of adipose tissue inflammation extend beyond insulin resistance to involve a series of metabolic derangements associated with metabolic syndrome. Dyslipidemia, characterized by elevated triglycerides, reduced high-density lipoprotein (HDL) cholesterol, and increased low-density lipoprotein (LDL) cholesterol, arises from impaired adipocyte lipid metabolism and increased hepatic lipid synthesis (Huerta-Delgado et al., 2020). Endothelial dysfunction, manifested by impaired vasodilation, increased vascular permeability, and heightened prothrombotic state, predisposes to cardiovascular complications, including atherosclerosis, hypertension, and coronary artery disease.

10.4.9 Neurodegenerative disorders

Chronic neuroinflammation consists of various neurodegenerative disorders, including Alzheimer's disease, Parkinson's disease, and multiple sclerosis. Activation of microglia and astrocytes within the central nervous system (CNS) drives the production of proinflammatory cytokines, oxidative stress, and neurotoxic mediators, culminating in neuronal injury and neurodegeneration. Furthermore, neuroinflammation exacerbates blood—brain barrier dysfunction, facilitating the infiltration of peripheral immune cells and perpetuating CNS inflammation and neuronal damage (Candelario-Jalil et al., 2022). Neuroinflammation, characterized by the activation of immune cells within the central nervous system (CNS), emerges as a prominent pathological feature of various neurodegenerative disorders, including Alzheimer's disease (AD), Parkinson's disease (PD), and multiple sclerosis (MS). Chronic activation of microglia and astrocytes drives a cascade of inflammatory events, contributing to neuronal injury, synaptic dysfunction, and progressive neurodegeneration (Teixeira et al., 2017). Microglia, the resident immune cells of the CNS, and astrocytes, the most abundant glial cells, play pivotal roles in orchestrating the neuroinflammatory response in neurodegenerative disorders (Tjalkens et al., 2017). In response to neuronal injury, protein aggregates, or other pathological stimuli, microglia and astrocytes undergo activation, adopting an inflammatory phenotype characterized by morphological changes, increased expression of surface markers, and secretion of proinflammatory cytokines and chemokines. This activation triggers a self-propagating cycle of inflammation, exacerbating neuronal damage and contributing to disease progression. Activated microglia and astrocytes release a plethora of proinflammatory mediators, including cytokines (e.g., TNF-α, IL-1β), chemokines, and ROS, which mediate neuroinflammatory processes and contribute to neuronal injury. Proinflammatory cytokines disrupt synaptic function, promote excitotoxicity, and induce neuronal apoptosis, leading to synaptic dysfunction and neuronal loss observed in neurodegenerative diseases. Additionally, ROS generated by activated glial cells contribute to oxidative stress, impairing cellular homeostasis, and exacerbating neurodegeneration (Nazmi et al., 2019; Tjalkens et al., 2017).

10.4.10 Cancer

Inflammation plays a dual role in cancer, by the development of both tumor promotion and antitumor immune responses (Padoan et al., 2019). Chronic inflammation within the tumor microenvironment promotes tumor initiation, progression, and metastasis through the induction of DNA damage, angiogenesis, and immune evasion mechanisms. Additionally, inflammatory mediators foster an immunosuppressive milieu, dampening antitumor immune responses and promoting tumor immune evasion. Conversely, inflammation can also stimulate antitumor immune responses, highlighting the complex interplay between inflammation and cancer immunosurveillance (Ginckels & Holvoet, 2022; Zhang et al., 2021).

10.4.11 Therapeutic strategies targeting inflammation

The therapeutic potential of modulating inflammatory pathways has yielded a diverse array of pharmacological and nonpharmacological interventions. Traditional antiinflammatory agents such as nonsteroidal antiinflammatory drugs (NSAIDs) and corticosteroids remain pivotal in managing acute and chronic inflammatory conditions. Additionally, biological agents targeting specific cytokines or cellular receptors have revolutionized the treatment landscape for autoimmune disorders (Bootz & Neri, 2015). Nonetheless, the quest for safer, more efficacious therapies persists, spurring research into novel pharmacological agents, including small molecule inhibitors and monoclonal antibodies. Furthermore, the emerging pattern of personalized medicine emphasizes the importance of therapeutic approaches to individual inflammatory profiles, including genetic predispositions and environmental factors. The research on therapeutic interventions targeting inflammation represents a basis of modern medicine, aiming to alleviate symptoms, prevent disease progression, and improve patient outcomes. Through a multifaceted approach incorporating pharmacological and nonpharmacological modalities, researchers and clinicians trying to modulate inflammatory pathways to restore immune homeostasis and mitigate the problem of inflammatory diseases (Engelen et al., 2022).

10.4.12 Traditional antiinflammatory agents

Nonsteroidal antiinflammatory drugs (NSAIDs) and corticosteroids are used for the acute and chronic antiinflammatory conditions. NSAIDs exert their antiinflammatory effects by inhibiting cyclooxygenase (COX) enzymes, thereby attenuating the synthesis of proinflammatory prostaglandins. Corticosteroids, on the other hand, act by suppressing the production of inflammatory cytokines and chemokines, dampening immune responses. While effective in alleviating symptoms, long-term use of these agents may be associated with adverse effects, underscoring the need for safer therapeutic alternatives (Li et al., 2021).

10.4.13 Biological agents

The advent of biological agents heralds a paradigm shift in the treatment landscape for autoimmune disorders, offering targeted interventions against specific cytokines or cellular receptors implicated in inflammation. Monoclonal antibodies targeting tumor necrosis factor-alpha (TNF-α), interleukin-6 (IL-6), and interleukin-17 (IL-17) have revolutionized the management of conditions such as rheumatoid arthritis, psoriasis, and inflammatory bowel disease (Chen et al., 2018; Dinarello, 2010). By neutralizing key mediators of inflammation, biological agents afford precise and potent therapeutic effects with reduced systemic toxicity compared to traditional immunosuppressive therapies.

10.4.14 Novel pharmacological agents

Small molecule inhibitors target intracellular signaling molecules, such as Janus kinase (JAK) inhibitors and phosphodiesterase, significantly modulating inflammatory responses with improved specificity and reduced off-target effects (Banerjee et al., 2017). Advances in drug delivery technologies facilitate the targeted delivery of antiinflammatory agents to inflamed tissues, enhancing therapeutic efficacy while minimizing systemic exposure (Hu et al., 2021).

10.4.15 Personalized medicine approach

The emerging pattern of personalized medicine emphasizes the importance of adapting therapeutic approaches to individual inflammatory profiles, including genetic predispositions, environmental factors, and disease heterogeneity (Dinarello, 2010). Biomarker-guided strategies enable the identification of patients likely to benefit from specific therapies, optimizing treatment selection and response monitoring. Integrated multiomics approaches, including genomics, transcriptomics, and proteomics, provide insights into the molecular mechanisms driving inflammation, facilitating the development of precision therapeutics tailored to individual patient needs ("A Current View on Inflammation," 2017; Dinarello, 2010).

The therapeutic strategies targeting inflammation incorporate a diverse array of modalities aimed at modulating the pathways to restore immune homeostasis and alleviate disease severity. From traditional antiinflammatory agents and biological therapies to novel pharmacological agents and personalized medicine approaches, more efficacious and safer therapies continue to drive innovation in the field of inflammatory disease management. By incorporating the therapeutic potential of inflammation modulation, clinicians hope to improve patient outcomes and enhance quality of life for individuals affected by inflammatory disorders.

10.5 Application of functional food on the mediation of inflammation

The immune system is largely regulated by inflammatory processes, which is a defensive reaction against pathogens, damaged cells, or irritants (Medzhitov, 2010). In addition, some diseases, including asthma, arthritis, cancers, and cardiovascular diseases, may cause inflammation. In response to an immediate (acute condition) pathogenic infection or foreign invaders or irritants, the innate immune system is activated by releasing macrophages, dendritic cells, mast cells, neutrophils, and lymphocytes (Abdulkhaleq et al., 2018). Depending on the type and nature of the stimulant, the inflammatory signaling pathway is significantly different. In bacterial infections or tissue damage/injury, the immune system activates the production of inflammatory mediators such as inflammatory cytokines; tumor necrosis factor (TNF), interleukin-1 (IL-1) and interleukin-6 (IL-6), and chemokines (Chen et al., 2018). As a result, the progression of inflammation accelerates by increasing the blood flow and vascular endothelial permeability, accompanying leukocytes and excess fluid accumulation into the site of infection (Abdulkhaleq et al., 2018). Often, inflammatory responses lead to excessive production of inflammatory cytokines, which facilitate recruiting of prostaglandins, thereby causing the onset of symptoms such as pain and fever (Abdulkhaleq et al., 2018). If acute inflammation is not controlled or if persistent, it can turn into a chronic stage (Murakami & Hirano, 2012). The underlying mechanism for chronic inflammation is not well elucidated, as our understanding of the pathological process has become complicated. However, chronic inflammations are believed to be mediated by the host's inflammatory response itself without the involvement of foreign invaders (Chen et al., 2018). Thus it is vital to understand the association of inflammation with the rapidly increasing chronic diseases such as atherosclerosis, obesity, type 2 diabetes, neurodegenerative diseases, and cancer, in modern society. For example, obesity can cause multiple chronic inflammations that lead to type 2 diabetes as obesity-induced insulin resistance (Ruze et al., 2023). Even, long-term inflammation results in stimulation of cancer risk due to the reaction of various types of inflammatory and proinflammatory mediators (Wen et al., 2022).

What you eat and what you are signify the vital role that diets play in the human body, as the type of nutrients can either control or trigger inflammation (Ricordi et al., 2015). For example, a high intake of refined carbohydrates and saturated fats may boost inflammation via a nuclear transcription factor-κB (NF-kB) signaling pathway (Ilich et al., 2014). Simultaneously, a high consumption of certain nutrients such as glucose, fructose, and lipids could promote an elevated risk of inflammation that may result in the progression of metabolic diseases, cardiovascular diseases, and cancers (Clemente-Suárez et al., 2022). For instance, an excessive intake causes obesity that results in an increase of white adipocytes leading to a stable state of inflammation (Oliveira et al., 2013). In this case, there are dietary options that could provide beneficial effects over synthetic pharmacological therapies. Mediterranean diets have been shown to have a positive impact on the prevention of these noncommunicable diseases (Tsigalou et al., 2020). However, some natural compounds present in foods such as bioactive peptides, fatty acids, phytosterol, flavonoids, curcumin, ascorbic acid, and tannin are claimed to exhibit antiinflammatory properties (Li et al., 2019; Sánchez & Vázquez, 2017; Teodoro, 2019). Therefore, based on the research findings, foods with these natural compounds have a wide range of bioactivities, including anticancer, antibacterial, and immunomodulating effects.

10.5.1 Functional foods for the control of inflammation

10.5.1.1 Bioactive peptides

Bioactive peptides (BPs) are specific protein fragments (2–20 amino acids) with sizes not exceeding 20 kDa, which play an important role in body functions, and, consequently may influence human health (Sánchez & Vázquez, 2017). BPs derived from plant and animal sources such as milk, pulses, eggs, and fish, have been shown to have a wide range of biological activities, including antioxidative, immunomodulatory, antimicrobial, and antihypertensive properties (Sánchez & Vázquez, 2017) (Fig. 10.1). Peptides are generated by suitable proteolytic enzymatic digestion, chemical hydrolysis, gastrointestinal digestion, or microbial fermentation through food processing (Daliri et al., 2017). Therefore the structural and functional characteristics of peptides differ based on the method of production, and the activity of

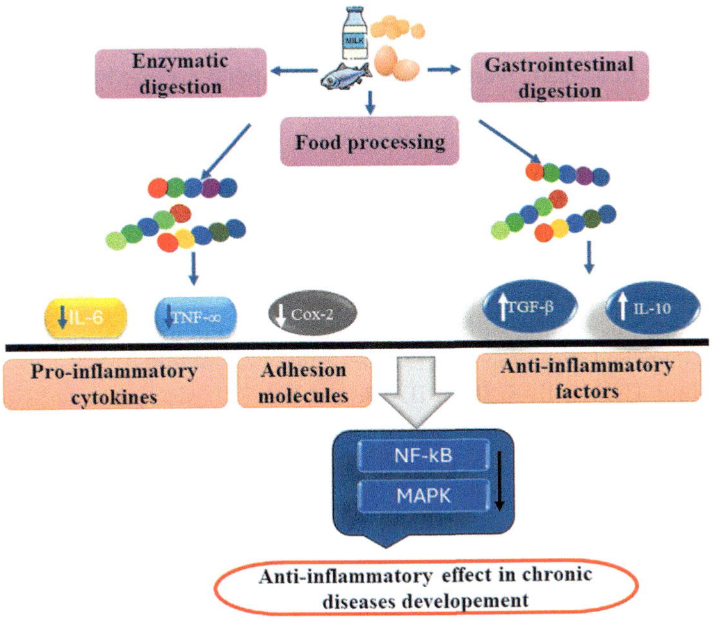

FIGURE 10.1 Antiinflammatory effect of bioactive peptides; (I) bioactive peptide production from enzymatic, gastrointestinal and food processing (ex: fermentation), (II) suppression of proinflammatory cytokines (IL-6-Interleukin-6, TNF-α-tumor necrosis factor-α, CoX-2- cyclooxygenase 2), (III) expression of antiinflammatory factors (TGF-β-transforming growth factor β, IL-10-Interleukin 10) (IV) antiinflammatory effect of peptides by suppressing the NF-kB-nuclear factor kappa B, MAPK-mitogen-activated protein kinase.

peptides is mainly determined by their amino acid composition and sequence (Guha & Majumder, 2019). However, certain properties, such as a relative ratio of a specific amino acid, hydrophobic properties, weight and length of the peptides, and type of residues at C- and N-terminals, also influence the biological activities of peptides 67. Nevertheless, the current understanding of structure–functional activity and molecular mechanism of the action of BPs in disease prevention is still in its early phases. However, recent studies have shown that peptides could exert an array of biological functions in human health. Recent in vitro and in vivo studies elucidated that the potential antiinflammatory activity is mostly due to modulation of transcription factors, kinases (NF-kB and mitogen-activated protein kinase [MAPK]) and/or either suppressing or inhibiting the tumor necrosis factor-α (TNF-α), interleukin-1 (IL-1) and interleukin-6 (IL-6) or chemokines (monocyte chemotactic protein-1 [MCP-1]) (Fig. 10.1) (Kwak et al., 2016; Majumder et al., 2016; Meza Márquez et al., 2022).

Plant-derived BPs have gained much interest in recent years as numerous in vitro studies have confirmed that they modulate the inflammatory signaling pathways (Zhang, Fu, et al., 2020; Zhang, Li, et al., 2020). However, there are a limited number of studies conducted in in vivo settings. Protein and peptide fractions extracted from chickpeas were found to have reduced levels of nitric oxide inhibition, interleukin-1, and tumor necrosis factor (Meza Márquez et al., 2022). BPs extracted from different plant protein sources, including soybean, beans, lupins, and cereals (wheat, rye barley), also exhibited antiinflammatory potential. López-Barrios *et al.* (2016) demonstrated that hydrolysates produced from germinated black bean (*Phaseolus vulgaris*) had a higher inhibitory effect on the nitric oxide (NO), compared to the raw sample. They further suggested that the antiinflammatory effect may be due to the peptide produced from the germination process. In addition, peptides from soybeans, lunasin (43 amino acids), which inhibit NF-kB activation, have been investigated in anticancer potential (Majumder et al., 2016). Based on the study conducted by Hsieh *et al.* (2010), lunasin also exhibited antitumorigenic effect by inhibiting the cell proliferation and foci formation on 12-dimethylbenz(*a*)anthracene (DMBA) and 3-methylcholanthrene-treated (MCA) fibroblast NIH/3T3 cells. In another study, tripeptides from soybean; FLV (Phe-Leu-Val) showed inhibition action on TNF-α, Il-6, and MCP-1 induced adipocytes cells and adipocytes/macrophage co-cultured cells (Kwak et al., 2016). Similarly, it was reported that VPY (Val-Pro-Tyr) peptide extracted from soybean inhibited the secretion of IL-8 from TNF-α induced colorectal adenocarcinoma (Caco-2 cells) (Kovacs-Nolan et al., 2012). The same peptide sequence from soybean was further shown to suppress the action of TNF-α, interferon-gamma (IFN-γ), and IL-1β in colitis of female BALB mice. In addition, food sources such as edible beans and yeast extract also exhibited significant antiinflammatory effects in intestinal epithelial cells (Caco-2 cells) through the γ-glutamyl dipeptides (Zhang, Zhang, et al., 2015).

Several peptides derived from animal proteins have been well-documented in both in vitro and in vivo studies. Milk, one of the main protein sources in human diet is reported to have peptides derived from whey and casein that exert biological activity on antiinflammatory effects (Chakrabarti et al., 2014). BPs generated from microbial fermentation of casein VPP (Val-Pro-Pro) and IPP (Ile-Pro-Pro) have been shown to have biological activity with multifunctional effects (Guha & Majumder, 2019). Reportedly, these two peptides were found to reduce the adipokine levels in 3T3-F442A murine preadipocytes and cytokine-induced proinflammatory changes (activation of NF-kB pathway) (Chakrabarti & Wu, 2015). The same peptides, VPP and IPP from milk, were shown to be beneficial for preventing atherosclerosis caused by hypercholesterolemia (Nakamura et al., 2013). In this case, reduced messenger RNA (mRNA) expressed inflammatory cytokines, such as IL-6 and IL-1β, oxidized low-density lipoprotein receptor, and transcription regulators in apolipoprotein E-deficient (apoE[− / −]) mice. Moreover, Piccolomini *et al.* (2012) demonstrated that hydrostatic pressure-treated whey protein hydrolysates had an inhibitory effect on the IL-8 secretion in intestinal epithelial cells (Caco-2).

Egg white proteins contain a variety of BPs derived from enzymatic hydrolysis, which could be used to alleviate the antiinflammation (Zhou et al., 2022). The peptides identified from egg white demonstrated decreased levels of proinflammatory cytokines and the extent of crypt damage in dextran sodium sulfate (DSS)-induced colitis model (Ge et al., 2021). Similarly, peptides isolated from simulated gastrointestinal digestion of preserved egg white inhibited IL-8 secretion and decreased gene expression significantly, including TNF-α, IL-8, IL-6, IL-1β, and IL-12. It also promoted IL-10 gene expression in Caco-2 cells in DSS-induced colitis mouse model (Zhang et al., 2018). In another study, peptides derived from cooked tuna juice, PRRTRMMNGGR (Pro-Arg-Arg-Thr-Arg-Met-Met-Asn-Gly-Gly-Arg), and MGPAMMRTMPG (Met-Gly-Pro-Ala-Met-Met-Arg-Thr-Met-Pro-Gly) exhibited an inhibitory action against the secretion of IL-2, TNF-α, and IFN-γ in LPS-induced RAW264.7 macrophage cells (Cheng et al., 2015).

10.5.2 Curcumin

Curcumin, derived from the rhizome of *Curcuma longa* L. (Turmeric), belongs to the *Zingiberaceae* family. Turmeric has long been used in the traditional *aurvedic* medicine for various treatments such as improvement of blood circulation, pain management, and inflammatory disorders (Peng et al., 2021). Turmeric contains active compounds, curcumin, demethoxycurcumin, bisdemethoxycurcumin, called "curcuminoids" and volatile oils (Fig. 10.2) (Peng et al., 2021; Shehzad et al., 2012). Curcumin is the major active compound, chemically known as 1,7-bis (4-hydroxy-3-methoxyphenyl)-1,6-hepta-diene-3, 5-dione, and is a strong hydrophobic compound that is fairly stable at lower pH (Priyadarsini, 2014), which has demonstrated various pharmacological benefits, including antioxidant, antiinflammatory, antitumor properties, and other biological activities.

Curcumin shows strong therapeutic potential for various chronic inflammatory diseases (Fig. 10.2). Curcumin may act as a natural radical scavenger due to its O−H phenolic group and C−H in the chemical structure (He et al., 2015). Currently, different mechanisms via multiple pathways by which curcumin can exert antiinflammatory activities have been reported. It was proposed that curcumin could act as a TNF blocker by binding to TNF directly, thereby suppressing the proinflammatory pathway. Further, it suggests that curcumin is a potent antioxidant, which alleviates oxidative stress in cells, and reduces the risk of inflammation through the nuclear factor erythroid-2-related factor 2 (Nrf2-keap1) pathway (Anthwal et al., 2014; Gupta et al., 2014).

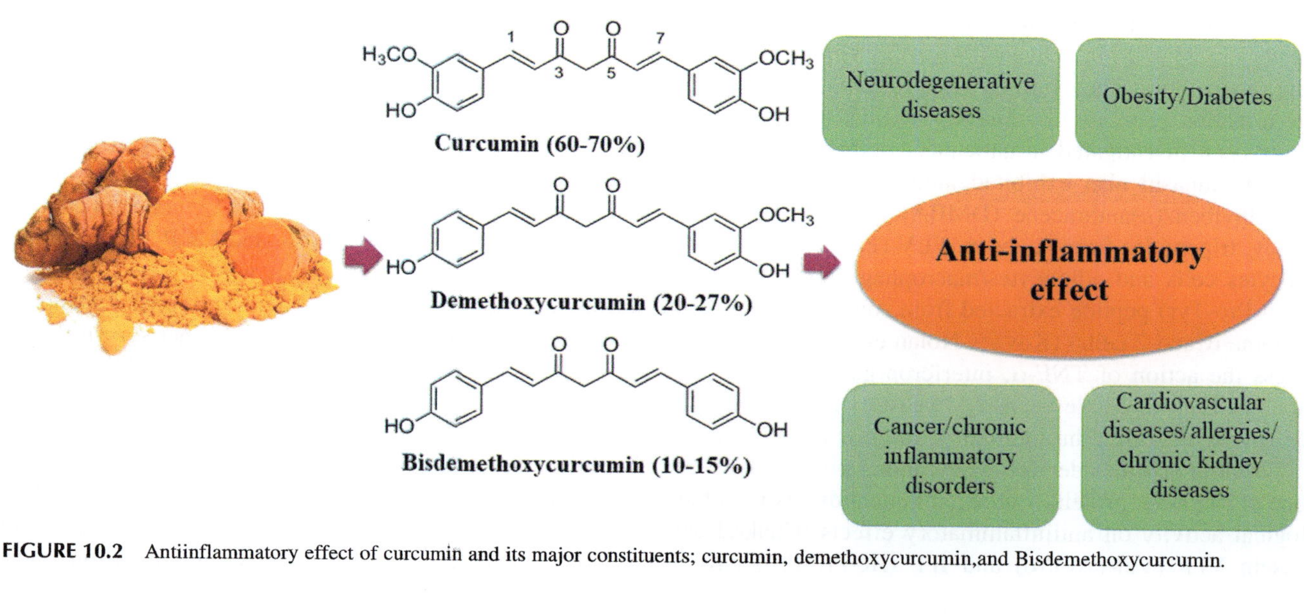

FIGURE 10.2 Antiinflammatory effect of curcumin and its major constituents; curcumin, demethoxycurcumin,and Bisdemethoxycurcumin.

Currently, chronic diseases are increasing at an alarming rate, of which cardiovascular diseases (CVDs) are a critical global health threat (Li et al., 2019). Based on the epidemiological and clinical data, risk of having CVDs has been strongly connected with the expression of inflammatory markers such as C-reactive proteins (CRP) and proinflammatory cytokines (Wongcharoen & Phrommintikul, 2009). Atherosclerosis is believed to be involved with the latter (He et al., 2015), which is a progressive problem of arteries leading to the development of pathologies related to other forms of CVDs, including hypertension, coronary heart disease, and ischemic stroke (Li et al., 2019). The therapeutic effect of curcumin was demonstrated in ApoE-knockout (ApoE$^{-/-}$) mice (0.2% curcumin *w*/w in diet, 4 months) by a 26% reduction in atherosclerosis lesions, leukocyte adhesion and transendothelial migration via changes of expression of genes (Coban et al., 2012). It was suggested that these changes were mediated by decreasing the binding capacity of NF-κB/DNA with stimulation of TNF-α and increased expression of inhibitor of NF-κB protein. Similarly, in another study using the same animal model, a curcumin supplemented diet (0.1% w/w, 16 weeks) significantly suppressed the development of atherosclerosis by downregulating the TLR4, and consequently the expression of IL-1β, TNF-α, vascular cell adhesion molecule 1 (VCAM-1) and intercellular adhesion molecule-1 (ICAM-1) and NF-kB activity (Zhang et al., 2018). In a recent study using an inflammation-induced- lipopolysaccharide (LPS) rat model, curcumin was reported to decrease the white blood cells (WBC) ameliorating the decreased level of malondialdehyde (MDA) while improving the oxidative stress (Ahmadabady et al., 2021).

Obesity is a risk factor, which is closely associated with CVD-related morbidity and mortality and impaired glucose metabolism (type 2 diabetes mellitus) (Bastard et al., 2006; Campbell et al., 2019) and other chronic diseases such as metabolic syndrome (Panahi et al., 2016), fatty liver (Jazayeri-Tehrani et al., 2019), and cancers (Mansouri et al., 2020). Excessive expansion of adipocytes (AC) resulted in obesity, disrupting the metabolic functions in AC cells by altering the balance between pro- and antiinflammatory markers (Varì et al., 2021). Consequently, increased levels of proinflammatory markers, adipocytokines, including leptin and decreased levels of antiinflammatory markers such as adiponectin, could lead to changes in the AC environment resulting in metabolic dysfunction and various disease states (Lee & Lee, 2013; Schwartz & Yehuda-Shnaidman, 2014; Wellen & Hotamisligil, 2003). The current literature showed delevated level of TNF-α and IL-6, simultaneously with decreased levels of antiinflammatory markers in obese individuals (Yamashita et al., 2018). Research performed on 30 obese individuals in a randomized cross-over trial reported that curcumin therapy with 1 g/day for 4 weeks, induced the reduction of serum IL-1β, IL-4, and VEGF, while no significant differences were found in concentrations of antiinflammatory markers (Ganjali et al., 2014). Moreover, 60 healthy adolescent girls tested in a randomized placebo-controlled clinical trial on a weight-loss diet for 10 weeks (curcumin 500 mg/day) showed a significant decrease in high-sensitive C-reactive proteins (hs-CRP) and IL-6, compared to the placebo group (Saraf-Bank et al., 2019). In another study, the administration of curcumin (1 g/day, 8 weeks) to obese/overweight males and females diagnosed with metabolic syndrome, reduced serum concentrations of TNFα, IL-6, and monocyte chemoattractant protein-1 (MCP-1) in comparison to placebo group (Panahi et al., 2016).

Similar results were reported in 84 obese patients with nonalcoholic fatty liver disease (NAFLD), who were fed two 40 mg capsules/day after meals for 3 months under a double-blind randomized controlled clinical trial (Jazayeri-Tehrani et al., 2019). In contrast, a double-blinded randomized controlled trial on obesity-associated CVDs (22 young obese men, curcumin 500 mg/day, 12 weeks) subjects revealed no significant difference in changes between the circulating concentrations of glucose, insulin, leptin, adiponectin, or oxidative stress biomarkers in the curcumin group with respect to the placebo group, accompanying with endothelial function, augmentation index, or central blood pressure. However, homocysteine levels were lower in the curcumin group compared to the placebo group (Campbell et al., 2019). Nonetheless, administration of high-fat diet with curcumin (20 mg/kg body weight) in a rat model demonstrated that the curcumin group had reduced risk of hyperglycemia and hyperlipidemia by improving the leptin and insulin resistance (Elwakf et al., 2013). Treatment with a high dose of curcumin (1500 mg/day) for subjects (both men and women, 6 months) diagnosed with type 2 diabetes mellitus, however, showed elevated levels of adiponectin and decreased leptin levels after the intervention (Chuengsamarn et al., 2014). In addition, many other interventions using animal models and in human clinical trials have investigated the effect of curcumin on insulin resistance and changes in inflammatory markers (Funamoto et al., 2019; Mokgalaboni et al., 2021; Pourhabibi-Zarandi et al., 2022; Weisberg et al., 2008).

Curcumin has also gained increasing attention in cancer therapies owing to its powerful anticancer properties. Despite the significant development in pharmacological agents, the efficacy of these chemotherapeutics is limited due to severe side effects. Therefore it is extremely important to identify novel efficacious therapeutic agents in cancer treatments. Currently, there are in vitro and in vivo clinical and animal studies examining the anticancer properties of curcumin (He et al., 2015) with the anticancer mechanisms involved in multiple cellular targets and signaling pathways well elucidated in the literature. Curcumin was found to downregulate multiple signaling pathways such as Wnt/β-catenin signaling, phosphoinositide 3-kinase (PI3K)/protein kinase B (Akt) pathway, Janus kinase (JAK)/signal transducer and activator of transcription (STAT) signaling pathway, mitogen-activated protein kinase (MAPK) pathway, p53 signaling and NF-κB pathway (Kunnumakkara et al., 2017; Wang et al., 2019). Clearly, curcumin is capable of effectively interfering with cancer cell growth, apoptosis, invasion, and metastasis. As a result, it suggests that curcumin can modulate various types of cancers (Hesari et al., 2019; Jalili-Nik et al., 2018). Curcumin appears to be an effective chemopreventive agent for inhibiting proinflammatory cytokines, CXCL1, and the development of breast cancer metastases (Kronski et al., 2014). Similar observations were reported by Killian *et al.*, (2012) for prostate carcinoma growth, apoptosis, and metastasis. They demonstrated the inhibitory action of curcumin on translocation of NFκB to the nucleus through downregulation of IκB-kinase. Kunnumakkara *et al.* (2009) investigated whether curcumin could potentiate the effect of capecitabine against the growth and metastasis of colorectal cancer cells (CRC) in both *in vitro* and nude mice models. In vitroresults suggested that curcumin was able to inhibit the proliferation of human CRC cell lines, NF-κB activation, and suppression NF-κB-regulated gene products, whereas in nude mice, the combination treatment of curcumin and capecitabine was found to be more effective in suppressing ascites and distant metastasis to the liver, intestines, lungs, rectum, and spleen accompanied by suppressed expression of activated NF-κB and NF-κB-regulated gene products. Moreover, curcumin was shown to be effective in downregulating the human papillomaviruses 18 (HPV18) transcription and activator protein-1 (AP-1) binding activity in Hela cells, suggesting a novel therapeutic approach for controlling pathogenic HPV infection (Prusty & Das, 2005).

Curcumin has also been evaluated for its effectiveness in treating a number of other chronic diseases, including the pathogenesis of neurodegenerative diseases, Parkinson's (Donadio et al., 2022; Fikry et al., 2022) and Alzheimer's diseases (Ringman et al., 2012; Voulgaropoulou et al., 2019; Xiong et al., 2011), kidney disease (Ghosh et al., 2014), and chronic inflammatory disorder, rheumatoid arthritis (Amalraj et al., 2017; Dai et al., 2018), allergy (Kinney et al., 2015), asthma (Yang et al., 2017), and bronchitis (Abidi et al., 2014; Memarzia et al., 2022). The broader investigation of curcumin has provided important insights into its antiinflammation therapy and further clinical design applications will assess its potential significance in disease prevention.

10.5.3 Polyphenol compounds

Polyphenolic compounds (PPCs) are diverse groups of naturally occurring secondary metabolites in plant (Handique & Baruah, 2002) as a part of their defense system in response to various stimulants, including insect and pathogen attacks, physical injuries, and UV radiation (Khoddami et al., 2013). Chemically, PPCs comprise one or more aromatic rings coupled to a single or more hydroxyl groups generating over 8000 heterogenous structural compounds. PPCs account for the color and taste of foods and can be found in many food sources such as fruits, vegetables, coffee, tea, wine, and legumes (Alara et al., 2021). PPCs can be classified into two major groups: flavonoids and nonflavonoids. Both groups can then be subdivided into many subclasses depending on the number of structural differences (Fig. 10.3) (Singla et al., 2019).

In recent years, PPCs have gained increasing interest among the consumers due to their broad range of bioactivities such as antioxidant, antimicrobial, antiinflammatory, antitumoral, and hepatoprotective effects (Caleja et al., 2017). With respect to antiinflammatory properties, dietary PPCs have been shown to exert beneficial effects in both in vitro and in vivo studies. Therefore PPCs may be used as a therapeutic tool in multiple chronic diseases. Currently, the immunomodulatory effects of PPCs have been explained by different signaling pathways: NF-kB signaling pathway, MAPK signaling pathway, and arachidonic signaling pathway, supported by in vivo and in vitro studies (Ambriz-Pérez et al., 2016; Yahfoufi et al., 2018). Interestingly, PPCs are capable of showing antiinflammatory properties in multiple ways compared to drugs. As evident by its suppression of LPS-induced NF-κB activations by kaempferol (Hämäläinen et al., 2007), inducible nitric oxide synthase (iNOS) expression and nitric oxide (NO) production (Hämäläinen et al., 2007), cyclooxygenase (COX-2) expression and prostaglandin E2 (PGE2) production (Yoon et al., 2013), aldosterone signaling and aldosterone-induced gene expression (Liu et al., 2013) and cytokines (TNF-α, IL-1β) production (Kong et al., 2013).

The classical antioxidant properties of PPCs can scavenge a wide range of ROS. The higher production of ROS is associated with oxidative stress, and its promotion of protein oxidation and the tissue damage (Berlett & Stadtman, 1997). As a result, it can initiate the inflammatory process leading to various onset of disease development (Naik & Dixit, 2011). The antioxidant capacity of PPCs has been shown to suppress low-density lipoprotein (LDL) oxidation modulating inflammatory CVDs. For example, quercetin (red wine) was shown to inhibit LDL oxidation with elevated paraoxonase, leading to reduction of atherogenic lesions in apo E deficient (E°) mice study (Aviram & Fuhrman, 2002). In addition, anthocyanins were reported to exert antihypertensive and endothelium-protective activity through multiple signaling pathways, targeting the (protein kinase/endothelial NOS) Akt/eNOS and NF-κB mediated vascular cell adhesion molecule (VCAM) and intercellular cell adhesion molecule (ICAM) expression (Domitrovic, 2011).

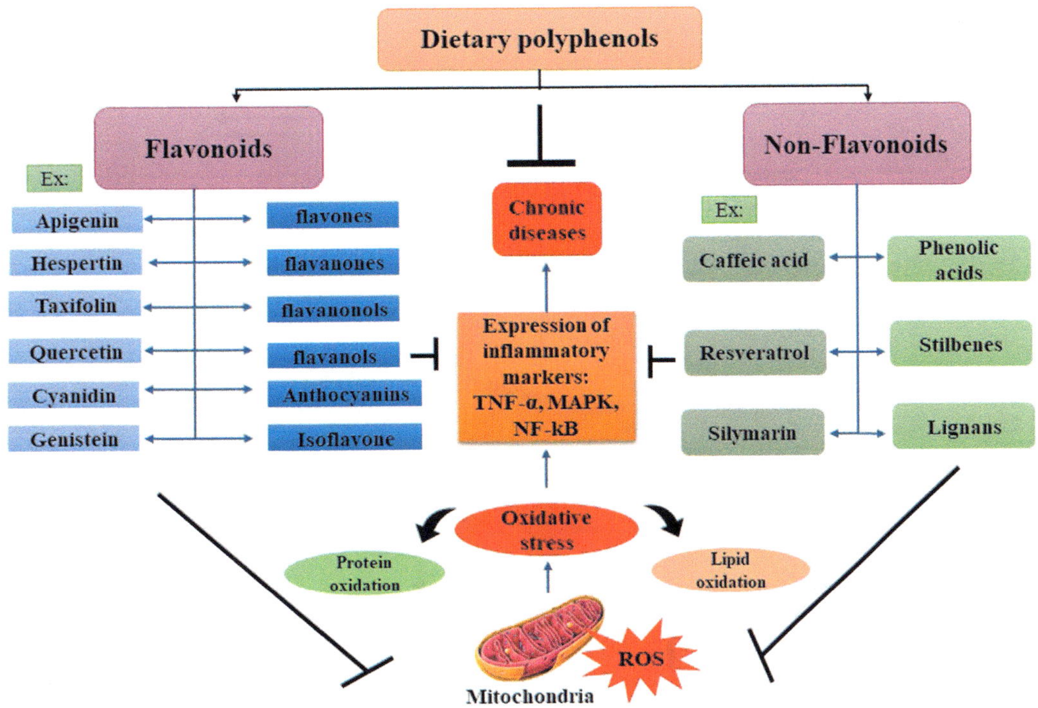

FIGURE 10.3 Dietary polyphenol classification and its antiinflammatory effect (I)- ROS causes the oxidative stress in mitochondria leading to lipid and protein oxidation, (II), expression of inflammatory markers; TNF-α-tumor necrosis factor-α, MAPK-mitogen-activated protein kinase and NF-kB-Nuclear factor kappa B, (III), chronic disease development, (IV), polyphenol compounds act as antioxidant suppressing the oxidative stress, thereby prevention of chronic disease development. *ROS*, Reactive oxygen species.

Growing evidence confirmed the beneficial effects of PPCs on the prevention of insulin resistance, obesity, neurodegenerative diseases, and cancers. Quercetin is known to have significant anti-diabetic effects affecting signaling pathways involved in insulin resistance through inhibiting the TNFα, NF-KB, AMPK, AKT, and NRF2 markers (Yan et al., 2023). In a study conducted by Chao et al. (2010), caffeic acid (CA) and ellagic acid (EA) (5%) were shown to diminish the renal activity of aldose reductase and sorbitol dehydrogenase, as well as suppressed renal aldose reductase mRNA expression in the kidney of diabetic mice. Further, CA and EA downregulated the renal levels of IL-6, IL-1β, TNF-α, and monocyte chemoattractant protein-1 (MCP-1). An improvement in insulin secretion by pancreatic β−cells by PPCs such as flavonoids was reported by Chu (2014). A study of pomegranate fruit peel, a rich source of PPCs, demonstrated that PPE supplementation (high-fat [HF]) diet with 6 mg/day, 4 weeks, attenuated the serum level of total cholesterol and LDL induced by HF feeding and counteracted the HF-induced expression of inflammatory markers both in the colon and the visceral adipose tissue (Neyrinck et al., 2013). A recent study in which pomegranate fruit pulp (PFP) fed to C57BL/6 J mice (HFD supplemented with PFP, 45% energy, 14 weeks) exhibited reduced HFD-induced body weight gain by 35.23%, steatosis scores by 50%, and insulin resistance by 56.84%, compared to mice fed HFD alone (Song et al., 2022).

Regarding the chemopreventive and anticancer efficacy of PPCs, they have the ability to inhibit the proliferation of different types of cancers (Yahfoufi et al., 2018). The chemotherapeutic efficacy of dietary polyphenols has been supported by effective inhibition of invasion, metastasis, and angiogenesis along with the inflammation-associated cancer initiation and progression. For example, the flavonoid quercetin (3, 3′, 4′, 5, 7-pentahydroxyflavone) induced apoptosis in colon cancer cells (Yerokun, 2014), and cervical Hela cancer cells (Vidya Priyadarsini et al., 2010) , and lymphoma cells 133. Similarly, epigallocatechin (EGCG) and genistein (4′,5,7-trihydroxyisoflavone) were found to exert anticancer properties in various cancer cell lines (Choudhari et al., 2020; H.-Q. Li et al., 2012). With respect to the association between chronic inflammation and cancer, many cancers are initiated and tumor progression results from inflammation (Patra et al., 2021). In this context, PPCs as an antioxidant agent, play a crucial role by suppression of proinflammatory markers such as ROS, ILs, TNF-α, and NF-κB. The polyphenol, curcumin, one of the potent antioxidants and antiinflammatory agents derived from *Curcuma longa*, discussed in the previous section, regulates the proinflammatory cytokines and transcription factors in several cancer cells (Fig. 10.4).

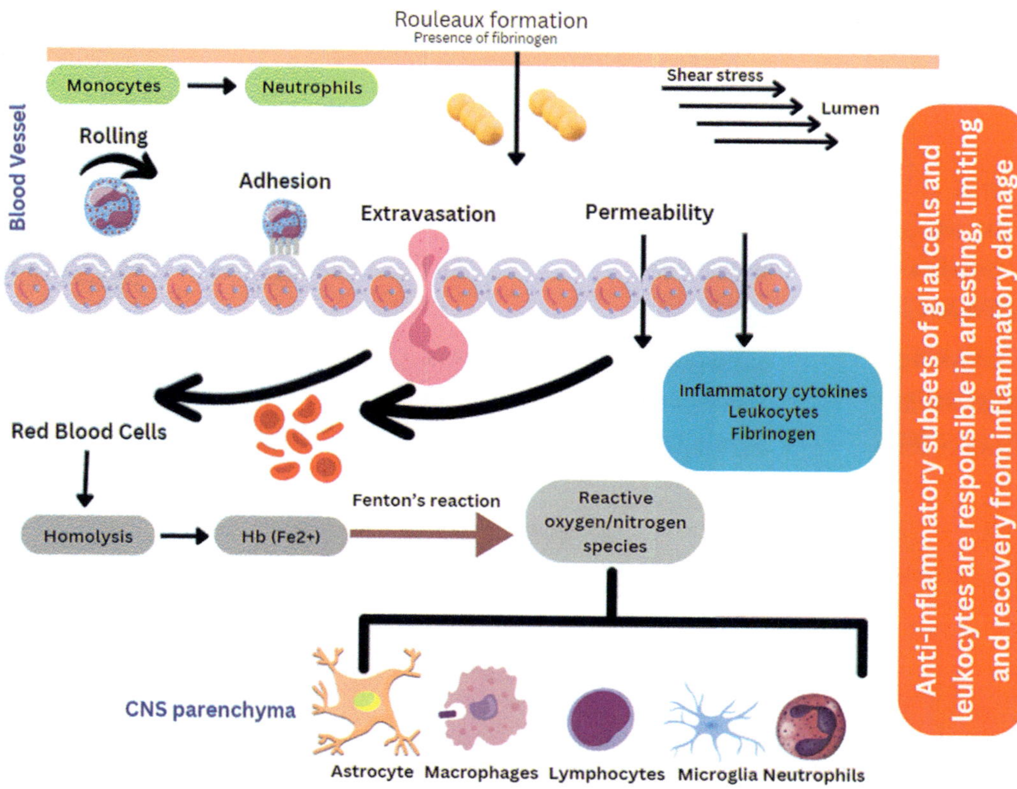

FIGURE 10.4 Progression of Inflammation.

The antiinflammatory effect of resveratrol is evident by its inhibition of TNF-α, NF-κB, AP-1, as well as TNF-induced NF-κB activation in myeloid cells (U37), lymphoid (Jurkat), and epithelial (HeLa and H4) cells (Manna et al., 2000). Short noncoding RNAs called MicroRNAs (miRNAs) regulate the expression of many target genes posttranscriptionally and have been implicated in inflammation leading to the development of cancer (Stefani & Slack, 2008). The most prominent of these are*miR-155*, *miR-21*, and *miR-125b*, which were found elevated in several human leukemias and lymphomas (Tili et al., 2009). Resveratrol was found to downregulate these MicroRNAs, *miR-155* and *miR-21* along with the inducing a tumor-suppressor, *miR-663, and* antiinflammatory microRNA (Tili & Michaille, 2011). Moreover, Zhang, Kovacs-Nolan, et al. (2015) demonstrated inhibitory expression of NF-κB in human colon cancer cells (CACO-2 and SW620) with subsequent induction of apoptosis while downregulating the B-cell lymphoma 2 (anti-apoptotic protein) and upregulation of Bax (pro-apoptotic protein) with quercetin. In addition, TNF-α, NF-κB, IL-1R, and inhibitors of kB kinase (IKKβ) in lung cancer cells (H460) were also reported by the same PPCs, (Youn et al., 2013).

Neurodegeneration (ND), manifested by loss of neurons in the central nervous system, can lead to many progressive neurological disorders, including Parkinson's and Alzheimer's diseases accompanied by dysfunction of cognition and motor activity. However, ND also is associated with other conditions such as multiple sclerosis, neurotrophic infections, spinal cord injury, stroke, and genetic disorders (Ambriz-Pérez et al., 2016). The pathogenic mechanism behind the neurodegenerative disease is believed to be associated with an increase in inflammatory markers such as the elevation of IL-1β, as well as IL-6 and TNF-α, and oxidative stress (Azizi et al., 2015). Based on evidence, inflammatory cytokine IL-1β, IL-6, soluble tumor necrosis factor receptor-1 (sTNFα-R1), and CRP blood/serum were elevated in patients suffering from Alzheimer's disease patients and mild cognitive impairment (Ambriz-Pérez et al., 2016; Walker et al., 2019). Three or more cups of tea with EGCG were recommended to reduce the risk of Parkinson's disease (PD) (Choi et al., 2002). According to Choi *et al.* (2002), administration of green tea with high levels of EGCG (25 mg EGCG/kg body weight) and tea (1 g of green tea) in 1-methyl-4-phenyl-1,2,3,6-tetrahydropyridine (MPTP)-induced PD mice revealed that both tea and EGCG had decreased expression of neuronal NO synthase (nNOS) *Substantia nigra.* Consequently, inhibition of NOS activity in the brain produces a neuroprotective effect against PD induced by MPTP (Choi et al., 2002). In AD pathogenesis, amyloid-beta peptide (Aβ) accumulation is the primary cause due to cell membrane perturbation and oxidative stress (Fändrich, 2012). Nine different food constituents (l-ascorbic acid, caffeic acid, caffeine, curcumin, EGCG, gallic acid, propyl gallate, resveratrol, and α-tocopherol) evaluated for the expression of Aβ in AD showed that PPCs: EGCG, gallic acid, and curcumin were multifunctional food constituents with free radicals scavenging abilities, and Aβ fibrillation inhibition (Chan et al., 2015). In another PD study, it was found that EGCG (2 mg/kg body weight per day) administration ameliorated the cognitive impairments, reduced the overexpression of Aβ and amyloid precursor protein (APP), and inhibited the neuronal apoptosis in the *APP/PS1* mice (Liu et al., 2014). In addition, many studies have been conducted on dietary polyphenols including, berberine (Simõ Es Pires et al., 2014), curcumin (El-Shamarka et al., 2023), resveratrol (Guo et al., 2016), quercetin (Suganthy et al., 2016), and genistein (Shi et al., 2023) in ND pathogenesis.

References

A current view on inflammation. (2017). *Nature Immunology, 18*(8), 825. Available from https://doi.org/10.1038/ni.3798, Nature Publishing Group.

Abdel Hammed, M. R., Elgendy, S. G., El-Mokhtar, M. A., Sayed, D., Mansour, S. M., & Darwish, A. M. (2022). T-lymphocytes Expression of Toll-like Receptors 2 and 4 in Acute Myeloid Leukemia Patients with Invasive Fungal Infections. *Mediterranean Journal of Hematology and Infectious Diseases, 14*(1). Available from https://doi.org/10.4084/MJHID.2022.022.

Abdulkhaleq, L. A., Assi, M. A., Abdullah, R., Zamri-Saad, M., Taufiq-Yap, Y. H., & Hezmee, M. N. M. (2018). The crucial roles of inflammatory mediators in inflammation: A review. *Veterinary World, 11*(5), 627.

Abidi, A., Gupta, S., Agarwal, M., Bhalla, H. L., & Saluja, M. (2014). Evaluation of Efficacy of Curcumin as an Add-on therapy in Patients of Bronchial Asthma. *Journal of Clinical and Diagnostic Research: JCDR, 8*(8), HC19.

Ahmadabady, S., Beheshti, F., Shahidpour, F., Khordad, E., & Hosseini, M. (2021). A protective effect of curcumin on cardiovascular oxidative stress indicators in systemic inflammation induced by lipopolysaccharide in rats. *Biochemistry and Biophysics Reports, 10*, 100908.

Alara, O. R., Abdurahman, N. H., & Ukaegbu, I. (2021). Extraction of phenolic compounds: A review. *Current Research in Food Science, 4*, 200–214.

Alberto, R., Frers, K., Otero-Losada, M., Herrera, M.I., Porta, S., Cosentino, V., Kerzberg, E., Udovin, L., & Capani, F. (2019). *Immune-Mediated Inflammation: Human T CD4 Helper Lymphocyte Diversity and Plasticity in Health and Disease*. www.intechopen.com

Amalraj, A., Varma, K., Jacob, J., Divya, C., Kunnumakkara, A. B., Stohs, S. J., & Gopi, S. (2017). A Novel Highly Bioavailable Curcumin Formulation Improves Symptoms and Diagnostic Indicators in Rheumatoid Arthritis Patients: A Randomized, Double-Blind, Placebo-Controlled, Two-Dose, Three-Arm, and Parallel-Group Study. *Journal of Medical Food, 20*(10), 1022–1030.

Ambriz-Pérez, D. L., Leyva-López, N., Gutierrez-Grijalva, E. P., & Heredia, J. B. (2016). Phenolic compounds: Natural alternative in inflammation treatment. A Review. *Cogent Food & Agriculture, 2*(1), 1131412.

Anthwal, A., Thakur, B. K., Rawat, M. S. M., Rawat, D. S., Tyagi, A. K., & Aggarwal, B. B. (2014). Synthesis, characterization and in vitro anticancer activity of C-5 curcumin analogues with potential to inhibit TNF-α-induced NF-κB activation. *BioMed Research International, 2014*, 524161.

Antunes, I., & Kassiotis, G. (2010). Suppression of Innate Immune Pathology by Regulatory T Cells during Influenza A Virus Infection of Immunodeficient Mice. *Journal of Virology, 84*(24), 12564–12575. Available from https://doi.org/10.1128/jvi.01559-10.

Aviram, M., & Fuhrman, B. (2002). Wine Flavonoids Protect against LDL Oxidation and Atherosclerosis. *Annals of the New York Academy of Sciences, 957*(1), 146–161.

Azizi, G., Navabi, S., Al-shukaili, A., Seyedzadeh, M. H., Yazdani, R., & Mirshafiey, A. (2015). The role of inflammatory mediators in the pathogenesis of Alzheimer's disease. *Sultan Qaboos University Medical Journal, 15*(3), e315–e316.

Babaeijandaghi, F., Paiero, A., Long, R., Tung, L.W., Smith, S.P., Cheng, R., Smandych, J., Kajabadi, N., Chang, C.-K., Ghassemi, A., Kennedy, W. D. M., Soliman, H., Schutz, P.W., & Rossi, F.M. V. (2022). *TNFα and IFNγ cooperate for efficient pro-to anti-inflammatory transition of macrophages during muscle regeneration*. https://doi.org/10.1073/pnas.

Banerjee, S., Biehl, A., Gadina, M., Hasni, S., & Schwartz, D. M. (2017). JAK–STAT Signaling as a Target for Inflammatory and Autoimmune Diseases: Current and Future Prospects. *Drugs, 77*(5), 521–546. Available from https://doi.org/10.1007/s40265-017-0701-9, Springer International Publishing.

Bartekova, M., Radosinska, J., Jelemensky, M., & Dhalla, N. S. (2018). Role of cytokines and inflammation in heart function during health and disease. *Heart Failure Reviews, 23*(5), 733–758. Available from https://doi.org/10.1007/s10741-018-9716-x, Springer New York LLC.

Bastard, J.-P., Maachi, M., Lagathu, C., Kim, M. J., Caron, M., Vidal, H., Capeau, J., & Feve, B. (2006). Recent advances in the relationship between obesity, inflammation, and insulin resistance. *Europian Cytokine Network, 17*(1), 4–12.

Berlett, B. S., & Stadtman, E. R. (1997). Protein oxidation in aging, disease, and oxidative stress. *Journal of Biological Chemistry, 272*(33), 20313–20316.

Blázquez-Prieto, J., López-Alonso, I., Huidobro, C., & Albaiceta, G. M. (2018). The emerging role of neutrophils in repair after acute lung injury. *American Journal of Respiratory Cell and Molecular Biology, Vol. 59*(Issue 3), 289–294. Available from https://doi.org/10.1165/rcmb.2018-0101PS, American Thoracic Society.

Boehncke, W. H. (2018). Systemic inflammation and cardiovascular comorbidity in psoriasis patients: Causes and consequences. *Frontiers in Immunology, Vol. 9*(APR). Available from https://doi.org/10.3389/fimmu.2018.00579, Frontiers Media S.A.

Bootz, F., & Neri, D. (2015). *Immunocytokines: a novel class of products for the treatment of chronic inflammation and autoimmune conditions.*

Boroumand, N., Samarghandian, S., & Hashemy, S. I. (2018). Immunomodulatory, anti-inflammatory, and antioxidant effects of curcumin. *Journal of Herbmed Pharmacology, 7*(4), 211–219.

Bretscher, P., Egger, J., Shamshiev, A., Trötzmüller, M., Köfeler, H., Carreira, E. M., Kopf, M., & Freigang, S. (2015). Phospholipid oxidation generates potent anti-inflammatory lipid mediators that mimic structurally related pro-resolving eicosanoids by activating Nrf2. *EMBO Molecular Medicine*, *7*(5), 593–607. Available from https://doi.org/10.15252/emmm.201404702.

Caleja, C., Ribeiro, A., Barreiro, M. F., & Ferreira, I. C. F. R. (2017). Phenolic compounds as nutraceuticals or functional food ingredients. *Current Pharmaceutical Design*, *23*(19), 2787–2806.

Campbell, M. S. D., Charnigo, R. J., Westgate, P. M., & Fleenor, B. S. (2019). Influence of enhanced bioavailable curcumin on obesity-associated cardiovascular disease risk factors and arterial function: A double-blinded, randomized, controlled trial. *Nutrition*, *62*, 135–139.

Candelario-Jalil, E., Dijkhuizen, R. M., & Magnus, T. (2022). Neuroinflammation, Stroke, Blood-Brain Barrier Dysfunction, and Imaging Modalities. *Stroke; a Journal of Cerebral Circulation*, *53*(5), 1473–1486. Available from https://doi.org/10.1161/STROKEAHA.122.036946, Lippincott Williams and Wilkins.

Chakrabarti, S., Jahandideh, F., & Wu, J. (2014). Food-derived bioactive peptides on inflammation and oxidative stress. *BioMed Research International*, *2014*, 608979.

Chakrabarti, S., & Wu, J. (2015). Milk-Derived Tripeptides IPP (Ile-Pro-Pro) and VPP (Val-Pro-Pro) Promote Adipocyte Differentiation and Inhibit Inflammation in 3T3-F442A Cells. *PLoS One*, *10*(2)e0117492.

Chan, S., Kantham, S., Rao, V. M., Kumar Palanivelu, M., Pham, H. L., Shaw, P. N., Mcgeary, R. P., & Ross, B. P. (2015). Metal chelation, radical scavenging and inhibition of Ab 42 fibrillation by food constituents in relation to Alzheimer's disease. *Food Chemistry*, *199*, 185–194.

Chao, C. Y., Mong, M. C., Chan, K. C., & Yin, M. C. (2010). Anti-glycative and anti-inflammatory effects of caffeic acid and ellagic acid in kidney of diabetic mice. *Molecular Nutrition & Food Research*, *54*(3), 388–395.

Chen, L., Deng, H., Cui, H., Fang, J., Zuo, Z., Deng, J., Li, Y., Wang, X., & Zhao, L. (2018). Inflammatory responses and inflammation-associated diseases in organs. *Oncotarget*, *9*(6), 7204.

Cheng, M. L., Wang, H. C., Hsu, K. C., & Hwang, J. S. (2015). Anti-inflammatory peptides from enzymatic hydrolysates of tuna cooking juice. *Food and Agricultural Immunology*, *26*(6), 770–781.

Chhikara, N., Panghal, A., & Chaudhary, G. (2021). Functional Foods. *Functional Foods*, 1–568. Available from https://doi.org/10.1002/9781119776345.

Choi, J.-Y., Park, C.-S., Kim, D.-J., Cho, M.-H., Jin, B.-K., Pie, J.-E., & Chung, W.-G. (2002). Prevention of Nitric Oxide-Mediated 1-Methyl-4-Phenyl-1,2,3,6-Tetrahydropyridine-Induced Parkinson's Disease in Mice by Tea Phenolic Epigallocatechin 3-Gallate. *Neurotoxilogy*, *23*(3), 367–374.

Choudhari, A. S., Mandave, P. C., Deshpande, M., Ranjekar, P., & Prakash, O. (2020). Phytochemicals in cancer treatment: From preclinical studies to clinical practice. *Frontiers in Pharmacology*, *10*, 497776.

Chu, A. J. (2014). Antagonism by bioactive polyphenols against inflammation: A systematic view. *Inflammation and Allergy - Drug Targets*, *13*(1), 34–64.

Chuengsamarn, S., Rattanamongkolgul, S., Phonrat, B., Tungtrongchitr, R., & Jirawatnotai, S. (2014). Reduction of atherogenic risk in patients with type 2 diabetes by curcuminoid extract: a randomized controlled trial. *The Journal of Nutritional Biochemistry*, *25*(2), 144–150.

Clemente-Suárez, V. J., Mielgo-Ayuso, J., Martín-Rodríguez, A., Ramos-Campo, D. J., Redondo-Flórez, L., & Tornero-Aguilera, J. F. (2022). The Burden of Carbohydrates in Health and Disease. *Nutrients*, *14*(18), 3809.

Coban, D., Milenkovic, D., Chanet, A., Khallou-Laschet, J., Sabbe, L., Palagani, A., Vanden Berghe, W., Mazur, A., & Morand, C. (2012). Dietary curcumin inhibits atherosclerosis by affecting the expression of genes involved in leukocyte adhesion and transendothelial migration. *Molecular Nutrition & Food Research*, *56*(8), 1270–1281.

Dai, Q., Zhou, D., Xu, L., & Song, X. (2018). Curcumin alleviates rheumatoid arthritis-induced inflammation and synovial hyperplasia by targeting mTOR pathway in rats. *Drug Design, Development and Therapy*, *12*, 4095–4105.

Daliri, E. B. M., Oh, D. H., & Lee, B. H. (2017). Bioactive Peptides. *Foods*, *6*(5), 32.

Dandona, P., Aljada, A., Chaudhuri, A., Mohanty, P., & Garg, R. (2005). Metabolic syndrome: A comprehensive perspective based on interactions between obesity, diabetes, and inflammation. *Circulation*, *111*(11), 1448–1454. Available from https://doi.org/10.1161/01.CIR.0000158483.13093.9D.

Dinarello, C. A. (2010). Anti-inflammatory Agents: Present and Future. *Cell*, *140*(6), 935–950. Available from https://doi.org/10.1016/j.cell.2010.02.043, Elsevier B.V.

Domitrovic, R. (2011). The Molecular Basis for the Pharmacological Activity of Anthocyans. *Current Medicinal Chemistry*, *18*(29), 4454–4469.

Donadio, V., Incensi, A., Rizzo, G., Fileccia, E., Ventruto, F., Riva, A., Tiso, D., Recchia, M., Vacchiano, V., Infante, R., Petrangolini, G., Allegrini, P., Avino, S., Pantieri, R., Mostacci, B., Avoni, P., & Liguori, R. (2022). The Effect of Curcumin on Idiopathic Parkinson Disease: A Clinical and Skin Biopsy Study. *Journal of Neuropathology & Experimental Neurology*, *81*(7), 545–552.

Ehteshamfar, S. M., Akhbari, M., Afshari, J. T., Seyedi, M., Nikfar, B., Shapouri-Moghaddam, A., Ghanbarzadeh, E., & Momtazi-Borojeni, A. A. (2020). Anti-inflammatory and immune-modulatory impacts of berberine on activation of autoreactive T cells in autoimmune inflammation. *Journal of Cellular and Molecular Medicine*, *24*(23), 13573–13588. Available from https://doi.org/10.1111/jcmm.16049, Blackwell Publishing Inc.

Ellis, E. (2022). *Functional Foods*. https://www.eatright.org/health/wellness/healthful-habits/functional-foods.

El-Shamarka, M. E. S., Abdel-Salam, O. M. E., Shafee, N., & Zeidan, H. M. (2023). Curcumin modulation of L-dopa and rasagiline-induced neuroprotection in rotenone model of Parkinson's disease. *Iranian Journal of Basic Medical Sciences*, *26*(2), 139.

Elwakf, A. M., El-Wakf, A. M., El-Habibi, E.-S. M., & Mogalli, A. (2013). Curcumin acts as Cardiovascular Protector via Improving Leptin and Insulin Resistance in Obese Male Rats. *Journal of American Science*, *9*(3), 397–405.

Engelen, S. E., Robinson, A. J. B., Zurke, Y. X., & Monaco, C. (2022). Therapeutic strategies targeting inflammation and immunity in atherosclerosis: how to proceed? *Nature Reviews Cardiology*, *19*(8), 522–542. Available from https://doi.org/10.1038/s41569-021-00668-4, Nature Research.

Ernandes, M.J., & Kagan, J.C. (2021). Interferon-Independent Restriction of RNA Virus Entry and Replication by a Class of Damage-Associated Molecular Patterns. https://doi.org/10.1128/mBio.

Fain, J. N. (2010). Release of inflammatory mediators by human adipose tissue is enhanced in obesity and primarily by the nonfat cells: A review. *Mediators of Inflammation*, *Vol. 2010*. Available from https://doi.org/10.1155/2010/513948.

Feijóo-Bandín, S., Aragón-Herrera, A., Moraña-Fernández, S., Anido-Varela, L., Tarazón, E., Roselló-Lletí, E., Portolés, M., Moscoso, I., Gualillo, O., González-Juanatey, J. R., & Lago, F. (2020). Adipokines and inflammation: Focus on cardiovascular diseases. *International Journal of Molecular Sciences*, *21*(20), 1–34. Available from https://doi.org/10.3390/ijms21207711, MDPI AG.

Feng, S.-W., Lin, W.-C., Lee, I.-T., Luo, S.-D., & Wang, C.-S. (2024). Ribonucleic Acid Sequencing Reveals the Upregulation and Resolution of Inflammation and Extracellular Matrix Remodeling in Lidocaine-Treated Human Acute Monocytic Leukemia Cell Line THP-1. *Biomedicines*, *12* (3), 509. Available from https://doi.org/10.3390/biomedicines12030509.

Fikry, H., Saleh, L. A., & Abdel Gawad, S. (2022). Neuroprotective effects of curcumin on the cerebellum in a rotenone-induced Parkinson's Disease Model. *CNS Neuroscience & Therapeutics*, *28*(5), 732–748.

Frejo, L., & Lopez-Escamez, J. A. (2022). Cytokines and Inflammation in Meniere Disease. *Clinical and Experimental Otorhinolaryngology*, *15*(1), 49–59. Available from https://doi.org/10.21053/ceo.2021.00920, Korean Society of Otolaryngology.

Fu, P., Ebenezer, D. L., Ha, A. W., Suryadevara, V., Harijith, A., & Natarajan, V. (2018). Nuclear lipid mediators: Role of nuclear sphingolipids and sphingosine-1-phosphate signaling in epigenetic regulation of inflammation and gene expression. *Journal of Cellular Biochemistry*, *119*(8), 6337–6353. Available from https://doi.org/10.1002/jcb.26707.

Funamoto, M., Shimizu, K., Sunagawa, Y., Katanasaka, Y., Miyazaki, Y., Kakeya, H., Yamakage, H., Satoh-Asahara, N., Wada, H., Hasegawa, K., & Morimoto, T. (2019). Clinical Study Effects of Highly Absorbable Curcumin in Patients with Impaired Glucose Tolerance and Non-Insulin-Dependent Diabetes Mellitus. *Journal of Diabete Research*, *2019*, 8208237.

Fändrich, M. (2012). Oligomeric Intermediates in Amyloid Formation: Structure Determination and Mechanisms of Toxicity. *Journal of Molecular Biology*, *421*(4-5), 427–440.

Ganjali, S., Sahebkar, A., Mahdipour, E., Jamialahmadi, K., Torabi, S., Akhlaghi, S., Ferns, G., Parizadeh, S. M. R., & Ghayour-Mobarhan, M. (2014). Investigation of the effects of curcumin on serum cytokines in obese individuals: A randomized controlled trial. *The Scientific World Journal*, *2014*, 898361.

Garg, A. D., Vandenberk, L., Fang, S., Fasche, T., Van Eygen, S., Maes, J., Van Woensel, M., Koks, C., Vanthillo, N., Graf, N., De Witte, P., Van Gool, S., Salven, P., & Agostinis, P. (2017). Pathogen response-like recruitment and activation of neutrophils by sterile immunogenic dying cells drives neutrophil-mediated residual cell killing. *Cell Death and Differentiation*, *24*(5), 832–843. Available from https://doi.org/10.1038/cdd.2017.15.

Ge, H., Cai, Z., Chai, J., Liu, J., Liu, B., Yu, Y., Liu, J., & Zhang, T. (2021). Egg white peptides ameliorate dextran sulfate sodium-induced acute colitis symptoms by inhibiting the production of pro-inflammatory cytokines and modulation of gut microbiota composition. *Food Chemistry*, *360*, 129981.

Ghosh, S. S., Gehr, T. W. B., & Ghosh, S. (2014). Curcumin and Chronic Kidney Disease (CKD): Major Mode of Action through Stimulating Endogenous Intestinal Alkaline Phosphatase. *Molecules (Basel, Switzerland)*, *19*(12), 20139–20156.

Ginckels, P., & Holvoet, P. (2022). Oxidative Stress and Inflammation in Cardiovascular Diseases and Cancer: Role of Non-coding RNAs. *YALE JOURNAL OF BIOLOGY AND MEDICINE*, *Vol. 95*.

Guha, S., & Majumder, K. (2019). Structural-features of food-derived bioactive peptides with anti-inflammatory activity: A brief review. *Journal of Food Biochemistry*, *43*(1)e12531.

Guo, Y. J., Dong, S. Y., Cui, X. X., Feng, Y., Liu, T., Yin, M., Kuo, S. H., Tan, E. K., Zhao, W. J., & Wu, Y. C. (2016). Resveratrol alleviates MPTP-induced motor impairments and pathological changes by autophagic degradation of α-synuclein via SIRT1-deacetylated LC3. *Molecular Nutrition & Food Research*, *60*(10), 2161–2175.

Gupta, S. C., Tyagi, A. K., Deshmukh-Taskar, P., Hinojosa, M., Prasad, S., & Aggarwal, B. B. (2014). Downregulation of tumor necrosis factor and other proinflammatory biomarkers by polyphenols. *Archives of Biochemistry and Biophysics*, *559*, 91–99.

Gómez-Ambrosi, J. (2023). Adipose Tissue Inflammation. *Cells*, *Vol. 12*(Issue 11). Available from https://doi.org/10.3390/cells12111484, MDPI.

Hall, S. C., & Agrawal, D. K. (2016). Toll-like receptors, triggering receptor expressed on myeloid cells family members and receptor for advanced glycation end-products in allergic airway inflammation. *Expert Review of Respiratory Medicine*, *10*(2), 171–184. Available from https://doi.org/10.1586/17476348.2016.1133303, Taylor and Francis Ltd.

Handique, J. G., & Baruah, J. B. (2002). P olyphenolic compounds: an overview. *Reactive & Functional Polymers*, *52*, 163–188.

He, Y., Yue, Y., Zheng, X., Zhang, K., Chen, S., & Du, Z. (2015). Curcumin, Inflammation, and Chronic Diseases: How Are They Linked? *Molecules (Basel, Switzerland)*, *20*(5), 9183–9213.

Hesari, A. R., Azizian, M., Sheikhi, A., Nesaei, A., Sanaei, S., Mahinparvar, N., Derakhshani, M., Hedayt, P., Ghasemi, F., & Mirzaei, H. (2019). Chemopreventive and therapeutic potential of curcumin in esophageal cancer: Current and future status. *International Journal of Cancer*, *144*(6), 1215–1226.

Hsieh, C. C., Hernández-Ledesma, B., & De Lumen, B. O. (2010). Soybean Peptide Lunasin Suppresses In Vitro and In Vivo 7,12-Dimethylbenz[a]anthracene-Induced Tumorigenesis. *Journal of Food Science, 75*(9), H311–H316.

Hu, X., li, J., Fu, M., Zhao, X., & Wang, W. (2021). The JAK/STAT signaling pathway: from bench to clinic. *Signal Transduction and Targeted Therapy, 6*(1). Available from https://doi.org/10.1038/s41392-021-00791-1, Springer Nature.

Huerta-Delgado, A. S., Roffe-Vazquez, D. N., Gonzalez-Gil, A. M., Villarreal-Calderón, J. R., Tamez-Rivera, O., Rodriguez-Gutierrez, N. A., Castillo, E. C., Silva-Platas, C., Garcia-Rivas, G., & Elizondo-Montemayor, L. (2020). Serum Irisin Levels, Endothelial Dysfunction, and Inflammation in Pediatric Patients with Type 2 Diabetes Mellitus and Metabolic Syndrome. *Journal of Diabetes Research, 2020*. Available from https://doi.org/10.1155/2020/1949415.

Hung, Y.-L., & Suzuki, K. (2017). The Pattern Recognition Receptors and Lipopolysaccharides (LPS)-induced Systemic Inflammation. *International Journal of Research Studies in Medical and Health Sciences, 2*(7).

Hämäläinen, M., Nieminen, R., Vuorela, P., Heinonen, M., & Moilanen, E. (2007). Anti-inflammatory effects of flavonoids: Genistein, kaempferol, quercetin, and daidzein inhibit STAT-1 and NF-κB activations, whereas flavone, isorhamnetin, naringenin, and pelargonidin inhibit only NF-κB activation along with their inhibitory effect on iNOS expression and NO production in activated macrophages. *Mediators of Inflammation, 2007*, 45673.

Ilich, J. Z., Kelly, O. J., Kim, Y., & Spicer, M. T. (2014). Low-grade chronic inflammation perpetuated by modern diet as a promoter of obesity and osteoporosis. *Arhiv za Higijenu Rada i Toksikologiju, 65*(2), 139–147.

Immler, R., Simon, S. I., & Sperandio, M. (2018). Calcium signalling and related ion channels in neutrophil recruitment and function. *European Journal of Clinical Investigation, Vol. 48*. Available from https://doi.org/10.1111/eci.12964, Blackwell Publishing Ltd.

Jalili-Nik, M., Soltani, A., Moussavi, S., Ghayour-Mobarhan, M., Ferns, G. A., Hassanian, S. M., & Avan, A. (2018). Current status and future prospective of Curcumin as a potential therapeutic agent in the treatment of colorectal cancer. *Journal of Cellular Physiology, 233*(9), 6337–6345.

Jasso, G. J., Jaiswal, A., Varma, M., Laszewski, T., Grauel, A., Omar, A., Silva, N., Dranoff, G., Porter, J. A., Mansfield, K., Cremasco, V., Regev, A., Xavier, R. J., & Graham, D. B. (2022). Colon stroma mediates an inflammation-driven fibroblastic response controlling matrix remodeling and healing. *PLoS Biology, 20*(1). Available from https://doi.org/10.1371/journal.pbio.3001532.

Jazayeri-Tehrani, S. A., Rezayat, S. M., Mansouri, S., Qorbani, M., Alavian, S. M., Daneshi-Maskooni, M., & Hosseinzadeh-Attar, M. J. (2019). Nano-curcumin improves glucose indices, lipids, inflammation, and Nesfatin in overweight and obese patients with non-alcoholic fatty liver disease (NAFLD): A double-blind randomized placebo-controlled clinical trial. *Nutrition and Metabolism, 16*(1), 1–13.

Jiang, Y., Zhang, J., Shi, C., Li, X., Jiang, Y., & Mao, R. (2023). *NF-κB: a mediator that promotes or inhibits angiogenesis in human diseases? Expert Reviews in Molecular Medicine* (Vol. 25). Cambridge University Press. Available from https://doi.org/10.1017/erm.2023.20.

Kang, H., Ma, J., Wu, D., Shen, W. H., & Zhu, Y. (2019). Functional coordination of the chromatin-remodeling factor AtiNO80 and the histone chaperones NRP1/2 in inflorescence meristem and root apical meristem. *Frontiers in Plant Science, 10*. Available from https://doi.org/10.3389/fpls.2019.00115.

Kany, S., Vollrath, J. T., & Relja, B. (2019). Cytokines in inflammatory disease. *International Journal of Molecular Sciences, 20*(23). Available from https://doi.org/10.3390/ijms20236008, MDPI AG.

Khoddami, A., Wilkes, M. A., & Roberts, T. H. (2013). Techniques for Analysis of Plant Phenolic Compounds. *Molecules (Basel, Switzerland), 18*(2), 2328–2375.

Killian, P., Kronski, E., Michalik, K. M., Barbieri, O., Astigiano, O., & Sommerhoff, C. P. (2012). Curcumin inhibits prostate cancer metastasis in vivo by targeting the inflammatory cytokines CXCL1 and -2. *Carcinogenesis, 33*(12), 2507–2519.

Kinney, S. R. M., Carlson, L., Ser-Dolansky, J., Thompson, C., Shah, S., Gambrah, A., Xing, W., Schneider, S. S., & Mathias, C. B. (2015). Curcumin Ingestion Inhibits Mastocytosis and Suppresses Intestinal Anaphylaxis in a Murine Model of Food Allergy. *PLoS One, 10*(7)e0132467.

Kong, L., Luo, C., Li, X., Zhou, Y., & He, H. (2013). The anti-inflammatory effect of kaempferol on early atherosclerosis in high cholesterol fed rabbits. *Lipids in Health and Disease, 12*(1), 1–12.

Kovacs-Nolan, J., Zhang, H., Ibuki, M., Nakamori, T., Yoshiura, K., Turner, P. V., Matsui, T., & Mine, Y. (2012). The PepT1-transportable soy tripeptide VPY reduces intestinal inflammation. *Biochimica et Biophysica Acta - General Subjects, 1820*(11), 1753–1763.

Kronski, E., Fiori, M. E., Barbieri, O., Astigiano, S., Mirisola, V., Killian, P. H., Bruno, A., Pagani, A., Rovera, F., Pfeffer, U., Sommerhoff, C. P., Noonan, D. M., Nerlich, A. G., Fontana, L., & Bachmeier, B. E. (2014). miR181b is induced by the chemopreventive polyphenol curcumin and inhibits breast cancer metastasis via down-regulation of the inflammatory cytokines CXCL1 and -2. *Molecular Oncology, 8*(3), 581.

Kunnumakkara, A. B., Bordoloi, D., Harsha, C., Banik, K., Gupta, S. C., & Aggarwal, B. B. (2017). Curcumin mediates anticancer effects by modulating multiple cell signaling pathways. *Clinical Science, 131*(15), 1781–1799.

Kunnumakkara, A. B., Diagaradjane, P., Anand, P., Kuzhuvelil, H. B., Deorukhkar, A., Gelovani, J., Guha, S., Krishnan, S., & Aggarwal, B. B. (2009). Curcumin sensitizes human colorectal cancer to capecitabine by modulation of cyclin D1, COX-2, MMP-9, VEGF and CXCR4 expression in an orthotopic mouse model. *International Journal of Cancer, 125*(9), 2187–2197.

Kwak, S. J., Kim, C. S., Choi, M. S., Park, T., Sung, M. K., Yun, J. W., Yoo, H., Mine, Y., & Yu, R. (2016). The Soy Peptide Phe-Leu-Val Reduces TNFα-Induced Inflammatory Response and Insulin Resistance in Adipocytes. *Journal of Medicinal Food, 19*(7), 678–685.

Lee, B.-C., & Lee, J. (2013). Cellular and molecular players in adipose tissue inflammation in the development of obesity-induced insulin resistance. *Biochimica et Biophysica Acta, 1842*(3), 446–462.

Li, H., Sureda, A., Devkota, H. P., Pittalà, V., Barreca, D., Sanches Silva, A., Tewari, D., Xu, S., & Nabavi, S. M. (2019). Curcumin, the golden spice in treating cardiovascular diseases. *Biotechnology Advances, 38*, 107343.

Li, H.-Q., Luo, Y., & Qiao, C.-H. (2012). The Mechanisms of Anticancer Agents by Genistein and Synthetic Derivatives of Isoflavone. *Mini-Reviews in Medicinal Chemistry*, *12*(4), 350–362.

Li, Y., Huang, H., Liu, B., Zhang, Y., Pan, X., Yu, X. Y., Shen, Z., & Song, Y. H. (2021). Inflammasomes as therapeutic targets in human diseases. *Signal Transduction and Targeted Therapy*, *6*(1). Available from https://doi.org/10.1038/s41392-021-00650-z, Springer Nature.

Liu, M., Chen, F., Sha, L., Wang, S., Tao, L., Yao, L., He, M., Yao, Z., Liu, H., Zhu, Z., Zhang, Z., Zheng, Z., Sha, X., & Wei, M. (2014). (-)-Epigallocatechin-3-gallate ameliorates learning and memory deficits by adjusting the balance of TrkA/p75NTR signaling in APP/PS1 transgenic mice. *Molecular Neurobiology*, *49*(3), 1350–1363.

Liu, Z. K., Xiao, H. B., & Fang, J. (2013). Anti-inflammatory properties of kaempferol via its inhibition of aldosterone signaling and aldosterone-induced gene expression. *The Canadian Journal of Physiology and Pharmacology*, *92*(2), 117–123.

Luo, R., Wan, Y., Luo, X., Liu, G., Li, Z., Chen, J., Su, D., Lu, N., & Luo, Z. (2022). A Rapid Self-Assembly Peptide Hydrogel for Recruitment and Activation of Immune Cells. *Molecules (Basel, Switzerland)*, *27*(2). Available from https://doi.org/10.3390/molecules27020419.

López-Barrios, L., Antunes-Ricardo, M., & Gutiérrez-Uribe, J. A. (2016). Changes in antioxidant and antiinflammatory activity of black bean (Phaseolus vulgaris L.) protein isolates due to germination and enzymatic digestion. *Food Chemistry*, *203*, 417–424.

Majumder, K., Mine, Y., & Wu, J. (2016). The potential of food protein-derived anti-inflammatory peptides against various chronic inflammatory diseases. *Journal of the Science of Food and Agriculture*, *96*(7), 2303–2311.

Manna, S. K., Mukhopadhyay, A., & Aggarwal, B. B. (2000). Resveratrol Suppresses TNF-Induced Activation of Nuclear Transcription Factors NF-κB, Activator Protein-1, and Apoptosis: Potential Role of Reactive Oxygen Intermediates and Lipid Peroxidation. *The Journal of Immunology*, *164*(12), 6509–6519.

Mansouri, K., Rasoulpoor, S., Daneshkhah, A., Abolfathi, S., Salari, N., Mohammadi, M., Rasoulpoor, S., & Shabani, S. (2020). Clinical effects of curcumin in enhancing cancer therapy: A systematic review. *BMC Cancer*, *20*(1), 1–11.

Martirosyan, D. M., & Singh, J. (2015). A new definition of functional food by FFC: what makes a new definition unique? *Functional Foods in Health and Disease*, *5*(6), 209–223. Available from https://doi.org/10.31989/FFHD.V5I6.183.

Medzhitov, R. (2010). Inflammation 2010: New Adventures of an Old Flame. *Cell*, *140*(6), 771–776.

Memarzia, A., Saadat, S., Behrouz, S., & Boskabady, M. H. (2022). Curcuma longa and curcumin affect respiratory and allergic disorders, experimental and clinical evidence: A comprehensive and updated review. *Biofactors (Oxford, England)*, *48*(3), 521–551.

Meza Márquez, O. G., Juárez-Chairez, M. F., Márquez-Flores, Y. K., Jiménez-Martínez, C., & Osorio-Revilla, G. (2022). In vitro anti-inflammatory and antioxidant activity of chickpea (Cicer arietinum L.) proteins hydrolysate fractions. *Biotecnia*, *24*(2), 59–68.

Mokgalaboni, K., Ntamo, Y., Ziqubu, K., Nyambuya, T. M., Nkambule, B. B., Mazibuko-Mbeje, S. E., Gabuza, K. B., Chellan, N., Tiano, L., & Dludla, P. V. (2021). Curcumin supplementation improves biomarkers of oxidative stress and inflammation in conditions of obesity, type 2 diabetes and NAFLD: updating the status of clinical evidence. *Food & Function*, *12*(24), 12235–12249.

Moyse, E., Krantic, S., Djellouli, N., Roger, S., Angoulvant, D., Debacq, C., Leroy, V., Fougere, B., & Aidoud, A. (2022). Neuroinflammation: A Possible Link Between Chronic Vascular Disorders and Neurodegenerative Diseases. *Frontiers in Aging Neuroscience*, *Vol. 14*. Available from https://doi.org/10.3389/fnagi.2022.827263, Frontiers Media S.A.

Murakami, M., & Hirano, T. (2012). The molecular mechanisms of chronic inflammation development. *Frontiers in Immunology*, *3*, 323.

Naik, E., & Dixit, V. M. (2011). Mitochondrial reactive oxygen species drive proinflammatory cytokine production. *Journal of Experimental Medicine*, *208*(3), 417–420.

Nailwal, H., & Chan, F. K. M. (2019). Necroptosis in anti-viral inflammation. *Cell Death and Differentiation*, *26*(1), 4–13. Available from https://doi.org/10.1038/s41418-018-0172-x, Nature Publishing Group.

Nakamura, T., Hirota, T., Mizushima, K., Ohki, K., Naito, Y., Yamamoto, N., & Yoshikawa, T. (2013). Milk-Derived Peptides, Val-Pro-Pro and Ile-Pro-Pro, Attenuate Atherosclerosis Development in Apolipoprotein E–Deficient Mice: A Preliminary Study. *Journal of Medicinal Food*, *16*(5), 396–403.

Nazmi, A., Field, R. H., Griffin, E. W., Haugh, O., Hennessy, E., Cox, D., Reis, R., Tortorelli, L., Murray, C. L., Lopez-Rodriguez, A. B., Jin, L., Lavelle, E. C., Dunne, A., & Cunningham, C. (2019). Chronic neurodegeneration induces type I interferon synthesis via STING, shaping microglial phenotype and accelerating disease progression. *Glia*, *67*(7), 1254–1276. Available from https://doi.org/10.1002/glia.23592.

Neyrinck, A. M., Van Hée, V. F., Bindels, L. B., De Backer, F., Cani, P. D., & Delzenne, N. M. (2013). Polyphenol-rich extract of pomegranate peel alleviates tissue inflammation and hypercholesterolaemia in high-fat diet-induced obese mice: potential implication of the gut microbiota. *British Journal of Nutrition*, *109*(5), 802–809.

Oliveira, M. C., Menezes-Garcia, Z., Henriques, M. C. C., Soriani, F. M., Pinho, V., Faria, A. M. C., Santiago, A. F., Cara, D. C., Souza, D. G., Teixeira, M. M., & Ferreira, A. V. M. (2013). Acute and sustained inflammation and metabolic dysfunction induced by high refined carbohydrate-containing diet in mice. *Obesity*, *21*(9), E396–E406.

Onalan, E., Bozkurt, A., Gursu, M. F., Yakar, B., & Donder, E. (2022). Role of Betatrophin and Inflammation Markers in Type 2 Diabetes Mellitus, Prediabetes and Metabolic Syndrome. *Journal of the College of Physicians and Surgeons Pakistan*, *32*(3), 303–307. Available from https://doi.org/10.29271/jcpsp.2022.03.303.

Padoan, A., Plebani, M., & Basso, D. (2019). Inflammation and pancreatic cancer: Focus on metabolism, cytokines, and immunity. *International Journal of Molecular Sciences*, *20*(3). Available from https://doi.org/10.3390/ijms20030676, MDPI AG.

Pahler, J. C., Tazzyman, S., Erez, N., Chen, Y. Y., Murdoch, C., Nozawa, H., Lewis, C. E., & Hanahan, D. (2008). Plasticity in tumor-promoting inflammation: Impairment of macrophage recruitment evokes a compensatory neutrophil response. *Neoplasia (New York, N.Y.)*, *10*(4), 329–339. Available from https://doi.org/10.1593/neo.07871.

Panahi, Y., Hosseini, S., Khalili, N., Naimi, E., Simental-Mendía, L.E., Majeed, M., & Sahebkar, A. (2016). Effects of curcumin on serum cytokine concentrations in subjects with metabolic syndrome: A post-hoc analysis of a randomized controlled trial. *Biomedicine & Pharmacotheraphy, 82*, 578-582

Park, J. Y., Chung, T. W., Jeong, Y. J., Kwak, C. H., Ha, S. H., Kwon, K. M., Abekura, F., Cho, S. H., Lee, Y. C., Ha, K. T., Magae, J., Chang, Y. C., & Kim, C. H. (2017). Ascofuranone inhibits lipopolysaccharideinduced inflammatory response via nfkappab and ap-1, p-ERK, TNF-α, IL-6 and IL-1β in RAW 264.7 macrophages. *PLoS One, 12*(2). Available from https://doi.org/10.1371/journal.pone.0171322.

Patra, S., Pradhan, B., Nayak, R., Behera, C., Das, S., Patra, S. K., Efferth, T., Jena, M., & Kumar Bhutia, S. (2021). Dietary polyphenols in chemoprevention and synergistic effect in cancer: Clinical evidences and molecular mechanisms of action. *Phytomedicine : International Journal of Phytotherapy and Phytopharmacology, 90*, 153554.

Pendurthi, U.R., Williams, J.T., Vijaya, L., & Rao, M. (1997). *Inhibition of Tissue Factor Gene Activation in Cultured Endothelial Cells by Curcumin Suppression of Activation of Transcription Factors Egr-1, AP-1, and NF-KB*. http://ahajournals.org.

Peng, Y., Ao, M., Dong, B., Jiang, Y., Yu, L., Chen, Z., Hu, C., & Xu, R. (2021). Anti-inflammatory effects of curcumin in the inflammatory diseases: Status, limitations and countermeasures. *Drug Design, Development and Therapy, 15*, 4503–4525.

Piccolomini, A. F., Iskandar, M. M., Lands, L. C., & Kubow, S. (2012). High hydrostatic pressure pre-treatment of whey proteins enhances whey protein hydrolysate inhibition of oxidative stress and IL-8 secretion in intestinal epithelial cells. *Food & Nutrition Research, 56*.

Pourhabibi-Zarandi, F., Rafraf, M., Zayeni, H., Asghari-Jafarabadi, M., & Ebrahimi, A. A. (2022). Effects of curcumin supplementation on metabolic parameters, inflammatory factors and obesity values in women with rheumatoid arthritis: A randomized, double-blind, placebo-controlled clinical trial. *Phytotherapy Research, 36*(4), 1797–1806.

Priyadarsini, K. I. (2014). The Chemistry of Curcumin: From Extraction to Therapeutic Agent. *Molecules (Basel, Switzerland), 19*(12), 20091.

Prusty, B. K., & Das, B. C. (2005). Constitutive activation of transcription factor AP-1 in cervical cancer and suppression of human papillomavirus (HPV) transcription and AP-1 activity in HeLa cells by curcumin. *International Journal of Cancer, 113*(6), 951–960.

Reinehr, T., & Roth, C. L. (2018). Inflammation Markers in Type 2 Diabetes and the Metabolic Syndrome in the Pediatric Population. *Current Diabetes Reports, 18*(12). Available from https://doi.org/10.1007/s11892-018-1110-5, Current Medicine Group LLC 1.

Reyes-Farias, M., & Carrasco-Pozo, C. (2019). The Anti-Cancer Effect of Quercetin: Molecular Implications in Cancer Metabolism. *International Journal of Molecular Sciences, 20*(13), 3177.

Ricordi, C., Garcia-Contreras, M., & Farnetti, S. (2015). Diet and Inflammation: Possible Effects on Immunity, Chronic Diseases, and Life Span. *Journal of the American College of Nutrition, 34*, 10–13.

Rigamonti, E., Zordan, P., Sciorati, C., Rovere-Querini, P., & Brunelli, S. (2014). Macrophage plasticity in skeletal muscle repair. *BioMed Research International, 2014*. Available from https://doi.org/10.1155/2014/560629, Hindawi Publishing Corporation.

Ringman, J. M., Frautschy, S. A., Teng, E., Begum, A. N., Bardens, J., Beigi, M., Gylys, K. H., Badmaev, V., Heath, D. D., Apostolova, L. G., Porter, V., Vanek, Z., Marshall, G. A., Hellemann, G., Sugar, C., Masterman, D. L., Montine, T. J., Cummings, J. L., & Cole, G. M. (2012). Oral curcumin for Alzheimer's disease: Tolerability and efficacy in a 24-week randomized, double blind, placebo-controlled study. *Alzheimer's Research and Therapy, 4*(5), 1–8.

Roberfroid, M. B. (2002). Global view on functional foods: European perspectives. *British Journal of Nutrition, 88*(S2), S133–S138. Available from https://doi.org/10.1079/BJN2002677.

Ruze, R., Liu, T., Zou, X., Song, J., Chen, Y., Xu, R., Yin, X., & Xu, Q. (2023). Obesity and type 2 diabetes mellitus: connections in epidemiology, pathogenesis, and treatments. *Frontiers in Endocrinology, 14*, 1161521.

Saraf-Bank, S., Ahmadi, A., Paknahad, Z., Maracy, M., & Nourian, M. (2019). Effects of curcumin supplementation on markers of inflammation and oxidative stress among healthy overweight and obese girl adolescents: A randomized placebo-controlled clinical trial. *Phytotherapy Research, 33* (8), 2015–2022.

Sato, T., Takeuchi, M., Karasawa, Y., Enoki, T., & Ito, M. (2018). Intraocular inflammatory cytokines in patients with neovascular age-related macular degeneration before and after initiation of intravitreal injection of anti-VEGF inhibitor. *Scientific Reports, 8*(1). Available from https://doi.org/10.1038/s41598-018-19594-6.

Schebb, N. H., Kühn, H., Kahnt, A. S., Rund, K. M., O'Donnell, V. B., Flamand, N., Peters-Golden, M., Jakobsson, P. J., Weylandt, K. H., Rohwer, N., Murphy, R. C., Geisslinger, G., FitzGerald, G. A., Hanson, J., Dahlgren, C., Alnouri, M. W., Offermanns, S., & Steinhilber, D. (2022). Formation, Signaling and Occurrence of Specialized Pro-Resolving Lipid Mediators—What is the Evidence so far? *Frontiers in Pharmacology, Vol. 13*. Available from https://doi.org/10.3389/fphar.2022.838782, Frontiers Media S.A.

Schwartz, B., & Yehuda-Shnaidman, E. (2014). Putative role of adipose tissue in growth and metabolism of colon cancer cells. *Frontiers in Oncology, 4*, 164.

Shehzad, A., Rehman, G., & Lee, Y. S. (2012). Review Article Curcumin in Inflammatory Diseases. *Biofactors (Oxford, England), 39*(1), 69–77.

Shi, B., Chen, M., Xia, Z., Tang, W., Li, Y., Qin, C., Ahmadi, A., Huang, C., & Xu, H. (2023). Genistein attenuates neuroinflammation and oxidative stress and improves cognitive impairment in a rat model of sepsis-associated encephalopathy: potential role of the Nrf2 signaling pathway. *Metabolic Brain Disease, 38*(1), 339–347.

Shimizu, K., Funamoto, M., Sunagawa, Y., Shimizu, S., Katanasaka, Y., Miyazaki, Y., Wada, H., Hasegawa, K., & Morimoto, T. (2019). Anti-inflammatory Action of Curcumin and Its Use in the Treatment of Lifestyle-related Diseases. *European Cardiology Review, 14*(2), 117.

Simõ Es Pires, E. N., Luiz Frozza, R., Hoppe, J. B., De, B., Menezes, M., & Salbego, G. (2014). Berberine was neuroprotective against an in vitro model of brain ischemia: Survival and apoptosis pathways involved. *Brain Research, 1557*, 26–33.

Singla, R. K., Dubey, A. K., Garg, A., Sharma, R. K., Fiorino, M., Ameen, S. M., Haddad, M. A., & Al-Hiary, M. (2019). Natural Polyphenols: Chemical Classification, Definition of Classes, Subcategories, and Structures. *Journal of AOAC International*, *102*(5), 1397–1400.

Song, H., Shen, X., Chu, Q., & Zheng, X. (2022). Pomegranate fruit pulp polyphenols reduce diet-induced obesity with modulation of gut microbiota in mice. *Journal of the Science of Food and Agriculture*, *102*(5), 1968–1977.

Song, Y., Li, Z., Gao, Q., Pavase, T. R., & Lin, H. (2016). Effect of malonaldehyde cross-linking on the ability of shrimp tropomyosin to elicit the release of inflammatory mediators and cytokines from activated RBL-2H3 cells. *Journal of the Science of Food and Agriculture*, *96*(12), 4263–4267. Available from https://doi.org/10.1002/jsfa.7637.

Stankov, S. V. (2012). Definition of Inflammation, Causes of Inflammation and Possible Anti-inflammatory Strategies. *The Open Inflammation Journal*, *5*.

Stefani, G., & Slack, F. J. (2008). Small non-coding RNAs in animal development. *Nature Reviews. Molecular Cell Biology*, *9*(3), 219–230.

Suganthy, N., Devi, K. P., Fazel Nabavi, S., Braidy, N., & Nabavi, S. M. (2016). Bioactive effects of quercetin in the central nervous system: Focusing on the mechanisms of actions. *Biomedicine & Pharmocotheraphy*, *84*, 892–908.

Suzuki, K. (2019). Characterization of Exercise-Induced Cytokine Release, the Impacts on the Body, the Mechanisms and Modulations. *International Journal of Sports and Exercise Medicine*, *5*(3). Available from https://doi.org/10.23937/2469-5718/1510122.

Swinbanks, D., & O'Brien, J. (1993). Japan explores the boundary between food and medicine. *Nature*, *364*(6434), 180. Available from https://doi.org/10.1038/364180A0.

Szade, A., Grochot-Przeczek, A., Florczyk, U., Jozkowicz, A., & Dulak, J. (2015). Cellular and molecular mechanisms of inflammation-induced angiogenesis. *IUBMB Life*, *67*(3), 145–159. Available from https://doi.org/10.1002/iub.1358.

Sánchez, A., & Vázquez, A. (2017). Bioactive peptides: A review. *Food Quality and Safety*, *1*(1), 29–46.

Teixeira, F. B., Saito, M. T., Matheus, F. C., Prediger, R. D., Yamada, E. S., Maia, C. S. F., & Lima, R. R. (2017). Periodontitis and alzheimer's disease: A possible comorbidity between oral chronic inflammatory condition and neuroinflammation. *Frontiers in Aging Neuroscience*, *9*(OCT). Available from https://doi.org/10.3389/fnagi.2017.00327.

Teodoro, A. J. (2019). Bioactive Compounds of Food: Their Role in the Prevention and Treatment of Diseases. *Oxidative Medicine and Cellular Longevity*, *2019*, 3765686.

Tilg, H., & Moschen, A. R. (2006). Adipocytokines: Mediators linking adipose tissue, inflammation and immunity. *Nature Reviews. Immunology*, *6* (10), 772–783. Available from https://doi.org/10.1038/nri1937.

Tili, E., Croce, C. M., & Michaille, J. J. (2009). MiR-155: On the crosstalk between inflammation and cancer. *International Reviews of Immunology*, *28*(5), 264–284.

Tili, E., & Michaille, J. J. (2011). Resveratrol, MicroRNAs, inflammation, and cancer. *Journal of Nucleic Acids*, *2011*, 102431.

Tjalkens, R. B., Popichak, K. A., & Kirkley, K. A. (2017). Inflammatory Activation of Microglia and Astrocytes in Manganese Neurotoxicity. *Advances in Neurobiology*, *18*, 159–181. Available from https://doi.org/10.1007/978-3-319-60189-2_8, Springer New York LLC.

Tsigalou, C., Konstantinidis, T., Paraschaki, A., Stavropoulou, E., Voidarou, C., & Bezirtzoglou, E. (2020). Mediterranean Diet as a Tool to Combat Inflammation and Chronic Diseases. An Overview. *Biomedicines*, *8*(7), 201.

Varì, R., Scazzocchio, B., Silenzi, A., Giovannini, C., & Masella, R. (2021). Obesity-Associated Inflammation: Does Curcumin Exert a Beneficial Role? *Nutrients*, *13*(3), 1021.

Vicentini, A., Liberatore, L., & Mastrocola, D. (2016). FUNCTIONAL FOODS: TRENDS AND DEVELOPMENT OF THE GLOBAL MARKET. *Italian Journal of Food Science*, *28*(2), 338–351. Available from https://doi.org/10.14674/1120-1770/IJFS.V211.

Vidya Priyadarsini, R., Senthil Murugan, R., Maitreyi, S., Ramalingam, K., Karunagaran, D., & Nagini, S. (2010). The flavonoid quercetin induces cell cycle arrest and mitochondria-mediated apoptosis in human cervical cancer (HeLa) cells through p53 induction and NF-κB inhibition. *European Journal of Pharmacology*, *649*(1–3), 84–91.

Viola, A., Munari, F., Sánchez-Rodríguez, R., Scolaro, T., & Castegna, A. (2019). The metabolic signature of macrophage responses. *Frontiers in Immunology*, *10*(JULY). Available from https://doi.org/10.3389/fimmu.2019.01462, Frontiers Media S.A.

Voulgaropoulou, S. D., Van Amelsvoort, T. A. M. J., Prickaerts, J., & Vingerhoets, C. (2019). The effect of curcumin on cognition in Alzheimer's disease and healthy aging: A systematic review of pre-clinical and clinical studies. *Brain Research*, *1725*, 146476.

Walker, K. A., Ficek, B. N., & Westbrook, R. (2019). Understanding the Role of Systemic Inflammation in Alzheimer's Disease. *ACS Chemical Neuroscience*, *10*(8), 3340–3342.

Wang, M., Jiang, S., Zhou, L., Yu, F., Ding, H., Li, P., Zhou, M., & Wang, K. (2019). Potential Mechanisms of Action of Curcumin for Cancer Prevention: Focus on Cellular Signaling Pathways and miRNAs. *International Journal of Biological Sciences*, *15*(6), 1200.

Wani, S. A., Singh, A., & Kumar, P. (2022). Spice Bioactive Compounds: Properties, Applications, and Health Benefits. *Spice Bioactive Compounds: Properties, Applications, and Health Benefits*, 1–360. Available from https://doi.org/10.1201/9781003215387.

Weisberg, S. P., Leibel, R., & Tortoriello, D. V. (2008). Dietary Curcumin Significantly Improves Obesity-Associated Inflammation and Diabetes in Mouse Models of Diabesity. *Endocrinology*, *149*(7), 3549–3558.

Wellen, K. E., & Hotamisligil, G. S. (2003). Obesity-induced inflammatory changes in adipose tissue. *The Journal of Clinical Investigation*, *112*(12), 1785–1788.

Wen, Y., Zhu, Y., Zhang, C., Yang, X., Gao, Y., Li, M., Yang, H., Liu, T., & Tang, H. (2022). Chronic inflammation, cancer development and immunotherapy. *Frontiers in Pharmacology*, *13*, 1040163.

Wongcharoen, W., & Phrommintikul, A. (2009). The protective role of curcumin in cardiovascular diseases. *International Journal of Cardiology*, *133*, 145–151.

Xiong, Z., Hongmei, Z., Lu, S., Li, Y., & Yu, L. (2011). Curcumin mediates presenilin-1 activity to reduce b-amyloid production in a model of Alzheimer's disease. *Pharmocological report, 63*(5), 1101–1108.

Yahfoufi, N., Alsadi, N., Jambi, M., & Matar, C. (2018). The Immunomodulatory and Anti-Inflammatory Role of Polyphenols. *Nutrients, 10*(11), 1618.

Yamashita, A. S., Belchior, T., Lira, F. S., Bishop, N. C., Wessner, B., Rosa, J. C., & Festuccia, W. T. (2018). Regulation of Metabolic Disease-Associated Inflammation by Nutrient Sensors. *Mediators of Inflammation, 2018*, 8261432.

Yan, L., Vaghari-Tabari, M., Malakoti, F., Moein, S., Qujeq, D., Yousefi, B., & Asemi, Z. (2023). Quercetin: an effective polyphenol in alleviating diabetes and diabetic complications. *Critical Reviews in Food Science and Nutrition, 63*(28), 9163–9186.

Yang, X., Lv, J. N., Li, H., Jiao, B., Zhang, Q. H., Zhang, Y., Zhang, J., Liu, Y. Q., Zhang, M., Shan, H., Zhang, J. Z., Wu, R. M., & Li, Y. L. (2017). Curcumin reduces lung inflammation via Wnt/β-catenin signaling in mouse model of asthma. *Journal of Asthma, 54*(4), 335–340.

Yerokun, T. (2014). Expression of C-Terminal Modified Serine Palmitoyltransferase-1 Alters Chemosensitivity of Inflammation-Associated Human Cancer Cell Lines. *Journal of Cancer Therapy, 05*(10), 902–919.

Yoon, H., Lee, E., Lee, H., Cho, I. J., Choi, Y. J., Sung, M. S., Yoo, H. G., & Yoo, W. H. (2013). Kaempferol inhibits IL-1β-induced proliferation of rheumatoid arthritis synovial fibroblasts and the production of COX-2, PGE2 and MMPs. *International Journal of Molecular Medicine, 32*(4), 971–977.

Youn, H. S., Jeong, J. C., Jeong, Y. S., Kim, E. J., & Um, S. J. (2013). Quercetin Potentiates Apoptosis by Inhibiting Nuclear Factor-kappaB Signaling in H460 Lung Cancer Cells. *Biological and Pharmaceutical Bulletin, 36*(6), 944–951.

Zatterale, F., Longo, M., Naderi, J., Raciti, G. A., Desiderio, A., Miele, C., & Beguinot, F. (2020). Chronic Adipose Tissue Inflammation Linking Obesity to Insulin Resistance and Type 2 Diabetes. *Frontiers in Physiology, Vol. 10.* Available from https://doi.org/10.3389/fphys.2019.01607, Frontiers Media S.A.

Zhang, H., Kovacs-Nolan, J., Kodera, T., Eto, Y., & Mine, Y. (2015). γ-Glutamyl cysteine and γ-glutamyl valine inhibit TNF-α signaling in intestinal epithelial cells and reduce inflammation in a mouse model of colitis via allosteric activation of the calcium-sensing receptor. *Biochimica et Biophysica Acta (BBA) - Molecular Basis of Disease, 1852*(5), 792–804.

Zhang, J., Fu, X., Li, W., Li, H., Ying, Z., Liu, X., & Yin, L. (2020). Enhancement of nutritional soy protein and peptide supplementation on skin repair in rats. *Journal of Functional Foods, 75.*

Zhang, J., Li, W., Ying, Z., Zhao, D., Yi, G., Li, H., & Liu, X. (2020). Soybean protein-derived peptide nutriment increases negative nitrogen balance in burn injury-induced inflammatory stress response in aged rats through the modulation of white blood cells and immune factors. *Food and Nutrition Research, 64*, 1–13.

Zhang, M., Zhao, Y., Yao, Y., Xu, M., Du, H., Wu, N., & Tu, Y. (2018). Isolation and identification of peptides from simulated gastrointestinal digestion of preserved egg white and their anti-inflammatory activity in TNF-α-induced Caco-2 cells. *The Journal of Nutritional Biochemistry, 63*, 44–53.

Zhang, S., Zou, J., Li, P., Zheng, X., & Feng, D. (2018). Curcumin Protects against Atherosclerosis in Apolipoprotein E-Knockout Mice by Inhibiting Toll-like Receptor 4 Expression. *Journal of Agricultural and Food Chemistry, 66*(2), 449–456.

Zhang, T., Ma, C., Zhang, Z., Zhang, H., & Hu, H. (2021). NF-κB signaling in inflammation and cancer. *MedComm, 2*(4), 618–653. Available from https://doi.org/10.1002/mco2.104, John Wiley and Sons Inc.

Zhang, X. A., Zhang, S., Yin, Q., & Zhang, J. (2015). Quercetin induces human colon cancer cells apoptosis by inhibiting the nuclear factor-kappa B Pathway. *Pharmacognosy Magazine, 11*(42), 404.

Zhou, N., Zhao, Y., Yao, Y., Wu, N., Xu, M., Du, H., Wu, J., & Tu, Y. (2022). Antioxidant Stress and Anti-Inflammatory Activities of Egg White Proteins and Their Derived Peptides: A Review. *Journal of Agricultural and Food Chemistry, 70*(1), 5–20.

Chapter 11

Functional foods and immune support: strengthening the body's defense

Gitanjali S. Deokar[1], Pooja A. Shinde[2], Sanjay J. Kshirsagar[1], Zyta M. Ziora[3] and Nilesh Prakash Nirmal[4]
[1]MET's Institute of Pharmacy, Bhujbal Knowledge City, Adgaon, Nashik, Maharashtra, India, [2]MET's Institute of Pharmacy, Nashik, Maharashtra, India, [3]Institute for Molecular Bioscience, The University of Queensland-Saint Lucia Campus, Brisbane, QLD, Australia, [4]Institute of Nutrition, Mahidol University, Salaya, Nakhon Pathom, Thailand

Abbreviations

gI	gastrointestinal
T Cell	T lymphocytes cell
B Cell	B lymphocytes cell
Th1,Th2, Th17	T helper
CD4 + FOXP3 + stands for regulatory T (TReg) cells	these cells are a subset of CD4 T cells that express CD25 and the transcription factor fork-head box P3 (FOXP3)
NFAT	nuclear factor of activated T cells
NFalphaB	nuclear factor alpha B
APC	antigen-presenting cell
rDCs	respiratory dendritic cells
IL-10	interleukin-10
TGF-β	transforming growth factor-beta
COX-2	cyclooxygenase 2
IgA, IgG, IgD, IgM, and IgE	immunoglobulin A, G, D, M, and E
SCFAs	short-chain fatty acids
GPR 41,43,81,91,109	pair of mammalian G protein–coupled receptors (GPCRs)
HDACs	histone deacetylases
TNF-α	tumor necrosis factor-α
TLRs	Toll-like receptors
NADPH	nicotinamide adenine dinucleotide phosphate
PXR	*pregnane X receptor*
AXR	abdominal X-rays
FXR	*farnesoid X receptor*
SXR	*steroid and xenobiotic receptor*
VDR	*vitamin D Receptor*
CAR	*constitutive androstane receptor*
TGR-5	Takeda G protein–coupled receptors
5HT	5 -hydroxytryptamine
GABA	gamma-aminobutyric acid
H2S	hydrogen sulfide
H2	hydrogen gas
CO2	carbondioxide
CH4	methane

Unleashing the Power of Functional Foods and Novel Bioactives. DOI: https://doi.org/10.1016/B978-0-443-28862-3.00011-X

NO	nitrogen
PKC	protein kinase C
NLR3	nod-like receptor

11.1 Introduction

People frequently look for specialized meals or vitamin supplements that are said to strengthen immunity during flu season or times of illness. Citrus fruits, chicken soup, and tea with honey are a few examples of common foods that include vitamin C (Harvard School of Public Health, 2020). But our immune system's composition is not greatly affected by diet alone, and especially not by any one food or vitamin. However, a balanced diet rich in a range of vitamins and minerals, together with healthy lifestyle choices like getting enough sleep, exercising regularly, and lowering stress, are effective methods for helping the body fight infections and diseases (Harvard School of Public Health, 2020; Shao et al., 2021). The demand for food ingredients that may boost immune response is currently trendy. Functional foods can control the immune system, strengthen host defenses against infection, and reduce allergies and inflammation by enhancing or inhibiting immunological responses (Ashaolu, 2020). Functional foods have emerged as viable alternatives for the prevention and treatment of several diseases as a result of research into bioactive substances from food to clarify their biological activity in the human body systems. According to research, stress and unhealthy lifestyles hurt the immune system, increasing the risk of infections, cancer, and a variety of cardiovascular and cerebrovascular diseases (Segerstrom & Miller, 2004). As people become more conscious of how diet affects their health, there has been a considerable rise in the demand for functional foods and nutraceuticals. Bioactive components have been added to functional foods, nutraceuticals, and pharmaceuticals for their antimicrobial properties humoral and cell-mediated immunological functions, where their biological activities can help with disease control and prevention (Mondal et al., 2021). According to the latest definition of FAO/WHO (Probiotics in food Health & nutritional properties and guidelines for evaluation, 2006), "Prebiotics are inert substances that stimulate the growth or activity of healthy microorganisms, whereas probiotics are live microorganisms (yeasts or bacteria) that, when given in sufficient proportions, offer health benefits to the host." To generate health advantages, probiotic products must include a sufficient quantity of live cells that can multiply and move in the digestive tract (Hill et al., 2014). These food items typically include prebiotic dietary fibers and probiotic bacteria. Probiotic products must have enough live cells to grow and colonize in the gut to produce health benefits. Ensuring the viability and functionality of probiotics and the effective modulation of microbiota through prebiotics, to provide the maximum health benefit to the host, is a complex and intriguing topic of investigation (Yanni, 2022). This chapter examines the relationship between functional foods and immune support, highlighting key dietary components and following significance.

11.1.1 Significance

In recent years, there has been an increasing emphasis on the role that functional foods play in improving general health and wellness. Among the many purposes functional foods fulfill, one of the most essential is that they maintain and build the body's immune system (Ajmera, 2020). This rising health awareness is driving a global increase in the consumption of functional foods. This chapter delves into the benefits of functional foods as potential natural means to modulate the host immune system to enhance defense mechanisms against microbial infections.

Worldwide well-known functional foods and food supplements are available in the market. While foods can be used as dietary supplements and are a significant source of important nutrients, functional foods are important for human health (Szakos et al., 2022). Functional food, as defined by various organizations such as the European Food Safety Authority (EFSA), the Functional Food Center (FFC), the Food and Drug Administration (FDA), the Institute of Food Technologists (IFT), and the International Life Sciences Institute (ILSI), refers to a type of food that goes beyond providing basic nutrition. It is a food that positively impacts specific functions within the body, contributing to improved health and well-being or reducing the risk of disease. Functional foods can be natural or modified through technological or biotechnological means and must demonstrate their beneficial effects in quantities typically consumed as part of a regular diet (Omer et al., 2022). Naturally, a variety of fruits, vegetables, grains, seafood, dairy products, and meat products are thought to be the main sources of functional food; also, each of these meals can nourish the host body with vitamins, minerals, antioxidants, and phytochemicals, which are frequently abundant in functional foods (Fig. 11.1). These elements are essential for keeping a strong immune system (Vigar et al., 2019). A balanced diet is essential for both physical and mental health, as it can sustain bodily functioning. It is significant for consumers throughout their lives (Plasek et al., 2020). Functional food benefits an organism's body; it can supply essential metabolic needs, guard

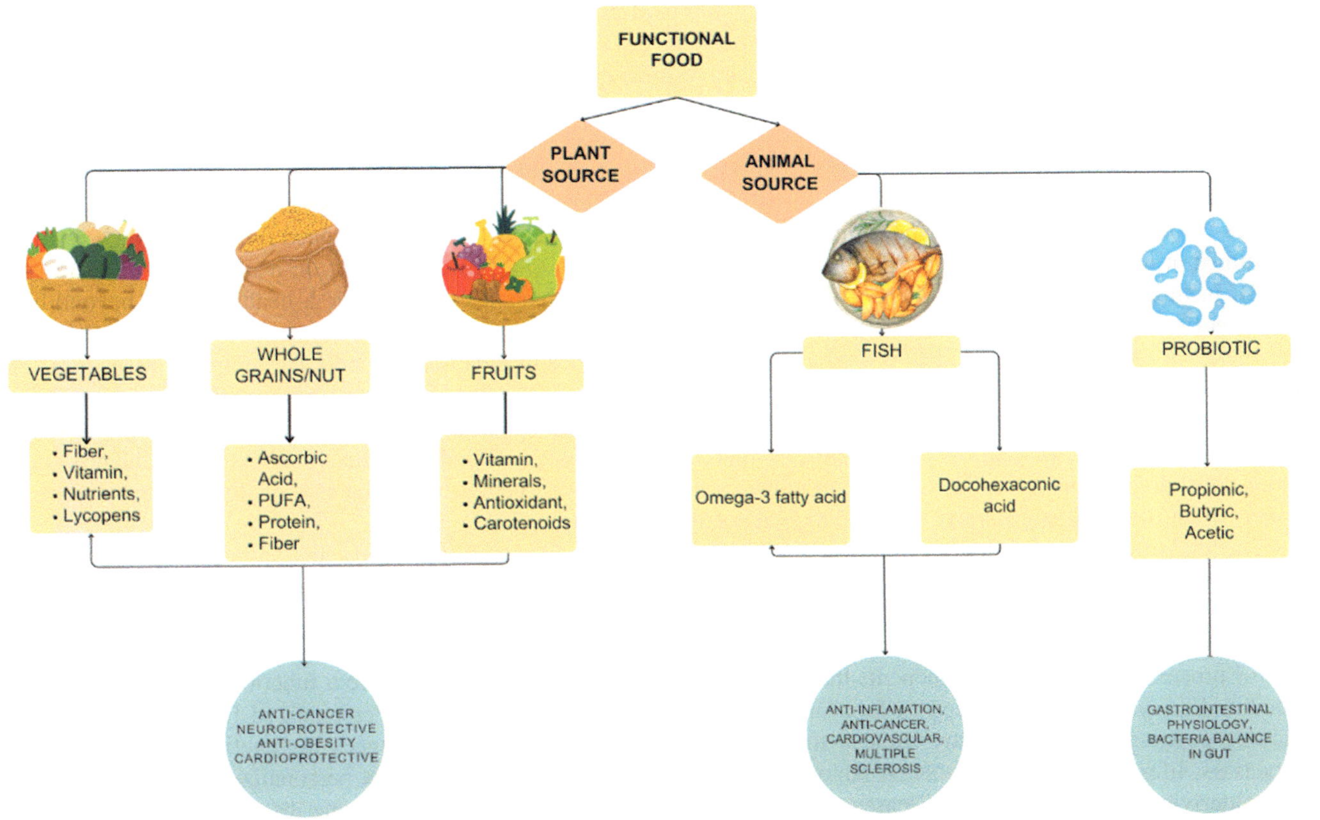

FIGURE 11.1 Functional food sources and immune health benefits.

the host body against numerous malnutrition-related ailments, and eliminate a variety of hazardous substances from the body (Topolska et al., 2021). According to studies, a dietary product is considered functional if it can raise the body's metabolic rate without interfering with its regular processes or maintaining the body's outward appearance (Qazi et al., 2023). Functional foods, including both whole foods and extracts, along with their low-molecular-weight phytochemicals, play a significant role in enhancing the health of the intestines. They achieve this by promoting the renewal of intestinal epithelial cells, strengthening the intestinal barrier, restoring healthy gut flora, reducing inflammation in the intestines, and impeding the growth of tumors. These beneficial effects contribute to improving intestinal health in both the small and large intestines, addressing various stages of intestinal ailments. Depending on the nature of the specific intestinal disease, consuming particular functional foods or their low-molecular-weight phytochemicals can alleviate symptoms and support the maintenance of intestinal balance to varying extents (Chen et al., 2021). A comprehensive and measurable approach was necessary to understand how various nutrients impact food choices, consumption, and overall animal health through homeostatic regulation. This necessity spurred the creation of nutritional geometry and its associated geometric model for nutrition, originating from the study of dietary patterns in insects (Sperfeld et al., 2017). Functional food formulations lead to beneficial adjustments in homeostasis, resulting in improved health outcomes (Raubenheimer et al., 2009).

11.1.2 Definition of functional foods

A substantial number of foods are referred to as "functional foods." The term is not well defined, nevertheless. One definition that is frequently applied is that they include ingredients that are beneficial to health "beyond basic nutrition." However, there are a few issues with this definition. The phrase "functional foods" frequently includes nutritious foods (Temple, 2022). These terms are used by the Food and Agriculture Organization (FAO) of the United Nations (www.fao.org, n.d.a). They define functional foods as foods that contain, in addition to nutrients, other components that may be beneficial to health. The phrase "functional foods" was initially used in Japan in the middle of the 1980s to describe processed foods that are both nutrient-dense and contain additives that support particular body processes. As of right now, only Japan has developed a unique regulatory approval procedure for functional foods. The Japanese Ministry of Health and Welfare has the authority to certify some foods as Foods for Specified Health Use (FOSHU) (www.mhlw.go.jp, n.d). Because they contain physiologically active food components, foods or food ingredients that offer health advantages beyond merely meeting basic nutritional demands are referred to as functional foods (i.e. bioactive compounds or bioactive food components). But in the United States, there is no precise definition for functional foods. Crucially, functional foods are not defined by statute and are not governed by the Food and Drug Administration (FDA) (FDA, 2019). Various reputable organizations have their definitions (Saarela, 2011). Academy of Nutrition and Dietetics defines "foods that are characterized as whole foods as well as fortified, enriched, or enhanced foods that, when regularly consumed at appropriate amounts as part of a balanced diet, may have a positive impact on health" (Crowe & Francis, 2013). Institute of Food Technologists defines "Foods and food components that provide a health benefit beyond basic nutrition (for the intended population) "(www.ift.org, n.d). International Life Sciences Institute defines "Foods that under the presence of physiologically active food components provide health benefits beyond basic nutrition" (M, n.d). The main types of functional foods that are covered by current definitions are conventional foods, modified foods, and food ingredients, although the term "functional foods" is not well defined. When a food contains a bioactive ingredient such as vitamins, minerals, protein, or phytochemicals such as polyphenols and prebiotic dietary fibers that influence one or more physiological processes in the body to enhance health and well-being, lower the risk of disease, or improve the course of an illness, it is generally regarded as functional food (Saarela, 2011).

The classification of functional food is given in Table 11.1. Conventional foods are unprocessed, whole foods that, depending on the bioactive substances they contain, may be useful. These substances often exert their effects in an additive or synergistic manner. Foods that have undergone modifications that are deemed functional foods have had their bioactive components' type, content, bioaccessibility, and/or bioavailability altered by aspects of food production and/or processing. Bioactive components that are employed in food products to provide a functional effect can be separated and/or synthesized and used as food ingredients (Dable-Tupas et al., 2020). Personalized functional medicine is gaining popularity as a healthcare strategy that acknowledges the individual differences in genetic makeup, metabolic processes, lifestyle, and environmental factors that influence health and disease. This personalized approach addresses the underlying causes of chronic diseases such as heart disease, diabetes, and autoimmune disorders rather than simply treating symptoms with medicine. It creates personalized treatment plans that empower patients to participate actively in their healthcare decisions by leveraging technological breakthroughs such as genetic testing and data analytics. PFM focuses on preventive medicine, identifying and addressing risk factors before they become disease, to reduce the burden of chronic illness and improve overall quality of life. The addition of functional meals improves this technique by offering targeted nutritional support to address specific health concerns (Kraus, 2018; Pizzorno, 2014).

11.1.2.1 Personalized functional medicine

Tailoring healthcare techniques to individual patients based on their unique genetic composition, lifestyle, environment, and other aspects contributing to their health and well-being is the core idea of adopting functional medicine as personalized medicine (www.gethealthie.com, n.d). The following explains how functional medicine and personalized medicine complement each other:

1. Personalized treatment activities: A key component of functional medicine is developing patient-specific treatment regimens. This entails being aware of the unique health issues, medical background, genetic predispositions, lifestyle

TABLE 11.1 Classification of Functional Food.

Classes	Description	Examples	References
Traditional food	Whole, unchanged meal that inherently contains health-promoting bioactive components	Vegetables, fruit, fish, and grain	www.ift.org (n.d), M (n.d), Dable-Tupas et al. (2020)
Modified food	Food products that have been improved, supplemented, or strengthened with useful food ingredients	Calcium-enriched fruit juices, breads enhanced with folate, plant-based beverages, and salt that has been iodized	Pizzorno (2014)
Synthetic food	Laboratories that synthesize functional components	Insulin-type fructans	Kraus (2018)

variables (such as stress levels, exercise, and diet), and environmental effects for each patient. Functional medicine practitioners strive to create complete treatment plans that target the underlying causes of illness rather than just treating its symptoms by taking these individualized factors into account (Yoshimura, 2023).

2. Incorporation of genomic medicine: In personalized medicine, genomic analysis is frequently used to find genetic differences that may affect a person's reaction to a given medication or their susceptibility to a particular disease. By employing genetic testing to identify putative genetic vulnerabilities or predispositions that may influence treatment choices, functional medicine integrates genomic medicine. Genetic testing, for instance, may identify gene variants that affect detoxification pathways, inflammatory processes, or nutrition metabolism. These variants can then be used to inform customized interventions, including dietary changes or targeted supplementation (The Regeneration Center, n.d).
3. Gut health optimization: Along the gastrointestinal tract, intestinal epithelial cells (IECs) create a barrier that keeps the internal body milieu and the outside world apart. Due to its ability to stop tissue damage, pathogen invasion, and disease development, this barrier is crucial for preserving gut health and general well-being. Bacterial translocation may occur when the intestinal barrier's integrity is weakened. Furthermore, the gut microbiota is critical to health because it influences the immune system, regulates metabolism, and preserves the integrity of the intestinal barrier. Any disruption in the gut microbiota's makeup, or dysbiosis, can result in several health issues (Wan et al., 2018). The gut microbiota and intestinal barrier play important roles in determining gut health. The digestive system is a complicated environment that is continually exposed to a wide range of food ingredients and friendly microorganisms. The concept of functional foods has emerged as dietary components are recognized for their various positive activities that extend beyond basic nourishment (Riaz Rajoka et al., 2021). Numerous dietary modifiers have been studied and found to have a positive impact on gut health and overall host well-being. These include probiotics (live bacteria), prebiotics (ingestible food constituents), and polyphenols or synbiotics (combinations of probiotics and prebiotics) (Szydłowska & Sionek, 2022).
4. Multidisciplinary approach: Functional medicine adopts a holistic approach to treatment, acknowledging the interdependence of all body systems and the impact of environmental and lifestyle factors on health outcomes. This holistic viewpoint is crucial to personalized medicine to comprehend how various facets of a person's life contribute to their overall health profile. Functional medicine seeks to optimize health and prevent disease progression in an individualized way by treating imbalances in diet, stress, sleep, exercise, exposure to toxins, and other lifestyle factors (www.mdpi.com, n.d).
5. Balance diet overall wellness: In personalized functional medicine (PFM), achieving overall wellness through a balanced diet is paramount. A balanced diet provides essential nutrients, supports metabolic processes, and helps maintain optimal health (Aguiar et al., 2019). PFM emphasizes tailoring dietary recommendations to individual needs based on factors such as genetics, biochemistry, lifestyle, and health goals. This personalized approach considers variations in nutrient requirements, food sensitivities, and metabolic tendencies among individuals (Essa et al., 2021). A balanced diet in PFM typically includes a variety of whole foods such as fruits, vegetables, whole grains, lean proteins, and healthy fats, while minimizing processed foods, sugar, and unhealthy fats (Vlaicu et al., 2023). Additionally, functional foods—rich in bioactive compounds with specific health benefits—are often incorporated to address individual health concerns. By promoting a balanced diet tailored to individual needs, PFM supports overall wellness, enhances energy levels, optimizes metabolic function, and reduces the risk of chronic diseases (de Brito Alves et al., 2023).
6. Focused on patient care: Patient-centered care, in which the patient's values, preferences, and goals are important to the decision-making process, is prioritized by both personalized medicine and functional medicine. Practitioners of functional medicine work closely with patients to jointly develop treatment regimens that are tailored to their particular requirements and situations. By encouraging a therapeutic alliance between the patient and the provider, this cooperative approach gives people the confidence to actively manage their health and well-being (Kong et al., 2022).

There is a close relationship between functional food components and personalized functional medicine. Functional food components are essential in delivering targeted nutritional support based on lifestyle factors, genetic predispositions, and individual health needs. Through the integration of these elements into customized therapy regimens, professionals can target underlying imbalances, encourage optimum health, and enable people to actively participate in their well-being (Beidelschies et al., 2019).

11.2 The immune system

The immune system defends the body against diseases such as bacteria, viruses, fungi, and parasites. Researchers can learn more about how diseases grow and spread by researching the immune system, which plays an important role in recognizing disease causes, creating vaccines, treating autoimmune illnesses, and enhancing cancer treatments. This understanding has significant implications for public health, medical care, and biomedical research (Nicholson, 2016).

11.2.1 Overview of the immune system

The immune system is a host defense system it comprises many biological structures of cells, tissues, and organs that play a critical role in protecting the body from harmful pathogens, such as bacteria, viruses, fungi, and parasites. The function of the immune system is to recognize and eliminate these foreign invaders while maintaining tolerance to the body's cells and tissues. In humans and most other vertebrates, the immune system consists of layered defenses that have increased specificity for particular pathogens or tumor cells. The layered defenses of the human immune system are usually classified into two subsystems called the innate immune system and the adaptive immune system (Biology LibreTexts, 2018). The mammalian immune system serves as a remarkable defense mechanism against pathogens. Throughout history, plagues have had devastating effects, and the COVID-19 pandemic exemplifies a global health crisis. While vaccines have saved lives, understanding the immune system remains complex. Animal models, particularly inbred mice, have yielded valuable insights but may not fully represent human diseases or immune responses. Direct studies of the human immune system hold great promise for scientific and medical advancements (Pulendran & Davis, 2020). Let us understand first the components of the immune system to safeguard our health so that we can correlate ahead the role of functional components in maintaining and boosting the immune system. The mammalian immune system is divided into two main parts: innate and adaptive as shown in Fig. 11.2.

11.2.2 Component of the immune system

Antigen are molecules or molecular structures that are foreign to the body. They generally induce an immune reaction, leading to the production of antibodies against them. In simpler terms, antigens can be anything that does not belong to

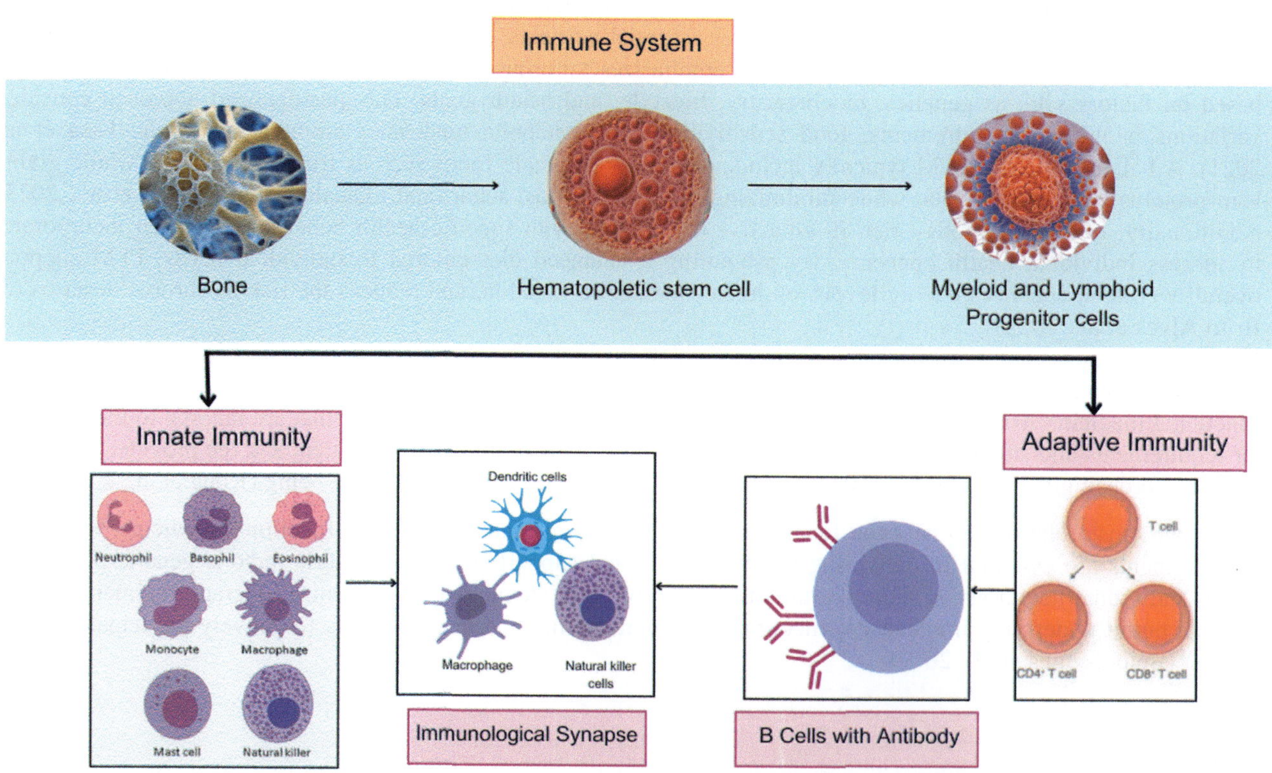

FIGURE 11.2 The mammalian immune system.

the body and is foreign. Some antigens are specifically termed immunogens, as they effectively trigger an immune response. The ability of antigens to elicit an immune response depends on specific regions called antigenic determinants. These determinants bind to receptor molecules on immune cells, initiating a response. Most antigens in humans are proteins, peptides, or polysaccharides. However, lipids and nucleic acids can also act as antigens when combined with proteins or polysaccharides (Charles et al., 2001a; MSD Manual Professional Edition, n.d; Sapkota, 2021).

Antibodies, also known as immunoglobulins (Ig), are special proteins created by white blood cells that can kill or weaken infection-causing organisms. These Y-shaped proteins are produced by the immune system in response to the presence of foreign substances called antigens, which could be pathogens such as bacteria, viruses, fungi, or toxins. Antibodies play a crucial role in the adaptive immune response, specifically in the humoral immune response, where they recognize and bind to specific antigens, thereby neutralizing or marking them for destruction by other immune cells. The immune system generates antibodies in response to encountering new pathogens or receiving vaccinations, enhancing protective immunity (Charles et al., 2001a; MSD Manual Professional Edition, n.d; Sapkota, 2021).

White blood cells (WBCs), also known as leukocytes, are a vital component of the immune system, playing a crucial role in defending the body against pathogens such as bacteria, viruses, fungi, and parasites. They are produced in the bone marrow and circulate throughout the bloodstream and lymphatic system, actively seeking out and destroying foreign invaders. There are several types of white blood cells, each with unique functions:

Neutrophils are the most abundant type of white blood cell and are typically the first responders to infections. They engulf and digest bacteria, fungi, and other foreign particles through a process called phagocytosis. Neutrophils are often found in pus, which is formed at the site of infection.

Lymphocytes are responsible for mounting specific immune responses against pathogens. There are two main types of lymphocytes: B cells (B lymphocytes)and T cells (T lymphocytes). B cells produce antibodies, which are proteins that recognize and bind to specific antigens on pathogens, marking them for destruction by other immune cells. T cells, on the other hand, directly attack infected cells and regulate the immune response.

Monocytes are large white blood cells that can differentiate into macrophages and dendritic cells. Macrophages engulf and digest pathogens and dead cells, playing a key role in both innate and adaptive immunity. Dendritic cells are specialized antigen-presenting cells that activate T cells, initiating adaptive immune responses.

Eosinophils are involved in combating parasitic infections and allergic reactions. They release toxic proteins that damage parasites, as well as inflammatory mediators that contribute to allergic responses.

Basophils release histamine and other inflammatory chemicals in response to allergens and parasitic infections. They play a role in the inflammatory response and help recruit other immune cells to the site of infection. These different types of white blood cells work together in a coordinated manner to detect, neutralize, and eliminate pathogens while also regulating immune responses to prevent damage to the body's tissues. For example, during a bacterial infection, neutrophils are recruited to the site of infection to engulf and destroy bacteria, while lymphocytes are activated to produce antibodies specific to the invading pathogen. Monocytes differentiate into macrophages, which further ingest and destroy bacteria, while dendritic cells activate T cells to coordinate the immune response. In the case of an allergic reaction, eosinophils and basophils release inflammatory mediators that trigger symptoms such as itching, swelling, and mucus production (Charles et al., 2001a; MSD Manual Professional Edition, n.d; Sapkota, 2021).

Lymphatic system: The network of veins, nodes, and organs that make up the lymphatic system is responsible for the movement of lymph, a clear fluid that contains white blood cells, throughout the body. Because lymph nodes filter the lymph to get rid of infections and contain immune cells, they are very significant (Zhao et al., 2011).

Bone marrow plays an important function in the immune system by creating numerous types of blood cells that are required to defend the body against pathogens and maintain overall health. Here is an explanation of how bone marrow works within the immune system. Hematopoiesis, or the process of producing blood cells, occurs mostly in the bone marrow. In the bone marrow, hematopoietic stem cells (HSCs) differentiate into many types of blood cells. However, accumulated evidence shows that immune cells such as regulatory T cells, conventional T cells, B cells, dendritic cells, natural killer (NK) T (NKT) cells, neutrophils, myeloid-derived suppressor cells, and mesenchymal stem cells are actively functioning and trafficking in the bone marrow (Zhao et al., 2011).

The spleen is the body's largest secondary lymphoid organ, and as such, it serves a variety of immunological obligations in addition to hematopoiesis and red cell clearance. The spleen's physical organization allows it to filter blood for pathogens and aberrant cells while also facilitating low-probability connections between antigen presentation cells (APCs) and relevant lymphocytes. Spleen-specific APCs regulate the T and B cell response to antigenic stimuli in the blood. The structure of the spleen consists of white pulp and red pulp, each serving different immune functions. White pulp aids in immunological monitoring and response. When infections enter the bloodstream, they are identified by immune cells in the white pulp, which activates immunological responses such as antibody production and cytotoxic T cells. For example, if someone is afflicted with a virus, such as influenza, the virus may enter their bloodstream. Immunological cells in the spleen's white pulp recognize viral antigens, triggering an immunological response that includes the generation of virus-specific antibodies. These antibodies contribute to the virus's neutralization and removal from the body. Red pulp serves as a blood filter, eliminating damaged or senescent (old) red blood cells, as well as foreign particles and pathogens in the bloodstream. It also functions as a blood reserve, releasing it as needed, such as after a hemorrhage. For example, in people with certain blood disorders, such as sickle cell anemia, the spleen may grow (splenomegaly) as it filters out aberrant blood cells. However, in some situations, this might result in an overwhelming destruction of both normal and aberrant red blood cells, causing anemia and other issues (Lewis et al., 2019).

The thymus is a primary lymphoid organ that is required for the development of T lymphocytes, which orchestrate adaptive immune responses. T cell development in the thymus is spatially regulated; key checkpoints in T cell maturation and selection occur in cortical and medullary regions to eliminate self-reactive T cells, establish central tolerance, and export naive T cells to the periphery with the potential to recognize diverse pathogens. Thymic output is also temporally regulated due to age-related thymus involvement combined with epithelial cell loss (Thapa & Farber, 2019).

The complement system comprises numerous distinct plasma proteins that interact to enhance the immune response against pathogens by marking them for destruction and triggering inflammatory reactions. Some of these proteins are enzymes known as zymogens, which require proteolytic cleavage for activation. Zymogens were initially identified in the digestive system, where they prevent self-digestion. For instance, the digestive enzyme pepsin is stored as an inactive form called pepsinogen within cells and is only converted to its active form, pepsin, in the acidic environment of the stomach, thus protecting the host from autodigestion (Charles et al., 2001b).

Cytokines, ranging from 8000 to 30,000 daltons, function as intercellular messengers within the immune system, akin to its "hormones." They exert diverse roles, including cell activation, effector function (such as killing virus-infected cells), immune suppression, and cell differentiation induction. Primarily, cytokines promote, sustain, and cease immunological responses relevant to the specific antigen or pathogen. They bind to specific receptors on target cells, which vary structurally and can increase in number or appear de novo upon cell activation. Cytokines exhibit pleiotropy, with each molecule possessing multiple biological functions, leading to their designation under the unified "interleukin" nomenclature. Redundancy is evident among cytokines, where several molecules share similar functions, ensuring robustness in immune responses. Moreover, cytokines often act synergistically, amplifying biological effects through cascading pathways. Understanding these principles is vital for studying cytokine interactions and their implications for health and disease (Research, 1999).

Mucosal immunity: The vulnerability of mucosal surfaces to infection arises from their thin and permeable nature due to physiological functions such as gas exchange, food absorption, sensory activities, and reproduction. The gut, acting as a primary entry point for foreign antigens from food, poses a challenge for the immune system to distinguish between harmless food antigens and pathogenic organisms. Moreover, the gut harbors a vast population of commensal microorganisms, which can be both beneficial and pathogenic. Gut-associated lymphoid tissue (GALT), including tonsils, adenoids, Peyer's patches, and solitary lymphoid follicles, plays a crucial role in mucosal immune responses. Peyer's patches, characterized by dome-like structures containing microfold (M) cells, facilitate antigen uptake via transcytosis and subsequent presentation to lymphocytes and antigen-presenting cells. Understanding the complex interactions within the mucosal immune system is essential for combating infections and maintaining homeostasis (Russell et al., 2015).

Innate immunity: The innate immune response, which predates the adaptive immune system, serves as the primary defense mechanism against environmental threats such as toxins and various pathogens across multicellular organisms. It comprises preexisting mechanisms, including natural barriers like skin and mucosa, and secretions, alongside adaptive immunity, which targets specific microorganisms or antigens upon recognition. Initially, the innate immune system detects new pathogens, followed by activating the adaptive response (Finnegan et al., 2023). Innate immunity acts rapidly (within minutes to hours) compared to the slower adaptive response (days to weeks). Components of innate immunity encompass physical barriers like skin-tight junctions and epithelial surfaces, as well as enzymatic defenses of epithelial and phagocytic cells, such as lysozyme. Additionally, it includes various immune cells such as phagocytes (neutrophils, monocytes, macrophages), inflammation-related serum proteins (complement, C-reactive protein), antimicrobial peptides (defensins, cathelicidin), microorganism-sensing cell receptors (Toll-like receptors), and cytokine-releasing cells (macrophages, mast cells, NK cells). Upon interaction with pathogens, a signaling cascade is initiated, amplifying the immune response and activating specific defense mechanisms. This innate response aims to prevent infection, eliminate pathogens, and stimulate the adaptive immune system (Stephen et al., 2023).

The immune system can be categorized into two main types: innate immunity and adaptive immunity. The innate defense system is an immediate nonspecific response mediated by various types of immune cells, including macrophages, NK cells, and dendritic cells (DCs). Macrophages are crucial cells of the innate immune system capable of removing pathogens through phagocytosis and recruiting other immune cells to combat invaders. Activated macrophages also secrete cytokines such as tumor necrosis factor (TNF)-α, which activates or recruits NK cells, neutrophils, and eosinophils. Furthermore, macrophages produce nitric oxide (NO) via inducible NO synthase (iNOS) to eliminate foreign microbial agents. Toll-like receptors (TLRs) are pattern recognition receptors that regulate the immune system in macrophages. Activation of TLR2 induces mitogen-activated protein kinase (MAPK) signaling pathways and nuclear factor κ-light-chain-enhancer of activated B cells (NF-κB), which control the immune response in macrophages. NK cells play a critical role in surveillance and defense against viral infections and malignant cells by secreting interferon (IFN)-γ to activate macrophages for phagocytosis, thereby enhancing the immune response. DCs, originating from hematopoietic bone marrow progenitor cells, are professional antigen-presenting cells that bridge the innate and adaptive immune systems by processing antigens and presenting them to T lymphocytes. In summary, these specialized immune cells constitute the first line of defense against external microbes as part of the innate immune system, identifying nonself-elements and generating cytotoxic effects (Kim et al., 2022; Porcelli, 2017).

Adaptive immunity: The adaptive immune system, also referred to as acquired or specific immunity, is a vital component of the body's defense mechanism against pathogens. Unlike the innate immune system, which provides broad and generic responses, the adaptive immune system is specialized and highly specific to encountered pathogens. Through processes like antibody production by B cells and cell-mediated responses by T cells, it targets and eliminates invading pathogens. Importantly, adaptive immunity creates immunological memory, enabling a more robust response upon subsequent encounters with the same pathogen. This phenomenon forms the basis of vaccination. The adaptive immune system is mediated by lymphocytes, including B and T cells, which undergo genetic alterations to generate a diverse repertoire of antigen receptors. These mechanisms ensure the system's adaptability and effectiveness in combating various pathogens. However, dysregulation of adaptive immunity can lead to conditions such as allergies or autoimmunity (Institute for Quality & Efficiency in Health Care, 2020).

11.2.3 Mechanism of the immune system

The immune system comprises two main branches: acquired and innate immunity (Weyh et al., 2020). The innate immune system's neutrophils and macrophages operate as a first line of defense against a variety of common pathogens and are crucial for the management of bacterial infections. The cells of the innate immune system, however, play a crucial part in the initiation and subsequent direction of adaptive immune responses, as well as participating in the removal of pathogens that have been targeted by an adaptive immune response. Upon first entering the body's epithelial surfaces, microorganisms like bacteria are instantly confronted by chemicals and cells capable of initiating an innate immune response shown in Fig. 11.3. Using surface receptors that can identify and bind common components of several bacterial surfaces, phagocytic macrophages carry out the fight against germs. The macrophage engulfs the bacterium and secretes physiologically active chemicals when bacteria attach to these receptors. Activated macrophages secret macrophages that influence the actions of other cells that have their receptors attached to them. Additionally, they emit chemokine-releasing proteins that draw bloodstream cells like neutrophils and monocytes that have chemokine receptors. Inflammation is brought on by the cytokines and chemokines that macrophages release in reaction to components of bacteria. The activation of adaptive immunity is significantly aided by the innate immune response Fig. 11.1. While complementing fragments on microbial surfaces and changes in cells that have taken up microorganisms provide signals that synergize in activating lymphocytes, the receptors of which bind to specific microbial antigens, the inflammatory response increases the flow of lymph-containing antigen and antigen-bearing cells into lymphoid tissue. T cells can also be triggered by active macrophages that have taken up pathogens (A et al., 2018). The research reports that CD4 + Foxp3 + regulatory T cells indicate regulatory T (Treg) cells. These cells are a group of CD4 T cells that express both CD25 and the transcription factor forkhead box (FOXP3) and are upregulated by probiotics or specific gut flora. In the (Kwon et al., 2010) study, it was discovered that probiotic combination administration caused downregulation of T helper (Th) 1, Th2, and Th17 cytokines without inducing apoptosis and generated hyporesponsiveness in both T cells and B cells. Additionally, it enhanced the suppressor activity of naturally occurring CD4 + CD25 + Tregs and stimulated the production of CD4 + Foxp3 + Tregs from the CD4 + CD25 − population. Regulatory dendritic cells (rDCs), which produce high quantities of interleukin-10 (IL-10), transforming growth factor-beta (TGF-β), cyclooxygenase 2 (COX-2), and indoleamine 2,3-dioxygenase, directly facilitate the conversion of T cells into Foxp3 + Tregs. *L. acidophilus (LA), L. casei (LC), Lactobacillus reuteri (LR), Bifidobacterium bifidium (BB), and Streptococcus thermophilus (ST)* were the probiotic strains used during the study (Kwon et al., 2010). Uncontrolled apoptosis is a condition in numerous human problems, including ischemia damage, autoimmune disorders, and neurodegenerative diseases,

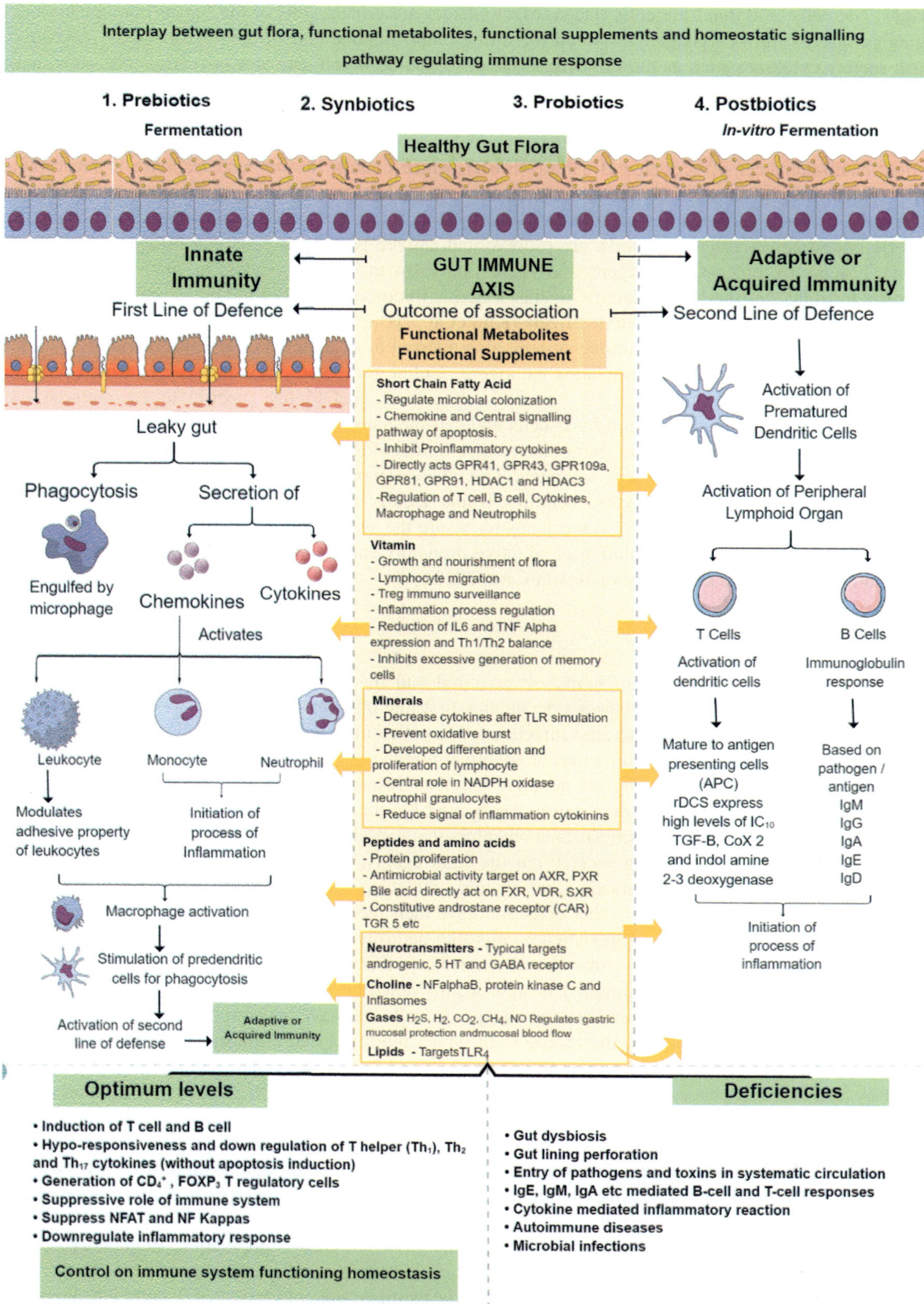

FIGURE 11.3 Interplay between gut flora, functional metabolites, functional supplements, and homeostatic signaling pathway regulating the immune response.

which are associated with inappropriate apoptosis, either too little or too much (Elmore, 2007). The forkhead transcription factor family includes FOXP3. In contrast to other members, it is primarily expressed by a fraction of CD4 + T-cells, which function as immune system suppressors. One of FOXP3 functions is inhibiting the nuclear factor of activated T cells (NFAT) and nuclear factor κB (NFκB) activity, suppressing the expression of numerous genes, including IL-2 and effector T-cell cytokines. In addition, FOXP3 functions as a transcription activator for a large number of genes, such as CD25, glucocorticoid-induced TNF receptor family gene (GITR), cytotoxic T-lymphocyte antigen 4 (CTLA4), and folate receptor 4. FOXP3 + T-cells are produced in the peripheral and thymus (Nagai et al., 2019). The thymus produces FOXP3 + T cells, which move to secondary lymphoid organs and prevent lymphocytes from priming them with antigens. After naive FOXPY and naive FOXP3-T-cells are primed with antigens, memory FOXP3 + T-cells are produced, which are effective in migrating to nonlymphoid regions. Therefore naive FOXP3 + T-cells are skilled at suppressing the early immunological responses in lymphoid tissues, while memory FOXP3 + T-cells are efficient in reducing effector T-cell function.

For the body as a whole to effectively maintain tolerance and prevent autoimmune disorders, naive and memory FOXP3 + T cells are needed. The production of FOXP3 + T cells is controlled by a variety of variables, including cytokines and noncytokine factors (Laissue, 2019; Passerini & Bacchetta, 2017). For example, retinoic acid, produced by the dendritic cells and epithelial cells in the intestine, works together with TGF-∼1 and promotes the generation of small intestine-homing FOXPY T cells by upregulating the expression of FOXP3 and gut-homing receptors. Wherein retinoic acid is made in the body from vitamin A and helps cells to grow and develop, especially in the embryo, and vitamin A is produced in cross-talk between prebiotics and probiotics. During development, T lymphocytes get survival signals from self-molecules on specialized epithelial cells in the thymus. These same molecules are also expressed by dendritic cells in the peripheral lymphoid organs (Czarnewski et al., 2017). The activation of adaptive immunity is significantly aided by the innate immune response. While complementing fragments on microbial surfaces and changes in cells that have taken up microorganisms provide signals that synergize in activating lymphocytes, the receptors of which bind to specific microbial antigens, the inflammatory response increases the flow of lymph-containing antigen and antigen-bearing cells into lymphoid tissue. T cells can also be triggered by active macrophages that have taken up pathogens. On the other hand, dendritic cells are the cells that are experts in presenting antigens to T lymphocytes and starting adaptive immunity shown in Fig. 11.3 (A et al., 2018). When a bacterium binds to these receptors, the dendritic cell is stimulated to engulf the pathogen and digest it intracellularly, just like it happens with neutrophils and macrophages. Dendritic cells are the cells that are experts in presenting antigens to T lymphocytes and starting adaptive immunity. When a pathogen is consumed by an immature dendritic cell in the infected tissue, the production of an adaptive immune response starts. Receptors on the surface of immature dendritic cells are capable of identifying shared characteristics with numerous pathogens, including bacterial cell wall proteoglycans. When a bacterium binds to these receptors, the dendritic cell is stimulated to engulf the pathogen and digest it intracellularly, just like it happens with neutrophils and macrophages. A dendritic cell migrates to a neighboring lymph node after becoming activated by a pathogen it has taken up in infected tissue. Upon activation, the dendritic cell undergoes modifications that allow it to activate pathogen-specific lymphocytes in the lymph node and grow into a highly potent antigen-presenting cell (APC) (A et al., 2018; Soto et al., 2020). Another important component of the adaptive immune response that gives mammals humoral immunity is the B cell, also known as the B lymphocyte (bursa-derived cell). In humans, the process of producing B cells begins in the fetal liver during pregnancy and continues in the bone marrow following delivery. Hematopoietic stem cells are the source of their development. The process of developing B cells includes every stage of early differentiation without antigen interaction up until maturity, antigen interaction, and the final stage of antibody manufacturing. B cells gain two key components of adaptive immunity through this process: memory (the capacity to remember prior interactions with antigens, which in turn prompts a more rapid response) and discrimination between self and nonself (the capacity of B cell to identify foreign antigens instead of self-antigens) (Althuwaiqeb & Bordoni, 2020). The antigen receptor on B cells is a functional component of cell surface multimolecular protein complexes. The multimolecular protein complex known as the B cell receptor (BCR) is noncovalently linked to other proteins. The membrane-bound immunoglobulin receptor (mIg), Ig-alpha (CD79a), and Ig-beta (CD79b) are involved in the function of BCR. Signal transduction molecules Ig-alpha and Ig-beta form a disulfide-linked heterodimeric complex with mIg. The immune receptor tyrosine-based activation motif (ITAM), which is present in both Ig-alpha and Ig-beta, is necessary for signal transduction in both B and T cells. Tyrosine amino acid (tyrosine amino acid) is phosphorylated by protein tyrosine kinases (PTKs) during cellular activation to interact with cytoplasmic signaling proteins. ITAM is important for transporting these activation signals from the cell surface to the cytoplasm. It is believed that due to genetic diversity and organization, there is sufficient B cell receptor antigen for every microorganism (Althuwaiqeb &

Bordoni, 2020; Tkachenko et al., 2024). After being stimulated by an antigen, B cells develop into plasma cells, which produce big amounts of five distinct antibody immunoglobulin classes (IgA, IgG, IgD, IgM, and IgE) (Fig. 11.3).

A clone of cells with the capacity to make immunoglobulin with the same antigen specificity is created when a B cell is activated and goes through mitotic division. Plasma cells are mostly what these cells will develop into. The first time a B cell comes into contact with an antigen, the initial immunological response is triggered. A small portion of this clone, though, will develop into memory cells, when exposed to that same antigen again, react quickly and cause a secondary immune response. The secondary immune response is substantially larger, happens a lot faster, and generates more IgG than IgM. The fundamental idea behind vaccinations and lifetime immunity is this phenomenon. B cells are critical for humoral immunity, but they also mediate or control a wide range of other immunological homeostasis-related processes (Justiz Vaillant et al., 2024; Schroeder et al., 2023). The initial antibody that engages with newly ingested bacteria and triggers a basic immune response is called immunoglobulin M (IgM). Because it acts as the immune system's initial line of defense and offers temporary protection, IgM is sometimes referred to as a natural antibody. These types of Ig enhance the elimination of pathogens, neutralize bacterial or viral toxins, and trigger the activation of the complement system. IgA antibodies protect the body from bacterial growth and colonization. Serum antibodies consist of less than 0.5% immunoglobulin D (IgD). It functions as the surface to receive a signal and is present on the surface of immature B cells (receptors). It belongs to the innate immune system as well. It is thought by researchers that IgD controls the activation of B cells and their development into plasma cells (Leduc & D, 2021). Certain antigens and ways in which antigens are presented to the immune system promote the generation of IgE. Allergens are substances that specifically activate TH2 cells, which initiate an IgE reaction. CD4 TH2 cells can change an antibody's isotype from IgM to IgE (A et al., 2010). Some of the literature reveals the relationship between particular subsets of gut microbial dysbiosis and IgE-mediated responses (Berin, 2021; Chiu et al., 2019).

11.3 Specific functional food components

11.3.1 Prebiotic

Prebiotics are all those substances and substrates that provide our gut bacteria with nutrition and promote healthy growth, which is necessary for their long-term survival in the gastrointestinal tract (Dahiya & Nigam, 2022). "A substrate that is selectively utilized by host microorganisms in the gut, conferring a health benefit" is the accepted definition of a prebiotic (Gibson et al., 2017). Prebiotic fibers may improve our gut and overall health. Prebiotics are naturally occurring in some foods and promote the growth of healthy bacteria in the gut. You can use prebiotic supplements with or without probiotics (Deokar et al., 2022). In addition to the known prebiotics, which are oligosaccharides such as fructooligosaccharides (FOS), galactooligosaccharides (GOS), inulin, and xylooligosaccharides (XOS) that are metabolized by gut microbes such as *Saccharomyces, bifidobacteria, eubacteria, and lactobacilli* instead of being broken down by enzyme activities, some substances have also been shown to have prebiotic qualities. These include proteins or peptides, unsaturated fatty acids, flavonoids, micronutrients, and macronutrients (Table 11.2) (Ashaolu et al., 2018). Prebiotics strengthen the immune system in several ways, which are linked to probiotic stimulation and the metabolites they create, such as branched- and short-chain fatty acids (SCFAs). The fermentation of prebiotics by gut bacteria produces SCFAs, particularly acetate, propionate, and butyrate. These SCFAs serve as an energy source for colonocytes (cells lining the colon), help maintain gut barrier integrity, regulate immune responses, and reduce inflammation in the gut. Other rare microbial categories, such as fecal bacteria, eubacteria, or roseburia, may also contribute to these effects (Guimarães et al., 2020; Neri-Numa & Pastore, 2020).

11.3.2 Probiotic

Probiotics are live microbial food supplements that provide numerous health benefits, such as maintaining great stability and composition of the intestinal microbiota and increasing resistance to pathogen infection (Ghosh et al., 2021). The Food and Agriculture Organization/World Health Organization defines probiotics as "Live microorganisms which, when administered in sufficient quantities, confer a health benefit on the host" (Amara & Shibl, 2015). Probiotics include some yeast strains from the *Saccharomyces genus*, including bacterial cultures, primarily *Lactobacillus, Bacillus, and Bifidobacterium* (Dahiya & Nigam, 2022), according to the consensus panel of the International Scientific Association for Probiotics and Prebiotics (ISAPP) (Venkataratnamma et al., 2017). Lactic acid bacteria (LAB), which are classified by the US Food and Drug Administration (FDA) as "Generally Recognized As Safe (GRAS)" microorganisms, are typically used as probiotics (Ipa Europe, 2021). LAB are classified as members of the class Bacilli, phylum Firmicutes, and

TABLE 11.2 Bioactive Component in Functional Foods With Potential Benefits.

Classification of functional food	Functional components	Source	Potential benefits	References
Prebiotic	Insulin, FOS, polydextrose	Whole grains, beans, oats, tomatoes, onions, soybeans, wheat, yacon root, dandelion greens, flaxseed, garlic, leeks, carrots, bananas, barley, berries, and chocolate, bread, cereal, cookies, and yogurt.	Enhances the flora in the gut, which relieves constipation, lowers the risk of heart disease and specific types of cancer, improves calcium absorption, and reduces blood lipids in hyperlipidemia.	Dahiya and Nigam (2022), Gibson et al. (2017), Ashaolu et al. (2018), Neri-Numa and Pastore (2020), Guimarães et al. (2020)
Probiotic	*Lactobacillus, Bifidobacteria, Yeast*	Yoghurt, pickles, kimchi, sauerkraut, cheese, kefir, and traditional buttermilk.	Enhancing digestive health, enhancing the function of the intestinal mucosal barrier, acting as antipathogens, and boosting immunity to increase the body's resilience.	Dahiya and Nigam (2022), Guimarães et al. (2020), Venkataratnamma et al. (2017), Ipa Europe (2021), International Scientific Association for Probiotics and Prebiotics ISAPP (n.d)
Postbiotic	Peptides, teichoic acids, peptidoglycan-derived muropeptides, polysaccharides, antioxidant enzymes, and short-chain fatty acids including acetic, propionic, and butyric acids	Yoghurt, kombucha, pickled veggies, and sauerkraut.	Short-chain fatty acids derived from gut microbes play crucial roles in immune regulation, gene expression modulation, pathogen prevention, intestinal health maintenance, infection, antiinflammatory, and immune-stimulating effects via Toll-like receptors.	Parte et al. (2020), Zheng et al. (2020)
Synbiotic	Probiotics, prebiotics, and postbiotics	Sauerkraut, tempeh, whole grains, kefir, and yoghurt.	Synbiotics can lower respiratory tract infections, sepsis, and newborn mortality in low-birth-weight babies. Enhance the viability of probiotic supplements in the gut, decrease colonic tumor occurrence, and hinder the proliferation of harmful bacteria.	www.optibacprobiotics.com (n.d), Sergeev et al. (2020)
Short-chain fatty acids	Propionate, acetate, butyrate	Oats, apple, pears, sweet potato, beet, garlic, onion, chia seeds, flaxseeds.	Regulate the host immune response to microbial colonization by regulating phagocytosis, chemokine, and central signaling pathways of cell growth and apoptosis.	Dimidi et al. (2019), McLoughlin et al. (2017), Ney et al. (2023)

(*Continued*)

TABLE 11.2 (Continued)

Classification of functional food	Functional components	Source	Potential benefits	References
Dietary fibers	Cellulose, pectin, lignin, and NSPs	Vegetables, berries, oats, brown rice, popcorn, nuts, baked potatoes with skin, whole grains and beans	May reduce the chance of breast and colon cancer reduce the risk of cardiovascular disease	Yegin et al. (2020), Shaikh (2022), Holscher (2017)
Omega-3 fatty acids	ALA, EPA, and DHA	Canola oils, flaxseeds, anchovies, walnuts, chia seeds, salmon, herring, oysters, soybeans, and sardines.	May enhance mental and visual abilities and lower the risk of cardiovascular disease, postbiotics impact the metabolism of cells and tissues.	ods.od.nih.gov (n.d), Surette (2008)
Vitamins	Vitamins A, B, C, D, E, and K	Liver and kidney, meat (chicken and red meat), citrus fruit (oranges and orange juice), strawberries, peppers, blackcurrants, brussels sprouts, black-eyed peas, mango, sweet red pepper, cantaloupe, dried apricots, pumpkin pie, tomato juice, and beef liver, cod liver oil.	Being beneficial in warding off colds and diseases, reducing bone loss, and preserving bone strength. It also aids in producing collagen, which facilitates wound healing, reduces stress and anxiety, and supports the well-being of blood vessels, bones, cartilage, and skin.	de et al. (2016), National Institutes of Health (2017a), Hanna et al. (2022), Frank (2015), Plantone et al. (2021), Gasperi et al. (2019), Rajasekaran (2017), National Institutes of Health (2021a), Lu et al. (2007), National Institutes of Health (2021b), Gholami et al. (2023)
Minerals	Folic acid, calcium, magnesium, zinc, iron, copper, and selenium	Mushrooms, Potato, Apple, Sunflower seeds, Pumpkin seeds, Banana, Yoghurt.	All functional components independently and in direct relation to each other to support this essential function and maintain homeostasis.	Weyh et al. (2022), Ştefanache et al. (2023), Barone et al. (2022)
Carotenoids	Beta-Carotene, alpha-carotene, lutein, lycopene, zeaxanthin	Fruits and vegetables, such as oranges, tomatoes, bell peppers, kale, spinach, cantaloupe, watermelon, and carrots, eggs, citrus, corn.	An increase in β-carotene concentration that has a prooxidant effect. Reduce the likelihood of muscular atrophy and intensify visual impairment, Reduce the possibility of getting prostate cancer.	Maoka (2019), Nagarajan et al. (2017), Olatunde et al. (2020), Crupi et al. (2023), Dhinaut et al. (2017)
Flavonoids	Anthocyanidins, flavanones, flavones, catechins	Red table wine, apples, peaches, dried parsley, aronia, green pepper, bilberries, chickpeas, blackcurrants, American bilberries, red cabbage, red currants, raspberries, and strawberries. Fresh capers, elderberry juice, dried parsley, sorrel, red onions, rocket lettuce, fresh cranberries, goji	The antioxidant and antibacterial properties of anthocyanidins are beneficial for neurological and noncommunicable diseases. It lessens the effects of chronic disorders like Alzheimer's disease. Removing free radicals to reduce the risk of	Panche et al. (2016), Atef et al. (2017), Abarikwu et al. (2016)

(Continued)

TABLE 11.2 (Continued)

Classification of functional food	Functional components	Source	Potential benefits	References
		berries, cooked asparagus, blackcurrants, dried oregano, grapefruit, lemons, orange juice, limes, oranges, grapefruit juice, artichokes, green tea, black tea, dried cocoa, dark chocolate, blackberries, cooked broad beans, pecan nuts, and pecan nuts.	cancer Tea catechins are beneficial for diabetes, obesity, and heart disease.	
Phenolic acids	Polyphenols, mono- and polysaccharides	Grains, legumes, oilseeds, fruits, vegetables, drinks, and herbs, blueberries Strawberry and grape pomace.	Reduce the risk of cardiovascular disease and improve neurological function.	Kasote et al. (2021), Călinoiu and Vodnar (2018), Liu et al. (2023)
Biles acids	Cholate, hyocholate, deoxycholate, taurohyocholate, ursodeoxycholate, taurocholate, tauro-αmuricholat	Flaxseeds, green tea, banana, garlic, onion, apple, oats	Improve lipid and vitamin absorption; regulate gut microbiota composition, gut hormones, intestinal immunity, intestinal electrolyte and fluid balance, gut motility, lipid homeostasis, glucose homeostasis, amino acid homeostasis, and circadian clocks; modify neurotransmission and physiology.	Xie et al. (2021), Xu et al. (2023)
Gases	H_2S, H_2, CO_2, CH_4, NO	Ginger, fennel seed, cucumber, carrots pappya, pineapple, rice, banana	No mediates gastric mucosal protection and regulates mucosal blood flow.	Kalantar-Zadeh et al. (2019), McCarville et al. (2020)

ALA, Alpha-linolenic acid; *DHA*, docosahexaenoic acid; *EPA*, eicosapentaenoic acid; *FOS*, fructooligosaccharides; *NSPs*, nonstarch polysaccharides.

order Lactobacillales (Table 11.2). They are made up of more than 300 species and are divided into over 50 genera arranged into 6 families, which include *Lactobacillus, Levilactobacillus, Lacticaseibacillus, Limosilactobacillus, Lactococcus, Pediococcus, Enterococcus, Leuconostoc, Oenococcus, Streptococcus, Tetragenococcus, Aerococcus, Carnobacterium, Weissella, Alloiococcus, Symbiobacterium, and Vagococcus* (International Scientific Association for Probiotics and Prebiotics ISAPP, n.d; Salminen et al., 2021; Scott et al., 2022). Furthermore, the microbial strains employed in food preparation or supplements need to have shown benefits to the host to be deemed effective probiotics. Probiotics instruct the immune system to distinguish between beneficial and harmful microbes, which aids in immune system function. Additionally, they aid in the digestion of certain fibers, which produce SCFAs, including butyrate, acetate, and propionate, influencing immune cell activity and inflammation in the intestines and throughout the body. They also create several vitamins that humans' metabolisms are unable to manufacture. Probiotics, which are primarily bacteria and some helpful yeast strains, are an effective approach to introducing a specific number and variety of advantageous microorganisms into the gastrointestinal tract (Dahiya & Nigam, 2022; Guimarães et al., 2020). Depending on the circumstances in these regions, the probiotics gradually remain in the small or large intestine. Once in place, the probiotics can outcompete any dangerous bacteria by vying for their food supplies and colonization space. Probiotics create various vitamins and SCFAs while they are living in the GIT, which is good for the hosts' health (Deokar et al., 2022).

11.3.3 Postbiotic

Postbiotics are an innovative type of biotics with potential health advantages. Unlike probiotics, postbiotics do not require living cells to produce health effects and are therefore exempt from the regulations governing food safety that are applicable to live microbes (Parte et al., 2020). "Preparation of inanimate microorganisms and/or their components that confer a health benefit on the host" is the definition of postbiotics (Koren & Rautava, 2020). The impact that certain short-chain fatty acids (SCFAs) have on the health of the gut environment, the effect that the presence of exopolysaccharides (EPS) can have on strengthening the gut barrier and reducing inflammation within the gut environment, and the effect that bacteriocins produced by specific bacteria have on promoting antimicrobial activity against gut pathogens are just a few of the endpoints of gut health that postbiotics compounds from a broad range of microbes can positively affect (Zheng et al., 2020). The gut microbiome's synthesis of the SCFAs butyrate, propionate, and acetate is essential for human health. Cross-feeding in the human colon and bacterial fermentation of food fibers are the two sources of SCFAs. Among other aspects, SCFAs protect against intestinal inflammation by stimulating G protein—coupled receptors (GPCRs), which are SCFA-sensing receptors and help maintain the intestinal epithelial barrier and regulate the immune system (Martin-Gallausiaux et al., 2020).

11.3.4 Synbiotic

Gibson and Roberfroid coined the term "synbiotics" in 1995 to describe an infusion of a probiotic and a prebiotic (Gibson & Roberfroid, 1995). Supporting overall gut health can be achieved with synbiotics, often with great success. The prebiotics in them nourish not just the probiotic bacteria in the supplement but also the naturally friendly bacteria that live in our stomachs (www.optibacprobiotics.com, n.d). "A mixture that benefits the host's health and consists of live microorganisms and substrate(s) that are specifically used by the host microorganisms." The microbiota that typically resides in the host GIT is indicated by the host microorganisms in the present scenario. This microbiota will also include the intake of externally cultivated microbes that are eaten through probiotic supplements. Within the synbiotic preparations, the substrate (prebiotic) may be directed towards either or both kinds of microflora. In the total dietary approach to lowering obesity, targeting the gut flora using synbiotics—probiotic supplements including prebiotic components—is emerging as a potential strategy (Sergeev et al., 2020). Li et al. (2023) conducted a study to investigate the immunomodulatory effects of synbiotics in healthy individuals, as there is limited evidence in this area. The study involved 106 healthy adults who were randomly assigned to receive either synbiotics or a placebo for 8 weeks in a double-blind, randomized, placebo-controlled trial. The synbiotic supplement contained *Bifidobacterium lactis* HN019, *Lactobacillus rhamnosus* HN001, and fructooligosaccharide. Results showed that participants who received synbiotic supplementation experienced greater reductions in plasma C-reactive protein and interferon-gamma levels, along with increased plasma interleukin-10 and stool secretory IgA levels compared to those in the placebo group. Moreover, synbiotic supplementation resulted in an enrichment of beneficial bacteria and functional pathways related to amino acids and short-chain fatty acids biosynthesis, while reducing potential proinflammatory bacteria such as Parabacteroides. Importantly, changes in antiinflammatory markers (IL-10 and sIgA) were found to be significantly associated with microbial variations induced by synbiotic supplementation. Stratification of participants based on their pretreatment Prevotella-to-bacteroides ratio revealed a more favorable effect of synbiotic supplements in individuals with a higher ratio. In conclusion, the study provided direct evidence supporting the beneficial effects of synbiotic supplementation on immune parameters, which were correlated with changes in the gut microbiota induced by synbiotics. These findings highlight the potential for personalized supplementation of symbiotics for immunomodulation (Li et al., 2023).

11.3.5 Short-chain fatty acids

The term "fermented foods" refers to "foods or beverages produced through controlled microbial growth, and the conversion of food components through enzymatic action" (Marco et al., 2017). Many foods have traditionally been fermented, including meat and fish, dairy, vegetables, soybeans, other legumes, grains, and fruits. The fermentation process involves various variables, including microorganisms, nutritional elements, and ambient conditions, which result in thousands of different types of fermented foods such as kefir, kombucha, sauerkraut, tempeh, natto, miso, kimchi, and sourdough bread (Dimidi et al., 2019). Short-chain fatty acids (SCFAs) such as acetate, butyrate, and propionate are physiologically active by-products produced by commensal bacteria in the colon through the fermentation of soluble dietary fiber and resistant starch. SCFA production can be influenced by various variables, including accessible fermentation substrates. Oligosaccharide soluble fibers, such as fructooligosaccharides (FOS), release more SCFA than long-4chain polysaccharide-soluble fibers such as pectin. SCFAs lower intestinal pH, promoting the growth of good bacteria such as *Lactobacillus and Bifidobacterium.* These bacteria are powerful SCFA makers that contribute to good immunological responses. Prebiotics are soluble fibers like FOS that promote the growth and activity of beneficial bacteria for the host. Probiotics can potentially modify the colonic microbiota. Live bacteria, mainly *Bifidobacterium and Lactobacillus species*, are delivered directly to the host through supplements or functional foods like yogurt. Synbiotics combine prebiotics and probiotics, resulting in synergistic effects (McLoughlin et al., 2017). Ney et al. (2023) Finding, In recent years, the field of immune metabolism has emerged, highlighting the intricate relationship between metabolism and the immune response. Short-chain fatty acids (SCFAs) have been recognized as potent regulators of innate immune cells like macrophages, monocytes, and neutrophils. They achieve this by altering metabolic pathways, inhibiting histone deacetylases (HDACs), and suppressing signaling via nuclear factor-kappa B (NF-κB). Regarding T cells, SCFAs, particularly butyrate, exert significant immunomodulatory effects. Butyrate indirectly influences T cells through its actions on macrophages and dendritic cells (DCs), regulating T cell homeostasis and differentiation into various subsets, including naive and regulatory T cells (Treg). SCFAs also modulate the release of key cytokines like IL-10 and IL-17, crucial in inflammatory bowel disease (IBD) pathogenesis. Furthermore, SCFAs control the immune response of cytotoxic T lymphocytes (CTL) and increase the number of Treg. They can selectively support the development of different T helper cell subsets depending on the cytokine milieu and immunological context. These regulatory pathways operate independently of specific receptors but rely on histone deacetylase (HDAC) inhibition and increased *mechanistic target of rapamycin* (mTOR) *ribosomal protein kinase (S6K)* (mTOR-S6K) activity.

SCFAs, especially butyrate, play a pivotal role in promoting the memory potential of antigen-activated CD8 + T cells by altering cellular metabolism. They promote oxidative phosphorylation (OXPHOS) and utilize various metabolic pathways, enhancing CD8 + T cell survival and antitumor activity. In adoptive T cell therapy (ATC), pretreatment with SCFAs enhances antigen-specific antitumor responses. Pentanoate, another SCFA, exhibits antiinflammatory effects and induces regulatory B-cell formation, offering potential therapeutic benefits in autoimmune conditions. The regulation of B cell responses is crucial in various conditions, including rheumatoid arthritis (RA). Changes in gut microbiota and SCFA formation have been linked to alleviating RA symptoms. SCFAs can also restore antibody responses in the gut, particularly against enterotoxins like cholera toxin (CT), highlighting their role in mucosal immunity. In macrophages, SCFAs influence polarization states, with butyrate shifting M2-polarized macrophages towards oxidative phosphorylation and fatty acid oxidation, promoting antimicrobial activity. Similarly, SCFAs enhance innate immune responses of neutrophils, promoting migration to inflammatory sites and coordinating antibacterial host responses. Overall, SCFAs play multifaceted roles in modulating immune responses, influencing various immune cell types and pathways. Their therapeutic potential in immune-related disorders continues to be explored, offering promising avenues (Ney et al., 2023).

11.3.6 Dietary fibers

Dietary fiber is described as "the edible sections of plants or comparable carbohydrates that are resistant to digestion and absorption in the human small intestine with complete or partial fermentation in the large intestine. "Prebiotic dietary fibers serve as carbon sources for the colon's primary and secondary fermentation pathways, benefiting digestive health in numerous ways. Fructooligosaccharides, inulin, and galactooligosaccharides are universally recognized prebiotics (Table 11.2) (Carlson et al., 2018). Any plant element that is resistant to enzymatic digestion is considered a dietary fiber. Examples of this include cellulose, hemicellulose, and other noncellulosic polysaccharides, pectin compounds, gums, mucilage, and lignin, which is a noncarbohydrate component. Diets rich in dietary fiber, such as those found in fruits, vegetables, nuts, and cereals, are beneficial to your health because they have been linked to a lower risk of many ailments (Yegin et al., 2020). Digested fibers in the colon produce short-chain fatty acids, which are very beneficial to health. Artificially created functional fibers are added to food products to provide similar health benefits without raising the calorie count. These consist of polydextrose, cellulose, maltodextrin, and inulin (Shaikh, 2022). Dietary and functional fiber consumption has several possible health benefits. In addition to lowering cholesterol and decreasing the risk of coronary and circulatory heart diseases, constipation, irritable bowel syndrome (IBS), colon cancer, diabetes, and breast cancer, fibers also prevent obesity and diabetes. Dietary fiber is present in many functional foods, such as beverages, baked items, and animal products. Different processing methods (canning, frying, grinding, boiling, and extrusion-cooking) alter the physicochemical properties of dietary fiber and increase its therapeutic value. Dietary fibers are plant-based polysaccharide components with a limited ability for absorption since they are resistant to digestion (Yegin et al., 2020).

In this study, the author says the health advantages of dietary fiber have long been recognized. Higher dietary fiber intakes have been associated with lower rates of cardiovascular disease, and fiber plays a role in gastrointestinal health, with many effective laxatives being fiber isolates. Higher fiber consumption is associated with decreased body weight. Originally, only polysaccharides were considered dietary fiber, but more current definitions include oligosaccharides as well, based on their physiological benefits rather than their chemical detection as dietary fiber using the standard total dietary fiber (TDF) method. Inulin, fructooligosaccharides, and other oligosaccharides are included as fiber on food labels in the United States. In addition, oligosaccharides are known as "prebiotics," "a selectively fermented ingredient that allows specific changes, both in the composition and/or activity in the gastrointestinal microflora that confers benefits upon host well-being and health." Too far, all known and suspected prebiotics are carbohydrate molecules, predominantly oligosaccharides that resist digestion in the human small intestine before reaching the colon and being fermented by gut microorganisms. According to studies, inulin and oligofructose (OF), lactulose, and resistant starch (RS) meet all of the definition's requirements, including stimulating *Bifidobacterium*, a beneficial bacterial genus. Other isolated carbohydrates and carbohydrate-containing meals include galactooligosaccharides (GOS), transgalactooligosaccharides (TOS), polydextrose, wheat dextrin, and acacia, gum, psyllium, banana, whole grain wheat, also have a prebiotic effect (Holscher, 2017).

11.3.7 Omega-3 fatty acids

Foods such as fish and flaxseed, as well as dietary supplements such as fish oil, contain omega-3 fatty acids. Alpha-linolenic acid (ALA), eicosapentaenoic acid (EPA), and docosahexaenoic acid (DHA) are the three primary omega-3 fatty acids (Table 11.2). The primary sources of ALA are plant oils like canola, soybean, and flaxseed oils. Fish and other seafood include DHA and EPA. Because ALA is an essential fatty acid—one that your body cannot produce on its own—you must obtain it from the foods and liquids you eat and drink. Only extremely tiny amounts of ALA can be converted by your body from EPA to DHA. Thus the only practical approach to increase your intake of EPA and DHA is to receive them from food or dietary supplements, is the only realistic method to raise your body's levels of these omega-3 fatty acids. Important constituents of the membranes enveloping every cell in your body are omega-3 fatty acids. The brain, sperm cells, and retina (eye) have very high DHA levels. In addition to giving your body energy in the form of calories, omega-3s help support numerous bodily systems, including the immune system, endocrine system, heart, blood vessels, and lungs (the network of hormone-producing glands) (ods.od.nih.gov, n.d; Surette, 2008). A 6-week randomized intervention trial was conducted by Vijay et al. (2020) proving the prebiotic potentials of omega-3 fatty acids consumed as functional food through various sources which in turn contributes positively to immune responses mediated via various mechanisms depicted above in Fig. 11.1 They conducted a 6-week dietary intervention in which they contrasted the effects of taking 500 mg of omega-3 supplementation daily with 20 g of inulin, a well-studied prebiotic. Bifidobacterium and Lachnospiraceae significantly increased in response to inulin intake. On the other hand, coprococcus and Bacteroides species showed notable increases with omega-3 treatment, while Collinsella species linked to fatty liver showed considerable declines. Conversely, the results of omega-3 supplementation showed large increases in isobutyrate and isovalerate and almost significant increases in butyrate, which was comparable to the effects of inulin supplementation, which produced significant increases in butyrate, isovalerate, and iso-butyrate. After controlling for confounders, coprococcus was found to be positively associated with isobutyric acid and negatively associated with triglyceride-rich lipoproteins like VLDL. Coprococcus was found to be considerably enhanced postsupplementation with omega-3 (Vijay et al., 2020).

11.3.8 Vitamins

Vitamins are necessary chemical compounds that must be consumed in modest amounts through a balanced diet for the human body to function properly. Water-soluble vitamins and fat-soluble vitamins are the two primary categories into which they are divided. Fat-soluble vitamins, such as A, D, E, and K, can be stored for future use in the body's fatty tissues and liver. Water-soluble vitamins, on the other hand, cannot be kept in the body for a long time. These include vitamin C and the B-complex vitamins, which comprise niacin (B3), riboflavin (B2), biotin (B7), thiamine (B1), pantothenic acid (B5), and folic acid (B9) as shown in Table 11.2 Sweat and urine are examples of body fluids that discharge excess water-soluble vitamin content. Consequently, to keep the levels of these vitamins appropriate, you must eat them every day (de et al., 2016).

11.3.8.1 Vitamin A

One of the most important groups of micronutrients, vitamin A is widely distributed in a wide range of foods and is essential for many body processes. Being a fat-soluble vitamin, it aids in immune system function, growth and development of the body, and appropriate vision. It is added to some items, including cereal and milk, and can be found naturally in a variety of dietary sources (Carazo et al., 2021). The recommended intake of vitamin A can be obtained by eating a wide variety of foods, such as fish (salmon, herring, and salmon), organ meats (beef liver, though intake of this meat should be limited due to its high cholesterol content), green leafy vegetables, and colorful vegetables (spinach, sweet potatoes, carrots, broccoli, and winter squash). Cantaloupe, mangoes, and apricots are among the fruits; dairy products, fortified cereals for breakfast, and eggs, which help increase vitamin A intake. This vital vitamin is necessary for healthy growth and skin and for the maintenance of the immune system, reproductive health, eyesight, and the correct operation of several organs, including the heart, kidneys, and lungs. In addition, vitamin A may be used therapeutically to treat retinitis pigmentosa, skin conditions, and leukemia, and possibly help prevent breast and lung cancer (National Institutes of Health, 2017a).

11.3.8.2 Vitamin B

B vitamins, collectively known as B-complex vitamins, are essential for both catabolic and anabolic metabolism. These water-soluble vitamins, including thiamine (B1), riboflavin (B2), niacin (B3), pantothenic acid (B5), pyridoxine (B6), biotin (B7), folate (B9), and cobalamin (B12), need to be replenished daily as they are excreted in urine (Hanna et al., 2022).

Thiamine, or vitamin B1, is naturally present in many foods, with whole grains, pork, fish, and yeast being particularly rich sources. Processed foods are often fortified with thiamine due to its partial removal during processing (Frank, 2015).

Riboflavin (B2) is found in eggs, dairy products, green vegetables, meat, mushrooms, and almonds. It is also added to certain staples like rice, corn, and flour (Plantone et al., 2021).

Niacin (B3) is present in both animal and plant-based foods such as soy, nuts, seeds, legumes, and grains. Many grain products and infant formulas are fortified with niacin (Gasperi et al., 2019).

Pantothenic acid (B5) is widely distributed in various foods, including fortified cereals, dried foods, mushrooms, eggs, fish, avocados, poultry, beef, pork, sunflower seeds, sweet potatoes, and lentils (Rajasekaran, 2017).

Pyridoxine (B6) is found in beef, poultry, starchy vegetables, noncitrus fruits, and fortified cereals (National Institutes of Health, 2017b).

Biotin (B7) is naturally occurring in organ meats, eggs, fish, seeds, soybeans, and nuts and is also available through supplementation (National Institute of Health, 2017).

Folate (B9) is abundant in dark green leafy vegetables, nuts, beans, dairy products, meat, poultry, grains, and Brussels sprouts (National Institutes of Health, 2022).

Cobalamin (B12) is primarily found in animal products and fortified foods (National Institutes of Health, 2024).

Each B vitamin serves unique biochemical functions in the body, aiding in processes such as DNA repair, energy metabolism, red blood cell production, and nerve function. Deficiencies in these vitamins can lead to various health issues, emphasizing the importance of consuming a balanced diet rich in B vitamin sources (Liu et al., 2022; PubChem, n.d).

11.3.8.3 Vitamin C

Since vitamin C is a necessary nutrient, your body is unable to synthesize it. Still, it plays a variety of roles and has been connected to several noteworthy health advantages. Numerous fruits and vegetables, such as oranges, strawberries, kiwi fruit, bell peppers, broccoli, kale, and spinach, contain this water-soluble substance (National Institutes of Health, 2021a). Vitamin C has strong antioxidant properties, which means that it helps shield cells from harm brought on by free radicals. Unstable chemicals known as free radicals can harm cells, accelerate aging, and cause several diseases. Through its ability to neutralize these free radicals, vitamin C enhances the immune system's general health (Wintergerst et al., 2006). Collagen is a protein that is vital to the development of skin, blood vessels, bones, and connective tissues. Collagen synthesis requires vitamin C. By serving as a barrier against pathogens, these tissues aid in the prevention of illnesses (Zelman, 2022). Neutrophils, lymphocytes, and phagocytes are examples of white blood cells whose functions are supported by vitamin C. These cells support the body's defenses against infections and foreign invasion reactions (Carr & Maggini, 2017).

11.3.8.4 Vitamin D

Oily fish (such as sardines, salmon, herring, and mackerel), liver, egg yolks, red meat, fortified foods (such as fat spreads and breakfast cereals), and liver are good sources of vitamin D, which is made up of calciferol (vitamin D2) and cholecalciferol (vitamin D3). Vitamin D has several essential roles in the human body. It helps maintain healthy teeth and bones, strengthens the immune system, supports the proper functioning of the brain and nerve system, and helps control diabetes by controlling insulin levels. It also improves cardiovascular health and lung function, and it affects the expression of genes linked to the development of cancer (Lu et al., 2007).

11.3.8.5 Vitamin E

There are several types of vitamin E, but the human body can only efficiently use alpha-tocopherol. It can be obtained from fruits, vegetables, nuts, seeds, and plant-based oils such as olive, soybean, maize, and sunflower. Vitamin E has been linked to several health benefits, including skin moisturization, wound healing assistance, cancer prevention, relief from skin conditions such as psoriasis, and dermatitis, reducing and preventing scars, wrinkle treatment, protection from sunburn, nail health, and immune system support. Furthermore, vitamin E is used in the management of dementia and diabetes (National Institutes of Health, 2021b).

11.3.8.6 Vitamin K

Among the many substances that make up vitamin K are vitamin K1 and vitamin K2. Leafy greens and other vegetables such as broccoli, cauliflower, cabbage, and Brussels sprouts are the main sources of vitamin K1. On the other hand, foods, including eggs, cheese, fish, meats, and liver, are good providers of vitamin K2. To prevent cardiovascular disease, vascular calcification, and osteoporosis, vitamin K is essential. It also supports heart health, cognitive function, and bone health (National Institutes of Health, 2021c). Gholami et al. (2023) suggest that not all cancer patients benefit from immunotherapy, and recent evidence hints at a connection between gut microbiota and treatment effectiveness. While various mechanisms linking microbial contributions to the immune response have been proposed, one likely role is the provision of essential co-factors to the host, including certain vitamins. While humans mainly obtain vitamins from external sources, bacteria, fungi, and plants can produce their vitamins. Surprisingly, the significance of microbial-derived vitamins as key immune system regulators has been overlooked in humans. These vitamins are often shared among gut bacteria, stabilizing bioenergetic pathways within microbial communities. Changes in gut microbiota composition can impact metabolic pathways, thereby influencing immune function. Conversely, the immune system plays a vital role in maintaining gut microbiota, which in turn affects vitamin production. The authors elucidate the immune-interactive mechanisms through which microbially derived vitamins may enhance the efficacy of immunotherapies in cancer. In the gastrointestinal (GI) tract, immune cells and vitamin-producing bacteria are distributed with varying frequencies. The gut-associated lymphoid tissue (GALT), comprising mesenteric lymph nodes (MLNs), isolated lymphoid follicles (ILFs), and Peyer's patches, is crucial for host immune defense, particularly in the small intestine. Gut microbes express pathogen-associated molecular patterns (PAMPs), recognized by immune cells via pattern recognition receptors (PRRs). Interaction between PAMPs and PRRs triggers maturation of antigen-presenting cells (APCs), leading to differentiation of naïve CD4 + T cells in MLNs and beyond, amplifying T- and B-cell responses. Th17 and Treg cells, predominant in the gut, exhibit an inverse concentration gradient along the tract. Bacterial abundance also varies along the GI tract, with the lowest in the duodenum and increasing towards the colon, dominated by Firmicutes and Bacteroides in healthy individuals. Most gut-derived vitamins are produced and absorbed in the large intestine, while dietary vitamins are absorbed in the small intestine. Vitamin K2 and several water-soluble B vitamins are among those produced by gut bacteria and play diverse roles in immune function. Additionally, certain carbohydrates and carbohydrate-containing foods possess prebiotic effects, such as galactooligosaccharides (GOS), transgalactooligosaccharides (TOS), polydextrose, wheat dextrin, acacia gum, psyllium, banana, and whole grain wheat. These compounds promote the antimicrobial activity of monocytes and macrophages (Coker & Madan, 2020; Gholami et al., 2023).

11.3.9 Minerals

Minerals are essential components of our diet, serving various functions such as bone structure, muscle and nerve function, and hormone and enzyme production. Some minerals also play crucial roles in immune system function, both innate and adaptive responses (Fig. 11.1) (Weyh et al., 2022). While a balanced diet typically provides adequate mineral intake to support immune health, certain vulnerable populations should ensure they obtain sufficient amounts of minerals such as magnesium, zinc, copper, iron, and selenium. Inadequate levels of these minerals can temporarily compromise immune function and disrupt the long-term regulation of inflammation. Therefore understanding mineral mechanisms and sources is vital. In cases of mineral deficiencies, supplementation may be necessary, but excessive intake can have adverse effects on the immune system and should be approached cautiously (Ştefanache et al., 2023). Barone et al. (2022) conducted a study on the critical role of the human gut microbiome in regulating mineral levels within the body. They found that enzymes produced by gut bacteria, such as phytases, help release essential minerals such as calcium, magnesium, iron, and phosphorous from dietary sources. Short-chain fatty acids (SCFAs), produced through the fermentation of polysaccharides by microbes, aid in mineral absorption, especially calcium, by lowering the pH in the gastrointestinal tract and increasing solubility. Administration of probiotics, such as *Enterococcus faecium*, has been linked to improved bone mineral density, likely due to increased SCFA production and enhanced phytase activity. However, iron supplementation, though necessary, can negatively impact the gut microbiome by reducing beneficial bacteria and promoting pathogenic growth, potentially leading to intestinal inflammation. Iron absorption is influenced by microbial metabolites, with SCFAs promoting absorption while other compounds hinder it. Zinc deficiency alters gut microbiome composition, reducing diversity and increasing inflammation markers, which can affect gut-brain signaling. Clinical trials on probiotic supplementation for zinc deficiency have shown mixed results, with some demonstrating significant increases in zinc levels, particularly when combined with zinc supplementation. Furthermore, animal studies suggest a connection between magnesium availability and gut microbiome composition. Magnesium also plays a role in the metabolism of vitamins B1 and D, particularly in conditions like metabolic syndrome, type 2 diabetes, and obesity (Barone et al., 2022).

11.3.10 Carotenoids

Carotenoids are crucial components of all photosynthetic organisms because of their superior photoprotective and antioxidant characteristics. However, carotenoids are not just found in plants, algae, and cyanobacteria; some fungi and nonphotosynthetic bacteria may also synthesize them, and many animals rely on foodborne carotenoids as visual pigments, antioxidants, or colorants (Maoka, 2019; Nagarajan et al., 2017). Carotenoids are hydrocarbon compounds that give fruits, vegetables, and seeds their reddish-pink hues (Table 11.2). They are made up of a conjugated double-bond structure. Depending on whether an oxygen molecule is present in their fundamental structure or not, carotenoids are divided into two categories. In nature, they are widely dispersed. Through phytoene, geranylgeranyl pyrophosphate is used in their production. This is followed by oxidation, epoxidation, cyclization, hydroxylation, dehydrogenation, and desaturation (Olatunde et al., 2020). The most studied carotenoids in diets are the three hydrocarbon carotenes (α-, β-, and lycopene) and the three oxygenated xanthophylls (lutein, zeaxanthin, and β-cryptoxanthin). Colorless carotenoids, such as phytoene and phytofluene, have also attracted a lot of attention lately because they are widely distributed in food and may have benefits for both health and appearance (Meléndez-Martínez et al., 2021). Many of the distinct pharmacological effects of carotenoids, such as their antiaging, anticancer, antidiabetic, immune-modulating, antiobesity, antioxidant, provitamin, osteoprotective, cardioprotective, and hepatoprotective qualities, have been attributed to their distinct chemical structure. Carotenoids are used in food and beverages as nutraceuticals and nutritional supplements due to a number of their health benefits (Crupi et al., 2023).

The most well-known mechanism of carotenoid action is its antioxidant activity. Individual oxygen species and peroxyl radicals are regularly produced in biological systems. These reactive species can affect cell membrane function and cause DNA single-strand breaks. β-Carotene and other carotenoids have been shown to have immunomodulatory effects in humans and animals. These carotenoids promote lymphocyte blastogenesis, increase the number of particular lymphocyte subsets, boost lymphocyte cytotoxicity, and stimulate the production of various cytokines. Furthermore, carotenoids increase the phagocytic and bacteria-killing abilities of blood neutrophils and peritoneal macrophages (Chew & Park, 2004). Dhinaut et al. (2017) performed an experimental study that found immunopathology refers to self-damage the inflammatory response caused by oxidizing chemicals created when the immune system is active. Immunopathology frequently contributes to age-related disorders and is thought to promote aging. Immunopathology is prevented through the use of endogenous antioxidant enzymes and the absorption of dietary antioxidants, including carotenoids like astaxanthin. Astaxanthin is currently gaining popularity as a powerful antioxidant and for its ability to alleviate age-related illnesses. Current in vitro and in vivo investigations show promising results for astaxanthin's immune-stimulating and antioxidant effects. However, it is unclear how much dietary astaxanthin can avoid long-term immunopathological consequences on longevity. We used the mealworm beetle, Tenebrio molitor, as a biological model to assess the effect of lifetime nutritional supplementation with exposure to inflammation early in life, astaxanthin improves longevity. While astaxanthin supplementation was shown to lower immunopathology costs on larval survival and insect lifespan, it also reduced immunity, growth rate, and survival of non-immune-challenged larvae. As a result, this study demonstrates that astaxanthin protects immunopathology by suppressing the immune system, which might harm growth (Dhinaut et al., 2017).

11.3.11 Flavonoids

Flavonoids are a class of naturally occurring compounds that have various phenolic structures that can be found in tea, wine, cereals, roots, flowers, fruits, and vegetables. The health benefits of these natural products are well known, and attempts are being undertaken to separate the components known as flavonoids. Nowadays, flavonoids are seen as an essential component of many pharmacological, cosmetic, nutraceutical, and medical uses. This is explained by their ability to modify the activity of important cellular enzymes and their antioxidative, antiinflammatory, antimutagenic, and anticarcinogenic qualities (Panche et al., 2016). Recent years have seen a significant amount of research done to investigate the processes by which foods high in flavonoids protect the body from pathological disorders (Waheed Janabi et al., 2020). It has been observed that certain flavonoids, such as quercetin, reduce ischemia-reperfusion injury by obstructing the action of inducible nitric oxide synthase (Atef et al., 2017). It has been claimed that flavonoids directly scavenge nitric oxide molecules, which can be thought of as radicals themselves. Thus it has been hypothesized that one of the ways flavonoids work as a medicine is through nitric oxide scavenging (Abarikwu et al., 2016). Although radical scavenging accounts for many of the benefits of flavonoids, they may also have an effect via interacting with different enzyme systems such as glutathione peroxidase, superoxide dismutase, and catalase (Abarikwu et al., 2016). Additionally, studies conducted in vitro have demonstrated the antiproliferative activity of flavonoids by inhibiting the biosynthesis of polyamines and signal transduction enzymes such as phosphoinositide 3-kinases (PI3K), protein tyrosine kinase (PTK), and protein kinase C (PKC). They have also been shown to induce apoptosis and cell cycle arrest at Gap (G1/G2), differentiate transformed cells, and restore cellular homeostasis (Oršolić & Jazvinšćak Jembrek, 2022; Waheed Janabi et al., 2020). One of the studies was conducted using flavonoid apigenin which is a yellow crystalline solid and its main nonpharmaceutical application is its use to dye wool. It was found that compared to other structurally related flavonoids, apigenin was a useful and health-promoting agent in recent years due to its low toxicity and significant effects on normal versus cancer cells. Antigen-presenting cells, activated T cells, and other cancer cell types all express programmed death ligand 1 (PD-L1). Breast cancer (BC) cells use constitutive and inducible PD-L1 expression to evade the immune system. Studies have indicated that the dietary phytochemical apigenin inhibited the upregulation of PD-L1 induced by interferon (IFN)-γ in triple-negative M.D. Anderson and metastasis breast cancer (MDA-MB-468 BC) cells, human epidermal growth factor receptor 2 HER2(+) SK-BR-3 BC cells, 4T1 mouse mammary carcinoma cells, and human mammary epithelial cells. However, apigenin did not affect triple-negative MDA-MB-231 BC cells' constitutive PD-L1 expression. Apigenin also prevented MDA-MB-468 cells from expressing PD-L1 in response to IFN-β. It was further proved that apigenin-mediated inhibition of IFN-γ-induced PD-L1 expression by MDA-MB-468 cells also increased proliferation and interleukin-2 synthesis by PD-1-expressing Jurkat T cells that were cocultured with MDA-MB-468 cells. Apigenin therefore has the potential to increase the vulnerability of BC cells to T cell—mediated antitumor immune responses (Ashrafizadeh et al., 2020; Coombs et al., 2016).

11.3.12 Phenolic acids

Phenolic acids (ferulic acid, ferulic, vanillic, p-coumaric, caffeic, protocatechuic, p-hydroxybenzoic, genetic, chlorogenic, and syringic acids), flavonoids (flavones, flavonols, isoflavones, flavanols, flavanones, anthocyanins), and avenanthramides are among the polyphenolic molecules found in cereal grains (Kasote et al., 2021). Since they account for 30% of the total phenolic acids in Mediterranean diets, phenolic acids are one of the majority of metabolites of cereal crops that have antioxidant effects on humans. A particular family of polyphenols known as phenolic acids is typically engaged in defense mechanisms against both biotic and abiotic stressors. The phenylpropanoid pathway uses phenylalanine as a substrate to start the production of phenolic acids. The biosynthetic route can be influenced by biotic and abiotic variables, such as agricultural practices and environmental concerns, which can change the concentration of phenolic acid. Furthermore, the genetic effect needs to be considered because genetic-environmental interactions can cause a significant variation in the phenolic content of cereal species and cultivars within the same species (Călinoiu & Vodnar, 2018). In one of the studies conducted using phenolic acid, plant-derived foods and beverages frequently include phenolic acids such as caffeic acid (CA) and chlorogenic acid (CGA). Their equivalent adducts with cysteine (Cys) have been found in coffee-containing beverages. Despite the well-documented antioxidant and antiinflammatory action of CA and CGA, the immunomodulatory properties of the Cys adducts (CA-Cys and CGA-Cys) remain unknown. The adducts were then synthesized, and their immunomodulatory effects in lipopolysaccharide (LPS)-treated RAW 264.7 cells were compared to the activity of the parent phenolic acids. CA and CGA usually suppress inflammatory reactions. However, RNA-sequencing showed that the LPS-induced pathways related to Toll-like receptor signaling, chemokine signaling, and NOD-like receptor signaling, as well as JAK-STAT/MAPK signaling pathways, were upregulated in adduct-treated cells relative to the parent phenolic acids, while neurodegenerative disorder-related pathways and metabolic pathway were downregulated. CA and CGA reduced the production of prostaglandin E2 (PGE2), interleukin-6, TNF-α, and reactive oxygen species (ROS) (all $P < .05$). Adduct-stimulated cells produced less PGE2 and TNF-α ($P < .05$), but more ROS. TNF-α levels in cells activated with 100 μM CGA and CGA-Cys adduct were 4.46 ± 0.23 and 1.61 ± 0.18 ng/mL, respectively. Thus adding the Cys moiety significantly affects the antiinflammatory effect of phenolic compounds (Liu et al., 2023).

11.3.13 Bile acids

Bile acids, originally known for their role in fat digestion, have gained new recognition as key signaling molecules in metabolic health (Xie et al., 2021). Recent discoveries have revealed their interaction with nuclear farnesoid X receptor (FXR) and membrane Takeda G protein–coupled receptor 5 (TGR5), leading to a reevaluation of their physiological functions. Bile acids now serve as regulators of blood glucose, lipid, and energy metabolism. FXR and TGR5 signaling influence various metabolic processes, including the secretion of gastrointestinal hormones such as glucagon-like peptide-1 (GLP-1) and peptide YY (PYY), hepatic gluconeogenesis, glycogen synthesis, energy expenditure, and the composition of the gut microbiome. These findings shed light on the mechanisms underlying the metabolic benefits observed with interventions like bile acid sequestrants, metformin, and bariatric surgery. Bile acids can act directly on nuclear receptors involved in immunological modulation, including FXR (farnesoid X receptor), SXR (steroid and xenobiotic receptor), and VDR (vitamin D receptor). Bile acids can activate these receptors, modulating inflammatory responses, and immune cell activity, and helping to maintain immunological homeostasis Fig. 11.1 (Xu et al., 2023). Prete et al. (2020) investigated how bile acid (BA) signatures, crucial for gut colonization and microbial survival during gastrointestinal transit, are altered in various disease states. They highlighted bile salt hydrolase (BSH) as a key enzyme for BA metabolism, primarily expressed by gut-associated microbes, providing them with an advantage in the gut environment. However, they discovered that certain food-associated strains of *Lactobacillus plantarum* possess the capability to metabolize bile acids, withstand associated stress, and proliferate, essential for survival in the gastrointestinal tract. Moreover, these food-associated strains exhibited the ability to selectively modify BA signatures in favor of receptor activation beneficial to humans. Specifically, they showed a preference for altering human glycol-conjugated BAs, with variations observed among strains. This study underscores the beneficial role of BA metabolism by nonpathogenic bacteria found in food, revealing an evolutionarily conserved trait previously thought to be unique to gut-residing microbes (Prete et al., 2020).

11.3.14 Gases

The intricate interplay between the human body and its microbiome within the intestines significantly impacts gut function and overall health; yet much about this interaction remains unclear. Within the gut, chemical reactions and microbial activity give rise to various gases such as carbon dioxide, hydrogen, methane, and hydrogen sulfide, alongside trace gases Fig. 11.1 Profiling these intestinal gases and observing their responses to dietary changes can unveil the activities and roles of gut microbiota in human health (Kalantar-Zadeh et al., 2019). Advanced techniques, including innovative gas-sensing capsule technology, have been developed to measure these gases accurately. Depending on their composition, concentration, and volume, intestinal gases can either trigger or alleviate abdominal symptoms and may also exert physiological, pathogenic, or therapeutic effects. Therefore understanding and manipulating intestinal gas profiles hold promise for disease prevention and treatment. Given that dietary intake profoundly influences gut microbiota composition and fermentation processes, dietary modification represents the primary therapeutic strategy for gastrointestinal disorders, as it directly affects gas profiles. Enhanced comprehension of the complex interactions driving gas production in the intestines will empower us to better prevent, diagnose, treat, and monitor a wide range of gastrointestinal conditions (McCarville et al., 2020). Sen (2017) researched hydrogen sulfide (H2S), a novel gasotransmitter produced endogenously by various enzymes that are expressed differently in peripheral tissues and the central nervous system. H_2S influences cellular signaling pathways and the sulfhydration of target proteins to regulate a wide range of physiological activities, including cardiovascular, neurological, immunological, respiratory, gastrointestinal, hepatic, and endocrine functions. This review focuses on recent advances in H_2S signaling, which affects mechanistic and functional aspects of a variety of biological processes including autophagy, inflammation, stem cell proliferation and differentiation, cell survival/death, and cellular metabolism under both physiological and pathologic conditions. Furthermore, we highlighted the interaction of nitric oxide (NO) with H_2S in numerous biological settings (Sen, 2017).

11.4 Strategies for Incorporating functional foods into the diet

Incorporating functional foods into one's diet involves adopting strategies aimed at making healthier choices and seamlessly integrating these foods. The concept of nutrition by design explores the relationship between poultry production, the utilization of dietary by-products to create functional foods, and their impact on human health. Functional foods are defined as products that go beyond basic nutritional value, offering potential benefits in disease prevention and management (Vlaicu et al., 2023). Various methods, including extraction, fermentation, enrichment, biotechnology, and nanotechnology, are employed to obtain bioactive compounds for functional foods. Obtaining functional foods requires a sophisticated interplay of methods and processing operations designed to unleash the full potential of natural ingredients. These techniques are crucial for enhancing the bioavailability of bioactive compounds, ensuring that functional foods can genuinely promote human health and well-being (Alongi & Anese, 2021). Several methods, such as extraction, encapsulation, and fortification, play pivotal roles in creating functional foods by concentrating bioactive components and enhancing their absorption within the human body. Among these methods and operations, technological methods are the easiest to use and apply. Milk and bakery products are among the most common and easily obtainable functional foods due to several reasons (Zhu et al., 2022). For example, fermentation is a natural, safe food preservation technology that improves the bioavailability and digestibility of nutrients in foods high in probiotics and beneficial bacteria. The most common fermentations include lactic acid homofermentation and heterofermentation, butyric acid, mixed acid, propionic acid, and acetic acid. Products include yogurt, kefir, sauerkraut, beans, legumes, flours, and various cereals (Sun et al., 2022). Sprouting seeds, grains, or legumes boosts their nutritional value, which includes vitamins, minerals, and antioxidants. This approach also improves the digestibility and sensory properties of sprouts while decreasing the quantities of antinutritional components. Products include vegetables, fruits, grains, and seasonings (Waliat et al., 2023). Incorporating functional foods into your diet to support immune health involves focusing on nutrient-rich options that provide vitamins, minerals, antioxidants, and other bioactive compounds known for their immune-boosting properties. Here are some dietary guidelines and strategies for incorporating functional foods into your diet to support immune health.

11.4.1 Dietary guidelines for functional foods in your diet to support immune health

The ongoing global pandemic has brought about widespread disruptions, illness, and unfortunately, loss of life. Even as various aspects of life, including scientific endeavors, continue to progress, the suffering and mortality caused by the pandemic remain a constant concern. Amidst these unprecedented and turbulent times, maintaining a healthy and balanced diet remains crucial for supporting the well-being of individuals and communities. Additionally, the global burden of noncommunicable diseases continues to pose significant challenges. The Functional Foods & Nutrition Special Issue presents nine review articles covering a range of topics within the food, nutrition, and health sciences. Each article, authored by experts in the field, explores how foods and food ingredients contribute to nutrition and underlying health and disease processes. For instance, curcumin has been shown to have physiological effects, but its low water solubility poses a challenge to its bioavailability and how colloids, such as nanoemulsions and Pickering emulsions, can be utilized to encapsulate curcumin. This encapsulation method enhances solubility, allows for a higher loading capacity, and enables controlled delivery of curcumin as a functional food ingredient. Such strategies are crucial for maximizing the potential benefits of curcumin and similar diet-derived compounds (Wright, 2022). As per the World Health Organization (WHO), a balanced and nutritious diet is essential for preventing various forms of malnutrition and noncommunicable diseases (NCDs) such as diabetes, heart disease, stroke, and cancer. Unhealthy eating habits and a sedentary lifestyle pose significant global health risks. Encouraging healthy dietary practices from an early age, such as breastfeeding, promotes proper growth, cognitive development, and long-term health benefits, including a reduced risk of obesity and NCDs in later life.

Caloric intake should align with energy expenditure to prevent unhealthy weight gain. It is recommended that total fat intake should not exceed 30% of total energy intake, with saturated fats making up less than 10% and trans-fats less than 1%. Prioritizing unsaturated fats over saturated and trans-fats is advised, to eliminate industrially produced trans-fats. Limiting the consumption of free sugars to less than 10% of total energy intake is part of a healthy diet, with additional health benefits suggested by further reducing this to less than 5%. Reducing salt intake to less than 5 g/day (equivalent to less than 2 g of sodium) helps prevent hypertension, heart disease, and stroke WHO Member States have committed to reducing global salt intake by 30% by 2025 and stopping the rise of diabetes, obesity, and childhood overweight by the same year (World Health Organization, 2020). The report begins by acknowledging the mounting evidence supporting the necessity for humanity to transition towards dietary patterns that not only promote health but also respect environmental boundaries according to the Food and Agriculture Organization of the United Nations (FAO). It asserts that diets that achieve positive outcomes in both areas are feasible. A significant way for governments to demonstrate their commitment to a sustainable and healthy future is by creating and disseminating Food-Based Dietary Guidelines (FBDG) that embody this integrated approach (www.fao.org, n.d.b). These guidelines can then serve as the foundation for policies aimed at encouraging such dietary patterns. With this objective in mind, the report aims to delve into the efforts of governments already taking steps to develop and endorse integrated guidelines (Food and Agriculture Organization of the United Nations, n.d). It seeks to understand the processes behind their creation and the content of these guidelines. The ultimate goal is to determine whether and how other countries could replicate the approaches adopted by these leading nations. The recommended dietary pattern emphasizes diversity, encompassing a wide range of foods. It stresses achieving a balance between energy intake and needs. The foundation of the diet revolves around minimally processed tubers, whole grains, legumes, and fruits and vegetables, particularly those that are field-grown, sturdy, and less reliant on rapid and energy-intensive transportation. Moderate consumption of meat, with utilization of all animal parts, is advised. Dairy products or alternatives, unsalted seeds and nuts, and small quantities of fish from certified sources are also included.

The guidelines advocate for very limited consumption of foods high in fat, sugar, or salt and low in micronutrients, such as crisps, confectionery, and sugary drinks. They recommend using oils and fats with a beneficial omega 3:6 ratio, such as rapeseed and olive oil, and prioritizing tap water over other beverages, particularly soft drinks (Plates, n.d). Nutrition is a fundamental human requirement crucial for a healthy life, supporting proper growth and development from early stages. Dietary guidelines serve as a translation of scientific knowledge into practical advice, outlining recommended nutrient allowances for populations to follow for nutritionally adequate diets and healthy lifestyles throughout life. To achieve these dietary goals, appropriate nutritional behavior and dietary choices are essential. The following 15 dietary guidelines offer a comprehensive framework for action:

1. Embrace dietary variety to maintain a balanced diet.
2. Provide additional food and healthcare support to pregnant and lactating women.
3. Advocate for exclusive breastfeeding for 6 months, with continued breastfeeding for up to 2 years or longer.
4. Introduce home-based semisolid foods to infants after 6 months.
5. Ensure children and adolescents receive adequate and suitable diets, both in health and illness.
6. Consume ample quantities of vegetables and fruits.
7. Use edible oils and animal foods moderately, minimizing the use of ghee/butter/vanaspati.
8. Avoid overeating to prevent overweight and obesity.
9. Engage in regular exercise and physical activity to maintain an ideal body weight.
10. Limit salt intake to a minimum.
11. Ensure the consumption of safe and hygienic foods.
12. Employ proper precooking techniques and suitable cooking methods.
13. Stay hydrated by drinking plenty of water and consuming beverages in moderation.
14. Reduce the consumption of processed foods high in salt, sugar, and fats.
15. Incorporate micronutrient-rich foods into the diets of elderly individuals to support their fitness and activity levels.

These guidelines underscore the importance of a diverse diet, appropriate nutrition for various life stages, and healthy lifestyle practices to promote overall well-being (https://www.nin.res.in/downloads/DietaryGuidelinesforNINwebsite.pdf).

11.5 Clinical studies and evidence of immune support

11.5.1 Case studies and experimental results on functional foods and immunity

Functional foods, defined as those providing additional health benefits beyond basic nutrition, have garnered significant attention for their potential role in supporting immune function. Numerous clinical studies have investigated the effects of various functional foods on immunity, focusing on enhancing immune response, reducing inflammation, and bolstering overall health. Below is an overview of some key clinical studies in this area;

1. A case report published in the *Journal of Dietary Supplements* examined the use of honey in wound healing and immune modulation. The report described a case of a patient with a chronic wound who experienced accelerated healing and reduced inflammation following the topical application of honey. The objective of this study was to evaluate the effectiveness and practicality of applying topical manuka honey to treat chronic nonhealing extraoral wounds with discharge. A total of 15 patients (9 males and 6 females, mean age: 38.06 years, range: 20–50 years) with

chronic nonhealing extraoral wounds were included in the study from January 2018 to January 2020. Following wound irrigation with normal saline, manuka honey was directly applied to the wound surface along with antibiotic treatment. The honey was covered with an absorbent layer to keep it in place. Dressings were changed every other day for a week until pus discharge ceased, after which the interval between dressings was extended to 1 week for 4 weeks. The discharge and depth of the wounds were assessed before the procedure and weekly for 4 weeks. The results showed a significant decrease in the average depth of wounds from 5.72 mm at the end of the first week to 0.88 mm by the fourth week, with complete wound epithelialization observed. No cases of allergy, pain, infection, inflammation, or swelling were reported during the study period. In conclusion, the use of manuka honey as a wound dressing material in this study demonstrated its ability to promote tissue growth, reduce inflammation, and facilitate rapid wound healing through autolytic debridement (Kapoor & Yadav, 2021).

2. A case study published in the *Journal of Evidence-Based Integrative Medicine* explored the use of *Echinacea* in treating upper respiratory tract infections. The study reported significant improvement in symptoms and a reduction in the duration of illness in a patient following *Echinacea* supplementation. *Echinacea* preparations are frequently used as general immune system regulators. Alcohol extracts from three commonly utilized *Echinacea* species, *Echinacea angustifolia, Echinacea pallida, and Echinacea purpurea*, were examined for their ability to modulate the immune system. These species exhibited notable differences in the concentrations of specific lipophilic amides and hydrophilic caffeic acid derivatives. In an experiment involving mice, each Echinacea extract (administered at a dose of 130 mg/kg) or a control vehicle was orally administered once daily for 7 days. The mice were then immunized with sheep red blood cells (RBC), and immune cell samples were collected for various immunological assays. The results indicated that all three Echinacea species induced similar yet distinct changes in the composition and function of immune cell populations, such as increased proportions of CD49 + and CD19 + lymphocytes in the spleen, as well as enhanced NK cell activity. Additionally, antibody responses to sRBC were significantly augmented by all three *Echinacea* extracts. Moreover, splenocytes stimulated with Concanavalin A exhibited increased T cell proliferation in mice treated with *E. angustifolia and E. pallida* extracts. Furthermore, cytokine production by mitogen-stimulated splenic cells was significantly altered by *Echinacea* treatment. Specifically, all three extracts increased interferon-γ production while suppressing the release of tumor necrosis factor-α and interleukin (IL)-1β. Furthermore, treatment with *E. angustifolia and E. pallida* extracts resulted in significantly higher levels of IL-4 and increased IL-10 production. In summary, these findings suggest that *Echinacea* possesses broad-spectrum immunomodulatory properties, impacting both innate and adaptive immune responses. Notably, *E. angustifolia and E. pallida* extracts may exhibit greater antiinflammatory potential compared to *E. purpurea* (Zhai et al., 2007).

3. Diabetes mellitus encompasses a diverse range of conditions characterized by elevated blood sugar levels, leading to various complications, including periodontal disease. The chronic hyperglycemia seen in diabetes exacerbates periodontal issues through increased inflammation triggered by advanced glycation end products and their receptor, RAGE. In this context, substances with antiinflammatory properties could potentially mitigate this harmful interaction. Among them, green tea stands out due to its polyphenol content, known for its antiinflammatory effects. This study aimed to understand how green tea could alleviate diabetes–induced periodontitis. To achieve this, the researchers induced diabetes in rats using streptozotocin (STZ) and divided them into groups receiving either water or green tea treatment. They analyzed the animals at various time points postdiabetes induction. Immunohistochemistry was employed to quantify the expression of inflammatory markers such as tumor necrosis factor-α (TNF-α), receptor activator of nuclear factor-kappa-B ligand (RANKL), osteoprotegerin (OPG), interleukin-10 (IL-10), and runt-related transcription factor 2 (RUNX-2) in the oral tissues. Morphometric measurements assessed bone loss. Results indicated significant bone loss and alterations in inflammatory marker expression in diabetic rats. However, those treated with green tea showed decreased expression of RANKL and TNF-α, while exhibiting increased levels of OPG, RUNX-2, and IL-10 compared to untreated diabetic rats. This suggests that green tea intake normalized the expression of proinflammatory and osteoclastogenic markers while enhancing antiinflammatory and osteogenic factors. In conclusion, green tea emerges as a potential therapeutic option for managing diabetes-related periodontal disease (Gennaro et al., 2015).

4. The effects of functional foods mixture on inflammatory cytokines and biochemical findings in hospitalized patients with COVID-19: The COVID-19 pandemic has highlighted the importance of nutritional recommendations, with some functional foods showing promise in aiding treatment. However, little is known about the combined effects of such foods on disease management. This study aimed to investigate the impact of a mixture of functional foods on inflammatory cytokines and biochemical markers in COVID-19 patients. Conducted at Baqiyatallah Al-Azam Hospital in Tehran, Iran, this randomized double-blind controlled trial involved 60 patients. Participants were randomly assigned to receive either a soup containing functional foods or a standard soup (control group).

Sociodemographic data were collected via a general questionnaire, while blood samples were analyzed for inflammatory markers and biochemical parameters using standard methods. The findings revealed that the functional food soup was more effective in controlling serum levels of D-dimer, blood urea nitrogen, and creatinine compared to the control group. Additionally, the intervention group exhibited significant improvements in interleukin (IL)-1β, IL-6, IL-17, IL-10, and tumor necrosis factor-α levels compared to the control group. Conversely, the control intervention betterregulated potassium levels and reduced quantitative C-reactive protein compared to the intervention group. In conclusion, the study suggests that a soup containing functional foods may help alleviate inflammation markers in COVID-19 patients. However, its impact on biochemical findings requires further investigation (Gouvarchinghaleh et al., 2023).

5. A double-blind, placebo-controlled trial published in JAMA Network Open investigated the effects of high-dose vitamin D supplementation on respiratory tract infections in older adults. The study found that vitamin D supplementation reduced the incidence of respiratory infections and the severity of symptoms. In a systematic review and metaanalysis conducted up to May 1, 2020, researchers aimed to reassess the relationship between vitamin D supplementation and the prevention of acute respiratory infections (ARIs), building upon a 2017 metaanalysis of 25 randomized controlled trials (RCTs) that indicated a protective effect of vitamin D. Their analysis included data from 46 RCTs involving 75,541 participants. The study found that a lower proportion of participants who received vitamin D supplementation experienced one or more ARIs compared to those who received a placebo. The odds ratio (OR) was 0.92, suggesting a modest reduction in ARI risk with vitamin D supplementation. Subgroup analyses revealed that daily dosing regimens, doses equivalent to 400–1000 IU/day, durations of 12 months or less, and enrollment ages of 1.00–15.99 years, were associated with protective effects of vitamin D supplementation against ARIs. However, no significant interaction was observed between vitamin D supplementation and dose, dose frequency, study duration, or age. The study concluded that vitamin D supplementation was generally safe and associated with a slight reduction in ARI risk, particularly with daily doses of 400–1000 IU for up to 12 months and among participants aged 1.00–15.99 years at enrollment. However, the relevance of these findings to COVID-19 specifically remains uncertain and requires further investigation (Jolliffe et al., 2021).

11.6 Future direction and research areas for functional foods and immune support

Expanding the scope of high-quality clinical trials is essential for establishing safe intake ranges of bioactive components, determining efficacy for disease prevention, and identifying optimal food sources. Additionally, it is crucial to develop defined categories and criteria for functional foods and supplements supported by scientific evidence. Creating financial incentives and allocating public funding for research on functional foods is necessary, considering the limitations of patents and exclusivity rights for natural products. Improving regulatory coordination domestically and globally is essential to enhance consistency, oversight efficiency, and transparency in the functional food industry. Establishing federal quality standards, implementing testing processes, monitoring adverse events, and enforcing marketing and health claims are crucial steps toward ensuring consumer safety. Consumer education campaigns should be optimized to guide appropriate selections and usage of functional foods and supplements, tailored to individual health histories. Moreover, studying the synergistic and additive effects of bioactive combinations across functional food groups can enhance understanding and efficacy. Addressing health disparities and improving prevention strategies in at-risk communities with elevated chronic disease rates are imperative. This involves exploring the impacts of functional foods on health disparities and identifying opportunities for intervention. Monitoring the ecological impacts of diversified sustainable agriculture required for supplying functional foods and nutraceuticals supported by science is essential. Cooperative initiatives across public health agencies, legislative bodies, scientific funding organizations, and stakeholders in the food and nutrition industries, as well as farming communities, are needed to guide responsible policies and advance dietary approaches leveraging functional foods in chronic disease prevention and health promotion.

11.7 Conclusion

This chapter highlights the importance of various immune modulators in maintaining and enhancing immune function, including macrophages, phagocytes, NK cells, DCs, neutrophils, B cells, and T cells. These components collectively contribute to the body's defense mechanisms against pathogens and play distinct roles in adaptive and innate immunity. Additionally, the body's nutritional status, along with other factors such as sleep, exercise, and stress levels, can impact the function of these immune cells. Among the key nutrients examined for their effects on the immune system are vitamins, probiotics, prebiotics, postbiotics, synbiotics, short-chain fatty acids, dietary fibers, omega-3 fatty acids, minerals, lipids, gases etc. These nutrients play essential roles in supporting various aspects of immune function, from cellular signaling to antibody production. Understanding the interactions between the gut microbiome and host metabolism has shed light on the importance of functional components in modulating immune health. Supplementing nutrients with synbiotics, which combine probiotics and prebiotics, can influence the composition and metabolic activity of the gut microbiota, thereby impacting immune function. These nutrients support various immune functions, including phagocytosis, cytokine production, and antibody synthesis. Supplementing these micronutrients can strengthen immunity and support the body's natural defenses against infections. Adopting these dietary rules and guidelines allows for the easy incorporation of functional foods, which improves general well-being and immunity. Clinical studies have extensively explored the effects of functional foods on immune function, aiming to enhance immune response, alleviate inflammation, and promote overall health, thereby highlighting their potential to provide additional health benefits beyond basic nutrition. In conclusion, a balanced intake of vitamins, minerals, probiotics, prebiotics, and omega-3 fatty acids, etc is essential for maintaining optimal immune function. By incorporating these nutrients into the diet or through supplementation, individuals can support their immune system and enhance their body's ability to fight off pathogens.

References

Abarikwu, S. O., Olufemi, P. D., Lawrence, C. J., Wekere, F. C., Ochulor, A. C., & Barikuma, A. M. (2016). Rutin, an antioxidant flavonoid, induces glutathione and glutathione peroxidase activities to protect against ethanol effects in cadmium-induced oxidative stress in the testis of adult rats. *Andrologia*, *49*(7), e12696. Available from https://doi.org/10.1111/and.12696.

Aguiar, L. M., Geraldi, M. V., Betim Cazarin, C. B., & Maróstica Junior, M. R. (2019). Functional food consumption and its physiological effects. *Bioactive Compounds*, 205–225. Available from https://doi.org/10.1016/b978-0-12-814774-0.00011-6.

Ajmera, R. (2020). Functional foods: Definition, benefits, and uses. [online] Healthline. Available at: https://www.healthline.com/nutrition/functional-foods.

Alongi, M., & Anese, M. (2021). Re-thinking functional food development through a holistic approach. *Journal of Functional Foods*, *81*104466. Available from https://doi.org/10.1016/j.jff.2021.104466.

Althuwaiqeb, S.A. and Bordoni, B. (2020). Histology, B Cell Lymphocyte. [online] PubMed. Available at: https://www.ncbi.nlm.nih.gov/books/NBK560905/.

Amara, A. A., & Shibl, A. (2015). Role of probiotics in health improvement, infection control and disease treatment and management. *Saudi Pharmaceutical Journal*, *23*(2), 107–114. Available from https://doi.org/10.1016/j.jsps.2013.07.001, [online].

Ashaolu, T. J. (2020). Immune boosting functional foods and their mechanisms: A critical evaluation of probiotics and prebiotics. *Biomedicine & Pharmacotherapy*, *130*110625. Available from https://doi.org/10.1016/j.biopha.2020.110625.

Ashaolu, T. J., Saibandith, B., Yupanqui, C. T., & Wichienchot, S. (2018). Human colonic microbiota modulation and branched chain fatty acids production affected by soy protein hydrolysate. *International Journal of Food Science & Technology*, *54*(1), 141–148. Available from https://doi.org/10.1111/ijfs.13916.

Ashrafizadeh, M., Bakhoda, M. R., Bahmanpour, Z., Ilkhani, K., Zarrabi, A., Makvandi, P., Khan, H., Mazaheri, S., Darvish, M., & Mirzaei, H. (2020). Apigenin as tumor suppressor in cancers: Biotherapeutic activity, nanodelivery, and mechanisms with emphasis on pancreatic cancer. *Frontiers in Chemistry*, *8*. Available from https://doi.org/10.3389/fchem.2020.00829.

Atef, Y., El-Fayoumi, H. M., Abdel-Mottaleb, Y., & Mahmoud, M. F. (2017). Quercetin and tin protoporphyrin attenuate hepatic ischemia reperfusion injury: role of HO-1. *Naunyn-Schmiedeberg's Archives of Pharmacology*, *390*(9), 871–881. Available from https://doi.org/10.1007/s00210-017-1389-9.

Barone, M., D'Amico, F., Brigidi, P., & Turroni, S. (2022). Gut microbiome–micronutrient interaction: The key to controlling the bioavailability of minerals and vitamins? *Biofactors (Oxford, England)*, *48*(2), 307–314. Available from https://doi.org/10.1002/biof.1835.

Beidelschies, M., Alejandro-Rodriguez, M., Ji, X., Lapin, B., Hanaway, P., & Rothberg, M. B. (2019). Association of the Functional medicine model of care with patient-reported health-related quality-of-life outcomes. *JAMA Network Open*, *2*(10), e1914017. Available from https://doi.org/10.1001/jamanetworkopen.2019.14017, [online].

Berin, M. C. (2021). Dysbiosis in food allergy and implications for microbial therapeutics. *Journal of Clinical Investigation*, *131*(2). Available from https://doi.org/10.1172/jci144994.

Biology LibreTexts. (2018). 20.2: Introduction to the Immune System. [online] Available at: https://bio.libretexts.org/Bookshelves/Human_Biology/Human_Biology_(Wakim_and_Grewal)/20%3A_Immune_System/20.2%3A_Introduction_to_the_Immune_System.

de Brito Alves, J. L., Souza, E. L., & de. (2023). Functional foods with modulating action on metabolic risk factors. *Foods*, *12*(21), 4043. Available from https://doi.org/10.3390/foods12214043, [online].

Carazo, A., Macáková, K., Matoušová, K., Krčmová, L. K., Protti, M., & Mladěnka, P. (2021). Vitamin A update: Forms, sources, kinetics, detection, function, deficiency, therapeutic use and toxicity. *Nutrients*, *13*(5), 1703. Available from https://doi.org/10.3390/nu13051703, [online].

Carlson, J. L., Erickson, J. M., Lloyd, B. B., & Slavin, J. L. (2018). Health effects and sources of prebiotic dietary fiber. *Current Developments in Nutrition*, *2*(3). Available from https://doi.org/10.1093/cdn/nzy005, [online].

Carr, A. C., & Maggini, S. (2017). Vitamin C and immune function. *Nutrients*, *9*(11), 1211, [online]. Available from https://www.ncbi.nlm.nih.gov/pmc/articles/PMC5707683/.

Charles A. Janeway, J., Travers, P., Walport, M. and Shlomchik, M.J. (2001a). The components of the immune system. Immunobiology: The Immune System in Health and Disease. 5th edition. [online] Available at: https://www.ncbi.nlm.nih.gov/books/NBK27092/#:~:text = The%20myeloid%20progenitor%20is%20the.

Charles A. Janeway, J., Travers, P., Walport, M. and Shlomchik, M.J. (2001b). The complement system and innate immunity. Immunobiology: The Immune System in Health and Disease. 5th edition. [online] Available at: https://www.ncbi.nlm.nih.gov/books/NBK27100/#:~:text = The%20complement%20system%20is%20made.

Chen, G., Li, Y., Li, X., Zhou, D., Wang, Y., Wen, X., Wang, C., Liu, X., Feng, Y., Li, B., & Li, N. (2021). Functional foods and intestinal homeostasis: The perspective of in vivo evidence. *Trends in Food Science & Technology*, *111*, 475–482. Available from https://doi.org/10.1016/j.tifs.2021.02.075.

Chew, B. P., & Park, J. S. (2004). Carotenoid action on the immune response. *The Journal of Nutrition*, *134*(1), 257S261S. Available from https://doi.org/10.1093/jn/134.1.257s, [online].

Chiu, C.-Y., Chan, Y.-L., Tsai, M.-H., Wang, C.-J., Chiang, M.-H., & Chiu, C.-C. (2019). Gut microbial dysbiosis is associated with allergen-specific IgE responses in young children with airway allergies. *World Allergy Organization Journal*, *12*(3)100021. Available from https://doi.org/10.1016/j.waojou.2019.100021, [online].

Coker, M. O., & Madan, J. C. (2020). The microbiome and immune system development. *The Developing Microbiome*, 43–66. Available from https://doi.org/10.1016/b978-0-12-820602-7.00003-9.

Coombs, M. R. P., Harrison, M. E., & Hoskin, D. W. (2016). Apigenin inhibits the inducible expression of programmed death ligand 1 by human and mouse mammary carcinoma cells. *Cancer Letters*, *380*(2), 424–433. Available from https://doi.org/10.1016/j.canlet.2016.06.023.

Crowe, K. M., & Francis, C. (2013). Position of the academy of nutrition and dietetics: Functional foods. *Journal of the Academy of Nutrition and Dietetics*, *113*(8), 1096–1103. Available from https://doi.org/10.1016/j.jand.2013.06.002, [online].

Crupi, P., Faienza, M. F., Naeem, M. Y., Corbo, F., Clodoveo, M. L., & Muraglia, M. (2023). Overview of the potential beneficial effects of carotenoids on consumer health and well-being. *Antioxidants*, *12*(5), 1069. Available from https://doi.org/10.3390/antiox12051069, [online].

Czarnewski, P., Das, S., Parigi, S. M., & Villablanca, E. J. (2017). Retinoic acid and its role in modulating intestinal innate immunity. *Nutrients*, *9*(1). Available from https://doi.org/10.3390/nu9010068, 68–68.

Călinoiu, L. F., & Vodnar, D. C. (2018). Whole grains and phenolic acids: A review on bioactivity, functionality, health benefits and bioavailability. *Nutrients*, *10*(11), 1615. Available from https://doi.org/10.3390/nu10111615.

Dable-Tupas, G., Otero, M. C. B., & Bernolo, L. (2020). Functional foods and health benefits. *Functional Foods and Nutraceuticals*, 1–11. Available from https://doi.org/10.1007/978-3-030-42319-3_1.

Dahiya, D., & Nigam, P. S. (2022). Probiotics, prebiotics, synbiotics, and fermented foods as potential biotics in nutrition improving health via microbiome-gut-brain axis. *Fermentation*, *8*(7), 303. Available from https://doi.org/10.3390/fermentation8070303.

de, C., Elia., Ana., Luis., Magalhães, A. I., Luis., & Soccol, C. R. (2016). *Vitamins and Nutraceuticals* (pp. 207–254). BENTHAM SCIENCE PUBLISHERS eBooks. Available from https://doi.org/10.2174/9781681082653116010008.

Deokar, G., Shinde, P., & Kshirsagar, S. (2022). In- vitro biorelevant media and time simulation probiotic proliferation methodology to determine prebiotic potentials of flaxseed powder. *Bioactive Carbohydrates and Dietary Fibre*, *28*100335. Available from https://doi.org/10.1016/j.bcdf.2022.100335.

Dhinaut, J., Balourdet, A., Teixeira, M., Chogne, M., & Moret, Y. (2017). A dietary carotenoid reduces immunopathology and enhances longevity through an immune depressive effect in an insect model. *Scientific Reports*, *7*. Available from https://doi.org/10.1038/s41598-017-12769-7, [online].

Dimidi, E., Cox, S. R., Rossi, M., & Whelan, K. (2019). Fermented foods: Definitions and characteristics, impact on the gut microbiota and effects on gastrointestinal health and disease. *Nutrients*, *11*(8), 1806. Available from https://doi.org/10.3390/nu11081806, [online].

Elmore, S. (2007). Apoptosis: A review of programmed cell death. *Toxicologic Pathology*, *35*(4), 495–516. Available from https://doi.org/10.1080/01926230701320337, [online].

Essa, M. M., Bishir, M., Bhat, A., Chidambaram, S. B., Al-Balushi, B., Hamdan, H., Govindarajan, N., Freidland, R. P., & Qoronfleh, M. W. (2021). Functional foods and their impact on health. *Journal of Food Science and Technology*. Available from https://doi.org/10.1007/s13197-021-05193-3.

FDA (2019). Food Labeling & Nutrition. [online] U.S. Food and Drug Administration. Available at: https://www.fda.gov/food/food-labeling-nutrition.

Finnegan, D., Tocmo, R., & Loscher, C. E. (2023). Targeted application of functional foods as immune fitness boosters in the defense against viral infection. *Nutrients*, *15*(15). Available from https://doi.org/10.3390/nu15153371, [online].

Food and Agriculture Organization of the United Nations. (n.d.). Nutrition. [online] Available at: https://www.fao.org/nutrition/en/.

Frank, L. L. (2015). Thiamin in clinical practice. *Journal of Parenteral and Enteral Nutrition*, *39*(5), 503–520. Available from https://doi.org/10.1177/0148607114565245.

Gasperi, V., Sibilano, M., Savini, I., & Catani, M. V. (2019). Niacin in the central nervous system: An update of biological aspects and clinical applications. *International Journal of Molecular Sciences*, *20*(4). Available from https://doi.org/10.3390/ijms20040974, [online].

Gennaro, G., Claudino, M., Cestari, T. M., Ceolin, D., Germino, P., Garlet, G. P., & de Assis, G. F. (2015). Green tea modulates cytokine expression in the periodontium and attenuates alveolar bone resorption in type 1 diabetic rats. *PLoS One*, *10*(8), e0134784. Available from https://doi.org/10.1371/journal.pone.0134784, [online].

Gholami, H., Chmiel, J. A., Burton, J. P., & Maleki Vareki, S. (2023). The role of microbiota-derived vitamins in immune homeostasis and enhancing cancer immunotherapy. *Cancers*, *15*(4), 1300. Available from https://doi.org/10.3390/cancers15041300.

Ghosh, A., Chandra, A., Dhar, A., Shukla, P., & Baishya, D. (2021). Multi-efficient thermostable endoxylanase from Bacillus velezensis AG20 and its production of xylooligosaccharides as efficient prebiotics with anticancer activity. *Process Biochemistry*, *109*, 59–71. Available from https://doi.org/10.1016/j.procbio.2021.06.011.

Gibson, G. R., Hutkins, R., Sanders, M. E., Prescott, S. L., Reimer, R. A., Salminen, S. J., Scott, K., Stanton, C., Swanson, K. S., Cani, P. D., Verbeke, K., & Reid, G. (2017). Expert consensus document: The International Scientific Association for Probiotics and Prebiotics (ISAPP) consensus statement on the definition and scope of prebiotics. *Nature Reviews Gastroenterology & Hepatology*, *14*(8). Available from https://doi.org/10.1038/nrgastro.2017.75, [online].

Gibson, G. R., & Roberfroid, M. B. (1995). Dietary modulation of the human colonic microbiota: Introducing the concept of prebiotics. *The Journal of Nutrition*, *125*(6), 1401–1412. Available from https://doi.org/10.1093/jn/125.6.1401.

Gouvarchinghaleh, H. E., Kiany, F., Parastouei, K., Alishiri, G. H., Jafari, N. J., Imani, A., Pargar, A., Ghazvini, A., Mirnejad, R., Raei, M., Olounabadi, A. S., Babaei, M., Heydari, S., Rostami, H., Shahriary, A., Farnoosh, G., Sobhani, V., Mazhari, M. M., & NajjarAsiabani, F. (2023). The effects of functional foods mixture on inflammatory cytokines and biochemical findings in hospitalized patients with COVID-19: A randomized double-blind controlled trial. *Trials*, *24*(1). Available from https://doi.org/10.1186/s13063-023-07481-z.

Guimarães, J. T., Balthazar, C. F., Silva, R., Rocha, R. S., Graça, J. S., Esmerino, E. A., Silva, M. C., Sant'Ana, A. S., Duarte, M. C. K. H., Freitas, M. Q., & Cruz, A. G. (2020). Impact of probiotics and prebiotics on food texture. *Current Opinion in Food Science*, *33*, 38–44. Available from https://doi.org/10.1016/j.cofs.2019.12.002, [online].

Hanna, M., Jaqua, E., Nguyen, V., & Clay, J. (2022). B vitamins: Functions and uses in medicine. *The Permanente Journal*, *26*(2), 89–97. Available from https://doi.org/10.7812/TPP/21.204, [online].

Harvard School of Public Health (2020). Nutrition and Immunity. [online] The Nutrition Source. Available at https://www.hsph.harvard.edu/nutritionsource/nutrition-and-immunity/.

Hill, C., Guarner, F., Reid, G., Gibson, G. R., Merenstein, D. J., Pot, B., Morelli, L., Canani, R. B., Flint, H. J., Salminen, S., Calder, P. C., & Sanders, M. E. (2014). Expert consensus document. The International Scientific Association for Probiotics and Prebiotics consensus statement on the scope and appropriate use of the term probiotic. *Nature reviews. Gastroenterology & hepatology*, *11*(8), 506–514. Available from https://doi.org/10.1038/nrgastro.2014.66, [online].

Holscher, H. D. (2017). Dietary fiber and prebiotics and the gastrointestinal microbiota. *Gut Microbes*, *8*(2), 172–184. Available from https://doi.org/10.1080/19490976.2017.1290756.

Institute for Quality and Efficiency in Health Care (2020). The innate and adaptive immune systems. [online] Nih.gov. Available at: https://www.ncbi.nlm.nih.gov/books/NBK279396/.

International Scientific Association for Probiotics and Prebiotics (ISAPP). (n.d.). Probiotics. [online] Available at: https://isappscience.org/for-scientists/resources/probiotics/.

Ipa Europe. (2021). IPA Europe - 20th Anniversary of the FAO/WTO definition of probiotic microorganisms in food and food supplements. [online] Available at: https://www.ipaeurope.org/fao-wto-definition-probiotics-microorganisms/ [Accessed 17 Mar. 2024].

Jolliffe, D. A., Camargo, C. A., Sluyter, J. D., Aglipay, M., Aloia, J. F., Ganmaa, D., Bergman, P., Bischoff-Ferrari, H. A., Borzutzky, A., Damsgaard, C. T., Dubnov-Raz, G., Esposito, S., Gilham, C., Ginde, A. A., Golan-Tripto, I., Goodall, E. C., Grant, C. C., Griffiths, C. J., Hibbs, A. M., & Janssens, W. (2021). Vitamin D supplementation to prevent acute respiratory infections: a systematic review and meta-analysis of aggregate data from randomised controlled trials. *The Lancet Diabetes & Endocrinology*, *9*(5), 276–292. Available from https://doi.org/10.1016/S2213-8587(21)00051-6, [online].

Justiz Vaillant, A.A., Jamal, Z., Patel, P. and Ramphul, K. (2024). Immunoglobulin. [online] PubMed. Available at: https://www.ncbi.nlm.nih.gov/books/NBK513460/#:~:text = of%20B%20lymphocytes.- [Accessed 19 Apr. 2024].

Kalantar-Zadeh, K., Berean, K. J., Burgell, R. E., Muir, J. G., & Gibson, P. R. (2019). Intestinal gases: influence on gut disorders and the role of dietary manipulations. *Nature Reviews Gastroenterology & Hepatology*, *16*(12), 733–747. Available from https://doi.org/10.1038/s41575-019-0193-z, [online].

Kapoor, N., & Yadav, R. (2021). Manuka honey: A promising wound dressing material for the chronic nonhealing discharging wounds: A retrospective study. *National Journal of Maxillofacial Surgery*, *12*(2), 233. Available from https://doi.org/10.4103/njms.njms_154_20.

Kasote, D., Tiozon, R. N., Sartagoda, K. J. D., Itagi, H., Roy, P., Kohli, A., Regina, A., & Sreenivasulu, N. (2021). Food processing technologies to develop functional foods with enriched bioactive phenolic compounds in cereals. *Frontiers in Plant Science*, *12*771276. Available from https://doi.org/10.3389/fpls.2021.771276, [online].

Kim, J. H., Kim, D. H., Jo, S., Cho, M. J., Cho, Y. R., Lee, Y. J., & Byun, S. (2022). Immunomodulatory functional foods and their molecular mechanisms. *Experimental & Molecular Medicine*, *54*(1), 1–11. Available from https://doi.org/10.1038/s12276-022-00724-0.

Kong, D., Yu, H., Sim, X., White, K., Shyong Tai, E., Wenk, M. R., & Kee, A. (2022). Multidisciplinary effort to drive precision-medicine for the future. *Frontiers in digital health*, 4. Available from https://doi.org/10.3389/fdgth.2022.845405.

Koren, O. and Rautava, S. (2020). The Human Microbiome in Early Life: Implications to Health and Disease. [online] Google Books. Academic Press. Available at: https://books.google.co.in/books?hl = en&lr = &id = tOneDwAAQBAJ&oi = fnd&pg = PP1&ots = nA-WrPx-Yp&sig = Ess5q80kjIuQ_OGiTP3XfMVM2jY&redir_esc = y#v = onepage&q&f = false [Accessed 17 Mar. 2024].

Kraus, W. E. (2018). *Personalized lifestyle medicine* (pp. 17–26). Elsevier eBooks. Available from https://doi.org/10.1016/b978-0-12-801812-5.00013-5.

Kwon, H.-K., Lee, C.-G., So, J.-S., Chae, C.-S., Hwang, J.-S., Sahoo, A., Nam, J. H., Rhee, J. H., Hwang, K.-C., & Im, S.-H. (2010). Generation of regulatory dendritic cells and CD4 + Foxp3 + T cells by probiotics administration suppresses immune disorders. *Proceedings of the National Academy of Sciences of the United States of America*, *107*(5), 2159–2164. Available from https://doi.org/10.1073/pnas.0904055107, [online].

Laissue, P. (2019). The forkhead-box family of transcription factors: Key molecular players in colorectal cancer pathogenesis. *Molecular Cancer*, *18*(1). Available from https://doi.org/10.1186/s12943-019-0938-x.

Leduc, D. C., & D, P. (2021). *Immunoglobulin types and their functions*. [online] AmeriPharma Specialty Care. Available at: https://ameripharmaspecialty.com/immunoglobulins-ig/.

Lewis, S. M., Williams, A., & Eisenbarth, S. C. (2019). Structure and function of the immune system in the spleen. *Science Immunology*, *4*(33) eaau6085. Available from https://doi.org/10.1126/sciimmunol.aau6085, [online].

Li, X., Huang, S., Yin, J., Peng, X., King, L., Li, L., Xu, Z., Zhou, L., Zhao, P., Ze, X., Zhang, X., Hou, Q., Shan, Z., & Liu, L. (2023). Effect of synbiotic supplementation on immune parameters and gut microbiota in healthy adults: A double-blind randomized controlled trial. *Gut microbes*, *15* (2). Available from https://doi.org/10.1080/19490976.2023.2247025.

Liu, J., Poojary, M. M., Zhu, L., Williams, A. R., & Lund, M. N. (2023). Phenolic acid–amino acid adducts exert distinct immunomodulatory effects in macrophages compared to parent phenolic acids. *Journal of Agricultural and Food Chemistry*. Available from https://doi.org/10.1021/acs.jafc.2c06658.

Liu, Z., Farkas, P., Wang, K., Kohli, M., & Fitzpatrick, T. B. (2022). B vitamin supply in plants and humans: The importance of vitamer homeostasis. *The Plant Journal*, *111*(3), 662–682. Available from https://doi.org/10.1111/tpj.15859, [online].

Lu, Z., Chen, T. C., Zhang, A., Persons, K. S., Kohn, N., Berkowitz, R., Martinello, S., & Holick, M. F. (2007). An evaluation of the vitamin D3 content in fish: Is the vitamin D content adequate to satisfy the dietary requirement for vitamin D? *The Journal of Steroid Biochemistry and Molecular Biology*, *103*(3-5), 642–644. Available from https://doi.org/10.1016/j.jsbmb.2006.12.010, [online].

M, A. (n.d.). Concepts of Functional Foods – ILSI Europe. [online] Available at: https://ilsi.eu/publication/concepts-of-functional-foods/.

Maoka, T. (2019). Carotenoids as natural functional pigments. *Journal of Natural Medicines*, *74*(1), 1–16. Available from https://doi.org/10.1007/s11418-019-01364-x, [online].

Marco, M., Heeney, D., Binda, S., Cifelli, C., Cotter, P., & Foligné, B. (2017). ScienceDirect. *Current Opinion in Biotechnology*, *44*. Available from https://doi.org/10.1016/j.copbio.2016.11.010, [online].

Martin-Gallausiaux, C., Marinelli, L., Blottière, H. M., Larraufie, P., & Lapaque, N. (2020). SCFA: mechanisms and functional importance in the gut. *Proceedings of the Nutrition Society*, *80*(1), 37–49. Available from https://doi.org/10.1017/S0029665120006916.

McCarville, J. L., Chen, G. Y., Cuevas, V. D., Troha, K., & Ayres, J. S. (2020). Microbiota metabolites in health and disease. *Annual Review of Immunology*, *38*(1), 147–170. Available from https://doi.org/10.1146/annurev-immunol-071219-125715.

McLoughlin, R. F., Berthon, B. S., Jensen, M. E., Baines, K. J., & Wood, L. G. (2017). Short-chain fatty acids, prebiotics, synbiotics, and systemic inflammation: A systematic review and meta-analysis. *The American Journal of Clinical Nutrition*. Available from https://doi.org/10.3945/ajcn.117.156265, p.ajcn156265.

Meléndez-Martínez, A. J., Mandić, A. I., Bantis, F., Böhm, V., Borge, G. I. A., Brnčić, M., Bysted, A., Cano, M. P., Dias, M. G., Elgersma, A., Fikselová, M., García-Alonso, J., Giuffrida, D., Gonçalves, V. S. S., Hornero-Méndez, D., Kljak, K., Lavelli, V., Manganaris, G. A., Mapelli-Brahm, P., & Marounek, M. (2021). A comprehensive review on carotenoids in foods and feeds: Status quo, applications, patents, and research needs. *Critical Reviews in Food Science and Nutrition*, 1–51. Available from https://doi.org/10.1080/10408398.2020.1867959.

Mondal, S., Soumya, N. P. P., Mini, S., & Sivan, S. K. (2021). Bioactive compounds in functional food and their role as therapeutics. *Bioactive Compounds in Health and Disease*, *4*(3), 24, [online]. Available from https://ffhdj.com/index.php/BioactiveCompounds/article/view/786/1395.

MSD Manual Professional Edition. (n.d.). Cellular Components of the Immune System - Immunology; Allergic Disorders. [online] Available at: https://www.msdmanuals.com/en-in/professional/immunology-allergic-disorders/biology-of-the-immune-system/cellular-components-of-the-immune-system [Accessed 23 Mar. 2024].

Nagai, Y., Lam, L., Greene, M. I., & Zhang, H. (2019). FOXP3 and its cofactors as targets of immunotherapies. *Engineering*, *5*(1), 115–121. Available from https://doi.org/10.1016/j.eng.2019.01.001.

Nagarajan, J., Ramanan, R.N., Raghunandan, M.E., Galanakis, C.M. and Krishnamurthy, N.P. (2017). Chapter 8 - Carotenoids. [online] ScienceDirect. https://doi.org/10.1016/B978-0-12-805257-0.00008-9.

National Institute of Health (2017). Office of Dietary Supplements - Biotin. [online] Nih.gov. Available at: https://ods.od.nih.gov/factsheets/Biotin-HealthProfessional/.

National Institutes of Health (2017a). Office of Dietary Supplements - Vitamin A. [online] Nih.gov. Available at: https://ods.od.nih.gov/factsheets/VitaminA-HealthProfessional/.

National Institutes of Health (2017b). Office of Dietary Supplements - Vitamin B6. [online] Nih.gov. Available at: https://ods.od.nih.gov/factsheets/vitaminB6-healthprofessional/.

National Institutes of Health (2021a). Vitamin C. [online] National Institutes of Health. Available at: https://ods.od.nih.gov/factsheets/VitaminC-HealthProfessional/.

National Institutes of Health (2021b). Office of Dietary Supplements - Vitamin E. [online] Nih.gov. Available at: https://ods.od.nih.gov/factsheets/VitaminE-HealthProfessional/.

National Institutes of Health (2021c). Office of Dietary Supplements - Vitamin K. [online] Nih.gov. Available at: https://ods.od.nih.gov/factsheets/vitaminK-HealthProfessional/.

National Institutes of Health (2022). Office of Dietary Supplements - Folate. [online] Nih.gov. Available at: https://ods.od.nih.gov/factsheets/Folate-HealthProfessional/.

National Institutes of Health (2024). Office of Dietary Supplements - Vitamin B12. [online] Nih.gov. Available at: https://ods.od.nih.gov/factsheets/VitaminB12-HealthProfessional/.

Neri-Numa, I. A., & Pastore, G. M. (2020). Novel insights into prebiotic properties on human health: A review. *Food Research International*, *131*108973. Available from https://doi.org/10.1016/j.foodres.2019.108973.

Ney, L.-M., M. Wipplinger, Grossmann, M., Engert, N., Wegner, V.D. and Mosig, A.S. (2023). Short chain fatty acids: key regulators of the local and systemic immune response in inflammatory diseases and infections. 13(3). https://doi.org/10.1098/rsob.230014.

Nicholson, L. B. (2016). The immune system. *Essays in Biochemistry, 60*(3), 275–301. Available from https://doi.org/10.1042/ebc20160017, [online].

ods.od.nih.gov. (n.d.). Office of Dietary Supplements - Omega-3 Fatty Acids. [online] Available at: https://ods.od.nih.gov/factsheets/Omega3FattyAcids-Consumer/#: ~ :text = Omega%2D3%20fatty%20acids%20are.

Olatunde, A., Tijjani, H., Ishola, A. A., Egbuna, C., Hassan, S., & Akram, M. (2020). *Carotenoids as functional bioactive compounds* (pp. 415–444). Springer eBooks. Available from https://doi.org/10.1007/978-3-030-42319-3_20.

Omer, A. K., Khorshidi, S., Mortazavi, N., & Rahman, H. S. (2022). A review on the antiviral activity of functional foods against COVID-19 and viral respiratory tract infections. *International Journal of General Medicine, Volume 15*, 4817–4835. Available from https://doi.org/10.2147/ijgm.s361001.

Oršolić, N., & Jazvinšćak Jembrek, M. (2022). Molecular and cellular mechanisms of propolis and its polyphenolic compounds against cancer. *International Journal of Molecular Sciences, 23*(18), 10479. Available from https://doi.org/10.3390/ijms231810479.

Panche, A. N., Diwan, A. D., & Chandra, S. R. (2016). Flavonoids: An overview. *Journal of Nutritional Science*, 5e47. Available from https://doi.org/10.1017/jns.2016.41.

Parte, A. C., Sardà Carbasse, J., Meier-Kolthoff, J. P., Reimer, L. C., & Göker, M. (2020). List of prokaryotic names with standing in nomenclature (LPSN) moves to the DSMZ. *International Journal of Systematic and Evolutionary Microbiology, 70*(11), 5607–5612. Available from https://doi.org/10.1099/ijsem.0.004332.

Passerini, L., & Bacchetta, R. (2017). Forkhead-Box-P3 gene transfer in human CD4 + T conventional cells for the generation of stable and efficient regulatory T cells, suitable for immune modulatory therapy. *Frontiers in Immunology, 8*. Available from https://doi.org/10.3389/fimmu.2017.01282.

Pizzorno, L. (2014). Jeffrey S. Bland, phd—The disease delusion: Conquering the causes of chronic illness for a healthier, longer and happier life. *Integrative Medicine: A Clinician's Journal, 13*(5), 52–56, [online]. Available from https://www.ncbi.nlm.nih.gov/pmc/articles/PMC4684103/.

Plantone, D., Pardini, M., & Rinaldi, G. (2021). Riboflavin in neurological diseases: A narrative review. *Clinical Drug Investigation, 41*(6), 513–527. Available from https://doi.org/10.1007/s40261-021-01038-1.

Plasek, B., Lakner, Z., Kasza, G., & Temesi, Á. (2020). Consumer evaluation of the role of functional food products in disease prevention and the characteristics of target groups. *Nutrients, 12*(1), 69. Available from https://doi.org/10.3390/nu12010069, [online].

Plates, pyramids, planet Developments in national healthy and sustainable dietary guidelines: a state of play assessment. (n.d.). Available at: https://www.fao.org/3/i5640e/i5640e.pdf.

Porcelli, S. A. (2017). Innate immunity. *Kelley and Firestein's Textbook of Rheumatology*, 274–287. Available from https://doi.org/10.1016/b978-0-323-31696-5.00017-6.

Prete, R., Long, S. L., Gallardo, A. L., Gahan, C. G., Corsetti, A., & Joyce, S. A. (2020). Beneficial bile acid metabolism from *Lactobacillus plantarum* of food origin. *Scientific Reports, 10*, 1165. Available from https://doi.org/10.1038/s41598-020-58069-5, [online].

Probiotics in food Health and nutritional properties and guidelines for evaluation. (2006). Available at: https://www.fao.org/3/a0512e/a0512e.pdf.

PubChem (n.d.). Pantothenic acid. [online] pubchem.ncbi.nlm.nih.gov. Available at: https://pubchem.ncbi.nlm.nih.gov/compound/Pantothenic-acid#section = Therapeutic-Uses.

Pulendran, B., & Davis, M. M. (2020). The science and medicine of human immunology. *Science (New York, N.Y.), 369*(6511). Available from https://doi.org/10.1126/science.aay4014, [online].

Qazi, A., Khoso, U., Ahmad, F., & Raza, A. (2023). Food as an ingredient of well-being: from food and well-being to food well-being (FWB): A comparative study. *International Journal of Pharmaceutical and Healthcare Marketing*. Available from https://doi.org/10.1108/IJPHM-01-2022-0010.

Rajasekaran, A. (2017). Nutraceuticals. *Comprehensive Medicinal Chemistry III*, 107–134. Available from https://doi.org/10.1016/B978-0-12-409547-2.12287-5.

Raubenheimer, D., Simpson, S. J., & Mayntz, D. (2009). Nutrition, ecology, and nutritional ecology: toward an integrated framework. *Functional Ecology, 23*(1), 4–16. Available from https://doi.org/10.1111/j.1365-2435.2009.01522.x.

Research, I. of M. (U.S.) C. on M.N. (1999). Cytokines and Nutritional Status: Possible Correlations and Investigations. [online] www.ncbi.nlm.nih.gov. National Academies Press (US). Available at: https://www.ncbi.nlm.nih.gov/books/NBK230989/.

Riaz Rajoka, M. S., Thirumdas, R., Mehwish, H. M., Umair, M., Khurshid, M., Hayat, H. F., Phimolsiripol, Y., Pallarés, N., Martí-Quijal, F. J., & Barba, F. J. (2021). Role of food antioxidants in modulating gut microbial communities: Novel understandings in intestinal oxidative stress damage and their impact on host health. *Antioxidants, 10*(10), 1563. Available from https://doi.org/10.3390/antiox10101563, [online].

Russell, M.W., Mestecky, J., Strober, W., Lambrecht, B.N., Kelsall, B.L. and Cheroutre, H. (2015). Chapter 1 - Overview: The Mucosal Immune System. [online] ScienceDirect. Available at: https://www.sciencedirect.com/science/article/abs/pii/B978012415847400001X [Accessed 4 Apr. 2024].

Saarela, M. (2011). Functional Foods: Concept to Product. [online] Google Books. Elsevier. Available at: https://books.google.co.in/books?hl = en&lr = &id = cXlwAgAAQBAJ&oi = fnd&pg = PP1&dq = Gibson + GR [Accessed 17 Mar. 2024].

Salminen, S., Collado, M. C., Endo, A., Hill, C., Lebeer, S., Quigley, E. M. M., Sanders, M. E., Shamir, R., Swann, J. R., Szajewska, H., & Vinderola, G. (2021). The International Scientific Association of Probiotics and Prebiotics (ISAPP) consensus statement on the definition and scope of postbiotics. *Nature Reviews Gastroenterology & Hepatology, 18*(9). Available from https://doi.org/10.1038/s41575-021-00440-6.

Sapkota, A. (2021). Antigen- Definition, Properties, Structure, Types, Examples. [online] Microbe Notes. Available at: https://microbenotes.com/antigen/.

Schroeder, H. W., Radbruch, A., & Berek, C. (2023). *B-cell development and differentiation* (pp. 107–119). Elsevier eBooks. Available from https://doi.org/10.1016/b978-0-7020-8165-1.00007-1.

Scott, E., De Paepe, K., & Van de Wiele, T. (2022). Postbiotics and their health modulatory biomolecules. *Biomolecules, 12*(11), 1640. Available from https://doi.org/10.3390/biom12111640, [online].

Segerstrom, S. C., & Miller, G. E. (2004). Psychological stress and the human immune system: A meta-analytic study of 30 years of inquiry. *Psychological Bulletin, 130*(4), 601–630. Available from https://doi.org/10.1037/0033-2909.130.4.601, [online].

Sen, N. (2017). Functional and molecular insights of hydrogen sulfide signaling and protein sulfhydration. *Journal of Molecular Biology, 429*(4), 543–561. Available from https://doi.org/10.1016/j.jmb.2016.12.015.

Sergeev, I. N., Aljutaily, T., Walton, G., & Huarte, E. (2020). Effects of synbiotic supplement on human gut microbiota, body composition and weight loss in obesity. *Nutrients, 12*(1), 222. Available from https://doi.org/10.3390/nu12010222.

Shaikh, S. (2022). *Sources and Health benefits of functional food components*. IntechOpen eBooks. Available from https://doi.org/10.5772/intechopen.104091.

Shao, T., Verma, H. K., Pande, B., Costanzo, V., Ye, W., Cai, Y., & Bhaskar, L. V. K. S. (2021). Physical activity and nutritional influence on immune function: An important strategy to improve immunity and health status. *Frontiers in Physiology, 12*(751374). Available from https://doi.org/10.3389/fphys.2021.751374.

Soto, J. A., Gálvez, N. M. S., Andrade, C. A., Pacheco, G. A., Bohmwald, K., Berrios, R. V., Bueno, S. M., & Kalergis, A. M. (2020). The role of dendritic cells during infections caused by highly prevalent viruses. *Frontiers in Immunology, 11*. Available from https://doi.org/10.3389/fimmu.2020.01513, [online].

Sperfeld, E., Wagner, N., Kuehn, K. A., Malishev, M., & Raubenheimer, D. (2017). Bridging Ecological Stoichiometry and Nutritional Geometry with homeostasis concepts and integrative models of organism nutrition. *Functional Ecology, 31*(2), 286–296. Available from https://doi.org/10.1111/1365-2435.12707.

Ştefanache, A., Lungu, I.-I., Butnariu, I.-A., Calin, G., Guţu, C., Marcu, C., Grierosu, C., Roxana, E., Duceac, L. D., Dabija, M. G., Popa, F. L., & Damir, D. (2023). Understanding how minerals contribute to optimal immune function. *Journal of immunology research, 2023*, 1–26. Available from https://doi.org/10.1155/2023/3355733.

Stephen, J., Manoharan, D., & Radhakrishnan, M. (2023). Immune boosting functional components of natural foods and its health benefits. *Food Production, Processing and Nutrition, 5*(1). Available from https://doi.org/10.1186/s43014-023-00178-5.

Sun, W., Shahrajabian, M. H., & Lin, M. (2022). Research progress of fermented functional foods and protein factory-microbial fermentation technology. *Fermentation, 8*(12), 688. Available from https://doi.org/10.3390/fermentation8120688, [online].

Surette, M. E. (2008). The science behind dietary omega-3 fatty acids. *Canadian Medical Association Journal, 178*(2), 177–180. Available from https://doi.org/10.1503/cmaj.071356.

Szakos, D., Ózsvári, L., & Kasza, G. (2022). Health-related nutritional preferences of older adults: A segmentation study for functional food development. *Journal of Functional Foods, 92*105065. Available from https://doi.org/10.1016/j.jff.2022.105065.

Szydłowska, A., & Sionek, B. (2022). Probiotics and postbiotics as the functional food components affecting the immune response. *Microorganisms, 11*(1), 104. Available from https://doi.org/10.3390/microorganisms11010104.

Temple, N. J. (2022). A rational definition for functional foods: A perspective. *Frontiers in Nutrition, 9*. Available from https://doi.org/10.3389/fnut.2022.957516, [online].

Thapa, P., & Farber, D. L. (2019). The role of the thymus in the immune response. *Thoracic Surgery Clinics, 29*(2), 123–131. Available from https://doi.org/10.1016/j.thorsurg.2018.12.001, [online].

The Regeneration Center. (n.d.). Applications in Functional Medicine & Personalized Healthcare. [online] Available at: https://stemcellthailand.org/functional-medicine/ [Accessed 17 Mar. 2024].

Tkachenko, A., Kupcova, K., & Havranek, O. (2024). B-cell receptor signaling and beyond: The role of Igα (CD79a)/Igβ (CD79b) in normal and malignant B cells. *International Journal of Molecular Sciences, 25*(1), 10. Available from https://doi.org/10.3390/ijms25010010, [online].

Topolska, K., Florkiewicz, A., & Filipiak-Florkiewicz, A. (2021). Functional food—Consumer motivations and expectations. *International Journal of Environmental Research and Public Health, 18*(10), 5327. Available from https://doi.org/10.3390/ijerph18105327, [online].

Travers, A. C., Walport, P. M. & Shlomchik, M. J. (2010). The production of IgE. [online] Nih.gov. Available at: https://www.ncbi.nlm.nih.gov/books/NBK27117/.

Travers, A. C., Walport, P. M. & Shlomchik, M. J. (2018). Principles of innate and adaptive immunity. [online] Nih.gov. Available at: https://www.ncbi.nlm.nih.gov/books/NBK27090/.

Venkataratnamma, V., Begum, P., Madhavi, G., Rajagopal, S., Viswanath, B., & Razak, M. (2017). Probiotics as functional foods: potential effects on human health and its impact on neurological diseases. *International Journal of Nutrition, Pharmacology, Neurological Diseases, 7*(2), 23. Available from https://doi.org/10.4103/ijnpnd.ijnpnd_90_16.

Vigar, V., Myers, S., Oliver, C., Arellano, J., Robinson, S., & Leifert, C. (2019). A systematic review of organic versus conventional food consumption: Is there a measurable benefit on human health? *Nutrients, 12*(1), 7. Available from https://doi.org/10.3390/nu12010007, [online].

Vijay, A., Astbury, S., Le Roy, C., Spector, T. D., & Valdes, A. M. (2020). The prebiotic effects of omega-3 fatty acid supplementation: A six-week randomised intervention trial. *Gut Microbes, 13*(1), 1–11. Available from https://doi.org/10.1080/19490976.2020.1863133.

Vlaicu, P. A., Untea, A. E., Varzaru, I., Saracila, M., & Oancea, A. G. (2023). Designing nutrition for health—Incorporating dietary by-products into poultry feeds to create functional foods with insights into health benefits, risks, bioactive compounds, food component functionality and safety regulations. *ProQuest*, 4001. Available from https://doi.org/10.3390/foods12214001, [online].

Waheed Janabi, A. H., Kamboh, A. A., Saeed, M., Xiaoyu, L., BiBi, J., Majeed, F., Naveed, M., Mughal, M. J., Korejo, N. A., Kamboh, R., Alagawany, M., & Lv, H. (2020). Flavonoid-rich foods (FRF): A promising nutraceutical approach against lifespan-shortening diseases. *Iranian Journal of Basic Medical Sciences*, *23*(2), 140–153. Available from https://doi.org/10.22038/IJBMS.2019.35125.8353, [online].

Waliat, S., Arshad, M. S., Hanif, H., Ejaz, A., Khalid, W., Kauser, S., & Al-Farga, A. (2023). A review on bioactive compounds in sprouts: Extraction techniques, food application and health functionality. *International Journal of Food Properties*, *26*(1), 647–665. Available from https://doi.org/10.1080/10942912.2023.2176001.

Wan, M. L. Y., Ling, K. H., El-Nezami, H., & Wang, M. F. (2018). Influence of functional food components on gut health. *Critical Reviews in Food Science and Nutrition*, *59*(12), 1927–1936. Available from https://doi.org/10.1080/10408398.2018.1433629.

Weyh, C., Krüger, K., Peeling, P., & Castell, L. (2022). The role of minerals in the optimal functioning of the immune system. *Nutrients*, *14*(3), 644. Available from https://doi.org/10.3390/nu14030644, [online].

Weyh, C., Krüger, K., & Strasser, B. (2020). Physical activity and diet shape the immune system during aging. *Nutrients*, *12*(3), 622. Available from https://doi.org/10.3390/nu12030622.

Wintergerst, E. S., Maggini, S., & Hornig, D. H. (2006). Immune-enhancing role of vitamin C and zinc and effect on clinical conditions. *Annals of Nutrition & Metabolism*, *50*(2), 85–94. Available from https://doi.org/10.1159/000090495, [online].

World Health Organization (2020). Healthy Diet. [online] World Health Organization. Available at: https://www.who.int/news-room/fact-sheets/detail/healthy-diet.

Wright, A. (2022). Editorial overview: Functional foods and nutrition: The science of foods for health—A year in review. *Current Opinion in Food Science*, *46*100862. Available from https://doi.org/10.1016/j.cofs.2022.100862.

www.fao.org. (n.d.a). Entry details | FAO TERM PORTAL | Food and Agriculture Organization of the United Nations. [online] Available at: https://www.fao.org/faoterm/viewentry/en/?entryId = 170967.

www.fao.org. (n.d.b). Document card | FAO | Food and Agriculture Organization of the United Nations. [online] Available at: https://www.fao.org/documents/card/en/c/d8dfeaf1-f859-4191-954f-e8e1388cd0b7/.

www.gethealthie.com. (n.d.). New Ways to Implement Functional Medicine Programs | Healthie. [online] Available at: https://www.gethealthie.com/blog/personalized-functional-medicine-plan#: ~ :text = A%20personalized%20functional%20medicine%20program [Accessed 17 Mar. 2024].

www.ift.org. (n.d.). The 411 on Functional Foods. [online] Available at: https://www.ift.org/career-development/learn-about-food-science/food-facts/food-facts-food-health-and-nutrition/the-411-on-functional-foods.

www.mdpi.com. (n.d.). Journal of Personalized Medicine. [online] Available at: https://www.mdpi.com/journal/jpm/special_issues/Personalized_Multidisciplinary_Clinical [Accessed 17 Mar. 2024].

www.mhlw.go.jp. (n.d.). Ministry of Health, Labour and Welfare: Food with Health Claims, Food for Special Dietary Uses, and Nutrition Labeling. [online] Available at: https://www.mhlw.go.jp/english/topics/foodsafety/fhc/02.html.

www.optibacprobiotics.com. (n.d.). What are Synbiotics? | Probiotics Learning Lab. [online] Available at: https://www.optibacprobiotics.com/learning-lab/about/prebiotics/what-are-synbiotics#: ~ :text = Synbiotics%20can%20be%20a%20very%20effective%20way [Accessed 17 Mar. 2024].

Xie, C., Huang, W., Young, R. L., Jones, K. L., Horowitz, M., Rayner, C. K., & Wu, T. (2021). Role of bile acids in the regulation of food intake, and their dysregulation in metabolic disease. *Nutrients*, *13*(4), 1104. Available from https://doi.org/10.3390/nu13041104.

Xu, H., Fang, F., Wu, K., Song, J., Li, Y., Lu, X., Liu, J., Zhou, L., Yu, W., Yu, F., & Gao, J. (2023). Gut microbiota-bile acid crosstalk regulates murine lipid metabolism via the intestinal FXR-FGF19 axis in diet-induced humanized dyslipidemia. *Microbiome*, *11*(1). Available from https://doi.org/10.1186/s40168-023-01709-5.

Yanni, A. (2022). Editorial: Functional Foods and Bioactive Compounds for Improving and Maintaining Digestive Health. https://doi.org/10.3389/fnut.2021.815370.

Yegin, S., Kopec, A., Kitts, D.D. and Zawistowski, J. (2020). Chapter 24 - Dietary fiber: a functional food ingredient with physiological benefits. [online] ScienceDirect. https://doi.org/10.1016/B978-0-12-816918-6.00024-X.

Yoshimura, H. (2023). Using Functional Medicine As Personalized Medicine. [online] Rupa Health. Available at: https://www.rupahealth.com/post/using-functional-medicine-as-personalized-medicine.

Zelman, K. (2022). The Benefits of Vitamin C. [online] WebMD. Available at: https://www.webmd.com/diet/features/the-benefits-of-vitamin-c.

Zhai, Z., Liu, Y., Wu, L., Senchina, D. S., Wurtele, E. S., Murphy, P. A., Kohut, M. L., & Cunnick, J. E. (2007). Enhancement of innate and adaptive immune functions by multiple echinacea species. *Journal of Medicinal Food*, *10*(3), 423–434. Available from https://doi.org/10.1089/jmf.2006.257.

Zhao, E., Xu, H., Wang, L., Kryczek, I., Wu, K., Hu, Y., Wang, G., & Zou, W. (2011). Bone marrow and the control of immunity. *Cellular & Molecular Immunology*, *9*(1), 11–19. Available from https://doi.org/10.1038/cmi.2011.47, [online].

Zheng, J., Wittouck, S., Salvetti, E., Franz, C. M. A. P., Harris, H. M. B., Mattarelli, P., O'Toole, P. W., Pot, B., Vandamme, P., Walter, J., Watanabe, K., Wuyts, S., Felis, G. E., Gänzle, M. G., & Lebeer, S. (2020). A taxonomic note on the genus Lactobacillus: Description of 23 novel genera, emended description of the genus Lactobacillus Beijerinck 1901, and union of Lactobacillaceae and Leuconostocaceae. *International Journal of Systematic and Evolutionary Microbiology*, *70*(4), 2782–2858. Available from https://doi.org/10.1099/ijsem.0.004107.

Zhu, X., Yang, T., Sanchez, C. A., Hamilton, J. M., & Fonseca, J. M. (2022). Nutrition by design: Boosting selenium content and fresh matter yields of salad greens with preharvest light intensity and selenium applications. *Frontiers in Nutrition*, *8*. Available from https://doi.org/10.3389/fnut.2021.787085.

Chapter 12

Functional foods for bone and joint health: building a solid foundation

Zahra Emam-Djomeh[1], Homa Behmadi[2], Elham Azarpazhooh[3] and Hosahalli S. Ramaswamy[4]

[1]Functional Food ResearchCore (FFRC), Transfer Phenomena Laboratory (TPL), College of Agriculture & Natural Resources, University of Tehran, Karaj Campus, Tehran, Iran, [2]Agricultural Engineering Research Institute, Agricultural Research, Education and Extension Organization (AREEO), Karaj, Iran, [3]Agricultural Engineering Research Department, Khorasan Razavi Agricultural and Natural Resources Research and Education Center, AREEO, Mashhad, Iran, [4]Department of Food Science, Macdonald Campus, McGill University, Ste Anne de Bellevue, QC, Canada

12.1 Introduction

Bone and joint-related diseases such as osteoarthritis, rheumatoid arthritis, psoriatic arthritis, gout, spondyloarthritis, osteoporosis, osteopenia and associated fragility fractures, and traumatic fractures are highly prevalent and affecting millions across the globe (WHO, 2022).

While medications like analgesics, antiinflammatory drugs, disease-modifying antirheumatic drugs (DMARDs), bisphosphonates, and supplements like calcium and vitamin D can help, they often have side effects or do not fully address the progression of bone and joint-related diseases. Many patients continue to experience joint degeneration and worsening discomfort over time (WHO, 2023b). There is an increasing interest in complementary integrative approaches such as specialized precision diets and functional foods that can modulate inflammatory pathways, promote cartilage repair, improve bone mineral density, and meet nutritional requirements for managing bone and joint disorders (Kciuk et al., 2024)

Several bioactive compounds present naturally in foods or added to dietary supplements have shown potential benefits for bone and joint health, usually through antiinflammatory, antioxidative, or anabolic mechanisms. These include omega-3 fatty acids, vitamins (A, K, D, etc.), minerals (Ca, Zn, etc.), phytochemicals such as polyphenols, fibers, proteins, and analytes such as glucosamine, chondroitin, collagen peptides, and hyaluronic acid. These specialized diets and foods, imbued with bioactive compounds, have demonstrated capabilities in modulating inflammatory responses, fostering cartilage repair, augmenting bone mineral density, and satisfying specific nutritional needs, offering a holistic approach to managing bone and joint disorders (Kciuk et al., 2024; Keservani and Ahire, 2024).

This chapter explores the current scenario of bone and joint diseases and outlines the principles, applications, and future potential of functional foods and novel bioactives for prevention and management of bone and joint-related disorders. The key statistics, risk factors, existing treatments, and their limitations will also be discussed along with principles of how targeted functional foods and bioactives can complement conventional treatment. Specific functional food applications in development, their availability, and adoption trends will be covered. Recent advances in improving bioavailability, exploring new raw materials, and progress towards personalized nutrition will also be analyzed to provide future perspectives in this rapidly evolving domain.

12.2 Current scenario and literature review

12.2.1 Statistics on global bone and joint diseases

Osteoarthritis is a prevalent form of arthritis in adults, characterized by chronic pain and mobility loss. It is most common after age 40 and increases with age. The World Health Organization (WHO) has designated 2021–30 as the decade of healthy aging, emphasizing the need to address conditions like osteoarthritis, which significantly impact functional ability and quality of life. Osteoarthritis can coexist with other chronic conditions and is a major health

Unleashing the Power of Functional Foods and Novel Bioactives. DOI: https://doi.org/10.1016/B978-0-443-28862-3.00012-1

expenditure, with the US alone contributing an estimated $80 billion in healthcare spending in 2016. The WHO Global Ageing and Health Report highlights osteoarthritis as a leading cause of disability in adults aged 60 and older. Preventing or mitigating osteoarthritis could prevent decades of reduced quality of life.(Steinmetz et al., 2023)

According to WHO factsheets (WHO, 2023a), in 2019, about 528 million people worldwide were living with osteoarthritis; an increase of 113% since 1990 (Steinmetz et al., 2023). About 73% of people living with osteoarthritis are older than 55 years, and 60% are female (Steinmetz et al., 2023). With a prevalence of 365 million, the knee is the most frequently affected joint, followed by the hip and the hand (Long et al., 2022). A total of 344 million people living with osteoarthritis experience severity levels (moderate or severe) that could benefit from rehabilitation (Cieza et al., 2020). *Osteoarthritis* and obesity are coexisting conditions, and the number of patients with these diseases is expected to increase, representing a serious medical and social problem (Dydykina et al., 2024). With aging populations and increasing rates of obesity and injury, the prevalence of osteoarthritis and other bone and joint-related diseases is expected to continue to increase globally. The prevalence of *Osteoarthritis* is anticipated to double in the next decade (Salahuddin Salih et al., 2024). Most of these diseases are not an evitable consequence of aging.

Osteoporosis affects approximately 30% of women globally between the ages of 40 and 50. This disease is among the top causes of death and disability among the elderly (Kha et al., 2024). Between 1,039,348 and 1,240,807 Irish men and women aged ≥50 years have low bone mass and between 308,474 and 498,104 men and women aged ≥50 years have osteoporosis. The burden of osteoporosis is expected to increase, necessitating national policies to reduce the illness burden (Carey et al., 2023).

In patients with end-stage chronic kidney disease (CKD), the incidence of fragility fractures is significantly higher compared to the general population (De Mauro et al., 2024).

Rheumatoid arthritis is also a chronic autoimmune disease, causing joint inflammation and affects multiple body systems, with the joints of hands, wrists, feet, ankles, knees, shoulders, and elbows being most affected (Long et al., 2022). It is characterized by joint pain, stiffness, tenderness, heat, and swelling. Risk factors include smoking, obesity, and exposure to air pollution. Women and older individuals are at a higher risk of developing Rheumatoid arthritis. If diagnosed early, symptoms and disease progression can be controlled with pharmacological treatment and rehabilitation. In severe cases, surgical procedures, such as joint replacement, may be necessary to restore movement or manage pain and maintain physical function (WHO, 2023b). In 2019, 18 million people worldwide lived with Rheumatoid arthritis, with 70% being women and 55% older than 55 years (Steinmetz et al., 2023).

Gout is the most common rheumatic disease in adults, with prevalence ranging from 0.1% to about 10% (Wojtania et al., 2024).

With greater life expectancy and aging populations across most countries, the incidence of bone and joint disorders is expected to rise further in the coming decades (Table 12.1). This highlights the urgent need to find better prevention and treatment approaches to curb the mounting public health and economic crisis posed by musculoskeletal diseases.

12.2.2 Risk factors

Common risk factors for bone and joint disorders include genetic predisposition, advanced age, female gender, obesity, sedentary lifestyle, smoking, repetitive occupational or sports injuries, and poor nutrition.

Genetic factors significantly influence the risk of developing bone and joint disorders. For instance, certain genetic loci are associated with increased susceptibility to conditions like juvenile idiopathic arthritis (Oberle et al., 2014).

TABLE 12.1 Key Statistics on Common Bone and Joint Diseases Worldwide, Prevalence, and Forecast.

Disease	Current Prevalence (2023)	Forecasted Trend	Key Factors
Osteoporosis	30% of women aged 40–50	Increasing	Aging population, lifestyle
Osteoarthritis	High, significant burden	Expected to double	Aging, obesity
Fragility fractures	Higher in CKD patients	Increasing	CKD prevalence
Gout	0.1%–10%	Stable to increasing	Lifestyle, diet

Aging is also a major risk factor for bone and joint disorders, as it leads to decreased regenerative potential and increased inflammation, contributing to conditions like osteoporosis and osteoarthritis (Cheng et al., 2023).

Women, especially postmenopausal, are at higher risk for osteoporosis due to hormonal changes, reduction in estrogen levels after menopause, that affect bone density (McClung et al., 2021)

Excess body weight increases the risk of osteoarthritis and other musculoskeletal disorders due to additional stress on joints and systemic inflammation (Roy et al., 2016).

Physical inactivity is linked to musculoskeletal disorders, including osteoporosis and osteoarthritis, due to reduced muscle strength and joint flexibility (Park et al., 2020).

Smoking negatively impacts bone health by reducing bone mass and impairing bone healing, increasing the risk of osteoporosis and fractures (Chang et al., 2020).

Repetitive stress and injuries from certain activities can lead to joint damage and increase the risk of osteoarthritis (Khan et al., 2023).

Inadequate intake of essential nutrients, such as calcium and vitamin D, can compromise bone health and increase the risk of osteoporosis (Ahmadieh and Arabi, 2011).

12.2.3 Current treatments and their limitations

Current management strategies for bone and joint-related diseases include exercise, physical therapy, assistive devices, home modifications, self-management educational programs, pain medication, surgical treatments, prescribing suitable diets, supplements, and bioactive and functional foods. Modifiable risk factors for osteoarthritis include high BMI, joint injury, physically demanding occupations, elite-level sports, surgery, joint anatomy, and muscle weakness (Steinmetz et al., 2023).

Bone is a specialized skeletal structure that mainly consists of a group of cells, scaffold proteins, and minerals. The dynamic cycle of bone growth and resorption driven by cells, minerals, vitamins, and hormonal regulations differs in individuals. The bone grows at the highest rate at a young age. Calcium has been well-accepted as a crucial element that accumulates in the bone and strengthens the skeleton when produced with its partner ions and some trace elements. The recommended daily requirement of calcium is different due to genetics, sex, and stages of life. Milk is a calcium-rich food and people worldwide consume it. Grains and vegetables are also the right answer. Furthermore, some aging people also find some panacea for joint mobility and support. In this chapter, a reader will learn the basis of bone metabolism, calcium homeostasis, and functional foods that can support bone and joint health during aging (Charoensin et al., 2023).

Common pharmacological treatments for musculoskeletal disorders include analgesics like NSAIDs, acetaminophen, and opioids, as well as nutritional supplements for bone and joint health. Disease-modifying antirheumatic drugs (DMARDs) such as methotrexate and biological agents block inflammatory cytokines for inflammatory types of arthritis (Hochberg et al., 2012; Smolen et al., 2020). Surgeries such as knee replacements aim to improve joint function but have risks of complications, limited durability, and do not repair cartilage or cure disease progression (Nikolaevich et al., 2023).

Rheumatoid arthritis is a chronic condition that impacts many aspects of life, and early diagnosis and management can reduce symptoms, slow the disease, and prevent disability. Therapeutic approaches help improve and maintain joint mobility and muscle strength, reduce pain, and increase exercise capacity. Assistive technologies, such as orthosis and assistive products for self-care, help people protect their joints and perform meaningful activities independently (Nikolaevich et al., 2023; Zhang, 2023).

There is an increasing need for alternative and complementary treatment approaches that not only provide symptomatic relief but also modulate underlying disease pathways to limit, delay, or prevent the progression of bone and joint disorders. The prescription of food supplements like calcium and vitamin D and other nutraceuticals such as resveratrol, anthocyanins, isoflavones, lycopene, curcumin, lutein, and β-carotene, personalized diets and the use of functional foods that proffer more than mere sustenance, aiming to turn the tide against inflammatory processes, stoke the repair of cartilage, prop up bone mineral density, and fulfill the nutritional armor required to combat bone and joint disorders are among the most important approaches in this regard.

12.2.4 Potential of functional foods

Because there is a direct link between food and health, different scientific research has been conducted to determine the impact of foods or dietary substances on key bodily functions. The phrase "functional food," which refers to foods that have distinct health benefits, was first used in Japan (Keservani & Ahire, 2024). Several natural compounds present in foods like fruits, vegetables, herbs, spices, and marine sources have exhibited protective effects for musculoskeletal health in human trials. Common examples with promising bone and joint benefits include omega-3 fatty acids from fish oil, antiinflammatory spices like turmeric and ginger, collagen peptides from animal bones and cartilage, glucosamine, and chondroitin from shellfish, prebiotics, and probiotics for gut health and a range of antioxidants and polyphenols from fruits and teas (Basak et al., 2024; Faienza et al., 2024; Sophocleous, 2023).

12.2.5 Common bioactives and functional food for bone and joint health

12.2.5.1 Bioactives

A variety of vitamins, minerals, fibers, healthy fats, proteins, polyphenols, and other compounds found naturally in foods or added to dietary supplements have shown beneficial effects for musculoskeletal health. These can be incorporated into functional foods and beverages to provide bone and joint benefits. Key examples include:

12.2.5.1.1 Glucosamine and chondroitin

Glucosamine and chondroitin are naturally occurring compounds found in the cartilage of animals. Glucosamine is typically derived from shellfish shells, such as shrimp, lobster, and crab, or synthesized in laboratories. Chondroitin sulfate is extracted from animal cartilage, including bovine, porcine, and shark cartilage (Santos et al., 2017).

These compounds are commonly used as dietary supplements to support joint health and manage symptoms of osteoarthritis. Glucosamine and chondroitin play crucial roles in maintaining the structural integrity and function of joints. Glucosamine is a precursor for glycosaminoglycans, which are essential components of the cartilage matrix. It stimulates the production of proteoglycans and hyaluronic acid, contributing to the formation and repair of cartilage (Kelly, 1998). Chondroitin sulfate, a major component of cartilage, provides resistance to compression and enhances the shock-absorbing properties of cartilage. It also inhibits enzymes that degrade cartilage and promotes water retention in the cartilage matrix, maintaining its elasticity and resilience (Kelly, 1998).

Numerous in vitro and in vivo studies have investigated the efficacy of glucosamine and chondroitin in bone and joint health (Fernández-Martín et al., 2021; Shen et al., 2023). In vitro studies have shown that glucosamine and chondroitin can stimulate the synthesis of glycosaminoglycans and inhibit the activity of degradative enzymes in cartilage cells (Lippiello et al., 2000). These findings suggest that these compounds can enhance cartilage repair and reduce cartilage degradation.

In vivo studies have provided further evidence of the benefits of glucosamine and chondroitin. There are several systematic reviews and metaanalysis of clinical trials about the safety and efficacy of glucosamine, chondroitin, and their combination supplementation significantly reduced pain and improved joint function in patients with knee osteoarthritis (Čeh & Šarabon, 2023; Meng et al., 2023). Another study found that a combination of glucosamine hydrochloride, chondroitin sulfate, and manganese ascorbate was more effective in reducing cartilage degeneration and improving joint health in a rabbit model of osteoarthritis compared to each agent alone (Lippiello et al., 2000).

Clinical trials have also shown that glucosamine and chondroitin can slow the progression of osteoarthritis. A comprehensive metaanalysis reported that glucosamine sulfate significantly reduced joint space narrowing and improved symptoms in patients with knee osteoarthritis, while chondroitin sulfate was effective in reducing pain and improving mobility (Richy et al., 2003). These findings suggest that glucosamine and chondroitin can provide both symptomatic relief and structural benefits in the management of osteoarthritis. To optimize the formulation and delivery methods, and enhance the safety, bioavailability, and therapeutic efficacy, the use of different salt forms of glucosamine, such as glucosamine sulfate and glucosamine hydrochloride, and a combination of glucosamine, chondroitin, and their salts with other bioactive compounds or antiinflammatory drugs, such as manganese ascorbate, were studied (Ivanovska & Dimitrova, 2011; Rabade et al., 2024; Lippiello et al., 2000). A recent metaanalysis revealed that the chondroitin sulfate (with decreased pain intensity and improvement in physical function) and glucosamine sulfate (with a significant reduction in the joint space narrowing) have significant therapeutic benefits. However, their combination did not significantly improve the symptoms or modify the disease (Rabade et al., 2024).

In conclusion, glucosamine and chondroitin are widely used nutraceuticals with significant potential for supporting bone and joint health. Their ability to stimulate cartilage synthesis, inhibit cartilage degradation, and reduce inflammation makes them valuable bioactive agents for managing osteoarthritis and other joint disorders. Continued research and clinical validation are essential to fully understand their mechanisms of action and optimize their use in clinical practice.

12.2.5.1.2 Methylsulfonylmethane

Methylsulfonylmethane (MSM) is a naturally occurring sulfur compound found in various foods, including fruits, vegetables, grains, and beverages such as coffee, tea, and beer. MSM is also present in cow's milk and certain plants, making it a bioavailable source of sulfur for human consumption (Butawan et al., 2017).

MSM has been extensively studied for its potential benefits in bone and joint health. It is known to alleviate symptoms of osteoarthritis, reduce inflammation, and promote collagen synthesis. MSM enhances the signaling pathways involved in bone growth and promotes the differentiation of mesenchymal stem cells (MSCs) into osteoblasts, which are crucial for bone formation. Additionally, MSM has been shown to inhibit osteoclastogenesis, thereby reducing bone resorption (McFarlin et al., 2023).

In vitro studies have demonstrated MSM's ability to enhance osteoblast differentiation and mineralization. For instance, MSM increases the expression of osteogenic markers and promotes autophagy in hepatoma cells, which is beneficial for metabolic-associated fatty liver disease (Han et al., 2023). Furthermore, MSM has shown antiinflammatory effects by inhibiting the release of proinflammatory cytokines in murine macrophages (McFarlin et al., 2023).

In vivo studies have corroborated the beneficial effects of MSM on bone health. For example, MSM supplementation in aging female mice increased bone density and reduced bone resorption markers (McFarlin et al., 2021). Additionally, MSM has demonstrated anticancer properties by inhibiting tumor growth and inducing apoptosis in various cancer models (McFarlin et al., 2023).

In summary, MSM is a versatile compound with multiple health benefits, particularly in bone and joint health. Its efficacy has been supported by both in vitro and in vivo studies, making it a promising candidate for further research and clinical applications.

12.2.5.1.3 Collagen and other bioactive peptides

Bioactive peptides derived from food proteins are recognized for their potential to promote bone health. These peptides can enhance bone formation and inhibit bone resorption, making them valuable ingredients in functional foods and nutraceuticals. However, their commercial use is limited by challenges related to bioavailability and stability during digestion (Amigo and Hernández-Ledesma, 2020). Research is ongoing to develop more effective delivery systems for these peptides.

Collagen peptides are derived from the hydrolysis of collagen, a structural protein found abundantly in animal connective tissues such as skin, bones, and cartilage. Common sources include bovine, porcine, and marine organisms. Bovine and porcine collagen peptides are typically extracted from skin and bones, while marine collagen is sourced from fish skin, scales, and bones (Rahaman et al., 2023). The extraction process involves demineralization, deproteinization, and enzymatic hydrolysis to produce bioactive peptides with low molecular weights, enhancing their bioavailability and bioactivity (Fu et al., 2019).

Collagen peptides play a significant role in maintaining and improving bone and joint health. They are known to enhance bone mineral density (BMD) and support the structural integrity of bones by promoting osteoblast activity and inhibiting osteoclast activity. This dual action helps in bone formation and reduces bone resorption, which is crucial for preventing osteoporosis and other bone-related diseases (Mukherjee et al., 2024). Additionally, collagen peptides improve joint health by reducing inflammation and pain associated with conditions such as osteoarthritis (OA) and rheumatoid arthritis (RA). They achieve this by modulating inflammatory cytokines and enhancing the synthesis of extracellular matrix components in cartilage (Kumar et al., 2015).

Numerous in vitro and in vivo studies have demonstrated the efficacy of collagen peptides in bone and joint health. In vitro studies have shown that collagen peptides can stimulate the proliferation and differentiation of osteoblasts, the cells responsible for the formation of bone, while inhibiting the activity of osteoclasts, the cells involved in bone resorption (Fu et al., 2019). These studies highlight the potential of collagen peptides to enhance bone regeneration and repair.

In vivo studies further support these findings. For instance, a double-blind, placebo-controlled clinical trial demonstrated that collagen peptides derived from pork skin and bovine bone significantly reduced pain and improved joint function in patients with knee osteoarthritis. The study reported significant reductions in Western Ontario McMaster Universities (WOMAC) and visual analog scale (VAS) scores, indicating improved quality of life and joint health (Kumar et al., 2015). Another study involving chicken bone collagen peptides showed that oral administration of these peptides alleviated skin aging and improved bone health by regulating collagen synthesis and degradation, inhibiting inflammation, and activating lysosomal pathways (Cao et al., 2022).

Recent research has focused on optimizing the extraction and characterization of collagen peptides to enhance their therapeutic potential. For example, studies have explored the use of different enzymes and processing parameters to produce collagen peptides with higher antioxidant and antiinflammatory activities (Aubry et al., 2023). Additionally, marine collagen peptides have gained attention due to their sustainability and unique bioactive properties, making them suitable for use in nutraceuticals and functional foods (Cadar et al., 2024).

Collagen peptides have shown potential in improving skin, wound healing, and cardiovascular health, making them potential components of dietary supplements and therapeutic interventions. Further research and clinical validation will further explore their therapeutic potential (Rahaman et al., 2023).

12.2.5.1.4 Hyaluronic acid

Hyaluronic acid (HA) is a naturally occurring glycosaminoglycan found in various tissues and fluids in the human body, including connective tissues, synovial fluid, and the vitreous humor of the eye. It is also present in certain bacterial capsules and can be extracted from animal sources such as rooster combs and umbilical cords (Galla et al., 2022). Its natural occurrence in various biological sources and its therapeutic potential in treating joint disorders make it valuable in medical and nutritional applications. Recent advancements have led to the development of plant-derived HA, such as GreenIuronic, which has shown promising results in maintaining joint homeostasis and preventing osteoarthritis (Galla et al., 2022).

Hyaluronic acid plays a crucial role in maintaining joint health by providing lubrication and shock absorption in synovial fluid, promoting cell proliferation, and enhancing tissue regeneration (Bonifacio et al., 2023). It helps in reducing inflammation and pain associated with osteoarthritis by modulating molecular mechanisms responsible for cartilage degradation and repair (Galla et al., 2022). HA also contributes to the viscoelastic properties of synovial fluid, which are essential for load-bearing and minimizing wear and tear in joints (Kakati et al., 2024).

In vitro studies have demonstrated that hyaluronic acid enhances osteoblast metabolism, proliferation, and differentiation, promoting bone repair and regeneration (Bonifacio et al., 2023). HA, when combined with amino acids, has been shown to boost osteoblasts' metabolic activity and cell cycle progression, increasing the expression of differentiation markers such as osteoprotegerin and osteonectin (Bonifacio et al., 2023). Additionally, HA has been found to improve the viability and proliferation of chondrocytes, supporting cartilage health (Asensio et al., 2021).

In vivo studies have further supported the benefits of hyaluronic acid in bone and joint health. For instance, HA-based hydrogels have been used as delivery systems for osteoinductive agents, showing positive effects on bone healing (Deng et al., 2023). Self-healing HA has demonstrated improved in vivo retention and function, mitigating cartilage degeneration in rodent models of anterior cruciate ligament injury (Gilpin et al., 2021). Moreover, HA supplemented with porous bioglass-derived granules has shown excellent bioactivity and fast bone formation in femoral defect models, indicating its potential as an injectable bone substitute for early bone regeneration (Im et al., 2021).

12.2.5.1.5 Omega-3 fatty acids

Polyunsaturated fatty acids (PUFAs), particularly omega-3 (*n*-3), and omega-6 (*n*-6) fatty acids are essential fats found in various foods, playing important roles in human health. Long-chain omega-3 PUFAs, such as alpha-linolenic acid (ALA), eicosapentaenoic acid (EPA), and docosahexaenoic acid (DHA), are primarily sourced from fish and fish oils, though alternative sources like algal oils and genetically modified plants are being explored for sustainability (Baker, 2024; Hegde et al., 2016). These fatty acids are vital for maintaining bone and joint health due to their antiinflammatory properties, which help reduce joint pain and stiffness, associated with conditions like osteoarthritis (Deckelbaum and Torrejon, 2012; Kuberskaya et al., 2023). Additionally, EPA and DHA contribute to bone health by promoting calcium absorption and bone density, potentially reducing the risk of osteoporosis (Ward and Singh, 2005).

Omega-6 PUFAs, such as linoleic acid (LA) and arachidonic acid (AA), are also essential but must be balanced with omega-3 intake to avoid proinflammatory effects (Montecillo-Aguado et al., 2023). Despite their benefits, the typical Western diet is often deficient in these valuable nutrients, necessitating dietary supplements or fortified foods to achieve optimal health outcomes (Cholewski et al., 2018).

In vitro studies have demonstrated that omega-3 PUFAs can enhance osteoblast differentiation and mineralization, promoting bone formation. For instance, EPA and DHA have been shown to increase the expression of osteogenic markers and reduce the production of proinflammatory cytokines in osteoblast cultures (Dou et al., 2022). Additionally, omega-3 PUFAs can modulate the activity of osteoclasts, the cells responsible for bone resorption, thereby maintaining a balance between bone formation and resorption (Islam et al., 2023).

In vivo studies have further supported the beneficial effects of PUFAs on bone and joint health. A systematic review and metaanalysis of randomized controlled trials found that omega-3 PUFA supplementation slightly enhances bone mineral density (BMD), particularly in postmenopausal women (Dou et al., 2022). Another study using a Mendelian randomization approach confirmed the positive causal relationship between omega-3 and omega-6 PUFAs and estimated bone mineral density (eBMD) (Tao et al., 2022).

Moreover, animal studies have shown that diets rich in omega-3 PUFAs can improve bone quality and reduce markers of bone resorption. For example, rats fed with a balanced blend of monounsaturated and polyunsaturated fatty acids exhibited improved bone mineral density and reduced inflammation and oxidative stress markers (Yang et al., 2022). These findings suggest that PUFAs can positively influence bone metabolism and overall bone health.

12.2.5.1.6 Antioxidant polyphenols

Polyphenols are a diverse group of naturally occurring compounds found in plants, known for their antioxidant properties. Polyphenols like anthocyanins in berries, ellagitannins in pomegranates, curcumin in turmeric and EGCG in green tea and quercetin as a flavonoid that is found in many fruits, vegetables have shown protective effects for cartilage, bone, and muscle tissue by reducing oxidative damage and inflammation.

Flavonoids: Flavonoids are found in fruits, vegetables, tea, and wine. Specific types include quercetin, kaempferol, and naringin. Enhance bone formation and inhibit bone resorption by affecting osteoblast and osteoclast activity. They modulate signaling pathways such as MAPK and NF-kB, which are crucial for bone remodeling (Ramesh et al., 2021).

Anthocyanins: Anthocyanins are present in red, purple, and blue fruits and vegetables like berries, grapes, and red cabbage (Li et al., 2021). Exhibit antiinflammatory and antioxidant properties, which help in reducing bone loss and improving bone density (Mattioli et al., 2020).

Stilbenes: Resveratrol is the most studied, found in grapes, red wine, and peanuts. Resveratrol has been shown to promote bone health by enhancing osteoblast activity and inhibiting osteoclastogenesis (Williamson and Manach, 2005).

Curcumin: It is the active compound in turmeric, widely used in Asian cuisine and traditional medicine. Known for its antiinflammatory properties, curcumin helps in reducing joint pain and inflammation, beneficial for conditions like arthritis (Miran et al., 2021; Zamani-Garmsiri et al., 2022).

Ginger: It contains gingerol and shogaol, used in culinary and medicinal applications. Exhibits antiinflammatory effects, which can help in managing joint pain and improving mobility (Serreli and Deiana, 2019).

Polyphenols have been shown to enhance osteoblast differentiation and activity and reduce osteoclast formation in cell cultures. For example, flavonoids like quercetin and kaempferol have demonstrated significant effects on bone cell activity (Ramesh et al., 2021).

Animal studies have shown that polyphenols can improve bone density and strength. For instance, blueberry polyphenols have been found to enhance bone health in rats by modulating gut microbiota and improving polyphenol bioavailability (Weaver et al., 2023). Further research, especially long-term human studies, is needed to fully understand their potential and optimize their use in clinical settings.

12.2.5.1.7 Carotenoids

Carotenoids are a class of naturally occurring pigments found in plants, algae, and photosynthetic bacteria. They are responsible for the red, yellow, and orange colors in many fruits and vegetables and are known for their antioxidant properties. Carotenoids are broadly classified into two categories: carotens include α-carotene, β-carotene, and lycopene, which are hydrocarbons and do not contain oxygen. And the second category, xanthophylls, include lutein, zeaxanthin, and β-cryptoxanthin, which contain oxygen and are more polar than carotenes (Zeb & Sultan, 2004; Ávila-Román et al., 2021).

Carotenoids are abundant in various foods, such as fruits and vegetables (carrots, pumpkins, sweet potatoes, tomatoes, and leafy greens, watermelon, papaya, pink grapefruit, oranges, tangerins) (Gebregziabher et al., 2023), marine microalgae, which are natural sources of carotenoids used in pharmaceutical, food, and cosmetic applications (Guedes et al., 2011) and some of nuts and seeds (Mandal and Domb, 2024).

Carotenoids have been shown to positively influence bone and joint health through various mechanisms The most important mechanisms are through antioxidant properties, which is crucial for maintaining bone health (Kulczyński et al., 2024; Sahni et al., 2009). Antiinflammatory effects help in reducing inflammation, which is beneficial for joint health (Khalil et al., 2021; Sharma et al., 2021) and bone remodeling. Carotenoids like β-carotene and lycopene enhance osteoblast activity and inhibit osteoclastogenesis, promoting bone formation and reducing bone resorption (Kulczyński et al., 2024). Carotenoids such as β-cryptoxanthin and lycopene have been shown to stimulate bone formation and mineralization in cell cultures (Ribeiro et al., 2010). Lycopene has demonstrated potential in reducing oxidative stress and promoting osteoblast differentiation (Walallawita et al., 2020).

Animal studies have demonstrated that carotenoids can improve bone density and strength. For instance, high serum carotenoid levels are associated with a lower risk for bone loss and osteoporosis in postmenopausal women (Sugiura et al., 2012; Walallawita et al., 2020). Additionally, dietary carotenoid intake has been linked to better bone mineral density and reduced fracture risk in elderly populations (Hayhoe et al., 2017; Kulczyński et al., 2024). Further research, especially long-term human studies, is needed to fully understand their potential and optimize their use in clinical settings.

12.2.5.1.8 Bromelain

Bromelain is a complex mixture of proteolytic enzymes obtained mainly from the pineapple plant (*Ananas comosus*). It is known for its antiinflammatory, antiedematous, and fibrinolytic properties. Bromelain is extracted from various parts of the pineapple plant, including stem, which is the main commercial source of bromelain, fruit, which contains a different composition of enzymes than the stem (Varilla et al., 2021) and leaves and roots, which also contain bromelain but are less commonly used for extraction (Sharma & Vimal, 2023).

Bromelain has been shown to have a positive effect on bone and joint health through various mechanisms. Bromelain has antiinflammatory properties and may reduce inflammation by modulating the arachidonate cascade and inhibiting proinflammatory mediators such as cyclooxygenase-2 (COX-2) and nuclear factor kappa B (NF-κB) (Bottega et al., 2021). Bromelain can help relieve joint pain, making it useful for conditions such as osteoarthritis (Quarta et al., 2022). By reducing inflammation and pain, bromelain can also improve joint mobility and function (Quarta et al., 2022).

Bromelain has demonstrated significant antiinflammatory effects in cell cultures. For example, it reduced inflammatory markers in human chondrocytes and other cell lines, suggesting its potential in treating joint inflammation (Bottega et al., 2021).

Animal studies have shown that bromelain can reduce joint inflammation and pain. In a study involving mice with induced osteoarthritis, bromelain treatment resulted in significant reductions in joint swelling and pain (Quarta et al., 2022). Additionally, bromelain has been shown to protect normal cells from radiation effects while sensitizing tumor cells to radiation, indicating its potential in reducing inflammation and promoting tissue repair (Mekkawy et al., 2020).

Although recent in vitro and in vivo studies support its therapeutic potential, further research, especially long-term human studies, is needed to fully understand its benefits and optimize its use in clinical settings.

12.2.5.1.9 Minerals and vitamins

Minerals and vitamins are essential nutrients that play critical roles in maintaining bone and joint health. Key minerals include calcium, phosphorus, magnesium, and silicon, while important vitamins include vitamin D, vitamin K, vitamin A, and vitamin C. Calcium is primarily sourced from dairy products, leafy green vegetables, and fortified foods. Phosphorus is found in meat, fish, dairy, and whole grains. Magnesium is abundant in nuts, seeds, whole grains, and green leafy vegetables. Silicon can be obtained from whole grains, cereals, beer, and some vegetables like green beans (Price et al., 2013).

Vitamin D is synthesized in the skin upon exposure to sunlight and can also be obtained from fatty fish, fortified dairy products, and supplements. Vitamin K is found in green leafy vegetables, fermented foods, and some animal products. Vitamin A is present in foods of animal origin (retinol) and plant origin (provitamin A carotenoids). Vitamin C is abundant in fruits and vegetables, particularly citrus fruits, strawberries, bell peppers, and broccoli (Van Ballegooijen et al., 2017; Yee et al., 2021).

Minerals and vitamins are crucial for bone formation, maintenance, and repair. Calcium and phosphorus are the primary components of hydroxyapatite, the mineral matrix that gives bones their strength and rigidity. Magnesium plays a role in bone mineralization and the regulation of calcium balance. Silicon is involved in collagen synthesis and bone mineralization, contributing to bone strength and density (Baeverfjord et al., 2019; Price et al., 2013).

Vitamins also play significant roles in bone health. Vitamin D enhances calcium absorption in the gut and maintains adequate serum calcium and phosphate levels for bone mineralization. Vitamin K is essential for the carboxylation of osteocalcin, a protein involved in bone formation. Vitamin A regulates bone remodeling by influencing osteoblast and osteoclast activity. Vitamin C is necessary for collagen synthesis, which is vital for the structural integrity of bones and cartilage (Ahmadieh & Arabi, 2011; Van Ballegooijen et al., 2017).

Numerous in vitro and in vivo studies have demonstrated the importance of minerals and vitamins in bone and joint health. In vitro studies have shown that calcium and phosphorus are essential for osteoblast differentiation and bone matrix formation. Magnesium deficiency has been linked to impaired bone growth and increased bone fragility in animal models (Baeverfjord et al., 2019). Silicon supplementation has been shown to enhance bone mineral density and improve bone strength in both animal and human studies (Price et al., 2013).

In vivo studies have provided substantial evidence of the benefits of vitamins in bone health. Clinical trials have demonstrated that vitamin D supplementation improves bone mineral density and reduces the risk of fractures in elderly populations. Vitamin K supplementation has been shown to enhance bone strength and reduce the risk of osteoporotic fractures by improving the carboxylation of osteocalcin (Van Ballegooijen et al., 2017). Vitamin A and its metabolites have been found to influence bone remodeling processes, with both beneficial and adverse effects depending on the dosage (Yee et al., 2021). Vitamin C has been shown to promote collagen synthesis and improve bone density in epidemiological studies (Ahmadieh and Arabi, 2011).

Recent research has focused on the synergistic effects of combined mineral and vitamin supplementation on bone health. Studies have shown that the combined supplementation of vitamins D and K is more effective in improving bone and cardiovascular health than either vitamin alone. This synergy enhances calcium metabolism and bone mineralization, providing a comprehensive approach to bone health management (Van Ballegooijen et al., 2017). Additionally, the role of vitamin D in modulating immune function and its potential benefits in autoimmune diseases and chronic inflammatory conditions affecting the joints are being explored (Szulc et al., 2023).

Innovative delivery methods and formulations are being developed to enhance the bioavailability and efficacy of these nutrients. For example, nanoencapsulation and liposomal delivery systems are being investigated to improve the absorption and targeted delivery of vitamins and minerals (de Wildt et al., 2022). Furthermore, the integration of these nutrients into functional foods and nutraceuticals offers a practical approach to improving bone and joint health through diet (Goggs et al., 2005). Continued research and clinical validation are essential to optimize their use in preventing and managing bone-related diseases, highlighting the importance of adequate nutrition and supplementation in promoting skeletal health.

12.2.5.1.10 Probiotics and prebiotics

Probiotics and prebiotics offer promising therapeutic potential for bone and joint health by modulating gut microbiota and influencing systemic inflammation and bone metabolism. The gut microbiota plays a crucial role in bone health through the gut-bone axis. Probiotics and prebiotics can modulate gut microbiota, influencing bone metabolism and reducing inflammation (Bhardwaj et al., 2022). They help maintain bone mineral density (BMD) and may prevent conditions such as osteoporosis by enhancing calcium absorption and modulating immune responses (de Sire et al., 2022).

Recent studies have highlighted the potential of probiotics and prebiotics in bone and joint health. In vitro studies have shown that probiotics can enhance osteoblast activity and inhibit osteoclastogenesis, promoting bone formation and reducing bone resorption (Zhang et al., 2023). In vivo studies using animal models have demonstrated that probiotics and prebiotics can reverse gut microbiota dysbiosis and rescue bone loss induced by osteoporosis (Li et al., 2021).

A systematic review of animal models revealed that interventions with probiotics, prebiotics, and other nutritional supplements positively affect bone health by improving BMD and bone quality (Li et al., 2021). Additionally, clinical trials are underway to assess the combined effects of synbiotic supplementation and exercise on bone biomarkers and gut microbiota in postmenopausal women, aiming to provide noninvasive approaches to manage osteoporosis (Ilesanmi-Oyelere et al., 2021). Further clinical trials are necessary to establish their efficacy and safety in human populations. Integrating these functional foods into daily diets could be a valuable strategy for enhancing bone health and preventing bone-related diseases.

12.2.5.2 Natural functional food

Natural functional foods such as honey, olive oil, tea, flaxseed, dried plums, and blueberries offer promising therapeutic potential for bone and joint health. Their bioactive compounds help in reducing inflammation, oxidative stress, and bone resorption while promoting bone formation. Further clinical trials are necessary to establish their efficacy and safety in human populations, but current evidence supports their integration into daily diets for enhancing bone health and preventing bone-related diseases (Faienza et al., 2024).

12.2.5.2.1 Honey

Honey is rich in antioxidants and antiinflammatory compounds, which contribute to bone health by reducing oxidative stress and inflammation. In vitro and in vivo studies have shown that honey can improve bone microstructure and strength and reduce bone loss in osteoporotic models (Martiniakova et al., 2023). Honey's polyphenols also help in managing metabolic syndrome, which indirectly benefits bone health by reducing oxidative damage and inflammation (Mohd Ramli et al., 2021).

12.2.5.2.2 Olive oil

Olive oil, a key component of the Mediterranean diet, contains monounsaturated fatty acids and polyphenols like hydroxytyrosol, which have antiinflammatory and antioxidant properties. These compounds help in maintaining bone density and reducing the risk of osteoporosis (Antonopoulou and Demopoulos, 2023). In vivo studies have shown that olive oil can improve bone mineral density and reduce bone resorption (Campo et al., 2024).

12.2.5.2.3 Tea

Tea, particularly green and black tea, contains polyphenols such as catechins and theaflavins, which have been shown to have antiinflammatory and antioxidant effects. These compounds help in reducing bone resorption and promoting bone formation (Xie et al., 2024). However, some studies suggest that the relationship between tea consumption and bone health is not conclusive and requires further investigation (Chen et al., 2022).

12.2.5.2.4 Flaxseed

Flaxseed is rich in alpha-linolenic acid, lignans, and dietary fiber, which contribute to its antiinflammatory and antioxidant properties. In vivo studies have shown that flaxseed can improve bone biomarkers and reduce bone loss in osteoporotic models (Nowak and Jeziorek, 2023). Flaxseed's polyphenols also exhibit antidiabetic and antiinflammatory effects, which indirectly benefit bone health (Mechchate et al., 2021).

12.2.5.2.5 Dried plums

Dried plums (prunes) are rich in polyphenols and have been shown to have osteoprotective effects. In vivo studies have demonstrated that dried plums can prevent and reverse bone loss in osteoporotic models by reducing inflammation and oxidative stress (Damani et al., 2022). Clinical trials have also shown that prune consumption can improve bone mineral density and bone biomarkers in postmenopausal women (George et al., 2022).

12.2.5.2.6 Blueberries

Blueberries are rich in anthocyanins and other polyphenols, which have antioxidant and antiinflammatory properties. In vitro and in vivo studies have shown that blueberries can improve bone health by reducing oxidative stress and inflammation and promoting bone formation (Weaver et al., 2023). Blueberries also have potential benefits in preventing age-related bone loss and improving gut microbiota, which indirectly supports bone health (Golovinskaia and Wang, 2021).

12.2.6 Mechanisms of action

The beneficial effects of most functional food bioactives for bone and joint health are exerted through various mechanisms.

12.2.6.1 Antiinflammatory effects

Functional food bioactives exert antiinflammatory effects by inhibiting proinflammatory cytokines like IL-1β, IL-6, and TNF-α and reducing COX and LOX eicosanoids. Bioactive peptides, polyphenols, and omega-3 fatty acids have been shown to modulate cell signaling pathways such as NF-κB and MAPK, which are crucial in chronic inflammation (Elbandy, 2022; Guha & Majumder, 2019; Jayarathne et al., 2017). Hesperidin, a flavonoid found in citrus fruits, has shown significant antiinflammatory effects by modulating the NF-κB pathway (Tejada et al., 2019). Similarly, bioactive peptides from edible mushrooms regulate the MAPK and NF-κB pathways, reducing inflammation (Li et al., 2023).

12.2.6.2 *Antioxidative effects*

Bioactives reduce cartilage degradation from oxidative damage by boosting antioxidants like superoxide dismutase (SOD) and glutathione. Peptides and polyphenols from various food sources exhibit significant antioxidative properties, protecting bone and joint tissues from oxidative stress (Ahn & Je, 2019; Chakrabarti et al., 2014; Zaky et al., 2022). Camel milk, for example, contains bioactive components such as lactoferrin and vitamin C, which exhibit strong antioxidant properties (Behrouz et al., 2022). Polyphenols from *Moringa oleifera* also demonstrate significant antioxidant activity, protecting joint tissues from oxidative stress (Hunthayung and Bhawamai, 2024).

12.2.6.3 *Stimulating anabolic pathways*

Bioactives stimulate anabolic pathways by increasing collagen, proteoglycans, and osteoblast and chondrocyte activity. Peptides derived from food proteins enhance bone formation and inhibit bone resorption, contributing to bone health (Ahn & Je, 2019; Kamaruzzaman et al., 2019; Yamaguchi, 2024). Creatine supplementation has also been shown to have anabolic effects on muscle and bone, enhancing bone remodeling processes (Cordingley et al., 2022).

12.2.6.4 *Regulating catabolic pathways*

Functional food bioactives prevent excessive osteoclastic bone resorption and metalloproteinase activity. They modulate pathways involved in bone remodeling, maintaining a balance between bone formation and resorption (Nosrati et al., 2017; Peng et al., 2020; Schwartz et al., 2003). Systemic drugs like bisphosphonates and selective estrogen receptor modulators (SERMs) have been shown to enhance bone mineral density and osseointegration, thus preventing bone loss (Apostu et al., 2017).

12.2.6.5 *Supporting nutritional balance*

Bioactives support nutritional balance by meeting the needs for calcium, magnesium, vitamin D, protein, and polyunsaturated fatty acids (PUFAs). Nutraceuticals and functional foods rich in these nutrients are essential for maintaining bone density and joint health (Faienza et al., 2024; Sharma et al., 2024; Teodoro, 2019).

12.2.6.6 *Gut microbiome modulation*

Bioactives modulate the gut microbiome by promoting the growth of antiinflammatory gut microbes and reducing gut permeability. Polyphenols and fibers from functional foods positively influence gut microbiota composition, which in turn supports bone and joint health (Bhattarai & Janaswamy, 2022; Moco et al., 2012; Nagpal et al., 2019).

12.2.6.7 *Synergistic mechanisms*

The combined effects of omega-3 fatty acids, vitamins, and peptides work synergistically to enhance bone and joint health. These bioactives interact to provide comprehensive benefits, including antiinflammatory, antioxidative, and bone remodeling effects(Faienza et al., 2024; Sharma et al., 2024).

In conclusion, functional food bioactives offer a multifaceted approach to enhancing bone and joint health through their antiinflammatory, antioxidant, and bone-remodeling properties. Continued research and clinical trials are essential to fully understand their mechanisms and optimize their use in dietary interventions for bone and joint health.

12.2.7 Developing functional foods and studying efficacy

The formulation and development of functional foods for bone and joint health involve several critical issues and criteria. These include the selection of bioactive compounds, ensuring bioavailability, maintaining stability during processing and storage, consumer acceptance, and regulatory compliance. Below, these aspects are explored in detail, supported by recent scientific sources.

12.2.7.1 *Selection of bioactive compounds*

The choice of bioactive compounds is fundamental to the efficacy of functional foods. Compounds such as glucosamine, chondroitin, collagen peptides, hyaluronic acid, omega-3 fatty acids, calcium, magnesium, vitamins D3, K1, and K2, and herbal extracts like *Boswellia serrata* are commonly used due to their proven benefits for bone and joint health

(Korhonen, 2002). The selection process involves identifying compounds that have demonstrated efficacy in clinical studies and can be effectively incorporated into food matrices.

12.2.7.2 Ensuring bioavailability

Bioavailability is a critical factor in the effectiveness of functional foods. It refers to the extent and rate at which the active ingredients are absorbed and utilized in the body. Techniques such as microencapsulation, nanoemulsion, and the use of bioenhancers can improve the bioavailability of bioactive compounds (Sharma et al., 2021). For instance, the bioavailability of curcumin can be significantly enhanced through nanoemulsion techniques.

12.2.7.3 Stability during processing and storage

Maintaining the stability of bioactive compounds during food processing and storage is essential to ensure their efficacy. Factors such as temperature, pH, and exposure to light and oxygen can affect the stability of these compounds. Advanced processing technologies, such as high-pressure processing and freeze-drying, can help preserve the bioactivity of functional ingredients (Sun-Waterhouse, 2011). Additionally, the use of natural antioxidants can help protect bioactive compounds from degradation.

12.2.7.4 Consumer acceptance

Consumer acceptance is essential for the success of functional foods. This involves not only the health benefits but also the sensory attributes such as taste, texture, and appearance. Functional foods must be palatable and appealing to consumers. The use of natural flavors, colors, and sweeteners can enhance the sensory properties of these products (Yakovleva et al., 2021). Market research and consumer testing are essential steps in the product development process to ensure that the final product meets consumer preferences.

12.2.7.5 Regulatory compliance

Regulatory compliance is a significant consideration in the development of functional foods. Different countries have varying regulations regarding health claims, ingredient safety, and labeling requirements. It is essential to ensure that this kind of functional food product complies with the relevant regulations in the target market (Sharma, 2005). This involves conducting thorough safety assessments and obtaining necessary approvals from regulatory bodies.

12.2.7.6 Technological advancements

Technological advancements play a vital role in the formulation of functional foods. Innovations in food processing and preservation technologies can enhance the stability and bioavailability of bioactive compounds. For example, the use of probiotics in functional beverages requires a careful selection of strains with strong technological properties to ensure viability during storage and consumption (Sharma et al., 2021).

12.2.7.7 Nutritional synergies

As mentioned earlier, functional foods often contain multiple bioactive compounds that work synergistically to enhance health benefits. Understanding the interactions between different ingredients is very important for optimizing the formulation. For instance, the combination of calcium, magnesium, and vitamins D3 and K2 can enhance bone mineralization and reduce the risk of osteoporosis (Weaver and Liebman, 2002). Similarly, the combination of omega-3 fatty acids, turmeric, and ginger can provide potent antiinflammatory effects (Corbo et al., 2014).

12.2.7.8 Evaluation of efficacy

The efficacy of functional foods must be evaluated through rigorous scientific studies. This includes in vitro studies to assess the stability and bioactivity of compounds in different food matrices, animal studies to understand the mechanisms of action, and human clinical trials to demonstrate health benefits (Davicco et al., 2016). Biomarkers of bone health, such as bone mineral density and biochemical markers of bone turnover, are commonly used to evaluate the effectiveness of functional foods (Weaver and Liebman, 2002). Human trials assessing pain levels, stiffness, joint mobility, and imaging biomarkers are conducted to demonstrate efficacy along with measuring circulating or urinary biomarkers. Reduced plasma CRP, interleukin-6, and cartilage oligomeric matrix protein (COMP) indicate lowered inflammation and cartilage breakdown. An increase in plasma P1NP (aminoterminal propeptide of type 1 procollagen) and osteocalcin levels denotes greater bone formation. Effects on bone mineral density and prevention of osteoporotic fractures are also evaluated in long-term studies (Judex et al., 2009). Medium- to large-scale double-blind placebo-controlled trials with validated subjective questionnaires like the WOMAC index for pain/stiffness and objective biomarkers are considered high-grade evidence. Mechanistic studies in cellular models and animal arthritis models also provide supporting data on chondroprotective, anabolic, or antiresorptive effects (Apostu et al., 2017).

12.2.7.9 Market trends and opportunities

The market for functional foods targeting bone and joint health is growing, driven by increasing consumer awareness and demand for preventive health solutions. Trends such as the preference for natural and plant-based ingredients, the rise of personalized nutrition, and the integration of digital health technologies are shaping the market (Sharma, 2005). Companies need to stay abreast of these trends and innovate continuously to meet evolving consumer needs.

In conclusion, the formulation and development of functional foods for bone and joint health involve a complex interplay of scientific, technological, and consumer-related factors. Selecting the right bioactive compounds, ensuring their bioavailability and stability, meeting consumer preferences, and complying with regulatory requirements are critical for the success of these products. Continued research and innovation are essential to address the challenges and leverage the opportunities in this dynamic market. For detailed visual representations and data, resources like Euromonitor International, Statista, and market research reports from companies like Grand View Research and Market Research Future can provide valuable insights.

12.3 Applications

12.3.1 Commercial Availability

Companies are constantly innovating in delivering bioactives through palatable powders, flavored functional waters, and convenient combined dosing systems. New formats like collagen peptide powders for smoothies and functional waters containing vitamins, minerals, and bioactives like glucosamine are being introduced. Convenient supplements combining multiple ingredients ensure patient adherence. There is a growing demand for natural and plant-based products, driven by increasing health consciousness and concerns about synthetic ingredients. Additionally, the convenience of functional beverages and ready-to-eat products is appealing to busy consumers (Corbo et al., 2014).

The bone and joint health supplements market is robust and growing (Fig. 12.1), driven by increasing consumer awareness and scientific validation of their benefits. The global bone and joint health supplements market size was estimated at USD 3.90 billion in 2023 and is expected to grow at a compound annual growth rate (CAGR) of 7.26% from 2024 to 2030 (https://www.grandviewresearch.com, 2022) (Fig. 12.2, Fig. 12.3).

Table 12.2 shows the market size of these supplements in terms of value and the currency used as USD.

Several evidence-based bone and joint health supplements are already available globally.

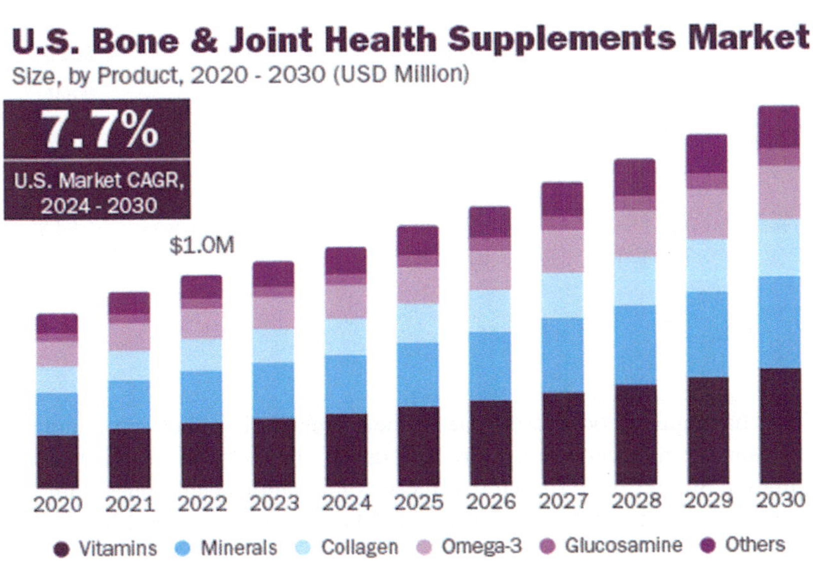

FIGURE 12.1 US bone and joint health supplement market size and growth rate, 2024–30 (https://www.grandviewresearch.com, 2022).

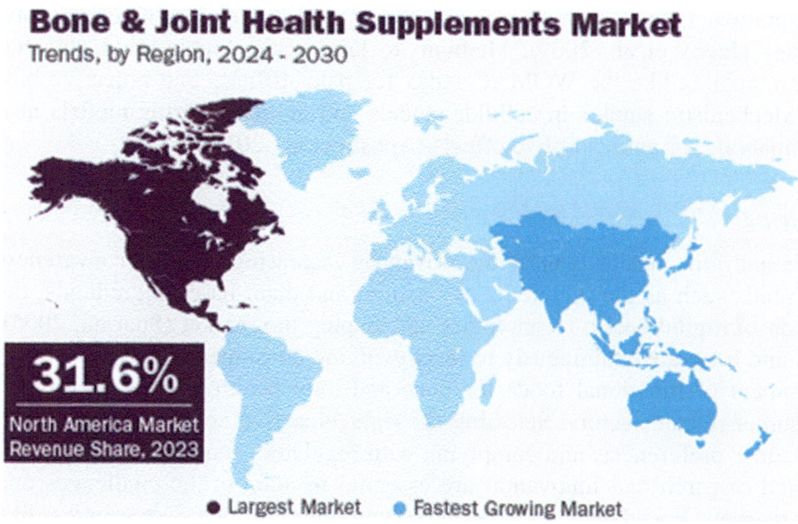

FIGURE 12.2 Bone and joint health supplements market, trends by region, 2024–30 (https://www.grandviewresearch.com, 2022). Map lines delineate study areas and do not necessarily depict accepted national boundaries.

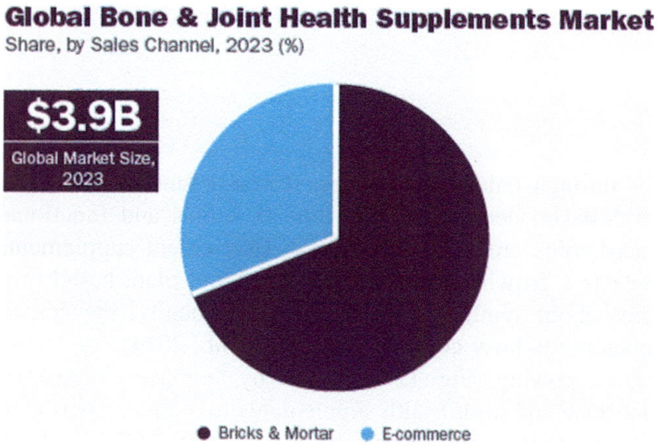

FIGURE 12.3 Global bone and joint health supplements market, share by sales channel, 2023 (%) (https://www.grandviewresearch.com, 2022).

TABLE 12.2 Bone and Joints Health Supplement Market Value; Based on USD Exchange Rates, 2017–21 (MarketsandMarkets, 2022).

Country/Region (Currency)	2017	2018	2019	2020	2021
Europe (EUR)	0.923	0.848	0.893	0.877	0.846
UK (GBP)	0.808	0.750	0.784	0.779	0.727
Denmark (DKK)	6.864	6.319	6.670	6.538	6.290
India (INR)	67.809	68.422	70.394	74.102	73.936
Japan (JPY)	116.667	110.424	109.008	106.725	109.817

Glucosamine + Chondroitin + MSM

Supplements combining these three ingredients have gained popularity due to their synergistic effects on maintaining cartilage integrity and joint flexibility. Glucosamine and chondroitin are natural components of cartilage, while MSM provides sulfur, essential for collagen synthesis. Studies have shown that these combinations can reduce pain and improve joint function in individuals with osteoarthritis (Venugopal, 2008). Products like Osteo Bi-Flex and Move Free are widely available in pharmacies and online stores.

Collagen Peptides + Hyaluronic Acid

These combinations exploit the moisture-retaining properties of hyaluronic acid alongside the tissue-rebuilding potential of collagen for improved joint mobility. These supplements are designed to improve joint mobility and reduce symptoms of osteoarthritis. Collagen peptides have been shown to stimulate collagen synthesis in cartilage, while hyaluronic acid helps maintain joint lubrication (Ahn and Je, 2019). Popular products include Vital Proteins Collagen Peptides and NeoCell Hyaluronic Acid.

Omega − 3 + Turmeric + Ginger

Capitalizing on the natural antiinflammatory properties, this trifecta is becoming increasingly popular for managing chronic joint conditions. Omega-3s reduce inflammation by modulating the production of inflammatory eicosanoids, while turmeric and ginger inhibit pro-inflammatory cytokines and enzymes (Corbo et al., 2014). Products like Nordic Naturals Omega Curcumin and Garden of Life Omega-3 with Turmeric are examples of such combinations.

Calcium + Magnesium + Vitamin D3 + K1 + K2

These supplements address the nutritional milieu necessary for optimal bone health, acting to mitigate the risk of osteoporosis. These nutrients work together to enhance calcium absorption, bone mineralization, and the regulation of bone remodeling. Vitamin K2, in particular, helps direct calcium to the bones and away from the arteries (Faienza et al., 2024). Examples of these products include Nature Made Calcium with Vitamin D3 and K2 and NOW Foods Calcium & Magnesium with Vitamin D3.

12.3.2 *Boswelliaserrata* extract

Boswellia serrata extract is an herbal supplement known for its potential to ease inflammatory processes within joints. It contains boswellic acids, which inhibit the 5-lipoxygenase enzyme, reducing the production of leukotrienes, compounds that cause inflammation (Weaver and Liebman, 2002). Products like Boswellia by Pure Encapsulations and Boswellia Complex by MediHerb are widely available.

12.3.3 Other formulated functional foods and beverages

Functional foods and beverages, such as fortified yogurts, cereals, and beverages containing bioactive compounds like omega-3 fatty acids, probiotics, and antioxidants, are gaining popularity among consumers (Vella et al., 2013). Companies like Danone and Nestlé have developed functional food lines targeting bone and joint health, aiming to improve overall musculoskeletal health. Current products include omega-3 fortified dairy, curcumin-fortified honey, collagen peptide beverages, calcium + vitamin D functional cereal, and omega-3 + polyphenol capsules. These products aim to reduce inflammation, improve pain management, and promote bone density. Advances in food technology have also allowed for turmeric infusion into honey.

12.4 Future perspectives

Progress in enhancing the bioavailability of functional ingredients, the exploration of novel sources for these bioactives, and the tailored approaches under the umbrella of personalized nutrition are also examined to understand their contribution to the domain's evolution. With each step, the vision of a future where the body's structural integrity and freedom of movement can be preserved and restored is built- not only through medicine but through the very sustenance derive from diets-a future where nourishment converges with healing, promising an enhanced quality of life for the aging population worldwide.

The future of managing bone and joint health through functional foods is poised on the precipice of significant breakthroughs, with an array of innovative strategies being developed to enhance the effectiveness of bioactive ingredients in diets. For this burgeoning field, advancements are anticipated across three primary domains: improving bioavailability, diversification of ingredient sources, and the nascent enterprise of personalized nutrition.

12.4.1 Improving bioavailability

Improving bioavailability stands as a cornerstone challenge in maximizing the efficacy of functional foods. Bioactives, such as curcumin, omega-3, and polyphenols, face challenges due to poor oral bioavailability, rapid metabolism, or excretion. Novel technologies like nanoencapsulations, emulsions, novel extraction techniques, and chemical modifications can improve the absorption and retention of these compounds. Personalized gut microbiome analysis can also help select prebiotics that are metabolized by an individual's unique microbial signature. Bioavailability is crucial for the functionality of bioactives, but many functional food components are not optimized for efficient absorption. To overcome these challenges, future strategies focus on innovative delivery systems. Nanoencapsulation, which encapsulates bioactive compounds within nanometer-sized vesicles, protects them from degradation and enhances their retention in the body. Emulsions and liposomes can increase solubility and uptake of hydrophobic compounds like omega-3 fatty acids. Chemical modifications, such as bonding bioactives to other molecules that the body absorbs more efficiently, can theoretically increase their presence in target tissues. This bioengineering of molecules could lead to a new class of enhanced functional foods with deeper therapeutic impacts.

12.4.2 Novel food sources

Beyond traditional ingredients such as oils, spices, and collagen peptides, researchers are now exploring novel food sources of bone and joint health compounds. These include bioactive peptides from egg whites, polysaccharides from mushrooms, omega-3-rich microalgae oils and antioxidants from fruit skins and seeds earlier discarded as waste.

Such novel materials can expand the portfolio of functional foods to prevent cartilage degeneration, stimulate bone remodeling, and reduce inflammatory pathways underlying common musculoskeletal disorders.

Research is diving into exploiting previously undervalued food sources—eggshell membranes, mushroom chitin, algae-based lipids, upcycled plant by-products—to introduce an abundance of untapped bioactives with bone and joint assertions. Such resourcefulness addresses not only human health but also ecological sustainability.

Moving beyond traditional extracts and compounds, researchers are pioneering the acquisition of bioactives from unconventional sources. Eggshell membrane, often discarded as waste, is now recognized as a repository of collagen and other joint-supportive nutrients. Similarly, the chitin in mushroom cell walls, once thought indigestible, is being transformed into bioavailable chitosan—a substance touted for its potential health benefits including support of joint and cartilage.

Additionally, there is an upsurge in leveraging biotechnological methods to cultivate omega-3-rich microalgae, providing a sustainable alternative to fish oils. Valorization of food waste also encourages the extraction of polyphenols and antioxidants from fruit peels and seeds, bolstering the repertoire of functional ingredients while simultaneously addressing environmental concerns.

12.4.3 Personalized nutrition

Instead of a one-size-fits-all approach, personalized or tailor-made functional foods based on individual risk factors (age, gender, genetics), disease state (osteopenia, osteoarthritis, etc.) and nutritional status are gaining interest.

For instance, calcium and vitamin D needs are higher for postmenopausal women at high fracture risk while omega-3 dosage can be tailored based on baseline eicosanoid and cytokine levels.

Such customization allows optimal efficacy alongside minimizing adverse effects, costs, and nutritional overload—ushering in the era of precision nutrition.

Personalized nutrition is the harbinger of a new dietary epoch, one that leverages an individual's specifics to prevent and mitigate musculoskeletal afflictions efficaciously. It embraces the concept of nutritional genomics, marrying diet with DNA to reveal profound insight into how one's body may respond to particular substances. This emergent paradigm is goal-directed towards precise nutrition rather than broad-spectrum dietary recommendations, thereby articulating a more coherent baseline for disease prevention and management.

Tailoring nutrition to the individual's biological makeup is a burgeoning frontier that promises to revolutionize the way diet and health are approached. Personalized nutrition examines a confluence of factors—genetic disposition, age, gender, lifestyle, and unique health status—to deliver optimized dietary interventions.

For instance, women may have specific calcium and vitamin D requirements tied to hormonal changes postmenopause, or an individual's genetic markers may indicate a particular susceptibility to reduced vitamin absorption. Advances in biotechnology and data analysis are enabling more sophisticated assessments of personal health, leading not only to customized supplement regimens but also to functional foods designed to meet these unique requirements.

Precision nutrition lifts the veil on the complex interplay between diet and wellness, offering new opportunities for preventing and managing musculoskeletal conditions through targeted nutritional strategies. This bespoke approach seeks to enhance nutritional adequacy, mitigate risk factors, and reduce the likelihood of adverse effects, all while steering clear of unnecessary or excessive intake.

12.5 Conclusion

Functional foods are emerging as a promising future for managing and potentially preventing bone and joint diseases through dietary means. Market trends confirm a societal pivot towards these natural adjuncts, with preclinical and clinical evidence supporting their efficacy in treating RA, osteoporosis, and osteoporosis. The functional food industry is paving the way for a holistic, integrative approach to health that aligns modern scientific advancements with natural nutritional wisdom.

Bone and joint diseases are becoming a significant public health concern due to the aging population and rising healthcare costs. Functional foods, rich in bioactive compounds like omega-3 fatty acids, polyphenols, vitamins, and minerals, have been identified as potential complements or alternatives to traditional drug therapies. Advancements in science, such as nanoencapsulation and novel chemical constructs, are improving the delivery and assimilation of bioactives, amplifying their impact on health.

The trend towards personalized nutrition is emerging, where dietary recommendations are tailored to individual profiles, taking into account genetic backgrounds, personal health states, and specific nutrient requirements. This precision nutrition extends beyond the one-size-fits-all approach, promising more targeted and effective management of bone and joint health.

In conclusion, the interface between functional foods and musculoskeletal disorders represents a critical juncture in health sciences and nutrition. Advances in oral bioavailability, food waste valorization, and personalized nutrition could increase the efficacy and adoption of these specialized functional foods.

References

Ahmadieh, H., & Arabi, A. (2011). Vitamins and bone health: Beyond calcium and vitamin D. *Nutrition Reviews*, *69*(10), 584–598. Available from https://doi.org/10.1111/j.1753-4887.2011.00372.x.

Ahn, C. B., & Je, J. Y. (2019). Bone health-promoting bioactive peptides. *Journal of Food Biochemistry*, *43*(1). Available from https://doi.org/10.1111/jfbc.12529, http://onlinelibrary.wiley.com/journal/10.1111/(ISSN)1745-4514.

Amigo, L., & Hernández-Ledesma, B. (2020). Current evidence on the bioavailability of food bioactive peptides. *Molecules (Basel, Switzerland)*, *25* (19), 4479. Available from https://doi.org/10.3390/molecules25194479.

Antonopoulou, S., & Demopoulos, C. A. (2023). Protective effect of olive oil microconstituents in atherosclerosis: Emphasis on PAF implicated atherosclerosis theory. *Biomolecules*, *13*(4), 700. Available from https://doi.org/10.3390/biom13040700.

Apostu, D., Lucaciu, O., Lucaciu, G. D. O., Crisan, B., Crisan, L., Baciut, M., Onisor, F., Baciut, G., Câmpian, R. S., & Bran, S. (2017). Systemic drugs that influence titanium implant osseointegration. *Drug Metabolism Reviews*, *49*(1), 92–104. Available from https://doi.org/10.1080/03602532.2016.1277737.

Asensio, G., Benito-Garzón, L., Ramírez-Jiménez, R. A., Guadilla, Y., Gonzalez-Rubio, J., Abradelo, C., Parra, J., Martín-López, M. R., Aguilar, M. R., Vázquez-Lasa, B., & Rojo, L. (2021). Biomimetic gradient scaffolds containing hyaluronic acid and Sr/Zn folates for osteochondral tissue engineering. *Polymers*, *14*, 12. Available from https://doi.org/10.3390/polym14010012.

Aubry, L., Sy, K., Sayd, T., & Ferraro, V. (2023). Collagen peptides-minerals complexes from the bovine bone by-product to prevent lipids peroxidation in meat and butter and to quench free radicals—influence of proteases and of steam sterilisation. *Applied Sciences*, *13*(6), 3979. Available from https://doi.org/10.3390/app13063979, https://www.mdpi.com/2076-3417/13/6/3979.

Ávila-Román, J., García-Gil, S., Rodríguez-Luna, A., Motilva, V., & Talero, E. (2021). Anti-inflammatory and anticancer effects of microalgal carotenoids. *Marine Drugs*, *19*(10), 531. Available from https://doi.org/10.3390/md19100531.

Baeverfjord, G., Antony Jesu Prabhu, P., Fjelldal, P. G., Albrektsen, S., Hatlen, B., Denstadli, V., Ytteborg, E., Takle, H., Lock, E. J., Berntssen, M. H. G., Lundebye, A. K., Åsgård, T., & Waagbø, R. (2019). Mineral nutrition and bone health in salmonids. *Reviews in Aquaculture*, *11*(3), 740–765. Available from https://doi.org/10.1111/raq.12255, http://onlinelibrary.wiley.com/journal/10.1111/(ISSN)1753-5131.

Baker, E. J. (2024). Alternative sources of bioactive omega-3 fatty acids: What are the options? *Current Opinion in Clinical Nutrition and Metabolic Care*, *27*(2), 106–115. Available from https://doi.org/10.1097/MCO.0000000000001006, http://journals.lww.com/co-clinicalnutrition/pages/default.aspx.

Basak, S., Hridayanka, K. S. N., & Duttaroy, A. K. (2024). Bioactives and their roles in bone metabolism of osteoarthritis: evidence and mechanisms on gut-bone axis. *Frontiers in Immunology*, *14*, 1323233. Available from https://doi.org/10.3389/fimmu.2023.1323233.

Behrouz, S., Saadat, S., Memarzia, A., Sarir, H., Folkerts, G., & Boskabady, M. H. (2022). The antioxidant, anti-inflammatory and immunomodulatory effects of camel milk. *Frontiers in Immunology*, *13*. Available from https://doi.org/10.3389/fimmu.2022.855342, https://www.frontiersin.org/journals/immunology#.

Bhardwaj, A., Sapra, L., Tiwari, A., Mishra, P. K., Sharma, S., & Srivastava, R. K. (2022). Osteomicrobiology": The nexus between bone and bugs. *Frontiers in Microbiology*, *12*. Available from https://doi.org/10.3389/fmicb.2021.812466, https://www.frontiersin.org/journals/microbiology#.

Bhattarai, S., & Janaswamy, S. (2022). The nexus of gut microbiota, diet, and health. *Functional Food Science-Online ISSN: 2767-3146*, *2*(2), 47–63. Available from https://doi.org/10.31989/ffs.v2i2.885, https://www.ffhdj.com/index.php/FunctionalFoodScience/article/view/885.

Bonifacio, M. A., Cassano, A., Vincenti, A., Vinella, A., Dell'Olio, F., Favia, G., & Mariggiò, M. A. (2023). In vitro evaluation of the effects of hyaluronic acid and an aminoacidic pool on human osteoblasts. *Biomedicines, 11*(3). Available from https://doi.org/10.3390/biomedicines11030751, www.mdpi.com/journal/biomedicines.

Bottega, R., Persico, I., De Seta, F., Romano, F., & Di Lorenzo, G. (2021). Anti-inflammatory properties of a proprietary bromelain extract (Bromeyal™) after in vitro simulated gastrointestinal digestion. *International Journal of Immunopathology and Pharmacology, 35*, 2058–7384. Available from https://doi.org/10.1177/20587384211034686.

Butawan, M., Benjamin, R. L., & Bloomer, R. J. (2017). Methylsulfonylmethane: Applications and safety of a novel dietary supplement. *Nutrients, 9* (3), 290. Available from https://doi.org/10.3390/nu9030290, https://www.mdpi.com/2072-6643/9/3/290.

Cadar, E., Pesterau, A.-M., Prasacu, I., Ionescu, A.-M., Pascale, C., Dragan, A.-M. L., Sirbu, R., & Tomescu, C. L. (2024). Marine antioxidants from marine collagen and collagen peptides with nutraceuticals applications: A review. *Antioxidants, 13*(8), 919. Available from https://doi.org/10.3390/antiox13080919, https://www.mdpi.com/2076-3921/13/8/919.

Campo, C., Gangemi, S., Pioggia, G., & Allegra, A. (2024). Beneficial effect of olive oil and its derivates: Focus on hematological neoplasm. *Life (Chicago, Ill.: 1978), 14*(5), 583. Available from https://doi.org/10.3390/life14050583.

Cao, C., Xiao, Z., Tong, H., Liu, Y., Wu, Y., & Ge, C. (2022). Oral intake of chicken bone collagen peptides anti-skin aging in mice by regulating collagen degradation and synthesis, inhibiting inflammation and activating lysosomes. *Nutrients, 14*(8), 1622. Available from https://doi.org/10.3390/nu14081622, https://www.mdpi.com/2072-6643/14/8/1622.

Carey, J. J., Erjiang, E., Wang, T., Yang, L., Dempsey, M., Brennan, A., Yu, M., Chan, W. P., Whelan, B., Silke, C., O'Sullivan, M., Rooney, B., McPartland, A., & O'Malley, G. (2023). Prevalence of low bone mass and osteoporosis in Ireland: the Dual-Energy X-Ray Absorptiometry (DXA) Health Informatics Prediction (HIP) Project. *JBMR Plus, 7*(10). Available from https://doi.org/10.1002/jbm4.10798, https://asbmr.onlinelibrary.wiley.com/journal/24734039.

Čeh, T., & Šarabon, N. (2023). Effects of adding glucosamine or glucosamine combined with chondroitin to exercise on pain and physical function in adults with knee osteoarthritis: a systematic review and meta-analysis. *European Journal of Translational Myology, 33*(4). Available from https://doi.org/10.4081/ejtm.2023.12013, https://pmc.ncbi.nlm.nih.gov/articles/PMC10811636/.

Chakrabarti, S., Jahandideh, F., & Wu, J. (2014). Food-derived bioactive peptides on inflammation and oxidative stress. *BioMed research international 2014, 1*, 608979. Available from https://doi.org/10.1155/2014/608979, https://onlinelibrary.wiley.com/doi/full/10.1155/2014/608979.

Chang, C. J., Jou, I. M., Wu, T. T., Su, F. C., & Tai, T. W. (2020). Cigarette smoke inhalation impairs angiogenesis in early bone healing processes and delays fracture union. *Bone and Joint Research, 9*(3), 99–107. Available from https://doi.org/10.1302/2046-3758.93.BJR-2019-0089.R1, https://online.boneandjoint.org.uk/doi/full/10.1302/2046-3758.93.BJR-2019-0089.R1.

Charoensin, S., Pothacharoen, P., Wanachewin, O., Kongtawelert, P., & Suttajit, M. (2023). *Functional foods in improving bone health during aging. in: Plant bioactives as natural panacea against age-induced diseases* (pp. 287–305). Elsevier. Available from https://doi.org/10.1016/B978-0-323-90581-7.00009-8.

Chen, S., Chen, T., Chen, Y., Huang, D., Pan, Y., & Chen, S. (2022). Causal association between tea consumption and bone health: A mendelian randomization study. *Frontiers in Nutrition, 9*. Available from https://doi.org/10.3389/fnut.2022.872451.

Cheng, M., Yuan, W., Moshaverinia, A., & Yu, B. (2023). Rejuvenation of mesenchymal stem cells to ameliorate skeletal aging. *Cells, 12*(7), 998. Available from https://doi.org/10.3390/cells12070998.

Cholewski, M., Tomczykowa, M., & Tomczyk, M. (2018). A comprehensive review of chemistry, sources and bioavailability of omega-3 fatty acids. *Nutrients, 10*(11), 1662. Available from https://doi.org/10.3390/nu10111662.

Cieza, A., Causey, K., Kamenov, K., Hanson, S. W., Chatterji, S., & Vos, T. (2020). Global estimates of the need for rehabilitation based on the Global Burden of Disease study 2019: a systematic analysis for the Global Burden of Disease Study 2019. *Lancet Publishing Group, Switzerland The Lancet, 396*(10267), 2006–2017. Available from https://doi.org/10.1016/S0140-6736(20)32340-0, http://www.journals.elsevier.com/the-lancet/.

Corbo, M. R., Bevilacqua, A., Petruzzi, L., Casanova, F. P., & Sinigaglia, M. (2014). Functional beverages: The emerging side of functional foods: Commercial trends, research, and health implications. *Comprehensive Reviews in Food Science and Food Safety, 13*(6), 1192–1206. Available from https://doi.org/10.1111/1541-4337.12109Italy, http://onlinelibrary.wiley.com/journal/10.1111/(ISSN)1541-4337.

Cordingley, D. M., Cornish, S. M., & Candow, D. G. (2022). Anti-inflammatory and anti-catabolic effects of creatine supplementation: A brief review. *Nutrients, 14*(3). Available from https://doi.org/10.3390/nu14030544, https://www.mdpi.com/2072-6643/14/3/544/pdf.

Damani, J. J., De Souza, M. J., VanEvery, H. L., Strock, N. C. A., & Rogers, C. J. (2022). The role of prunes in modulating inflammatory pathways to improve bone health in postmenopausal women. *Advances in Nutrition, 13*(5), 1476–1492. Available from https://doi.org/10.1093/advances/nmab162, https://www.sciencedirect.com/journal/advances-in-nutrition.

Davicco, M. J., Wittrant, Y., & Coxam, V. (2016). Berries, their micronutrients and bone health. *Current Opinion in Clinical Nutrition and Metabolic Care, 19*(6), 453–457. Available from https://doi.org/10.1097/MCO.0000000000000324, http://journals.lww.com/co-clinicalnutrition/pages/default.aspx.

De Mauro, D., De Luca, G., Marino, S., Smakaj, A., Rovere, G., Liuzza, F., Covino, M., Fulignati, P., Grandaliano, G., & El Ezzo, O. (2024). Fragility fractures in end-stage chronic kidney disease (CKD) population: Patient-related and CKD-related factor analysis—A single-center experience. *Journal of Clinical Medicine, 13*(8), 2430. Available from https://doi.org/10.3390/jcm13082430.

de Sire, A., de Sire, R., Curci, C., Castiglione, F., & Wahli, W. (2022). Role of dietary supplements and probiotics in modulating microbiota and bone health: The gut-bone axis. *Cells, 11*(4), 743. Available from https://doi.org/10.3390/cells11040743.

de Wildt, B. W. M., van der Meijden, R., Bartels, P. A. A., Sommerdijk, N. A. J. M., Akiva, A., Ito, K., & Hofmann, S. (2022). Bioinspired silk fibroin mineralization for advanced in vitro bone remodeling models. *Advanced Functional Materials*, *32*(41). Available from https://doi.org/10.1002/adfm.202206992, http://onlinelibrary.wiley.com/journal/10.1002/(ISSN)1616-3028.

Deckelbaum, R. J., & Torrejon, C. (2012). The omega-3 fatty acid nutritional landscape: Health benefits and sources. *The Journal of Nutrition*, *142*(3), 587S. Available from https://doi.org/10.3945/jn.111.148080.

Deng, H., Wang, J., & An, R. (2023). Hyaluronic acid-based hydrogels: As an exosome delivery system in bone regeneration. *Frontiers in Pharmacology*, *14*. Available from https://doi.org/10.3389/fphar.2023.1131001.

Dou, Y., Wang, Y., Chen, Z., Yu, X., & Ma, D. (2022). Effect of n-3 polyunsaturated fatty acid on bone health: A systematic review and meta-analysis of randomized controlled trials. *Food Science & Nutrition*, *10*(1), 145–154. Available from https://doi.org/10.1002/fsn3.2655, https://onlinelibrary.wiley.com/doi/pdfdirect/10.1002/fsn3.2655.

Dydykina, I. S., Kovalenko, P. S., & Kovalenko, A. A. (2024). Effect of weight loss and exercise on joint pain in patients with osteoarthritis and obesity. *Meditsinskiy sovet = Medical Council*, *18*(3), 168–176. Available from https://doi.org/10.21518/ms2024-132.

Elbandy, M. (2022). Anti-inflammatory effects of marine bioactive compounds and their potential as functional food ingredients in the prevention and treatment of neuroinflammatory disorders. *Molecules*, *28*(1), 2. Available from https://doi.org/10.3390/molecules28010002, https://www.mdpi.com/1420-3049/28/1/2.

Faienza, M. F., Giardinelli, S., Annicchiarico, A., Chiarito, M., Barile, B., Corbo, F., & Brunetti, G. (2024). Nutraceuticals and functional foods: A comprehensive review of their role in bone health. *International Journal of Molecular Sciences*, *25*(11), 5873. Available from https://doi.org/10.3390/ijms25115873.

Fernández-Martín, S., González-Cantalapiedra, A., Muñoz, F., García-González, M., Permuy, M., & López-Peña, M. (2021). Glucosamine and chondroitin sulfate: is there any scientific evidence for their effectiveness as disease-modifying drugs in knee osteoarthritis preclinical studies?—A systematic review from 2000 to 2021. *Animals*, *11*(6), 1608.

Fu, Y., Therkildsen, M., Aluko, R. E., & Lametsch, R. (2019). Exploration of collagen recovered from animal by-products as a precursor of bioactive peptides: Successes and challenges. *Critical Reviews in Food Science and Nutrition*, *59*(13), 2011–2027. Available from https://doi.org/10.1080/10408398.2018.1436038, https://www.researchgate.net/profile/Yu-Fu-17/publication/322907017_Exploration_of_collagen_recovered_from_animal_by-products_as_a_precursor_of_bioactive_peptides_Successes_and_challenges/links/5a993d5b45851535bce1e5c8/Exploration-of-collagen-recovered-from-animal-by-products-as-a-precursor-of-bioactive-peptides-Successes-and-challenges.pdf.

Galla, R., Ruga, S., Aprile, S., Ferrari, S., Brovero, A., Grosa, G., Molinari, C., & Uberti, F. (2022). New hyaluronic acid from plant origin to improve joint protection—An in vitro study. *International Journal of Molecular Sciences*, *23*(15), 8114. Available from https://doi.org/10.3390/ijms23158114.

Gebregziabher, B. S., Gebremeskel, H., Debesa, B., Ayalneh, D., Mitiku, T., Wendwessen, T., Habtemariam, E., Nur, S., & Getachew, T. (2023). Carotenoids: Dietary sources, health functions, biofortification, marketing trend and affecting factors – A review. *Journal of Agriculture and Food Research*, *14*, 100834. Available from https://doi.org/10.1016/j.jafr.2023.100834.

George, K. S., Munoz, J., Ormsbee, L. T., Akhavan, N. S., Foley, E. M., Siebert, S. C., Kim, J. S., Hickner, R. C., & Arjmandi, B. H. (2022). The short-term effect of prunes in improving bone in men. *Nutrients*, *14*(2). Available from https://doi.org/10.3390/nu14020276, https://www.mdpi.com/2072-6643/14/2/276/pdf.

Gilpin, A., Zeng, Y., Hoque, J., Ryu, J. H., Yang, Y., Zauscher, S., Eward, W., & Varghese, S. (2021). Self-healing of hyaluronic acid to improve in vivo retention and function. *Advanced Healthcare Materials*, *10*(23). Available from https://doi.org/10.1002/adhm.202100777, http://onlinelibrary.wiley.com/journal/10.1002/(ISSN)2192-2659.

Goggs, R., Vaughan-Thomas, A., Clegg, P. D., Carter, S. D., Innes, J. F., Mobasheri, A., Shakibaei, M., Schwab, W., & Bondy, C. A. (2005). Nutraceutical therapies for degenerative joint diseases: A critical review. *Critical Reviews in Food Science and Nutrition*, *45*(3), 145–164. Available from https://doi.org/10.1080/10408690590956341.

Golovinskaia, O., & Wang, C.-K. (2021). Review of functional and pharmacological activities of berries. *Molecules (Basel, Switzerland)*, *26*(13), 3904. Available from https://doi.org/10.3390/molecules26133904.

Guedes, A. C., Amaro, H. M., & Malcata, F. X. (2011). Microalgae as sources of carotenoids. *Marine Drugs*, *9*(4), 625–644. Available from https://doi.org/10.3390/md9040625, http://www.mdpi.com/1660-3397/9/4/625/pdf.

Guha, S., & Majumder, K. (2019). Structural-features of food-derived bioactive peptides with anti-inflammatory activity: A brief review. *Journal of Food Biochemistry*, *43*(1), e12531. Available from https://doi.org/10.1111/jfbc.12531, https://onlinelibrary.wiley.com/doi/pdf/10.1111/jfbc.12531?casa_token = qjKAm6Afeo8AAAAA%3ATjB_R2VDK0D-UszQjRPrnVVpMDg2_UcBfcEynOYfawDj6VxYSDbUXfAOpMuooowOfBhUWpga3jt_.

Han, D., Kim, D., Kim, H., Lee, J., Lyu, J., Kim, J. S., Shin, J., Kim, J. S., Kim, D. K., & Park, H. W. (2023). Methylsulfonylmethane ameliorates metabolic-associated fatty liver disease by restoring autophagy flux via AMPK/mTOR/ULK1 signaling pathway. *Frontiers in Pharmacology*, *14*. Available from https://doi.org/10.3389/fphar.2023.1302227, http://www.frontiersin.org/Pharmacology.

Hayhoe, R. P. G., Lentjes, M. A. H., Mulligan, A. A., Luben, R. N., Khaw, K. T., & Welch, A. A. (2017). Carotenoid dietary intakes and plasma concentrations are associated with heel bone ultrasound attenuation and osteoporotic fracture risk in the European Prospective Investigation into Cancer and Nutrition (EPIC)-Norfolk cohort. *British Journal of Nutrition*, *117*(10), 1439–1453. Available from https://doi.org/10.1017/S0007114517001180, http://journals.cambridge.org/BJN.

Hegde, M. V., Zanwar, A. A., & Adekar, S. P. (2016). Preface. *Omega-3 Fatty Acids: Keys to Nutritional Health*, 5–7. Available from https://doi.org/10.1007/978-3-319-40458-5, http://doi.org/10.1007/978-3-319-40458-5.

Hochberg, M. C., Altman, R. D., April, K. T., Benkhalti, M., Guyatt, G., McGowan, J., Towheed, T., Welch, V., Wells, G., & Tugwell, P. (2012). American College of Rheumatology 2012 recommendations for the use of nonpharmacologic and pharmacologic therapies in osteoarthritis of the hand, hip, and knee. *Arthritis Care and Research*, *64*(4), 465–474. Available from https://doi.org/10.1002/acr.21596.

https://www.grandviewresearch.com. (2022). Bone Jt. Health Suppl. Mark. Rep. 2030 Rep. ID GVR-4-68039-974-6. 2022. https://www.grandviewresearch.com/industry-analysis/bone-joint-health-supplements-market-report.

Hunthayung, K., & Bhawamai, S. (2024). Polyphenol compounds of freeze-dried Moringa oleifera Lam pods and their anti-inflammatory effects on RAW 264.7 macrophages stimulated with lipopolysaccharide. *Bioactive Compounds in Health and Disease - Online ISSN: 2574-0334; Print ISSN: 2769-2426*, *7*(4), 185–198. Available from https://doi.org/10.31989/bchd.v7i4.1356.

Ilesanmi-Oyelere, B. L., Roy, N. C., & Kruger, M. C. (2021). Modulation of bone and joint biomarkers, gut microbiota, and inflammation status by synbiotic supplementation and weight-bearing exercise:human study protocol for a randomized controlled trial. *JMIR Research Protocols*, *10*(10). Available from https://doi.org/10.2196/30131, https://www.researchprotocols.org/2021/10/e30131/PDF.

Im, S. B., Tripathi, G., Le, T. T. T., & Lee, B. T. (2021). Early-stage bone regeneration of hyaluronic acid supplemented with porous 45s5 bioglass-derived granules: An injectable system. *Biomedical Materials (Bristol)*, *16*(4). Available from https://doi.org/10.1088/1748-605X/ac058f, https://iopscience.iop.org/article/10.1088/1748-605X/ac058f.

Islam, F., Imran, A., Nosheen, F., Fatima, M., Arshad, M. U., Afzaal, M., Ijaz, N., Noreen, R., Shilpa, M., Biswas, S., Ul Rasoo, I. F., Aslam, M. A., Usman, I., Zahra, S. M., Segueni, N., & Amer Ali, Y. (2023). Functional roles and novel tools for improving-oxidative stability of polyunsaturated fatty acids: A comprehensive review. *Food Science & Nutrition*, *11*(6), 2471–2482. Available from https://doi.org/10.1002/fsn3.3272, https://onlinelibrary.wiley.com/doi/pdfdirect/10.1002/fsn3.3272.

Ivanovska, N., & Dimitrova, P. (2011). Bone resorption and remodeling in murine collagenase-induced osteoarthritis after administration of glucosamine. *Arthritis research & therapy*, *13*, 1–13, R44. Available from https://doi.org/10.1186/ar3283, https://link.springer.com/article/10.1186/ar3283.

Jayarathne, S., Koboziev, I., Park, O.-H., Oldewage-Theron, W., Shen, C.-L., & Moustaid-Moussa, N. (2017). Anti-inflammatory and anti-obesity properties of food bioactive components: effects on adipose tissue. *Preventive nutrition and food science*, *22*(4), 251–262. Available from https://doi.org/10.3746/pnf.2017.22.4.251, https://pmc.ncbi.nlm.nih.gov/articles/PMC5758087/.

Judex, S., Gupta, S., & Rubin, C. (2009). Regulation of mechanical signals in bone. *Orthodontics & Craniofacial Research*, *12*(2), 94–104. Available from https://doi.org/10.1111/j.1601-6343.2009.01442.x.

Kakati, N., Ahari, D., Parmar, P. R., Deshmukh, O. S., & Bandyopadhyay, D. (2024). Lactic acid-induced colloidal microrheology of synovial fluids. *ACS Biomaterials Science and Engineering*, *10*(5), 3378–3386. Available from https://doi.org/10.1021/acsbiomaterials.3c01846, http://pubs.acs.org/journal/abseba.

Kamaruzzaman, M. A., Chin, K.-Y., & Mohd Ramli, E. S. (2019). A review of potential beneficial effects of honey on bone health. *Evidence-Based Complementary and Alternative Medicine*, *1*, 8543618. Available from https://doi.org/10.1155/2019/8543618, https://onlinelibrary.wiley.com/doi/pdf/10.1155/2019/8543618.

Kciuk, M., Garg, A., Rohilla, M., Chaudhary, R., Dhankhar, S., Dhiman, S., Bansal, S., Saini, M., Singh, T. G., Chauhan, S., Mujwar, S., Gielecińska, A., & Kontek, R. (2024). Therapeutic potential of plant-derived compounds and plant extracts in rheumatoid arthritis—Comprehensive review. *Antioxidants*, *13*(7), 775. Available from https://doi.org/10.3390/antiox13070775.

Kelly, G. S. (1998). The role of glucosamine sulfate and chondroitin sulfates in the treatment of degenerative joint disease. *Alternative Medicine Review: A Journal of Clinical Therapeutic*, *3*(1), 27–39.

Keservani, R. K., & Ahire, E. D. (2024). *Applications of functional foods in disease prevention, First edition. ed, AAP advances in nutraceuticals*. Apple Academic Press.

Kha, M. S., Kibria, M. G., Hossain, F., Ferdous, J., Shihab, H. M., & Faisal, S. M. (2024). Unveiling the burden of osteoporosis: exploring the prevalence and risk factors among postmenopausal women in north central Bangladesh. *Central Medical College Journal*, *7*(1), 32–40. Available from https://doi.org/10.3329/cemecj.v7i1.70940.

Khalil, A., Tazeddinova, D., Aljoumaa, K., Kazhmukhanbetkyzy, Z. A., Orazov, A., & Toshev, A. D. (2021). Carotenoids: Therapeutic strategy in the battle against viral emerging diseases, COVID-19: An overview. *Preventive Nutrition and Food Science*, *26*(3), 241–261. Available from https://doi.org/10.3746/PNF.2021.26.3.241, http://www.pnfs.or.kr/journal/view.html?doi = 10.3746/pnf.2021.26.3.241.

Khan, A., Jamil, M., Butti, S., Ahmad, I., Ullah, H., Khan, A., & Imitaz. (2023). Causes, precautions and management of risk factors associated with sports injuries. *THE THERAPIST (Journal of Therapies & Rehabilitation Sciences)*, 56–58.

Korhonen, H. (2002). Technology options for new nutritional concepts. *International Journal of Dairy Technology*, *55*(2), 79–88. Available from https://doi.org/10.1046/j.1471-0307.2002.00050.x.

Kuberskaya, A. P., Podgurskaya, V. V., & Omsk State Medical University. (2023). Omega-3 fatty acids: promising plant sources and effects on the human body. *Scientific Bulletin of the Omsk State Medical University*, *3*, 95–107. Available from https://doi.org/10.61634/2782-3024-2023-9-95-107.

Kulczyński, B., Sidor, A., Brzozowska, A., & Gramza-Michałowska, A. (2024). The role of carotenoids in bone health—A narrative review. *Nutrition (Burbank, Los Angeles County, Calif.)*, *119*, 112306. Available from https://doi.org/10.1016/j.nut.2023.112306.

Kumar, S., Sugihara, F., Suzuki, K., Inoue, N., & Venkateswarathirukumara, S. (2015). A double-blind, placebo-controlled, randomised, clinical study on the effectiveness of collagen peptide on osteoarthritis. *Journal of the Science of Food and Agriculture*, *95*(4), 702–707. Available from https://doi.org/10.1002/jsfa.6752, https://scijournals.onlinelibrary.wiley.com/doi/full/10.1002/jsfa.6752?casa_token = s91aerOJHpcAAAAA%3AmlNeW3QBFJV4iKHLR3FnTcAuGFeeFGmdBD5J_57b2ZJauDmC7M71becmoX-dzDBDWte9Fw6_zgPRng.

Li, J., Ho, W. T. P., Liu, C., Chow, S. K. H., Ip, M., Yu, J., Wong, H. S., Cheung, W. H., Sung, J. J. Y., & Wong, R. M. Y. (2021). The role of gut microbiota in bone homeostasis. *Bone and Joint Research, 10*(1), 51–59. Available from https://doi.org/10.1302/2046-3758.101.BJR-2020-0273.R1, https://online.boneandjoint.org.uk/doi/10.1302/2046-3758.101.BJR-2020-0273.R1.

Li, B., Wang, L., Chen, W., Chen, F., & Shu, C. (2021). *Anthocyanins: Chemistry, processing, bioactivity*. Springer Singapour.

Li, H., Gao, J., Zhao, F., Liu, X., & Ma, B. (2023). Bioactive peptides from edible mushrooms—The preparation, mechanisms, structure—Activity relationships and prospects. *Foods, 12*, 2935. Available from https://doi.org/10.3390/foods12152935.

Lippiello, Louis, Woodward, John, Karpman, Robert, & Hammad, Tarek A. (2000). In vivo chondroprotection and metabolic synergy of glucosamine and chondroitin sulfate. *Clinical Orthopaedics and Related Research (1976–2007), 381*, 229–240. Available from http://www.vetanco.com/pdf/cosequin/condroprotection.pdf.

Long, H., Liu, Q., Yin, H., Wang, K., Diao, N., Zhang, Y., Lin, J., & Guo, A. (2022). Prevalence trends of site-specific osteoarthritis from 1990 to 2019: Findings From the Global Burden of Disease Study 2019. *Arthritis & Rheumatology, 74*(7), 1172–1183. Available from https://doi.org/10.1002/art.42089.

Mandal, M. K., & Domb, A. J. (2024). Antimicrobial activities of natural bioactive polyphenols. *Pharmaceutics, 16*(6). Available from https://doi.org/10.3390/pharmaceutics16060718, http://www.mdpi.com/journal/pharmaceutics.

MarketsandMarkets, 2022. Bone and Joint Health Supplements Market Size, Share, Trends [Latest]. MarketsandMarkets Available at: https://www.marketsandmarkets.com/Market-Reports/bone-joint-health-supplements-market-67838616.html.

Martiniakova, M., Kovacova, V., Mondockova, V., Zemanova, N., Babikova, M., Biro, R., Ciernikova, S., & Omelka, R. (2023). Honey: A promising therapeutic supplement for the prevention and management of osteoporosis and breast cancer. *Antioxidants, 12*(3), 567. Available from https://doi.org/10.3390/antiox12030567.

Mattioli, R., Francioso, A., Mosca, L., & Silva, P. (2020). Anthocyanins: A comprehensive review of their chemical properties and health effects on cardiovascular and neurodegenerative diseases. *Molecules (Basel, Switzerland), 25*(17), 3809. Available from https://doi.org/10.3390/molecules25173809.

McClung, M. R., Pinkerton, J., Blake, J., Cosman, F., Lewiecki, E., & Shapiro, M. (2021). Management of osteoporosis in postmenopausal women: The 2021 position statement of The North American. *Menopause Society*. Available from https://doi.org/10.1097/GME.0000000000001831.

McFarlin, B. K., Hill, D. W., Vingren, J. L., Curtis, J. H., & Tanner, E. A. (2021). Dietary polyphenol and methylsulfonylmethane supplementation improves immune, DAMP signaling, and inflammatory responses during recovery from all-out running efforts. *Frontiers in Physiology, 12*, 712731. Available from https://doi.org/10.3389/fphys.2021.712731.

McFarlin, B. K., Vingren, J. L., Hill, D. W., & Bridgeman, E. A. (2023). MSM supplementation is associated with reduced inflammation and improved innate immune response following in vitro LPS-stimulation in humans after a bout of downhill running. *Muscles, 2*, 204–217. Available from https://doi.org/10.3390/muscles2020015.

Mechchate, H., Es-safi, I., Conte, R., Hano, C., Amaghnouje, A., Jawhari, F. Z., Radouane, N., Bencheikh, N., Grafov, A., & Bousta, D. (2021). In vivo and in vitro antidiabetic and anti-inflammatory properties of flax (*Linum usitatissimum* L.) seed polyphenols. *Nutrients, 13*(8), 2759. Available from https://doi.org/10.3390/nu13082759.

Mekkawy, M. H., Fahmy, H. A., Nada, A. S., & Ali, O. S. (2020). Study of the Radiosensitizing and Radioprotective Efficacy of Bromelain (a Pineapple Extract): In Vitro and In Vivo. *Integrative Cancer Therapies, 19*. Available from https://doi.org/10.1177/1534735420950468, http://ict.sagepub.com/.

Meng, Z., Liu, J., & Zhou, N. (2023). Efficacy and safety of the combination of glucosamine and chondroitin for knee osteoarthritis: a systematic review and meta-analysis. *Archives of Orthopaedic and Trauma Surgery, 143*(1), 409–423. Available from https://doi.org/10.1007/s00402-021-04326-9, https://link.springer.com/article/10.1007/s00402-021-04326-9.

Miran, M., Salami, M., Emam-Djomeh, Z., & Ghaffari, S.-B. (2021). Recent achievements in the improvement of oral bioavailability of curcumin and its health benefits. *Canadian Journal of Clinical Nutrition*, 1–6. Available from https://doi.org/10.14206/canad.j.clin.nutr.2021.02.01.

Moco, S., Martin, F.-P. J., & Rezzi, S. (2012). Metabolomics view on gut microbiome modulation by polyphenol-rich foods. *Journal of Proteome Research, 11*(10), 4781–4790. Available from https://doi.org/10.1021/pr300581s, https://pubs.acs.org/doi/pdf/10.1021/pr300581s?casa_token = o_wqAvQOfhwAAAAA:Gw45IlXHe3PvQ1df5dt3PzI1lIMge1i-lvMpTf7QvhH-UnPQa7lzjvRPTwusPz-ySRsU5-To0ul4Nw.

Mohd Ramli, E. S., Sukalingam, K., Kamaruzzaman, M. A., Soelaiman, I. N., Pang, K.-L., & Chin, K.-Y. (2021). Direct and indirect effect of honey as a functional food against metabolic syndrome and its skeletal complications. *Diabetes Metab. Syndr. Obes. Targets Ther., Volume 14*, 241–256. Available from https://doi.org/10.2147/DMSO.S291828.

Montecillo-Aguado, M., Tirado-Rodriguez, B., & Huerta-Yepez, S. (2023). The involvement of polyunsaturated fatty acids in apoptosis mechanisms and their implications in cancer. *International Journal of Molecular Sciences, 24*(14), 11691. Available from https://doi.org/10.3390/ijms241411691, https://www.mdpi.com/1422-0067/24/14/11691.

Mukherjee, A. N., Londhe, S., Prasad, P. V. S., Shetty, N., Shetty, S., Kumar, N., Jinsiwale, A. K., Ponnanna, K. M., Balamurugan, R., Rathod, N., Katoch, S., Mittal, V., Thacker, H., Garg, M. R., & Desai, A. (2024). Specific collagen peptides in osteoporosis management: Unraveling therapeutic potential through expert perspectives and scientific insights. *International Journal of Orthopaedics Sciences, 10*(1), 165–171. Available from https://doi.org/10.22271/ortho.2024.v10.i1c.3513, https://www.orthopaper.com/archives/2024/vol10issue1/PartC/10-1-9-644.pdf.

Nagpal, R., Shively, C. A., Register, T. C., Craft, S., & Yadav, H. (2019). Gut microbiome-Mediterranean diet interactions in improving host health. *F1000Res., 8*, 699. Available from https://doi.org/10.12688/f1000research.18992.1, https://pmc.ncbi.nlm.nih.gov/articles/PMC7359750/.

Nikolaevich, T. A., Leonidovna, U. I., Shamsidinovich, M. D., & Valery Mikhailovich, K. (2023). Total Joint replacement and joint-saving techniques for the treatment of knee osteoarthritis: The problems of decision-making. *RA JOURNAL OF APPLIED RESEARCH, 09*(04). Available from https://doi.org/10.47191/rajar/v9i4.05.

Nosrati, N., Bakovic, M., & Paliyath, G. (2017). Molecular mechanisms and pathways as targets for cancer prevention and progression with dietary compounds. *International journal of molecular sciences, 18*(10), 2050. Available from https://doi.org/10.3390/ijms18102050, https://www.mdpi.com/1422-0067/18/10/2050.

Nowak, W., & Jeziorek, M. (2023). The role of flaxseed in improving human health. *Healthcare, 11*(3), 395. Available from https://doi.org/10.3390/healthcare11030395.

Oberle, E. J., Harris, J. G., & Verbsky, J. W. (2014). Polyarticular juvenile idiopathic arthritis – Epidemiology and management approaches. *Clinical Epidemiology*, 379–393. Available from https://doi.org/10.2147/CLEP.S53168.

Park, J. H., Moon, J. H., Kim, H. J., Kong, M. H., & Oh, Y. H. (2020). Sedentary lifestyle: Overview of updated evidence of potential health risks. *Journal of Family Medicine, 41*(6), 365–373. Available from https://doi.org/10.4082/KJFM.20.0165, http://koreamed.org/JournalVolume.php?id = 1&code = 0001KJFM.

Peng, M., Tabashsum, Z., Anderson, M., Truong, A., Houser, A. K., Padilla, J., Akmel, A., Bhatti, J., Rahaman, S. O., & Biswas, D. (2020). Effectiveness of probiotics, prebiotics, and prebiotic-like components in common functional foods. *Comprehensive Reviews in Food Science and Food Safety, 19*(4), 1908–1933. Available from https://doi.org/10.1111/1541-4337.12565, https://ift.onlinelibrary.wiley.com/doi/pdf/10.1111/1541-4337.12565?casa_token = MW2CU-9TOcsAAAAA:442sNGu4KmfZQ28oSCxeuMFUGabmFkcze4fPyrJqzROzmutSF2b6_Itk8EbKY_nbSgEb665vPY48.

Price, C. T., Koval, K. J., & Langford, J. R. (2013). Silicon: A review of its potential role in the prevention and treatment of postmenopausal osteoporosis. *International Journal of Endocrinology, 2013*. Available from https://doi.org/10.1155/2013/316783.

Quarta, S., Santarpino, G., Carluccio, M. A., Calabriso, N., Scoditti, E., Siculella, L., Damiano, F., Maffia, M., Verri, T., De Caterina, R., & Massaro, M. (2022). Analysis of the anti-inflammatory and anti-osteoarthritic potential of Flonat Fast®, a Combination of Harpagophytum Procumbens DC. ex Meisn., Boswellia Serrata Roxb., Curcuma longa L., Bromelain and Escin (Aesculus hippocastanum), Evaluated in In Vitro Models of Inflammation Relevant to Osteoarthritis. *Pharmaceuticals, 15*(10), 1263. Available from https://doi.org/10.3390/ph15101263.

Rabade, A., Viswanatha, G. L., Nandakumar, K., & Kishore, A. (2024). Evaluation of efficacy and safety of glucosamine sulfate, chondroitin sulfate, and their combination regimen in the management of knee osteoarthritis: A systematic review and meta-analysis. *Inflammopharmacology, 32*, 1759–1775. Available from https://doi.org/10.1007/s10787-024-01460-9, https://link.springer.com/article/10.1007/s10787-024-01460-9.

Rahaman, M., Das, S., Sahu, S., Karmakar, A., & Debnath, B. (2023). Extraction, isolation and characterization of collagen peptide from fish and recent biological activities of the collagen peptides. *Journal of Survey in Fisheries Sciences, 10*(2), 1450–1465. Available from https://doi.org/10.53555/sfs.v10i2.2719.

Ramesh, P., Jagadeesan, R., Sekaran, S., Dhanasekaran, A., & Vimalraj, S. (2021). Flavonoids: Classification, function, and molecular mechanisms involved in bone remodelling. *Frontiers in Endocrinology, 12*. Available from https://doi.org/10.3389/fendo.2021.779638.

Ribeiro, H. S., Schuchmann, H. P., Engel, R., Walz, E., & Briviba, K. (2010). *Encapsulation of carotenoids. Encapsulation Technologies for Active Food Ingredients and Food Processing* (pp. 211–252). United Kingdom: Springer New York. Available from http://www.springerlink.com/openurl.asp?genre = book&isbn = 978-1-4419-1007-3, 10.1007/978-1-4419-1008-0_8.

Richy, F., Bruyere, O., Ethgen, O., Cucherat, M., Henrotin, Y., & Reginster, J.-Y. (2003). Structural and symptomatic efficacy of glucosamine and chondroitin in knee osteoarthritis: a comprehensive meta-analysis. *Archives of Internal Medicine, 163*(13), 1514–1522. Available from https://doi.org/10.1001/archinte.163.13.1514, https://jamanetwork.com/journals/jamainternalmedicine/fullarticle/215809.

Roy, B., Curtis, M. E., Fears, L. S., Nahashon, S. N., & Fentress, H. M. (2016). Molecular mechanisms of obesity-induced osteoporosis and muscle atrophy. *Frontiers in Physiology, 7*. Available from https://doi.org/10.3389/fphys.2016.00439, http://journal.frontiersin.org/article/10.3389/fphys.2016.00439/full.

Sahni, S., Hannan, M. T., Blumberg, J., Cupples, L. A., Kiel, D. P., & Tucker, K. L. (2009). Protective effect of total carotenoid and lycopene intake on the risk of hip fracture: A 17-year follow-up from the Framingham Osteoporosis Study. *Journal of Bone and Mineral Research, 24*(6), 1086–1094. Available from https://doi.org/10.1359/jbmr.090102.

Salahuddin Salih, S., Mustafa Alsalihi, R., Esam Mahboub, N., Yasir Jasim, N., & Ali Almutawa, R. (2024). Assessment of public knowledge and awareness of knee osteoarthritis among individuals aged 18-65 in the United Arab Emirates (UAE). *Cureus*. Available from https://doi.org/10.7759/cureus.52134.

Santos, G. R. C., Piquet, A. A., Glauser, B. F., Tovar, A. M. F., Pereira, M. S., Vilanova, E., & Mourão, P. A. S. (2017). Systematic analysis of pharmaceutical preparations of chondroitin sulfate combined with glucosamine. *Pharmaceuticals, 10*(2), 38. Available from https://doi.org/10.3390/ph10020038, https://www.mdpi.com/1424-8247/10/2/38.

Schwartz, M. W., Woods, S. C., Seeley, R. J., Barsh, G. S., Baskin, D. G., & Leibel, R. L. (2003). Is the energy homeostasis system inherently biased toward weight gain? *Diabetes, 52*(2), 232–238. Available from https://citeseerx.ist.psu.edu/document?repid = rep1&type = pdf&doi = 719bec936f3c822776a85992a59075dfec20b178.

Serreli, G., & Deiana, M. (2019). In vivo formed metabolites of polyphenols and their biological efficacy. *Food & Function, 10*(11), 6999–7021. Available from https://doi.org/10.1039/c9fo01733j.

Sharma, G., & Vimal, A. (2023). Bromelain: An enzyme expanding its horizon from food to pharmaceuticalindustry. *Current Pharmaceutical Biotechnology, 24*, 1715–1726. Available from https://doi.org/10.2174/1389201024666230331115338.

Sharma, D., Chaubey, P., & Suvarna, V. (2021). Role of natural products in alleviation of rheumatoid arthritis—A review. *J. Food Biochem., 45*. Available from https://doi.org/10.1111/jfbc.13673.

Sharma, S., Singh, A., Sharma, S., Kant, A., Sevda, S., Taherzadeh, M. J., & Garlapati, V. K. (2021). Functional foods as a formulation ingredients in beverages: technological advancements and constraints. *Bioengineered*, *12*(2), 11055–11075. Available from https://doi.org/10.1080/21655979.2021.2005992, http://www.tandfonline.com/loi/kbie20.

Sharma, M., Vidhya, C. S., Ojha, K., Yashwanth, B. S., Barinderjit, S., Gupta, S., & Pandey, S. K (2024). The role of functional foods and nutraceuticals in disease prevention and health promotion. *European Journal of Nutrition & Food Safety*, *16*(2), 61–83. Available from https://doi.org/10.9734/ejnfs/2024/v16i21388, http://public.paper4promo.com/id/eprint/1858/1/Vidhya1622024EJNFS112340.pdf.

Sharma, R. (2005). Australia Market trends and opportunities for functional dairy beverages. *Australian Journal of Dairy Technology*, *60*(2), 195–198.

Shen, Q., Guo, Y., Wang, K., Zhang, C., & Ma, Y. (2023). A review of chondroitin sulfate's preparation, properties, functions, and applications. *Molecules*, *28*(20), 7093. Available from https://doi.org/10.3390/molecules28207093, https://www.mdpi.com/1420-3049/28/20/7093.

Smolen, J. S., Landewé, R. B. M., Bijlsma, J. W. J., Burmester, G. R., Dougados, M., Kerschbaumer, A., McInnes, I. B., Sepriano, A., van Vollenhoven, R. F., de Wit, M., Aletaha, D., Aringer, M., Askling, J., Balsa, A., Boers, M., den Broeder, A. A., Buch, M. H., Buttgereit, F., Caporali, R., ... van der Heijde, D. (2020). EULAR recommendations for the management of rheumatoid arthritis with synthetic and biological disease-modifying antirheumatic drugs: 2019 update. *Annals of the Rheumatic Diseases*, *79*(6), 685–699. Available from https://doi.org/10.1136/annrheumdis-2019-216655.

Sophocleous, A. (2023). The role of nutrition in osteoarthritis development. *Nutrients*, *15*(20), 4336. Available from https://doi.org/10.3390/nu15204336.

Steinmetz, J. D., Culbreth, G. T., Haile, L. M., Rafferty, Q., Lo, J., Fukutaki, K. G., Cruz, J. A., Smith, A. E., Vollset, S. E., Brooks, P. M., Cross, M., Woolf, A. D., Hagins, H., Abbasi-Kangevari, M., Abedi, A., Ackerman, I. N., Amu, H., Antony, B., Arabloo, J., ... Kopec, J. A. (2023). Global, regional, and national burden of osteoarthritis, 1990–2020 and projections to 2050: A systematic analysis for the Global Burden of Disease Study 2021. *Lancet Rheumatol*, *5*, e508–e522. Available from https://doi.org/10.1016/S2665-9913(23)00163-7.

Sugiura, M., Nakamura, M., Ogawa, K., Ikoma, Y., Yano, M., & Smith, B. (2012). High serum carotenoids associated with lower risk for bone loss and osteoporosis in post-menopausal japanese female subjects: Prospective cohort study. *PLoS One*, *7*(12), e52643. Available from https://doi.org/10.1371/journal.pone.0052643.

Sun-Waterhouse, D. (2011). The development of fruit-based functional foods targeting the health and wellness market: A review. *International Journal of Food Science & Technology*, *46*(5), 899–920. Available from https://doi.org/10.1111/j.1365-2621.2010.02499.x.

Szulc, M., Świątkowska-Stodulska, R., Pawłowska, E., & Derwich, M. (2023). Vitamin D3 metabolism and its role in temporomandibular joint osteoarthritis and autoimmune thyroid diseases. *International Journal of Molecular Sciences*, *24*(4), 4080. Available from https://doi.org/10.3390/ijms24044080.

Tao, S.-S., Wang, P., Wang, X.-Y., Yin, K.-J., Yang, X.-K., Wang, Z.-X., Wang, D.-G., & Pan, H.-F. (2022). Causal effect of polyunsaturated fatty acids on bone mineral density and fracture. *Frontiers in Nutrition*, *9*, 1014847. Available from https://doi.org/10.3389/fnut.2022.1014847, https://www.frontiersin.org/journals/nutrition/articles/10.3389/fnut.2022.1014847/full.

Tejada, S., Pinya, S., Martorell, M., Capó, X., Tur, J. A., Pons, A., & Sureda, A. (2019). Potential anti-inflammatory effects of hesperidin from the genus citrus. *Current Medicinal Chemistry*, *25*(37), 4929–4945. Available from https://doi.org/10.2174/0929867324666170718104412.

Teodoro, A. J. (2019). Bioactive compounds of food: Their role in the prevention and treatment of diseases. *Oxidative medicine and cellular longevity*. Available from https://doi.org/10.1155/2019/3765986, https://pmc.ncbi.nlm.nih.gov/articles/PMC6432691/.

Van Ballegooijen, A. J., Pilz, S., Tomaschitz, A., Grübler, M. R., & Verheyen, N. (2017). The synergistic interplay between vitamins D and K for bone and cardiovascular health: A narrative review. *International Journal of Endocrinology*, *2017*. Available from https://doi.org/10.1155/2017/7454376, http://www.hindawi.com/journals/ije/.

Varilla, C., Marcone, M., Paiva, L., & Baptista, J. (2021). Bromelain, a group of pineapple proteolytic complex enzymes (Ananas comosus) and their possible therapeutic and clinical effects. A summary. *Foods*, *10*(10), 2249. Available from https://doi.org/10.3390/foods10102249.

Vella, M. N., Stratton, L. M., Sheeshka, J., & Duncan, A. M. (2013). Exploration of functional food consumption in older adults in relation to food matrices, bioactive ingredients, and health. *Journal of Nutrition in Gerontology and Geriatrics*, *32*(2), 122–144. Available from https://doi.org/10.1080/21551197.2013.781419.

Venugopal, V. (2008). *Marine products for healthcare: Functional and bioactive nutraceutical compounds from the ocean Marine Products for Healthcare: Functional and Bioactive Nutraceutical Compounds from the Ocean* (pp. 1–527). CRC Press. Available from https://www.taylorfrancis.com/books/e/9781420052640.

Walallawita, U. S., Wolber, F. M., Ziv-Gal, A., Kruger, M. C., & Heyes, J. A. (2020). Potential role of lycopene in the prevention of postmenopausal bone loss: Evidence from molecular to clinical studies. *International Journal of Molecular Sciences*, *21*(19), 1–21. Available from https://doi.org/10.3390/ijms21197119, https://www.mdpi.com/1422-0067/21/19/7119/pdf.

Ward, O. P., & Singh, A. (2005). Omega-3/6 fatty acids: Alternative sources of production. *Process Biochemistry*, *40*(12), 3627–3652. Available from https://doi.org/10.1016/j.procbio.2005.02.020.

Weaver, C. M., & Liebman, M. (2002). Biomarkers of bone health appropriate for evaluating functional foods designed to reduce risk of osteoporosis. *British Journal of Nutrition*, *88*(2), S225–S232S225. Available from https://doi.org/10.1079/bjn2002687, http://journals.cambridge.org/BJN.

Weaver, C. M., Ferruzzi, M. G., Maiz, M., Cladis, D. P., Nakatsu, C. H., McCabe, G. P., & Lila, M. A. (2023). Crop, host, and gut microbiome variation influence precision nutrition: An example of blueberries. *Antioxidants*, *12*(5). Available from https://doi.org/10.3390/antiox12051136, www.mdpi.com/journal/antioxidants.

WHO (2022). *Musculoskeletal health*. WHO.

WHO (2023a). *Osteoarthritis*.

WHO (2023b). *Rheumatoid-arthritis*.

Williamson, G., & Manach, C. (2005). Bioavailability and bioefficacy of polyphenols in humans. II. Review of 93 intervention studies. *The American Journal of Clinical Nutrition, 81*(1). Available from https://doi.org/10.1093/ajcn/81.1.243s.

Wojtania, J., Płeska, K., Łepik, M., Uszok, Z., Rosiak, K., Reguła, K., Waloch, K., Piaszczyński, S., Czajka, A., & Szymański, B. (2024). Gout and its impact on physical activity. *Quality in Sport, 21*, 51463. Available from https://doi.org/10.12775/qs.2024.21.51463.

Xie, X., Fu, J., Gou, W., Qin, Y., Wang, D., Huang, Z., Wang, L., & Li, X. (2024). Potential mechanism of tea for treating osteoporosis, osteoarthritis, and rheumatoid arthritis. *Frontiers in Medicine, 11*. Available from https://doi.org/10.3389/fmed.2024.1289777.

Yakovleva, T. V., Gorlov, S. M., Pershakova, T. V., & Rybnikova, A. O. (2021). Formulating functional drinks using natural colors. *New Technologies, 17*(3), 59–70. Available from https://doi.org/10.47370/2072-0920-2021-17-3-59-70.

Yamaguchi, M. (2024). The marine alga sargassum horneri Is a functional food with high bioactivity. *Nutraceuticals, 4*(2), 181–189. Available from https://doi.org/10.3390/nutraceuticals4020012, https://www.mdpi.com/1661-3821/4/2/12.

Yang, L., Yang, C., Chu, C., Wan, M., Xu, D., Pan, D., Xia, H., Wang, S. K., Shu, G., Chen, S., & Sun, G. (2022). Beneficial effects of monounsaturated fatty acid-rich blended oils with an appropriate polyunsaturated/saturated fatty acid ratio and a low n-6/n-3 fatty acid ratio on the health of rats. *Journal of the Science of Food and Agriculture, 102*(15), 7172–7185. Available from https://doi.org/10.1002/jsfa.12083, https://scijournals.onlinelibrary.wiley.com/doi/full/10.1002/jsfa.12083?casa_token = H4g11d-0kGcAAAAA%3A_ARGMLge1Kb6PBB89qrMKLVowOQKvx-iHOrAIDrUB_w9SUNG-kUf7Mbkq19Io1e7ha850EHrcuQ9yg.

Yee, M. M. F., Chin, K. Y., Ima-Nirwana, S., & Wong, S. K. (2021). Vitamin a and bone health: A review on current evidence. *Molecules (Basel, Switzerland), 26*(6). Available from https://doi.org/10.3390/molecules26061757, https://www.mdpi.com/1420-3049/26/6/1757/pdf.

Zaky, A. A., Simal-Gandara, J., Eun, J.-B., Shim, J.-H., & El-Aty, A. M. A (2022). Bioactivities, applications, safety, and health benefits of bioactive peptides from food and by-products: A review. *Frontiers in Nutrition, 8*, 815640. Available from https://doi.org/10.3389/fnut.2021.815640, https://www.frontiersin.org/journals/nutrition/articles/10.3389/fnut.2021.815640/full.

Zamani-Garmsiri, F., Emamgholipour, S., Rahmani Fard, S., Ghasempour, G., Jahangard Ahvazi, R., & Meshkani, R. (2022). Polyphenols: Potential anti-inflammatory agents for treatment of metabolic disorders. *Phytotherapy Research, 36*(1), 415–432. Available from https://doi.org/10.1002/ptr.7329.

Zeb, A., & Sultan, M. (2004). Carotenoids contents from various sources and their potential health applications. *Pakistan Journal of Nutrition, 3*, 199–204. Available from https://doi.org/10.3923/pjn.2004.199.204.

Zhang, Y.-W., Cao, M.-M., Li, Y.-J., Dai, G.-C., Lu, P.-P., Zhang, M., Bai, L.-Y., Chen, X.-X., Zhang, C., Shi, L., & Rui, Y.-F. (2023). The regulative effect and repercussion of probiotics and prebiotics on osteoporosis: Involvement of brain-gut-bone axis. *Critical Reviews in Food Science and Nutrition, 63*, 7510–7528. Available from https://doi.org/10.1080/10408398.2022.2047005.

Zhang, J. (2023). Investigation of early diagnosis and treatment for rheumatoid arthritis. *Highlights in Science, Engineering and Technology, 36*, 1083–1087. Available from https://doi.org/10.54097/hset.v36i.6179.

Chapter 13

Bioactive compounds and cancer prevention: a nutritional approach

Sarra Akermi[1], Moufida Chaari[1], Khaoula Elhadef[1], Ashwani Sharma[2], Abira Dey[3], Altaf Choudhary[4], Subrata Sinha[5], Roberto Festuccia[6], Lotfi Mellouli[1] and Slim Smaoui[7]

[1]*Laboratory of Microbial Biotechnology, Enzymatic and Biomolecules, Center of Biotechnology of Sfax (CBS), University of Sfax, Sfax, Tunisia,* [2]*Insight Biosolutions, Biopole Rennes, Rennes, France,* [3]*Moldoc Biotech Private, SINE Limited Business Center, IIT Bombay, Mumbai, Maharashtra, India,* [4]*Pharma Department, Dr APJ Abdul Kalam Technical University, AKTU CDRI RD, Lucknow, Uttar Pradesh, India,* [5]*Department of Computational Sciences, Brainware University, Kolkata, West Bengal, India,* [6]*Department of Ecological and Biological Sciences, Tuscia University, Viterbo, Italy,* [7]*Laboratory of Microbial, Enzymes Biotechnology and Biomolecules (LMEBB), Centre of Biotechnology of Sfax (CBS), University of Sfax, Sfax, Tunisia*

13.1 Introduction

Cancer is an epidemic and malignant disease that has claimed the lives of millions throughout the globe and over many years. This hazardous disease is exclusively marked by the difficulty of its early detection and the shortage of efficient treatments that could cure advanced stages (Crosby et al., 2022). Additionally, the cancerous cells have developed drug resistance mechanisms toward the existent treatments which were already proven, in their turn, to engender multiple side effects and poor prognosis due to their nonselective properties and cytotoxicity (Li et al., 2021). Recently, the advancements in genetic engineering, nanotechnology, and bioinformatics tools facilitated the process of drug discovery and development of effective antiproliferative agents by extracting bioactive compounds from natural sources such as plants. Oncologists suggested that the usage of those compounds could overcome cancer risks and malignant cells resistance.

Bioactive compounds could be defined as the functional components in various food matrices such as vegetables and fruits. Those compounds could comprise flavonoids, anthocyanins, tannins, carotenoids, and plant sterols that provide beneficial biological properties and protective effects against a myriad of diseases and metabolic disorders (Walia et al., 2019). In fact, the term "bioactive compounds" englobes the secondary metabolites of plants that play an important ecological role in plant defense, adaptation strategies to their local environments, attraction, and signaling pathways (Yeshi et al., 2022). Moreover, owing to their diversity, plant secondary metabolites (PSMs) exert a wide range of pharmacological as well as toxicological effects against other living organisms making them a skeletal framework in drug discovery and development (Sharma et al., 2022). Based on their chemical structure, number of carbons, and number of aromatic rings, bioactive compounds could be classified into diverse groups that have tremendous biological activities on human health besides their nutritional values, including the prevention of chronic diseases, such as diabetes, cancer, and neurodegenerative diseases that are the main causes of death worldwide, according to the World Health Organization (Budreviciute et al., 2020). These diseases have a multifactorial etiology and are still, until the present moment, not having a definitive therapy (Ortega et al., 2019). Furthermore, plant-based compounds hold other multiple biological properties, as shown by the, such as antibacterial, antioxidant (against reactive oxygen species (ROS) that increase cancer susceptibility and genetic mutations), antidiabetic, antiinflammatory, neuroprotective, antiviral, and antifungal activities (Banwo et al., 2021). However, in the present book chapter, we aimed to only focus on the anticancer properties of plant-based bioactive compounds, their possible biological targets, and the relationship between nutrition, lifestyle, and diet in cancer prevention (Fig. 13.1, Fig. 13.2, Fig. 13.3, Fig. 13.4).

Part of your document could not be imported as it contained an unsupported element. For more information about unsupported elements, please visit the Support Cent

Unleashing the Power of Functional Foods and Novel Bioactives. DOI: https://doi.org/10.1016/B978-0-443-28862-3.00013-3

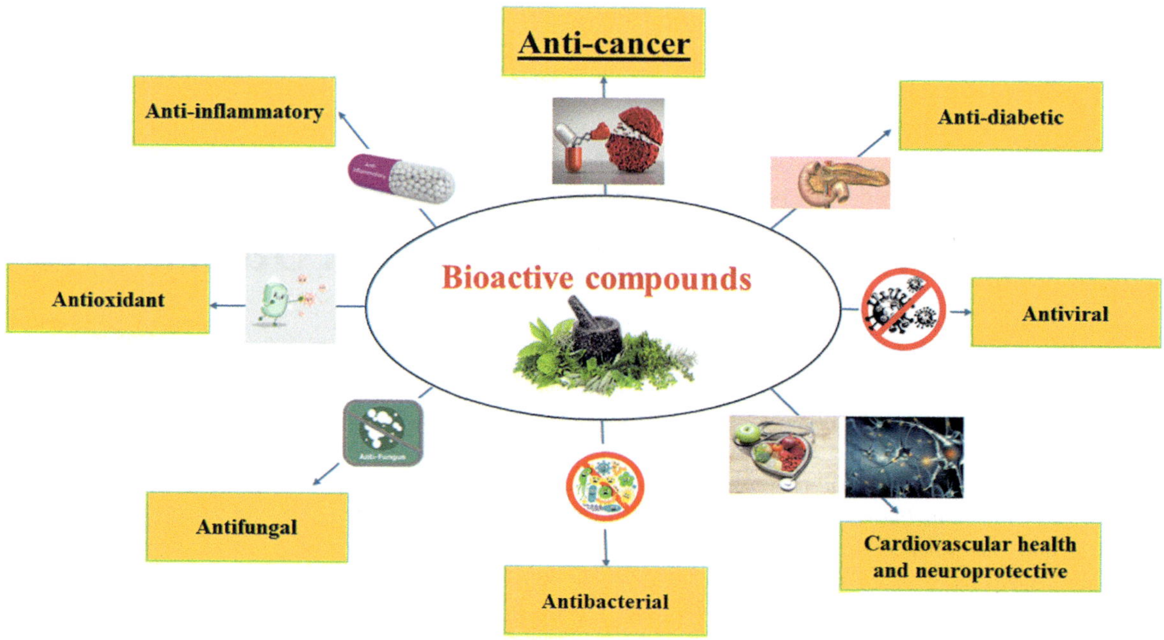

FIGURE 13.1 The biological properties of bioactive compounds.

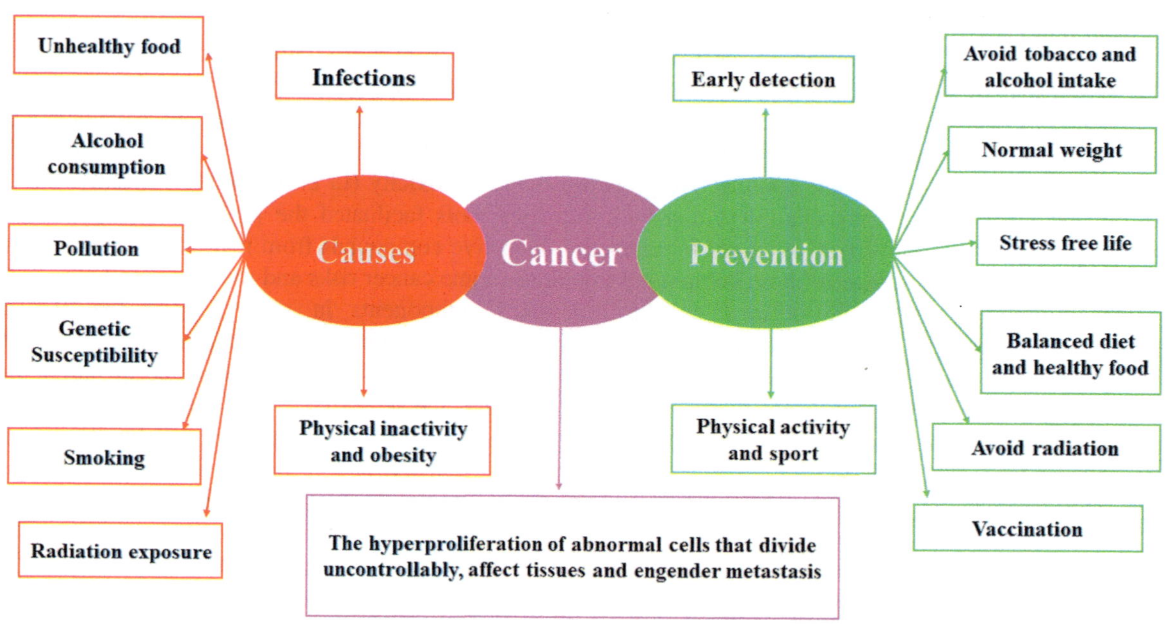

FIGURE 13.2 Major cancer causes and prevention attitudes and behaviors.

13.2 Cancer hallmarks and metabolic pathways involved in tumor growth

Cancer hallmarks designate the hyperproliferation and the development of malignant cells that have a great capacity to divide rapidly and uncontrollably and to invade other tissues resulting in metastasis (Hanahan, 2022).

There exist several causes that lead to cancer; among them we mention the chromosomal and genomic instability which induce alterations in the genetic structure of cancer cells and modulate their behavior and their response to treatment (Chen, Linstra, et al., 2022). To find effective therapeutical and curative strategies to treat cancer disease, it is better to start by analyzing and understanding its molecular markers and genetic processes and focusing on the main reasons. Mutations are among the causes coming into the light, and they could occur due to external environmental

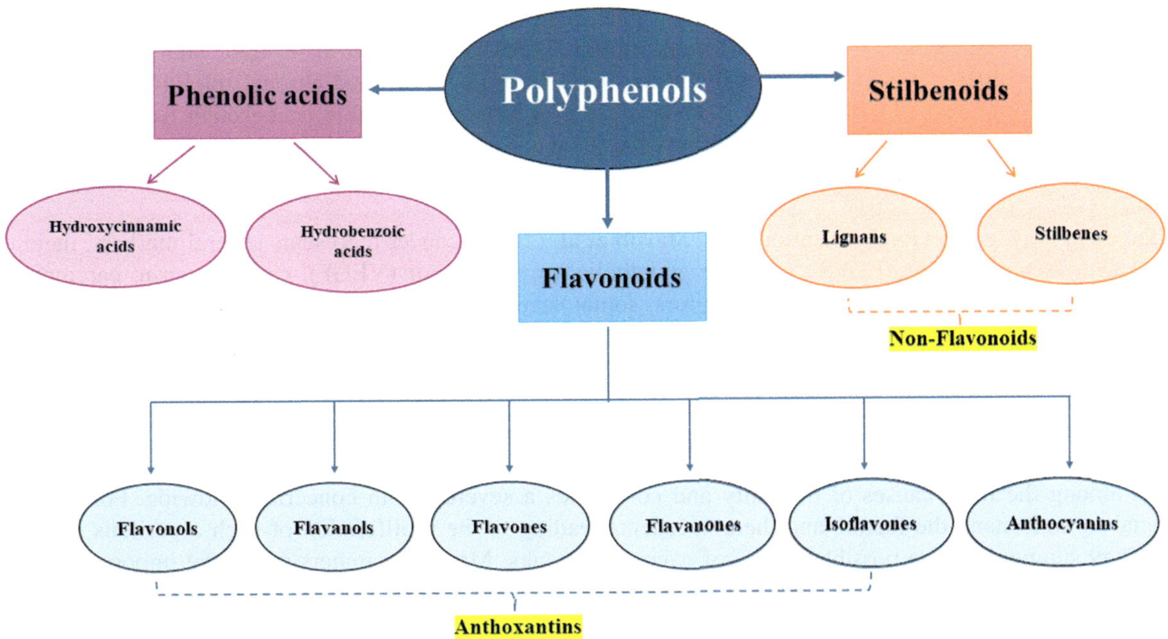

FIGURE 13.3 Different polyphenols classes.

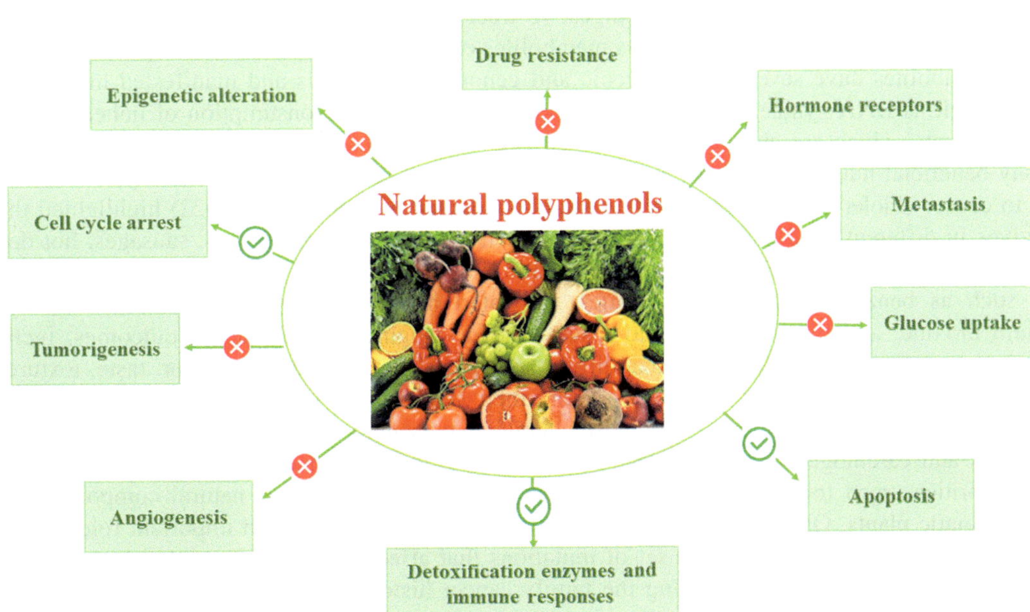

FIGURE 13.4 Antiproliferative and preventive effects of polyphenols.

factors, including pollution, prolonged exposure to ultraviolet UV light, and contamination by chemical carcinogens (McTigue et al., 2022). Furthermore, somatic mutations as well as sensitivity and permanent exposure to mutagenic agents and the deficit in DNA repair mechanisms could engender mutations and severe damages in DNA structure and function (Nohmi, 2018). Previous studies showed that cancer could be the consequence of dysregulation of multiple signaling pathways leading to the overexpression of various factors including EGFR, cyclooxygenase-2 (COX-2), nuclear factor (NF)-κB, interleukin (IL)-6, and IL-1, prostaglandins, cyclin D1 and cyclin E, vascular endothelial growth factor (VEGF), matrix metalloproteinases, Bcl-2, Bcl-X_L, survivin, and XIAP, cMyc, and AP-1 involved in cellular invasion, proliferation, and survival (Shoaib et al., 2023). The second major antecedent of cancer is inflammation which promotes tumor growth, proliferation, migration, invasion, and malignant transformation by upregulating hypoxia-inducible factor-1 (HIF-1), signal transducer and activator of transcription 3 (STAT3), NF-κB, IL-6, IL-1, and tumor necrosis factor (TNF) (Singh et al., 2019). It is crucial to mention that apart from mutations and chronic inflammation, immunocompromised persons could face elevated cancer risks because they present a suitable background for the proliferation of malignancies and the infection by oncogenic viruses due to the weakness of the immune system defense and surveillance (Ilham et al., 2023). This situation may engender apoptosis inhibition and induce tumor vascularization and metastasis.

On the other way, as previously mentioned by Shoaib et al. (2023), cancer represents several markers, including epidermal growth factor receptor (EGFR), vascular endothelial growth factor (VEGF), αvβ3 integrin, carcinoembryonic antigen (CEA), folate receptors, transferrin receptors, somatostatin receptors, and prostate stimulating membrane antigen (PSMA). Targeting those markers could be a promising strategy to treat cancer, to increase survival rate, and to tackle drug resistance.

13.3 Relation between lifestyle, diet, and cancer risk

Cancer is among the main causes of mortality and constitutes a severe health concern worldwide. For that reason, it was crucial to understand the factors and the antecedents leading to the proliferation of such a perilous and hazardous disease. They summarized the possible causes of cancer outbreaks. Many researchers stated the importance of diet and lifestyle behaviors in cancer prevention as well as treatment. A previous study indicated that there was a noticeable link and strong connection between smoking and cancer risk and showed that the steady heavy smokers displayed higher larynx and lung cancer incidence and mortality rate as compared to nonsmokers individuals (Luu et al., 2022). It also proposed that smoking cessation and quitting could significantly reduce cancer risks and mortality. In addition, Rumgay et al. (2021) demonstrated that alcohol consumption is associated with 740 000 new cancer cases annually and could induce seven types of cancer such as upper aerodigestive tract, liver, colorectal, and breast cancers. Heavy episodic drinking habits of alcohol lead to the increase of its metabolites especially the ethanol which generates, in turn, the acetaldehyde. Both metabolites have several carcinogenic and genotoxic properties and manifested higher probabilities of DNA damage as well as DNA synthesis and repair blocking. Moreover, the consumption of unhealthy food, including ultraprocessed products, which are characterized by their high contents of saturated fat, salt, and added sugar and do not provide any beneficial nutritional value due to their deficiency in fibers and vitamins, may lead to harmful effects and give rise to cancer (Fiolet et al., 2018). Another study conducted by Supe et al. (2022) highlighted the side effects of using additives in different food matrices such as processed meats (luncheon, salami, sausages, hot dogs, and hamburgers), carbonated beverages, pastries, and ready-to-eat and heat products. It showed that the employment of chemical preservatives such as benzoic acid, nitrites, sulfites, butylated hydroxy anisole (BHA), butylated hydroxytoluene (BHT), titanium dioxide, and bisphenol A could result in wide-ranging adverse health outcomes, including cancer, severe allergies, and endocrine disorders. Those additives are mainly used to enhance flavor, taste, texture, odor, color, and the appearance of food products as well as to extend their shelf life by limiting protein and lipid oxidations processes and microbial proliferation. Nevertheless, these chemicals presented harmful complications and were considered food contaminants and carcinogen agents. Consequently, their usage was banned by various European countries, and many health authorities urged food industries to find novel alternatives and to use natural compounds extracted from medicinal and aromatic plants. On the other side, the genetic susceptibility played an important role in the proliferation of malignant tumors. It could be defined as a set of mutations that affect cellular differentiation, growth, and survival. These mutations could be detected by analyzing the family cancer history. McGee and Nichols (2016) underlined that the existence of a positive family cancer history is one of the strongest and most recognized indicators of cancer genetic susceptibility syndrome. It also suggested the obligation of data collection from different relatives to facilitate cancer diagnosis and early detection by checking consanguinity and ancestry. Regarding pollution nuisances, it is well known that prolonged exposures to pollutants have destructive health consequences. Dehghani et al. (2023) stipulated that permanent exposure to air pollutant mixtures could have adverse effects and a direct cause of cancer by provoking estrogen-like effects and genetic mutations resulting in ovarian tumorigenesis. Another study indicated that the exposure to toxic heavy metals, such as copper, cadmium, nickel, plomb, zinc, and manganese, through inhalation, skin contact, and ingestion could pose harmful effects, including the increase of breast cancer risks probability (Ali et al., 2024). Similarly, radiation and chronic exposure to solar ultraviolet rays, especially UV-A and UV-B, were found to initiate oxidative stress and to cause skin damage. Moreover, this photooxidative stress was shown to affect the composition and activity of skin microbiota and could alter cellular response and immunological function which may pose the risk of melanoma (Verma et al., 2024). On the other side, viral infections caused by human papillomaviruses (HPVs) and hepatitis virus's types B and C are associated with great number of cancer cases. The previously cited viruses could engender cervical and hepatocellular malignancies (Schiller & Lowy, 2021). Several research studies indicated that infections by oncoviruses, including Epstein–Barr virus (EBV), Kaposi's sarcoma herpesvirus (KSHV), human T-cell leukemia virus (HTLV-I), and Merkel cell polyoma virus (MCPyV), hold carcinogenic potential in humans manifested by a decrease in various pathways involved in tumor suppressor signaling, apoptosis, metastasis, and angiogenesis (Sobhi Amjad et al., 2023). Finally, the consumption of unhealthy food accompanied by physical inactivity could constitute a major cause of cancer proliferation. In fact, the excessive consumption of fats, carbohydrates, salt, and processed foods could induce an excess in caloric intake and the sedentary behavior could make the situation worst by causing obesity and overweight-related problems. Physical inactivity may affect biological pathways by modulating insulin sensitivity and exerting influence on the production of metabolic hormones resulting in the occurrence of 13 different cancers, including gastrointestinal tract cancers (ardim et al., 2023). Therefore consuming fruits and vegetables rich in polyphenols, keeping healthy weight, practicing physical activities, and avoiding food contaminants, tobacco, and alcohol consumption could be the keys to longevity and cancer prevention.

Part of your document could not be imported as it contained an unsupported element. For more information about unsupported elements, please visit the Support Center.

13.4 Importance of the nutritional approach on cancer prevention and mode of action of bioactive compounds on antitumor targets

The knowledge of the molecular process of cancer and its possible interactions with bioactive molecules could support the arsenal of oncologists in drug design and development steps (Ahmed et al., 2024). Besides, dietary practices could have a pivotal impact on cancer prevention as the consumptions of appropriate and healthy food options have demonstrated suitable effects on different life stages and were considered effective alternative to fight cancer disease by diminishing its incidence and aggressiveness (Rowles & Erdman, 2020). In this context, a study conducted by Bahrami (2023) showed that adequate consumption of natural unprocessed raw dry fruits and fresh vegetables and fruits, including almonds, lemons, dates, mangoes, figs, grapes, garlic, red onions, green leafy vegetables, tomatoes, carrots, celery, cucumbers, sprouted wheat, sprouted peas, olive oil, spices, and ginger, could be important sources of essential vitamins, minerals, enzymes, beneficial bacteria (probiotics), and antioxidants with protective anticancer properties. These effects could be attributed to the richness of the consumed fruits and vegetables in natural polyphenols which can limit the initiation and the progression of specific cancers (Patra et al., 2021). For that reason, polyphenols were prescribed as nutraceuticals and pharmaceuticals in human medicine to treat certain diseases, including cancer (Piccolella et al., 2019).

Polyphenols family is derived from the biosynthesis of phenylalanine amino acid via the shikimate pathway. This group is characterized by their specific chemical structure that contain an aromatic ring with one or more hydroxyl groups (Zagoskina et al., 2023). They include a large class of subgroups such as flavonoids, phenolic acids and their derivatives, and nonflavonoids, including lignans and stilbenes (Zagoskina et al., 2023).

13.4.1 Phenolic acids

Phenolic acid is an important class of plant secondary metabolites that have tremendous nutritional properties, as well as pleasant taste and smell (Palko-Łabuz et al., 2021). The consumption of plant phenolics is reputed to engender numerous health benefits owing to their antioxidant activities and their capability to neutralize reactive oxygen species (ROS) (Kiokias et al., 2020). Phenolic acids could be categorized into two main groups. The first group is the hydroxybenzoic acids, which are composed of several compounds such as gallic, p-hydroxybenzoic, vanillic, and syringic acids (Kalinowska, Gołębiewska, Świderski, et al., 2021). A previous study reported that the isoferulic acid was demonstrated to hold an anticancer activity against HaCaT human immortalized keratinocyte cell line (Kalinowska, Gołębiewska, Mazur, et al., 2021). Another study spotlighted the powerful anticancer activities of gallic acid in the treatment of various malignancies by affecting various biological pathways associated with tumorigenesis and cellular growth (Jiang et al., 2022). In addition, vanillic acid was found to impede tumor growth in a xenografted tumor model by targeting hypoxia-inducible factor-1 (HIF-1) and suppressing (mTOR)/p70 ribosomal protein S6 kinase (p70S6K)/(4E-BP1) and Raf/extracellular signal-regulated kinase (ERK) kinase (MEK)/ERK signaling pathways involved in colon cancer (Gong et al., 2019). On the other hand, the second group is the hydroxy-cinnamic acids. This group contains several examples, including ferulic, caffeic, p-coumaric, chlorogenic, and sinapic acid. Coffee, lettuce, carrots, berries, sweet potatoes, prunes, peaches, apples, tomatoes, and grapes are the main sources of this group of phenolics. A recent research conducted by Tehami et al. (2023) indicated that p-coumaric acid could be used as a potent cure for preventing and managing colorectal cancer owing to its antiinflammatory and antitumorigenic effects by inducing pro-apoptotic signaling pathways. Additionally, caffeic acid and the chlorogenic acid were employed as adjuvants to the FDA-approved drug Bortezomib to alleviate its side effects (neurotoxicity) and to improve its anticancer potential against multiple myeloma (Matsuda et al., 2022). Sinapic acid stipulated various health-promoting properties, including its effective antiproliferative effects by inducing the apoptosis of several cell lines collected from prostate, pancreatic, and colon cancers (Eroğlu et al., 2018; Huang, Chen, et al., 2022; Taştemur et al., 2023).

13.4.2 Flavonoids

Flavonoids are the most abundant and diversified polyphenols in diet that could be found in many nutrients, including onions, cherries, apples, broccoli, cabbage, tomatoes, berries, tea, red wine, cumin, and buckwheat (Garg et al., 2019). This group is classified into two main subgroups. The first one is known as anthoxanthins, which comprise various categories, including flavones, flavonols, flavanols, flavanones, and isoflavones, and the second one is known as anthocyanins (Kopustinskiene et al., 2020). The chemical structure of flavonoids is basically composed of phenylbenzopyrone with two aromatic rings, and they could exist in two different forms, free and conjugated, and their biosynthesis arises via two biological pathways, including the shikimate pathway and the acetate pathway (Desam & Al-Rajab, 2022; Nabavi et al., 2020). The structural differences between all the previously indicated classes could be attributed to the degree of hydroxylation and substitution in their basic skeleton (Shen et al., 2022). Tiwari and Mishra (2020) discussed the use of flavonoids as radioprotectors and radiosensitizers agents by killing malignant tumor cells without affecting the normal cells. Another study showed that flavonoids could impede the proliferation of cancer cells by inhibiting the epidermal growth factor receptor/mitogen-activated protein kinase (EGFR/MAPK), protein kinase B (Akt), and the phosphatidylinositide 3-kinases (PI3K) (Rodríguez-García et al., 2019). They could also promote apoptotic actions by inducing caspases and Bcl-2 family proteins involved in cell death pathways (Abotaleb et al., 2019).

13.4.2.1 Flavanones

Flavanones are a subclass of flavonoids group, distinguished by a saturate, heterocyclic, and oxidized C ring (Bose et al., 2018). These phytochemical compounds are largely available in citrus fruits, grapes, and other botanical families such as *Rutaceae*, *Rosaceae,* and *Leguminosae* (Khajuria & Shalini Singh, 2019). Among the principal compounds belonging to flavanones class, we cite naringenin, hesperidin, eriodictyol, taxifolin, didymin, and eriocitrin (Cháirez-Ramírez et al., 2021). A previous study described the antitumor potential of naringenin which manifested pleiotropic effects dictated by the modulation of cellular signaling pathways, the inhibition of growth factor production, and the arrest of malignant cell cycle (Stabrauskiene et al., 2022). Another study depicted that the same compound embellished the anticancer activity of cyclophosphamide against MDA-MB-231 breast cancer cells via hindering the STAT3 signaling pathway (Noori et al., 2020). Moreover, hesperidin exhibited powerful antiproliferative properties by engendering various inhibitory effects on different cell lines, including breast, colon, lung, and prostate cancers. Interestingly, hesperidin showed an interesting mode of action by influencing the apoptosis, cell cycle, angiogenesis, and impeding cellular metastasis as well as reversing cells resistance (Aggarwal et al., 2020; Pandey & Khan, 2021; Rahmani et al., 2023; Sulaiman et al., 2020; Yap et al., 2021). Concerning the plant compound taxifolin, Butt et al. (2021) stated that it could have chemoprotective and pro-apoptotic impacts against hepatocellular carcinoma cell line HepG2 and Huh7. It also conquered the progression of gastric and cervical cancers by regulating the AhR/CYP1A1 pathway and inhibiting E6-mediated p53 protein, respectively (Gomes et al., 2022; Xie et al., 2021). In addition, eriodictyol was found to repress PI3K/Akt pathway involved in breast cancer and to induce PI3K/Akt/NF-κB associated with the apoptosis phenomena of glioma (He et al., 2022; Li et al., 2020). It also affects many other pathways of upper and lower gastrointestinal tract (Huang, He, et al., 2022; Shan et al., 2022; Tang, Qin, et al., 2020).

13.4.2.2 Flavanols

Flavanol is a subclass of flavonoids that have a special chemical structure characterized by the absence of the double bond between C2 and C3 and carbonyl group on the C ring and the presence of an hydroxyl group(s) on C3 or C-4 (Luo et al., 2022). Catechin, epicatechin, epigallocatechin, epicatechin gallate, and epigallocatechin gallate (EGCG) are among the most well-known examples of flavanols compounds. These latter could be found in tea, apples, berries, cocoa, and catechu. Sun et al. (2020) demonstrated that catechin could induce cyclin kinase inhibitor p21 and suppress cyclin E1 and P-AKT of lung carcinoma cells. Han et al. (2021) revealed that the same bioactive molecule could be used as an adjuvant drug to reduce chemoresistance to 5-fluorouracil by restricting the activity of the glycolysis-related enzyme lactate dehydrogenase A in colon cancer. On the other side, epigallocatechin gallate (EGCG) exhibited powerful suppressive and protective effects against endometrial, breast, and ovarian cancers by interacting with DNA methyltransferases and histone deacetylases involved in the occurrence of epigenetic modifications (Huang et al., 2020). Another study reported that (EGCG) nanoparticles showed an impressive chemotherapeutical activity against lung cancer cells (Zhang et al., 2020). Moreover, it manifested a promising anticancer potential by its application in in vitro 3D spheroid model of prostate cancer (Alserihi et al., 2023).

13.4.2.3 Flavones

Flavones subclass is largely found in leaves, rinds, barks, and pollens. Luteolin, apigenin, nobiletin, and tangeritin are the main examples representing this group. A study conducted by Ganai et al. (2021) stipulated that luteolin exhibited an antineoplastic effect by targeting histone deacetylases and DNA methylation regulator enzymes. It also showed an antitumor effect against gastric cancer cells by inhibiting cancer cell cycle arrest and proliferation and inducing apoptosis regulators (Pu et al., 2018). In addition, apigenin could be used as a potent chemotherapeutic agent against cervical cancer cells by downregulating FAK and PI3K/AKT signaling pathways (Chen, Wu, et al., 2022). This phytochemical compound could also enhance DNA damage and cell death in cancerous cells and prevent normal cells from genomic instability (Moslehi et al., 2023).

13.4.2.4 Isoflavones

This class is largely distributed in many plant species that belong to *Leguminosae* botanical family (Aboushanab et al., 2022; Aboushanab et al., 2023). Daidzein, genistein, and glycitein are examples of bioactive compounds that belong to this subclass. Daidzein improved the anticancer effect of topotecan by reversing BCRP-mediated drug resistance in breast cancer (Guo et al., 2019). On the other hand, genistein could inhibit Polo-like kinase 1 (PLK1) protein involved in cancer disease (Chae et al., 2019).

13.4.2.5 Flavonols

Flavonols are another subclass of flavonoids characterized by a double bond between C2 and C3 and the presence of a ketone group at the ring C in the fourth position (Kubina et al., 2021). Fisetin, kaempferol, and quercetin are examples of bioactive molecules that belong to flavonols group. Many previous studies examined their antitumor effects. The anticancer capacity of quercetin was evaluated in vitro, and it showed good cytotoxic effect against colon carcinoma CT-26 cells, prostate adenocarcinoma LNCaP cells, and acute lymphoblastic leukemia MOLT-4 T-cells (Hashemzaei et al., 2017). It has been reported that it could modulate PI3K/Akt/mTOR, Wnt/β-catenin, and MAPK/ERK1/2 pathways which are crucial promoters of cell cycle arrest and apoptosis (Reyes-Farias et al., 2019). Regarding kaempferol, Guo et al. (2017) proved its chemoprotective effect by promoting hepatocarcinoma cell death via ER stress and CHOP-autophagy signaling pathway. These authors demonstrated that both compounds could exert anti-cancer effects by impeding the proliferation, migration, and colony formation of cancer cells.

Part of your document could not be imported as it contained an unsupported element. For more information about unsupported elements, please visit the Support Center.

The antiproliferative potential of polyphenols against different tumor cell lines is tightly linked to their antioxidant and antiinflammatory properties (Rudrapal et al., 2022). Briguglio et al. (2020) highlighted the multiple mechanisms of these valuable plant-derived compounds, including the modulation of molecular and signaling pathways, impeding the proliferation, differentiation, migration, angiogenesis, and hormonal activities as well as inducing detoxification enzymes, immune responses, and cell cycle arrest. Table 13.1 represents examples of other phytochemical bioactive compounds and their possible antitumor markers and targets.

Part of your document could not be imported as it contained an unsupported element. For more information about unsupported elements, please visit the Support Center.

13.5 Challenges and perspectives toward the employment of bioactive compounds in cancer treatment

The treatment of cancer without recourse to chemotherapy, surgery, and radiotherapy, the overcoming of malignant cells resistance to existent medications, and the immense increase in mortality rates required the search for novel

TABLE 13.1 Examples of bioactive compounds and their antitumor targets and pathways.

Bioactive compounds	Plant	Antitumor markers and targets	Main findings	References
Tiliroside	*Rosa brunonii*	• Vascular endothelial growth factor D • Human Myosin 9b RhoGAP domain	• Tiliroside exhibited a powerful antiproliferative activity against both studied targets with free energies of binding equal to −13.8 kcal/mol and −14.9 kcal/mol, respectively	Khanum et al. (2024)
Paeonol	*Paeonia suffruticosa*	• Human nonsmall cell lung cancer cell lines	• Paeonol exerted noticeable antineoplastic effects via suppressing the AKT signaling pathway by upregulating TNNC1 and SCARA5 expression	Zhang, Zhang, and Guo (2024)
Biochanin A	Peanuts, cabbage, and red clover	• Serine/threonine protein kinase (AKT1) • Transmembrane glycoprotein (EGFR) • Caspase-3 (CASP3) • Matrix Metallopeptidase 9 (MMP9)	• Biochanin promoted Glioblastoma cell apoptosis by upregulating cleaved CASP3 expression and downregulating p-AKT, EGFR, and MMP9 expression	Ge et al. (2024)
– Milrinone I – Dehydromiltirone – Neocryptotanshinone II	*Salvia miltiorrhiza*	• Proto-oncogene (SRC) • Interleukin-6 (IL-6) • Insulin gene (INS)	• *Salvia miltiorrhiza* components could efficiently impede the progression of colorectal cancer via regulating the INS/SRC/IL-6 pathways	Jiang and Xun (2024)
Neoclerodane diterpenoid	*Ajuga nipponensis*	• Aldo-keto reductase family 1, member 10 (AKR1B10)	• It impeded the activity of KR1B10 involved in the process of tumor occurrence and development	Sun et al. (2024)
Betulinic acid	Jujube fruits, papaya, and persimmon	Glucose metabolism and NF-κB signaling pathways	Betulinic acid improved breast cancer cells sensitivity to paclitaxel and reduce its deleterious side effects.	Mu et al. (2023)
Myricetin	*Myrica rubra*	Human hypoxia-inducible factor-1 subunit alpha (HIF-1α)	Myricetin mitigated formaldehyde-enhanced Warburg effect in tumor cells through HIF-1α inhibition.	Li et al. (2022)
Luteolin	Broccoli, pepper, thyme, and celery	p53 wild-type cells	Luteolin inhibits the growth of HCT116 colon cancer cells through p53-dependent regulation of apoptosis and cell cycle arrest	Yoo et al. (2022)
Genistein	*Genista tinctoria*	• Caspase-3 enzyme • p38 mitogen-activated protein kinase (p38MAPK)	Genistein induced apoptosis, inhibited cell proliferation and suppressed metastatic effect of prostate cancer cells	Shafiee et al. (2022)
Apigenin	Parsley, chamomile, celery, vine-spinach and artichokes	IFN-γ induced PD-L1 expression	Apigenin significantly inhibited lung cancer cell growth, induced cell apoptosis by affecting the IFN-γ-induced PD-L1 expression by hindering the phosphorylation of STAT3	Jiang et al. (2021)

(Continued)

TABLE 13.1 (Continued)

Bioactive compounds	Plant	Antitumor markers and targets	Main findings	References
Artemisinin	*Artemisia annua*	MDA-MB-231 cisplatin-resistant breast cancer cells.	Artemisinin had dose-dependent antiproliferative effects on MDA-MB-231 cisplatin-resistant breast cancer cells with less toxicity in normal cell line	Guan and Guan (2020)
Cytisine	*Laburnum watereri*	• Human tongue squamous carcinoma cells (SCC-25) • Human pharyngeal squamous carcinoma cells (FaDu) • Human triple-negative breast adenocarcinoma cell line (MDA-MB-231) • Human breast adenocarcinoma cell line (MCF-7)	Cytisine had the strongest toxic activity against SCC-25 cell line. It showed the lowest viability (only 0.64%).	Petruczynik et al. (2020)
Quercetin	*Camellia sinensis*	Glycolytic and mitochondrial pathways for ATP production	Quercetin could cause a dose-dependent inhibitory effect on cellular bioenergetics of murine melanoma cells	Tang, Deng, et al. (2020)
Curcumin	*Curcuma longa*	Dual-specificity tyrosine-regulated kinase 2 (DYRK2).	Curcumin complexed with DYRK2, a regulator of the 26 S proteasome, exhibited a high specificity by binding to the ATP-binding domain. It significantly reduced tumor burden in immunocompromised mice.	Banerjee et al. (2018)

insights and the discovery of targeted cancer therapies by finding effective, safe, and powerful alternatives to save millions of lives. In this regard, the employment of bioactive compounds was suggested in the development of new pharmaceuticals especially the anticancerous drugs. However, their use for cancer treatment is still limited due to their low solubility, high volatility, low absorption, and moderate bioavailability (Garcia-Oliveira et al., 2021). Thus we encourage the use of innovative strategies as drug delivery systems to enhance their availability, including nano-formulations, liposomes, and nanoparticles. There exist trends toward the use of smart nanocarrier-based delivery of bioactive compounds by incorporating several biodegradable and biocompatible polymers such as chitosan and hyaluronic acid which could improve plant compounds efficacy by enhancing their solubility and pharmacokinetic profiles, increasing their half-life, and controlling their release in sustained manner (Gorain et al., 2023). Additionally, it is crucial to mention that regulations systems, guidance, and quality control are still needed to deal with the toxicity issues of phytochemicals by focusing on clinical and preclinical outcomes. Indeed, standardized platforms for patient-reported outcome assessment selection, delivery, and data collection and interpretation are highly recommended (Mao et al., 2022).

Furthermore, scientists have been venturing more in-depth into the advanced tools and approaches offered by artificial intelligence (AI) and machine learning methods. In this context, the introduction of the next-generation sequencing (NGS) platforms provides several clinical applications that are crucial for risk predictor and early detection of cancer by the identification of molecular biomarkers and the possible therapeutic targets for novel drug discovery (Dlamini et al., 2020). Moreover, structure-based virtual screening models allowed the modelization and the analysis of the binding-conformation between a ligand and a target enzyme/protein involved in cancer proliferation pathway by using the molecular docking approach (Arjmand et al., 2022). Nevertheless, specialized computing softwares are still being updated to find the accurate targets and the most effective phytoconstituents for cancer treatment.

13.6 Conclusion

Nowadays, the burden of cancer and the hazardous side effects as well as the nonselectivity of conventional chemotherapies imposed a serious challenge and extensive efforts from oncologists to reduce mortality rates. Searching for therapeutics from nature was one of the suggested strategies to treat one of the leading causes of death worldwide in recent years. In this sense, the present book chapter compiled the necessary information about the novel insights toward using phytochemicals as promising candidates in cancer treatment and prevention. Owing to their richness, beneficial properties, and safety compared to conventional chemotherapies, bioactive compounds have attracted researchers to study and assess the anticancer potency of herbal medicines to increase survival rates in cancer patients and to provide efficient prevention and life quality enhancement. In line with these findings, this chapter discussed cancer hallmarks and its risky causes. Additionally, it highlights the beneficial health-promoting effects and anticancerous effects of consuming nutrients rich in powerful bioactive compounds. Finally, it spotlighted their effect by targeting different pathways involved in tumor proliferation, apoptosis, and other markers.

References

Abotaleb, M., Samson, M. S., Elizabeth, V., Sharon, V., Peter, K., Alena, L., & Dietrich, B. (2019). 'Flavonoids in cancer and apoptosis'. *Cancers, 11* (1), 28. Available from https://doi.org/10.3390/cancers11010028.

Aboushanab, S. A., Khedr, S. M., Gette, I. F., Danilova, I. G., Kolberg, N. A., Ravishankar, G. A., Ambati, R. R., & Kovaleva, E. G. (2023). Isoflavones derived from plant raw materials: bioavailability, anti-cancer, anti-aging potentials, and microbiome modulation. *Critical Reviews in Food Science and Nutrition, 63*(2), 261–287. Available from https://doi.org/10.1080/10408398.2021.1946006.

Aboushanab, S. A., Khedr, S. M., Gette, I. F., Danilova, I. G., Kolberg, N. A., Ravishankar, G. A., Ambati, R. R., & Kovaleva, E. G. (2022). Isoflavones derived from plant raw materials: Bioavailability, anti-cancer, anti-aging potentials, and microbiome modulation. *Critical Reviews in Food Science and Nutrition, 63*, 261–287. Available from https://doi.org/10.1080/10408398.2021.1946006.

Aggarwal, V., Tuli, H. S., Thakral, F., Singhal, P., Aggarwal, D., Srivastava, S., Pandey, A., Sak, K., Varol, M., Khan, M. A., & Sethi, G. (2020). Molecular mechanisms of action of hesperidin in cancer: Recent trends and advancements. *Experimental Biology and Medicine, 245*(5), 486–497. Available from https://doi.org/10.1177/1535370220903671.

Ahmed, M. H., Karkush, S. I., Ali, S. A., & Ali, A. M. (2024). Phytochemicals: A new arsenal in drug discovery. *International Journal of Medical Science and Dental Health, 10*(01), 29–44. Available from https://doi.org/10.55640/ijmsdh-10-01-03.

Ali, A. S., Nazar, M. E., Mustafa, R. M., Hussein, S., Qurbani, K., & Ahmed, S. K. (2024). Impact of heavy metals on breast cancer (Review). *World Academy of Sciences Journal, 6*(1). Available from https://doi.org/10.3892/wasj.2023.219, https://www.spandidos-publications.com/10.3892/wasj.2023.219.

Alserihi, R. F., Shait Mohammed, M. R., Kaleem, M., Khan, M. I., Sechi, M., Zughaibi, T. A., & Tabrez, S. (2023). 'Comparative efficacy of epigallocatechin gallate and its nano-formulation in prostate cancer 3D spheroids model'. *Journal of King Saud University - Science, 35*, 102627. Available from https://doi.org/10.1016/j.jksus.2023.102627.

Arjmand, B., Hamidpour, S. K., Alavi-Moghadam, S., Yavari, H., Shahbazbadr, A., Tavirani, M. R., Gilany, K., & Larijani, B. (2022). Molecular docking as a therapeutic approach for targeting cancer stem cell metabolic processes. *Frontiers in Pharmacology, 13*. Available from https://doi.org/10.3389/fphar.2022.768556.

Bahrami, H. (2023). Nutrition for cancer prevention and control: A review of dietary risk factors and protective measures. *Cancer Screening and Prevention, 2*(4), 250–259. Available from https://doi.org/10.14218/CSP.2023.00008S.

Banerjee, S., Ji, C., Mayfield, J. E., Goel, A., Xiao, J., Dixon, J. E., & Guo, X. (2018). 'Ancient drug curcumin impedes 26S proteasome activity by direct inhibition of dual-specificity tyrosine-regulated kinase 2'. *Proceedings of the National Academy of Sciences, 115*(32), 8155–8160. Available from https://doi.org/10.1073/pnas.1806797115.

Banwo, K., Olojede, A. O., Adesulu-Dahunsi, A. T., Verma, D. K., Thakur, M., Tripathy, S., Singh, S., Patel, A. R., Gupta, A. K., Aguilar, C. N., & Lara Utama, G. (2021). Functional importance of bioactive compounds of foods with Potential Health Benefits: A review on recent trends. *Food Bioscience, 43*101320. Available from https://doi.org/10.1016/j.fbio.2021.101320.

Bose, S., Sarkar, D., Bose, A., Subhash, C., & Mandal. (2018). *Natural Flavonoids and Its Pharmaceutical Importance, 2018.*

Briguglio, G., Costa, C., Pollicino, M., Giambò, F., Catania, S., & Fenga, C. (2020). Polyphenols in cancer prevention: New insights (Review). *International Journal of Functional Nutrition, 1*(2), 1. Available from https://doi.org/10.3892/ijfn.2020.9, –1.

Budreviciute, A., Damiati, S., Sabir, D. K., Onder, K., Schuller-Goetzburg, P., Plakys, G., Katileviciute, A., Khoja, S., & Kodzius, R. (2020). Management and prevention strategies for non-communicable diseases (NCDs) and their risk factors. *Frontiers in Public Health, 8*. Available from https://doi.org/10.3389/fpubh.2020.574111.

Butt, S. S., Khan, K., Badshah, Y., Rafiq, M., & Shabbir, M. (2021). 'Evaluation of pro-apoptotic potential of taxifolin against liver cancer'. *PeerJ*, *9* (May), e11276. Available from https://doi.org/10.7717/peerj.11276.

Chae, H.-S., Xu, R., Won, J.-Y., Chin, Y.-W., & Yim, H. (2019). 'Molecular targets of genistein and its related flavonoids to exert anticancer effects'. *International Journal of Molecular Sciences*, *20*, 2420. Available from https://doi.org/10.3390/ijms20102420.

Chen, M., Linstra, R., & van Vugt, M. A. T. M. (2022). Genomic instability, inflammatory signaling and response to cancer immunotherapy. *Biochimica et Biophysica Acta (BBA) - Reviews on Cancer*, *1877*188661. Available from https://doi.org/10.1016/j.bbcan.2021.188661.

Chen, Y.-H., Wu, J.-X., Yang, S.-F., Yang, C.-K., Chen, T.-H., & Hsiao, Y.-H. (2022). 'Anticancer effects and molecular mechanisms of apigenin in cervical cancer cells'. *Cancers*, *14*(7), 1824. Available from https://doi.org/10.3390/cancers14071824.

Cháirez-Ramírez, M. H., de la Cruz-López, K. G., & García-Carrancá, A. (2021). Polyphenols as antitumor agents targeting key players in cancer-driving signaling pathways. *Frontiers in Pharmacology*, *12*. Available from https://doi.org/10.3389/fphar.2021.710304.

Crosby, D., Bhatia, S., Brindle, K. M., Coussens, L. M., Dive, C., Emberton, M., Esener, S., et al. (2022). Early detection of cancer. *Science (New York, N.Y.)*, *375*(6586)eaay9040. Available from https://doi.org/10.1126/science.aay9040.

Dehghani, S., Moshfeghinia, R., Ramezani, M., Vali, M., Oskoei, V., Amiri-Ardekani, E., & Hopke, P. (2023). Exposure to air pollution and risk of ovarian cancer: a review. *Reviews on Environmental Health*, *38*(3), 439–450. Available from https://doi.org/10.1515/reveh-2021-0129.

Desam, N. R., & Al-Rajab, A. J. (2022). *Herbal biomolecules: Anticancer agents. Herbal biomolecules in healthcare applications* (pp. 435–474). Elsevier. Available from https://www.sciencedirect.com/book/9780323858526, 10.1016/B978-0-323-85852-6.00001-9.

Dlamini, Z., Francies, F. Z., Hull, R., & Marima, R. (2020). 'Artificial intelligence (AI) and big data in cancer and precision oncology'. *Computational and Structural Biotechnology Journal*, *18*(January), 2300–2311. Available from https://doi.org/10.1016/j.csbj.2020.08.019.

Eroğlu, C., Avcı, E., Vural, H., & Kurar, E. (2018). 'Anticancer mechanism of sinapic acid in PC-3 and LNCaP human prostate cancer cell lines'. *Gene*, *671*(September), 127–134. Available from https://doi.org/10.1016/j.gene.2018.05.049.

Fiolet, T., Srour, B., Sellem, L., Kesse-Guyot, E., Allès, B., Méjean, C., Deschasaux, M., et al. (2018). Consumption of ultra-processed foods and cancer risk: Results from NutriNet-Santé prospective cohort. *BMJ 360 (February*, k322. Available from https://doi.org/10.1136/bmj.k322.

Ganai, S. A., Sheikh, F. A., Baba, Z. A., Mir, M. A., Mantoo, M. A., & Yatoo, M. A. (2021). Anticancer activity of the plant flavonoid luteolin against preclinical models of various cancers and insights on different signalling mechanisms modulated. *Phytotherapy Research*, *35*, 3509–3532. Available from https://doi.org/10.1002/ptr.7044.

Garcia-Oliveira, P., Otero, P., Pereira, A. G., Chamorro, F., Carpena, M., Echave, J., Fraga-Corral, M., Simal-Gandara, J., & Angel Prieto, M. (2021). Status and challenges of plant-anticancer compounds in cancer treatment. *Pharmaceuticals*, *14*, 157. Available from https://doi.org/10.3390/ph14020157.

Garg., Kumar, S., Shukla, A., & Choudhury, S. (2019). Polyphenols and flavonoids. In R. C. Gupta, A. Srivastava, & R. Lall (Eds.), *Nutraceuticals in veterinary medicine* (edited by, pp. 187–204). Springer International Publishing. Available from https://doi.org/10.1007/978-3-030-04624-8_13.

Ge, W., Yuan, G., Wang, D., & Dong, L. (2024). 'Exploring the therapeutic mechanisms and prognostic targets of biochanin A in glioblastoma via integrated computational analysis and in vitro experiments'. *Scientific Reports*, *14*, 3783. Available from https://doi.org/10.1038/s41598-024-53442-0.

Gomes, D., Yaduvanshi, S., Silvestre, S., Duarte, A. P., Santos, A. O., Soares, C. P., Kumar, V., Passarinha, L., & Sousa, Â. (2022). Taxifolin and lucidin as potential E6 Protein inhibitors: P53 function re-establishment and apoptosis induction in cervical cancer cells. *Cancers*, *14*, 2834. Available from https://doi.org/10.3390/cancers14122834.

Gong, J., Zhou, S., & Yang, S. (2019). 'Vanillic acid suppresses HIF-1α expression via inhibition of mTOR/p70S6K/4E-BP1 and Raf/MEK/ERK pathways in human colon cancer HCT116 Cells'. *International Journal of Molecular Sciences*, *20*, 465. Available from https://doi.org/10.3390/ijms20030465.

Gorain, B., Karmakar, V., Sarkar, B., Dwivedi, M., Leong, J. T. L., Toh, J. H., Seah, E., et al. (2023). Biomacromolecule-based nanocarrier strategies to deliver plant-derived bioactive components for cancer treatment: A recent review. *International Journal of Biological Macromolecules*, *253* (December))126623. Available from https://doi.org/10.1016/j.ijbiomac.2023.126623.

Guan, X., & Guan, Y. (2020). Artemisinin induces selective and potent anticancer effects in drug-resistant breast cancer cells by inducing cellular apoptosis and autophagy and G2/M cell cycle arrest. *Zerbinis Publications, ChinaJournal of B.U.ON.*, *25*(3), 1330–1337. Available from http://jbuon.com/archive/25-3-1330.pdf.

Guo, H., Lin, W., Zhang, X., Zhang, X., Hu, Z., Li, L., Duan, Z., Zhang, J., & Ren, F. (2017). 'Kaempferol induces hepatocellular carcinoma cell death via endoplasmic reticulum stress-CHOP-autophagy signaling pathway'. *Oncotarget*, *8*, 82207–82216. Available from https://doi.org/10.18632/oncotarget.19200.

Guo, J., Wang, Q., Zhang, Y., Sun, W., Zhang, S., Li, Y., Wang, J., & Bao, Y. (2019). 'Functional daidzein enhances the anticancer effect of topotecan and reverses BCRP-mediated drug resistance in breast cancer'. *Pharmacological Research*, *147*(September), 104387. Available from https://doi.org/10.1016/j.phrs.2019.104387.

Hanahan, D. (2022). Hallmarks of cancer: New dimensions. *Cancer Discovery*, *12*, 31–46. Available from https://doi.org/10.1158/2159-8290.CD-21-1059.

Han, J. H., Kim, M., Kim, H. J., Jang, S. B., Bae, S.-J., Lee, I.-K., Ryu, D., & Ha, K.-T. (2021). 'Targeting lactate dehydrogenase A with catechin resensitizes SNU620/5FU gastric cancer cells to 5-fluorouracil'. *International Journal of Molecular Sciences*, *22*, 5406. Available from https://doi.org/10.3390/ijms22105406.

Hashemzaei, M., Far, A. D., Yari, A., Heravi, R. E., Tabrizian, K., Taghdisi, S. M., Sadegh, S. E., et al. (2017). Anticancer and apoptosis-inducing effects of quercetin in vitro and in vivo. *Oncology Reports*, *38*, 819–828. Available from https://doi.org/10.3892/or.2017.5766.

He, J., Fu, H., Li, C., Deng, Z., & Chang, H. (2022). 'Eriodictyol inhibits breast carcinogenesis by targeting Circ_0007503 and repressing PI3K/Akt pathway'. *Phytomedicine: International Journal of Phytotherapy and Phytopharmacology*, *102*(July), 154159. Available from https://doi.org/10.1016/j.phymed.2022.154159.

Huang, Z., Chen, H., Tan, P., Huang, M., Shi, H., Sun, B., Cheng, Y., et al. (2022). Sinapic Acid inhibits pancreatic cancer proliferation, migration, and invasion via downregulation of the AKT/Gsk-3β signal pathway. *Drug Development Research*, *83*, 721–734. Available from https://doi.org/10.1002/ddr.21904.

Huang, H., He, Y., Li, Y., Gu, M., Wu, M., & Ji, L. (2022). Eriodictyol suppresses the malignant progression of colorectal cancer by downregulating tissue specific transplantation antigen P35B (TSTA3) expression to restrain fucosylation'. *Bioengineered*, *13*, 5551–5563. Available from https://doi.org/10.1080/21655979.2022.2039485.

Huang, Y.-J., Wang, K.-L., Chen, H.-Y., Chiang, Y.-F., & Hsia, S.-M. (2020). 'Protective effects of epigallocatechin gallate (EGCG) on endometrial, breast, and ovarian cancers'. *Biomolecules*, *10*, 1481. Available from https://doi.org/10.3390/biom10111481.

Ilham, S., Willis, C., Kim, K., Chung, K. C., Wood, B. M., Tan, M. S., Tan, C. J., Nguyen, D. T., Brixner, D. I., & Stenehjem, D. D. (2023). Cancer incidence in immunocompromised patients: A single-center cohort study. *BMC Cancer*, *23*, 33. Available from https://doi.org/10.1186/s12885-022-10497-4.

Jardim, S. R., de Souza, L. M. P., & Pereira de Souza, H. S. (2023). The rise of gastrointestinal cancers as a global phenomenon: Unhealthy behavior or progress? *International Journal of Environmental Research and Public Health*, *20*, 3640. Available from https://doi.org/10.3390/ijerph20043640.

Jiang, Y., Pei, J., Zheng, Y., Miao, Y.-J., Duan, B.-Z., & Huang, L.-F. (2022). 'Gallic acid: A potential anti-cancer agent'. *Chinese Journal of Integrative Medicine*, *28*, 661–671. Available from https://doi.org/10.1007/s11655-021-3345-2.

Jiang, Z.-B., Wang, W.-J., Xu, C., Xie, Y.-J., Wang, X.-R., Zhang, Y.-Z., Huang, J.-M., et al. (2021). Luteolin and its derivative apigenin suppress the inducible PD-L1 expression to improve anti-tumor immunity in KRAS-mutant lung cancer. *Cancer Letters*, *515*(September)), 36–48. Available from https://doi.org/10.1016/j.canlet.2021.05.019.

Jiang, Y.-L., & Xun, Y. (2024). 'Molecular mechanism of salvia miltiorrhiza in the treatment of colorectal cancer based on network pharmacology and molecular docking technology'. *Drug Design, Development and Therapy*, *18*(December), 425–441. Available from https://doi.org/10.2147/DDDT.S443102.

Kalinowska, M., Gołębiewska, E., Mazur, L., Lewandowska, H., Pruszyński, M., Świderski, G., Wyrwas, M., Pawluczuk, N., & Lewandowski, W. (2021). Crystal structure, spectroscopic characterization, antioxidant and cytotoxic activity of new Mg(II) and Mn(II)/Na(I) complexes of isoferulic acid. *Materials*, *14*(12), 3236. Available from https://doi.org/10.3390/ma14123236.

Kalinowska, M., Gołębiewska, E., Świderski, G., Męczyńska-Wielgosz, S., Lewandowska, H., Pietryczuk, A., Cudowski, A., et al. (2021). Plant-derived and dietary hydroxybenzoic acids—A comprehensive study of structural, anti-/pro-oxidant, lipophilic, antimicrobial, and cytotoxic activity in MDA-MB-231 and MCF-7 cell lines. *Nutrients*, *13*, 3107. Available from https://doi.org/10.3390/nu13093107.

Khajuria, R., Singh, S., & A, B. (2019). General introduction and sources of flavonoids. In H. Singh Tuli (Ed.), *Current aspects of flavonoids: Their role in cancer treatment* (pp. 1–7). Singapore: Springer. Available from https://doi.org/10.1007/978-981-13-5874-6_1.

Khanum, A., Bibi, Y., Khan, I., Mustafa, G., Attia, K. A., Mohammed, A. A., Yang, S. H., & Qayyum, A. (2024). 'Molecular docking of bioactive compounds extracted and purified from selected medicinal plant species against covid-19 proteins and in vitro evaluation'. *Scientific Reports*, *14*, 3736. Available from https://doi.org/10.1038/s41598-024-54470-6.

Kiokias, S., Proestos, C., & Oreopoulou, V. (2020). 'Phenolic acids of plant origin—A review on their antioxidant activity in vitro (O/W Emulsion Systems) along with their in vivo health biochemical properties'. *Foods*, *9*, 534. Available from https://doi.org/10.3390/foods9040534.

Kopustinskiene, D. M., Jakstas, V., Savickas, A., & Bernatoniene, J. (2020). 'Flavonoids as anticancer agents'. *Nutrients*, *12*, 457. Available from https://doi.org/10.3390/nu12020457.

Kubina, R., Iriti, M., & Kabała-Dzik, A. (2021). 'Anticancer potential of selected flavonols: Fisetin, kaempferol, and quercetin on head and neck cancers'. *Nutrients*, *13*, 845. Available from https://doi.org/10.3390/nu13030845.

Li, W., Du, Q., Li, X., Zheng, X., Lv, F., Xi, X., Huang, G., Yang, J., & Liu, S. (2020). 'Eriodictyol inhibits proliferation, metastasis and induces apoptosis of glioma cells via PI3K/Akt/NF-κB signaling pathway'. *Frontiers in Pharmacology*, *11*. Available from https://www.frontiersin.org/journals/pharmacology/articles/10.3389/fphar.2020.00114.

Li, L., Ma, H., Li, D., Shu, Q., Wang, T., Song, X., & Xu, H. (2022). 'Myricetin alleviates the formaldehyde-enhanced warburg effect in tumor cells through inhibition of HIF-1α'. *Toxicology and Applied Pharmacology*, *454*(November), 116246. Available from https://doi.org/10.1016/j.taap.2022.116246.

Li, Y., Wang, Z., Ajani, J. A., & Song, S. (2021). 'Drug resistance and cancer stem cells'. *Cell Communication and Signaling*, *19*, 19. Available from https://doi.org/10.1186/s12964-020-00627-5.

Luo, Y., Jian, Y., Liu, Y., Jiang, S., Muhammad, D., & Wang, W. (2022). 'Flavanols from nature: A phytochemistry and biological activity review'. *Molecules (Basel, Switzerland)*, *27*, 719. Available from https://doi.org/10.3390/molecules27030719.

Luu., Minh, N., Han, M., Bui, T. T., Tran, P. T. T., Lim, M.-K., & Oh, J. K. (2022). 'Smoking trajectory and cancer risk: A population-based cohort study'. *Tobacco Induced Diseases*, *20*(August), 1–10. Available from https://doi.org/10.18332/tid/152137.

Mao, J. J., Pillai, G. G., Andrade, C. J., Ligibel, J. A., Basu, P., Cohen, L., Khan, I. A., et al. (2022). Integrative oncology: Addressing the global challenges of cancer prevention and treatment. *CA: a Cancer Journal for Clinicians*, *72*, 144–164. Available from https://doi.org/10.3322/caac.21706.

Matsuda, R., Sakagami, H., Amano, S., Iijima, Y., Sano, M., Uesawa, Y., Tamura, N., Oishi, Y., & Takeshima, H. (2022). 'Inhibition of neurotoxicity/anticancer activity of bortezomib by caffeic acid and chlorogenic acid'. *Anticancer Research*, *42*, 781–790. Available from https://doi.org/10.21873/anticanres.15536.

McGee, R. B., & Nichols, K. E. (2016). Introduction to cancer genetic susceptibility syndromes. *Hematology (Amsterdam, Netherlands), 2016*, 293–301. Available from https://doi.org/10.1182/asheducation-2016.1.293.

McTigue, Madeline, J. Goelzer, and W. Ranahan. 2022. 'Medicinal Plants and Herbs for Cancer Prevention'. Research Symposium, July. https://digitalshowcase.oru.edu/research_symposium/2022/cose/1.

Moslehi, M., Rezaei, S., Talebzadeh, P., Ansari, M. J., Jawad, M. A., Jalil, A. T., Rastegar-Pouyani, N., Jafarzadeh, E., Taeb, S., & Najafi, M. (2023). Apigenin in cancer therapy: Prevention of genomic instability and anticancer mechanisms. *Clinical and Experimental Pharmacology and Physiology, 50*, 3–18. Available from https://doi.org/10.1111/1440-1681.13725.

Mu, H., Sun, Y., Yuan, B., & Wang, Y. (2023). 'Betulinic acid in the treatment of breast cancer: Application and mechanism progress'. *Fitoterapia, 169*(September), 105617. Available from https://doi.org/10.1016/j.fitote.2023.105617.

Nabavi, S. M., Šamec, D., Tomczyk, M., Milella, L., Russo, D., Habtemariam, S., Suntar, I., et al. (2020). Flavonoid biosynthetic pathways in plants: Versatile targets for metabolic engineering. *Biotechnology Advances, New advances in biotechnology of dietary phytochemicals, 38*(January)) 107316. Available from https://doi.org/10.1016/j.biotechadv.2018.11.005.

Nohmi, T. (2018). Thresholds of Genotoxic and Non-Genotoxic Carcinogens. *Toxicological Research, 34*, 281–290. Available from https://doi.org/10.5487/TR.2018.34.4.281.

Noori, S., Tavirani, M. R., Deravi, N., Rabbani, M. I. M., & Zarghi, A. (2020). 'Naringenin enhances the anti-cancer effect of cyclophosphamide against MDA-MB-231 breast cancer cells via targeting the STAT3 signaling pathway'. *Iranian Journal of Pharmaceutical Research : IJPR, 19*, 122. Available from https://doi.org/10.22037/ijpr.2020.113103.14112.

Ortega, M., Armando, M., & Campos, M. R. S. (2019). Chapter 13 - Bioactive compounds as therapeutic alternatives. In M. R. S. Campos (Ed.), *In* Bioactive compounds (edited by, pp. 247–264). Woodhead Publishing. Available from https://doi.org/10.1016/B978-0-12-814774-0.00013-X.

Palko-Łabuz, A., Gliszczyńska, A., Skonieczna, M., Poła, A., Wesołowska, O., & Środa-Pomianek, K. (2021). 'Conjugation with phospholipids as a modification increasing anticancer activity of phenolic acids in metastatic melanoma—In vitro and in silico studies'. *International Journal of Molecular Sciences, 22*, 8397. Available from https://doi.org/10.3390/ijms22168397.

Pandey, P., & Khan, F. (2021). 'A mechanistic review of the anticancer potential of hesperidin, a natural flavonoid from citrus fruits'. *Nutrition Research, 92*(August), 21–31. Available from https://doi.org/10.1016/j.nutres.2021.05.011.

Patra, S., Pradhan, B., Nayak, R., Behera, C., Das, S., Patra, S. K., Efferth, T., Jena, M., & Bhutia, S. K. (2021). Dietary polyphenols in chemoprevention and synergistic effect in cancer: Clinical evidences and molecular mechanisms of action. *Phytomedicine International Journal of Phytotherapy and Phytopharmacology, 90*(September))153554. Available from https://doi.org/10.1016/j.phymed.2021.153554.

Petruczynik, A., Wróblewski, K., Misiurek, J., Plech, T., Szalast, K., Wojtanowski, K., Mroczek, T., Szymczak, G., Waksmundzka-Hajnos, M., & Tutka, P. (2020). 'Determination of cytisine and N-methylcytisine from selected plant extracts by high-performance liquid chromatography and comparison of their cytotoxic activity'. *Toxins, 12*, 557. Available from https://doi.org/10.3390/toxins12090557.

Piccolella, S., Crescente, G., Candela, L., & Pacifico, S. (2019). 'Nutraceutical polyphenols: New analytical challenges and opportunities'. *Journal of Pharmaceutical and Biomedical Analysis, 175*(October), 112774. Available from https://doi.org/10.1016/j.jpba.2019.07.022.

Pu, Y., Zhang, T., Wang, J., Mao, Z., Duan, B., Long, Y., Xue, F., Liu, D., Liu, S., & Gao, Z. (2018). 'Luteolin exerts an anticancer effect on gastric cancer cells through multiple signaling pathways and regulating miRNAs'. *Journal of Cancer, 9*, 3669–3675. Available from https://doi.org/10.7150/jca.27183.

Rahmani, A. H., Babiker, A. Y., & Anwar, S. (2023). 'Hesperidin, a bioflavonoid in cancer therapy: A review for a mechanism of action through the modulation of cell signaling pathways'. *Molecules (Basel, Switzerland), 28*, 5152. Available from https://doi.org/10.3390/molecules28135152.

Reyes-Farias., Marjorie., & Carrasco-Pozo, C. (2019). 'The anti-cancer effect of quercetin: Molecular implications in cancer metabolism'. *International Journal of Molecular Sciences, 20*, 3177. Available from https://doi.org/10.3390/ijms20133177.

Rodríguez-García, C., Sánchez-Quesada, C., & Gaforio, J. J. (2019). Dietary flavonoids as cancer chemopreventive agents: An updated review of human studies. *Antioxidants, 8*, 137. Available from https://doi.org/10.3390/antiox8050137.

Rowles, J. L., & Erdman, J. W. (2020). Carotenoids and their role in cancer prevention. *Biochimica et Biophysica Acta (BBA) - Molecular and Cell Biology of Lipids, Carotenoids recent advances in cell and molecular biology, 1865*158613. Available from https://doi.org/10.1016/j.bbalip.2020.158613.

Rudrapal, M., Shubham, J. K., Khan, J., Dukhyil, A. B., Ansari, M. A., Alomary, M. N., Alshabrmi, F. M., Palai, S., Deb, P. K., & Devi, R. (2022). Dietary polyphenols and their role in oxidative stress-induced human diseases: Insights into protective effects, antioxidant potentials and mechanism(s) of action. *Frontiers in Pharmacology, 13*. Available from https://www.frontiersin.org/journals/pharmacology/articles/10.3389/fphar.2022.806470.

Rumgay., Harriet., Shield, K., Charvat, H., Ferrari, P., Sornpaisarn, B., Obot, I., Islami, F., Lemmens, V. E. P. P., Rehm, J., & Soerjomataram, I. (2021). Global burden of cancer in 2020 attributable to alcohol consumption: A population-based study'. *The Lancet Oncology, 22*, 1071–1080. Available from https://doi.org/10.1016/S1470-204500279-5.

Schiller, J. T., & Lowy, D. R. (2021). *An introduction to virus infections and human cancer. Viruses and human cancer* (pp. 1–11). Springer. Available from https://doi.org/10.1007/978-3-030-57362-1_1.

Shafiee, G., Saidijam, M., Tayebinia, H., & Khodadadi, I. (2022). 'Beneficial effects of genistein in suppression of proliferation, inhibition of metastasis, and induction of apoptosis in PC3 prostate cancer cells'. *Archives of Physiology and Biochemistry, 128*, 694–702. Available from https://doi.org/10.1080/13813455.2020.1717541.

Shan, H., Zhang, X., Mi, Y., Jia, J., Wang, B., & Yang, Q. (2022). 'Eriodictyol suppresses gastric cancer cells via inhibition of PI3K/AKT pathway'. *Pharmaceuticals, 15*, 1477. Available from https://doi.org/10.3390/ph15121477.

Sharma, A., Sharma, S., Kumar, A., Kumar, V., & Sharma, A. K. (2022). Plant secondary metabolites: An introduction of their chemistry and biological significance with physicochemical aspect. In A. K. Sharma, & A. Sharma (Eds.), *Plant Secondary Metabolites: Physico-Chemical Properties and Therapeutic Applications* (edited by, pp. 1–45). Singapore: Springer Nature. Available from https://doi.org/10.1007/978-981-16-4779-6_1.

Shen, N., Wang, T., Gan, Q., Liu, S., Wang, L., & Jin, B. (2022). 'Plant flavonoids: Classification, distribution, biosynthesis, and antioxidant activity'. *Food Chemistry, 383*(July), 132531. Available from https://doi.org/10.1016/j.foodchem.2022.132531.

Shoaib., Shoaib., Ansari, M. A., Ghazwani, M., Hani, U., Jamous, Y. F., Alali, Z., Wahab, S., et al. (2023). Prospective epigenetic actions of organo-sulfur compounds against cancer: Perspectives and molecular mechanisms. *Cancers, 15*, 697. Available from https://doi.org/10.3390/cancers15030697.

Singh, N., Baby, D., Rajguru, J. P., Patil, P. B., Thakkannavar, S. S., & Pujari, V. B. (2019). 'Inflammation and cancer'. *Annals of African Medicine, 18*, 121–126. Available from https://doi.org/10.4103/aam.aam_56_18.

Sobhi Amjad, Z., Shojaeian, A., Nahand, J. S., Bayat, M., Taghizadieh, M., Rostamian, M., Babaei, F., & Moghoofei, M. (2023). 'Oncoviruses: Induction of cancer development and metastasis by increasing anoikis resistance'. *Heliyon, 9*, e22598. Available from https://doi.org/10.1016/j.heliyon.2023.e22598.

Stabrauskiene, J., Dalia, M. K., Lazauskas, R., & Bernatoniene, J. (2022). 'Naringin and naringenin: Their mechanisms of action and the potential anticancer activities'. *Biomedicines, 10*, 1686. Available from https://doi.org/10.3390/biomedicines10071686.

Sulaiman., Ghassan, M., Hanaa, M. W., Jabir, M. S., Khazaal, S. H., Dewir, Y. H., & Naidoo, Y. (2020). 'Hesperidin loaded on gold nanoparticles as a drug delivery system for a successful biocompatible, anti-cancer, anti-inflammatory and phagocytosis inducer model'. *Scientific Reports, 10*, 9362. Available from https://doi.org/10.1038/s41598-020-66419-6.

Sun, N., Ma, S., Jin, L., Wang, Y., Zhou, C., Zhang, X., Kang, H., Zhou, M., Yang, H., & Shu, P. (2024). 'Development of AKR1B10 inhibitors from *Ajuga Nipponensis* based on diseases and targets'. *Fitoterapia, 172*(January), 105742. Available from https://doi.org/10.1016/j.fitote.2023.105742.

Sun, H., Yin, M., Hao, D., & Shen, Y. (2020). 'Anti-cancer activity of catechin against A549 lung carcinoma cells by induction of cyclin kinase inhibitor P21 and lin E1 and P–AKT'. *Applied Sciences, 10*, 2065. Available from https://doi.org/10.3390/app10062065.

Supe, U. R., Menghani, Y. R., Trivedi, R. V., Umekar, M. J., Supe, U. R., Menghani, Y. R., Trivedi, R. V., & Umekar, M. J. (2022). 'Consumption of ultra-processed foods and their link with increasing risk of cancer'. *GSC Biological and Pharmaceutical Sciences, 20*, 006–016. Available from https://doi.org/10.30574/gscbps.2022.20.3.0339.

Tang, S.-M., Deng, X.-T., Zhou, J., Li, Q.-P., Ge, X.-X., & Miao, L. (2020). 'Pharmacological basis and new insights of quercetin action in respect to its anti-cancer effects'. *Biomedicine & Pharmacotherapy, 121*(January), 109604. Available from https://doi.org/10.1016/j.biopha.2019.109604.

Tang, L., Qin, Y., Ling, K., & Wan, H. (2020). Eriodictyol inhibits the growth of CNE1 human nasopharyngeal cancer growth by targeting MEK/ERK signalling pathway, inducing cellular autophagy and inhibition of cell migration and invasion'. *Journal of B.U.ON., 25*, 2389–2394.

Taştemur, Ş., Hacısüleyman, L., Karataş, Ö., Yulak, F., & Ataseven, H. (2023). 'Anticancer activity of sinapic acid by inducing apoptosis in HT-29 human colon cancer cell line'. *Canadian Journal of Physiology and Pharmacology, 101*, 361–368. Available from https://doi.org/10.1139/cjpp-2022-0523.

Tehami, W., Nani, A., Khan, N. A., & Hichami, A. (2023). 'New insights into the anticancer effects of P-coumaric acid: Focus on colorectal cancer'. *Dose-Response, 21*. Available from https://doi.org/10.1177/15593258221150704, 15593258221150704.

Tiwari, P., & Mishra, K. P. (2020). 'Flavonoids sensitize tumor cells to radiation: Molecular mechanisms and relevance to cancer radiotherapy'. *International Journal of Radiation Biology, 96*, 360–369. Available from https://doi.org/10.1080/09553002.2020.1694193.

Verma, A., Zanoletti, A., Kareem, K. Y., Adelodun, B., Kumar, P., Ajibade, F. O., Silva, L. F. O., et al. (2024). Skin protection from solar ultraviolet radiation using natural compounds: A review. *Environmental Chemistry Letters, 22*, 273–295. Available from https://doi.org/10.1007/s10311-023-01649-4.

Walia., Aanchal., Gupta, A. K., & Sharma, V. (2019). *Role of Bioactive Compounds in Human Health.*

Xie, J., Pang, Y., & Wu, X. (2021). 'Taxifolin suppresses the malignant progression of gastric cancer by regulating the AhR/CYP1A1 signaling pathway'. *International Journal of Molecular Medicine, 48*, 1–9. Available from https://doi.org/10.3892/ijmm.2021.5030.

Yap, K. M., Sekar, M., Wu, Y. S., Gan, S. H., Rani, N. N. I. M., Seow, L. J., Subramaniyan, V., Fuloria, N. K., Fuloria, S., & Teng Lum, P. (2021). Hesperidin and its aglycone hesperetin in breast cancer therapy: A review of recent developments and future prospects. *Saudi Journal of Biological Sciences, 28*, 6730–6747. Available from https://doi.org/10.1016/j.sjbs.2021.07.046.

Yeshi, K., Crayn, D., Ritmejerytė, E., & Wangchuk, P. (2022). 'Plant secondary metabolites produced in response to abiotic stresses has potential application in pharmaceutical product development'. *Molecules (Basel, Switzerland), 27*, 313. Available from https://doi.org/10.3390/molecules27010313.

Yoo, H. S., Won, S. B., & Hye Kwon, Y. (2022). Luteolin induces apoptosis and autophagy in HCT116 colon cancer cells via P53-dependent pathway. *Nutrition and Cancer, 74*, 677–686. Available from https://doi.org/10.1080/01635581.2021.1903947.

Zagoskina, N. V., Zubova, M. Y., Nechaeva, T. L., Kazantseva, V. V., Goncharuk, E. A., Katanskaya, V. M., Baranova, E. N., & Aksenova, M. A. (2023). Polyphenols in plants: Structure, biosynthesis, abiotic stress regulation, and practical applications (review). *International Journal of Molecular Sciences, 24*, 13874. Available from https://doi.org/10.3390/ijms241813874.

Zhang, L., Chen, W., Tu, G., Chen, X., Lu, Y., Wu, L., & Zheng, D. (2020). 'Enhanced chemotherapeutic efficacy of PLGA-encapsulated epigallocatechin gallate (EGCG) against human lung cancer'. *International Journal of Nanomedicine, 15*(June), 4417–4429. Available from https://doi.org/10.2147/IJN.S243657.

Zhang, C., Zhang, J., & Guo, K. (2024). 'Paeonol upregulates expression of tumor suppressors TNNC1 and SCARA5, exerting anti-tumor activity in non-small cell lung cancer cells'. *Naunyn-Schmiedeberg's Archives of Pharmacology, January.* Available from https://doi.org/10.1007/s00210-024-02963-6.

Chapter 14

Functional food for cancer management: integrating complementary approaches

Azime Özkan Karabacak[1,2], Burcu Saygıdeğer Demir[3], Canan Ece Tamer[4], Yasemin Saygideger[5] and Özge Süfer[6]

[1]Bursa Uludag University, Gemlik Asim Kocabiyik Vocational School, Food Technology Program, Gemlik, Bursa, Türkiye, [2]Bursa Uludag University, Science and Technology Application and Research Center, Bursa, Türkiye, [3]Department of Biotechnology, Insititute of Natural and Applied Sciences, Cukurova University, Sarıcam, Adana, Türkiye, [4]Department of Food Engineering, Faculty of Agriculture, Bursa Uludag University, Gorukle, Bursa, Türkiye, [5]Department of Pulmonary, Department of Translational Medicine, Faculty of Medicine, Cukurova University, Adana, Türkiye, [6]Food Engineering Department, Osmaniye Korkut Ata University, Osmaniye, Türkiye

14.1 Introduction

Cancer can be defined as a condition in which cells lose their inherent ability to regulate their growth and division. Certain types of cancer manifest as tumors, whereas others, like leukemia, do not exhibit localized growth but can instead disseminate throughout the body via blood circulation or lymph vessels (Rahman et al., 2020). This disease ranks as the second primary contributor to mortality in prosperous nations. In the year 2024, it is projected that the United States will witness a total of 2,001,140 new cases of cancer and 611,720 deaths caused by this disease, projecting a financial burden of approximately $458 billion by the year 2030. More than half of all cancer occurrences and fatalities are avoidable. The disease control priorities series emphasizes the implementation of efficacious healthcare measures that curtail mortality and debilitation at a reasonable expense. Functional foods, known for their supplementary health advantages beyond basic nourishment, have been associated with cancer prevention. These foods not only provide important nutrients, but they also help slow down the progression of cancer. They have the ability to fight against cancer in different ways, such as preventing its spread and protecting against oxidative damage. Especially, the consumption of functional foods can hinder the growth of gastric and prostate cancer cells, even at lower consumption levels (Aghajanpour et al., 2017; Dizon & Kamal, 2024; Gupta, 2020). Although several commercial chemotherapeutic agents are currently available, the development of new anticancer agents is urgently required, due to the emergence of tumor drug resistance and the accompanying side effects. Bioactive foods and their derivatives have exhibited promising potential in cancer treatment, offering the advantage of reduced adverse effects and therefore serving as potential alternatives to novel anticancer drugs (Gupta, 2020; Riganti et al., 2015; Zeng et al., 2013) (Fig. 14.1).

The Mediterranean diet is widely acknowledged as a highly beneficial dietary pattern for cancer prevention, thanks to its abundant inclusion of fish, vegetables, fruits, nuts, legumes, whole grains, and extra virgin olive oil. This specific combination of food groups possesses remarkable preventive and therapeutic properties that contribute to reducing the risk of cancer. By incorporating this diet into one's lifestyle, individuals can effectively combat inflammation, oxidative harm, metabolic syndrome, and excessive weight, all of which are known to contribute to the development of chronic illnesses. Notably, the Mediterranean diet has been found to be particularly advantageous in preventing breast and colon cancers, making it a highly recommended dietary choice for those seeking to safeguard their health (Islam & Siddiqua, 2020).

On the other hand, studies indicate that cancer patients often do not consume adequate amounts of essential nutrients, including vitamin E, vitamin D, dietary fiber, potassium, and calcium. Insufficient levels of vitamin D have been associated with lower survival rates, particularly in breast cancer patients. The lack of attention to nutrition in the existing outpatient oncology model in the United States is a significant concern. It is imperative to conduct further research to develop effective approaches for incorporating diet and nutrition into current oncology care to enhance the nutrient

Unleashing the Power of Functional Foods and Novel Bioactives. DOI: https://doi.org/10.1016/B978-0-443-28862-3.00014-5

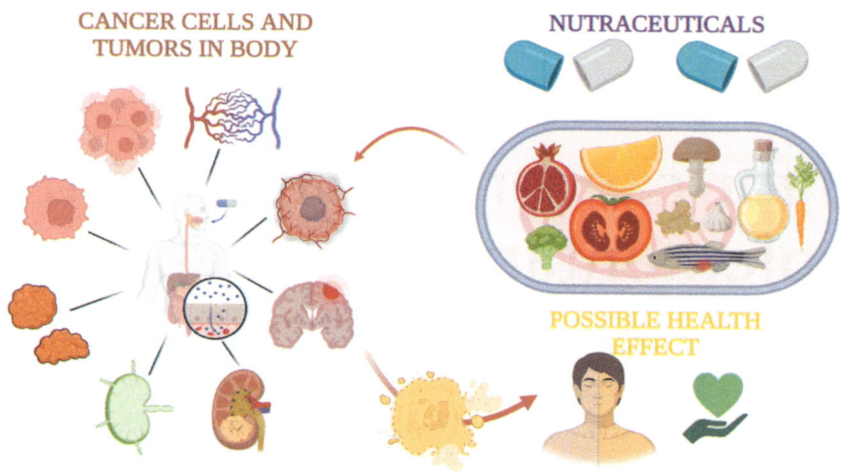

FIGURE 14.1 Functional (bioactive) foods can contribute a good health. *(created with Biorender.com)*

intake of cancer patients. Additional research is required to devise successful strategies for addressing the nutritional requirements of individuals with cancer (Gacche, 2021a; Kim & Je, 2014; Zhang et al., 2015a).

This chapter aims to (1) define functional foods as a supplementary method for managing cancer, (2) investigate different food categories with cancer-fighting properties, (3) study the mechanisms through which functional foods combat cancer, (4) assess epidemiological studies and intervention trials, (5) tackle obstacles related to the use of functional foods in managing cancer, and (6) offer forthcoming suggestions for standardization, personalized nutrition, and incorporation with traditional treatments.

14.2 Functional foods with anticancer properties

Chemoprevention refers to the ability to prevent the development of cancer by using natural or synthetic drugs. Recent scientific discoveries have shown that certain substances found in food, even in small amounts, can have a significant impact on regulating cancer mechanisms. These bioactive foods can be categorized based on their source (plants or animals), their anticancer action (preventing metastasis or angiogenesis, acting as antioxidants, etc.), and the specific chemical components they contain (such as phenolic compounds or carotenoids) (Gupta, 2020; Tripathi et al., 2005).

14.2.1 Fruits and vegetables

Edible fruits and vegetables serve as abundant sources of antioxidants with diverse capabilities. The inclusion of plant-based foods in the human diet yields approximately 8–9 times higher antioxidant capacity, compared to animal-based foods (Grosso et al., 2017; Wall-Medrano & Olivas-Aguirre, 2020). Phytochemicals derived from fruits and vegetables, such as polyphenols, flavonoids, stilbenes, carotenoids, and acetogenins, have demonstrated potential efficacy against cancer cells in both laboratory and animal studies. These natural compounds can impact protein expression through their interaction with transcription factors, as well as potentially influence cellular response, signaling pathways, and epigenetic changes (Kubczak et al., 2021).

According to Table 14.1, several antioxidant assays (ABTS, DPPH, FRAP, BBT, ORAC, TRAP, and so on) have been conducted for determining antioxidant activities of fruits and vegetables. Although the results have been expressed as different antioxidant equivalents, the common one is trolox. Comparing those which have same units among themselves, the maximum antioxidant potential has been detected in cranberry, black chokeberry and cortex of apple (μmol TE/g) (Denev et al., 2018, 2019; Oszmianski et al., 2017; Sethi et al., 2020); zucchini (μg/ml) (Sicari et al., 2022); pineapple (mg/ml) (Huang et al., 2021); cauliflower and apricot (%) (Saeed et al., 2021; Saeedi et al., 2021).

14.2.2 Mushrooms

Mushrooms are often consumed as a functional food, because of their high protein content, low fat content, and low calorie content. They contain various minerals such as iron and phosphorus, as well as vitamins like riboflavin, thiamine, ergosterol (precursor of vitamin D_2), niacin, and ascorbic acid. Additionally, mushrooms contain bioactive compounds such as secondary metabolites and polysaccharides. These bioactive components have been found to possess

TABLE 14.1 Reported Antioxidant Activities of Several Fruits and Vegetables.

Sample	Antioxidant Potential	References
Apple	Peel/cortex: 50.47–192.02/71.79–137.66 μmol TE/g (FRAP) 190.68–411.83/0.48–11.69 μmol TE/g (DPPH) 47.99–185.95/22.94–57.65 μmol TE/g (CUPRAC)	Sethi et al. (2020)
Apricot	51.74%–94.25% (DPPH) 16.86%–60.97% (H_2O_2) 163–379.2 mg AAE/100 g (PMA) 176.8–265.6 mg GAE/100 g (FRAP) 1.018–4.707 mmol TE/100 g (ORAC)	Saeed et al. (2021)
Banana	IC_{50}: 41.2–49.2 μg/mL (in petroleum ether) (DPPH) IC_{50}: 44.4–51.6 μg/mL (in methanol) (DPPH) IC_{50}: 46.4–54.8 μg/mL (in water) (DPPH)	Siji and Nandini (2017)
Blackberry	30.855–48.900 μmol TE/g (TEAC) 201.05–241.06 μmol FE^{+2}/g DM (FRAP) 16.06–51.35 μmol TE/g (ABTS)	Gündogdu et al. (2016); Schulz et al. (2019); Guedes et al. (2017)
Black chokeberry	IC_{50}: 24.6 μg/mL (DPPH) 138.9 μmol TE/g (ORAC) 146.3 μmol TE/g (TRAP) 110.5–191.1 μmol TE/g (ORAC)	Strugala et al. (2016); Denev et al., 2019, 2018)
Blueberry	2627–6747 μmol TE/100 g (ORAC) 859–1754 μmol AAE/100 g (PSC)	Wang et al. (2017)
Broccoli	6.37 μmol TE/g (DPPH) 22.46 μmol TE/g (ABTS) 18.82 μmol FE^{+2}/g (FRAP)	López-Hernández et al. (2022)
Cauliflower	14% (DPPH, Clapton cv.) 129% (DPPH, Graffiti cv.)	Saeedi et al. (2021)
Cranberry	214–320 μmol TE/g DM (DPPH) 189–264 μmol TE/g DM (ABTS) 93.25–139 μmol TE/g DM (FRAP)	Oszmianski et al. (2017)
Eggplant	IC_{50}: 1.24–3.50 mmol TEAC/g (ABTS) IC_{50}: 2.84–3.64 mg/mL (DPPH)	Nwanna et al. (2019)
Grape	8.2–24.4 mM TE/100 g DM (ABTS) 17.7–43.6 mM TE/100 g DM (ORAC)	Samoticha et al. (2018)
Grapefruit	EC_{50}: 5.61–7.21 mg/mL (DPPH, freeze-dried) EC_{50}: 7.60–8.61 mg/mL (DPPH, spray-dried) 270 days after fruit set: Juice: 60.94%–73.69% (DPPH) Peel: 72.58%–83.43% (DPPH) Pulp: 39.82%–54.64% (DPPH)	Agudelo et al. (2017), Singh et al. (2021)
Hawthorn	IC_{50}: 45.9 (DPPH)	Strugala et al. (2016)
Kiwifruit	1.29–5.02 μmol TE/g (DPPH, ascorbic acid extract) 4.31–11.96 μmol TE/g (DPPH, phenol extract) 5.73–25.92 μmol TE/g (FRAP, ascorbic acid extract) 6.22–17.69 μmol TE/g (FRAP, phenol extract)	Zhang et al. (2020)
Leek	6.48–7.04 mM FE^{+2}/g DM (FRAP) 0.90–0.91 mM TE/g DM (DPPH)	Salta et al. (2022)
Lemon	3.10–7.96 μM RE/g (DPPH) 8.79–13.09 μM RE/g (ABTS) 1.08–3.65 μM RE/g (FRAP)	Xi et al. (2017)

(Continued)

TABLE 14.1 (Continued)

Sample	Antioxidant Potential	References
Mandarin	Peel: 11.19–44.40 mg AAE/g DM (DPPH) 64.24–97.31 mg AAE/g DM (ABTS) Pulp residue: 2.13–4.47 mg AAE/g DM (DPPH) 6.75–16.95 mg AAE/g DM (ABTS) Juice: 5.84–28.84 mg AAE/g DM (DPPH) 12.95–47.84 mg AAE/g DM (ABTS)	Zhang et al. (2018)
Orange	IC_{50}: 26.66–38.34 μL (DPPH)	Rapisarda et al. (2008)
Pineapple	EC_{50}: 0.98–5.6 mg/mL (ABTS) 0.66–4.9 mg/mL (DPPH)	Huang et al. (2021)
Pomegranate	Peel: 45%–58% (BBT) Seed: 26%–54% (BBT) Juice: 9%–10% (BBT) Juice: 25.4–69.1 μmol TE/mL (DPPH) 18.4–39.7 μmol TE/mL (FRAP) 14.29–48.83 μmol TE/mL (ABTS)	Derakhshan et al. (2018) and Esposto et al. (2021)
Potato	EC_{50}: 41.815–58.195 mg/mL (DPPH)	Hesam et al. (2012)
Pumpkin	14.41%–24.18% (DPPH)	Abbas et al. (2020)
Rosehip	IC_{50}: 33.5 μg/mL (DPPH)	Strugala et al. (2016)
Sweet potato	3.58–20.15 mg AAE/g DM (DPPH) 0.16–18.71 mg TE/g DM (FRAP) 14.61–26.11 mg AAE/g DM (ABTS)	Kourouma et al. (2020)
Zucchini	41.82% (DPPH) IC_{50}: 20.45 μg/mL (ABTS)	Sicari et al. (2022)

hepatoprotective, immune-stimulating, anticancer, antiviral, and hypocholesterolemic properties. Despite these advantages, mushrooms are not fully utilized, and researchers are currently exploring environment-friendly methods to extract bioactive compounds from edible mushrooms (Kumar et al., 2021). Respecting Nowakowski et al. (2021)'s study, mushroom extracts sourced from a diverse range of 92 species and processed with 12 distinct solvents demonstrated potential for reducing the viability of 38 different types of cancer cells. Breast cancer was found to be responsive to the largest quantity of mushroom extracts.

In Table 14.2, antioxidant potentials of many mushrooms were listed. Mostly, their antioxidant behaviors were given as EC_{50} or IC_{50} values. The EC_{50} value, a measure indicating the concentration required to achieve a 50% antioxidant effect, is frequently employed in the evaluation of antioxidant activity and the comparison of effectiveness among different compounds (Chen et al., 2013). On the other hand, the IC_{50} refers to the concentration of a substance containing antioxidants needed to eliminate half of the initial DPPH/ABTS radicals. A lower IC_{50} value indicates a higher potency in scavenging DPPH/ABTS, thus suggesting a stronger antioxidant activity (Olugbami et al., 2014). *A. bisporus, C. cylindracea, L. squarrosulus, L. tigrinus,* and *Pleurotus* sp. are the edible mushroom varieties with the highest antioxidant activity.

14.2.3 Whole grains

Whole grains have been processed in a way that maintains their original components, such as the starchy endosperm, germ, and bran, in their natural proportions. This procedure involves removing any inedible parts like hulls and husks, while ensuring minimal losses during preparation (Ross et al., 2017; Tieri et al., 2020). Consuming whole grains has been found to be associated with a reduced risk of several types of cancers and overall mortality. The positive effects of whole grains are particularly notable in the gastrointestinal tract, where their consumption is inversely linked to the

TABLE 14.2 Reported Antioxidant Activities of Several Mushroom Types.

Sample	Antioxidant Potential	References
Agaricus bisporus	EC_{50}: 0.083−0.245 mg/mL (DPPH) EC_{50}: 4.83 mg/mL (DPPH) 18.38 μM TE/g DM (ABTS)	Krüzselyi et al. (2020), Fogarasi et al. (2020), Gasecka et al. (2018)
Armillaria mellea	IC_{50}: 1.06−1.32 mg/mL (DPPH)	Erbiai et al. (2021)
Auricularia auricula-judae	IC_{50}: 187.8 μg/mL (DPPH) EC_{50}: 4.60 mg/mL (DPPH)	Gasecka et al. (2018) and Ao and Deb (2019)
Auricularia polytricha	IC_{50}: 130.1 μg/mL (DPPH)	Ao and Deb (2019)
Boletus edulis	97.09 μM TE/g DM (ABTS)	Fogarasi et al. (2020)
Cantharellus cibarius	12.50 μM TE/g DM (ABTS) EC_{50}: 4.84 mg/mL (DPPH)	Fogarasi et al. (2020) and Gasecka et al. (2018)
Cyclocybe cylindracea	EC_{50}: 0.058−0.089 mg/mL (DPPH)	Krüzselyi et al. (2020)
Flammulina velutipes	EC_{50}: 5.129−19.57 mg/mL (DPPH)	Krüzselyi et al. (2020)
Grifola frondosa	0.19 μmol TE/mg (ORAC) 13.9 μmol Fe^{2+}/g (FRAP) EC_{50}: 4.57 mg/mL (DPPH)	Gasecka et al. (2018) and Sharpe et al. (2021)
Hericium erinaceus	0.026 μmol TE/mg (ORAC) 3.5 μmol Fe^{2+}/g (FRAP)	Sharpe et al. (2021)
Inonotus obliquus	0.63 μmol TE/mg (ORAC) 81.6 μmol Fe^{2+}/g (FRAP)	Sharpe et al. (2021)
Lactarius piperatus	11.15 μM TE/g DM (ABTS)	Fogarasi et al. (2020)
Lactifluus piperatus	IC_{50}: 157.7 μg/mL (DPPH)	Ao and Deb (2019)
Laetiporus sulphureus	IC_{50}: 95.1 μg/mL (DPPH)	Ao and Deb (2019)
Leccinum duriusculum	EC_{50}: 0.103−0.266 mg/mL (DPPH)	Krüzselyi et al. (2020)
Lentinula edodes	EC_{50}: 0.129−0.213 mg/mL (DPPH) 0.030 μmol TE/mg (ORAC) 1.7 μmol Fe^{2+}/g (FRAP) IC_{50}: 137.4 μg/mL (DPPH)	Krüzselyi et al. (2020), Ao and Deb (2019), and Sharpe et al. (2021)
Lentinus sajor-caju	IC_{50}: 137.9 μg/mL (DPPH)	Ao and Deb (2019)
Lentinus squarrosulus	IC_{50}: 82.6 μg/mL (DPPH)	Ao and Deb (2019)
Lentinus tigrinus	IC_{50}: 47.5 μg/mL (DPPH)	Ao and Deb (2019)
Macrolepiota procera	EC_{50}: 3.55 mg/mL (DPPH)IC_{50}: 1.19−1.31 mg/mL (DPPH)	Gasecka et al. (2018) and Erbiai et al. (2021)
Morchella esculenta	EC_{50}: 3.09 mg/mL (DPPH)	Gasecka et al. (2018)
Pleurotus eryngii	EC_{50}: 0.171−6.331 mg/mL (DPPH)	Krüzselyi et al. (2020)
Pleurotus levis	EC_{50}: 0.51 μg/mL (DPPH) EC_{50}: 0.50 μg/mL (ABTS)	Adebayo et al. (2018)
Pleurotus ostreatus	EC_{50}: 0.246−13.91 mg/mL (DPPH) EC_{50}: 0.63−1.05 μg/mL (DPPH) EC_{50}: 0.24−0.42 μg/mL (ABTS) 27.17 μM TE/g DM (ABTS)	Krüzselyi et al. (2020), Fogarasi et al. (2020), and Adebayo et al. (2018)
Pleurotuspulmonarius	EC_{50}: 0.49−0.70 μg/mL (DPPH) EC_{50}: 0.35−0.37 μg/mL (ABTS)	Adebayo et al. (2018)
Pleurotus tuber-regium	EC_{50}: 1.68 μg/mL (DPPH) EC_{50}: 0.50 μg/mL (ABTS)	Adebayo et al. (2018)
Schizophyllum commune	IC_{50}: 153.1 μg/mL (DPPH)	Ao and Deb (2019)
Termitomyces heimii	IC_{50}: 107.2 μg/mL (DPPH)	Ao and Deb (2019)
Trametes versicolor	0.036 μmol TE/mg (ORAC) 0.2 μmol Fe^{2+}/g (FRAP)	Sharpe et al. (2021)

TABLE 14.3 Reported Antioxidant Activities of Some Whole Grains.

Sample	Antioxidant Potential	References
Barley	0.251–0.354 μmol ABTS/g DM (30 min) 274–581.19 μmol TE/100 g (DPPH) 351.30–843.54 μmol TE/100 g (FRAP) 64%–69% (winter) (DPPH) 56%–65% (spring) (DPPH)	Gamel and Abdel-Aal (2012), Rao et al. (2020), and Horvat et al. (2020)
Corn	37%–45% (DPPH) 2.46–5.17 μmol TE/g flour (FRAP) 7.85–11.94 μmol TE/g flour (CUPRAC)	Horvat et al. (2020) and Capocchi et al. (2017)
Millet	2.1–6.6 μmol TE/g DM (finger) (TEAC) 0.8–5.2 μmol TE/g DM (foxtail) (TEAC) 0.3–2.5 μmol TE/g DM (proso) (TEAC)	Kumari et al. (2017)
Oat	149.81–239.65 μmol TE/100 g (DPPH) 104.58–298.76 μmol TE/100 g (FRAP)	Rao et al. (2020)
Rice	0.05–0.19 μmol TE/g (white, free) (DPPH) 0.19–1.66 μmol TE/g (red, free) (DPPH) 1.04–3.72 μmol TE/g (black, free) (DPPH) 0.13–0.25 μmol TE/g (white, free) (ABTS) 0.27–2.66 μmol TE/g (red, free) (ABTS) 1.89–6.19 μmol TE/g (black, free) (ABTS)	Pang et al. (2018)
Rye	302.30–1570.49 mg TE/kg (ABTS) 120.68–3041.34 mg TE/kg (DPPH) 2277–5365.82 mg TE/kg (FRAP) 879.69–20104.58 mg TE/kg (RP)	Kulichová et al. (2019)
Wheat	13%–15% (DPPH) 42.4–47.6 μmol TE/g DM (ABTS)	Horvat et al. (2020) and Ma et al. (2015)

occurrence of colorectal tumors. This can be ascribed to the existence of advantageous components such as dietary fiber and polyphenolic compounds, which are often lost during the milling process. Despite the acknowledged health advantages, whole grains are not consumed in sufficient quantities in the majority of countries (Tullio et al., 2021).

In Table 14.3, antioxidant measurements conducted in cereal whole grains were summarized. Depending on their types, cultivars, harvest times, and testing methods, bioactivity of cereals varied. Barley and wheat have strikingly high antioxidant activity, when compared to other cereals, and among rice varieties, black one stands out for its high antioxidant capacity.

14.2.4 Marine products

Marine organisms such as algae, seaweeds, corals, and ascidians are important sources of bioactive compounds and potential drug candidates. These organisms, which make up over 90% of oceanic biomass, provide a wide range of pharmacologically active and unique chemical compounds, presenting a significant opportunity for the discovery of new anticancer agents. These marine environments harbor powerful molecules that contribute to life sustainability and act as natural defenses against various microorganisms and organisms. Despite their abundance, the potential of marine flora and fauna in the context of anticancer properties remains largely unexplored. Nevertheless, in recent times, significant advancements have been made in isolating, characterizing, and evaluating marine compounds for their potential use in treating cancer (Wali et al., 2019).

Omega-3 fatty acids are essential polyunsaturated fats known for their antiinflammatory properties, specifically eicosapentaenoic acid (EPA) and docosahexaenoic acid (DHA) found in marine sources (Table 14.4). Research suggests that EPA and DHA may be beneficial in reducing the risk of breast, colon, and prostate cancers by reducing inflammation, inhibiting aromatase activity, inducing cell differentiation and apoptosis, and improving insulin sensitivity. The ideal ratio of EPA to DHA for cancer prevention and the minimum effective dose have not been definitively

TABLE 14.4 Reported Omega-3 Amounts of Some Marine Products (Cretton et al., 2023).

Sample	Omega-3 Fatty Acid Content (mg/100 g)	References
Atlantic mackerel	EPA: 420–1700 EPA_{liver}: 420 DHA: 420–1000 DHA_{liver}: 1430	Rincón-Cervera et al. (2009) and Guil-Guerrero et al. (2011)
Atlantic salmon	EPA: 330–960 DHA: 650–1050	Rincón-Cervera et al. (2009) and Kolanowski (2021)
European anchovy	EPA: 1067 EPA_{liver}: 840 DHA: 1071 DHA_{liver}: 1738	Guil-Guerrero et al. (2011) and Tufan et al. (2011)
Microalgae (*Crypthecodinium cohni, Nannochloropsis* sp., *Phaeodactylum tricornutum, Schizochytrium* sp., *Tisochrysis lutea, Ulkenia* sp.)	EPA: 2250–4000 DHA: <50–2700	Paz et al. (2020), Durmaz et al. (2007), Chang et al. (2014), Cui et al. (2021), Hu et al. (2019), Zittelli et al. (1999)
Mussel	EPA: 260 DHA: 338	Cherifi et al. (2018)
Oyster	EPA: 794 DHA: 957	Abdulkadir and Tsuchiya (2008)

Adapted from Cretton, M., Malanga, G., Sobczuk, T. M., & Mazzuca, M. (2023). Marine lipids as a source of high-quality fatty acids and antioxidants. *Food Reviews International, 39*, 4941–4964.

established, but it is likely to be greater than 600 mg/day, significantly higher than the current average intake in the United States (Fabian & Kimler, 2013).

14.2.5 Spices

Throughout history, spices and herbs have been recognized for their traditional taste, scent, and medicinal attributes. The growing prevalence of chronic and widespread medical conditions and the rising expenses associated with modern pharmaceutical treatments have sparked a significant research interest in investigating the diverse properties of herbal spices (Kammath et al., 2021). The bioactive compounds present in these spices exhibit properties as antioxidants (Table 14.5), antiinflammatory agents, modulators of immune function, and inducers of apoptosis in tumor cells. These compounds have the potential to be beneficial as standalone treatments or as supplementary agents. Their biological effects are attributed to their capacity to induce epigenetic alterations, including methylation, acetylation, ubiquitination, and inhibition of lipid peroxidation. The favorable aspect of these spices lies in their low toxicity, making them promising candidates as chemopreventive agents (Gao et al., 2021).

14.2.6 Olive oil

Olive oil, a highly intricate composition, is a quintessential element of the Mediterranean diet. It serves as the primary source of fats and is utilized in the culinary preparation of dishes, whether as a raw ingredient in recipes or for cooking purposes (Battino et al., 2019). Olive oil demonstrates various chemopreventive effects associated with the stages of carcinogenesis, attributed to the biological properties of its bioactive components such as hydroxytyrosol, squalene, oleanolic acid, and polyphenols. These compounds have the ability to mitigate cellular oxidative stress and DNA damage caused by reactive oxygen metabolites, as well as regulate cellular mechanisms and signaling pathways pertinent to carcinogenesis (Battino et al., 2019; López-Miranda et al., 2010; Warleta et al., 2010). Multiple studies have demonstrated the antiproliferative and pro-apoptotic properties of oleuropein and hydroxytyrosol on a range of cancer types, such as breast, colorectal, lung, leukemia, and prostate cancer cell lines. Furthermore, oleocanthal has exhibited the ability to induce cell death or impede proliferation and migration in diverse cancer cell lines, including multiple

TABLE 14.5 Reported Antioxidant Activities of Some Spices.

Sample	Antioxidant Potential	References
Cardamom	9.24–21.90 μmol TE/g DM (ethanol, CUPRAC) 3.83–9.28 μmol TE/g DM (ethyl acetate, CUPRAC)	Nurcholis et al. (2021)
Chili pepper	IC_{50}: 0.2174 ppm (DPPH)	Akor et al. (2024)
Cinnamon	IC_{50}: $0.0162 + 7.5 \times 10^{-4}$ mg/mL (ethanol, DPPH) IC_{50}: $0.1069 + 1.7 \times 10^{-3}$ mg/mL (ethanol-acetone, DPPH) IC_{50}: $0.0397 + 7.0 \times 10^{-4}$ mg/mL (acetone, DPPH)	Rahayu et al. (2022)
Cloves	45%–52% (DPPH)	Alexandru et al. (2013)
Garlic	0.13 mg AAE/g (DPPH) 0.05 mg AAE/g (FRAP) 0.32 mg AAE/g (ABTS)	Yang et al. (2020)
Ginger	0.22 mg AAE/g (DPPH) 0.08 mg AAE/g (FRAP) 1.15 mg AAE/g (ABTS)	Yang et al. (2020)
Saffron	Leaves: 62.7–64.6 mg AAE/g (FRAP) IC_{50}: 488–560 μg/mL (DPPH)	Lahmass et al. (2018)
Turmeric	70.9 mg/L GAE (DPPH)	Permatananda et al. (2021)

myeloma cells. These discoveries underscore the promising therapeutic potential of oleuropein and hydroxytyrosol for cancer treatment, while preserving the integrity of normal cells (Akl et al., 2014; Boss et al., 2016; Casapullo et al., 2016; Farooqi et al., 2017; LeGendre et al., 2015; Nan et al., 2014; Rafehi et al., 2012; Ray et al., 2019).

14.3 Mechanisms of action

14.3.1 Antioxidant effects

Reactive oxygen species (ROS) encompass various oxygen-containing chemicals that react with lipids, proteins, and DNA, with different types exhibiting distinct reactivities and biological targets. Mitochondria and NADPH oxidases (NOXs) are primary sources of ROS, particularly generating superoxide which can be converted to hydrogen peroxide (H_2O_2) (Fig. 14.2). While superoxide is produced within mitochondria via complexes I, II, and III of the electron transport chain, NOX_2 generates superoxide extracellularly by transferring electrons from NADPH to oxygen. H_2O_2, a stable form of ROS, can modulate cellular signaling by interacting with specific cysteine residues on target proteins and readily diffuses through membranes, unlike superoxide and hydroxyl radicals. Mitochondria and NOX proteins can localize to ROS-responsive signaling proteins, influencing cellular responses to produced ROS (Cockfield & Schafer, 2019; Glasauer & Chandel, 2014).

ROS play a role in cancer genesis by regulating cell signaling processes (Fig. 14.2). In the process of cancer progression, a persistent condition of oxidative stress occurs due to decreased levels of endogenous antioxidants, such as superoxide dismutase and glutathione peroxidase, as well as exogenous antioxidants like vitamins A, C, E, β-carotene, and selenium (Bavatharani, 2023; Fuchs-Tarlovsky, 2013). Oxidative stress has the potential to impact various functions of cancer cells, such as their ability to multiply, their genetic stability and mutation patterns, changes in their responsiveness towards anticancer drugs, invasion capabilities, and potential for metastasis (Serna-Thomé et al., 2018). Oxidative stress induces tumor angiogenesis by promoting the upregulation of angiogenic factors such as interleukin-8 and vascular endothelial growth factor, as well as the release of matrix metalloproteinase-1, which are facilitated by the presence of ROS. In a study conducted on patients diagnosed with bladder cancer, it was noted that an imbalance in redox status exhibited a significant association with the severity and progression of the disease. This association was attributed to a reduction in the concentrations of antioxidant vitamins and enzymes. The process of chemoradiotherapy treatment induces an increment in oxidative stress levels, subsequently resulting in detrimental consequences that undermine the overall well-being and satisfaction of the patient. The levels of antioxidants are diminished during the period of cancer detection and during the course of treatment, potentially impacting the functioning of vital organs like the

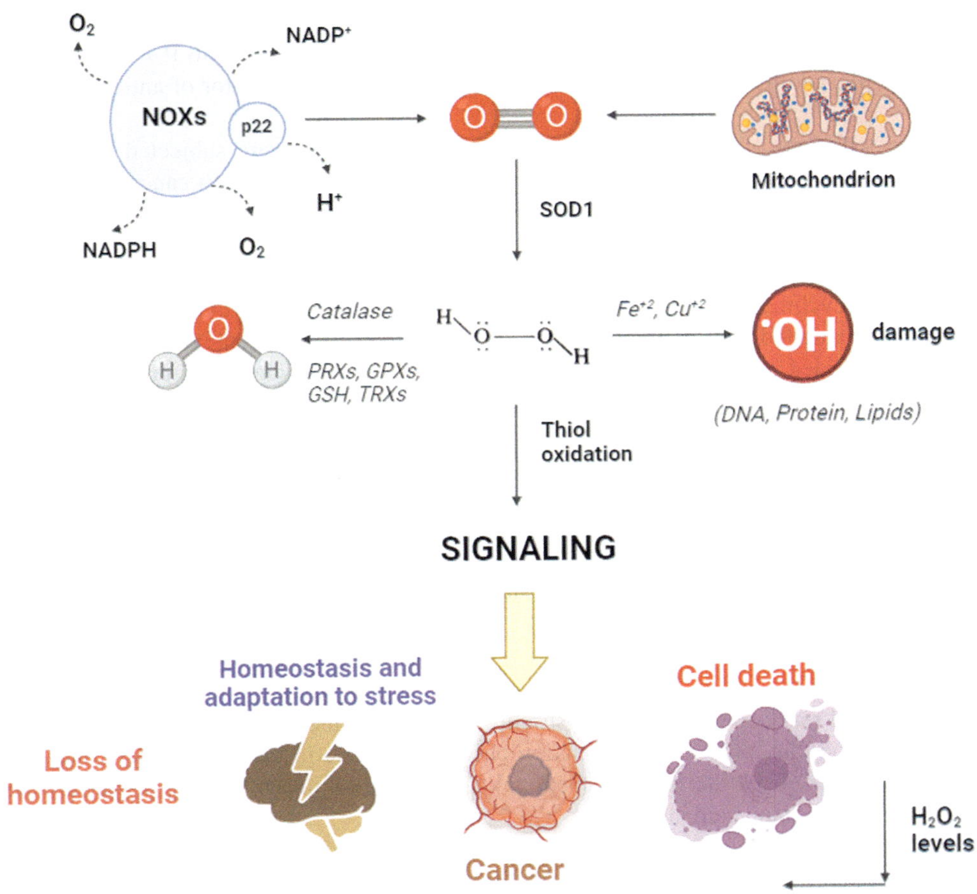

FIGURE 14.2 The origins, control mechanisms, and biological effects of ROS. *(Adapted from Glasauer, A., & Chandel, N. S. (2014). Targeting antioxidants for cancer therapy.* Biochemical Pharmacology, 92, *90–101, created with Biorender.com)*

heart, lungs, and central nervous system (Bavatharani, 2023). Therefore the use of antioxidants as preventative measures in the prevention and treatment of cancer has been suggested, and they may also mitigate the adverse effects of treatment and enhance the overall well-being of patients (Fuchs-Tarlovsky, 2013).

However, significant controversies about this matter as numerous clinical trials have yielded conflicting findings regarding the effectiveness of antioxidants in the treatment of cancer. While some researches indicate that, antioxidants or antioxidant supplements should not be employed as replacements for cancer treatments due to their potential impact on treatment efficacy, alternative studies propose that antioxidants, specifically vitamins C and E, could potentially improve the efficacy of chemotherapy and radiation therapy, while also ameliorating therapy-induced adverse effects, thereby improving overall quality of life (Khurana et al., 2013). Nevertheless, the potential involvement of cellular DNA and cell membrane degradation through oxidative processes, which is considered an essential aspect of the anticancer drug mechanism, cannot be disregarded (Guo et al., 2014; Yang et al., 2015). Significantly, the utilization of antioxidants has been linked to cancer survivors for the purpose of addressing a range of disorders and pathophysiologies. Some studies have revealed the efficacy of antioxidants as palliative agents and their ability to mitigate the toxic adverse effects of cancer therapy (Bavatharani, 2023). Moreover, extensive researches demonstrate that consuming a diet abundant in fruits and vegetables, primarily due to the presence of natural polyphenols, may potentially reduce the possibility of cancer genesis (Bavatharani, 2023; Gacche, 2021b; Zhang et al., 2016a).

In a study involved 43 patients recently diagnosed with solid tumors, who were administered a ginger extract supplement alongside moderate-to-high emetogenic adjuvant chemotherapy. The findings revealed that, ginger extract supplementation led to an increase in blood levels of antioxidant enzymes and a reduction in oxidative stress. Importantly, no serious adverse effects were observed with the daily intake of ginger extract as a supplement during the treatment (Danwilai et al., 2017). Similarly in (Ma et al. (2014) research, clinical research involving 27 ovarian cancer patients, vitamin C supplementation was explored during paclitaxel and carboplatin treatment. The results indicated a reduction in chemotherapy-related toxicities with the administration of vitamin C. However, despite this positive outcome, no statistically significant improvement in overall survival was observed. In a study conducted by Paredes-Gonzalez et al. (2014), the regulatory effects of apigenin on oxidative stress were investigated. The researchers observed that, apigenin could reverse hypermethylation occurring at 15 CpG sites within the promoter region of the Nrf2 gene in JB6 P + skin epidermal cells. This hypermethylation was implicated in the silencing of the Nrf2 gene, a critical modulator of antioxidant and detoxification enzymes.

In another study, resveratrol along with two of its derivatives, viniferin and labruscol, were subjected to in vitro experimentation using melanoma cells (Kim et al., 2016). The properties of resveratrol in relation to cancer have been extensively investigated, revealing significant antiinflammatory, antioxidant, and antiproliferative effects (Lançon et al., 2016). Initially, a cytostatic effect was observed, succeeded by a cytotoxic response, leading to subsequent apoptosis and necrosis specifically targeting tumor cells while sparing fibroblasts. Notably, resveratrol was found to downregulate cyclin D1 expression while upregulating cyclin A2, E1, Cdk1, and Cdk2, thereby causing cell cycle arrest at the S phase. The two derivatives of resveratrol exhibited similar albeit less pronounced effects in this context.

The review by Vance et al. (2013) provided a comprehensive overview of dietary antioxidants and prostate cancer, highlighting the potential protective effects of tea and coffee against advanced prostate cancer. This review contributes to the understanding of specific dietary antioxidants and their impact on prostate cancer, offering valuable insights into the potential role of antioxidant-rich beverages in prostate cancer prevention.

In a study by Yong et al. (2013), the antioxidant and antiproliferative properties of *Clinacanthus nutans* extracts were investigated, demonstrating their potential as adjunctive regimens for cancer prevention or treatment. This study contributes to the growing body of evidence supporting the antioxidant and antiproliferative effects of natural compounds, offering promising avenues for complementary approaches in cancer management.

14.3.2 Antiinflammatory effects

Inflammation is a complicated physiological reaction to detrimental stimuli, including pathogens, cellular injury, or irritants (He et al., 2022a). It is well understood that, chronic inflammation plays a vital role in the development and progression of different diseases, such as cancer. Thus the use of functional foods with antiinflammatory properties has been explored as a possible strategy for cancer management.

Polyphenols and phytochemicals derived from plants have been shown to have antiinflammatory impacts through various molecular signaling pathways (Upadhyay & Dixit, 2015). It has been indicated that, these compounds possess the ability to eliminate ROS and enhance antioxidant levels, consequently mitigating the functioning of NF-κB and inhibiting the production of inflammatory cytokines and chemokines (Tian et al., 2021). Additionally, compounds such as calophyllolide, isolated from *Calophyllum inophyllum* Linn, have demonstrated antiinflammatory and wound-healing activities (Nguyen et al., 2017). The antiinflammatory activity of calophyllolide is based on its ability to reduce inflammation mediators and modulate gene expression related to inflammation (Nguyen et al., 2017).

Furthermore, natural ingredients such as scandoside and velvet bean leaf extract have been found to exert antiinflammatory impacts by suppressing NF-κB and MAPK signaling pathways (Fadilaturahmah et al., 2023; He et al., 2018). Similarly, chitooligosaccharides and chitobiose have been shown to modulate inflammatory signaling in macrophages, highlighting their potential as antiinflammatory agents (Hao et al., 2023; Jitprasertwong et al., 2021). These findings suggest that, functional foods containing these bioactive compounds may offer promising antiinflammatory effects for cancer management.

Moreover, the review of Brazilian medicinal plants has corroborated their antiinflammatory activities, indicating the potential of plant extracts in managing inflammation-related conditions (Ribeiro et al., 2018). Additionally, the antiinflammatory effects of docosahexaenoic acid (DHA) have been demonstrated in studies on carrageenan-induced paw edema in rats, further supporting the role of specific dietary components in modulating inflammation (Singhal et al., 2020).

In conclusion, the antiinflammatory effects of functional foods play a vital role in cancer management. The bioactive compounds present in these foods have been shown to modulate various inflammatory signaling pathways, scavenge ROS, and suppress the expression of inflammatory mediators. These outcomes underscore the potential of functional foods as a complementary approach to cancer management through their antiinflammatory properties.

14.3.3 Immune modulation (immunoregulation)

Immune modulation, also known as immunoregulation, refers to the process of regulating the immune system's activity to maintain homeostasis and prevent excessive immune responses (He et al., 2022b). This regulation involves a complex interplay of various factors, including cytokines, immune cells, and regulatory molecules, to ensure an appropriate response to pathogens and other challenges while avoiding autoimmunity and hypersensitivity reactions (Huaux, 2021).

The immune system's ability to modulate its responses is crucial for overall health and plays a significant role in various physiological and pathological conditions, including cancer management (Criscitiello et al., 2014).

Functional foods, such as those containing polyphenols and probiotics, have been studied for their potential immunomodulatory effects. Polyphenols, found in red wine grapes and nuts, have been shown to possess antiinflammatory properties, which can modulate immune responses (Buljeta et al., 2023). Similarly, probiotics have been recognized for their ability to modulate immune function, particularly in the gastrointestinal tract, and have shown beneficial effects in modulating diverse immune disorders (Tenta et al., 2017). Panax ginseng has been studied for their immunoregulatory effects and has also been shown to possess immunoregulatory activity, which can modulate the immune response through its interaction with macrophages (Hao et al., 2019). Additionally, the microbiota composition, diet, and antibiotic use have been identified as contributing factors to immunoregulation, highlighting the intricate relationship between diet and the immune system (Rook et al., 2014). Furthermore, the complement system, a key component of the immune response, has been implicated in modulating tumor growth, antitumor immunity, and angiogenesis, emphasizing its role in immunoregulation and cancer progression (Kolev & Markiewski, 2018).

Furthermore, the microbiota, particularly certain indigenous intestinal bacteria, has been implicated in the induction of regulatory T cells that are essential for maintaining immune homeostasis and preventing excessive inflammation. This highlights the intricate relationship between the gut microbiota and immune regulation, with potential implications for cancer management (Zheng et al., 2020).

In addition to dietary factors, parasitic infections, such as helminth infections, have been associated with immunoregulatory effects. Studies have suggested that, helminth infections may have beneficial effects on chronic immune disorders, including allergies, autoimmune diseases, and alloimmune responses. The immunomodulatory properties of helminths underscore the complex interactions between the immune system and parasitic organisms, with potential implications for cancer immunotherapy (McSorley & Maizels, 2012).

Exosomes, small extracellular vesicles, have also been recognized for their involvement in immunoregulation in the context of cancer. Tumor-derived exosomes have been found to affect immunoregulation mechanisms, including immune activation and suppression, to support neoplastic growth and metastasis (Zhang et al., 2016c). Moreover, the neddylation pathway has been identified as playing a pivotal role in immune-related diseases, such as infection, inflammation and cancer, further underscoring the intricate regulatory mechanisms involved in immunoregulation (Lu & Yang, 2020).

Moreover, the role of cytokines and growth factors, such as those belonging to the TGF-β superfamily, in immunoregulation has, been extensively studied. These signaling molecules play crucial roles in modulating immune responses in the context of infection, inflammation, and cancer. The dysregulation of these immunoregulatory pathways can have profound implications for cancer progression and the tumor microenvironment (Sanjabi et al., 2017).

In the context of cancer management, understanding tissue-specific immunoregulation, or "tissue-specific immunostats," has been highlighted as crucial for advancing cancer treatments (Pao et al., 2018). Additionally, research has investigated the potential of schistosome-associated factors to act as therapeutic agents in modulating the immune system, indicating that specific infections may offer therapeutic benefits in the management of chronic immune disorders such as allergies and autoimmune diseases (Li et al., 2020).

In summary, immunoregulation encompasses a complex network of interactions and regulatory mechanisms that are essential for maintaining immune homeostasis. The references provided offer insights into the diverse aspects of immunoregulation, ranging from the effects of functional foods and microbiota composition to the potential therapeutic implications for cancer management and other immune-related disorders.

14.4 Clinical evidence (epidemiological studies and interventional trials)

Epidemiological studies investigate the link between functional food consumption and cancer risk. Due to confounding variables, including diet adherence and carcinogen exposure, observational research on functional foods may generate erroneous results. These researches cannot prove causation. Rare randomized controlled trials (RCTs) that seek causal links have ambiguous consequences. RCTs are the best way to establish causal linkages, despite the challenges of long-term patient follow-up. Many RCTs are needed to determine functional meal effects. Epidemiological research and interventional trials on functional diets or its components are summarized in Fig. 14.3.

14.4.1 Polyphenols

Polyphenols are found in many foods such as tea, green tea, red wine, cocoa, berries, cranberries, pomegranates, and papaya. There is evidence that, they influence tumor development and carcinogenesis (Adhami et al., 2009).

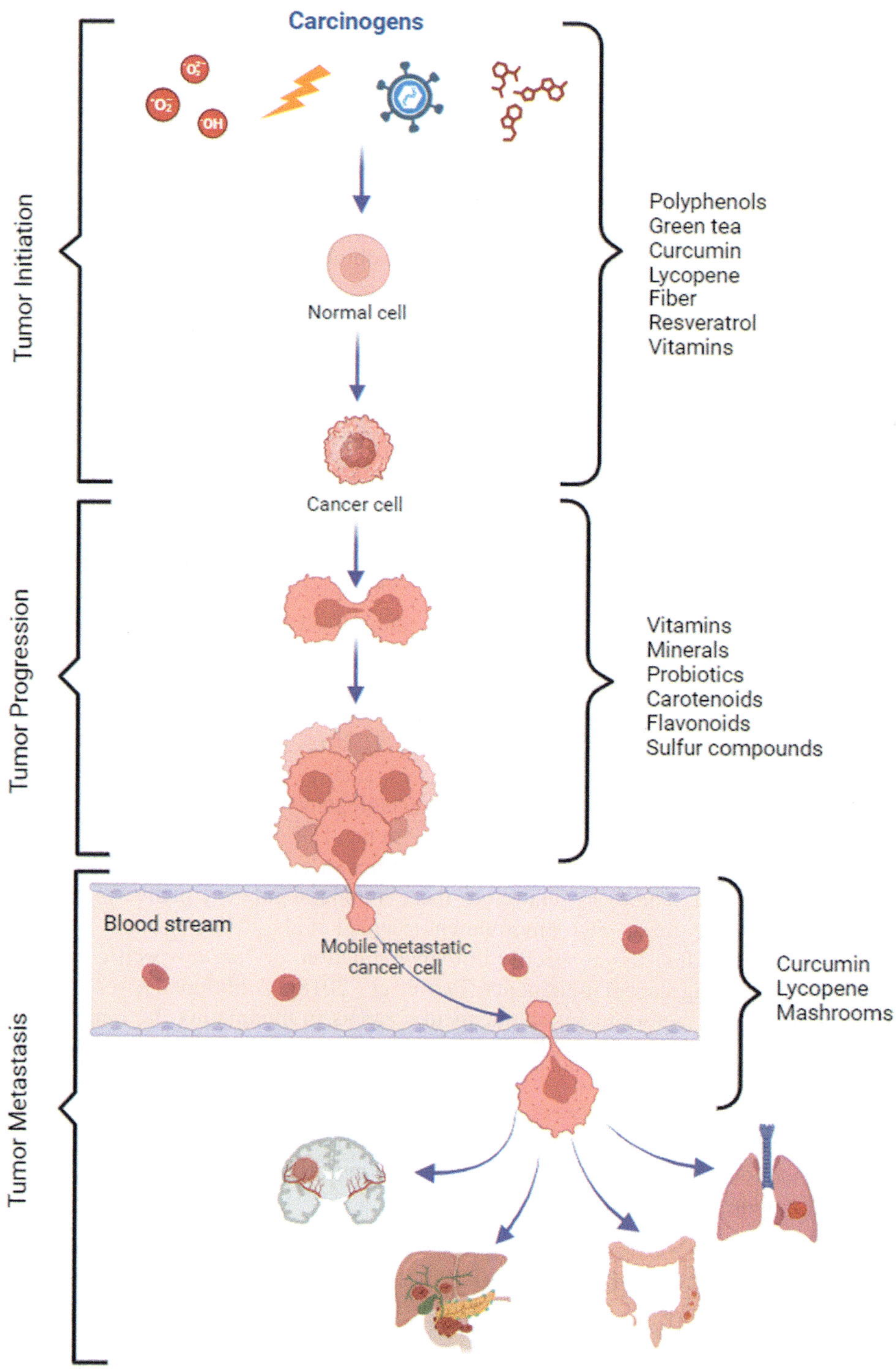

FIGURE 14.3 Potential anticancer roles of certain functional foods. *(Adapted from Islam, S. R., & Siddiqua, T. J. (2020). Functional foods in cancer prevention and therapy: Recent epidemiological findings.* Functional Foods in Cancer Prevention and Therapy, *405–433, Created with Biorender.com)*

14.4.1.1 Curcumin

There is a limited number of human investigations on curcumin, which is a polyphenol found in turmeric. As a result, our understanding of its mechanisms in relation to cancer is incomplete (Lao et al., 2006). Nevertheless, via a multitude of in vivo and in vitro investigations, it has been discovered that, there are inhibitory effects on the growth of tumors, the formation of new blood vessels, and the spread of cancer cells through the regulation of several cellular signaling pathways (Kumar et al., 2016; Shanmugam et al., 2015). Furthermore, another study has demonstrated that it can enhance the efficacy of chemotherapy and safeguard healthy cells against oxidative harm caused by radiation therapy

(Verma, 2016). A meta analysis of five randomized clinical studies revealed that, the consumption of curcumin resulted in certain favorable outcomes, while it did not have a substantial impact on survival (De Waure et al., 2023). Curcumin, when used as an additional treatment, has been shown to enhance remission in patients with myeloma (Santosa et al., 2022), improve outcomes in patients with advanced metastatic breast cancer, when combined with paclitaxel (Saghatelyan et al., 2020), and produce much superior results compared to placebo in a phase II research involving patients with oral leukoplakia (Kuriakose et al., 2016), with a success rate of 75%. Negligible toxicity was observed in phase 1 human investigation, when individuals were administered single oral dosages of up to 12 g/day or oral intakes of 8 g daily for a duration of 3 months (Mahran et al., 2017; Ono et al., 2015). Although human studies reported few negative effects, certain animals exhibited carcinogenic effects such as hepatic adenomas and interstitial intestinal cancer. Consequently, further research on safety is required (Kumar et al., 2016).

14.4.1.2 Green tea

The advantageous properties of green tea are ascribed to its polyphenol content, particularly catechin and epigallocatechin-3-gallate (EGCG) (Lee et al., 2014; Yuan, 2013; Zheng et al., 2017). Epidemiological evidence indicates that, consuming green tea has a positive effect in preventing the development of oral-digestive tract cancer or precancerous lesions in the oral cavity (Yuan, 2013). A population-based meta analysis study involving 163,810 individuals has revealed that consuming green tea has a beneficial impact on breast cancers (Lee et al., 2014). A case control research found that, women who consumed high amounts of green tea had a 19% reduced likelihood of developing breast cancer compared to those who consumed low amounts of green tea (Zheng et al., 2017). The findings of clinical or epidemiological studies investigating the impact of green tea on cancer have been inconclusive. This may be attributed to confounding factors associated with the preparation and consumption of tea, as well as the patient's lifestyle and dietary habits.

14.4.2 Stilbenes

Grapes, berries, peanuts, and Japanese knotweed roots contain resveratrol, specifically trans-3,5,4-trihydroxystilbene. Resveratrol's effects on cancer signaling pathways have been studied in vitro and in vivo (Iskandar & Hodgson, 2013; Wu et al., 2004). Due to its antioxidant properties, resveratrol may prevent cancer, according to these researches. Epidemiological models of breast, colon, prostate, liver, and pancreatic cancers provide inconsistent data (Sporn et al., 2011).

14.4.3 Carotenoids

The most well-known carotenoids that lower cancer risk are lycopene, alpha-, and beta-carotene (Boyanapalli & Kong, 2015; Hyun et al., 2006). Through antioxidant, antiproliferative, and immunological modulation, it possesses anticancer effects (Jiang et al., 2013). It is abundant in carrots (alpha and beta-carotenes) and tomatoes (lycopene). Tomato eating and its derivatives are inversely associated with stomach cancer risk in 11 and 6 cohort studies. Tomato products lowered stomach cancer risk by 27% in high-dose consumers (Yore et al., 2011). A phase II study found that lycopene affects prostate cancer patients' PSA levels (Petiwala & Johnson, 2015). Eight prospective breast cancer trials using carotenoids show encouraging results. Alpha-carotene reduced risk by 22%, beta-carotene by 13%, lycopene by 17%, and total carotenoids by 19% at the greatest and lowest intakes, respectively (Jin et al., 2016). For 20 years, 18,743 women were examined for plasma carotenoid levels in a case control study. Women with high carotenoid levels had a reduced risk of breast cancer by 18%–28% and recurrence by 68% (Dou et al., 2015). A study of ER-negative breast cancer patients found a 59% risk reduction in those with high beta-carotene levels and a 39% reduction in those with high alpha-carotene levels. Alpha-carotene lowered lung cancer risk by 34% and beta-carotenes by 16% (Boyanapalli & Kong, 2015). Pancreatic cancer risk is reduced by 26% with carotenoid intake (Hyun et al., 2006). However, some carotenoid research has found unfavorable results. After four years of giving 30 mg/day of beta-carotene and 25,000 IU of retinol palmitate to over 18,000 people at high risk of lung cancer due to smoking or asbestos exposure, the study was stopped, because the supplement increased the risk of death (Grover & Samson, 2010).

14.4.4 Flavonoids

14.4.4.1 Epigallocatechin gallate

One of the most studied flavonoids in green tea is EGCG. In vivo and in vitro studies have demonstrated that EGCG can affect EGFR, JAK/STAT, PI3K/AKT/mTOR, MAPK, and other signaling pathways in many cancer types

(Kciuk et al., 2023). EGCG targets epigenetic modulators to regulate DNA methylation and histone changes (Kciuk et al., 2023). EGCG clinical and epidemiological investigations are inconclusive. EGCG intake has been linked to high tea or green tea intake in various studies. Zhang et al. (2015b) found that, EGCG intake did not significantly reduce the risk of numerous malignancies, but it did reduce mouth cancer risk. Large tea drinking has also been linked to a lower bladder cancer risk in Western countries (Zhang et al., 2015b). Some Asian studies link green tea drinking to mortality (Shin et al., 2022). Positive results coexist with inefficient or erratic ones. A 400-mg daily EGCG supplement did not lower prostate cancer risk in men with high-grade prostatic intraepithelial neoplasia (Kumar et al., 2015). Epidemiological studies have revealed confusing effects of green tea on colorectal, esophageal, and stomach cancers (Kim et al., 2019; Sang et al., 2013; Zhou et al., 2008).

14.4.4.2 Soybeans (daidzein, genistein, and glycitein)

Soybean (*Glycine max*) isoflavones are best recognized for their competitive agonist activity against the estrogen receptor (ER) due to their chemical structures comparable to real estrogen. Many studies have demonstrated that isoflavone-rich soy products may reduce the risk of many malignancies, notably hormone-dependent tumors (Messina et al., 1994). The greatest soybean dose in breast cancer patients reduced death risk by 14% and recurrence risk by 26% (Chi et al., 2013). In an interventional research, a soy supplement with 154 mg/day of isoflavones for one month reduced breast cancer biomarkers estrogen and progesterone (Messina & Loprinzi, 2001). A prospective cohort study of 70,578 Chinese women followed for 13.2 years found an inverse relationship between soybean dietary intake and breast cancer risk. The greatest dose of soy protein, 16.4 g/day, reduced risk by 22% for women. The effect was considerably stronger for pre-menopausal women (54% risk reduction) (Baglia et al., 2016). In another trial, soy consumption reduced breast cancer risk by 28% for postmenopausal women with ER + /EP + and 54% for pre-menopausal women with ER − /EP − .

14.4.5 Mushrooms

Common medicinal mushrooms include *Ganoderma lucidum* (reishi), *Trametes (Coriolus) versicolor* (turkey tail), *Lentinus edodes* (shiitake), and *Grifola frondosa* (maitake). Polysaccharide K (PSK), a well-known bioactive ingredient in Turkey tail mushroom, is licensed for treating stomach, breast, colorectal, and lung cancers in Japan (Integrative & Alternative, 2019). Most medicinal fungi have immunomodulatory properties (Blagodatski et al., 2018). Multi-functional mushroom anticancer effects have been shown in preclinical and clinical trials. According to their findings, medicinal fungi increase tumor cell death and metastasis through immunomodulation and other indirect routes (Ayeka, 2018).

14.4.6 Fibers

Fiber-rich meals such as whole grains, fruits, vegetables, nuts, and seeds can prevent various cancers (Dreher, 2018; Sangaramoorthy et al., 2018). A case-control research found that, bean fiber, beans, and grains reduced ER-negative breast cancer risk (Calado et al., 2018; Sangaramoorthy et al., 2018). Despite poor diet adherence and a short follow-up period (2—4 years), randomized clinical trials suggest that, fiber consumption lowers colorectal cancer recurrence in males (Carraro et al., 2012). Human and animal studies demonstrate that, high-fiber flaxseed prevents colon cancers (Bommareddy et al., 2006). Nuts, which contain fiber, have been linked to gastric, colorectal, pancreatic, esophageal, anal and endometrial cancer (Glei et al., 2017). Compared to low-fiber diets, high-fiber diets reduce colon cancer risk, gut microbiota modification, and butyrate synthesis (Chen & Vitetta, 2018).

14.4.7 Sulfur compounds

According to research, broccoli, cabbage, cauliflower, Brussels sprouts, and other vegetables high in organosulfur compounds (isothiocyanates, indoles, etc.) may cut cancer risk (Liu & Lv, 2013; Liu et al., 2012; Liu et al., 2013a; Wu et al., 2013a, 2013b). Isothiocyanates reduce the risk of some cancers by 18% in colorectal cancer (24 case-control studies and 11 prospectives) (Wu et al., 2013a), 19% in gastric cancer (16 case-control studies and 6 prospective studies) (Wu et al., 2013b), 10% in prostate cancer (6 case controls) (Liu et al., 2012), 15% in breast cancer (11 cases in control and 2 cohorts) (Goulao et al., 2018), 28% in kidney cancer (7 case controls) (Liu et al., 2013a), and 20% in bladder cancer (5 cohort studies and 5 case control) (Liu et al., 2013b). Rates of statistically significant risk reductions have been reported. Consuming large amounts of *Allium* vegetables (onions, garlic, shallots, chives, and leeks) lowered stomach cancer risk by 46% (Zhou et al., 2011). Garlic intake reduced esophageal, head, and neck cancer risk by 26% and onion intake by 28% in case-control studies (Guercio et al., 2016). Additionally, garlic and onions protect against oral cavity cancer (39% and 86% risk reduction), with risk reductions in the esophagus (57% and 88%), colorectum (26% and 56%), larynx (44% and 83%), endometrium (38% and 60%), and ovaries (22% and 73%) (Turati et al., 2015). In contrast, a metaanalysis of a case study and five prospective studies indicated no connection between garlic consumption and colon cancer risk (Hu et al., 2014).

14.4.8 Vitamins and minerals

14.4.8.1 Vitamin D and calcium

Epidemiological studies show that, low 25(OH)D levels may increase cancer incidence, progression, and mortality (Feng et al., 2017; Goulao et al., 2018). In a meta analysis, vitamin D supplementation alone reduced cancer incidence or mortality (Goulao et al., 2018). Two large prospective cohort studies found that 700–800 mg of calcium per day decreases colon cancer risk (Wu et al., 2002). Breast cancer incidence was unaffected by calcium and vitamin D consumption (Chlebowski et al., 2008). Prediction studies on prostate cancer and calcium consumption are inconsistent. A 6-year randomized clinical trial found a tendency to protect calcium intake against prostate cancer, but 10.3 years showed no protective effect (Baron et al., 2005). Prospective studies reveal that, milk and calcium consumption marginally raises prostate cancer risk (Gao et al., 2005).

14.4.8.2 B vitamins

A meta analysis of randomized controlled studies showed that, vitamin B supplementation may have a detrimental effect on the overall occurrence of cancer (Zhang et al., 2016b). Even though the results indicate that, folic acid supplementation improves numerous cancer types (Heine-Broring et al., 2015; Tio et al., 2014), elevated blood folate levels in men have been associated with a heightened susceptibility to prostate and lung cancer in certain studies (Qin et al., 2015; Zhang et al., 2014). Insufficient consensus on B vitamins and folic acid indicates the necessity for more studies.

14.5 Challenges and future recommendations

14.5.1 Standardization of functional foods

To evaluate the anticancer properties of functional foods, in vitro studies and animal models provide information only regarding functionality and cannot establish a cause-and-effect relationship in humans. Randomized controlled clinical trials (RCTs) and placebo controls are essential for the validity and reliability of clinical trials (Weaver & Miller, 2017). Foods or products generated from them, however, that have the hypothesis of functionality and causality demonstrated by these investigations, can be certified or labeled using food standardization standards recognized by the states. Furthermore, the results should be published in a peer-reviewed scientific journal for critical examination by scientific authorities (Kamioka et al., 2019). The systematic evaluation of foods or functional substances, whose efficacy has already been researched and proven through meta-analysis also contributes to safety. The results of all these clinical and, if any, systematic and scientific studies are approved by experts of organizations such as the Food and Drug Administration or European Food Safety Authority, through a consensus-based agreement (Frestedt, 2017; Lenssen et al., 2018).

RCTs have some challenges. A substantial amount of money and people subjects are needed. Due to budget constraints, studies of this kind are rare. RCTs should consist of diverse cooperation (food engineering, chemistry, agriculture, pharmacology, dieticians), hence experienced and competent researchers, who are prepared to collaborate are needed (Granato et al., 2017).

Standardizing functional foods also faces production issues. Positively identifying and eliminating medicine and excipient additives is essential. Although manufacturers take great care to include the components they are supposed to, the danger of unknown or unexpected substances is low. Testing functional foods and food ingredients, according to USP-NF, FCC, and DSC standards, will protect public health from new additives and pollutants from raw material sources or processing methods. The law does not require food ingredient identification tests before marketing. Public health would benefit from manufacturers, distributors, exporters, importers, and consumers participating in USP's Food Chemicals Codex Forum standard-setting efforts (USP, 2024).

14.5.2 Personalized nutrition approaches

Cancer patients should be screened for mutations before choosing a treatment, because individual differences affect treatment goals and prognosis. A truly individualized therapy approach should analyze genetic and lifestyle factors such as inflammation, immunological health, nutrition, stress management, and exercise. A tailored cancer therapy strategy stresses patient-centered, multi-intervention planning that covers physical, mental, emotional, and environmental consequences (Block & Gyllenhaal, 2014).

Costs and therapeutic resistance are the primary issues with personalized, targeted cancer treatments. Cancers can have genetic heterogeneity in one patient (Vogelstein et al., 2013) or develop therapy resistance by switching growth pathways (Zahreddine & Borden, 2013). The discovery of therapeutic medicines that target several growth pathways requires significant effort, adverse effects, and costs (Jochems et al., 2014; Ringash et al., 2014). Supplementing existing treatments requires broader spectrum techniques.

Clinically, nutritional genomics for customized nutrition seems promising. Nutritional genetics includes nutrigenetics and nutrigenomics. Nutrigenetics explores how nutrition affects genes, while Nutrigenomics studies how nutrition affects gene expression. Numerous comprehensive reviews and metaanalyses have shown that the rs9939609 variation affects alpha-ketoglutarate-dependent dioxygenase in macro and micronutrient consumption (Livingstone et al., 2015) and diet-related weight reduction (de Luis et al., 2015; Xiang et al., 2016). MTHFR variants, especially the C677T variation, are the most common genetic factors affecting micronutrient response (Molloy et al., 1997). Vitamin B12 absorption, vitamin D biosynthesis or bioavailability, serum lycopene levels, and circulating carotenoid levels have significant relationships with the FUT2 variant (Hazra et al., 2008), VDR, CYP2R1, and CYP27B1 variants (Miller, 2017; Yao et al., 2017; Zhu et al., 2013), and a common variant in the SETD7 gene (C.R. D'Adamo et al., 2016).

The onset and progression of cancer depend on genomic instability. The genome is safeguarded by checkpoints throughout the cell cycle in normal cells, but in cancer, one or more fail. This picture may induce cancer growth. Grape seed resveratrol may improve this regulatory mechanism (Lee et al., 2010; Rusin et al., 2009). Small alterations in proto-oncogenes or tumor suppressor genes affect gene product function. Toxins, food, and smoking affect these tiny alterations. The cell must properly repair environmental DNA damage. Epigenetic changes in cancer etiology cause DNA mutations that synthesize proteins that promote cancer growth, suggesting that nutrition may prevent or treat cancer (Ho et al., 2011). Genetic or epigenetic state of DNA repair genes and nutraceuticals that modify them (Ferguson & Schlothauer, 2012) helps forecast, diagnose, and cure certain malignancies. Food elements that fight genomic instability include vitamins D and B, selenium, carotenoids, PARP inhibitors, resveratrol, and isothiocyanates. These components prevent cancer cells from establishing replicative immortality and growth-inhibiting signals, diminish tumor-forming inflammation, and may block or reduce other oncogenic metabolic processes (Hopkins et al., 2011; Lee et al., 2010; Sharp et al., 2013; Zhang et al., 2013).

Reversible histone acetylation regulates genes, and histone acetylation patterns change during cancer growth (Marks et al., 2001). Epigenomic clinical trials with hydroxamic acid-based (HDAC) inhibitors are promising. Sulforaphane, a cruciferous phytochemical similar to pharmacological HDAC inhibitors, inhibits HDAC in prostate cancer by increasing histone acetylation, DNA methylation, histone methylation, noncoding RNA, suppression of P21 and Bax, and cell cycle arrest/apoptosis (Clarke et al., 2011; Myzak et al., 2007). In a breast cancer clinical trial, broccoli sprout extracts reduced HDAC activity and MK167 expression (Atwell et al., 2015). B vitamins, S-adenosyl-L-methionine (SAM-e), choline, epigallocatechin-3-gallate (EGCG), and sulforaphane work as methyl donors (Anderson et al., 2012) and HDAC inhibitors (Bassett & Barnett, 2014) for DNA methylation and histone deacetylation.

An international study conducted by 180 scientists examined tailored nutrition and targeted medicines and addressed tumor genetic heterogeneity. They found 74 target genes, chemicals, or pathways that impact cancer phenotypes and tumor microenvironment events by examining cancer biology from numerous aspects. We proposed low-toxicity phytochemicals for these targets and reviewed the literature. According to the literature, 67% of goal-distinguishing feature correlations were complementary, with few or no contradictory or mixed impacts. Block & Gyllenhaal (2014) review the details of the study and lists these characteristics, objectives and functional foods or phytochemicals. Table 14.6 (Block & Gyllenhaal, 2014) lists these characteristics, objectives, and functional foods or phytochemicals.

Thus early molecular engagement in persistent proliferative signaling pathways reduces drug resistance. In continuous proliferative signaling pathways, target molecules include HIF-1, NF-B, PI3K/Akt, IGF-1R, CDKs/cyclins, androgen receptors, and estrogen receptors. Curcumin, genistein, and resveratrol can be used to treat these pathways. However, natural antigrowth signal activation methods are crucial. EGCG, luteolin, curcumin, genistein, resveratrol, withaferin A, and deguelin phytochemicals target antigrowth signaling molecules such RB, p53, PTEN, Hippo, 15 (GDF15), ARID1A, Notch, and IGF-1R. hTERT, mTOR, CDK4/6, CDK 1/2/5/9, Akt, and PI3K pathways need more study. Imetelstat, genistein, perillyl alcohol, palbociclib, dinaciclib, curcumin, and EGCG may be effective in these combined treatments, although this has not been clinically established. *Agaricus blazei, Albatrellus confluens, Cordyceps militaris, Ganoderma lucidum, Poria cocos, and Silybum marianum* inactivate gamma-linolenic acid and eicosapentaenoic acid activator protein 1 (AP-1) and matrix metalloproteinase 9 (MMP-9) and disrupt E-cadherin and tight junctions, urokinase-type

TABLE 14.6 Targeted Functional Foods in Cancer Treatment (Block & Gyllenhaal, 2014).

Hallmarks	Targets	Functional Foods/Phytochemicals
Proliferative signaling pathways	HIF1, NF-B, PI3K/Akt, IGF-1R, CDKs/cyclins, AR, ER	Curcumin, genistein, resveratrol
Antigrowth signals and tumor suppressor genes	RB, p53, PTEN, Hippo, 15 (GDF15), ARID1A, Notch, IGF-1R	EGCG, luteolin, curcumin, genistein, resveratrol, withaferin A and deguelin
Replicative immortality	Telomerase, hTERT, mTOR, CDK4/6, CDK 1/2/5/9, Akt, and PI3K	İmetelstat, genistein, perillyl alcohol, palbociclib, dinaciclib, curcumin, and EGCG
Tissue invasion and metastasis-related processes	AP-1, MMP-9, E-cadherin, tight junctions, urokinase-type plasminogen activator, PI3K/AKT, focal adhesion kinase, TGF	*Agaricus blazei, Albatrellus confluens, Cordyceps militaris, Ganoderma lucidum, Poria cocos,* and *Silybum marianum,* inactivation of the fatty acids gamma-linolenic acid and eicosapentaenoic acid
Cancer-related inflammation	Macrophage migration inhibitory factor, (COX-2), NF-B, (TNFα), (iNOS), Akt, and chemokines	Resveratrol, curcumin, genistein, EGCG, lycopene and anthocyanins
Tumor angiogenesis and vascular dysfunction	Endothelial cell migration, hypoxia, lymphangiogenesis, tumor-inducing inflammation disabling, tumor-promoting fibroblasts	Kaempferol, melatonin, oleanoic acid, EGCG, curcumin, tripterin, silibinin, withaferin A, enterolactone and resveratrol
Tumor microenvironment (senescence mechanism)	Tumorigenesis ROS Macrophage conversion IDO Regulation of dendritic cells Cholesterol synthesis Fibrosis İnflammation and immune signaling Jak signaling	Berberine, Resveratrol, desoxyrhapontigenin, Onionin A, EGCG, Genistein, Naringenin, Piperine, Zerumbone

AP-1, Eicosapentaenoic acid activator protein 1; *AR,* androgen reseptor; *CDKs,* cyclin-dependent kinases; *COX-2,* cyclooxygenase-2; *EGCG,* epigallocatechin-3-gallate; *ER,* estrogen reseptor; *HIF-1,* hypoxia-inducible factor-1; *IDO,* indolamine 2,3-dioxygenase; *IGF-1R,* insulin-like growth factor receptor; *iNOS,* inducible nitric oxide synthesis; *MMP-9,* matrix metalloproteinase 9; *PTEN,*; *TNFα,* tumor necrosis factor-alpha.

plasminogen activator Inflammation is another cancer therapy concern. Phytochemicals such as resveratrol, curcumin, genistein, EGCG, lycopene, and anthocyanins can target macrophage migration inhibitory factor, COX-2, NF-B, TNFα, iNOS, Akt, and chemokines due to their antiinflammatory properties. Kaempferol, melatonin, oleanoic acid, EGCG, curcumin, tripterin, silibinin, withaferin A, enterolactone, and resveratrol may reduce endothelial cell migration, hypoxia, lymphangiogenesis, tumor-inducing inflammation, and tumor-promoting fibroblasts. Comprehensive studies should examine their effects. Distinct phytochemicals may have distinct anticancer mechanisms. Berberine affects tumor growth and the tumor microenvironment, while phytochemicals affect specific pathways. EGCG targets dendritic cell indoleamine 2,3-dioxygenase (IDO) regulation, genistein targets cholesterol synthesis, naringenin targets fibrosis, piperine targets inflammation and immune signaling, and zerumbone targets JAK signaling (Table 14.6), (Block & Gyllenhaal, 2014).

Studies indicate that, phytochemicals may alter epigenetics to prevent or treat cancer. More proof is needed to use tailored dietary genetics to minimize oncogene expression and promote tumor suppressor gene expression. When a phytochemical alone is not enough, combining them can provide broader benefits. We require in vitro, in vivo, and human phase investigations on which functional dietary supplements should be utilized to prevent or treat which metabolic condition, their bioavailability, and adverse effects. This will strengthen the case for a tailored functional diet approach to cancer. It may be able to examine each patient's genome and epigenetically modify mutations with focused functional food consumption in the future.

14.5.3 Integration with conventional cancer treatments

Using dietary supplements during cancer therapy is contentious. While taking methotrexate, it is dangerous to mistakenly ingest functional foods with high folate content (Schattner & Shike, 2006). Many food supplements exceed phytochemical limits (Monsen, 2000; National Research Council, 2010). Numerous oncologists reject limiting dietary supplements during or after traditional cancer therapy. Radiation and some chemotherapies kill cancer cells by oxidative damage. Antioxidants, a subclass of functional foods, may reduce oxidative damage during chemotherapy and radiotherapy (Lawenda et al., 2008). Some experts believe this is a hypothetical and that antioxidants protect healthy cells from these therapies (Greenlee et al., 2004; Prasad et al., 1999). Therefore cancer patients should use food supplements cautiously. Until accurate and reliable scientific data are produced, functional foods with particular content under control should be used, if there is a substantial deficit or major adverse effects like osteoporosis.

Many cancer patients use complementary and alternative treatments, including surgery, chemotherapy, and radiation (Pihlak et al., 2014). Functional meals in combination with standard cancer treatments are rarely studied due to clinical and intervention research limitations. Synergy studies sometimes use laboratory in vitro cell culture experiments or observational research without a scientific or defined procedure. There are studies on functional foods or their constituents to reduce hunger and weight loss in advanced cancer patients and improve quality of life.

The American Institute for Cancer Research (Norman et al., 2003), the American Cancer Society (Rock et al., 2012), and the European Society for Clinical Nutrition and Metabolism- ESPEN (Arends et al., 2017) recommend multivitamin and multimineral supplements, due to conventional cancer treatments' side effects and patients' appetite and body composition loss. Low vitamin D has been linked to muscle loss and cancer (Arends et al., 2017). Vitamin D administration may reduce muscle loss in cancer patients, but more research is needed. In certain intervention studies, EPA (eicosapentaenoic acid) improved cancer patients' calorie and protein consumption (Lavriv et al., 2018; Papallardo et al., 2015). Some studies imply that, n-3 fatty acids decrease cancer cell growth (Hering et al., 2007), reduce chemotherapy toxicity (Murphy et al., 2012), and prevent muscle mass loss (Arends et al., 2017). RCT research should consider cancer type, stage, dose, and homogeneous patient group.

Red beet (*Beta vulgaris* L.) extract plus doxorubicin synergistically inhibited breast and prostate cancer cell growth in vitro (Kapadia et al., 2013). Wheatgrass (*Triticum aestivum* L.) extract and cisplatin synergistically modulated genes involved in growth inhibition, apoptosis, and proliferation in a breast cancer cell line (Hussain et al., 2014). A clinical investigation found that 400 mg of EGCG isolated from green tea three times a day for 2–8 weeks enhanced radiation efficacy and had an antimetastatic impact on breast cancer patients (Zhang et al., 2012). Another clinical trial indicated that, Chinese herbs improved metastatic breast cancer patients' treatment survival (Mao et al., 2017). There is little research on using functional diet or phytochemicals with standard cancer treatment. More clinical or preclinical investigations are needed to determine functional foods' synergistic or detrimental effects.

14.6 Conclusion

Functional foods are promising for the prevention, management, and treatment of cancer with the bioactive chemicals they contain. Research findings from both experimental and observational studies have indicated that, the utilization of nutritional supplements may potentially serve as a preventive measure against the development of cancer. Nevertheless, epidemiological research has yet to definitively demonstrate the protective effects of any nutritional substance against cancer. Sustainable healthy living conditions and a diet rich in functional foods can decrease the risk of cancer formation and progression and even help improve the conventional treatment process by reducing the side effects associated with cancer chemotherapy.

References

Abbas, H. M. K., Huang, H. X., Huang, W. J., Xue, S. D., Yan, S. J., Wu, T. Q., Li, J. X., & Zhong, Y. J. (2020). Evaluation of metabolites and antioxidant activity in pumpkin species. *Natural Product Communications*, *15*(4), 1–11.

Abdulkadir, S., & Tsuchiya, M. (2008). One-step method for quantitative and qualitative analysis of fatty acids in marine animal samples. *Journal of Experimental Marine Biology and Ecology*, *354*(1), 1–8.

Adebayo, E. A., Martínez-Carrera, D., Morales, P., Sobal, M., Escudero, H., Meneses, M. E., Avila-Nava, A., Castillo, I., & Bonilla, M. (2018). Comparative study of antioxidant and antibacterial properties of the edible mushrooms *Pleurotus levis, P. ostreatus, P. pulmonarius* and *P. tuber-regium*. *International Journal of Food Science and Technology*, *53*, 1316–1330.

Adhami, V. M., Khan, N., & Mukhtar, H. (2009). Cancer chemoprevention by pomegranate: Laboratory and clinical evidence. *Nutrition and Cancer*, *61*(6), 811–815.

Aghajanpour, M., Nazer, M. R., Obeidavi, Z., Akbari, M., Ezati, P., & Kor, N. M. (2017). Functional foods and their role in cancer prevention and health promotion: A comprehensive review. *American Journal of Cancer Research*, *7*(4), 740–769.

Agudelo, C., Barros, L., Santos-Buelga, C., Martínez-Navarrete, N., & Ferreira, I. (2017). Phytochemical content and antioxidant activity of grapefruit (Star Ruby): A comparison between fresh freeze-dried fruits and different. *LWT-Food Science and Technology*, *80*, 106–112.

Akl, M. R., Ayoub, N. M., Mohyeldin, M. M., Busnena, B. A., Foudah, A. I., Liu, Y. Y., & Sayed, K. A. (2014). Olive phenolics as c-met inhibitors: (-)-Oleocanthal attenuates cell proliferation, invasiveness, and tumor growth in breast cancer models. *PLoS One*, *9*(5), e97622.

Akor, J., Onyeyilim, E. L., Ugwu, J. E., & Chinweike, E. C. (2024). Evaluation of antioxidant activity of methanol extract of *Capsicum annum* (Red Bell Pepper), *Capsicum frutescens* (Chili Pepper), and *Capsicum annum* (Green Bell Pepper). *Journal of Food and Nutrition Sciences*, *12*(1), 20–26.

Alexandru, L., Cravotto, G., Giordana, L., Binello, A., & Chemat, F. (2013). Ultrasound-assisted extraction of clove buds using batch- and flow-reactors: A comparative study on a pilot scale. *Innovative Food Science & Emerging Technologies*, *20*, 167–172.

Anderson, O. S., Sant, K. E., & Dolinoy, D. C. (2012). Nutrition and epigenetics: An interplay of dietary methyl donors, one-carbon metabolism and DNA methylation. *Journal of Nutritional Biochemistry*, *23*(8), 853–859.

Ao, T., & Deb, C. R. (2019). Nutritional and antioxidant potential of some wild edible mushrooms of Nagaland, India. *Journal of Food Science and Technology-Mysore*, *56*(2), 1084–1089.

Arends, J., Bachmann, P., Baracos, V., Barthelemy, N., Bertz, H., Bozzetti, F., Fearon, K., Hütterer, E., Isenring, E., Kaasa, S., Krznaric, Z., Laird, B., Larsson, M., Laviano, A., Mühlebach, S., Muscaritoli, M., Oldervoll, L., Ravasco, P., Solheim, T., Strasser, F., de van der Schueren, M., & Preiser, J. C. (2017). ESPEN guidelines on nutrition in cancer patients. *Clinical Nutrition*, *36*(1), 11–48.

Atwell, L. L., Zhang, Z., Mori, M., Farris, P., Vetto, J. T., Naik, A. M., Oh, K. Y., Thuillier, P., Ho, E., & Shannon, J. (2015). Sulforaphane bioavailability and chemopreventive activity in women scheduled for breast biopsy. *Cancer Prevention Research (Philadelphia)*, *8*(12), 1184–1191.

Ayeka, P. A. (2018). Potential of mushroom compounds as immunomodulators in cancer immunotherapy a review. *Evidence-Based Complementary and Alternative Medicine*, 7271509.

Baglia, M. L., Zheng, W., Li, H., Yang, G., Gao, J., Gao, Y. T., & Shu, X. O. (2016). The association of soy food consumption with the risk of subtype of breast cancers defined by hormone receptor and HER2 status. *International Journal of Cancer*, *139*(4), 742–748. Available from https://doi.org/10.1002/ijc.30117.

Baron, J. A., Beach, M., Wallace, K., Grau, M. V., Sandler, R. S., Mandel, J. S., Heber, D., & Greenberg, E. R. (2005). Risk of prostate cancer in a randomized clinical trial of calcium supplementation. *Cancer Epidemiology Biomarkers & Prevention*, *14*(3), 586–589.

Bassett, S. A., & Barnett, M. P. (2014). The role of dietary histone deacetylases (HDACs) inhibitors in health and disease. *Nutrients*, *6*(10), 4273–4301.

Battino, M., Forbes-Hernández, T. Y., Gasparrini, M., Afrin, S., Cianciosi, D., Zhang, J., Manna, P. P., Reboredo-Rodríguez, P., Varela Lopez, A., Quiles, J. L., Mezzetti, B., Bompadre, S., Xiao, J., & Giampieri, F. (2019). Relevance of functional foods in the Mediterranean diet: The role of olive oil, berries and honey in the prevention of cancer and cardiovascular diseases. *Critical Reviews in Food Science and Nutrition*, *59*(6), 893–920.

Bavatharani, R. (2023). Chapter-3 Antioxidants and their impact on childhood cancer survivors. *Chief Editor*, *47*.

Blagodatski, A., Yatsunskaya, M., Mikhailova, V., Tiasto, V., Kagansky, A., & Katanaev, V. L. (2018). Medicinal mushrooms as an attractive new source of natural compounds for future cancer therapy. *Oncotarget*, *9*(49), 29259–29274.

Block, K. I., & Gyllenhaal, C. (2014). Chapter 6: Nutritional interventions in cancer. In D. Abrams, & A. Weil (Eds.), *Integrative oncology* (pp. 120–159). Oxford University Press.

Bommareddy, A., Arasada, B. L., Mathees, D. P., & Dwivedi, C. (2006). Chemopreventive effects of dietary flax seed on colon tumor development. *Nutrition and Cancer*, *54*(2), 216–222.

Boss, A., Bishop, K. S., Marlow, G., Barnett, M. P. G., & Ferguson, L. R. (2016). Evidence to support the anti-cancer effect of olive leaf extract and future directions. *Nutrients*, *8*(8), 513.

Boyanapalli, S. S. S., & Kong, A. N. T. (2015). Curcumin, the king of spices: Epigenetic regulatory mechanisms in the prevention of cancer, neurological, and inflammatory diseases. *Current Pharmacology Reports*, *1*(2), 129–139.

Buljeta, I., Pichler, A., Šimunović, J., & Kopjar, M. (2023). Beneficial effects of red wine polyphenols on human health: Comprehensive review. *Current Issues in Molecular Biology*, *45*(2), 782–798.

Calado, A., Neves, P. M., Santos, T., & Ravasco, P. (2018). The effect of flaxseed in breast cancer: A literature review. *Frontiers in Nutrition*, *5*, 4.

Capocchi, A., Bottega, S., Spanò, C., & Fontanini, D. (2017). Phytochemicals and antioxidant capacity in four Italian traditional maize (*Zea mays* L.) varieties. *International Journal of Food Sciences and Nutrition*, *68*(5), 515–524.

Carraro, J., Dantas, M. I. D. S., Espeschit, A., Martino, H., & Ribeiro, S. (2012). Flaxseed and human health: Reviewing benefits and adverse effects. *Food Reviews International*, *28*(2), 203–230.

Casapullo, A., Del Gaudio, F., Capolupo, A., Cassiano, C., & Chiara Monti, M. (2016). Multi-target profile of oleocanthal, an extra-virgin olive oil component. *Current Bioactive Compounds*, *12*(1), 3–9.

Chang, K. J. L., Nichols, C. M., Blackburn, S. I., Dunstan, G. A., Koutoulis, A., & Nichols, P. D. (2014). Comparison of thraustochytrids Aurantiochytrium sp., Schizochytrium sp., Thraustochytrium sp., and Ulkenia sp for production of biodiesel, long-chain omega-3 Oils, and exopolysaccharide. *Marine Biotechnology*, *16*(4), 396–411.

Chen, J., & Vitetta, L. (2018). Inflammation-modulating effect of butyrate in the prevention of colon cancer by dietary fiber. *Clinical Colorectal Cancer*, *17*(3), 541–544.

Chen, Z., Bertin, R., & Froldi, G. (2013). EC50 estimation of antioxidant activity in DPPH· assay using several statistical programs. *Food Chemistry*, *138*(1), 414–420.

Cherifi, H., Ajjabi, L. C., & Sadok, S. (2018). Nutritional value of the Tunisian mussel Mytilus galloprovincialis with a special emphasis on lipid quality. *Food Chemistry*, *268*(1), 307–314.

Chi, F., Wu, R., Zeng, Y. C., Xing, R., Liu, Y., & Xu, Z. G. (2013). Post-diagnosis soy food intake and breast cancer survival: A meta-analysis of cohort studies. *Asian Pacific Journal of Cancer Prevention*, *14*(2), 2407–2412.

Chlebowski, R. T., Johnson, K. C., Kooperberg, C., Pettinger, M., Wactawski-Wende, J., Rohan, T., Rossouw, J., Lane, D., O'Sullivan, M. J., Yasmeen, S., Hiatt, R. A., Shikany, J. M., Vitolins, M., Khandekar, J., & Hubbell, F. A., Women's Health Initiative Investigators. (2008). Calcium plus vitamin D supplementation and the risk of breast cancer. *Journal of the National Cancer Institute*, *100*(22), 1581–1591.

Clarke, J. D., Hsu, A., Yu, Z., Dashwood, R. H., & Ho, E. (2011). Differential effects of sulforaphane on histone deacetylases, cell cycle arrest and apoptosis in normal prostate cells versus hyperplastic and cancerous prostate cells. *Molecular Nutrition & Food Research*, *55*(7), 999–1009.

Cockfield, J. A., & Schafer, Z. T. (2019). Antioxidant defenses: A context-specific vulnerability of cancer cells. *Cancers*, *11*(8), 1208.

Cretton, M., Malanga, G., Sobczuk, T. M., & Mazzuca, M. (2023). Marine lipids as a source of high-quality fatty acids and antioxidants. *Food Reviews International*, *39*(8), 4941–4964.

Criscitiello, C., et al. (2014). Immune approaches to the treatment of breast cancer, around the corner? *Breast Cancer Research*, *16*(204), 1–8.

Cui, Y., Thomas-Hall, S. R., Chua, E. T., & Schenk, P. M. (2021). Development of high-level omega-3 eicosapentaenoic acid (EPA) production from *Phaeodactylum tricornutum*. *Journal of Phycology*, *57*(1), 258–268.

D'Adamo, C. R., D'Urso, A., Ryan, K. A., Yerges-Armstrong, L. M., Semba, R. D., Steinle, N. I., Mitchell, B. D., Shuldiner, A. R., & McArdle, P. F. (2016). A common variant in the SETD7 gene predicts serum lycopene concentrations. *Nutrients*, *8*(2), 82.

Danwilai, K., Konmun, J., Sripanidkulchai, B.-O., & Subongkot, S. (2017). Antioxidant activity of ginger extract as a daily supplement in cancer patients receiving adjuvant chemotherapy: a pilot study. *Cancer Management and Research*, *9*, 11–18.

Denev, P., Kratchanova, M., Petrova, I., Klisurova, D., Georgiev, Y., Ognyanov, M., & Yanakieva, I. (2018). Black chokeberry (*Aronia melanocarpa* (Michx.) Elliot) fruits and functional drinks differ significantly in their chemical composition and antioxidant activity. *Journal of Chemistry*, 9574587.

Denev, P., Ciz, M., Kratchanova, M., & Blazheva, D. (2019). Black chokeberry (*Aronia melanocarpa*) polyphenols reveal different antioxidant, antimicrobial and neutrophil-modulating activities. *Food Chemistry*, *284*, 108–117.

Derakhshan, Z., Ferrante, M., Tadi, M., Ansari, F., Heydari, A., Hosseini, M. S., Conti, G. O., & Sadrabad, E. K. (2018). Antioxidant activity and total phenolic content of ethanolic extract of pomegranate peels, juice and seeds. *Food and Chemical Toxicology*, *114*, 108–111.

Dizon, D. S., & Kamal, A. H. (2024). Cancer statistics 2024: All hands on deck. *Ca-a Cancer Journal for Clinicians*, *74*(1), 8–9.

Dou, J., et al. (2015). Solubility and stability of curcumin in poly (lactic acid) fibers: Effects of copolymers and chemical structure. *Industrial Engineering Chemistry Research*, *54*, 3291–3298.

Dreher, M. L. (2018). Fiber and colorectal cancer. In *Dietary Fiber in Health and Disease*, (pp. 333–362). USA: Humana Press.

Durmaz, Y., Monteiro, M., Bandarra, N., Gökpinar, S., & Isik, O. (2007). The effect of low temperature on fatty acid composition and tocopherols of the red microalga, Porphyridium cruentum. *Journal of Applied Phycology*, *19*, 223–227.

Erbiai, E., da Silva, L. P., Saidi, R., Lamrani, Z., Esteves da Silva, J. C. G., & Maouni, A. (2021). Chemical composition, bioactive compounds, and antioxidant activity of two wild edible mushrooms *Armillaria mellea* and *Macrolepiota procera* from Two Countries (Morocco and Portugal). *Biomolecules*, *11*(4), 575.

Esposto, S., Veneziani, G., Taticchi, A., Urbani, S., Selvaggini, R., Sordini, B., Daidone, L., Gironi, G., & Servili, M. (2021). Chemical composition, antioxidant activity, and sensory characterization of commercial pomegranate juices. *Antioxidants*, *10*(9), 1381.

Fabian, C. J., & Kimler, B. F. (2013). Marine-derived omega-3 fatty acids: fishing for clues for cancer prevention. *American Society of Clinical Oncology Educational Book*, *33*, 97–101.

Fadilaturahmah, F., Rahayu, R., & Santoso, P. (2023). In silico study on anti-inflammatory effect of bioactive compounds of velvet bean (*Mucuna pruriens*) leaves against NF-kB activation pathway. *Jurnal Sains Farmasi & Klinis*, *9*(sup), 168–174.

Farooqi, A. A., Fayyaz, S., Silva, A. S., Sureda, A., Nabavi, S. F., Mocan, A., Nabavi, S. M., & Bishayee, A. (2017). Oleuropein and cancer chemoprevention: The link is hot. *Molecules (Basel, Switzerland)*, *22*(5), 705.

Feng, Q., Zhang, H., Dong, Z., Zhou, Y., & Ma, J. (2017). Circulating 25-hydroxyvitamin D and lung cancer risk and survival: A dose-response meta-analysis of prospective cohort studies. *Medicine*, *96*(45), e8613.

Ferguson, L., & Schlothauer, R. (2012). The potential role of nutritional genomics tools in validating high-health foods for cancer control: Broccoli as an example. *Molecular Nutrition & Food Research*, *56*(1), 126–146.

Fogarasi, M., Diaconeasa, Z. M., Pop, C. R., Fogarasi, S., Semeniuc, C. A., Fărcaş, A. C., Ţibulcă, D., Sălăgean, C.-D., Tofană, M., & Socaci, S. A. (2020). Elemental composition, antioxidant and antibacterial properties of some wild edible mushrooms from Romania. *Agronomy-Basel*, *10*(12), 1972.

Frestedt, J. L. (2017). Similarities and differences between clinical trials for foods and drugs. *Austin Journal of Nutrition and Food Sciences*, *5*(1), 1086.

Fuchs-Tarlovsky, V. (2013). Role of antioxidants in cancer therapy. *Nutrition (Burbank, Los Angeles County, Calif.)*, *29*(1), 15–21.

Gacche, R. N. (2021a). Functional foods, nutraceuticals and dietary supplements in cancer prevention. In *Dietary Research and Cancer*, (pp. 121–130). Singapore: Springer. Available from https://doi.org/10.1007/978-981-16-6050-4_12.

Gacche, R. N. (2021b). Do antioxidants really help cancer patients? The puzzle of benefits and perils. In *Dietary Research and Cancer*, (pp. 131–146). Singapore: Springer. Available from https://doi.org/10.1007/978-981-16-6050-4_13.

Gamel, T. H., & Abdel-Aal, E. M. (2012). Phenolic acids and antioxidant properties of barley wholegrain and pearling fractions. *Agricultural and Food Science*, *21*, 118–131.

Gao, J., Mamouni, K., Zhang, L., & Lokeshwar, B. L. (2021). *In* Evolutionary Diversity as a Source for Anticancer Molecules (pp. 275–308). Elsevier.

Gao, X., Lavalley, M. P., & Tucker, K. L. (2005). Prospective studies of dairy product and calcium intakes and prostate cancer risk: A meta-analysis. *Journal of the National Cancer Institute*, *97*(23), 1768–1777.

Gasecka, M., Siwulski, M., & Mleczek, M. (2018). Evaluation of bioactive compounds content and antioxidant properties of soil-growing and wood-growing edible mushrooms. *Journal of Food Processing and Preservation*, *42*, e13386.

Glasauer, A., & Chandel, N. S. (2014). Targeting antioxidants for cancer therapy. *Biochemical Pharmacology*, *92*(1), 90–101.

Glei, M., Ludwig, D., Lamberty, J., Fischer, S., Lorkowski, S., & Schlörmann, W. (2017). Chemopreventive potential of raw and roasted pistachios regarding colon carcinogenesis. *Nutrients*, *9*(12), 1368.

Goulao, B., Stewart, F., Ford, J. A., MacLennan, G., & Avenell, A. (2018). Cancer and vitamin D supplementation: A systematic review and meta-analysis. *The American Journal of Clinical Nutrition*, *107*(4), 652–663.

Granato, D., Nunes, D. S., & Barba, F. J. (2017). An integrated strategy between food chemistry, biology, nutrition, pharmacology, and statistics in the development of functional foods: A proposal. *Trends in Food Science & Technology*, *62*, 13–22.

Greenlee, H., White, E., Patterson, R. E., & Kristal, A. R. (2004). Vitamins and Lifestyle (VITAL) Study Cohort. Supplement use among cancer survivors in the Vitamins and Lifestyle (VITAL) study cohort. *Journal of Alternative and Complementary Medicine*, *10*(4), 660–666.

Grosso, G., Godos, J., Galvano, F., & Giovannucci, E. L. (2017). Coffee, caffeine, and health outcomes: An umbrella review. *Annual Review of Nutrition*, *37*, 131–156.

Grover, A. K., & Samson, S. E. (2010). Antioxidant defense mechanisms in the aging kidney. *Nephron. Experimental Nephrology*, *114*, 95–99.

Guedes, M. N. S., Pio, R., Maro, L. A. C., Lage, F. F., Abreu, C. M. P. D., & Saczk, A. A. (2017). Antioxidant activity and total phenol content of blackberries cultivated in a highland tropical climate. *Acta Scientiarum-Agronomy*, *39*(1), 43–48.

Guercio, V., Turati, F., La Vecchia, C., Galeone, C., & Tavani, A. (2016). Allium vegetables and upper aerodigestive tract cancers a meta-analysis of observational studies. *Molecular Nutrition Food Research*, *60*(1), 212–222.

Guil-Guerrero, J. L., Venegas-Venegas, E., Rincón-Cervera, M. A., & Suárez, M. D. (2011). Fatty acid profiles of livers from selected marine fish species. *Journal of Food Composition and Analysis*, *24*(2), 217–222.

Guo, R., Li, W., Liu, B., Li, S., Zhang, B., & Xu, Y. (2014). Resveratrol protects vascular smooth muscle cells against high glucose-induced oxidative stress and cell proliferation *in vitro*. *Medical Science Monitor Basic Research*, *20*, 82–92.

Gupta, P. (2020). Targeted cancer therapy with bioactive foods and their products. In *Functional Foods in Cancer Prevention and Therapy*, (pp. 33–46). Elsevier.

Gündogdu, M., Kan, T., & Canan, I. (2016). Bioactive and antioxidant characteristics of blackberry cultivars from East Anatolia. *Turkish Journal of Agriculture and Forestry*, *40*(3), 344–351.

Hao, J., Hu, H., Liu, J., Wang, X., Niu, M., et al. (2019). Integrated metabolomics and network pharmacology study on immunoregulation mechanisms of Panax ginseng through macrophages. *Evidence-Based Complementary and Alternative Medicine*, 630260.

Hao, W., Li, K., Liu, S., Yu, H., Li, P., & Xing, R. (2023). Pleiotropic modulation of chitooligosaccharides on inflammatory signaling in LPS-induced macrophages. *Polymers*, *15*, 1613.

Hazra, A., Kraft, P., Selhub, J., Giovannucci, E. L., Thomas, G., Hoover, R. N., Chanock, S. J., & Hunter, D. J. (2008). Common variants of FUT2 are associated with plasma vitamin B12 levels. *Nature Genetics*, *40*(10), 1160–1162.

He, J., Li, J., Liu, H., Yang, Z., Zhou, F., Wei, T., Dong, Y., Xue, H., Tang, L., & Liu, M. (2018). Scandoside exerts anti-inflammatory effect via suppressing NF-κB and MAPK signaling pathways in LPS-induced RAW 264.7 macrophages. *International journal of molecular sciences*, *19*(2), 457.

He, T., Liu, W., & Shen, C. (2022a). Anti-inflammatory properties of pigment epithelium-derived factor. *European Journal of Inflammation*, *20*. Available from https://doi.org/10.1177/1721727X221138857.

He, M. M., Lo, C. H., Wang, K., Polychronidis, G., Wang, L., Zhong, R., Knudsen, M. D., Fang, Z., & Song, M. (2022b). Immune-mediated diseases associated with cancer risks. *JAMA oncology*, *8*, 209–219.

Heine-Broring, R. C., Winkels, R. M., Renkema, J. M., Kragt, L., van Orten-Luiten, A. C., Tigchelaar, E. F., Chan, D. S., Norat, T., & Kampman, E. (2015). Dietary supplement use and colorectal cancer risk: A systematic review and meta-analyses of prospective cohort studies. *International Journal of Cancer*, *136*(10), 2388–2401.

Hering, J., Garrean, S., Dekoj, T. R., Razzak, A., Saied, A., Trevino, J., Babcock, T. A., & Espat, N. J. (2007). Inhibition of proliferation by omega-3 fatty acids in chemoresistant pancreatic cancer cells. *Annals of Surgical Oncology*, *14*(12), 3620–3628.

Hesam, F., Balali, G. R., & Tehrani, R. T. (2012). Evaluation of antioxidant activity of three common potato (*Solanum tuberosum*) cultivars in Iran. *Avicenna Journal of Phytomedicine*, *2*(2), 79–85.

Ho, E., Beaver, L. M., Williams, D. E., & Dashwood, R. H. (2011). Dietary factors and epigenetic regulation for prostate cancer prevention. *Advances in Nutrition*, *2*(6), 497–510.

Hopkins, M. H., Owen, J., Ahearn, T., Fedirko, V., Flanders, W. D., et al. (2011). Effects of supplemental vitamin D and calcium on biomarkers of inflammation in colorectal adenoma patients: A randomized, controlled clinical trial. *Cancer Prevention Research*, *4*(10), 1645–1654.

Horvat, D., Šimić, G., Drezner, G., Lalić, A., Ledenčan, T., et al. (2020). Phenolic acid profiles and antioxidant activity of major cereal crops. *Antioxidants*, *9*, 527.

Hu, J. X., Lu, W., Lv, M., Wang, Y., Ding, R., et al. (2019). Extraction and purification of astaxanthin from shrimp shells and the effects of different treatments on its content. *Revista Brasileira De Farmacognosia-Brazilian Journal of Pharmacognosy*, *29*(1), 24–29.

Hu, J. Y., Hu, Y. W., Zhou, J. J., Zhang, M. W., Li, D., et al. (2014). Consumption of garlic and risk of colorectal cancer: An updated meta-analysis of prospective studies. *World Journal of Gastroenterology*, *20*(41), 15413–15422.

Huang, C. W., Lin, I. J., Liu, Y. M., & Mau, J. L. (2021). Composition, enzyme and antioxidant activities of pineapple. *International Journal of Food Properties*, *24*(1), 1244–1251.

Huaux, F. (2021). Interpreting immunoregulation in lung fibrosis: A new branch of the immune model. *Frontiers in Immunology, 12*, 690375.

Hussain, A., Gheewala, T. M., Vas, A. J., Shah, K., Goala, P., et al. (2014). Growth inhibitory and adjuvant therapeutic potential of aqueous extract of Triticum aestivum on MCF-7 and HeLa cells. *Experimental Oncology, 36*(1), 9–16.

Hyun, D. H., Emerson, S. S., Jo, D. G., Mattson, M. P., & de Cabo, R. (2006). Calorie restriction up-regulates the plasma membrane redox system in brain cells and suppresses oxidative stress during aging. *Proceedings of the National Academy of Sciences USA, 103*(52), 19908–19912.

Iskandar, A. R., & Hodgson, J. M. (2013). Mechanism for the action of sulforaphane as a radioprotective agent. *Radiation Research, 179*, 521–530.

Islam, S. R., & Siddiqua, T. J. (2020). Functional foods in cancer prevention and therapy: Recent epidemiological findings. *Functional Foods in Cancer Prevention and Therapy*, 405–433.

Jiang, W., Zhu, Z., McGinley, J. N., El Bayoumy, K., Manni, A., Thompson, H. J., et al. (2013). Identification of a molecular signature underlying inhibition of mammary carcinoma growth by dietary N-3 fatty acids. *Cancer Research, 72*(15), 3795–3806.

Jin, H. H., Lu, Q., & Jiang, J. G. (2016). Curcumin liposomes prepared with milk fat globule membrane phospholipids and soybean lecithin. *Food Science and Technology Research, 99*(3), 1780–1790.

Jitprasertwong, P., Khamphio, M., Petsrichuang, P., Eijsink, V. G. H., Poolsri, W., et al. (2021). Anti-inflammatory activity of soluble chito-oligosaccharides (CHOS) on VitD3-induced human THP-1 monocytes. *PLoS One, 16*(2), e0246381.

Jochems, C., Tucker, J. A., Tsang, K. Y., Madan, R. A., Dahut, W. L., et al. (2014). A combination trial of vaccine plus ipilimumab in metastatic castration-resistant prostate cancer patients: Immune correlates. *Cancer Immunology, Immunotherapy, 63*(4), 407–418.

Kamioka, H., Tsutani, K., Origasa, H., Yoshizaki, T., Kitayuguchi, J., et al. (2019). Quality of systematic reviews of the foods with function claims in Japan: Comparative before-and after-evaluation of verification reports by the consumer affairs agency. *Nutrients, 11*(7), 1583.

Kammath, A. J., Nair, B., Sreelekshmi, P., & Nath, L. R. (2021). Curry versus cancer: Potential of some selected culinary spices against cancer with *in vitro, in vivo*, and human trials evidences. *Journal of Food Biochemistry, 45*(3), e13285.

Kapadia, G. J., Rao, G. S., Ramachandran, C., ida, A., Suzuki, N., Tokuda, H., et al. (2013). Synergistic cytotoxicity of red beetroot (*Beta vulgaris* L.) extract with doxorubicin in human pancreatic, breast and prostate cancer cell lines. *Journal of Complementary and Integrative Medicine, 10*, 10.

Kciuk, M., Alam, M., Ali, N., Rashid, S., Głowacka, P., et al. (2023). Epigallocatechin-3-gallate therapeutic potential in cancer: Mechanism of action and clinical implications. *Molecules (Basel, Switzerland), 28*(13), 5246.

Khurana, S., Venkataraman, K., Hollingsworth, A., Piche, M., & Tai, T. (2013). Polyphenols: benefits to the cardiovascular system in health and in aging. *Nutrients, 5*(10), 3779–3827.

Kim, C.-W., Hwang, K. A., & Choi, K.-C. (2016). Anti-metastatic potential of resveratrol and its metabolites by the inhibition of epithelial-mesenchymal transition, migration, and invasion of malignant cancer cells. *Phytomedicine: International Journal of Phytotherapy and Phytopharmacology, 23*(14), 1787–1796.

Kim, H., Lee, J., Oh, J. H., Chang, H. J., Sohn, D. K., et al. (2019). Protective effect of green tea consumption on colorectal cancer varies by lifestyle factors. *Nutrients, 11*(11), 2612.

Kim, Y., & Je, Y. (2014). Vitamin D intake, blood 25(OH)D levels, and breast cancer risk or mortality: a meta-analysis. *British Journal of Cancer, 110*(11), 2772–2784.

Kolanowski, W. (2021). Salmonids as natural functional food rich in omega-3 PUFA. *Applied Sciences-Basel, 11*, 2409.

Kolev, M., & Markiewski, M. M. (2018). Targeting complement-mediated immunoregulation for cancer immunotherapy. In *Seminars in Immunology*, (37, pp. 85–97). Elsevier.

Kourouma, V., Mu, T. H., Zhang, M., & Sun, H. N. (2020). Comparative study on chemical composition, polyphenols, flavonoids, carotenoids and antioxidant activities of various cultivars of sweet potato. *International Journal of Food Science and Technology, 55*(1), 369–378.

Krüzselyi, D., Móricz, A. M., & Vetter, J. (2020). Comparison of different morphological mushroom parts based on the antioxidant activity. *LWT-Food Science and Technology, 127*, 109436.

Kubczak, M., Szustka, A., & Rogalinska, M. (2021). Molecular targets of natural compounds with anti-cancer properties. *International Journal of Molecular Sciences, 22*(24), 13659.

Kulichová, K., Jozef, S., Peter, N., Mária, M., Tibor, M., et al. (2019). Phenolic compounds and biological activities of rye (*Secale cereale* L.) grains. *Open Chemistry, 17*(1), 988–999.

Kumar, G., Mittal, S., Sak, K., & Tuli, H. S. (2016). Molecular mechanisms underlying chemopreventive potential of curcumin: Current challenges and future perspectives. *Life Sciences, 148*, 313–328.

Kumar, K., Mehra, R., Guiné, R. P. F., Lima, M. J., Kumar, N., et al. (2021). Edible mushrooms: A comprehensive review on bioactive compounds with health benefits and processing aspects. *Foods, 10*(12), 2996.

Kumar, N. B., Pow-Sang, J., Egan, K. M., Spiess, P. E., Dickinson, S., et al. (2015). Randomized, placebo-controlled trial of green tea catechins for prostate cancer prevention. *Cancer Prevention Research, 8*(10), 879–887.

Kumari, D., Madhujith, T., & Chandrasekara, A. (2017). Comparison of phenolic content and antioxidant activities of millet varieties grown in different locations in Sri Lanka. *Food Science & Nutrition, 5*(3), 474–485.

Kuriakose, M. A., Ramdas, K., Dey, B., Iyer, S., Rajan, G., et al. (2016). A randomized double-blind placebo-controlled phase IIB trial of curcumin in oral leukoplakia. *Cancer Prevention Research, 9*(8), 683–691.

Lahmass, I., Ouahhoud, S., Elmansuri, M., et al. (2018). Determination of antioxidant properties of six by-products of *Crocus sativus* L. (Saffron) plant products. *Waste and Biomass Valorization, 9*, 1349–1357.

Lançon, A., Frazzi, R., & Latruffe, N. (2016). Anti-oxidant, anti-inflammatory and anti-angiogenic properties of resveratrol in ocular diseases. *Molecules (Basel, Switzerland), 21*(3), 304.

Lao, C. D., Ruffin, M. T., Normolle, D., Heath, D. D., Murray, S. I., et al. (2006). Dose escalation of a curcuminoid formulation. *MC Complementary Medicine and Therapies*, *6*, 10.

Lavriv, D. S., Neves, P. M., & Ravasco, P. (2018). Should omega-3 be used in cancer cachexia? *Clinical Nutrition ESPEN*, *25*, 18–25.

Lawenda, B. D., Kelly, K. M., Ladas, E. J., Sagar, S. M., Vickers, A., & Blumberg, J. B. (2008). Should supplemental antioxidant administration be avoided during chemotherapy and radiation therapy? *Journal of the National Cancer Institute*, *100*(11), 773–783.

Lee, A. H., Fraser, M. L., & Binns, C. W. (2014). Breastfeeding and the risk of breast cancer. *The Open Epidemiology Journal*, *4*, 60–67.

Lee, S. C., Chan, J. Y., & Pervaiz, S. (2010). Spontaneous and 5-fluorouracil-induced centrosome amplification lowers the threshold to resveratrol-evoked apoptosis in colon cancer cells. *Cancer Letters*, *288*(1), 36–41.

LeGendre, O., Breslin, P. A. S., & Foster, D. A. (2015). (-)-Oleocanthal rapidly and selectively induces cancer cell death via lysosomal membrane permeabilization. *Molecular & Cellular Oncology*, *2*(4), e1006077.

Lenssen, K. G. M., Bast, A., & De Boer, A. (2018). Clarifying the health claim assessment procedure of EFSA will benefit functional food innovation. *Journal of Functional Foods*, *47*, 386–396.

Li, J., Liu, H., Jiang, J., She, X., Niu, Y., Ming, Y., et al. (2020). The potential role of schistosome-associated factors as therapeutic modulators of the immune system. *Infection and Immunity*, *88*(8), e00754–19. Available from https://doi.org/10.1128/iai.00754-00719.

Liu, B., Mao, Q., Wang, X., Zhou, F., Luo, J., Wang, C., Lin, Y., Zheng, X., & Xie, L. (2013a). Cruciferous vegetables consumption and risk of renal cell carcinoma: a meta-analysis. *Nutrition and Cancer*, *65*(5), 668–676.

Liu, B., Mao, Q., Lin, Y., Zhou, F., & Xie, L. (2013b). The association of cruciferous vegetables intake and risk of bladder cancer: A meta-analysis. *World Journal of Urology*, *31*, 127–133.

Liu, B., Mao, Q., Cao, M., & Xie, L. (2012). Cruciferous vegetables intake and risk of prostate cancer: A meta-analysis. *International Journal of Urology*, *19*(2), 134–141.

Liu, X., & Lv, K. (2013). Cruciferous vegetables intake is inversely associated with risk of breast cancer: A meta-analysis. *The Breast*, *22*, 309–313.

Livingstone, K. M., Celis-Morales, C., Lara, J., Ashor, A. W., Lovegrove, J. A., et al. (2015). Associations between FTO genotype and total energy and macronutrient intake in adults: A systematic review and meta-analysis. *Obesity Reviews*, *16*(8), 666–678.

Lu, Y., & Yang, X. (2020). The pivotal roles of neddylation pathway in immunoregulation. *Immunity, Inflammation and Disease*, *8*(4), 782–792.

de Luis, D. A., Aller, R., Izaola, O., Primo, D., Urdiales, S., Romero, E., et al. (2015). Effects of a high-protein/low-carbohydrate diet versus a standard hypocaloric diet on weight and cardiovascular risk factors: Role of a genetic variation in the rs9939609 FTO gene variant. *Journal of Nutrigenetics and Nutrigenomics*, *8*(3), 128–136.

López-Hernández, A. A., Ortega-Villarreal, A. S., Rodríguez, J. A. V., Lomelí, M. L. C., & González-Martínez, B. E. (2022). Application of different cooking methods to improve nutritional quality of broccoli (*Brassica oleracea* var. italica) regarding its compounds content with antioxidant activity. *International Journal of Gastronomy and Food Science*, *28*, 100510.

López-Miranda, J., Pérez-Jiménez, F., Ros, E., De Caterina, R., et al. (2010). Olive oil and health: Summary of the II international conference on olive oil and health consensus report, Jaen and Cordoba (Spain) 2008. *Nutrition Metabolism and Cardiovascular Diseases*, *20*(4), 284–294.

Ma, D. Y., Sun, D., Li, Y., Wang, C., Xie, Y., Guo, T., et al. (2015). Effect of nitrogen fertilisation and irrigation on phenolic content, phenolic acid composition, and antioxidant activity of winter wheat grain. *Journal of the Science of Food and Agriculture*, *95*(5), 1039–1046.

Ma, Y., Chapman, J., Levine, M., Polireddy, K., Drisko, J., Chen, Q., et al. (2014). High-dose parenteral ascorbate enhanced chemosensitivity of ovarian cancer and reduced toxicity of chemotherapy. *Science Translational Medicine*, *6*(222), 222ra18.

Mahran, R. I., Hagras, M. M., Sun, D., & Brenner, D. E. (2017). Bringing curcumin to the clinic in cancer prevention: A review of strategies to enhance bioavailability and efficacy. *The American Association of Pharmaceutical Scientists Journal*, *19*(1), 54–81.

Mao, Y., Hao, J., Jin, Z. Q., Niu, Y. Y., Yang, X., Liu, D., Cao, R., Wu, X. Z., et al. (2017). Network pharmacology-based and clinically relevant prediction of the active ingredients and potential targets of Chinese herbs in metastatic breast cancer patients. *Oncotarget*, *8*(16), 27007–27021.

Marks, P., Rifkind, R. A., Richon, V. M., Breslow, R., Miller, T., Kelly, W. K., et al. (2001). Histone deacetylases and cancer: Causes and therapies. *Nature Reviews. Cancer*, *1*(3), 194–202.

McSorley, H. J., & Maizels, R. M. (2012). Helminth infections and host immune regulation. *Clinical Microbiology Reviews*, *25*(4), 585–608.

Messina, M. J., & Loprinzi, C. L. (2001). Soy for breast cancer survivors: A critical review of the literature. *The Journal of Nutrition*, *131*(11 Suppl), 3095–3108.

Messina, M. J., Persky, V., Setchell, K. D., & Barnes, S. (1994). Soy intake and cancer risk a review of the *in vitro* and *in vivo* data. *Nutrition and Cancer*, *21*(2), 113–131.

Miller, W. L. (2017). Genetic disorders of vitamin D biosynthesis and degradation. *The Journal of Steroid Biochemistry and Molecular Biology*, *165* (Part A), 101–108.

Molloy, A. M., Daly, S., Mills, J. L., Kirke, P. N., Whitehead, A. S., et al. (1997). Thermolabile variant of 5,10-methylenetetrahydrofolate reductase associated with low red-cell folates: Implications for folate intake recommendations. *The Lancet*, *349*(9065), 1591–1593.

Monsen, E. R. (2000). Dietary Reference Intakes for the antioxidant nutrients: Vitamin C, vitamin E, selenium, and carotenoids. *Journal of the American Dietetic Association*, *100*, 637–640.

Murphy, R. A., Mourtzakis, M., & Mazurak, V. C. (2012). n-3 polyunsaturated fatty acids: The potential role for supplementation in cancer. *Current Opinion in Clinical Nutrition and Metabolic Care*, *15*(3), 246–251.

Myzak, M. C., Tong, P., Dashwood, W. M., Dashwood, R. H., & Ho, E. (2007). Sulforaphane retards the growth of human PC-3 xenografts and inhibits HDAC activity in human subjects. *Experimental Biology and Medicine (Maywood)*, *232*(2), 227–234.

Nan, J. N., Ververis, K., Bollu, S., Rodd, A. L., Swarup, O., Karagiannis, T. C., et al. (2014). Biological effects of the olive polyphenol, hydroxytyrosol: An extra view from genome-wide transcriptome analysis. *Hellenic Journal of Nuclear Medicine, 17*(Suppl 1), 62–69.

National Research Council. (2010). *Dietary Reference Intakes for Calcium and Vitamin D*. National Academies Press.

Nguyen, V. L., Truong, C. T., Nguyen, B. C. Q., Vo, T. V., Dao, T. T., et al. (2017). Anti-inflammatory and wound healing activities of calophyllolide isolated from *Calophyllum inophyllum* Linn. *PLoS One, 12*(10), e0185674.

Norman, H. A., Butrum, R. R., Feldman, E., Heber, D., Nixon, D., et al. (2003). The role of dietary supplements during cancer therapy. *Journal of Nutrition, 133*(11 Suppl 1), 3794S–3799S.

Nowakowski, P., Markiewicz-Żukowska, R., Bielecka, J., Mielcarek, K., Grabia, M., & Socha, K. (2021). Treasures from the forest: Evaluation of mushroom extracts as anti-cancer agents. *Biomedicine & Pharmacotherapy, 143*, 112106.

Nurcholis, W., Putri, D. N. S., Husnawati, H., Aisyah, S. I., & Priosoeryanto, B. P. (2021). Total flavonoid content and antioxidant activity of ethanol and ethyl acetate extracts from accessions of Amomum compactum fruits. *Annals of Agricultural Science, 66*(1), 58–62.

Nwanna, E. E., Adebayo, A. A., Ademosun, A. O., & Oboh, G. (2019). Phenolic distribution, antioxidant activity, and enzyme inhibitory properties of eggplant (*Solanum aethiopicum*) cultivated in two different locations within Nigeria. *Journal of Food Biochemistry, 43*(6), e12797.

Olugbami, J., Gbadegesin, M., & Odunola, O. (2014). *In vitro* evaluation of the antioxidant potential, phenolic and flavonoid contents of the stem bark ethanol extract of *Anogeissus leiocarpus. African Journal of Medicine and Medical Sciences, 43*(Suppl 1), 101–109.

Ono, M., Takeshima, M., & Nakano, S. (2015). Mechanism of the anticancer effect of lycopene (tetraterpenoids). *Enzymes, 37*, 139–166.

Oszmianski, J., Kolniak-Ostek, J., Lachowicz, S., Gorzelany, J., & Matlok, N. (2017). Phytochemical compounds and antioxidant activity in different cultivars of cranberry (*Vaccinium macrocarpon* L). *Journal of Food Science, 82*(11), 2569–2575.

Pang, Y., Ahmed, S., Xu, Y., Beta, T., Zhu, Z., et al. (2018). Bound phenolic compounds and antioxidant properties of whole grain and bran of white, red and black rice. *Food Chemistry, 240*, 212–221.

Pao, W., Ooi, C. H., Birzele, F., Ruefli-Brasse, A., Cannarile, M. A., et al. (2018). Tissue-Specific Immunoregulation: A Call for Better Understanding of the "Immunostat" in the Context of Cancer. *Cancer Discovery, 8*(4), 395–402.

Papallardo, G., Almeida, A., & Ravasco, P. (2015). Eicosapentaenoic acid in cancer: Does it improve body composition and modulate metabolism? *Nutrition, 31*(4), 549–555.

Paredes-Gonzalez, X., Fuentes, F., Su, Z.-Y., & Kong, A.-N. T. (2014). Apigenin reactivates Nrf2 anti-oxidative stress signaling in mouse skin epidermal JB6 P+ cells through epigenetics modifications. *The AAPS Journal, 16*(4), 727–735.

Paz, A., Karnaouri, A., Templis, C. C., Papayannakos, N., & Topakas, E. (2020). Valorization of exhausted olive pomace for the production of omega-3 fatty acids by *Crypthecodinium cohnii. Waste Management, 118*, 435–444.

PDQ Integrative, Alternative, and Complementary Therapies (2019). Medicinal Mushrooms (PDQ®): Available from https://www.ncbi.nlm.nih.gov/books/NBK424937/ (Access date: January, 2024).

Permatananda, P. A. N. K., et al. (2021). *In* Journal of Physics: Conference Series (1869). IOP Publishing012035.

Petiwala, S. M., & Johnson, J. J. (2015). Diterpenes from rosemary Rosmarinus officinalis defining their potential for anti-cancer activity. *Cancer Letters, 367*(2), 93–102.

Pihlak, R., Liivand, R., Trelin, O., Neissar, H., Peterson, I., et al. (2014). Complementary medicine use among cancer patients receiving radiotherapy and chemotherapy: Methods, sources of information and the need for counselling. *European Journal of Cancer Care (English), 23*(2), 249–254.

Prasad, K. N., Kumar, A., Kochupillai, V., & Cole, W. C. (1999). High doses of multiple antioxidant vitamins: Essential ingredients in improving the efficacy of standard cancer therapy. *Journal of the American College of Nutrition, 18*(1), 13–25.

Qin, T., Du, M., Du, H., Shu, Y., Wang, M., & Zhu, L. (2015). Folic acid supplements and colorectal cancer risk: Meta-analysis of randomized controlled trials. *Scientific Reports, 5*, 12044.

Rafehi, H., Smith, A. J., Balcerczyk, A., Ziemann, M., Ooi, J., et al. (2012). Investigation into the biological properties of the olive polyphenol, hydroxytyrosol: mechanistic insights by genome-wide mRNA-Seq analysis. *Genes and Nutrition, 7*(2), 343–355.

Rahayu, D. U. C., Hakim, R. A., Mawarni, S. A., & Satriani, A. R. (2022). Indonesian Cinnamon (*Cinnamomum burmannii*): Extraction, flavonoid content, antioxidant activity, and stability in the presence of ascorbic acid. *Cosmetics, 9*(3), 57.

Rahman, M. A., Bulbul, M. R. H., & Kabir, Y. (2020). *In* Functional Foods in Cancer Prevention and Therapy (pp. 237–259). Elsevier.

Rao, S. W., Santhakumar, A. B., Chinkwo, K. A., & Blanchard, C. L. (2020). Investigation of phenolic compounds with antioxidant activity in barley and oats affected by variation in growing location. *Cereal Chemistry, 97*(4), 772–782.

Rapisarda, P., Lo Bianco, M., Pannuzzo, P., & Timpanaro, N. (2008). Effect of cold storage on vitamin C, phenolics and antioxidant activity of five orange genotypes *Citrus sinensis* (L.) Osbeck. *Postharvest Biology and Technology, 49*(3), 348–354.

Ray, N. B., Hilsabeck, K. D., Karagiannis, T. C., & McCord, D. E. (2019). Bioactive olive oil polyphenols in the promotion of health. *Role of Functional Food Security in Global Health*, 623–637.

Ribeiro, V. P., Arruda, C., Abd El-Salam, M., & Bastos, J. K. (2018). Brazilian medicinal plants with corroborated anti-inflammatory activities: a review. *Pharmaceutical Biology, 56*(1), 253–268.

Riganti, C., Mini, E., & Nobili, S. (2015). Editorial: Multidrug resistance in cancer: Pharmacological strategies from basic research to clinical issues. *Frontiers in Oncology, 5*, 105.

Rincón-Cervera, M. A., Suárez-Medina, M. D., & Guil-Guerrero, J. L. (2009). Fatty acid composition of selected roes from some marine species. *European Journal of Lipid Science and Technology, 111*(9), 920–925.

Ringash, J., Au, H. J., Siu, L. L., Shapiro, J. D., Jonker, D. J., et al. (2014). Quality of life in patients with K-RAS wild-type colorectal cancer: The CO.20 phase 3 randomized trial. *Cancer, 120*(2), 181–189.

Rock, C. L., Doyle, C., Demark-Wahnefried, W., Meyerhardt, J., Courneya, K. S., et al. (2012). Nutrition and physical activity guidelines for cancer survivors. *CA: a Cancer Journal for Clinicians, 62*(2), 242–274.

Rook, G. A., Raison, C. L., & Lowry, C. A. (2014). *Microbial endocrinology: The microbiota-gut-brain axis in health and disease* (pp. 319–356). , Microbiota, immunoregulatory old friends and psychiatric disorders.

Ross, A. B., van der Kamp, J. W., King, R., Lê, K. A., Mejborn, H., et al. (2017). Perspective: A Definition for whole-grain food products-recommendations from the healthgrain forum. *Advances in Nutrition, 8*(4), 525–531.

Rusin, M., Zajkowicz, A., & Butkiewicz, D. (2009). Resveratrol induces senescence-like growth inhibition of U-2 OS cells associated with the instability of telomeric DNA and upregulation of BRCA1. *Mechanisms of Ageing and Development, 130*(8), 528–537.

Saeed, I., Guo, X., Azeem, M., Elshikh, M. S., Zainab, B., et al. (2021). Comparative assessment of polyphenolics' content, free radicals' scavenging and cellular antioxidant potential in apricot fruit. *Journal of King Saud University Science, 33*(5), 101459.

Saeedi, M., Soltani, F., Babalar, M., Izadpanah, F., Wiesner-Reinhold, M., & Baldermann, S. (2021). Selenium fortification alters the growth, antioxidant characteristics and secondary metabolite profiles of cauliflower (*Brassica oleracea* var. *botrytis*) cultivars in hydroponic culture. *Plants-Basel, 10*(8), 1537.

Saghatelyan, T., Tananyan, A., Janoyan, N., Tadevosyan, A., Petrosyan, H., et al. (2020). Efficacy and safety of curcumin in combination with paclitaxel in patients with advanced, metastatic breast cancer: A comparative, randomized, double-blind, placebo-controlled clinical trial. *Phytomedicine: International Journal of Phytotherapy and Phytopharmacology, 70*, 153218.

Salta, A., Nurzynska-Wierdak, R., Kalisz, A., & Moreno-Ramón, H. (2022). Impacts of alexandrian clover living mulch on the yield, phenolic content, and antioxidant capacity of leek and shallot. *Agronomy-Basel, 12*(11), 2602.

Samoticha, J., Jara-Palacios, M. J., Hernández-Hierro, J. M., Heredia, F. J., & Wojdylo, A. (2018). Phenolic compounds and antioxidant activity of twelve grape cultivars measured by chemical and electrochemical methods. *European Food Research and Technology, 244*, 1933–1943.

Sang, L. X., Chang, B., Li, X. H., & Jiang, M. (2013). Green tea consumption and risk of esophageal cancer a meta-analysis of published epidemiological studies. *Nutrition and Cancer, 65*(6), 802–812.

Sangaramoorthy, M., Koo, J., & John, E. M. (2018). Intake of bean fiber, beans, and grains and reduced risk of hormone receptor-negative breast cancer: The San Francisco Bay Area Breast Cancer Study. *Cancer Medicine, 7*(5), 2131–2144.

Sanjabi, S., Oh, S. A., & Li, M. O. (2017). Regulation of the immune response by TGF-β: From conception to autoimmunity and infection. *Cold Spring Harbor perspectives in biology, 9*(6), a022236.

Santosa, D., Suharti, C., Riwanto, I., Dharmana, E., Pangarsa, E. A., et al. (2022). Curcumin as adjuvant therapy to improve remission in myeloma patients: A pilot randomized clinical trial. *Caspian Journal of Internal Medicine, 13*(2), 375–384.

Schattner, M., & Shike, M. (2006). Nutrition support of the patient with cancer. In M. E. Shils, M. Shike, A. C. Ross, B. Cabellero, & R. J. Cousins (Eds.), *Modern Nutrition in Health and Disease* (10th ed., pp. 1290–1313). Philadelphia, PA: Lippincott Williams & Wilkins.

Schulz, M., eraglio, S. K. T., Della Betta, F., Nehring, P., Valese, A. C., et al. (2019). Blackberry (*Rubus ulmifolius* Schott): Chemical composition, phenolic compounds and antioxidant capacity in two edible stages. *Food Research International, 122*, 627–634.

Serna-Thomé, G., Castro-Eguiluz, D., Fuchs-Tarlovsky, V., Sánchez-López, M., Delgado-Olivares, L., et al. (2018). Use of functional foods and oral supplements as adjuvants in cancer treatment. *Revista de investigacion clinica, 70*(3), 136–146.

Sethi, S., Josh, A., Arora, B., et al. (2020). Significance of FRAP, DPPH, and CUPRAC assays for antioxidant activity determination in apple fruit extracts. *European Food Research and Technology, 246*, 591–598.

Shanmugam, M. K., Rane, G., Kanchi, M. M., Arfuso, F., Chinnathambi, A., et al. (2015). The multifaceted role of curcumin in cancer prevention and treatment. *Molecules, 20*(2), 2728–2769.

Sharp, L., Carsin, A. E., Cantwell, M. M., Anderson, L. A., & Murray, L. J., FINBAR Study Group. (2013). Intakes of dietary folate and other B vitamins are associated with risks of esophageal adenocarcinoma, Barrett's esophagus, and reflux esophagitis. *The Journal of Nutrition, 143*(12), 1966–1973.

Sharpe, E., Farragher-Gnadt, A. P., Igbanugo, M., Huber, T., Michelotti, J. C., et al. (2021). Comparison of antioxidant activity and extraction techniques for commercially and laboratory prepared extracts from six mushroom species. *Journal of Agriculture and Food Research, 4*, 100130.

Shin, S., Lee, J. E., Loftfield, E., Shu, X. O., Abe, S. K., et al. (2022). Coffee and tea consumption and mortality from all causes, cardiovascular disease and cancer: A pooled analysis of prospective studies from the Asia Cohort Consortium. *International Journal of Epidemiology, 51*(2), 626–640.

Sicari, V., Romeo, R., Leporini, M., et al. (2022). Comparison of traditional hot water and vacuum assisted blanching methods on the physico-chemical quality parameters and antioxidant activity of zucchini (*Cucurbita pepo* L.) slices. *Journal of Food Measurement and Characterization, 16*, 281–294.

Siji, S., & Nandini, P. (2017). Antioxidants and antioxidant activity common eight banana varieties in Kerala. *International Journal of Advanced Engineering Research and Science, 4*, 118–123.

Singh, V., Chahal, T. S., Grewal, S. K., & Gill, P. S. (2021). Effect of fruit development stages on antioxidant properties and bioactive compounds in peel, pulp and juice of grapefruit varieties. *Journal of Food Measurement and Characterization, 15*, 2531–2539.

Singhal, T., Chansoria, A., & Kothari, S. (2020). Evaluation of anti-inflammatory activity of docosahexaenoic acid on carrageenan induced paw oedema in rats. *International Journal of Basic & ClinicalPharmacology, 9*(5), 718–721.

Sporn, M. B., Liby, K. T., Yore, M. M., Fu, L., Lopchuk, J. M., Gribble, G. W., et al. (2011). New synthetic triterpenoids: Potent agents for prevention and treatment of tissue injury caused by inflammatory and oxidative stress. *Journal of Natural Products, 74*(3), 396–400.

Strugala, P., Gladkowski, W., Kucharska, A. Z., Sokól-Letowska, A., & Gabrielska, J. (2016). Antioxidant activity and anti-inflammatory effect of fruit extracts from blackcurrant, chokeberry, hawthorn, and rosehip, and their mixture with linseed oil on a model lipid membrane. *European Journal of Lipid Science and Technology, 118*(3), 461–474.

Tenta, R., Fragopoulou, E., Tsoukala, M., Xanthopoulou, M., Skyrianou, M., et al. (2017). Antiproliferative effects of red and white wine extracts in PC-3 prostate cancer cells. *Nutrition and Cancer*, *69*(6), 952–961.

Tian, G., Gu, X., Bao, K., Yu, X., Zhang, Y., et al. (2021). Anti-inflammatory effects and mechanisms of pudilan antiphlogistic oral liquid. *ACS Omega*, *6*(50), 34512–34524.

Tieri, M., Ghelfi, F., Vitale, M., Vetrani, C., Marventano, S., et al. (2020). Whole grain consumption and human health: An umbrella review of observational studies. *International Journal of Food Sciences and Nutrition*, *71*(6), 668–677.

Tio, M., Andrici, J., Cox, M. R., & Eslick, G. D. (2014). Folate intake and the risk of upper gastrointestinal cancers: A systematic review and meta-analysis. *Journal of Gastroenterology and Hepatology*, *29*(2), 250–258.

Tripathi, Y. B., Tripathi, P., & Arjmandi, B. H. (2005). Nutraceuticals and cancer management. *Frontiers in Bioscience-Landmark*, *10*, 1607–1618.

Tufan, B., Koral, S., & Köse, S. (2011). Changes during fishing season in the fat content and fatty acid profile of edible muscle, liver and gonads of anchovy (Engraulis encrasicolus) caught in the Turkish Black Sea. *International Journal of Food Science and Technology*, *46*(4), 800–810.

Tullio, V., Gasperi, V., Catani, M. V., & Savini, I. (2021). The Impact of Whole Grain Intake on Gastrointestinal Tumors: A Focus on Colorectal, Gastric, and Esophageal Cancers. *Nutrients*, *13*(1), 81.

Turati, F., Rossi, M., Pelucchi, C., Levi, F., & La Vecchia, C. (2015). Fruit and vegetables and cancer risk a review of southern European studies. *British Journal of Nutrition*, *113*(Suppl 2), 102–110.

Upadhyay, S., & Dixit, M. (2015). Role of polyphenols and other phytochemicals on molecular signaling. *Oxidative Medicine and Cellular Longevity*, *2015*, 504253.

USP, (2024). Food Chemicals Codex Forum. Available: https://login.usp.org/cas/login?service = https%3A%2F%2Fonline.foodchemicalscodex.org%2Fcas%2Flogin (Access date: February, 2024).

Vance, T. M., Su, J., Fontham, E. T., Koo, S. I., & Chun, O. K. (2013). Dietary antioxidants and prostate cancer: A review. *Nutrition and Cancer*, *65* (6), 793–801.

Verma, V. (2016). Relationship and interactions of curcumin with radiation therapy. *World Journal of Clinical Oncology*, *7*(3), 275–283.

Vogelstein, B., Papadopoulos, N., Velculescu, V. E., Zhou, S., Diaz, L. A. Jr, & Kinzler, K. W. (2013). Cancer genome landscapes. *Science (New York, N.Y.)*, *339*(6127), 1546–1558.

Wali, A. F., Majid, S., Rasool, S., Shehada, S. B., Abdulkareem, S. K., et al. (2019). Natural products against cancer: Review on phytochemicals from marine sources in preventing cancer. *Saudi Pharmaceutical Journal*, *27*(6), 767–777.

Wall-Medrano, A., & Olivas-Aguirre, F. J. (2020). Antioxidant phytochemicals in cancer prevention and therapy—An update. In *Functional Foods in Cancer Prevention and Therapy*, (pp. 195–220). Elsevier.

Wang, H. L., Guo, X., Hu, X., Li, T., Fu, X., & Liu, R. H. (2017). Comparison of phytochemical profiles, antioxidant and cellular antioxidant activities of different varieties of blueberry (Vaccinium spp.). *Food Chemistry*, *217*, 773–781.

Warleta, F., Campos, M., Allouche, Y., Sánchez-Quesada, C., Ruiz-Mora, J., et al. (2010). Squalene protects against oxidative DNA damage in MCF10A human mammary epithelial cells but not in MCF7 and MDA-MB-231 human breast cancer cells. *Food and chemical toxicology*, *48*(4), 1092–1100.

De Waure, C., Bertola, C., Baccarini, G., Chiavarini, M., & Mancuso, C. (2023). Exploring the contribution of curcumin to cancer therapy: A systematic review of randomized controlled trials. *Pharmaceutics*, *15*(4), 1275.

Weaver, C. M., & Miller, J. W. (2017). Challenges in conducting clinical nutrition research. *Nutrition Reviews*, *75*(7), 491–499.

Wu, K., Willett, W. C., Fuchs, C. S., Colditz, G. A., & Giovannucci, E. L. (2002). Calcium intake and risk of colon cancer in women and men. *Journal of the National Cancer Institute*, *94*(6), 437–446.

Wu, L., Noyan Ashraf, M. H., Facci, M., Wang, R., Paterson, P. G., et al. (2004). Dietary approach to attenuate oxidative stress, hypertension, and inflammation in the cardiovascular system. *Proceedings of the National Academy of Sciences USA*, *101*(18), 7094–7099.

Wu, Q. J., Yang, Y., Vogtmann, E., Wang, J., Han, L. H., Li, H. L., & Xiang, Y. B. (2013a). Cruciferous vegetables intake and the risk of colorectal cancer: a meta-analysis of observational studies. *Annals of Oncology*, *24*(4), 1079–1087.

Wu, Q. J., Yang, Y., Wang, J., Han, L. H., & Xiang, Y. B. (2013b). Cruciferous vegetable consumption and gastric cancer risk: A meta-analysis of epidemiological studies. *Cancer Science*, *104*(8), 1067–1073.

Xi, W. P., Lu, J. F., Qun, J. P., & Jiao, B. N. (2017). Characterization of phenolic profile and antioxidant capacity of different fruit part from lemon (*Citrus limon* Burm.) cultivars. *Journal of Food Science and Technology-Mysore*, *54*(5), 1108–1118.

Xiang, L., Wu, H., Pan, A., Patel, B., Xiang, G., et al. (2016). FTO genotype and weight loss in diet and lifestyle interventions: A systematic review and meta-analysis. *The American Journal of Clinical Nutrition*, *103*(4), 1162–1170.

Yang, D. W., Dunshea, F. R., & Suleria, H. A. R. (2020). LC-ESI-QTOF/MS characterization of Australian herb and spices (garlic, ginger, and onion) and potential antioxidant activity. *Journal of Food Processing and Preservation*, *44*(7), e14497.

Yang, O., Kim, H. L., Weon, J.-I., & Seo, Y. R. (2015). Endocrine-disrupting chemicals: review of toxicological mechanisms using molecular pathway analysis. *Journal of Cancer Prevention*, *20*(1), 12–24.

Yao, P., Sun, L., Lu, L., Ding, H., Chen, X., et al. (2017). Effects of genetic and nongenetic factors on total and bioavailable 25(OH)D responses to vitamin D supplementation. *The Journal of Clinical Endocrinology & Metabolism*, *102*(1), 100–110.

Yong, Y. K., Tan, J. J., Teh, S. S., Mah, S. H., Ee, G. C., et al. (2013). Clinacanthus nutans extracts are antioxidant with antiproliferative effect on cultured human cancer cell lines. *Evidence-Based Complementary and Alternative Medicine*, *2013*, 462751.

Yore, M. M., Kettenbach, A. N., Sporn, M. B., & Gerber, S. A. (2011). Stapled peptides for intracellular drug targets. *Methods Enzymology*, *503*, 3–33.

Yuan, J. M. (2013). Cancer prevention by green tea, evidence from epidemiologic studies. *The American Journal of Clinical Nutrition, 98*(6 Suppl), 1676S–1681S.

Zahreddine, H., & Borden, K. L. B. (2013). Mechanisms and insights into drug resistance in cancer. *Frontiers in Pharmacology, 4*, 28.

Zeng, Y. W., Yang, J. Z., Pu, X. Y., Du, J., Yang, T., et al. (2013). Strategies of functional food for cancer prevention in human beings. *Asian Pacific Journal of Cancer Prevention, 14*(3), 1585–1592.

Zhang, F. F., Liu, S. S., John, E. M., Must, A., & Demark-Wahnefried, W. (2015a). Diet quality of cancer survivors and noncancer individuals: Results from a national survey. *Cancer, 121*(23), 4212–4221.

Zhang, Y. F., et al. (2014). Association between folate intake and the risk of lung cancer: A dose-response meta-analysis of prospective studies. *PLoS One*, 9e93465.

Zhang, Y. F., Xu, Q., Lu, J., Wang, P., Zhang, H. W., Zhou, L., Ma, X. Q., & Zhou, Y. H. (2015b). Tea consumption and the incidence of cancer: A systematic review and meta-analysis of prospective observational studies. *European Journal of Cancer Prevention, 24*(4), 353–362.

Zhang, X. H., Ma, J., Smith-Warner, S., Lee, J., & Giovannucci, E. (2013). Vitamin B6 and colorectal cancer: Current evidence and future directions. *World Journal of Gastroenterology, 19*, 1005–1010.

Zhang, G., Wang, Y., Zhang, Y., Wan, X., Li, J., et al. (2012). Anti-cancer activities of tea epigallocatechin-3-gallate in breast cancer patients under radiotherapy. *Current Molecular Medicine, 12*(2), 163–176.

Zhang, H., Liu, Q., Lin, J., Wang, Y., Chen, S., et al. (2016a). GW27-e0657 Resveratrol Protects against oxidized LDL-induced foam cells formation and apoptosis through inhibition of ER stress and downregulation of CD36. *Journal of the American College of Cardiology, 68*(16), C26.

Zhang, S. L., Chen, T. S., Ma, C. Y., Meng, Y. B., Zhang, Y. F., Chen, Y. W., & Zhou, Y. H. (2016b). Effect of vitamin B supplementation on cancer incidence, death due to cancer, and total mortality: A PRISMA-compliant cumulative meta-analysis of randomized controlled trials. *Medicine, 95*(31), e3485.

Zhang, X., Pei, Z., Chen, J., Ji, C., Xu, J., Zhang, X., & Wang, J. (2016c). Exosomes for immunoregulation and therapeutic intervention in cancer. *Journal of Cancer, 7*(9), 1081–1087.

Zhang, H., Yang, Y. F., & Zhou, Z. Q. (2018). Phenolic and flavonoid contents of mandarin (Citrus reticulata Blanco) fruit tissues and their antioxidant capacity as evaluated by DPPH and ABTS methods. *Journal of Integrative Agriculture, 17*(1), 256–263.

Zhang, H., Zhao, Q., Lan, T., Geng, T., Gao, C., et al. (2020). Comparative Analysis of Physicochemical Characteristics, Nutritional and Functional Components and Antioxidant Capacity of Fifteen Kiwifruit (*Actinidia*) Cultivars-Comparative Analysis of Fifteen Kiwifruit (*Actinidia*) Cultivars. *Foods, 9*(9), 1267.

Zheng, D., Liwinski, T., & Elinav, E. (2020). Interaction between microbiota and immunity in health and disease. *Cell Research, 30*(6), 492–506.

Zheng, J., Zhou, Y., Li, S., Zhang, P., Zhou, T., et al. (2017). Effects and mechanisms of fruit and vegetable juices on cardiovascular diseases. *International Journal of Molecular Sciences, 18*(3), 555.

Zhou, Y., Li, N., Zhuang, W., Liu, G., Wu, T., et al. (2008). Green tea and gastric cancer risk: Meta-analysis of epidemiologic studies. *Asia Pacific Journal of Clinical Nutrition, 17*(1), 159–165.

Zhou, Y., Zhuang, W., Hu, W., Liu, G. J., Wu, T. X., et al. (2011). Consumption of large amounts of Allium vegetables reduces risk for gastric cancer in a meta-analysis. *Gastroenterology, 141*(1), 80–89.

Zhu, J. G., Ochalek, J. T., Kaufmann, M., Jones, G., & Deluca, H. F. (2013). CYP2R1 is a major, but not exclusive, contributor to 25-hydroxyvitamin D production in vivo. *Proceedings of the National Academy of Sciences of the United States of America, 110*(39), 15650–15655.

Zittelli, G. C., Lavista, F., Bastianini, A., Rodolfi, L., Vincenzini, M., et al. (1999). Production of eicosapentaenoic acid by Nannochloropsis sp cultures in outdoor tubular photobioreactors. *Journal of Biotechnology, 70*(1-3), 299–312.

Chapter 15

Functional foods and skin health: radiance from within

Sena Bakir[1,2], Zeynep Begum Kalyoncu-Atasoy[3], Zehra Gulsunoglu-Konuskan[3] and Zakir Showkat Khan[4]

[1]Tourism Faculty, Department of Gastronomy and Culinary Arts, Recep Tayyip Erdogan University, Ardesen, Rize, Türkiye, [2]Blueberry Application and Research Center, Recep Tayyip Erdogan University, Pazar, Rize, Türkiye, [3]Faculty of Health Sciences, Department of Nutrition and Dietetics, Istanbul Aydin University, Kucukcekmece, Istanbul, Türkiye, [4]Department of Food Technology, School of Applied and Life Sciences, Uttaranchal University, Dehradun, Uttarakhand, India

Abbreviations

FA:	Fatty acids
GI:	Glycemic index
LPO:	Lipid peroxidation
PUFA:	Polyunsaturated fatty acids
RNS:	Reactive nitrogen species
ROS:	Reactive oxygen species
UV-B:	Ultraviolet B
UVR:	Ultraviolet radiation

15.1 Introduction

From ancient times to the present, people have always been interested in learning more about the relationship between nutrition and skin health, specifically how diet affects skin aging. This curiosity has made the topic of study fascinating for scientists as well as the general public. The skin's inherent aging process affects it like all internal organs, symbolizing aging in time. Extrinsic aging of the skin refers to the aging of the skin as a result of environmental conditions and external variables, such as smoking, pollution, sleep deprivation, improper diet, exceptionally prolonged sun exposure and light ultraviolet radiation (UVR) exposure. Scientists have discovered that specific phytonutrients, such as carotenoids, tocopherols, and flavonoids, together with vitamins A, C, D, and E, omega-3 fatty acids (FA), certain proteins, and lactobacilli, function as antioxidants and can support skin health and beauty (Hiticas et al., 2019).

The functional food industry offers anything from prepared dishes to foods and beverages that have been fortified. Traditional dairy and nondairy food categories, such as oil products, baked goods, confections, and drinks, now offer foods and beverages with additional beneficial components like fiber, omega-3 FA, antioxidants, and probiotics (Sun-Waterhouse, 2011). In terms of health, skin protection is crucial since it can avert illnesses that could develop into dangerous problems. Furthermore, since skin appearance—particularly that of the face—conveys information that impacts on socioeconomic status, it is a feature of tremendous value in signaling. This chapter will outline the foods which should eat to expand the well-being of our skin.

15.2 Skin: organs, degenerations, regeneration, and aging

The skin is the largest organ throughout the body, and it functions as a connector between internal structures and the environment. Hence, it must be waterproof and resistant to environmental factors (Lizardo & Tavaria, 2022). It is a continually forming organ comprising three primary layers—the epidermis, dermis, and hypodermis—and maintains a constant activity state to fulfill its protective function (Fig. 15.1) (Kim et al., 2022). The epidermis determines skin

Unleashing the Power of Functional Foods and Novel Bioactives. DOI: https://doi.org/10.1016/B978-0-443-28862-3.00015-7

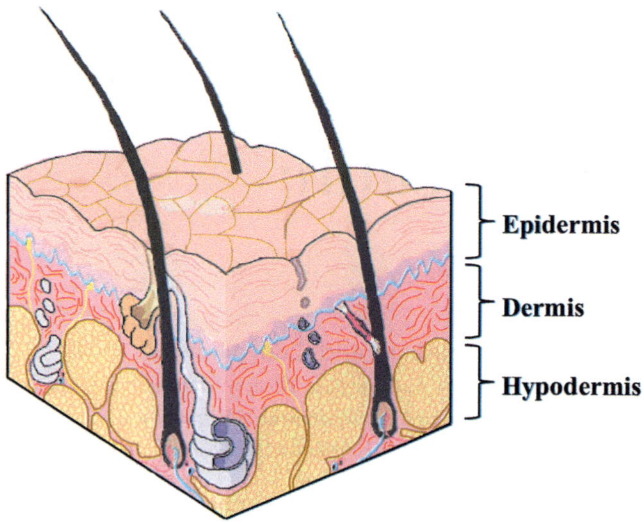

FIGURE 15.1 Representation of human skin layers.

characteristics such as color, texture, and moisture, and the outermost layer primarily comprises keratinocytes (accounting for 90%–95%) (Lizardo & Tavaria, 2022). Its thickness varies depending on where it is on the body; for instance, the eyelids are thin and the palms and soles are thick. According to the morphology and location of the keratinocytes, the epidermis is constructed of four layers: the stratum corneum (the outermost layer), stratum granulosum (granular layer), stratum spinosum, and basal layer. The dermis is located beneath the epidermis and supplies the skin with blood vessels. This layer comprises mostly fibroblasts, myeloid cells, and lymphoid immune cells. A layer of fat and collagen lies beneath the dermis, known as the hypodermis. The skin has many other anatomical structures, such as hair follicles, nails, sweat glands, and sebaceous glands (Kim et al., 2022).

The aging of the skin can be due to endogenous aging, which occurs naturally, and exogenous aging, which occurs from the sun. Aging results in thinner, drier, wrinkled, uneven pigmentation, liver spots in the skin, and delayed wound healing can be observed. Skincare and treatments aim to prevent skin aging and improve wrinkles and pigmentation with minimal adverse effects (Xu et al., 2018). A variety of factors can cause damage to the skin, including intrinsic and extrinsic factors. It is believed that intrinsic factors such as genetics cause physiological aging, dry skin, dermal atrophy, wrinkles, angiogenesis, an increase in skin permeability, decreased immune function, and decreased sweat production, while extrinsic factors include humidity, environmental pollution, UVR, smoking, and poor nutrition (Flores-Balderas et al., 2023). As a result of chronic exposure to UVR, wrinkles, skin relaxation, and other photoaging characteristics develop on the skin; during photoaging, skin structure changes, such as epidermal stratum corneum integrity, hydration and lipidation, thickness, and color (Xu et al., 2018).

Various chronic conditions can also negatively affect skin health, the most common of which are inflammatory skin diseases (Pasparakis et al., 2014). Skin and subcutaneous diseases rank as the 18th greatest cause of disability-adjusted life years worldwide, accounting in 2013. Skin conditions were the 4th most common cause of disability globally, excluding mortality (Mengist Dessie et al., 2022). Some skin illnesses and their incidences are represented at Table 15.1 Skin illnesses can be brought on by allergies, irritants, genetics, specific diseases, and issues with the immune system according to National Institution of Health (NIH, 2023).

Treatment for these skin diseases is available pharmacologically, which includes immunosuppressant drugs; however, most patients do not fully recover or experience negative effects (Flores-Balderas et al., 2023). Therefore patients frequently seek natural treatments, whether topical or nontopical. In addition to conventional treatments for skin disorders, dietary changes such as functional-based diets have become more popular as an alternative therapy.

15.3 Functional foods: from past to present

One of the main factors influencing consumers is the increasing desire for healthier living. Research has identified numerous factors influencing consumers' consumption and buying behaviors. Certain research has identified numerous factors that influence consumers' consumption and buying behaviors. These include the label's nutrition information, the stage of healthiness of diet, and the presence of particular requirements relating to health issues (Annunziata & Vecchio, 2012).

TABLE 15.1 Common Skin Diseases and Their Incidence.

Illnesses	Definition	Incidence	References
Acne	A common skin ailment caused by blocked hair follicles beneath the skin	Many teens and young adults suffer with acne, which typically starts during puberty. Between the ages of 12 and 24, 85% of people have at least mild acne.	Bhate and Williams (2013)
Atopic Dermatitis	It is a skin condition that causes itchiness, redness, swelling, splitting, leaking clear fluid, crusting, and scaling are the results of scratching	90% of those with this illness develop it before the age of five, and an estimated 60% of them do it in their first year of life	Eichenfield et al. (2014)
Psoriasis	It induces scaly, red skin that might feel hot, puffy, or painful	All age groups can get psoriasis, however, risk groups between the ages of 45 and 64 have the highest prevalence.	AADA (2017)
Rosacea	A chronic inflammatory skin disease that typically affects the nose and cheeks, resulting in flushed skin and a rash	It is more common in people aged 30–60 and had fair skin, blond hair and blue eyes	NIAMS (2024)
Skin cancer	The unusual proliferation of skin cells, which primarily appears on sun-exposed skin	An estimated 9,500 or more Americans receive a skin cancer diagnosis each day in the United States	Rogers et al. (2015)

Uncertainty persists about the meaning of "health" in functional food development and health promotion. However, the generally accepted idea is that functional foods have qualities that positively impact one or more physiological processes in addition to their nutritional qualities. This characteristic is connected to bioactive chemicals and is influenced by the different food-technological procedures (Arvanitoyannis & Van Houwelingen-Koukaliaroglou, 2005).

Scientific and technological advancements and direct customer demand drive food innovations. It requires a lot of money to develop a new functional food. Before launching any product onto the market, quantitative and qualitative marketing research must be conducted since product creation necessitates in-depth understanding of the items and the customers. The biggest problem is ensuring the functional components will last and continue to be "active" and "bioavailable" following processing and storage (Day et al., 2009).

15.4 The role of functional foods in skin health

The quantity of active substances that consumers should ingest to benefit from food intake is the main concern in functional food design. While there is a place for products designed to reduce sickness, there is also a movement toward items that offer "daily health benefits," such as healthy, attractive skin. In this part of chapter, food ingredients used in functional food design are evaluated and their effects on skin health are presented.

15.4.1 Fats

Fats, also known as lipids, are a group of macronutrients that play essential roles in the body's structure and function. They are composed of FA and serve as a concentrated energy source, providing more than twice the energy per gram compared to other macronutrients (i.e., carbohydrates and proteins). Fats absorb fat-soluble A, D, E, and K vitamins, produce hormones, maintain cell membrane integrity, and regulate inflammation and immune function.

Dietary fats are particularly relevant to skin health due to their influence on skin structure, hydration, and appearance (Insel et al., 2017). The quantity and quality of dietary fat intake affect skin health since fat consumption impacts the adipose tissue of body and skin's lipid composition (Cao et al., 2020). A high-fat diet is illustrated with skin aging and damage to skin matrix remodeling, as the increased content of fat delays skin healing through elevated inflammatory responses and oxidative stress (Rosa et al., 2018). Skin inflammation caused by a high-fat diet is illustrated with skin cancer by engendering the expression of inflammatory factors such as tumor necrosis factor in the skin by UV-B. A high-fat diet led to an upregulation of the epidermal FA binding protein in mice and caused a formation of lipid droplets that increased skin lesions (Zhang et al., 2015).

Understanding the dietary fat saturation levels is crucial in comprehending its impact on skin health, as consuming a balance of unsaturated and saturated fats has been shown to maintain skin barrier function, hydration, and overall radiance. Omega-6 and omega-3 FA are classified as "essential" due to the mammalian cells' inability to synthesize them endogenously, necessitating their acquisition through dietary sources to support dermatological well-being (Kalyoncu et al., 2022; Pappas et al., 2016). Both omega-6 and omega-3 are polyunsaturated fatty acids (PUFA) with multiple carbon double bonds. Eicosapentaenoic acid, which has three double bonds, is an omega-3 FA that produces eicosanoids that reduce inflammation. Linoleic acid, an omega-6 FA, is an essential constituent of skin barrier structures called ceramides. To begin with, a diet deficient in PUFA could increase transepidermal water loss, decrease skin barrier function, and increase the levels of proliferative keratins (Woodby et al., 2020). Rats that were fed a diet deficient in dietary fats developed scaly skin with increased transepidermal water loss. Secondly, PUFA has been shown to play critical roles in skin barrier function and integrity. Multiple in vivo studies have shown that PUFA intake enhances skin barrier function when faced with essential FA deficiency or skin disorders (Torrissen et al., 2023). Also, optimum dietary intake of omega-3 FA inhibits cutaneous oxidative inflammation (Valacchi et al., 2018; Woodby et al., 2020). Moreover, a high intake of omega-3 FA was associated with increased elasticity and ameliorated the impact of photoaging in both males and females (Latreille et al., 2013). However, an interaction between omega-6 FA and contaminants in the skin leads to the membrane phospholipids oxidation, which initiates proinflammatory cascade. Supplementation with omega-3 FA offers protection by enhancing antioxidant enzyme activity, such as superoxide dismutase (Huang et al., 2018). Research findings indicate enhanced blister epithelization in groups supplemented with omega-3 FA compared to control groups, suggesting improved wound healing and decreased incidence of wound infections in humans (Wesley Alexander & Dorothy, 2014).

In parallel, consumption of foods abundant in healthy fats, including fatty fish like salmon and mackerel, nuts and seeds such as walnuts and flaxseeds, as well as avocados and olive oil, has been linked to improved skin health due to their beneficial effects on skin barrier function and hydration.

On the other hand, excessive consumption of saturated and trans fats, commonly found in processed and fried foods, may promote inflammation and oxidative stress, contributing to skin conditions such as aging, dullness, and acne. Therefore limiting the intake of unhealthy fats, while incorporating healthy fats into the diet may contribute to skin radiance and overall skin health.

Acne, a common skin condition characterized by pimples, blackheads, whiteheads, and nodules primarily occurring on the face, neck, chest, back, and shoulders, is also affected by nutrition (AADA, 2024). Since acne is caused by the blockage and inflammation of hair follicles and their accompanying sebaceous due to excess oil production, hormonal changes and bacteria fat intake are associated with acne development (Sutaria et al., 2023). Research studies, such as the Growing Up Today Study from the United States, have shed light on this relationship. Findings from this study, which enrolled over 25,000 participants, demonstrated a significant association between teenage acne and milk consumption. Specifically, teenagers who consume milk, particularly low-fat and skim milk varieties, exhibited a higher prevalence of acne. This correlation posits that the water-soluble male hormones androgens present in milk may stimulate glandular tissue such as the sebaceous glands in the skin. Whole milk consumption is less strongly associated with acne than low-fat and skim milk. Hence, removing fat from milk in low-fat and skim milk varieties may exacerbate acne development by eliminating fat-soluble female hormones known as estrogens. Estrogens are thought to counteract the acne-inducing effects of androgens. These results highlight the potential impact of dietary fat intake, especially from milk sources, on acne occurrence among adolescents (Adebamowo et al., 2005).

Consistent with the study above, in a retrospective study that included 47,355 participants, acne was shown to be 44% more common in women who consumed two or more glasses of skim milk each day (Adebamowo et al., 2005). Also, in a case-control study that was conducted in Italy with patients with moderate-to-severe acne, cow's milk consumption was the only significant difference associated with acne (Di Landro et al., 2012).

Additionally, a systematic review of 35 articles reported that in addition to dairy fat-containing foods, chocolate was also associated with acne promotion (Dall'Oglio, Nasca, Fiorentini, & Micali, 2021). An increase of 17 g of fat and 50 g of carbohydrate intake is illustrated with a higher chance of skin atrophy and wrinkles (Cosgrove et al., 2007). Overall, by choosing nutrient-rich sources of fats and maintaining a balanced diet, individuals can support the health and vitality of their skin in the form of a glowing complexion and youthful appearance.

15.4.2 Carbohydrates

Carbohydrates are macronutrients in various foods, including grains, fruits, vegetables, and dairy products. They serve as the body's primary energy source and are broken down into glucose that fuels cellular processes (Insel et al., 2017).

TABLE 15.2 Glycemic Index Classification (Insel et al., 2017).

Classification Categories	Glycemic Index	Examples of Foods
Low GI	55 or less	Lentils, black-eyed peas, skim milk, bran, bulgur
Medium GI	56–69	White rice, pineapple, raisin, sweet corn, muesli, French fries
High GI	70 or more	White bread, baked potatoes, candies, cakes, muffins

Carbohydrates could be categorized according to the glycemic index (GI) measure. GI measures how quickly carbohydrates in food raise blood glucose levels after ingestion (Table 15.2). GI could be considered the percentage value ranging from 1 to 100 and categorized into low GI, medium GI, and high GI (Kalyoncu et al., 2022). While foods with a high GI cause a rapid strike in blood glucose levels followed by a quick drop, foods with a low GI lead to a slower and more gradual increase and then decrease in blood glucose levels (Wolever et al., 1991).

GI has gained attention for its potential impact on skin health. High GI foods trigger a cascade of hormonal changes, such as increased insulin levels and inflammation, that may deteriorate skin conditions like acne, wrinkles, and atrophy. In contrast, choosing carbohydrates with a low GI, such as whole grains, legumes, fruits, and vegetables, may contribute to healthier skin by maintaining a more stable blood glucose level. Therefore selecting healthier carbohydrate sources with a low GI could be a strategy for improving skin radiance as part of overall skin health.

Research findings suggest that adopting a low GI diet may lead to a reduction in acne severity. Studies conducted in various countries provide evidence for the efficacy of low GI diets in managing acne (Association, 2024). In the United States, a study involving 2258 people on a low GI diet for weight loss revealed a notable reduction in acne. While 87% of the participants reported a decrease in acne severity, 91% were documented to require less acne medication (El Moutaoui et al., 2009). Similarly, in Australia, a 12-week trial involving 43 male participants showed that those following a low GI diet experienced significantly less acne than those on their regular diet (Smith et al., 2007).

Furthermore, research conducted in Korea and Türkiye further supported these findings. Results demonstrated that individuals adhering to a low GI diet exhibited reduced acne symptoms compared to those consuming a regular or high GI diet (Çerman et al., 2016; Kwon et al., 2012). Last but not least, another study that was conducted in Saudi Arabia found that female participants who ate sweets and snacks under stress were documented to have a significantly higher percentage of severe acne (Basfar et al., 2023). Therefore prioritizing whole grains like oats, barley, and quinoa, as well as fruits and vegetables rich in fiber and nutrients, may support the appearance and vitality of the skin.

Fruits such as grapes, mulberries, raspberries, tomatoes, strawberries, and nuts contain resveratrol. Resveratrol's neuroprotective, antioxidant, antiinflammatory, and antiproliferative properties have been confirmed in numerous studies. In a randomized controlled trial involving 36 participants, a decrease in facial wrinkle depth was reported with the daily consumption of 85 grams of mango. However, daily consumption of 250 grams was associated with increased wrinkle length and depth in postmenopausal women (Fam et al., 2020).

15.4.3 Proteins

Proteins are macromolecules composed of 20 different amino acids considered the building blocks. They play a fundamental role in virtually every biological process in the body by serving as structural components, enzymes, hormones, antibodies, and transporters. Structurally, proteins consist of long chains of amino acids folded into complex three-dimensional shapes, which determine their function and specificity. Dietary proteins are indispensable for the growth, repair, and maintenance of tissues, including muscles, bones, and organs, and they play a crucial role in maintaining the health and integrity of the skin.

Collagen, the most abundant protein in the body, provides structural support and elasticity to the skin to maintain its firmness and smoothness. Another protein found in the skin, called elastin, contributes to the skin's flexibility and resilience, allowing it to stretch and return to its original shape. Furthermore, proteins are essential for repairing and regenerating skin cells, facilitating wound healing and tissue renewal. Therefore consuming adequate protein through a balanced diet is necessary for optimal skin function and appearance. Including protein-rich foods such as fish, poultry, legumes, nuts, seeds, lean meats, and dairy products other than milk can help to support optimal skin health and radiance by providing the necessary building blocks for collagen synthesis and repair processes.

Collagen, the primary protein of structure in the skin, provides over 75% of the extracellular matrix's body weight in total. Natural collagen from a variety of fish, chicken, and pork sources is hydrolyzed through enzymes to produce hydrolyzed collagen, which is utilized in oral supplements. During digestion, collagen is broken down into dipeptides and tripeptides, absorbed through the gastrointestinal system into the bloodstream, and accumulates significantly in the skin. These dipeptides stimulate fibroblast proliferation, migration, and metabolism, increasing collagen and hyaluronic acid production.

Despite the nineteen different types of collagen, types 1 and 3 constitute 70% of the skin. Especially type 1 collagen, the most abundant type, plays a crucial role in the formation of bone, cartilage, connective tissue, teeth, and skin structure. Type 3 collagen is a significant component of the organs and skin extracellular matrix. It supports muscles, organs, blood vessels, and skin.

To support collagen formation in the body, many supplements are sold in the form of tablets, capsules, powders, liquids, gummies, gum, etc. Hydrolyzed collagen peptides, broken down into amino acids during digestion and having the best absorption, are preferred for increased bioavailability. Hydrolyzed collagen peptides have been shown to penetrate the skin more rapidly and stimulate fibroblast cells, which produce collagen in the skin. The recommended daily intake of hydrolyzed collagen peptides is at least 2–2.5 g in 2–3-month periods throughout the year by giving breaks of similar duration. Other supplements that support collagen synthesis may contain copper, zinc, and vitamin C. Studies done with collagen generally show a decrease in facial wrinkles, improved hydration, and skin elasticity posttreatment, with benefits that continue for 30 days after treatment without significant side effects. However, meta analysis findings are limited due to heterogeneity in compound composition, concentration, and physical forms of collagen.

Another supplement used for skin radiance is glucosamine, commonly used in arthritis. Glucosamine is necessary for synthesizing glycoproteins, glycolipids, glycosaminoglycans, and proteoglycans. A study with eight participants demonstrated that applying 250 mg of glucosamine for eight weeks increased hyaluronan synthesis and expression of types 1 and 3 collagens. In a randomized controlled trial (n:53), oral dietary supplements, glucosamine, minerals, and antioxidants have been shown to significantly reduce facial wrinkles and fine lines.

Lastly, gluten may cause skin rashes and acne-like eruptions in some individuals who have nonceliac gluten sensitivity. Celiac disease is an autoimmune disorder characterized by an intolerance to gluten, a protein found in wheat, barley, and rye. In individuals with celiac disease, exposure to gluten triggers an abnormal immune response that leads to inflammation and damage to intestinal villi, resulting in malabsorption of nutrients. Individuals with gluten sensitivity should adhere to a gluten-free diet to manage symptoms associated with gluten sensitivity (Vats et al., 2023).

15.4.4 Micronutrients and hydration

Optimal skin health relies on external skincare practices and macronutrients and further internal factors such as adequate nutrition through micronutrients and hydration (Park, 2015). Micronutrients refer to essential nutrients, vitamins, and minerals the body requires in small amounts for various physiological functions. Micronutrients are essential for properly functioning of enzymes, hormones, and other biochemical processes in the body, including those involved in skin health and maintenance. Vitamins are organic compounds crucial in metabolism, growth, and immune function. Vitamins B complex and C are soluble in water, while vitamins A, D, E, and K are soluble in fat (Insel et al., 2017). Micronutrients, including vitamins, minerals, and antioxidants, play crucial roles in supporting skin health at the cellular level. To begin with, vitamins A, C, and E are potent antioxidants that protect skin from oxidative damage that is caused by free radicals, thereby preventing premature aging and promoting a youthful appearance (Lim et al., 2022).

Vitamins A, C, D, and E, green tea polyphenols, niacinamide, and trace elements such as zinc may help alleviate signs of skin aging. Vitamin E is protective against photodamage and effective in regulating skin moisture, but it is not as potent as an antioxidant as vitamin C (Rattanawiwatpong et al., 2020). Almonds, especially the non-roasted ones, consumed in the diet contain high amounts of vitamin E in a way that ¼ of a cup provides close to 30% of the daily value (Insel et al., 2017). In two randomized controlled trials (n:91 and n:31), participants who consumed almonds equivalent to 20% of their daily energy intake reported significant improvement in facial pigmentation and skin wrinkles (Foolad et al., 2019). Another vitamin that plays a key role in the antioxidant network and exhibits synergistic antioxidant effects with vitamin E is vitamin C. It is best obtained through a natural diet, as supplements may pose a risk of kidney stone formation, although most excess amounts are excreted in the urine. Vitamin C helps increase the synthesis of type 1 and 3 collagens and inhibits collagen breakdown (Lis & Baar, 2019). Also, vitamin C is associated with decreased hyperpigmentation and a radiant skin appearance. Both internal consumption and topical use of vitamin C are effective in brightening the skin, repairing fine lines and wrinkles, reducing skin discoloration, and lightening blemishes. It also alleviates acne and scars. In a large cohort study that included 4025 people, high vitamin C and linoleic acid intake were observed to have beneficial effects on facial wrinkles and skin dryness (Al-Niaimi & Chiang, 2017; Wang et al., 2018).

Another compound that functions similarly to a vitamin and is synthesized by the body endogenously is called coenzyme Q10. It plays a crucial role in cellular energy production and is a powerful antioxidant, protecting cells from oxidative damage. Coenzyme Q10 is recognized for its essential role in various physiological processes, including skin health. Oral coenzyme Q10 possesses both antioxidant and antiinflammatory properties. Improvement in wrinkles and skin smoothness was observed in a pair of double-blind randomized controlled trials involving 33 participants. However, the supplement was ineffective in skin hydration and increasing dermal thickness (Žmitek et al., 2017; Žmitek, Žmitek, Rogl Butina, & Pogačnik, 2020).

Conversely, minerals are inorganic elements critical for bone health, nerve function, muscle contraction, and fluid balance (Insel et al., 2017). Minerals like zinc and selenium are involved in collagen synthesis and wound healing, thus contributing to skin strength and resilience. Nevertheless, overdosing on zinc can exert adverse effects, including immune system suppression, impaired wound healing, taste and smell perception alterations, hair loss, and skin issues (Glutsch et al., 2019).

Deficiencies or imbalances in micronutrients can lead to various health issues, including skin disorders, impaired wound healing, and compromised immune function. Therefore consuming a balanced diet rich in micronutrient-dense foods is essential for optimal skin health and well-being.

Despite all the effects above of micronutrients, the evidence level for systematic treatments remains limited. Studies often feature small sample sizes, predominantly female cohorts, single-center designs, involvement of similar researchers, short durations of study, follow-up, and heterogeneity in methodology and assessment criteria. These limitations lead to a lack of consensus on which outcome measures are clinically valid. Furthermore, oral nutritional supplements may be associated with certain side effects, especially in countries where their regulation is heavily influenced by industry lobbying efforts.

Additionally, hydration is paramount for maintaining skin elasticity, moisture balance, and overall hydration levels. Adequate water intake supports proper skin hydration from within and prevents dryness, dullness, and irritation. Therefore in addition to external treatments and optimal nutrition, proper hydration should be maintained for skin health (Akdeniz et al., 2018).

Water aids in preserving the ideal moisture balance in the extracellular matrix and skin cells. For the stratum corneum in particular, proper hydration is crucial to avoiding dehydration, dryness, and early aging. The stratum corneum, the outermost layer of the epidermis, acts as a barrier to stop the body from losing water, which is how it largely regulates skin moisture (Wilhelm et al., 1991).

Further, being hydrated helps to maintain the structure and function of elastin fibers, which maintain skin suppleness. It also facilitates correct circulation and nutrient delivery to skin cells, which aid in cellular regeneration and repair as well as the body's excretion of waste materials. Drinking enough water each day and eating meals high in water content, like fruits and vegetables, are recommended to maintain good skin hydration and suppleness (Liska et al., 2019).

15.4.5 Carotenoids

Carotenoids are mainly derived from food, fruit, and vegetables because the body cannot synthesize them from scratch (Alaluf et al., 2002). Human health and interpersonal attractiveness may be influenced by carotenoids. It is conceivable that carotenoids influence human health and attraction to others. Although they cannot be manufactured by animals, carotenoids are found naturally in plants. Therefore like other animal species, humans get carotenoids from their food (Perrett et al., 2020).

The presence or absence of oxygen allows for the classification of carotenoids. Most of the time, oxygen is found in hydroxyl or epoxide groups (Srivastava, 2021). Oxygen-containing carotenoids are referred to as xanthophylls, where oxygen atoms are in the form of a hydroxyl group or epoxides, while no oxygen-containing carotenoids are known as carotenes. Human plasma, milk, and other tissues, such as the skin, are routinely found to contain certain carotenoids. The primary carotenoids are typically lycopene, α-carotene, β-carotene, lutein, zeaxanthin, β-cryptoxanthin, phytoene, and phytofluene (Meléndez-Martínez et al., 2017).

Bloodborne carotenoids are absorbed and then released onto the skin, giving it a yellow-orange color by contributing to the B* values of human skin (Alaluf et al., 2002; Coetzee & Perrett, 2014). It is seen as appealing and healthy (Lefevre & Perrett, 2015). Skin deposition of carotenoids may aid in photoprotection by lowering the degree of UV light–induced skin damage and raising the threshold of UV exposure needed to produce sunburn (Bouilly-Gauthier et al., 2010). In guinea pigs, injections of phytoene prevented UVR-induced erythema, according to one of the earliest studies highlighting the protective function of carotenoids in skin health (Mathews Roth et al., 1975). The first (Mathews-Roth, 1982) reported that giving mice phytoene over an extended period decreased the number and appearance of skin tumors caused by UV-B light. The fact that there was no discernible anticarcinogenic activity when the tumors were artificially produced was another important discovery of this investigation.

Besides a seasonal increase in carotenoid consumption during summer or autumn and/or consuming the same quantity of carotenoids throughout the year, the accumulation of carotenoids in human skin is dependent on the freshness and ripeness of fruits and vegetables (Lademann et al., 2011). The elastin and collagen fibers in polygene fibers are also destroyed by the free radicals created by UVR, which limits their repair (Kawaguchi et al., 1997). Before they cause harm, a high concentration of carotenoids and other antioxidants effectively neutralizes already-existing free radicals.

It may be shown that the volunteers' skin carotenoid content reflects their lifestyle. While stress factors like sickness, excessive sun exposure, alcohol intake, and smoking lower the number of carotenoids in the skin, carotenoids, like most antioxidants, can only be absorbed through a balanced diet rich in fruits and vegetables. A high concentration of carotenoids in the skin is the best defense against skin aging (Lademann et al., 2011). According to Chung et al. (2006), young women's judgments to eat fruit and vegetables are largely driven by the assumption that doing so will make them look better. Stephen et al. (2011) connect skin carotenoid coloration to a healthy appearance, which may thus send a strong message about the importance of eating a balanced diet and consuming more fruits and vegetables to meet the government's often ignored requirements. When volunteers with high carotenoid concentrations in their skin were compared to those with low concentrations, the former group showed fewer wrinkles and furrows (DARVIN et al., 2008).

The possibility of having a beautiful skin tone could inspire people to exercise, eat more fruits and vegetables, cut back on calories, manage their stress, and maintain proper sleeping habits. Such a comprehensive approach to living a healthy lifestyle, as opposed to a narrow concentration on one aspect, like weight, aligns nicely with health recommendations (Perrett et al., 2020). Enhanced skin yellowing, a sign of elevated carotenoid levels in the skin, was linked to low body fat, enhanced exercise, less stress, and improved sleep (Perrett et al., 2020). Exposure to the sun, skin conditions, age, or hormonal imbalances is associated with an increase in melanin deposition in certain areas of the skin, resulting in dark patches and freckles. The use of whitening treatments is motivated by the fact that dark patches have significance that extends beyond aesthetic considerations, as they can occasionally result in cancer (Von Oppen-Bezalel & Shaish, 2009). Topical formulations rich in phytoene and phytofluene have positive benefits on the skin, including skin whitening and antiaging and antiwrinkling properties (Oppen-Bezalel et al., 2014). Concerns were raised about the usage of canthaxanthin supplements after it was discovered that, in certain situations, taking large amounts of the carotenoid continuously (starting at 30 mg/day) could cause crystals to grow in the eye. However, these crystals could vanish if the use of the product was stopped (Mortensen, 2009).

15.4.6 Antioxidant-rich foods

The largest organ in the body, the skin, serves as a vital conduit between the environment and the body, shielding it from physical, chemical, and microbiological threats that could otherwise change the skin's composition and functionality by generating reactive oxygen species (ROS) and nitrogen (RNS). It has been demonstrated that phenolic compounds and extracts from a variety of plants, including blueberries, green tea, grapes, pomegranates, and various marine algae, are effective at reducing cellular oxidative stress.

Sunlight-induced UVR is a vital environmental risk factor in the development of skin cancer (Ichihashi et al., 2003; Narendhirakannan & Hannah, 2013). The creation of ROS and RNS from UVR is linked to the beginning, encouragement, and advancement of carcinogenesis (Narendhirakannan & Hannah, 2013). Lipid peroxidation (LPO), which is brought on by ROS, is accountable for alterations in membrane permeability, disruption of the cell membrane structure, malfunctioning metabolite exchange pathways, and in severe cases, cellular death (Vasconcelos et al., 2007).

Antioxidants should be applied to the skin before sun exposure. When administered topically before UVR exposure, research studies on humans have clearly shown that both synthetic and "natural" antioxidants have significant photoprotective effects. Despite several tries, there was no discernible protective impact of melatonin and antioxidants (vitamins E and C), either applied separately or in combination, following UVR exposure (Poljsak et al., 2013). Since oxidative damage brought on by ROS can cause some skin illnesses, antioxidants are a wonderful therapeutic option for treating these conditions. Thus some sunscreen creams contain antioxidants such as vitamin E, vitamin C, phenolic compounds, flavonoids, and carotenoids. These antioxidants primarily function by scavenging free radicals, neutralizing ROS, shielding cell membranes from oxidative stress, and absorbing UV rays. In certain situations, they also stop high collagen and elastase production (Ngoc et al., 2019).

Following a 12-week course of treatment, the dietary supplement fortified with polyphenols showed notable enhancements over the placebo in every clinically measurable efficacious parameter, including skin lipoperoxides. Positive results were observed after just two weeks of product use, including lessened wrinkle depth, enhanced elasticity and firmness, improved skin barrier function, and decreased dark spots (Nobile et al., 2021).

Because of its high potential for antioxidant activity and minimal cytotoxicity, coffee silverskin—a food by-product of the coffee roasting industry—has been investigated as an active component for skincare products by Rodrigues et al. (2016). After 180 days in storage, the formulation maintained its physical characteristics and antioxidant activity. Two skin cell lines (fibroblasts and keratinocytes) were used to screen for in vitro toxicity, and any toxicity was reported. The results of the in vivo test demonstrated that the Coffee silverskin Medicago sativa formulation is safe for topical administration regarding irritating effects and that after 30 days of use, skin hydration had improved. Furthermore, in light of customer acceptability, over 90% of participants said it was pleasant.

15.4.7 Phytoestrogens

Estrogens have a significant impact on a wide range of critical processes, including homeostasis, cell division and death, liver protein expression, lipid metabolism, energy balance, glucose metabolism, immunological and cardiovascular regulation, gonadotrophin feedback and gametogenesis, brain-neuronal development, memory processing, repair and regeneration, bone growth, and skin health, particularly in women with estrogen-deficient skin (Lephart & Naftolin, 2021). Regardless of age, gender, or region, everyone in the world is exposed to and eats phytoestrogens like resveratrol and equol on a daily basis (Lephart, 2021).

One major factor contributing to the reduction in skin functioning during menopause and climacteric is the drop in serum estrogen levels. Insufficient estrogen weakens the body's ability to fend off oxidative stress; the skin gets thinner, loses suppleness and collagen, wrinkles more easily, becomes drier, and has less vascularity (Sirotkin & Halim Harrath, 2014). Aging is linked to reduced wound healing, hair loss, pigmentary changes, and a higher risk of skin cancer as its protective function is undermined (Thornton, 2013).

Therefore hormone replacement therapy with estrogen or phytoestrogens has a positive impact on the skin's quality and functions in a number of ways. It promotes antiaging action by preventing the loss of collagen concentration, restoring skin elasticity, and increasing skin hydration. It also plays a critical role in accelerating the healing of wounds. Estrogen has several beneficial benefits on the skin; however, systemic hormone replacement therapy should not be used as a stand-alone treatment for skin aging (Carneiro et al., 2020).

15.4.8 Probiotics

The probiotic term is defined as "*live microorganisms that, when administrated in adequate amounts, confer a health benefit on the host*" (FAO/WHO, 2006). The most commonly used probiotics are lactic acid bacteria and *Bifidobacterium*. As these microorganisms colonize the host, they can perform biological functions while regulating the microbiome and contributing to health. Since probiotics alter the intestinal microbiota, they have been broadly marketed and consumed as functional foods and supplements (Lizardo & Tavaria, 2022). The action of these compounds is mediated by epithelial repair, increased gut barrier function, and immune modulation. Moreover, prenatal and postnatal supplementation of probiotic bacteria has been shown to prevent the development of eczema in newborns (Kim et al., 2010). Probiotics can produce antimicrobial peptides, called bacteriocins, and organic acids. It promotes the antiinfective activity of probiotics, and it is associated with a low pH and neutralization of some pathogen toxins (Pawar & Tiwari, 2022). The studies about the probiotic intake is alleviating skin diseases are shown in Table 15.3

There is evidence to suggest that commensal microorganisms in the gut modulate systemic immunity and therefore influence skin homeostasis. In recent years, several skin diseases, including atopic dermatitis, allergic rhinitis, and wound healing, have been prevented and treated with probiotics as part of intervention studies. In a study, when the head-killed cells of *Lactococcus lactis* H61 strain were supplemented on middle-aged women (31−62 years), an improvement on skin elasticity, more hydration, and improved hair follicles was observed (Kimoto-Nira et al., 2012). Similarly, in another study, when orally supplemented with heat-killed *Lactobacillus casei* subsp. *casei* 327 to 64 subjects, an improvement was observed in skin barrier functions (Saito et al., 2017). Moreover, oral intakes of *Lactobacillus plantarum* HY7714 by 110 volunteers aged 41−59 years for 12 weeks found to increase skin moisture, decrease wrinkle depth, and improve overall skin gloss and elasticity (Lee et al., 2015). Probiotics can also be used to

TABLE 15.3 The Effect of Probiotics on Skin Diseases.

Probiotics	Skin Disease	Duration	Treatment Group	Main Results	References
Lactobacillus acidophilus	Acne[1], Eczema[2]	12 weeks[1], 12 months[2]	Human	Decreased in total lesion, Reduction of development eczema in infants	Kim et al. (2010) and Rodrigues et al. (2016)
L. acidophilus	Allergic contact dermatitis	5 weeks	Mice	Increase the level of Foxp3, IL-10, TGF-β	Shah et al. (2012)M
L. casei	Skin conditions	8 weeks	Human	Reduction in skin flakiness, improvement in skin barrier functions	Saito, Mihara, Maruyama, Saito, and Ikeda (2017)
L. delbrueckii subs. bulgaricus	Acne	12 weeks	Human	Reduction of acne symptoms	Chan et al. (2021)
L. plantarum	Photoaging	12 weeks	Human	Reduction in wrinkle, skin gloss improved, skin elasticity improved	Lee et al. (2015)
L. rhamnosus	Atopic dermatitis	12 weeks	Human	ECP and IL-31 decrease	Jeong et al. (2020)
Lactococcus lactis	Skin conditions	8 weeks	Human	Improvement of skin elasticity	Kimoto-Nira et al. (2012)
Bifidobacterium bifidum	Acne[1], Eczema[2]	12 weeks[1], 12 months[2]	Human	Reduction of acne symptoms, reduction of development eczema in infants	Day et al. (2009) and Kim et al. (2010)
B. lactis	Eczema	12 months	Human	Reduction of development eczema in infants	Kim et al. (2010)

ECP, Eosinophil cationic protein; *Foxp3*, forkhead box P3; *IL-10*, interleukin-10, *IL-31*, interleukin-31; *TGF-β*, transforming growth factor-β.

reduce the side effects of antibiotics used in skin diseases. Probiotics are reported to reduce negative effects illustrated with chronic antibiotic use, and they may also play an interdependent role with antibiotics in treating acne by modulating inflammation and immune function (Jung et al., 2013).

Various bioactive compounds are found in vegetables and fruits, which play a key role in the prevention of diseases like cancer, aging, and oxidative stress. Adding lactic acid bacteria to vegetables and fruits can increase their nutritional value and function by enhancing their functional properties. Fermentation is the primary method used by researchers to produce probiotic vegetables and fruits. Chan et al. (2022) investigated the skin antiaging properties of fermented pomegranate products with *Saccharomyces cerevisiae* and *L. plantarum*. According to obtained data, fermented pomegranate drink improved the brightness, collagen density, elasticity, and moisture of the skin of subjects for 8 weeks of treatment. Another study conducted by Chan et al. (2021) showed that fermented apple juice with *S. cerevisiae* and *Streptococcus thermophilus* promoted collagen synthesis and delayed the aging of skin for 30 subjects aged between 35 and 55 years old. Moreover, a study has shown that when soymilk fermented with *L. casei* Shirota is administrated orally for 12 weeks, improvements in skin conditions like coarseness, dryness, elasticity, moisture, pigmentation, and stratum corneum morphology were observed (Nagino et al., 2018).

15.5 Future perspective

Natural dietary supplements known as antioxidants, proteins, and carotenoids have been demonstrated to have health-promoting effects, and their importance in nutricosmetics is only increasing. Evaluation of the markers of oxidative stress in people who had nonmelanoma skin cancer resulted in healthy people associating with habitual food intake relative to antioxidant nutrients. Before starting or stopping an antioxidant treatment, it is important to take into account while assessing each person's oxidative status. Based on existing research, it is suggested that eating a diet high in foods high in health-related compounds and avoiding stressors can improve skin health and attractiveness, with potential systemic benefits as well.

The primary function of antioxidative compounds in cosmetic formulations is obtained from Final Report Elmore (2005) of the safety assessment of these ingredients. However, the antioxidative potential of skincare products cannot be assessed using a commonly used and standardized approach that would make it easier for consumer to select skincare products.

Besides abovementioned health-related compounds, skin hydration and suppleness are vitally dependent on proper hydration and water consumption, which aid in preserving the ideal moisture balance in the extracellular matrix and skin cells. Skin hydration was significantly improved by the formulation containing the extracts in the human volunteers' clinical investigations of diets high in antioxidants. When the goal is skin hydration and protection, the efficacy of cosmetic formulations, including these extracts, is confirmed objectively by the improvement in skin conditions demonstrated by the efficacy studies.

Additionally, probiotics help lessen the negative effects of antibiotics used to treat skin conditions. Probiotics have been shown to help mitigate the negative effects of long-term antibiotic treatment.

15.6 Conclusion

Traditional approaches to food preparation based on specific nutrients are challenged by functional foods and their wider range of health advantages. According to epidemiological research, eating more fruits on a daily basis may improve overall health and well-being and lower the chance of developing chronic illnesses. As a result, there has been a surge of research from academic, corporate, and government institutions in an effort to incorporate fruit goodness into popular consumer goods. Different diets that boost food's antioxidant potential can delay photoaging in elderly European ancestors who have moderate-to-high levels of sun exposure and are vulnerable to UV damage. To fully understand how diets affect skin photoaging in younger adults and vulnerable adults who receive less ambient sun exposure, more extensive long-term research is needed. Since the industry has long recognized the importance of nutrition for skin health and beauty, it has made attempts to develop in the areas of cosmetics, cosmeceuticals, nutricosmetics, functional foods, and nutraceuticals.

AI disclosure

During the preparation of this work, the author(s) used QuillBot and Grammarly to AI applications were used to prepare Grammarly appropriate and readable chapter manuscript. After using this tool/service, the author(s) reviewed and edited the content as needed and take(s) full responsibility for the content of the publication.

References

AADA. (2017). *Burden of Skin Disease*. American Academy of Dermatology. Available from https://www.aad.org/member/clinical-quality/clinical-care/bsd.

AADA. (2024). *A low-glycemic diet may lead to fewer pimples*. American Academy of Dermatology. Available from https://www.aad.org/public/diseases/acne/causes/diet.

Adebamowo, C. A., Spiegelman, D., Danby, F. W., Frazier, A. L., Willett, W. C., & Holmes, M. D. (2005). High school dietary dairy intake and teenage acne. *Journal of the American Academy of Dermatology*, *52*(2), 207–214. Available from https://doi.org/10.1016/j.jaad.2004.08.007.

Akdeniz, M., Tomova-Simitchieva, T., Dobos, G., Blume-Peytavi, U., & Kottner, J. (2018). Does dietary fluid intake affect skin hydration in healthy humans? A systematic literature review. *Skin Research and Technology*, *24*(3), 459–465.

Alaluf, S., Heinrich, U., Stahl, W., Tronnier, H., & Wiseman, S. (2002). Dietary carotenoids contribute to normal human skin color and UV photosensitivity. *The Journal of Nutrition*, *132*(3), 399–403. Available from https://doi.org/10.1093/jn/132.3.399, http://jn.nutrition.org.

Al-Niaimi, F., & Chiang, N. Y. Z. (2017). Topical vitamin C and the skin: mechanisms of action and clinical applications. *The Journal of Clinical and Aesthetic Dermatology*, *10*(7), 14.

Annunziata, A., & Vecchio, R. (2012). Consumer perception of functional foods: A conjoint analysis with probiotics. *Food Quality and Preference*, *28*, 348–355.

Arvanitoyannis, I. S., & Van Houwelingen-Koukaliaroglou, M. (2005). Functional foods: A survey of health claims, pros and cons, and current legislation. *Critical Reviews in Food Science and Nutrition*, *45*(5), 385–404. Available from https://doi.org/10.1080/10408390590967667.

Basfar, A. S., Jawhari, A. M., Alotaibi, M. N., Alzahrani, E. S., Aseeri, I. A., & Atalla, A. A. (2023). Severity of acne, stress, and food habits of medical students at Taif University, Saudi Arabia. *Journal of Family and Community Medicine*, *30*(2), 131–136. Available from https://doi.org/10.4103/jfcm.jfcm_396_22, www.jfcmonline.com.

Bhate, K., & Williams, H. C. (2013). Epidemiology of acne vulgaris. *British Journal of Dermatology, 168*(3), 474–485. Available from https://doi.org/10.1111/bjd.12149.

Bouilly-Gauthier, D., Jeannes, C., Maubert, Y., Duteil, L., Queille-Roussel, C., Piccardi, N., Montastier, C., Manissier, P., Piérard, G., & Ortonne, J.-P. (2010). Clinical evidence of benefits of a dietary supplement containing probiotic and carotenoids on ultraviolet-induced skin damage. *British Journal of Dermatology, 163*(3), 536–543. Available from https://doi.org/10.1111/j.1365-2133.2010.09888.x.

Cao, C., Xiao, Z., Wu, Y., & Ge, C. (2020). Diet and skin aging—From the perspective of food nutrition. *Nutrients, 12*(3), 870.

Carneiro, J., Cunha, M., Haddad, A., & Neto, M. (2020). The Effects of estrogens and phytoestrogens on human skin and its topical use for prevention of skin ageing-Literature review. *Surg Cosmet Dermatol, 12*, 11–15.

Çerman, A. A., Aktaş, E., Altunay, I. K., Arici, J. E., Tulunay, A., & Ozturk, F. Y. (2016). Dietary glycemic factors, insulin resistance, and adiponectin levels in acne vulgaris. *Journal of the American Academy of Dermatology, 75*(1), 155–162. Available from https://doi.org/10.1016/j.jaad.2016.02.1220, http://www.elsevier.com/inca/publications/store/6/2/3/3/7/0/index.htt.

Chan, L. P., Tseng, Y. P., Liu, C., & Liang, C. H. (2022). Fermented pomegranate extracts protect against oxidative stress and ageing of skin. *Journal of Cosmetic Dermatology, 21*(5), 2236–2245. Available from https://doi.org/10.1111/jocd.14379.

Chan, L.-P., Tseng, Y.-P., Liu, C., & Liang, C.-H. (2021). Anti-oxidant and anti-ageing activities of fermented vegetable-fruit drink. *Journal of Food and Nutrition Research, 9*(5), 240–250. Available from https://doi.org/10.12691/jfnr-9-5-1.

Chung, S.-J., Hoerr, S., Levine, R., & Coleman, G. (2006). Processes underlying young women's decisions to eat fruits and vegetables. *Journal of Human Nutrition and Dietetics, 19*, 287–298.

Coetzee, V., & Perrett, D. I. (2014). Effect of beta-carotene supplementation on African skin. *Journal of Biomedical Optics, 19*(2). Available from https://doi.org/10.1117/1.JBO.19.2.025004.

Cosgrove, M. C., Franco, O. H., Granger, S. P., Murray, P. G., & Mayes, A. E. (2007). Dietary nutrient intakes and skin-aging appearance among middle-aged American women. *The American Journal of Clinical Nutrition, 86*(4), 1225–1231.

Dall'Oglio, F., Nasca, M. R., Fiorentini, F., & Micali, G. (2021). Diet and acne: Review of the evidence from 2009 to 2020. *International Journal of Dermatology, 60*(6), 672–685.

Darvin, M., Patzelt, A., Gehse, S., Schanzer, S., Benderoth, C., Sterry, W., & Lademann, J. (2008). Cutaneous concentration of lycopene correlates significantly with the roughness of the skin. *European Journal of Pharmaceutics and Biopharmaceutics, 69*(3), 943–947. Available from https://doi.org/10.1016/j.ejpb.2008.01.034.

Day, L., Seymour, R. B., Pitts, K. F., Konczak, I., & Lundin, L. (2009). Incorporation of functional ingredients into foods. *Trends in Food Science and Technology, 20*(9), 388–395. Available from https://doi.org/10.1016/j.tifs.2008.05.002.

Di Landro, A., Cazzaniga, S., Parazzini, F., Ingordo, V., Cusano, F., Atzori, L., Tripodi Cutrì, F., Letizia Musumeci, M., Zinetti, C., Pezzarossa, E., Bettoli, V., Caproni, M., Lo Scocco, G., Bonci, A., Bencini, P., & Naldi, L. (2012). Family history, body mass index, selected dietary factors, menstrual history, and risk of moderate to severe acne in adolescents and young adults. *Journal of the American Academy of Dermatology, 67*(6), 1129–1135. Available from https://doi.org/10.1016/j.jaad.2012.02.018.

Eichenfield, L. F., Tom, W. L., Chamlin, S. L., Feldman, S. R., Hanifin, J. M., Simpson, E. L., Berger, T. G., Bergman, J. N., Cohen, D. E., Cooper, K. D., Cordoro, K. M., Davis, D. M., Krol, A., Margolis, D. J., Paller, A. S., Schwarzenberger, K., Silverman, R. A., Williams, H. C., Elmets, C. A., … Sidbury, R. (2014). Guidelines of care for the management of atopic dermatitis: Section 1. Diagnosis and assessment of atopic dermatitis Work Group. *Journal of the American Academy of Dermatology, 70*(2), 338–351. Available from https://doi.org/10.1016/j.jaad.2013.10.010.

Elmore, A. R. (2005). Final report of the safety assessment of L-Ascorbic Acid, Calcium Ascorbate, Magnesium Ascorbate, Magnesium Ascorbyl Phosphate, Sodium Ascorbate, and Sodium Ascorbyl Phosphate as used in cosmetics. *International Journal of Toxicology, 24*, 51–111.

Fam, V. W., Holt, R. R., Keen, C. L., Sivamani, R. K., & Hackman, R. M. (2020). Prospective evaluation of mango fruit intake on facial wrinkles and erythema in postmenopausal women: A randomized clinical pilot study. *Nutrients, 12*(11), 3381.

FAO/WHO. (2006). Probiotics in food, Health and nutritional properties and guidelines for evaluation. *Chemical and Functional Properties of Food Components, 2006*, 413–426.

Flores-Balderas, X., Peña-Peña, M., Rada, K. M., Alvarez-Alvarez, Y. Q., Guzmán-Martín, C. A., Sánchez-Gloria, J. L., Huang, F., Ruiz-Ojeda, D., Morán-Ramos, S., Springall, R., & Sánchez-Muñoz, F. (2023). Beneficial effects of plant-based diets on skin health and inflammatory skin diseases. *Nutrients, 15*(13), 2842. Available from https://doi.org/10.3390/nu15132842, http://www.mdpi.com/journal/nutrients/.

Foolad, N., Vaughn, A. R., Rybak, I., Burney, W. A., Chodur, G. M., Newman, J. W., … Sivamani, R. K. (2019). Prospective randomized controlled pilot study on the effects of almond consumption on skin lipids and wrinkles. *Phytotherapy Research, 33*(12), 3212–3217. Available from https://doi.org/10.1002/ptr.6495, http://onlinelibrary.wiley.com/journal/10.1002/(ISSN)1099-1573.

El Moutaoui, L., Rochd, U.I., Benchikhi, H., Khadir, K., & Ibn, U. (2009). Comparative efficacy and tolerability results of tretinoin microsphere gel pump 0.04% and tazarotene cream 0.05% in the treatment of mild to moderate facial acne vulgaris. *Journal of the American Academy of Dermatology*, 60(3), AB14. Available from https://doi.org/10.1016/j.jaad.2008.11.088.

Glutsch, V., Hamm, H., & Goebeler, M. (2019). Zinc and skin: An update. *JDDG: Journal der Deutschen Dermatologischen Gesellschaft, 17*(6), 589–596.

Hiticas, V. V., Butnariu, M., & Sarac, I. (2019). Essential compounds in skin health. *EC Nutrition, 14*(11), 50–57.

Huang, T.-H., Wang, P.-W., Yang, S.-C., Chou, W.-L., & Fang, J.-Y. (2018). Cosmetic and therapeutic applications of fish oil's fatty acids on the skin. *Marine Drugs, 16*(8), 256.

Ichihashi, M., Ueda, M., Budiyanto, A., Bito, T., Oka, M., Fukunaga, M., Tsuru, K., & Horikawa, T. (2003). UV-induced skin damage. *Toxicology, 189*(1-2), 21–39. Available from https://doi.org/10.1016/s0300-483x(03)00150-1.

Insel, P., Ross, D., McMahon, K., & Bernstein, M. (2017). *Nutrition. Cathy L. Esperti (publisher). Johns&Bartlett Learning* (6th edition). Massachuset, USA: LLC.

Jeong, K., Kim, M., Jeon, S. A., Kim, Y. H., & Lee, S. (2020). A randomized trial of Lactobacillus rhamnosus IDCC 3201 tyndallizate (RHT3201) for treating atopic dermatitis. *Pediatric Allergy and Immunology*, *31*(7), 783–792. Available from https://doi.org/10.1111/pai.13269.

Jung, G. W., Tse, J. E., Guiha, I., & Rao, J. (2013). Prospective, randomized, open-label trial comparing the safety, efficacy, and tolerability of an acne treatment regimen with and without a probiotic supplement and minocycline in subjects with mild to moderate acne. *Journal of Cutaneous Medicine and Surgery*, *17*(2), 114–122. Available from https://doi.org/10.2310/7750.2012.12026.

Kalyoncu, Z. B., Norde, M. M., & Özel, H. G. (2022). Nutritional management of pediatric ENT infections. *Pediatric ENT Infections*, 1063–1083.

Kawaguchi, Y., Tanaka, H., Okada, T., Konishi, H., Takahashi, M., Ito, M., & Asai, J. (1997). Effect of reactive oxygen species on the elastin mRNA expression in cultured human dermal fibroblasts. *Free Radical Biology and Medicine*, *23*(1), 162–165. Available from https://doi.org/10.1016/s0891-5849(96)00570-9.

Kim, J. H., Ahamed, A., Chen, K., Lebig, E. G., Petros, B., Saeed, S., & Martins-Green, M. (2022). *Skin microbiota and its role in health and disease with an emphasis on wound healing and chronic wound development* Microbiome. *Immunity, Digestive Health and Nutrition* (pp. 297–311). Academic Press.

Kim, J. Y., Kwon, J. H., Ahn, S. H., Lee, S. I., Han, Y. S., Choi, Y. O., & Ji, G. E. (2010). Effect of probiotic mix (*Bifidobacterium bifidum, Bifidobacterium lactis, Lactobacillus acidophilus*) in the primary prevention of eczema: A double-blind, randomized, placebo-controlled trial. *Pediatric Allergy and Immunology*, *21*(2), 386–393. Available from https://doi.org/10.1111/j.1399-3038.2009.00958.x, *21(2 PART 2)*.

Kimoto-Nira, H., Aoki, R., Sasaki, K., Suzuki, C., & Mizumachi, K. (2012). Oral intake of heat-killed cells of lactococcus lactis strain h61 promotes skin health in women. *Journal of Nutritional Science*, *1*(7), 1. Available from https://doi.org/10.1017/jns.2012.22.

Kwon, H. H., Yoon, J. Y., Hong, J. S., Jung, J., Park, M. S., & Suh, D. H. (2012). Clinical and histological effect of a low glycaemic load diet in treatment of acne vulgaris in Korean patients: A randomized, controlled trial. *Acta Dermato-Venereologica*, *92*(3), 241–246. Available from https://doi.org/10.2340/00015555-1346South, http://www.medicaljournals.se/acta/content/download.php?doi = 10.2340/00015555-1346, Korea.

Lademann, J., Meinke, M. C., Sterry, W., & Darvin, M. E. (2011). Carotenoids in human skin. *Experimental Dermatology*, *20*(5), 377–382. Available from https://doi.org/10.1111/j.1600-0625.2010.01189.x.

Latreille, J., Kesse-Guyot, E., Malvy, D., Andreeva, V., Galan, P., Tschachler, E., Hercberg, S., Guinot, C., & Ezzedine, K. (2013). Association between dietary intake of n-3 polyunsaturated fatty acids and severity of skin photoaging in a middle-aged Caucasian population. *Journal of Dermatological Science*, *72*(3), 233–239. Available from https://doi.org/10.1016/j.jdermsci.2013.07.006.

Lee, D. E., Huh, C. S., Ra, J., Choi, I. D., Jeong, J. W., Kim, S. H., & Ahn, Y. T. (2015). Clinical evidence of effects of Lactobacillus plantarum HY7714 on skin aging: A randomized, double blind, placebo-controlled study. *Journal of Microbiology and Biotechnology*, *25*(12), 2160–2168. Available from https://doi.org/10.4014/jmb.1509.09021, http://www.jmb.or.kr/journal/download.php?Filedir = ./submission/Journal/025/&num = 7338.

Lefevre, C. E., & Perrett, D. I. (2015). Fruit over sunbed: Carotenoid skin colouration is found more attractive than melanin colouration. *Quarterly Journal of Experimental Psychology*, *68*(2), 284–293. Available from https://doi.org/10.1080/17470218.2014.944194, http://journals.sagepub.com/loi/qjpd.

Lephart, E. D. (2021). Phytoestrogens (resveratrol and equol) for estrogen-deficient skin—controversies/misinformation versus anti-ageing in vitro and clinical evidence via nutraceutical-cosmetics. *International Journal of Molecular Sciences*, *22*(20), 11218.

Lephart, E. D., & Naftolin, F. (2021). Menopause and the skin: Old favorites and new innovations in cosmeceuticals for estrogen deficient skin. *Dermatology and Therapy*, *11*, 53–69.

Lim, H. W., Kohli, I., Ruvolo, E., Kolbe, L., & Hamzavi, I. H. (2022). Impact of visible light on skin health: The role of antioxidants and free radical quenchers in skin protection. *Journal of the American Academy of Dermatology*, *86*(3), S27–S37.

Lis, D. M., & Baar, K. (2019). Effects of different Vitamin C-enriched collagen derivatives on collagen synthesis. *International Journal of Sport Nutrition and Exercise Metabolism*, *29*(5), 526–531. Available from https://doi.org/10.1123/ijsnem.2018-0385, https://journals.humankinetics.com/view/journals/ijsnem/29/5/article-p526.xml.

Liska, D., Mah, E., Brisbois, T., Barrios, P. L., Baker, L. B., & Spriet, L. L. (2019). Narrative review of hydration and selected health outcomes in the general population. *Nutrients*, *11*(1), 70. Available from https://doi.org/10.3390/nu11010070, https://www.mdpi.com/2072-6643/11/1/70/pdf.

Lizardo, M. V. P., & Tavaria, F. K. (2022). *Probiotics and skin health Probiotics: Advanced Food and Health Applications* (pp. 389–405). Elsevier, https://www.sciencedirect.com/book/9780323851701 10.1016/B978-0-323-85170-1.00020-8.

Mathews Roth, M. M., Pathak, M. A., Mathews-Roth, M. M., & Pathak, M. A. (1975). Phytoene as a protective agent against sunburn (>280nm) radiation in guinea pigs. *Photochemistry and Photobiology*, *21*, 261–263.

Mathews-Roth, M. M. (1982). Antitumor activity of β-carotene, canthaxanthin and phytoene. *Oncology (Switzerland)*, *39*(1), 33–37. Available from https://doi.org/10.1159/000225601.

Meléndez-Martínez, A. J., Pérez-Gálvez, A., Roca, M., Estévez Santiago, R., Olmedilla Alonso, B., Mercadante, A. Z., & Jesús Ornelas-Paz, J. D. (2017). Biodisponibilidad de carotenoides, factores que la determinan y métodos de estimación. In A. J. Meléndez-Martínez (Ed.), *Carotenoides en Agroalimentación y Salud* (pp. 574–608). México: Ciudad de México.

Mengist Dessie, A., Fenta Feleke, S., Getaye Workie, S., Getinet Abebe, T., Mossu Chanie, Y., & Kassa Yalew, A. (2022). Prevalence of skin disease and its associated factors among primary schoolchildren: A cross-sectional study from a Northern Ethiopian Town. *Clinical, Cosmetic and Investigational Dermatology*, *15*, 791–801. Available from https://doi.org/10.2147/ccid.s361051.

Mortensen, A. (2009). Supplements. *Nutrition and Health.*, *5*, 67–82, 2009.

Nagino, T., Kaga, C., Kano, M., Masuoka, N., Anbe, M., Moriyama, K., Maruyama, K., Nakamura, S., Shida, K., & Miyazaki, K. (2018). Effects of fermented soymilk with Lactobacillus casei Shirota on skin condition and the gut microbiota: A randomised clinical pilot trial. *Beneficial Microbes*, *9*(2), 209–218. Available from https://doi.org/10.3920/bm2017.0091.

Narendhirakannan, R. T., & Hannah, M. A. C. (2013). Oxidative stress and skin cancer: An overview. *Indian Journal of Clinical Biochemistry*, *28*(2), 110–115. Available from https://doi.org/10.1007/s12291-012-0278-8.

Ngoc, L. T. N., Tran, V. V., Moon, J. Y., Chae, M., Park, D., & Lee, Y. C. (2019). Recent trends of sunscreen cosmetic: An update review. *Cosmetics*, *6*(4), 64. Available from https://doi.org/10.3390/COSMETICS6040064, https://res.mdpi.com/d_attachment/cosmetics/cosmetics-06-00064/article_deploy/cosmetics-06-00064-v2.pdf.

NIAMS. (2024). Rosacea. National Institute of Arthritis and Musculoskeletal and Skin Diseases. https://www.niams.nih.gov/health-topics/rosacea#tab-risk.

NIH. (2023). *National Institute of Arthritis and Musculoskeletal and Skin Diseases*. Available from https://www.niams.nih.gov/health-topics/skin-diseases).

Nobile, V., Schiano, I., Peral, A., Giardina, S., Spartà, E., & Caturla, N. (2021). Antioxidant and reduced skin-ageing effects of a polyphenol-enriched dietary supplement in response to air pollution: A randomized, double-blind, placebo-controlled study. *Food & Nutrition Research*, *65*. Available from https://doi.org/10.29219/fnr.v65.5619.

Park, K. (2015). Role of micronutrients in skin health and function. *Biomolecules & Therapeutics*, *23*(3), 207–217. Available from https://doi.org/10.4062/biomolther.2015.003.

Pappas, A., Liakou, A., & Zouboulis, C. C. (2016). Nutrition and skin. *Reviews in Endocrine and Metabolic Disorders*, *17*, 443–448.

Pasparakis, M., Haase, I., & Nestle, F. O. (2014). Mechanisms regulating skin immunity and inflammation. *Nature Reviews. Immunology*, *14*(5), 289–301. Available from https://doi.org/10.1038/nri3646.

Pawar, A., & Tiwari, S. K. (2022). Bacteriocin-producing probiotic lactic acid bacteria in controlling dysbiosis of the gut microbiota. *Frontiers in Cellular and Infection Microbiology*, *12*, 1–11. Available from https://doi.org/10.3389/fcimb.2022.851140.

Perrett, D. I., Talamas, S. N., Cairns, P., & Henderson, A. J. (2020). Skin color cues to human health: Carotenoids, aerobic fitness, and body fat. *Frontiers in Psychology*, *11*, 392. Available from https://doi.org/10.3389/fpsyg.2020.00392, http://www.frontiersin.org/Psychology.

Poljsak, B., Dahmane, R., & Godic, A. (2013). Skin and antioxidants. *Journal of Cosmetic and Laser Therapy*, *15*(2), 107–113. Available from https://doi.org/10.3109/14764172.2012.758380.

Rattanawiwatpong, P., Wanitphakdeedecha, R., Bumrungpert, A., & Maiprasert, M. (2020). Anti-aging and brightening effects of a topical treatment containing vitamin C, vitamin E, and raspberry leaf cell culture extract: A split-face, randomized controlled trial. *Journal of Cosmetic Dermatology*, *19*(3), 671–676.

Rodrigues, F., Sarmento, B., Amaral, M. H., & Oliveira, M. B. P. (2016). Exploring the antioxidant potentiality of two food by-products into a topical cream: Stability, in vitro and in vivo evaluation. *Drug Development and Industrial Pharmacy*, *42*(6), 880–889. Available from https://doi.org/10.3109/03639045.2015.1088865, http://www.tandfonline.com/loi/iddi20#.Vmuk8Lfovcs.

Rogers, H. W., Weinstock, M. A., Feldman, S. R., & Coldiron, B. M. (2015). Incidence estimate of nonmelanoma skin cancer (keratinocyte carcinomas) in the US population. *JAMA Dermatol.*

Rosa, D. F., Sarandy, M. M., Novaes, R. D., Freitas, M. B., do Carmo Gouveia Pelúzio, M., & Gonçalves, R. V. (2018). High-fat diet and alcohol intake promotes inflammation and impairs skin wound healing in Wistar rats. *Mediators of Inflammation*, *2018*(1), 4658583. Available from https://doi.org/10.1155/2018/4658583, http://www.hindawi.com/journals/mi/.

Saito, Y., Mihara, T., Maruyama, K., Saito, J., Ikeda, M., Tomonaga, A., & Kumagai, T. (2017). Effects of intake of Lactobacillus casei subsp. casei 327 on skin conditions: a randomized, double-blind, placebo-controlled, parallel-group study in women. *Bioscience of Microbiota, Food and Health*, *36*(3), 111–120. Available from https://doi.org/10.12938/bmfh.16-031.

Shah, M. M., Saio, M., Yamashita, H., Tanaka, H., Takami, T., Ezaki, T., & Inagaki, N. (2012). Lactobacillus acidophilus strain L-92 induces CD4 + CD25 + Foxp3 + regulatory T cells and suppresses allergic contact dermatitis. *Biological and Pharmaceutical Bulletin*, *35*(4), 612–616. Available from https://doi.org/10.1248/bpb.35.612Japan, http://www.jstage.jst.go.jp/article/bpb/35/4/612/_pdf.

Sirotkin, A. V., & Halim Harrath, A. (2014). Phytoestrogens and their effects. *European Journal of Pharmacology*, *741*, 230–236. Available from https://doi.org/10.1016/j.ejphar.2014.07.057.

Smith, R. N., Mann, N. J., Braue, A., Mäkeläinen, H., & Varigos, G. A. (2007). The effect of a high-protein, low glycemic–load diet versus a conventional, high glycemic–load diet on biochemical parameters associated with acne vulgaris: A randomized, investigator-masked, controlled trial. *Journal of the American Academy of Dermatology*, *57*(2), 247–256.

Srivastava, R. (2021). Physicochemical, antioxidant properties of carotenoids and its optoelectronic and interaction studies with chlorophyll pigments. *Scientific Reports*, *11*(1). Available from https://doi.org/10.1038/s41598-021-97747-w.

Stephen, I. D., Coetzee, V., & Perrett, D. I. (2011). Carotenoid and melanin pigment coloration affect perceived human health. *Evolution and Human Behavior*, *32*(3), 216–227.

Sun-Waterhouse, D. (2011). The development of fruit-based functional foods targeting the health and wellness market: A review. *International Journal of Food Science & Technology*, *46*(5), 899–920.

Sutaria, A. H., Masood, S., Saleh, H. M., & Schlessinger, J. (2023). *Acne vulgaris* StatPearls [Internet]. StatPearls Publishing.

Thornton, M. J. (2013). Estrogens and aging skin. *Dermato-Endocrinology*, *5*(2), 264–270. Available from https://doi.org/10.4161/derm.23872United, https://www.landesbioscience.com/journals/dermatoendocrinology/article/22678/, Kingdom.

Torrissen, M., Ytteborg, E., Svensen, H., Stoknes, I., Nilsson, A., Østbye, T.-K., Marit Berge, G., Bou, M., & Ruyter, B. (2023). Investigation of the functions of n -3 very-long-chain PUFAs in skin using in vivo Atlantic salmon and in vitro human and fish skin models. *British Journal of Nutrition, 130*(11), 1915–1931. Available from https://doi.org/10.1017/s0007114523001150.

Valacchi, G., Virgili, F., Cervellati, C., & Pecorelli, A. (2018). OxInflammation: From subclinical condition to pathological biomarker. *Frontiers in physiology, 9*, 858.

Vasconcelos, S. M. L., Goulart, M. O. F., Moura, J. B. D. F., Manfredini, V., Benfato, M. D. S., & Kubota, L. T. (2007). Reactive oxygen and nitrogen species, antioxidants and markers of oxidative damage in human blood: Main analytical methods for their determination. *Química Nova, 30*, 1323–1338. Available from https://doi.org/10.1590/s0100-40422007000500046, http://www.scielo.br/pdf/qn/v30n5/a46v30n5.pdf.

Vats, V., Makineni, P., Hemaida, S., Haider, A., Subramani, S., Kaur, N., Naveed Butt, A., Scott-Emuakpor, R., Zahir, M., Mathew, M., & Iqbal, J. (2023). Gluten intolerance and its association with skin disorders: A narrative review. *Cureus*. Available from https://doi.org/10.7759/cureus.44549.

Von Oppen-Bezalel, L., Havas, F., Ramot, O., Kalo, E., & Fishbein, D. (2014). Ben-Chítrit, phytoene and phytofluene for (photo) protection, anti ageing, lightening and evening of skin tone. *SOFW J, 140*, 8–12, 2014.

Von Oppen-Bezalel, L., & Shaish, A. (2009). Application of the colorless carotenoids, phytoene, and phytofluene in cosmetics, wellness, nutrition, and therapeutics. In A. Ben-Amotz, J. Polle, & S. Rao (Eds.), *The alga Dunaliella: Biodiversity, Physiology, Genomics & Biotechnology* (pp. 423–444). Science Publishers.

Wang, K., Jiang, H., Li, W., Qiang, M., Dong, T., & Li, H. (2018). Role of vitamin C in skin diseases. *Frontiers in Physiology, 9*. Available from https://doi.org/10.3389/fphys.2018.00819.

Wesley Alexander, J., & Dorothy, M. (2014). Supp, Role of arginine and omega-3 fatty acids in wound healing and infection. *Advances in Wound Care, 3*(11), 682–690. Available from https://doi.org/10.1089/wound.2013.0469.

Wilhelm, K.-P., Cua, A. B., & Maibach, H. I. (1991). Skin aging: Effect on transepidermal water loss, stratum corneum hydration, skin surface pH, and casual sebum content. *Archives of Dermatology, 127*(12), 1806–1809.

Wolever, T. M., Jenkins, D., Jenkins, A. L., & Josse, R. G. (1991). The glycemic index: Methodology and clinical implications. *The American Journal of Clinical Nutrition, 54*(5), 846–854.

Woodby, B., Penta, K., Pecorelli, A., Lila, M. A., & Valacchi, G. (2020). Skin health from the inside out. *Annual Review of Food Science and Technology, 11*(1), 235–254. Available from https://doi.org/10.1146/annurev-food-032519-051722, http://www.annualreviews.org/journal/food.

Xu, H., Zheng, Y.-W., Liu, Q., Liu, L.-P., Luo, F.-L., Zhou, H.-C., Isoda, H., Ohkohchi, N., & Li, Y.-M. (2018). *Reactive oxygen species in skin repair, regeneration, aging, and inflammation*. IntechOpen. Available from 10.5772/intechopen.72747.

Zhang, Y., Li, Q., Rao, E., Sun, Y., Grossmann, M. E., Morris, R. J., & Li, B. (2015). Epidermal fatty acid binding protein promotes skin inflammation induced by high-fat diet. *Immunity, 42*(5), 953–964. Available from https://doi.org/10.1016/j.immuni.2015.04.016, www.immunity.com.

Žmitek, K., Pogačnik, T., Mervic, L., Žmitek, J., & Pravst, I. (2017). The effect of dietary intake of coenzyme Q10 on skin parameters and condition: Results of a randomised, placebo-controlled, double-blind study. *Biofactors (Oxford, England), 43*(1), 132–140.

Žmitek, K., Žmitek, J., Rogl Butina, M., & Pogačnik, T. (2020). Effects of a combination of water-soluble coenzyme Q10 and collagen on skin parameters and condition: results of a randomised, placebo-controlled, double-blind study. *Nutrients, 12*(3), 618.

Chapter 16

The assessment of the safety and toxicity of the functional foods and nutraceuticals

Elahesadat Hosseini[1,2], Rafael Audino Zambelli[3], Pantea Ghalambor[4] and Parisa Shamsaie[4]

[1]Department of Chemical Engineering, Payame Noor University, Tehran, Iran, [2]Department of Food Science and Technology, National Nutrition Sciences and Food Technology Research Institute, Faculty of Nutrition Sciences and Food Technology, Shahid Beheshti University of Medical Sciences, Tehran, Iran, [3]Food Engineering Department, Federal University of Ceará, Fortaleza, Brazil, [4]Department of Food Science and Technology, Science and Research Branch, Islamic Azad University, Tehran, Iran

16.1 Introduction

Functional foods, as defined by Health Canada, mimic traditional foods with proven physiological benefits, while nutraceuticals, take medicinal forms like pills and potions, also providing physiological benefits (Nutraceuticals/Functional Foods and Health Claims on Foods: Policy Paper, 1998). Health Canada has integrated nutraceuticals into a new category under natural health products, which encompasses herbal and other natural products. While functional foods and nutraceuticals are frequently confused, the overarching emphasis, globally, is on enhancing health and preventing disease through these specialized products. This alignment emphasizes the shared goal of improving overall well-being and health outcomes. There is a clear link between the increasing attention toward functional foods and nutraceuticals and the necessity for comprehensive safety evaluations. As these bioactive compounds gain popularity for their potential health benefits and become essential components of modern diets, it becomes imperative to establish robust assessment criteria to guarantee their safety. The recognition of the importance of these products is directly tied to health promotion, disease risk reduction, and the potential to lower healthcare costs. Consumers, increasingly conscious of their well-being, are seeking ways to enhance their health through dietary choices. This shift in consumer behavior underscores the importance of ensuring the safety and toxicity of functional foods and nutraceuticals. Establishing comprehensive assessment criteria involves rigorous evaluation processes to ascertain the potential risks and benefits associated with the consumption of these products. To conclude, the parallel rise in the popularity of functional foods and the need for safety evaluations highlights the pivotal role that comprehensive assessment criteria play in maintaining the health and wellness of individuals. This chapter offers a concise overview of the functional foods and nutraceuticals domain, focusing particularly on evaluating the safety and toxicity of these products.

16.2 Difference between functional foods and nutraceuticals

The terms "nutraceuticals" and "functional foods" describe categories of health- and nutrition-promoting products (El Sohaimy, 2012). The differentiation between nutraceuticals and functional foods stems from their composition, form, and intended use. Nutraceuticals refer to isolated, purified, and formulated healthful products commonly available in medicinal forms like capsules, pills, or tablets. They are separate from regular foods and often come with specific health claims. Conversely, functional foods are integrated into everyday dietary habits and not in a dose form (Jones, 2002). Nutraceuticals, according to Otles and Gokgunnec (2024), are associated with medical claims, aiming to prevent and cure diseases, including dietary supplements and other specialized foods. In contrast, functional foods, considered ordinary foods, primarily aim to reduce the risk of diseases rather than preventing or curing them. Essential nutrients required for healthy survival, such as vitamins, proteins, fats, and carbohydrates, fall under the category of functional foods. However, when a functional food is specifically utilized for preventing and/or curing diseases, excluding anemia, it is termed a nutraceutical (Espín et al., 2007). In understanding these terms, it becomes evident that definitions vary,

Unleashing the Power of Functional Foods and Novel Bioactives. DOI: https://doi.org/10.1016/B978-0-443-28862-3.00016-9

emphasizing the necessity for proven health benefits beyond nutritional advantages. Some widely accepted definitions assert that these products must demonstrate significant health advantages.

16.3 Functional foods classification

Functional foods represent an array of products designed to go beyond basic nutrition, offering health benefits. Emerging in the early 1900s in the United States, the idea of using food for health promotion began with iodine-fortified salt to combat goiter. Presently, functional foods and nutraceuticals strive to enhance a healthy lifestyle, falling into three categories: Nutraceuticals/Functional Foods and Health Claims on Foods: Policy Paper (1998) fortified foods addressing deficiency-based diseases; El Sohaimy (2012) foods with beneficial microorganisms for internal flora health; and Jones (2002) foods affecting regular metabolic pathways, including genetically modified options. Examples encompass dietary fibers, probiotics, and fatty acids for cardiac, digestive, mental, and immune health. Emerging functional foods like carotenoids, isothiocyanates, and polyphenols offer physiological support with antiinflammatory, antimicrobial, and antimutagenic properties (Gaur & Agnihotri, 2014). The spotlight is on zinc for immune system support against colds and flu (Bigliardi & Galati, 2013). This evolving field continually explores new nutritional combinations, playing a vital role in promoting overall well-being and health.

16.4 Regulatory standards for functional foods and nutraceutical ingredients

Consumers are showing an increasing awareness and interest in the purported health benefits of functional foods and nutraceutical ingredients. Hence, it is essential to ensure that claims linked with these products do not deceive consumers. Additionally, it is essential that the scientific evidence supporting these claims establishes the effectiveness of the materials at levels achievable within a normal dietary regimen.

To address this concern, various regulatory systems have been established by authorities worldwide, outlining the permissible health claims and providing guidelines for obtaining approval for functional food products. Notable examples include the European Authority of Food Safety (EFSA) in Europe, the Food and Drug Administration (FDA) in the USA, and the Ministry of Health, Labour, and Welfare (MHLW) in Japan.

These regulatory bodies have defined specific procedures that manufacturers must adhere to when seeking approval for health claims linked to these products. The purpose is to maintain transparency, accuracy, and reliability in the information provided to consumers. The implementation of such regulatory frameworks ensures that claims are grounded in sound scientific evidence and that the stated benefits are realistically attainable within normal dietary practices.

16.4.1 European regulation

In Europe, there is an absence of a defined regulatory framework and statutory definition for functional foods and nutraceuticals. Nevertheless, the legal obligations imposed on these functional products vary depending on their composition. These products may incorporate substances subject to clear regulations in the European market. Hence, functional foods and nutraceuticals incorporating nutritional and health assertions in their labeling, presentation, and/or advertising must adhere to precise criteria outlined in Regulation (EC) 1924/2006. As per the Regulation, a claim encompasses any message or depiction, whether mandated by community or domestic laws or not, including visual representations, that indicates, suggests, or implies specific attributes of a food. These assertions must be consistent with dietary practices and established fundamentals of nutrition and health. It is crucial to avoid promoting overconsumption of specific products, as a diverse and balanced diet is deemed sufficient to provide the necessary nutrients for the body.

Claims in food marketing (e.g., advertising, labeling, or presentation) are allowed under firm conditions:

- Applicable to ready-to-eat (RTE) products.
- Nutrient/ingredient in question must have a proven beneficial effect and be absorbable.
- The claimed benefits should be easily comprehensible to the average consumer, considering social and cultural factors.

Claims are required to be clear and beneficial to protect consumers, prevent misunderstandings, and encourage innovation and equitable competition in the food industry (Domínguez Díaz et al., 2020).

Following a collaborative initiative reinforced by the European Commission (EC) known as the "process for the assessment of scientific support for claims on foods" (PASSCLAIM), the European Regulation on nutrition and health claims became applicable in January 2007. This project aimed to assess the scientific landscape in diet and health, identifying key areas for health claims and establishing universally applicable criteria for scientifically substantiating these claims. The provided guidance is instrumental in fulfilling the prerequisites for health claims according to European legislation. You can find detailed information and resources on this subject by visiting the following link: http://www.ilsi.org/Europe/Pages/PASSCLAIM_Pubs.aspx. Classified by European regulatory framework, claims fall into two categories. The initial classification, "Nutrition claims," signifies that a food item boasts advantageous nutritional properties attributed to its energy content or nutrient composition (EU regulation 1924/2006). An example would be a claim of "reduced fat," which requires the product to meet specific nutritional criteria. For instance, a product labeled reduced fat must adhere to the criterion of "no more than 3 grams of fat per 100 grams for solids." Other claims falling into this category include "source of fiber" or "high in polyunsaturated fatty acids," each requiring compliance with specified nutrient levels. The second one is "health claims," which encompass statements indicating a connection between a food item or its components and potential health advantages. Article 13 addresses additional health claims, mandating that they must be substantiated by "scientific evidence widely accepted" and comprehensible to the average consumer. Claims associated with disease risk reduction or children's development and health are dealt with in specific articles of the European Union (EU) regulations (Article 14 1a, Article 14 1b) (Table 16.1). The process of authorizing health claims in the EU is governed by Regulation 1924/2006, which emphasizes the necessity for a rigorous scientific assessment. EFSA assesses the data for health claims, with the ultimate decision resting with the EC. For instance, out of the 44,000 health claims submitted to the EC in 2008, only 4637 underwent scientific evaluation by EFSA. Subsequently, EFSA assessed 2758 claims, and only 222 health claims were approved for use in December 2012 (http://www.efsa.europa.eu/en/topics/topic/article13.htm). Table 16.2 presents a selection of examples of claims regarding disease risk reduction that were approved by EFSA.

16.4.2 American regulation

In the United States, the regulation of functional foods is diverse, with products potentially classified as regular food items, medical foods, food additives, drugs, dietary supplements, or foods intended for special dietary purposes. The product's classification is contingent on the manufacturer's marketing approach, particularly the nature of claims featured on the package label (Crowe & Francis, 2013). These categorizations are governed by the Federal Food, Drug, and Cosmetic Act of 1938 (FDCA), which does not provide a precise definition for functional foods. In this regard, the generally recognized as safe (GRAS) system, established in 1958 under the FDCA, is utilized to evaluate and approve food ingredients.

A substance attains GRAS status when experts with scientific qualifications and experience reach a consensus regarding its safety. This consensus is established through scientific procedures. In cases where a substance was used in food before January 1, 1958, the consensus may also be grounded on scientific procedures or experience derived from general use in food. The GRAS expert panel meticulously surveys relevant data concerning a substance's safe usage, encompassing test data, consumption patterns, manufacturing specifics, and specifications. GRAS is categorized into three types:

- FDA's affirmation of GRAS
- Self-affirmation of GRAS

TABLE 16.1 Categorization of Health Claims in the European Regulation.

Article 13: Regulation pertains to health claims that do not specifically address the reduction of disease risk or children's development and health.
Article 13.1: Describing or referencing The role of a nutrient or other substances in growth, development, and the functions of the body. Addressing physiological or behavioral functions. Covering topics related to slimming or weight control, reduction in the sense of hunger, increase in the sense of satiety, or the reduction of available energy in the diet, with consideration given to Directive 96/8/EC
Article 13.5: Allowing for claims based on newly developed scientific evidence and/or those involving the protection of proprietary data
Article 14: Focuses on claims related to the reduction of disease risk and those referring to children's development and health

TABLE 16.2 Reduction of Disease Risk Claims Authorized by European Authority of Food Safety (EFSA).

Nutrient, substance, food, or food category	EFSA opinion reference/journal reference
Monounsaturated and/or polyunsaturated fatty acids	Scientific Opinion on the substantiation of a health claim related to "low fat and low trans spreadable fat rich in unsaturated and omega-3 fatty acids" and reduction of LDL-cholesterol concentrations pursuant to Article 14 of Regulation (EC) No 1924 (2006)
Plant stanol esters	Scientific Opinion on the substantiation of a health claim related to 3 g/day plant sterols/stanols and lowering blood LDL-cholesterol and reduced risk of coronary heart disease pursuant to Article 19 of Regulation EC No 1924 (2006)
Plant sterols/plant stanol esters	Scientific Opinion on the substantiation of a health claim related to 3 g/day plant sterols/stanols and lowering blood LDL-cholesterol and reduced risk of coronary heart disease pursuant to Article 19 of Regulation EC No 1924 (2006)
Plant sterols: sterols extracted from plants, free or esterified with food grade fatty	Plant EFSA (2006)
Barley beta-glucans	Scientific Opinion on the substantiation of a health claim related to barley beta-glucans and lowering of blood cholesterol and reduced risk of coronary heart disease pursuant to Article 14 of Regulation EC No 1924 (2006);
Oat beta-glucan	Scientific Opinion on the substantiation of a health claim related to oat beta glucan and lowering blood cholesterol and reduced risk of coronary heart disease pursuant to Article 14 of Regulation EC No 1924 (2006)
Calcium	Scientific Opinion in relation to the authorisation procedure for health claims on calcium and vitamin D and the reduction of the risk of osteoporotic fractures by reducing bone loss pursuant to Article 14 of Regulation EC No 1924 (2006)
Calcium and vitamin D	Scientific Opinion on the substantiation of a health claim related to vitamin D and risk of falling pursuant to Article 14 of Regulation EC No 1924 (2006)
Folate	Scientific Opinion on the substantiation of a health claim related to increasing maternal folate status by supplemental folate intake and reduced risk of neural tube defects pursuant to Article 14 of Regulation EC No 1924 (2006)
Chewing gum sweetened with 100% xylitol	Scientific Opinion on the substantiation of health claims related to sugar free chewing gum and reduction of dental plaque ID 3084 pursuant to Article 131 of Regulation EC No 1924 (2006)
Sugar-free chewing gum	Scientific Opinion on the substantiation of health claims related to sugar free chewing gum and reduction of dental plaque ID 3084 pursuant to Article 131 of Regulation EC No 1924 (2006)

- Notification of GRAS

  The GRAS evaluation encompasses several elements, including

1. History of use:
   - o Components: Includes factors such as the frequency of consumption, epidemiological data, the type of product, and consideration of specific subpopulations.
   - o Significance: Examines the historical use of the substance, helping to establish its safety based on real-world consumption patterns.
2. Specification of product:
   - o Components: Involves categorization and quantification of the product, specifying its identity, composition, analytical details, and addressing potential contamination concerns.
   - o Significance: Ensures a clear understanding of the product's characteristics and quality control measures.
3. Manufacturing process:
   - o Components: Encompasses a detailed flow diagram of the manufacturing process, compliance with Good Manufacturing Practices (GMP), and release procedures.

- o Significance: Evaluates the consistency and reliability of the manufacturing process to maintain product safety.

4. Reproducibility of process:
   - o Components: Requires data from at least five production batches to assess the consistency and reproducibility of the manufacturing process.
   - o Significance: Ensures that the production process reliably yields a product meeting specified standard.
5. Safety:
   - o Data sources: Involves toxicology data, clinical studies, and mechanism studies to comprehensively assess the safety profile.
   - o Consumption calculation: Includes calculating consumption at the 90th percentile to capture potential high-end exposures.
   - o Exposure comparison: Compares actual exposure levels to the no observed adverse effect level (NOAEL) identified in toxicology assessments.

Health claims in the United States are broadly grouped into three clusters: nutrient content claims, structure/function claims, and health claims (Ellwood et al., 2010).

1. **Nutrient content claims:** These claims directly indicate the level (low, high, lite, reduced, etc.) of a specific nutrient in the product. Such claims imply that the nutrient's presence at this level may support the maintenance of a healthy dietary practice. For instance, a claim such as "high in fiber" might be linked to promoting good digestive health, whereas "low in fat" could be associated with benefits for body weight management or cardiovascular health. These claims are applicable exclusively to nutrients for which there is a defined daily reference intake, as outlined by the food labeling regulations.
2. **Structure/Function claims:** These claims characterize the impacts of a food or substance on the body's structure or function. The Dietary Supplement Health and Education Act of 1994 introduced regulatory standards and protocols overseeing the utilization of three categories of these claims, including:
   - o **Claims describing the function of a nutrient or dietary ingredient:** These claims elucidate the role of a nutrient or dietary ingredient with the intention of positively influencing the human body's normal functions. For example, a statement such as "calcium builds strong bones" directly communicates the effect of calcium on the structural integrity of the body.
   - o **Claims characterizing the means by which a nutrient or dietary ingredient acts:** This category encompasses claims that characterize the mechanisms through which nutritional ingredients operate to reserve a particular structure or function in the body. An illustration could be a claim such as "fiber maintains bowel regularity," which specifies how the nutrient contributes to the maintenance of a specific bodily function.
   - o **Claims supporting generalized well-being or addressing nutrient deficiency benefits:** This type of claim either promotes overall well-being or links a benefit to the correction of a nutrient deficiency. An example is "vitamin D for the treatment of rickets," highlighting the nutrient's role in addressing a specific deficiency-related health condition.

Health claims: These claims, as outlined, encompass statements, symbols, or similar representations on a product label that establish the connection between a constituent and health-related condition. These claims are designed to inform consumers about how a specific food or ingredient may impact their health. Within the United States, the Food and Drug Administration Modernization Act of 1997 (FDAMA) implements a framework for the authorization of health claims in food labeling. This process necessitates the submission of a statement to FDA, reinforced by "a credible statement" from specific scientific bodies within the US government or the National Academy of Sciences (NAS) or any of its subdivisions (FDMA health claims) (FDA, Authorized Health Claims That Meet the Significant Scientific Agreement SSA Standard & FDA, 2019). It is important to note that this regulatory pathway for health claims is not applicable to dietary supplements, underlining the distinct regulatory frameworks governing food items and dietary supplements in the United States.

Exclusive to food products, the ability to comprise health claims in labeling is contingent on the product having an appropriate nutritional profile. Specifically, food items must hold a minimum of 10% of the daily value for at least one essential nutrient, such as calcium and vitamin D, per reference amount customarily consumed (RACC). Before intentionally adding any nutrients, the food product must meet this nutritional threshold. Furthermore, health claims must be communicated in a manner (Bagchi, 2019):

- Emphasizes the consequence of the claim effect in the overall daily diet.
- Easily understandable for consumers.

TABLE 16.3 FDA-Approved Health Claims Based on SSA Health Claims and FDMA Health Claims (https://www.fda.gov/Food/LabelingNutrition/ucm2006876.htm#approved; https://www.fda.gov/FoodLabelingGuide).

SSA Health Claims		
Ingredient	**Associated disease**	**Claim statement(s)**
Calcium, vitamin D	Osteoporosis	Adequate calcium and vitamin D as part of a balanced diet may reduce the risk of osteoporosis
Dietary lipids	Risk of cancer	A low-fat diet may reduce the risk of certain cancers, as cancer development is influenced by various factors
Dietary saturated fat and cholesterol	Risk of coronary heart disease	Low-saturated fat, low-cholesterol diets may reduce heart disease risk
Dietary noncariogenic carbohydrate sweeteners	Dental caries	Frequent snacking on sugary and starchy foods can cause tooth decay. However, [name of food] with sugar alcohols does not promote dental issues
Fiber-containing grain products, fruits and vegetables	Risk of cancer	Reducing cancer risk involves low-fat diets with fiber-rich grains, fruits, and vegetables, considering various contributing factors
Fruits and vegetables	Risk of cancer	Reducing cancer risk is associated with low-fat diets rich in fruits and vegetables, which may provide dietary fiber, vitamin A, or vitamin C. Cancer is influenced by various factors.
Folic acid	Neural tube defects	Eating a healthy diet with sufficient folate may lower the risk of birth defects in the brain or spinal cord for women
Fruits, vegetables, and grain products especially soluble fiber	Risk of coronary heart disease	Eating [name of food product], rich in soluble fiber, as part of a low-saturated fat, low-cholesterol diet, can reduce the risk of heart disease. One serving provides_ grams of the recommended daily soluble fiber intake from [name of soluble fiber source].
Sodium	Hypertension	Reducing sodium intake in diets may lower the risk of high blood pressure, a condition influenced by various factors
Soluble fiber from certain foods (barely, whole oat, psyllium seed husk)	Risk of coronary heart disease	Consuming soluble fiber, like that found in [name of soluble fiber source or specific food product], as part of a low-saturated fat, low-cholesterol diet, can lower the risk of heart disease. A serving of [name of food product] provides_ grams of the recommended daily soluble fiber intake from [name of soluble fiber source] for this benefit.
Soy protein	Risk of coronary heart disease	Diets low in saturated fat and cholesterol, with 25 g of soy protein daily, may reduce the risk of heart disease. One serving of [name of food] provides__ grams of soy protein
Stanols/Sterols	Risk of coronary heart disease	Consuming at least 0.65 g of vegetable oil sterol esters twice a day, with a daily total intake of at least 1.3 g as part of a low-saturated fat and low-cholesterol diet, may lower the risk of heart disease. A serving of [name of food] provides__ grams of vegetable oil sterol esters
FDMA health claims		
Whole grain food	Risk of heart disease and certain cancers	Eating whole grain foods and plant-based diets low in total fat, saturated fat, and cholesterol may lower the risk of heart disease and certain cancers
Saturated fat, cholesterol, and trans fat	Risk of heart disease	Reducing saturated fat and cholesterol intake, and minimizing trans-fat consumption, may lower the risk of heart disease
Fluoridated water	Risk of dental caries	Consuming fluoridated water may lower the risk of dental caries or tooth decay
Potassium	Risk of high blood pressure and stroke	Eating diets rich in potassium and low in sodium may lower the risk of high blood pressure and stroke
Unsaturated fatty acids replacement	Risk of heart disease	Substituting saturated fat with equivalent amounts of unsaturated fats may lower the risk of heart disease. To realize this benefit, total daily calorie intake should remain unchanged

TABLE 16.4 Summary of Qualified Health Claims in US (http://www.fda.gov/Food/IngredientsPackagingLabeling/LabelingNutrition/ucm073992.htm).

Components/Ingredients	Associated Disease
100% whey protein partially hydrolyzed infant formula	Atopic dermatitis
Tomatoes and/or tomato sauce	Risk of prostate, ovarian, gastric, and pancreatic cancer
Calcium and colon	Risk of rectal cancer and recurrent colon/rectal polyps.
Green tea	Risk of cancer
Selenium	Risk of cancer
Antioxidant vitamins	Risk of cancer
Nuts	Heart disease
Omega-3 fatty acids	Coronary heart disease
B Vitamins	Vascular disease
Monounsaturated fatty acids from olive oil	Coronary heart disease
Unsaturated fatty acids from canola oil	Coronary heart disease
Corn oil	Heart disease
Phosphatidylserine	Cognitive dysfunction and dementia
Psyllium husk	Diabetes
Chromium picolinate	Diabetes
Folic acid	Neural tube birth defects

Originally, health claims in the USA needed FDA approval, classified as either authorized health claims grounded in significant scientific agreement (SSA health claims) or NAS, or its subdivisions (FDAM health claims) (Table 16.3). However, due to a legal challenge in 1999, the introduction of "qualified health claims" took place (http://www.fda.gov/Food/IngredientsPackagingLabeling/LabelingNutrition/ucm073992.htm). These claims specifically address associations between constituents and diseases or the risk of disease, for which a less rigorous level of evidence is considered acceptable (Bagchi, 2019; FDA, Authorized Health Claims That Meet the Significant Scientific Agreement SSA Standard & FDA, 2019; FDA, 2019). In the case of qualified health claims, there is a requirement to include explanatory statements that explicitly outline the limitations of the scientific evidence supporting the link between the ingredient and the claimed health advantage (Table 16.4). This ensures transparency and provides consumers with a clear understanding of the accuracy of scientific support for the health claim associated with the product.

16.4.3 Japanese regulation

In Japan, the regulatory landscape for nutritional claims on food is distinctly structured, deviating from the United States. The system comprises only three approved nutrition claim categories: "rich in," "low," and "does not contain," each accompanied by precise nutrient limits. These regulations are stipulated in several acts, including the Act on standardization and proper labeling of the government of Japan (1947, modern Tables 16.1–16.5, Fig. 16.1 amendment in 2018) (Japan Government Of, Food Sanitation Act, 1947), the Act on food sanitation (1950, newest amendment in 2009) (Standardization and proper quality labelling of agricultural and forestry products Act, 1950), and the government of Japan Act (2002, up-to-date amendment in 2018) (Health Promotion Act, 2002).

To qualify for nutritional claims, products must align with standards set by the minister of consumer affairs agency. Such compliant products can be designated as falling into categories like food for specified health use (FOSHU) or food with nutrient function claims. This regulatory framework ensures a focused and standardized approach to nutritional information on food labels in Japan (Health Promotion Act, 2002). The FOSHU system, established by the MHLW, plays a crucial role as a regulatory framework for verifying claims regarding the impacts of food on human

TABLE 16.5 Summary of Approved FOSHU Products (https://www.mhlw.go.jp/english/topics/foodafety/fhc/02.html).

Dental hygiene Paratinose, Maltotriose, Erythritol, etc.
Mineral absorption Calcium citrated malate, Casein phosphopeptide, Hem iron, Fructooligosaccharide, etc.
Osteogenesis Soybean isoflavone, Milk basic protein (MBP), etc.
Blood sugar levels Indigestible dextrin, Wheat albumin, Guava tea polyphenol, L-arabinose, etc.
Blood pressure Lactotripeptide, Casein dodecapeptide, Tochu leaf glycoside (geniposidic acid), Sardine peptide, etc.
Triacylglycerol Middle chain fatty acid, etc.
Blood cholesterol level Chitosan, Soybean protein, Degraded sodium alginate
Cholesterol plus gastrointestinal conditions, triacylglycerol plus cholesterol Degraded sodium alginate, Dietary fiber from psyllium seed husk, etc.
Modify gastrointestinal conditions Oligosaccharides, Lactose, Bifidobacteria, Lactic acid bacteria, Dietary fiber 8 ingestible dextrin, Polydextrol, Guar gum, Psyllium seed coat, etc.

health. The initial FOSHU products, including nonallergenic rice and low-phosphorus milk, gained approval in 1993 for individuals with specific dietary needs. However, these products were later reclassified as "food for illness" since they could not substantiate health-related claims employing such terms as "prevent," "cure," or "treat." The oversight of the FOSHU structure transitioned to the consumer commission and cabinet office, marking a significant change in 2009. Table 16.5 presents the official empowerment of FOSHU to make medical claims regarding physiological results on the human body. In Japan, rigorous evaluation is imperative for FOSHU marketing, covering both safety and efficacy. Comprehensive information on the assessment procedures and requirements for FOSHU approval can be accessed on the MHLW's official website at http://www.mhlw.go.jp/english/topics/foodsafety/fhc/02.html. This regulatory framework guarantees that foods making health claims meet stringent standards before receiving authorization for commercialization in Japan (Food with health claims, 2019).

FOSHU products undergo meticulous assessments by the Japanese government before reaching the market, with categories including "regular FOSHU," "qualified FOSHU," "standardized FOSHU," and "reduction of disease risk

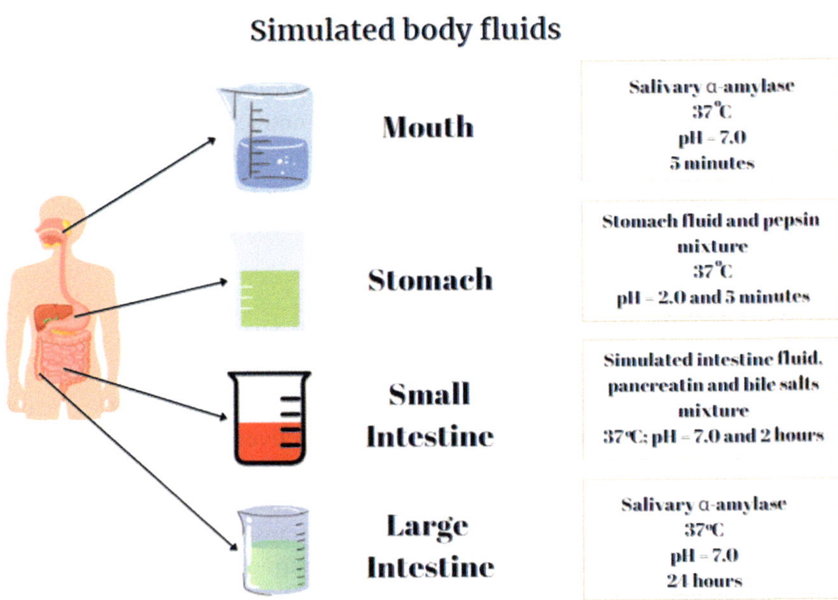

FIGURE 16.1 In vitro testing within simulated body fluids designed to replicate the conditions found in the gastrointestinal tract.

FOSHU" (Shimizu, 2003). The latter is the sole category authorized to claim disease risk reduction, backed by clinical and nutritional evidence. Nutrient function claims, focusing on specific minerals and vitamins, do not require premarketing approval. Additionally, products approved for defined dietary uses are considered "food for special dietary uses," encompassing formulations for specific groups such as pregnant women, infants, elderly individuals with swallowing difficulties, medical food, and FOSHU (Food with health claims, 2019).

16.4.4 Other global insights into functional food regulations

In various regions across the globe, legislation plays a vital role in overseeing the safety and nutritional quality of food products and their ingredients. In Canada, for example, the Food and Drugs Act stands as the principal legal framework governing these aspects. The act's purview extends to a comprehensive spectrum, encompassing food labeling, advertising, and claims, as well as stipulating food standards, compositional requirements, and fortification protocols. It also addresses foods intended for special dietary uses, oversees the use of food additives, and handles various areas, including microbial hazards, packaging materials, chemical, veterinary drug residues, and pesticides. The legal framework in Canada, detailed at http://laws-lois.justice.gc.ca/eng/acts/F-27/index.html, demonstrates the dedication to guaranteeing the safety, nutritional value, and authenticity of food items accessible to consumers. Such legislative measures not only uphold standards but also contribute to fostering public health and well-being.

In the Australasian region, specifically Australia and New Zealand, the oversight of foods is entrusted to the food standards code, accessible at http://www.foodstandards.gov.au/code/Pages/default.aspx. This regulatory framework meticulously governs various aspects of food standards and ensures adherence to quality and safety protocols. On the other hand, Russian legislation focuses on food supplements with biological activity, with manufacturers taking responsibility not only for the quality and safety of their products but also for their effectiveness. The federal law on food quality and safety highlights the importance of providing accurate and comprehensive information about these supplements (Tutelyan et al., 2019).

In Latin America, the regulatory landscape for functional foods and their health claims is not uniformly established, with Brazil standing out as the only country with well-defined legislation in this regard. In Brazil, functional foods are perceived as regular food items that offer additional health benefits, although there is no official definition for them. The National Health Surveillance Agency (ANVISA) in Brazil plays a critical role in this context by evaluating health claims on a case-by-case basis. ANVISA emphasizes scientific validation, ensuring that claims are reinforced by robust scientific evidence. Additionally, the agency prioritizes transparent communication with consumers, aiming to provide clear and accurate information on the health benefits of functional foods. This approach contributes to consumer awareness and helps build trust in the safety and efficacy of these products (Kurihayashi et al., 2022).

On a worldwide level, the Codex Alimentarius Commission (CAC), established by the Food and Agriculture Organization (FAO) and the World Health Organization (WHO), takes charge of formulating universal food standards (http://www.codexalimentarius.org/). For a comprehensive exploration of food regulations worldwide, Magnuson et al. (2013) offer valuable insights (Magnuson et al., 2013), and additional understandings into nutraceutical and functional food regulations can be found in "Nutraceutical and Functional Food Regulations in the United States and Around the World" by Bagchi (2019). This intricate network of regulations and standards underscores the concerted efforts on an international level to confirm the safety, quality, and transparency of the products.

16.5 Safety assessment of functional foods and nutraceuticals

In the contemporary landscape, food safety hazards have emerged as a critical global threat to public health. Given the several emergencies in food safety experienced on a worldwide, local, and national scale and their significant repercussions on the well-being of consumers, it becomes imperative to thoroughly appraise the effectiveness of risk communication strategies in each country. Recognizing the diverse challenges presented by various food safety problems, it is essential to develop robust and tailored communication approaches that are attuned to the specific contexts of individual nations. This not only involves identifying and addressing potential risks but also fosters transparent and informative communication channels among regulatory bodies, the food industry, and the public. Furthermore, integrating technological advancements and efficient data-sharing mechanisms can enhance these strategies, fostering a proactive and collaborative stance in addressing the global challenges associated with food safety (Tong et al., 2022).

The safety assessment of functional foods involves evaluating their potential risks and benefits to ensure that they are safe for human consumption. Ensuring the efficacy and safety of functional foods is crucial for consumer acceptance and trust. Rigorous clinical studies support health claims, and scientific validation ensures the integrity of these claims. Transparent labeling provides consumers with clear information on functional ingredients and potential health benefits (AbuMweis et al., 2010). Comprehensive safety assessments and stringent quality control measures are vital to identify and mitigate risks. However, despite some regulatory frameworks, global consistency remains a challenge. This lack of harmonization may contribute to consumer hesitancy or a lack of awareness about the benefits of functional foods. Efforts to educate both consumers and healthcare professionals are necessary to build trust and understanding, ultimately promoting the safe and effective integration of functional foods into diets (Lisa Clodoveo et al., 2022).

In this context, the key steps and considerations in the safety assessment of functional foods are as follows:

1. Identification of bioactive compound.
2. Toxicology studies.
3. Dose–response relationship.
4. Human clinical trials.
5. Allergenicity assessment.
6. Microbiological safety.
7. Quality control.
8. Regulatory compliance.
9. Postmarket surveillance.
10. Risk–benefit analysis.

It should be emphasized that the safety assessment process may differ depending on the exact functional food and its intended use. Additionally, collaboration with regulatory agencies, scientific experts, and stakeholders is essential for a comprehensive safety evaluation.

The identification and characterization of bioactive compounds in functional foods are pivotal steps in unraveling their potential health benefits. These compounds encompass a diverse array, including essential vitamins, minerals, antioxidants, probiotics, prebiotics, phytochemicals, and other functional ingredients (Bortolini et al., 2022). For example, vitamins, micronutrients vital for various physiological processes, contribute to functional foods such as vitamin C, acting as an antioxidant to bolster the immune system and promote skin health. Minerals, essential inorganic elements like calcium and iron, are often incorporated to support bone health, oxygen transport, and immune function (Gombart et al., 2020). The understanding of these bioactive compounds enables researchers to explore their mechanisms of action, paving the way for safety assessments and clinical studies to validate associated health claims. Analytical techniques like chromatography and spectrometry are employed to identify and quantify these compounds, forming the foundation for advancing the field of functional foods and their potential impact on human health (Valdés et al., 2022).

Toxicology studies are pivotal in assessing the safety of bioactive compounds in functional foods. These investigations encompass evaluating acute toxicity, which assesses immediate effects of high doses, and chronic toxicity, which examines prolonged exposure to lower doses, mimicking regular consumption. Genotoxicity studies explore the potential damage to genetic material, particularly DNA, while carcinogenicity assessments focus on determining if the compound induces cancer. Establishing a dose–response relationship is crucial to identifying safe consumption levels. The route of exposure, such as oral ingestion or dermal exposure, is considered, and species-specific effects are examined, recognizing variations in responses among different animals. These comprehensive studies provide essential data for regulatory decisions, ensuring the safe incorporation of functional foods into consumer diets (Kurek et al., 2022; Sandhya Rani et al., 2023).

Establishing a robust dose–response relationship is a crucial aspect in the comprehensive safety assessment of bioactive compounds within functional foods. This systematic exploration involves meticulously studying varying doses to ascertain the threshold at which these compounds bestow benefits while averting potential harm. The primary objective is to define an optimum range of intake, ensuring that the functional food manifests its intended health advantages without adverse effects. Critical considerations encompass understanding threshold effects, determining the maximum tolerable dose, and accounting for cumulative effects, all of which contribute to delineating a safety margin that accommodates population variability. The insights derived from dose–response studies yield evidence-based guidelines, shaping regulatory decisions and informing precise product labeling. This knowledge empowers consumers to make judicious dietary choices, maximizing the health benefits derived from functional foods while safeguarding against any potential risks (Konstantinidi & Koutelidakis, 2019; Martirosyan & Sanchez, 2022).

Undertaking well-designed human clinical trials is a critical step in evaluating the safety and efficacy of functional foods within the intended population. These trials are meticulously crafted to translate preclinical findings into real-world scenarios, offering valuable insights into the specific health outcomes associated with functional food consumption. Throughout these trials, participants are carefully monitored for potential adverse effects, and the impact on predetermined health parameters is rigorously assessed. This comprehensive approach ensures a thorough understanding of the safety profile of the functional food and its efficiency in delivering anticipated health benefits. The robust data derived from such human clinical trials not only aid in regulatory submissions but also play a pivotal role in establishing the scientific foundation supporting the integration of functional foods into a health-conscious lifestyle (Brown et al., 2018; Mattes et al., 2022).

Conducting an allergenicity assessment is a crucial measure in ensuring the safety of functional foods, particularly when incorporating novel ingredients or facing potential cross-reactivity with known allergens. This assessment entails a thorough identification and evaluation of the allergenic potential of the functional food components. In situations where the food introduces new elements or holds the risk of cross-reactivity with established allergens, rigorous testing becomes imperative. The primary goal is to pinpoint any substances that might provoke allergic reactions in sensitive individuals. By meticulously examining allergenicity, manufacturers and regulatory bodies can make informed decisions about labeling, providing essential information to consumers with allergies, and contributing to a more transparent and secure food product environment (Mazzucchelli et al., 2018).

Microbiological safety is a paramount consideration in guaranteeing the quality and safety of functional foods, especially those containing probiotics or other live microorganisms. The rigorous assessment involves ensuring that the functional food is devoid of harmful microorganisms such as bacteria, viruses, and fungi. This meticulous evaluation is crucial to prevent potential health risks related to the consumption of contaminated products. For functional foods with live microorganisms, the focus extends beyond the nutritional aspects to encompass the safety and viability of these beneficial microbes. Stringent quality control measures are implemented to meet microbiological safety standards, reducing the risk of infections or adverse effects. This commitment to microbiological safety not only aligns with regulatory requirements but also upholds consumer confidence in the integrity and health-promoting properties of functional foods (Siciliano et al., 2021).

The execution of a risk–benefit analysis is an important element in the assessment of the overall safety and suitability of functional foods. This analytical process entails a thorough evaluation, where the potential health benefits of the product are carefully balanced against any identified risks associated with its consumption. By systematically weighing the positive health outcomes against potential drawbacks, decision-makers can derive informed insights into the holistic impact of the functional food on consumer well-being. This comprehensive approach provides understanding of the safety profile of the product, considering both immediate and long-term implications. Ultimately, a well-conducted risk–benefit analysis serves as a valuable tool for shaping regulatory decisions, guiding product development, and assisting consumers in making judicious choices regarding the integration of functional foods into their dietary routines, effectively navigating the equilibrium between potential advantages and associated risks (Boué et al., 2022).

16.5.1 Hazard identification

The risk assessment process comprises four key components:

- Hazard identification,
- Hazard characterization,
- Exposure assessment,
- Risk characterization.

In hazard identification, the goal is to qualitatively understand the adverse effects caused by a contaminant, such as genotoxicity, carcinogenicity, or neurotoxicity. The risk assessment procedure, which involves determining the likelihood of potential adverse effects of consuming a food ingredient, must rely on robust scientific data and adhere to globally recognized transparency standards. This is vital for maintaining consumer trust in the safety of the food supply, especially when dealing with internationally traded foods. The conventional risk assessment approach for food additives typically involves toxicology testing through both in vitro and in vivo assays (Baba & Esfandiari, 2023).

In the safety evaluation of functional foods, hazard identification stands out as a critical phase dedicated to recognizing and comprehending potential risks associated with the consumption of these products. This systematic process involves identifying any biological, chemical, or physical elements that could pose a threat to human health when present in functional foods. Factors such as the characteristics of bioactive compounds, allergenic potential, potential contaminants, and the microbiological safety of the product are carefully considered (Rout & Sikdar, 2017).

Biological hazards may include harmful microorganisms, allergens, or toxins produced by microorganisms. For biological hazards, a thorough assessment involves evaluating the potential presence of pathogenic bacteria, viruses, or parasites that could compromise food safety. Rigorous testing ensures that these microorganisms remain viable and safe for consumption, and it helps prevent the introduction of harmful bacteria or fungi during the production process (Bonadonna et al., 2017).

Chemical hazards encompass the presence of detrimental substances like pesticides, heavy metals, or food additives. The assessment involves determining the levels of these substances and comparing them to established safety standards. Ensuring compliance with regulations and guidelines helps mitigate potential health risks associated with exposure to harmful chemicals (Yaqub et al., 2018).

Physical hazards involve tangible contaminants, such as foreign objects or insufficient packaging. In the case of physical hazards, the evaluation extends to examining the overall quality control measures in place during the production and packaging of functional foods. This includes assessing the potential presence of foreign objects, ensuring proper labeling, and verifying that packaging materials meet safety standards to prevent contamination (Onyeaka et al., 2023).

Thorough hazard identification sets the stage for subsequent risk assessment and management, enabling scientists, regulatory bodies, and manufacturers to implement effective strategies for mitigating or eliminating identified risks. This comprehensive approach ensures the overall safety of functional foods, promoting consumer confidence in their consumption. On the other hand, this multidimensional approach not only considers potential risks but also aims to establish preventive measures and quality control protocols, contributing to the overall safety and quality assurance of functional food products (Sanz-Serrano et al., 2021).

16.5.2 Hazard characterization

Originally designed for chemicals, the risk assessment process encounters substantial challenges when extended to microbial pathogens. Consequently, a majority of microbial risk assessments presently adopt a qualitative foundation. Nevertheless, there has been a notable surge of attention in nonquantitative methods to microbial food safety in recent years. This heightened interest has led to the development of quantitative models for specific pathogen/food combinations within various circles. While the qualitative base remains predominant, the evolving landscape reflects a growing acknowledgment of the need for more nuanced and quantitative assessments to comprehensively address microbial risks in the realm of food safety. This shift underscores the dynamic nature of risk assessment methodologies and the ongoing efforts to enhance precision and applicability in the evaluation of microbiological hazards in the food supply chain.

Hazard characterization then delves into establishing the connection between the dose of the contaminant and the occurrence of the adverse effect. This is often achieved through the examination and establishment of dose–response relationships, elucidating how varying doses correlate with the likelihood of specific effects. The hazard characterization phase plays a critical role in informing risk assessment, risk management, and the establishment of safety standards for functional foods. It provides a comprehensive understanding of the potential risks connected with identified hazards, facilitating the development of strategies to mitigate these risks and ensure food safety for consumers (Barlow et al., 2015).

Hazard characterization constitutes a vital process that involves identifying populations at risk and quantifying their exposures. In essence, exposure assessments aim to delineate real-life scenarios by (Nutraceuticals/Functional Foods and Health Claims on Foods: Policy Paper, 1998) identifying populations that may potentially be exposed (El Sohaimy, 2012), pinpointing the potential pathways through which exposure may occur, and (Jones, 2002) quantifying the magnitude, frequency, and duration of chemical intakes or potential doses. This comprehensive approach allows for a thorough understanding of the dynamics surrounding exposure, ensuring that potential risks are assessed in a nuanced manner. By evaluating the different facets of exposure, including the identification of exposed populations and the quantification of exposure paths, hazard characterization contributes significantly to informed decision-making and risk management strategies in diverse contexts.

Various methods can be employed to model exposure, including point estimates or probabilistic modeling. Point estimates provide a single value to represent the expected exposure level, offering a straightforward assessment. On the other hand, probabilistic modeling considers the variability in factors influencing exposure, providing a distribution of potential exposure levels. This method accounts for uncertainties and variations in the data, offering a more comprehensive and realistic depiction of the range of possible exposures. The choice between these modeling approaches depends on the existing data, the difficulty of the exposure scenario, and the degree of accuracy needed in the hazard characterization for a thorough understanding of the potential risks associated with any substance (Dey et al., 2016).

Three important functional ingredients, such as rutin, α-tocopherol, and docosahexaenoic acid (DHA), were evaluated for their in vitro genotoxicity on *Salmonella typhimurium* strains to evaluate the presence of premutagenic lesions. In this context, DHA and rutin showed interaction with DNA at the chromosomal level, in addition to presenting possible mutations. On the other hand, no genotoxic activity was observed for α-tocopherol (Sanz-Serrano et al., 2021).

16.5.3 Exposure assessment

Exposure assessment in the context of functional foods involves evaluating the extent to which individuals or populations come into contact with the bioactive components present in these foods and involves quantifying the levels of bioactive compounds in functional foods and determining how much of these compounds individuals or populations are exposed to through their diet. This can include measuring the concentrations of specific nutrients or bioactive substances in the functional foods (Barroso et al., 1988).

Conducting food consumption surveys is a common method for gathering data on dietary habits. Surveys may include information on the types and amounts of functional foods consumed, frequency of consumption, and variations among different demographic groups. Food consumption surveys employ various methodologies to collect data, including interviews, questionnaires, and food diaries. These methods capture information on the types and quantities of foods consumed, as well as the frequency of consumption (Bailey, 2021). Surveys often include tools or visual aids to help participants accurately report portion sizes. This is crucial for obtaining precise information about how much functional food is consumed (Nikolić et al., 2018).

The search for new functional foods, especially in the context of nonconventional food plants, must be carried out with caution, especially for plant species that are not present in the traditional consumption of populations.

Understanding how often individuals consume functional foods provides insights into dietary patterns. This information helps researchers and health professionals assess the regularity of exposure to bioactive compounds present in these foods. By categorizing individuals as habitual or occasional consumers, researchers can identify trends, potential variations, and shifts in dietary habits, contributing to a comprehensive understanding of exposure dynamics. These data are particularly important for evaluating compliance with dietary recommendations, customizing guidance, and communicating potential risks or benefits associated with bioactive compounds. Additionally, population-level analyses help inform public health policies, while long-term studies contribute to our understanding of the association between dietary patterns and chronic health outcomes. Overall, examining the frequency of functional food consumption provides behavioral insights, supports nutritional epidemiology, and aids in developing targeted interventions for promoting health and preventing potential risks (Dixit et al., 2023).

The computation of dietary intake concerning bioactive compounds necessitates a meticulous procedure that integrates data pertaining to food consumption patterns with comprehensive information on the composition of functional foods. Through a thorough analysis of both the types and quantities of functional foods consumed, coupled with a detailed examination of the specific bioactive compounds inherent in these foods, researchers can derive estimations for daily or weekly exposure levels within individuals or entire populations. This methodological approach ensures a precise assessment of the extent to which individuals incorporate bioactive components into their diets. Notably, this process considers the inherent variability in dietary practices, thereby providing a nuanced comprehension of exposure levels over delineated time periods. This insightful information is paramount for discerning the potential health implications and safety considerations associated with the functional food consumption (Ortea, 2022).

The exploration of the bioavailability and metabolism of functional ingredients constitutes a cornerstone in unraveling the intricate mechanisms governing their interaction with the human body. Bioavailability, a measure of how readily a nutrient or bioactive compound is absorbed and made available for utilization, involves a complex interplay of factors, including absorption dynamics, bloodstream transport, and potential tissue storage. This process is nuanced, influenced by the molecular structure of the compound, its interactions with other nutrients, and the presence of dietary fibers (Rein et al., 2013).

Importantly, not all bioactive compounds follow uniform pathways of absorption and utilization within the body. Variability arises due to diverse molecular structures and solubilities. The metabolic journey, encompassing absorption, distribution, biotransformation, and excretion, adds another layer of intricacy. Individual variations in metabolism, influenced by genetic factors, age, health status, and lifestyle choices, contribute to diverse metabolic pathways and rates of bioactive compound transformation. Notably, the liver's role in first-pass metabolism introduces unique challenges, impacting the bioactivity of compounds before they enter systemic circulation. Understanding these complexities isparamount for formulating effective functional foods and tailoring dietary recommendations to accommodate the individual differences in absorption and metabolism. Recognizing biomarkers of exposure and metabolic activity further enhances the precision of assessing bioavailability, offering invaluable insights for research and regulatory considerations within the framework of dietary guidelines (Kim et al., 2022).

After that, the harmonious integration of exposure data with both toxicity and efficacy information emerges as a crucial phase in formulating a comprehensive risk–benefit profile for functional foods. This method involves merging insights into the prevalence and patterns of exposure to bioactive compounds with a discerning analysis of their potential adverse effects and health benefits. Such a holistic approach is indispensable for regulators and healthcare professionals as they navigate decisions concerning the safety and potential advantages associated with the inclusion of specific functional foods in dietary practices.

In the scrutiny of the risk–benefit profile, the toxicological considerations encompass a thorough examination of potential adverse effects. This involves meticulous evaluation of factors such as dosage, duration of exposure, and the varying susceptibility of diverse population groups. Simultaneously, the efficacy component delves into the therapeutic or health-promoting attributes of functional ingredients. This dual perspective enables a balanced assessment, facilitating a nuanced determination of whether the potential benefits outweigh any associated risks. This integrated approach forms the bedrock for the development of regulatory frameworks, dietary guidelines, and well-informed healthcare recommendations. Ultimately, it enhances the capacity to strike an equitable balance between health promotion and risk mitigation in the context of functional food consumption (Pereira & Valado, 2023).

16.5.4 Risk characterization and risk assessment

Risk assessment and risk characterization are integral components in evaluating the safety and potential health benefits of functional foods. These processes are systematic and comprehensive approaches employed by researchers, regulatory bodies, and health professionals to understand and manage the potential risks associated with the consumption of these foods. Following this, exposure assessment quantifies the extent to which individuals or populations are likely to be exposed to these hazards based on dietary patterns. Hazard characterization then delves into understanding the nature and magnitude of potential adverse health effects associated with these identified hazards, considering factors like toxicity and allergenicity (Ashbolt et al., 2013).

Risk characterization integrates the data from hazard identification, exposure assessment, and hazard characterization to offer a comprehensive view of potential risks associated with functional foods. This step may involve quantitative risk estimation, assigning numerical values to the probability and severity of identified risks and providing a more precise understanding of the risk landscape. Additionally, consideration of uncertainty and variability in the data is crucial, ensuring a nuanced approach that acknowledges the limitations of available information.

The outcomes of risk assessment and risk characterization guide regulatory decision-making, influencing the establishment of safety standards, permissible exposure levels, and guidelines for the production and marketing of functional foods. Effective risk management includes transparent communication of risks and benefits to the public, educating consumers, healthcare professionals, and the food industry to facilitate informed decision-making. Continuous monitoring through surveillance systems and periodic reassessment of risk assessments is essential for adapting to emerging scientific evidence, changing consumption patterns, and updating safety standards to ensure the ongoing safety and regulatory compliance of functional foods in the market (Cheftel, 2011).

In the realm of ensuring global food safety, various organizations within the United Nations are at the forefront of conducting rigorous risk assessments. Among these, the Codex Alimentarius holds a prominent position, overseeing committees dedicated to food additives (Codex Committee on Food Additives: CCFA), food contaminants (Codex Committee on Contaminants in Food: CCCF), and pesticide residues (Codex Committee on Pesticide Residues: CCPR). Working on a global scale, these committees are instrumental in safeguarding consumer health, fostering optimum actions for universal food trade, and harmonizing procedures for launching international standards.

Within the risk analysis framework, the subsequent phase is risk management, a comprehensive process encompassing identification of risk, information acquisition, risk assessment, and the initiation of actions. It involves a meticulous series of steps, including the identification, appraisal, assortment, execution, monitoring, and adjustment of measures aimed at altering the level of unacceptable risk to one that is either tolerable or deemed acceptable. This multifaceted approach is designed to provide empirically grounded, economically viable, and integrated measures geared toward reducing risks. Importantly, risk management extends beyond the purely scientific realm, considering a spectrum of factors such as environmental, economic, social, political, cultural, and legal ethical considerations (Tummala & Schoenherr, 2011).

In the context of risk management, problem identification serves as the foundational step, recognizing potential issues that may pose risks. Information requests involve gathering relevant data to comprehensively understand the nature and extent of these identified risks. The subsequent risk assessment evaluates the magnitude and potential consequences of these risks, setting the stage for informed decision-making. Once risks are assessed, actions are initiated, involving the strategic identification, evaluation, and implementation of measures to mitigate or control risks. Continuous monitoring ensures that implemented measures are effective, and modification is undertaken as necessary based on evolving information (Aven, 2016).

This holistic approach to risk management not only addresses the scientific dimensions of risk but also acknowledges the broader societal and ethical implications. By integrating various factors into the decision-making process, risk management strives to strike a balance between minimizing risks and considering the diverse impacts on the environment, economy, society, politics, culture, and legal ethics. This nuanced and inclusive methodology is fundamental in developing resilient and adaptable risk management strategies within the complex landscape of global food safety and public health.

16.5.5 Clinical assessment

In the clinical assessment of functional foods, researchers aim to identify and evaluate any adverse health effects that may arise from the consumption of specific compounds present in these products. This assessment includes detailed studies on the distribution, metabolism, absorption, and excretion of bioactive components to determine their potential toxicity. Clinical trials may be designed to observe the effects of functional foods on various physiological parameters, such as organ function, blood markers, and overall health status (Balentine et al., 2015).

Clinical assessments often incorporate observational studies and epidemiological research to monitor the health outcomes of individuals who regularly consume functional foods over an extended period. Longitudinal studies contribute valuable data on the potential development of chronic conditions or adverse effects, providing a comprehensive understanding of the products safety (Balentine et al., 2015). In one illustrative case, a longitudinal study might meticulously track the incidence of age-related macular degeneration in individuals regularly incorporating lutein- and zeaxanthin-rich foods into their diet (Ma et al., 2012).

This thorough evaluation encompasses diverse facets, ranging from bioavailability studies, which scrutinize the absorption and utilization of bioactive compounds, to clinical trials exploring metabolic and physiological implications. For instance, investigations into omega-3 fatty acids from fish oil supplements may unfold in clinical trials, shedding light on their effects on lipid profiles and cardiovascular health in individuals with hyperlipidemia (Dyerberg et al., 2010).

The clinical assessment paradigm extends to trials focusing on specific health conditions, exemplified by research evaluating the impact of probiotic-rich yogurt on alleviating gastrointestinal symptoms in individuals grappling with irritable bowel syndrome (IBS). Simultaneously, it aims to pinpoint any potential adverse effects, ensuring the safety of functional foods. An investigation could scrutinize the safety aspects of high-dose vitamin supplementation and potential adverse reactions, such as toxicity.

A classic example of functional foods is based on the growing popularity of essential oils as food supplements have brought about a heightened need for a comprehensive assessment of their oral safety. Whether these oils are used individually or in various combinations, ensuring their safety for oral consumption is paramount. This imperative arises from the overarching principle that the risk associated with the consumption of food supplements should be maintained at the lowest possible level (Sartori Tamburlin et al., 2021). Essential oils are concentrated extracts derived from plants, and they often contain potent bioactive compounds with various therapeutic properties. When used as food supplements, individuals may incorporate them into their diets for reasons such as purported health benefits, flavor enhancement, or aromatic appeal. However, the ingestion of essential oils raises concerns related to their potential toxicity, allergenicity, and the overall impact on oral health.

To assess the oral safety of essential oils as food supplements, several factors come into play. First, the chemical composition of the oils needs to be thoroughly examined, considering the presence and concentration of specific compounds. Certain essential oils may contain components that, when ingested in excessive amounts, could lead to adverse reactions or toxicity. Additionally, consideration should be given to individual variations in response, as factors like age, preexisting health conditions, and medications may influence how individuals metabolize and react to essential oils. Rigorous clinical trials and observational studies are essential to monitor the effects of oral consumption over time and to identify any potential side effects or adverse reactions (Zhang & Yao, 2019).

Furthermore, the assessment of oral safety involves examining the overall impact on oral health, including potential effects on the mucous membranes, teeth, and gums. Some essential oils may have antimicrobial properties that can influence oral hygiene positively, while others may have abrasive or irritating effects (Radu et al., 2023).

Regulatory bodies often play a vital role in establishing guidelines and safety standards for the oral consumption of essential oils as food supplements. These guidelines may include recommended dosages, labeling requirements, and warnings about potential risks. As the popularity of essential oils in the realm of food supplements continues to rise, ongoing research and regulatory oversight are crucial to strike a balance between the potential benefits and risks associated with their oral use.

The utilization of nanocellulose has witnessed a substantial surge in the food industry. Subtypes such as cellulose nanofibrils or bacterial cellulose have garnered considerable attention due to their properties as a source of insoluble fiber, bringing forth significant benefits for human health. This trend is rooted in the remarkable characteristics of nanocellulose, which include its biocompatibility, biodegradability, and the capacity to modify the texture and viscosity of food products. Cellulose nanofibrils, characterized by their nanoscale dimensions, contribute to the enhancement of structural integrity in various food formulations. The incorporation of cellulose nanofibrils into food products has demonstrated positive effects on their rheological properties, stability, and texture. Furthermore, the insoluble fiber derived from nanocellulose, particularly when sourced from bacterial cellulose, has been linked to several health benefits. The presence of nanocellulose in the diet has been associated with improved digestive health, offering a substrate for beneficial gut microflora. Moreover, its ability to modulate water-holding capacity and viscosity can influence satiety and nutrient absorption, contributing to weight management and overall well-being (Zhang et al., 2022).

The assessment of the biological impacts of nanocellulose fibers on human health extends beyond a simplistic evaluation based solely on their chemical characteristics. This complexity arises from the understanding that factors such as size, shape, aggregation properties, and numerous other yet undiscovered elements play a pivotal role in determining how these nanocellulose fibers interact with cells and other living organisms. Nanocellulose, with its nanoscale dimensions, introduces a unique set of considerations when exploring its biological effects. The intricate interplay of these physical attributes may influence cellular responses, biodistribution, and potential toxicity. Researchers acknowledge that comprehensive investigations encompassing these nuanced factors are imperative for a thorough comprehension of the biological impact of nanocellulose fibers (Cañas-Gutiérrez et al., 2024).

Furthermore, the biomedical applications of nanocellulose have garnered attention, extending beyond its role in the food industry. As a biomaterial, nanocellulose demonstrates promise in drug delivery, wound healing, and tissue engineering. However, a cautious approach is warranted, considering the potential biological interactions that may vary based on the specific application and intended biological target. In the pursuit of safe and effective utilization, ongoing research endeavors are aimed at unraveling the intricacies of nanocellulose interactions with biological systems. This involves exploring its biocompatibility, cellular uptake mechanisms, and potential immunological responses. As our understanding evolves, this knowledge will not only inform regulatory considerations but also facilitate the development of guidelines for the responsible incorporation of nanocellulose into various applications, ensuring both innovation and safety in its utilization (Mishra et al., 2022). Fig. 16.1 presents one of the ways to clinically evaluate, in vitro, the effects of functional ingredients on the human body.

In vitro testing using simulated body fluids that replicate the conditions found within the gastrointestinal tract is a crucial aspect of research and development in various fields. This methodology allows researchers to simulate and study the complex environment of the digestive system outside of a living organism. Such testing is particularly valuable for assessing how substances, such as drugs or food components, may interact with the gastrointestinal environment, providing insights into their behavior, solubility, and potential effects. Researchers use these simulated conditions to gain a deeper understanding of processes like absorption, dissolution, and degradation that occur within the gastrointestinal tract, contributing valuable data to advancements in pharmaceuticals, food science, and related disciplines (Naissinger da Silva et al., 2021).

16.5.6 Human studies

Human studies in functional foods toxicology involve investigating the impact of consuming functional foods on human health, with a focus on determining whether there are any harmful effects or unintended consequences associated with their consumption. These studies are pivotal in establishing a dose–response relationship and determining safe and effective doses that deliver desired health benefits without causing harm. Bioavailability studies delve into how the body absorbs, distributes, metabolizes, and eliminates the bioactive compounds in these foods, shedding light on whether these compounds reach their intended target tissues.

Clinical trials, designed with randomization, control groups, and blinding, play a significant role in evaluating the safety and efficacy of functional foods across diverse populations. Long-term studies are essential for understanding cumulative or delayed toxic effects, providing insights into the sustained impact of these foods on health over extended periods. Biomarker analysis is often employed to assess the influence of functional foods on specific physiological processes, identifying potential markers of toxicity or beneficial effects (Staudacher et al., 2017). In this context, clinical trials employ rigorous methodologies to assess their safety and efficacy across diverse populations. Randomization, control groups, and blinding are key design elements used to minimize bias and ensure the reliability of study results.

The randomization involves randomly assigning participants to different groups within the study. This process helps distribute potential confounding factors evenly among the groups, making the comparison between the groups more reliable. In the context of functional foods, randomization ensures that any detected effects are more likely to be attributed to the intervention rather than other variables.

Clinical trials typically include a control group that does not receive the functional food intervention. This group serves as a baseline for comparison, permitting researchers to isolate and evaluate the specific effects of the functional food. The comparison with a control group helps determine whether observed changes are due to the intervention or would have occurred naturally (AbuMweis et al., 2010). In turn, blinding involves concealing information about the intervention from both participants and researchers. In a double-blind study, both the participants and the researchers are unaware of who is receiving the functional food and who is in the control group until the study concludes. Blinding helps prevent bias and ensures that the assessment of outcomes is objective (Monaghan et al., 2021). The long-term studies go beyond short-term effects and provide insights into cumulative or delayed toxic effects that may not be immediately apparent. Long-term observations allow researchers to assess the safety profile of functional foods over time, addressing concerns related to prolonged exposure (Konstantinidi & Koutelidakis, 2019). Biomarker analysis is a valuable tool employed in clinical trials to assess the influence of functional foods on specific physiological processes. Biomarkers are measurable indicators that reflect biological responses to the intervention. In the context of functional food toxicology, researchers use biomarker analysis to identify potential markers of toxicity or beneficial effects. This approach provides objective and quantifiable data, enhancing the understanding of how functional foods interact with the body at a molecular level (Ahmad et al., 2023). Another approach to human studies consists of population studies that involve large and diverse cohorts and help researchers discern patterns and associations between functional food consumption and health outcomes. This approach is crucial for understanding the effects across different demographic groups and identifying potential risks specific to certain populations. Adverse event monitoring is integral to these studies, ensuring the systematic collection and reporting of any negative incidents related to the consumption of functional foods. Compliance with regulatory guidelines and ethical standards is paramount to maintaining the validity and reliability of study results (Townsend et al., 2022).

16.6 Present and future trends

Current and ongoing growth areas for continued advancements in the functional foods encompass the development of genetically modified options, botanical/natural, and aquatic products, leveraging sensory demand and integrating nanotechnologies. In parallel, efforts by national and global food and law agencies are intensifying, aimed at enhancing surveillance of food distribution networks to combat threats of adulteration and bioterrorism.

Additionally, a deeper understanding of physiological mechanisms underlying individualized nutrition and targeted interventions holds promise for addressing health challenges associated with obesity and mental health on a global scale with an attention to sustainable food production to meet the requests of a growing population. Entrepreneurial ventures are driving innovations in agriculture technology.

Traditional farming practices are being revolutionized by robotic systems, which are now utilized for tasks such as lettuce harvesting and optimizing grass production for livestock. Moreover, there is a growing momentum in the development of meat and poultry substitutes, which aim to reduce dependence on chemicals and hormones while also addressing the challenge of foodborne illnesses.

In light of concerns about potential food shortages resulting from climate change, advancements in agricultural technology (Ag-tech) are positioned to exceed the influence and growth of even the telecommunications industry. Looking toward the future, the cultivation of edible insects arises as a sustainable and nutritious protein source, albeit encountering hurdles concerning consumer acceptance and regulatory frameworks.

16.7 Conclusion

The current trend of consumers actively engaging in safeguarding their health has spurred a proliferation of products in the market containing dietary ingredients aimed at positively impacting consumer well-being. These components are integrated into products marketed as "functional foods" or "nutraceuticals." These products, eligible for individual or combined use in food or beverages, serve specific technological purposes or health aids and must demonstrate a sufficient safety profile for human consumption. The movement toward safer approaches to health management is a response to concerns about potential risks linked with nutraceuticals and functional foods.

References

AbuMweis, S. S., Jew, S., & Jones, P. J. H. (2010). Optimizing clinical trial design for assessing the efficacy of functional foods. *Nutrition Reviews*, *68* (8), 485–499. Available from https://doi.org/10.1111/j.1753-4887.2010.00308.x, http://onlinelibrary.wiley.com/journal/10.1111/(ISSN)1753-4887.

Ahmad, A., Imran, M., & Ahsan, H. (2023). Biomarkers as biomedical bioindicators: Approaches and techniques for the detection, analysis, and validation of novel biomarkers of diseases. *Pharmaceutics*, *15*(6). Available from https://doi.org/10.3390/pharmaceutics15061630, http://www.mdpi.com/journal/pharmaceutics.

Ashbolt, N. J., Amézquita, A., Backhaus, T., Borriello, P., Brandt, K. K., Collignon, P., Coors, A., Finley, R., Gaze, W. H., Heberer, T., Lawrence, J. R., Larsson, D. G. J., McEwen, S. A., Ryan, J. J., Schönfeld, J., Silley, P., Snape, J. R., Van den Eede, C., & Topp, E. (2013). Human health risk assessment (HHRA) for environmental development and transfer of antibiotic resistance. *Environmental Health Perspectives*, *121*(9), 993–1001. Available from https://doi.org/10.1289/ehp.1206316, http://ehp.niehs.nih.gov/wp-content/uploads/121/9/ehp.1206316.pdf, United States.

Aven, T. (2016). Risk assessment and risk management: Review of recent advances on their foundation. *European Journal of Operational Research*, *253*(1), 1–13. Available from https://doi.org/10.1016/j.ejor.2015.12.023.

Baba, F. V., & Esfandiari, Z. (2023). Theoretical and practical aspects of risk communication in food safety: A review study. *Heliyon*, *9*(7). Available from https://doi.org/10.1016/j.heliyon.2023.e18141, http://www.journals.elsevier.com/heliyon/.

Bagchi, D. (2019). *Nutraceutical and functional food regulations in the United States and around the world* (pp. 1–678). Elsevier. Available from http://www.sciencedirect.com/science/book/9780128164679, https://doi.org/10.1016/C2018-0-00112-7.

Bailey, R. L. (2021). Overview of dietary assessment methods for measuring intakes of foods, beverages, and dietary supplements in research studies. *Current Opinion in Biotechnology*, *70*, 91–96. Available from https://doi.org/10.1016/j.copbio.2021.02.007, http://www.elsevier.com/locate/copbio.

Balentine, D. A., Dwyer, J. T., Erdman, J. W., Ferruzzi, M. G., Gaine, P. C., Harnly, J. M., & Kwik-Uribe, C. L. (2015). Recommendations on reporting requirements for flavonoids in research. *American Journal of Clinical Nutrition*, *101*(6), 1113–1125. Available from https://doi.org/10.3945/ajcn.113.071274, http://ajcn.nutrition.org/content/101/6/1113.full.pdf + html.

Barlow, S. M., Boobis, A. R., Bridges, J., Cockburn, A., Dekant, W., Hepburn, P., Houben, G. F., König, J., Nauta, M. J., Schuermans, J., & Bánáti, D. (2015). The role of hazard- and risk-based approaches in ensuring food safety. *Trends in Food Science and Technology*, *46*(2), 176–188. Available from https://doi.org/10.1016/j.tifs.2015.10.007, http://www.elsevier.com/wps/find/journaldescription.cws_home/601278/description#description.

Barroso, M. G. R. S. R., Diez, L. M., & Rodrigues, G. V. (1988). Comparative study of spectrofluorimetric and spectrophotometric methods for anionic surfactants determination in wastewater. *An. Quim. Ser. B.*, *1988*, 361–365.

Bigliardi, B., & Galati, F. (2013). Innovation trends in the food industry: The case of functional foods. *Trends in Food Science and Technology*, *31*(2), 118–129. Available from https://doi.org/10.1016/j.tifs.2013.03.006.

Bonadonna, L., Briancesco, R., & Coccia, A. M. (2017). *Analysis of microorganisms in hospital environments and potential risks. SpringerBriefs in Public Health* (pp. 53–62). Springer International Publishing. Available from http://www.springer.com/series/10138, https://doi.org/10.1007/978-3-319-49160-8_5.

Bortolini, D. G., Maciel, G. M., Fernandes, I. D. A. A., Pedro, A. C., Rubio, F. T. V., Branco, I. G., & Haminiuk, C. W. I. (2022). Functional properties of bioactive compounds from Spirulina spp.: Current status and future trends. *Food Chemistry: Molecular Sciences*, *5*. Available from https://doi.org/10.1016/j.fochms.2022.100134, www.journals.elsevier.com/food-chemistry-molecular-sciences.

Boué, G., Ververis, E., Niforou, A., Federighi, M., Pires, S. M., Poulsen, M., Thomsen, S. T., & Naska, A. (2022). Risk–Benefit assessment of foods: Development of a methodological framework for the harmonized selection of nutritional, microbiological, and toxicological components. *Front. Nutr.*, *9*. Available from https://doi.org/10.3389/FNUT.2022.951369/BIBTEX2022.

Brown, L., Caligiuri, S. P. B., Brown, D., & Pierce, G. N. (2018). Clinical trials using functional foods provide unique challenges. *Journal of Functional Foods*, *45*, 233–238. Available from https://doi.org/10.1016/j.jff.2018.01.024, http://www.elsevier.com/wps/find/journaldescription.cws_home/717426/description#description.

Cañas-Gutiérrez, A., Gómez Hoyos, C., Velásquez-Cock, J., Gañán, P., Triana, O., Cogollo-Flórez, J., Romero-Sáez, M., Correa-Hincapié, N., & Zuluaga, R. (2024). Health and toxicological effects of nanocellulose when used as a food ingredient: A review. *Carbohydrate Polymers*, *323*, 121382. Available from https://doi.org/10.1016/j.carbpol.2023.121382.

Cheftel, J. C. (2011). Emerging risks related to food technology. *Science for Peace and Security Series A: Chemistry and Biology*, 223–254. Available from https://doi.org/10.1007/978-94-007-1100-6_13, http://www.springer.com/series/7106.

Crowe, K. M., & Francis, C. (2013). Position of the academy of nutrition and dietetics: Functional foods. *Journal of the Academy of Nutrition and Dietetics*, *113*(8), 1096–1103. Available from https://doi.org/10.1016/j.jand.2013.06.002, http://www.elsevier.com/wps/find/journaldescription.cws_home/727057/description#description.

Dey, S., Carr, G. J., Li, L., Brink, S., & Zhou, S. (2016). Probabilistic Monte Carlo estimation for quantitative exposure assessment of lotion transfer via baby wipes usage. *Regulatory Toxicology and Pharmacology*, *79*, 54–63. Available from https://doi.org/10.1016/j.yrtph.2016.05.006, http://www.elsevier.com/inca/publications/store/6/2/2/9/3/9/index.htt.

Dixit, V., Joseph Kamal, S. W., Bajrang Chole, P., Dayal, D., Chaubey, K. K., Pal, A. K., Xavier, J., Manjunath, B. T., & Bachheti, R. K. (2023). Functional foods: Exploring the health benefits of bioactive compounds from plant and animal sources. *Journal of Food Quality*, *2023*. Available from https://doi.org/10.1155/2023/5546753, https://www.hindawi.com/journals/jfq/.

Domínguez Díaz, L., Fernández-Ruiz, V., & Cámara, M. (2020). An international regulatory review of food health-related claims in functional food products labeling. *Journal of Functional Foods*, *68*. Available from https://doi.org/10.1016/j.jff.2020.103896, http://www.elsevier.com/wps/find/journaldescription.cws_home/717426/description#description.

Dyerberg, J., Madsen, P., Møller, J. M., Aardestrup, I., & Schmidt, E. B. (2010). Bioavailability of marine n-3 fatty acid formulations. *Prostaglandins, Leukotrienes, and Essential Fatty Acids*, *83*(3), 137–141. Available from https://doi.org/10.1016/j.plefa.2010.06.007.

Ellwood, K. C., Trumbo, P. R., & Kavanaugh, C. J. (2010). How the US food and drug administration evaluates the scientific evidence for health claims. *Nutrition Reviews*, *68*(2), 114–121. Available from https://doi.org/10.1111/j.1753-4887.2009.00267.x.

El Sohaimy, S. (2012). Functional foods and nutraceuticals-modern approach to food science. *World Applied Sciences Journal*, *20*(5), 691–708. Available from https://doi.org/10.5829/idosi.wasj.2012.20.05.66119, http://idosi.org/wasj/wasj20%285%2912/12.pdf, Egypt.

Espín, J. C., García-Conesa, M. T., & Tomás-Barberán, F. A. (2007). Nutraceuticals: Facts and fiction. *Phytochemistry*, *68*(22-24), 2986–3008. Available from https://doi.org/10.1016/j.phytochem.2007.09.014.

FDA, Authorized Health Claims That Meet the Significant Scientific Agreement (SSA) Standard | FDA. (2019), 2019.

FDA, Label Claims for Food & Dietary Supplements. (2019), 2019.

Food with health claims, food for special dietary uses, and nutrition labeling. MHLW, MHLW, (2019), 2019.

Gaur, S., & Agnihotri, R. (2014). Green tea: A novel functional food for the oral health of older adults. *Geriatrics and Gerontology International*, *14*(2), 238–250. Available from https://doi.org/10.1111/ggi.12194.

Gombart, A. F., Pierre, A., & Maggini, S. (2020). A review of micronutrients and the immune system—working in harmony to reduce the risk of infection. *Nutrients*, *12*(1). Available from https://doi.org/10.3390/nu12010236, https://www.mdpi.com/2072-6643/12/1/236/pdf.

Health Promotion Act. Act. (2002), 2002.

Japan Government Of, Food Sanitation Act. Act No. 233 (1947), 1947.

Jones, P. J. (2002). Clinical nutrition: 7. Functional foods - More than just nutrition. *CMAJ. Canadian Medical Association Journal.*, *166*(12), 1555–1563. Available from http://www.cmaj.ca/.

Kim, E., Cui, J., Zhang, G., & Lee, Y. (2022). Physiological effects of green-colored food-derived bioactive compounds on cardiovascular and metabolic diseases. *Applied Sciences*, *12*(4), 1879. Available from https://doi.org/10.3390/app12041879.

Konstantinidi, M., & Koutelidakis, A. E. (2019). Functional foods and bioactive compounds: A review of its possible role on weight management and obesity's metabolic consequences. *Medicines*, *6*(3), 94. Available from https://doi.org/10.3390/medicines6030094.

Kurek, M., Benaida-Debbache, N., Garofulić, I. E., Galić, K., Avallone, S., Voilley, A., & Waché, Y. (2022). Antioxidants and bioactive compounds in food: Critical review of issues and prospects†. *Antioxidants*, *11*(4). Available from https://doi.org/10.3390/antiox11040742, https://www.mdpi.com/2076-3921/11/4/742/pdf.

Kurihayashi, A. Y., Palombo, C. N. T., Duarte, L. S., & Fujimori, E. (2022). Food commercialization in schools: Analysis of the regulatory process in Brazil. *Revista de Nutricao*, *35*, 1–18. Available from https://doi.org/10.1590/1678-9865202235E210094, http://www.scielo.br/scielo.php?script = sci_serial&pid = 1415-5273&lng = en&nrm = iso.

Lisa Clodoveo, M., Tarsitano, E., Crupi, P., Pasculli, L., Piscitelli, P., Miani, A., & Corbo, F. (2022). Towards a new food labelling system for sustainable food production and healthy responsible consumption: The Med Index Checklist. *Journal of Functional Foods, 98*. Available from https://doi.org/10.1016/j.jff.2022.105277, http://www.elsevier.com/wps/find/journaldescription.cws_home/717426/description#description.

Magnuson, B., Munro, I., Abbot, P., Baldwin, N., Lopez-Garcia, R., Ly, K., McGirr, L., Roberts, A., & Socolovsky, S. (2013). Review of the regulation and safety assessment of food substances in various countries and jurisdictions. *Food Additives and Contaminants - Part A, 30*(7), 1147–1220. Available from https://doi.org/10.1080/19440049.2013.795293, http://www.tandfonline.com/toc/tfac20/current.

Martirosyan, D., & Sanchez, S. S. (2022). Quantum theory of functional food science: Establishment of dosage of bioactive compounds in functional food products. *Funct. Food Sci.*, 79–93. Available from https://doi.org/10.31989/FFS.V2I3.9152022.

Mattes, R. D., Rowe, S. B., Ohlhorst, S. D., Brown, A. W., Hoffman, D. J., Liska, D. J., Feskens, E. J. M., Dhillon, J., Tucker, K. L., Epstein, L. H., Neufeld, L. M., Kelley, M., Fukagawa, N. K., Sunde, R. A., Zeisel, S. H., Basile, A. J., Borth, L. E., & Jackson, E. (2022). Valuing the diversity of research methods to advance nutrition science. *Advances in Nutrition, 13*(4), 1324–1393. Available from https://doi.org/10.1093/advances/nmac043, http://advances.nutrition.org/.

Mazzucchelli, G., Holzhauser, T., Cirkovic Velickovic, T., Diaz-Perales, A., Molina, E., Roncada, P., Rodrigues, P., Verhoeckx, K., & Hoffmann-Sommergruber, K. (2018). Current (food) allergenic risk assessment: Is it fit for novel foods? Status quo and identification of gaps. *Molecular Nutrition & Food Research, 62*(1). Available from https://doi.org/10.1002/mnfr.201700278.

Ma, L., Dou, H. L., Wu, Y. Q., Huang, Y. M., Huang, Y. B., Xu, X. R., Zou, Z. Y., & Lin, X. M. (2012). Lutein and zeaxanthin intake and the risk of age-related macular degeneration: A systematic review and meta-analysis. *British Journal of Nutrition, 107*(3), 350–359. Available from https://doi.org/10.1017/S0007114511004260.

Mishra, P. K., Pavelek, O., Rasticova, M., Mishra, H., & Ekielski, A. (2022). Nanocellulose-based biomedical scaffolds in future bioeconomy: A techno-legal assessment of the state-of-the-art. *Frontiers in Bioengineering and Biotechnology, 9*. Available from https://doi.org/10.3389/fbioe.2021.789603, http://journal.frontiersin.org/journal/bioengineering-and-biotechnology#archive.

Monaghan, T. F., Agudelo, C. W., Rahman, S. N., Wein, A. J., Lazar, J. M., Everaert, K., & Dmochowski, R. R. (2021). Blinding in clinical trials: Seeing the big picture. *Medicina (Lithuania), 57*(7). Available from https://doi.org/10.3390/medicina57070647, https://www.mdpi.com/1648-9144/57/7/647/pdf.

Naissinger da Silva, M., Tagliapietra, B. L., Flores, V. D. A., & Pereira dos Santos Richards, N. S. (2021). In vitro test to evaluate survival in the gastrointestinal tract of commercial probiotics. *Current Research in Food Science, 4*, 320–325. Available from https://doi.org/10.1016/j.crfs.2021.04.006, https://www.journals.elsevier.com/current-research-in-food-science.

Nikolić, M., Milešević, J., Zeković, M., Gurinović, M., & Glibetić, M. (2018). The development and validation of food atlas for portion size estimation in the Balkan Region. *Frontiers in Nutrition, 5*. Available from https://doi.org/10.3389/fnut.2018.00078, journal.frontiersin.org/journal/nutrition.

Nutraceuticals/Functional Foods and Health Claims on Foods: Policy Paper. Hc-sc.gc.ca. Health Canada. (1998), 1998.

Onyeaka, H., Jalata, D. D., & Mekonnen, S. A. (2023). Mitigating physical hazards in food processing: Risk assessment and preventive strategies. *Food Science and Nutrition*. Available from https://doi.org/10.1002/fsn3.3727, onlinelibrary.wiley.com/journal/10.1002/%28ISSN%292048-7177.

Ortea, I. (2022). Foodomics in health: Advanced techniques for studying the bioactive role of foods. *TrAC Trends in Analytical Chemistry, 150*, 116589. Available from https://doi.org/10.1016/j.trac.2022.116589.

Otles, S., & Gokgunnec, L. (2024). *Safety considerations in developing functional foods and nutraceuticals*. Elsevier BV. Available from https://doi.org/10.1016/b978-0-12-822521-9.00156-8.

Pereira, L., & Valado, A. (2023). Algae-derived natural products in diabetes and its complications—Current advances and future prospects. *Life (Chicago, Ill.: 1978), 13*(9). Available from https://doi.org/10.3390/life13091831, www.mdpi.com/journal/life/.

Plant EFSA, Plant Stanols, Sterols, LDL-Cholesterol Blood, Scientific Opinion of the Panel on Dietetic Products Nutrition and Allergies on a request from the European Commission and a similar request from France in relation to the authorization procedure for health claims on plant stanols and plant sterols and lowering/reducing blood LDL-cholesterol pursuant to Article 14 of Regulation (EC) No 1924. EFSA J. 7 (2006). Available from https://doi.org/10.2903/J.EFSA.2009.11752006.

Radu, C.-M., Radu, C. C., Bochiş, S.-A., Arbănaşi, E. M., Lucan, A. I., Murvai, V. R., & Zaha, D. C. (2023). Revisiting the therapeutic effects of essential oils on the oral microbiome. *Pharmacy, 11*(1), 33. Available from https://doi.org/10.3390/pharmacy11010033.

Rein, M. J., Renouf, M., Cruz-Hernandez, C., Actis-Goretta, L., Thakkar, S. K., & da Silva Pinto, M. (2013). Bioavailability of bioactive food compounds: A challenging journey to bioefficacy. *British Journal of Clinical Pharmacology, 75*(3), 588–602. Available from https://doi.org/10.1111/j.1365-2125.2012.04425.x.

Rout, B. K., & Sikdar, B. K. (2017). Hazard identification, risk assessment, and control measures as an effective tool of occupational health assessment of hazardous process in an iron ore pelletizing industry. *Indian Journal of Occupational and Environmental Medicine, 21*(2), 56–76. Available from https://doi.org/10.4103/ijoem.IJOEM_19_16, http://www.ijoem.com/.

Sandhya Rani, S., Vedavijaya, T., Sree, P. K., Shanmugasundaram, J., Deepalatha, C., Raju, M. G., & Babu Sayana, S. (2023). A comprehensive analysis of phytochemical composition, acute toxicity assessment, and antioxidant potential of ethanolic extract of carica papaya seeds. *Cureus*. Available from https://doi.org/10.7759/cureus.49686.

Sanz-Serrano, J., Vettorazzi, A., Muruzabal, D., Azqueta, A., & de Cerain, A. L. (2021). In vitro genotoxicity assessment of functional ingredients: Betaine, choline, and taurine. *Foods, 10*(2). Available from https://doi.org/10.3390/foods10020339, https://www.mdpi.com/2304-8158/10/2/339/pdf.

Sartori Tamburlin, I., Roux, E., Feuillée, M., Labbé, J., Aussaguès, Y., El Fadle, F. E., Fraboul, F., & Bouvier, G. (2021). Toxicological safety assessment of essential oils used as food supplements to establish safe oral recommended doses. *Food and Chemical Toxicology, 157*. Available from https://doi.org/10.1016/j.fct.2021.112603, www.elsevier.com/locate/foodchemtox.

Scientific Opinion in relation to the authorisation procedure for health claims on calcium and vitamin D and the reduction of the risk of osteoporotic fractures by reducing bone loss pursuant to Article 14 of Regulation (EC) No 1924. EFSA J. 8 (2006). Available from https://doi.org/10.2903/J.EFSA.2010.16092006.

Scientific Opinion on the substantiation of a health claim related to 3 g/day plant sterols/stanols and lowering blood LDL-cholesterol and reduced risk of (coronary) heart disease pursuant to Article 19 of Regulation (EC) No 1924. EFSA J. 10 (2006). Available from https://doi.org/10.2903/J.EFSA.2012.26932006.

Scientific Opinion on the substantiation of a health claim related to barley beta-glucans and lowering of blood cholesterol and reduced risk of (coronary) heart disease pursuant to Article 14 of Regulation (EC) No 1924. EFSA J. 9 (2006). Available from https://doi.org/10.2903/J.EFSA.2011.24702006.

Scientific Opinion on the substantiation of a health claim related to oat beta glucan and lowering blood cholesterol and reduced risk of (coronary) heart disease pursuant to Article 14 of Regulation (EC) No 1924. EFSA J. 8 (2006). Available from https://doi.org/10.2903/J.EFSA.2010.18852006.

Scientific Opinion on the substantiation of a health claim related to increasing maternal folate status by supplemental folate intake and reduced risk of neural tube defects pursuant to Article 14 of Regulation (EC) No 1924. EFSA J. 11 (2006). Available from https://doi.org/10.2903/J.EFSA.2013.33282006.

Scientific Opinion on the substantiation of a health claim related to vitamin D and risk of falling pursuant to Article 14 of Regulation (EC) No 1924. EFSA J. 9 (2006). Available from https://doi.org/10.2903/J.EFSA.2011.23822006.

Scientific Opinion on the substantiation of a health claim related to "low fat and low trans spreadable fat rich in unsaturated and omega-3 fatty acids" and reduction of LDL-cholesterol concentrations pursuant to Article 14 of Regulation (EC) No 1924. EFSA J. 9 (2006). Available from https://doi.org/10.2903/J.EFSA.2011.21682006.

Scientific Opinion on the substantiation of health claims related to sugar free chewing gum and reduction of dental plaque (ID 3084) pursuant to Article 13(1) of Regulation (EC) No 1924. EFSA J. 8 (2006). Available from https://doi.org/10.2903/J.EFSA.2010.14802006.

Shimizu, T. (2003). Health claims on functional foods: The Japanese regulations and an international comparison. *Nutrition Research Reviews*, *16*(2), 241–252. Available from https://doi.org/10.1079/NRR200363.

Siciliano, R. A., Reale, A., Mazzeo, M. F., Morandi, S., Silvetti, T., & Brasca, M. (2021). Paraprobiotics: A new perspective for functional foods and nutraceuticals. *Nutrients*, *13*(4). Available from https://doi.org/10.3390/nu13041225, https://www.mdpi.com/2072-6643/13/4/1225/pdf.

Standardization and proper quality labelling of agricultural and forestry products Act. (1950), 1950.

Staudacher, H. M., Irving, P. M., Lomer, M. C. E., & Whelan K. (2017). The challenges of control groups, placebos and blinding in clinical trials of dietary interventions. *Proceedings of the Nutrition Society*, *76*(3), 203–212. Available from http://journals.cambridge.org/PNS, https://doi.org/10.1017/S0029665117000350.

Tong, S., Bambrick, H., Beggs, P. J., Chen, L., Hu, Y., Ma, W., Steffen, W., & Tan, J. (2022). Current and future threats to human health in the Anthropocene. *Environment International*, *158*. Available from https://doi.org/10.1016/j.envint.2021.106892, www.elsevier.com/locate/envint.

Townsend, R. F., Woodside, J. V., Prinelli, F., O'Neill, R. F., & McEvoy, C. T. (2022). Associations between dietary patterns and neuroimaging markers: A systematic review. *Frontiers in Nutrition*, *9*. Available from https://doi.org/10.3389/fnut.2022.806006, https://journal.frontiersin.org/journal/nutrition.

Tummala, R., & Schoenherr, T. (2011). Assessing and managing risks using the Supply Chain Risk Management Process (SCRMP). *Supply Chain Management*, *16*(6), 474–483. Available from https://doi.org/10.1108/13598541111171165.

Tutelyan, V. A., Sukhanov, B. P., Kochetkova, A. A., Sheveleva, S. A., & Smirnova, E. A. (2019). *Russian regulations on nutraceuticals, functional foods, and foods for special dietary uses Nutraceutical and Functional Food Regulations in the United States and around the World* (pp. 399–416). Elsevier. Available from http://www.sciencedirect.com/science/book/9780128164679, https://doi.org/10.1016/B978-0-12-816467-9.00026-5.

Valdés, A., Álvarez-Rivera, G., Socas-Rodríguez, B., Herrero, M., Ibáñez, E., & Cifuentes, A. (2022). Foodomics: Analytical opportunities and challenges. *Analytical Chemistry*, *94*(1), 366–381. Available from https://doi.org/10.1021/acs.analchem.1c04678, http://pubs.acs.org/journal/ancham.

Yaqub, G., Ilyas, F., Idrees, M., & Mariyam, V. (2018). Monitoring and risk assessment due to presence of heavy metals and pesticides in tea samples. *Food Science and Technology (Brazil)*, *38*(4), 625–628. Available from https://doi.org/10.1590/fst.07417, http://www.scielo.br/pdf/cta/v38n4/0101-2061-cta-fst07417.pdf.

Zhang, X., Wang, D., Liu, S., & Tang, J. (2022). Bacterial cellulose nanofibril-based pickering emulsions: Recent trends and applications in the food industry. *Foods*, *11*(24). Available from https://doi.org/10.3390/foods11244064, www.mdpi.com/journal/foods.

Zhang, N., & Yao, L. (2019). Anxiolytic effect of essential oils and their constituents: A review. *Journal of Agricultural and Food Chemistry*, *67*(50), 13790–13808. Available from https://doi.org/10.1021/acs.jafc.9b00433, http://pubs.acs.org/journal/jafcau.

Chapter 17

Functional foods for oral and dental health

Ahmadreza Abedinia[1,2], Rafael Audino Zambelli[3] and Elahesadat Hosseini[4,5]

[1]Department of Food Engineering, Inonu University, Malatya, Turkey, [2]Department of Food Science and Technology, Damghan Branch, Islamic Azad University, Damghan, Iran, [3]Food Engineering Department, Federal University of Ceará, Fortaleza, Brazil, [4]Department of Chemical Engineering, Payame Noor University, Tehran, Iran, [5]Department of Food Science and Technology, National Nutrition Sciences and Food Technology Research Institute, Faculty of Nutrition Sciences and Food Technology, Shahid Beheshti University of Medical Sciences, Tehran, Iran

17.1 Introduction

Fluoridation of water, salt, and milk stands as a widely embraced practice in dentistry, pivotal in preventing tooth decay and oral diseases. Despite such measures, oral diseases continue to burden individuals both physically and socio-economically from an early age. A diet abundant in fermentable carbohydrates significantly contributes to this issue. Microorganisms with cariogenic properties are found in dental biofilm, metabolizing fermentable carbohydrates rapidly and producing acids that demineralize teeth (Takahashi & Nyvad, 2011). Consequently, World Health Organization (WHO) advocates for limiting daily sugar intake to less than 10% of total caloric intake. Furthermore, they suggest that reducing sugar consumption to 5% or lower would offer even greater benefits for oral health (World Health Organization, 2015). Recognizing the intimate link between oral care and lifestyle, there emerges a compelling need to explore dietary interventions with therapeutic benefits for promoting oral health. While traditional oral care practices like regular brushing and dental visits remain cornerstone habits, recent research underscores the potential of foods that counteract or diminish the effects of cariogenic microorganisms, such as milk, cacao, some fruits like grapes, and propolis, among others, or foods enriched with bioactive compounds tailored for specific oral health benefits (Hasler, 2009; Van Loveren et al., 2012). These functional foods, surpassing basic nutritional requirements, offer additional preventive and therapeutic strategies against oral diseases (Hasler, 2009; Van Loveren et al., 2012; Angarita-Díaz, Arias, et al., 2020; Angarita-Díaz, Forero-Escobar, et al., 2020). The efficacy of functional foods in oral health lies in their diverse mechanisms of action. From exhibiting antibacterial effects to modulating oral microbiota and possessing antiinflammatory properties, these foods exert multifaceted influences conducive to oral well-being. Functional foods span a wide array of categories, encompassing whole grains, dairy products, beverages, fruits, and vegetables, as well as fortified or enhanced foods. Traditional foods are increasingly acknowledged for their functional attributes, while innovation drives the development of new food products incorporating beneficial components. This chapter delves into the potential benefits of developing functional foods specifically targeted at dental caries prevention. By offering insights into the potential of functional foods in preventing dental caries, this overview explores how dietary components like antioxidants, probiotics, polyphenols, phytochemicals, and sugar alcohols can impact oral health and aid in disease prevention.

17.2 Common oral health problems

17.2.1 Oral health plaque and microbiome

The global landscape of oral epidemiology has undergone considerable transformations in recent years, with oral cancer, cleft lip and palate, dental caries, oral manifestations of HIV, oro-dental trauma, prevalent oral disorders, and periodontal disease. These conditions can substantially influence an individual's quality of life leading to pain, impaired function, and diminished overall well-being. The oral cavity hosts a rich and diverse community of microorganisms, commonly recognized as the oral microbiome. The oral microbiome is a dynamic system that maintains a delicate balance between beneficial and harmful bacteria. In a healthy mouth, the beneficial bacteria outnumber the harmful ones,

Unleashing the Power of Functional Foods and Novel Bioactives. DOI: https://doi.org/10.1016/B978-0-443-28862-3.00017-0

promoting oral health. However, when this balance is disrupted, the harmful bacteria can proliferate, resulting in the onset of related oral diseases. This intricate microbiome plays a crucial function in maintaining oral health, with plaque, a sticky biofilm composed primarily of bacteria, acting as its central hub. Plaque plays a pivotal role in the occurrence of oral diseases, such as dental caries and periodontal disease (Rouzi et al., 2023). The direct and indirect interaction of the oral microbiota on the intestinal microbiota is shown in Fig. 17.1.

17.2.1.1 Formation and composition of plaque

Plaque formation begins when food particles and bacteria adhere to the teeth and gums. Plaque is a complex microbial biofilm consisting of a dense accumulation of bacteria, extracellular matrix, a small number of white blood cells, shed epithelial cells, and food particles. Unlike individual bacteria that can easily be washed away by water, plaque forms a

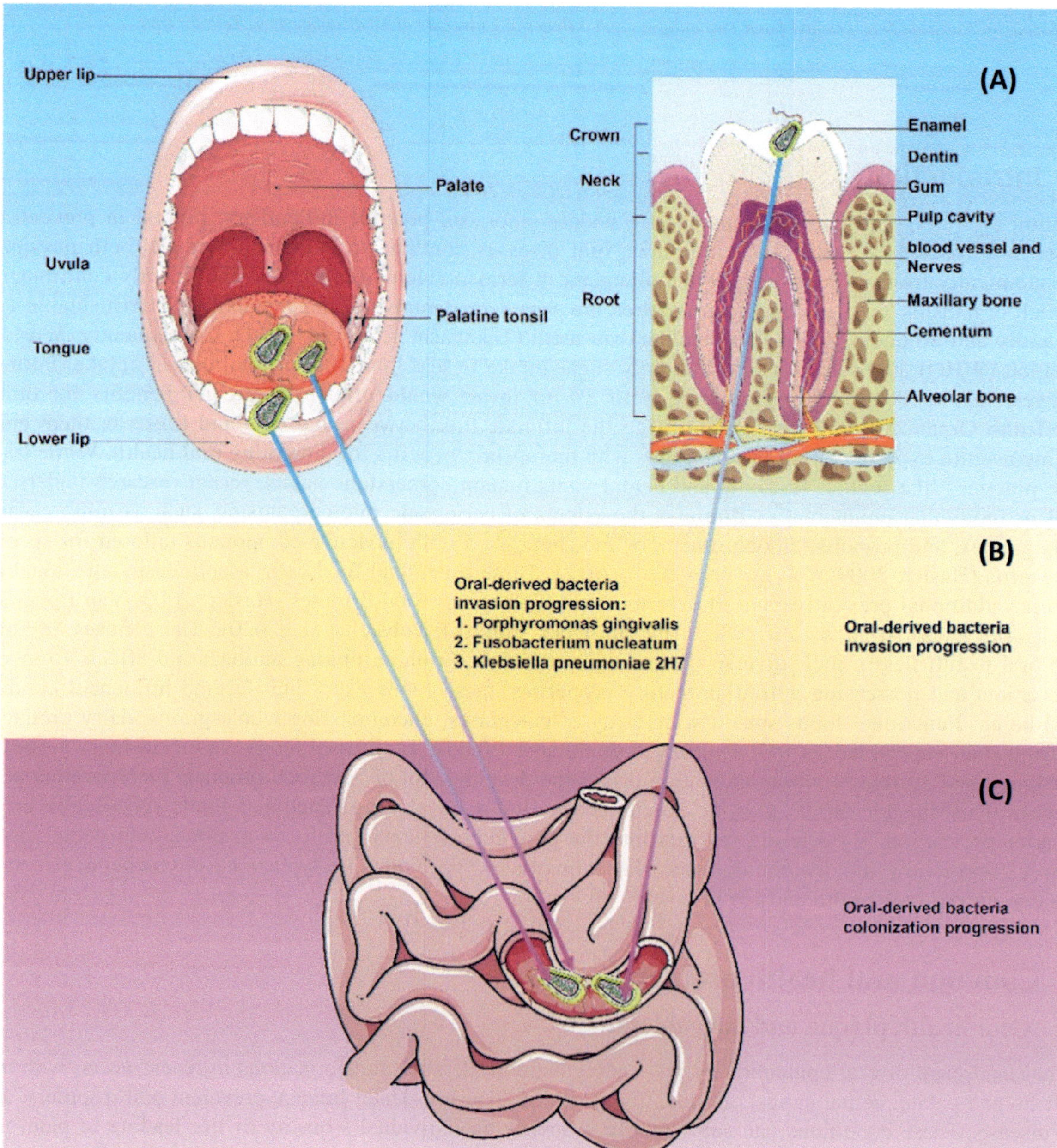

FIGURE 17.1 Directly and indirectly interaction of oral microbiota on gut microbiota. (A) Oral cavity's basic structure. (B) Advancement of oral bacteria's invasion. (C) Development of bacterial colonization originates in the mouth (Lu et al., 2019).

tenacious biofilm that adheres tightly to tooth surfaces, making it difficult to remove through regular brushing and flossing. As bacteria accumulate, they secrete extracellular polysaccharides, forming a matrix that traps additional bacteria and components (Huang et al., 2021).

17.2.1.2 Bacterial composition of plaque

The composition of plaque varies depending on individual oral hygiene practices, diet, and overall health status. However, certain bacteria are consistently found in plaque, including

- ***Streptococcus mutans***: This gram-positive bacterium is the primary cause of dental caries. It uses glycosyltransferases (GTFs) for glucan production, collaborates with *S. gordonii* for biofilm formation, and aids secondary attachment with acid-producing bacteria such as *S. sanguinis* and *S. salivarius* (Kim et al., 2023).
- ***Lactobacillus* spp.**: These gram-positive bacteria mainly *L. gasseri, L. fermentum, L. vaginalis,* and *L. casei* are recognized for their involvement in dental caries progression. They ferment carbohydrates, producing lactic acid, which contributes to enamel demineralization (Lamont et al., 2018).
- ***Actinomyces* spp.**: These gram-positive bacteria, notably *A. naeslundii* and *A. viscosus*, are linked to the advancement of dental caries in humans, particularly root caries and periodontal disease. They secrete enzymes that degrade connective tissue and bone, resulting in gum recession and tooth loss (Dame-Teixeira et al., 2016).

17.3 Impact of oral hygiene

Consistent brushing and flossing are vital for upholding excellent oral hygiene and averting plaque formation. These habits remove plaque bacteria and disrupt the biofilm, preventing its accumulation and reducing the risk of oral diseases. Mouth rinses and chewing gum are two additional methods for removing plaque. Mouth rinses cleanse the mouth by flushing it, and they contain antiinflammatory compounds that can treat oral diseases. Seawater mouthwash is an effective alternative to chlorhexidine mouthwash, which can cause tooth staining. Chewing gum stimulates saliva secretion, which aids in rinsing the mouth and removing dietary fermentable carbohydrates, along with plaque buildup. Sugar-free chewing gum can significantly reduce plaque production, but it has not been shown to improve gingivitis. Adding functional ingredients to chewing gum, such as quercetin, can potentially deliver bioactive molecules that can resist *S. mutans* strains and have anticaries effects. Besides mechanical cleaning, diet, natural agents, and nutrition play an indirect role in maintaining periodontal health and fighting alveolar bone resorption (Huang et al., 2021; Komara et al., 2023). Comparative studies conducted examining the effectiveness of manual and electric toothbrushes in plaque control (Silva et al., 2020; Vajawat et al., 2015). They found that electric toothbrushes significantly reduced clinical parameters in individuals compared to manual toothbrushes. Effective brushing is deemed to result in plaque reduction of 60% or more, with combined manual and electric methods exceeding 70% effectiveness.

17.4 Role of Saliva multilayer characteristics and its function in food oral processing

Within the oral cavity, saliva forms a unique bio-interface that is indispensable for efficient food processing. During the mastication and deglutition of food, the saliva bio-interface facilitates several essential mechanisms, including moistening and blending food particles, creating a unified food bolus, facilitating colloidal and enzymatic interactions among food components, lubricating the oral mucosa, and dispersing flavor compounds. These processes are all critically dependent on the intricate multilayered microstructure of the saliva bio-interface, with each layer playing a distinct functional role. Saliva plays a critical role in oral health by containing antimicrobial compounds, such as lactoferrin, lysozyme, and histatin, that inhibit the growth of harmful bacteria and plaque formation. Saliva also mechanically removes bacteria and food debris from the oral cavity (Mu & Chen, 2023).

It can also be effective in diseases caused by poor oral and dental health. For example, after the Covid-19 epidemic, the importance of oral hygiene has been noticed more than ever in the oral cavity. Saliva is one of the entry gates for viruses. Saliva is a potential reservoir of SARS-CoV-2, and if there is a gap in the mouth, the risk of infection increases. This allows the virus to enter the vascular system through the gingival or periodontal pocket, possibly into the pulmonary environment and then into the pulmonary vasculature by interaction with endothelial surface receptors that cause pulmonary vasoconstriction and lung injury due to endothelial dysfunction (Kumar et al., 2023).

17.5 Multilayered microstructure of the saliva bio-interface

17.5.1 Precursor layer

This layer consists of mucins, which are long, sticky molecules that form a gel-like matrix. It is a preliminary layer comprising saliva proteins that bind directly and firmly to the dental or mucosal epithelial layer. This is the outermost layer and is responsible for lubricating the oral mucosa and preventing food particles from sticking to the teeth (Fig. 17.2).

17.5.1.1 Tightly bound protein layer

The sublayer L2 of the saliva bio-interface is densely packed with low molecular weight proteins, including statherin, proline, and cystatins. These molecules exhibit strong affinity toward constituents present in L1, suggesting that L1 and L2 are two stable and firmly attached sublayers of the saliva bio-interface. This layer is a subphase of the lamellar layer and is composed of different types of polysaccharides. It plays a role in maintaining the viscoelastic properties of saliva and in preventing food particles from aggregating.

17.5.1.2 Surface-anchored mucin layer

The third layer (L3) of the saliva bio-interface consists of surface-bound mucins (MUC5B/MUC7), forming mucin brushes and loops anchored to the surface. These structures primarily serve as boundary lubricants during food processing. The continuous exchange of biopolymers with the bulk saliva layer (L4) maintains the high load-bearing capacity of L3.

17.5.1.3 Liquid bulk layer

It comprises supramolecular structures of MUC5B mucin and MUC7 mucin, which are responsible for the viscosity and adhesiveness of saliva and for the transport of molecules across the oral mucosa.

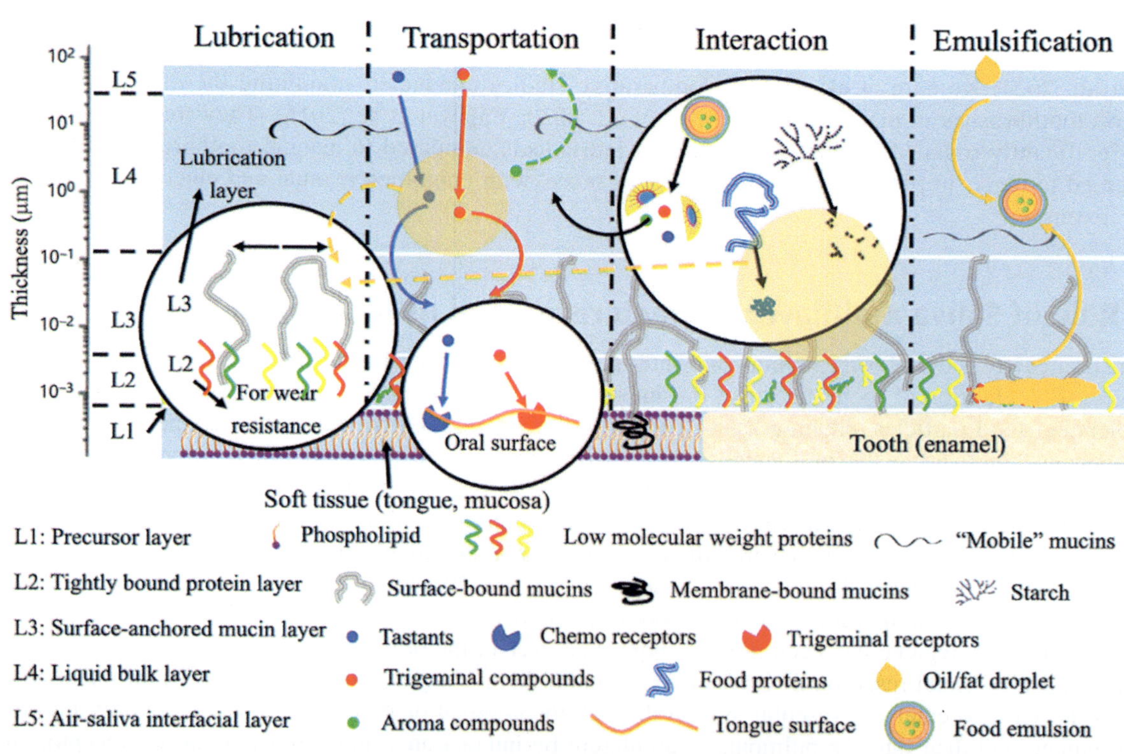

FIGURE 17.2 A five-layered film (SCF) representing the saliva in the mouth cavity is shown as a schematic of oral bio-interfaces (Mu & Chen, 2023).

17.5.1.4 Air-saliva interfacial layer

This layer serves as the outermost boundary of the saliva bio-interface and is where the food bolus is formed. It consists of proteinaceous material located at the interface and in close proximity to the bulk saliva or directly exposed to the air (Yakubov et al., 2015).

17.6 Methods of evaluating the impact of functional foods/bioactive ingredients in dental caries control

Functional foods and active ingredients play a pivotal role in dental caries control, necessitating robust methodologies for their assessment. Various approaches have been employed, each with distinct advantages and limitations. Herein, we delineate a comprehensive methodology integrating key aspects from existing protocols while addressing inherent challenges (Matsukubo & Takazoe, 2006).

- **In vitro models:** In vitro models provide a controlled environment for studying the effects of functional foods/active ingredients on oral bacteria. These models assess parameters such as growth, acid production, and biofilm formation. However, replicating intraoral conditions accurately poses challenges, diminishing their predictive value for cariogenicity.
- **Animal models:** Animal experiments, typically employing laboratory rats orally infected with human oral bacteria, simulate dietary patterns. However, ethical concerns and evolving regulatory frameworks underscore the need for alternative methods due to societal sensitivities towards animal research.
- **In vivo monitoring (human plaque pH method):** Human plaque pH monitoring offers a relatively simple yet informative approach. Through methods like plaque sampling, touch electrodes, or interproximal telemetry, it evaluates acidogenic potential. A product demonstrating a plaque pH profile statistically similar to a noncariogenic control (e.g., sorbitol rinse) is deemed noncariogenic. However, further in situ cariogenicity tests may be warranted for borderline cases.
- **Intraoral cariogenicity tests:** In situ caries models, utilizing intraoral appliances, mimic clinical conditions closely. These models enable comprehensive assessment under realistic scenarios, including changes in tooth mineral status. Notably, the critical pH for dentine and cementum remains to be determined, emphasizing the need for continued research in this domain.
- **Integration and advancement:** Synthesizing insights from diverse methodologies enhances the comprehensive evaluation of functional foods/active ingredients in dental caries control. By refining existing techniques and exploring novel approaches, we can improve the accuracy and reliability of assessments, thus advancing preventive dental care strategies.

Finally, a multifaceted methodology incorporating in vitro, in vivo, and in situ approaches is essential for comprehensively assessing the impact of functional foods and active ingredients in dental caries control. Through continued research and innovation, we can optimize preventive strategies, promoting oral health and well-being.

17.7 Functional food interaction in the oral environment

The oral environment serves as a dynamic interface where food, saliva, and microorganisms interact. Sugar consumption, inadequate oral care, and the presence of cavity-causing bacteria contribute to the initiation and progression of dental caries. Prevention and management strategies often involve a combination of dietary modifications, regular oral hygiene practices, and professional dental interventions. In the context of oral health and the prevention of dental caries and periodontal diseases, the incorporation of functional foods can play a significant role. Incorporating functional foods into diet can be a practical and enjoyable way to enhance overall health and well-being. Functional foods are those that offer additional health benefits beyond basic nutrition (Vlaicu et al., 2023). The intricate relationship between diet and oral health emphasizes the importance of maintaining a well-balanced and nutrient-rich diet throughout life. Adequate nutrition not only influences the prevention of malformations but also plays a crucial role in supporting the overall health and resilience of the oral cavity (Moynihan & Petersen, 2004).

Recognizing the connection between diet and oral health underscores the importance of adopting a holistic approach to well-being. Beyond the immediate impact on oral hygiene, a balanced diet contributes to overall systemic health, reducing the risk of chronic diseases and promoting a healthier lifestyle. Regular dental check-ups, combined with a nutrient-rich diet and proper oral hygiene practices, form a powerful preventive measure against both oral and systemic health issues (Folayan & Tantawi, 2023).

The exploration of the human oral microbiome has garnered increasing attention owing to its pivotal role in fostering overall health, as underscored by numerous studies. Diverse factors, including hygiene practices, genetic predispositions, and environmental influences, contribute to shaping the composition of the oral microbiota. Among these factors, diet emerges as a paramount external element that actively modulates the oral microbiota, consequently influencing the delicate equilibrium between host health and susceptibility to diseases. While the dynamic nature of the oral microbiota implies a continuous state of flux, maintaining a delicate balance between commensal bacteria and potential pathogens is essential for determining oral health status (Willis & Gabaldón, 2020). Understanding the impact of diet on the oral microbiome is crucial for comprehending the intricate interplay between external factors and microbial communities within the oral cavity. Dietary choices, encompassing the types of foods consumed and their nutritional content, can significantly influence the abundance and diversity of oral bacteria. Research suggests that a diet rich in sugars and processed foods may create an environment conducive to the proliferation of pathogenic bacteria, potentially leading to oral health issues such as dental caries and periodontal diseases (Santonocito et al., 2022). Overall, functional foods have the potential to improve oral health through various mechanisms that highlight their importance in oral care (Qamar et al., 2021; Quelemes et al., 2023).

17.7.1 Food containing vitamins

Vitamins are crucial micronutrients that play a crucial role in sustaining oral health by supporting various physiological processes and regulating the oral microbiome. Their diverse functions contribute to the inhibition of oral diseases such as tooth decay, periodontal disease, and oral-related diseases such as cancer (Cagetti et al., 2020).

Vitamin deficiencies can manifest as nonspecific oral disorders like glossitis, stomatitis, and mucosal ulceration. Linear lesions in glossitis may indicate early vitamin B12 deficiency (Kim et al., 2016). Inadequate vitamin D levels contribute to diminish bone density, osteoporosis, and worsened periodontal disease progression. Also, vitamin D exhibiting immunomodulatory, antiinflammatory, and antiproliferative properties contribute to their ability to regulate the immune system, reduce inflammation, and inhibit excessive cell growth (Botelho et al., 2020; Varela-López et al., 2018).

Vitamins possessing antioxidant properties and influencing the immune system appear to have the potential to prevent or ameliorate periodontal disease. Vitamins like E, which can counteract oxidative stress and modulate immune responses, demonstrate promise for promoting oral health (Varela-López et al., 2018).

Vitamin C is essential for collagen synthesis, a structural protein that strengthens connective tissues, including gingival tissue. Healthy gingiva is crucial for plaque resistance and periodontal health. Contrarily, chewable vitamin C tablets have been discovered to have a pH of around 2, falling below the critical pH threshold of 5.5 for enamel dissolution. This suggests a potential link between vitamin C and enamel erosion, with a relative risk of 1.16 (Varela-López et al., 2018). Vitamin A promotes salivary gland function, ensuring adequate saliva production. Saliva serves as a natural cleanser, buffer, and antimicrobial agent, protecting against oral bacteria and maintaining oral health. This vitamin with zinc has also effected taste and smell perception (Varela-López et al., 2018).

Vitamin B complex, particularly vitamin B3, may help alleviate dry mouth symptoms by promoting salivary gland function. Adequate saliva production is essential for maintaining oral health and comfort (Varela-López et al., 2018).

17.7.2 Food containing probiotics

Recently, the concept of bacteriotherapy, utilizing probiotic bacteria as a promising and cost-effective prophylactic approach with the ability to inhibit oral pathogens, has gained attention. Probiotics are live microorganisms defined as offering health benefits to the host when administered in adequate quantities. Regular consumption of probiotics has been suggested to play a vital role in preventing and treating various oral diseases (Chugh et al., 2020).

There are various sources of probiotics for maintaining oral health, including both natural and synthesized forms. Natural sources such as yogurt, kefir, soybean, and sauerkraut have probiotic bacteria (Jain & Sharma, 2012). Alternatively, probiotic food products can be found in the market, comprising formulated probiotics with different strains of *Streptococcus* and *Lactobacillus*. These products are commonly available as tablets or powdered supplements (Chugh et al., 2020; Sivamaruthi et al., 2020). Probiotic bacteria offer potential benefits for oral health through four primary mechanisms. First, they can compete with oral pathogens for adhesion sites, nutrients, and growth factors, thereby inhibiting the colonization of oral pathogens in the oral cavity. Second, probiotic bacteria can modify the oral environment, particularly by utilizing the arginine deiminase pathway to release alkali and raise the pH of the oral cavity, restoring pH homeostasis and reducing the risk of carious lesions. Third, probiotics can produce substances like bacteriocins, acids, or peroxide that can alter pH levels and inhibit the growth of oral bacteria. Lastly, certain oral probiotics, such as *Streptococcus salivarius*, have been shown to stimulate antiinflammatory activity by inhibiting the transportation of proinflammatory cytokines induced by oral pathogens (How & Yeo, 2021).

17.7.3 Food containing antioxidant

An excessive accumulation of free radicals, including reactive oxygen species, can lead to oxidative stress, a condition implicated in various systemic and localized disorders, such as periodontal diseases, rheumatoid arthritis, diabetes, atherosclerosis, and masticatory system dysfunctions. The oral cavity is exposed to various sources of free radicals, including air, water, food components, stimulants, medications, and xenobiotic (Tóthová et al., 2015). Consequently, the oral cavity has developed inherent antioxidant defense mechanisms to counteract free radicals-induced oxidative stress. Additionally, incorporating antioxidants, such as polyphenols, carotenoids, flavonoids, mineral element, and vitamins C and E into the oral environment, can effectively mitigate oxidative stress and promote oral health (Dąbrowska et al., 2020).

Flavonoids, polyphenols, carotenoids, mineral elements like zinc, and vitamins E and C have been studied for their effects on oral and dental health. Flavonoids and polyphenols, which are abundant in fruits, vegetables, tea, and red wine, are known for their antioxidant and antinflammatory properties. These compounds can help mitigate the risk of periodontal diseases and oral cancers. Carotenoids, found in fruits and vegetables like carrots and tomatoes, contribute to oral mucosal health and may protect against oral cancer. Zinc, a mineral element, plays a crucial role in maintaining oral tissue integrity and antioxidant defense. Vitamin E and C, known antioxidants, help protect oral tissues from oxidative damage and support gum health. Collectively, these antioxidant compounds have the potential to promote oral and dental health by combating oxidative stress, inflammation, and certain oral diseases (Kaur et al., 2016). On the other hand, saliva serves as the initial protective barrier against oxidative stress under its inherent antioxidants, which encompass salivary peroxidase (Px), catalase (CAT), myeloperoxidase (MPO), and nonenzymatic antioxidant uric acid (UA). These components play a crucial role in combating free radicals and reactive oxygen species, thereby providing defense against oxidative damage (Małgorzata & Słotwińska, 2011).

17.7.4 Food containing bioactive compounds

Foods contain biologically active components that can provide beneficial physiological effects. Oral diseases are often associated with lifestyle choices, and diet plays a significant role in their development. Certain foods have been identified for their potential to improve oral health. These foods contain specific properties that can positively impact oral well-being. These foods contain bioactive compounds that can elicit desirable physiological effects. Oral diseases, which are influenced by lifestyle factors, can be influenced by dietary choices. Certain foods have been found to contribute to better oral health outcomes (Vikneshan et al., 2016).

17.7.5 Zinc

Zinc plays a crucial role in various physiological processes, including its antioxidant properties. Its antioxidative effect stems from multiple mechanisms, such as the direct binding of zinc ions to thiol groups, safeguarding them against oxidation (Dąbrowska et al., 2020). Zinc also contributes to the structure of antioxidant proteins and regulates the induction of metallothionein. Zinc-rich food sources include animal products like oysters, meat, liver, and eggs alongside plant-based options like wheat germ, pumpkin, wheat bran, sunflower, garlic, and onions (Oteiza, 2012). In a study conducted by Kostecka-Sochoń et al., it was observed that zinc supplementation effectively decreased oxidative stress in the sublingual tissue of salivary glands. This reduction was evident through the inhibition of cadmium-induced lipid peroxidation (LPO), as well as the decrease in hydrogen peroxide (H2O2) levels and increase in glutathione (GSH) levels (Kostecka-Sochoń et al., 2018).

17.7.6 Flavonoids

Flavonoids a group of bioactive organic compounds act as antioxidants within the oral cavity. Over 4,000 flavonoids, including saponin, tannins, catechins, triterpenoids, and steroids, have been identified in plants and fruits,

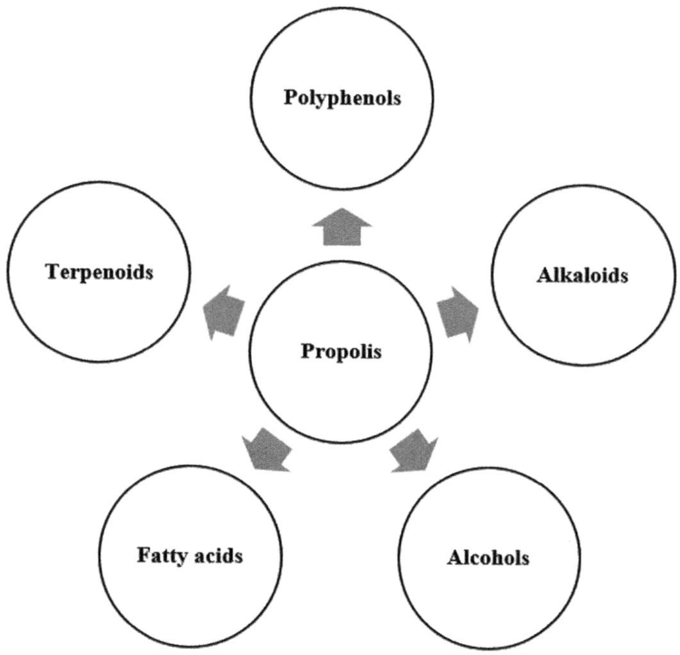

FIGURE 17.3 Propolis' chemical groups for its pharmacological properties and health uses.

predominantly found in red wine, citrus fruits, tea, seeds, olive oil, chocolate, and propolis (Dąbrowska et al., 2020). Pharmacologically, flavonoids exhibit antiviral, antiallergic, anticancerous, antifungal effects antiinflammatory, and wound-healing. Their high antioxidant capacity plays a role in oral health by inhibiting free radicals, which contribute to the inflammatory progression of periodontal diseases. Tannins present in flavonoid extracts can bind to salivary proteins, potentially affecting salivary bacteria (Mu & Chen, 2023). Notably, certain flavonoids like myricetin and rutin are recognized antifungal agents that hinder fungal growth through mechanisms such as RNA and protein synthesis, plasma membrane dysfunction, cell division, inhibition of cell wall formation, and suppression of efflux-mediated pumping systems. These flavonoids show promise as antifungal treatments for oral candidiasis (Goiana et al., 2022). Propolis, a natural resin harvested by bees from plants to seal gaps and fissures in their hives, boasts a rich profile of medicinal properties. The wide range of chemically active molecules found in propolis extracts contributes to their diverse pharmacological properties and various health-related applications (Fig. 17.3). Its impressive attributes include robust antibacterial, antiviral, antiinflammatory, wound-healing, and anticancer properties. For centuries, humans have leveraged the therapeutic potential of propolis, incorporating it into various remedies. Among its notable applications is the treatment of dental caries and oral infections. The multifaceted nature of propolis makes it a versatile and valuable resource in natural medicine. Its antibacterial qualities make it effective against a spectrum of harmful microorganisms, contributing to oral health. Additionally, propolis's antiinflammatory and wound-healing properties are particularly beneficial in addressing dental issues and promoting overall oral well-being. As an ancient remedy, propolis has stood the test of time in human therapeutic practices. Its historical use in treating dental caries and mouth infections underscores its efficacy in oral care. Modern research continues to unveil the intricate mechanisms behind propolis's medicinal properties, reinforcing its relevance as a natural solution for oral health concerns. Incorporating propolis into oral care routines or exploring its potential in dental products could offer a complementary and natural approach to maintaining a healthy mouth. The rich legacy of propolis in traditional medicine aligns with contemporary efforts to harness nature's remedies for holistic well-being, especially in the realm of oral health (Altabbal et al., 2023; Simone-Finstrom & Spivak, 2010; Zulhendri et al., 2019).

17.7.7 Polyphenols

Polyphenols, a diverse group of secondary plant metabolites distinguished by a benzene ring bearing multiple hydroxyl groups (−OH) and a functional side chain, are widely distributed in various dietary sources (Dąbrowska et al., 2020). Grapefruits, tea, ginger, blueberries, olive oil, red wine, rosemary, and hops (*Humulus lupulus* L.) are exceptional dietary sources of phenolic compounds, as well as vitamins, minerals, and anthocyanins (Abiko & Paudel, 2022; Esteban-

TABLE 17.1 Primary mechanisms of action of polyphenols.

Mechanisms of action	Description
Direct free radical scavenging	Polyphenols act as direct scavengers, donating electrons to ROS, neutralizing their oxidative potential, and converting them into harmless molecules
Enzymatic inhibition	Polyphenols can inhibit the activity of enzymes responsible for generating ROS, such as NADPH oxidase and COX-2, thereby reducing the overall ROS burden in the body
Enhancement of other antioxidant defense systems	Polyphenols can interact with and enhance the activity of other antioxidant molecules, such as vitamins C and E, amplifying the overall antioxidant capacity of the biological system

COX-2, Cyclooxygenase-2; *ROS*, reactive oxygen species.

Fernández et al., 2017). Extensive studies have linked dietary polyphenols to a plethora of health benefits, including antioxidant and antimicrobial properties, antiinflammatory effects, and modulation of the human microbiota composition and functionality. Recent investigations have established a connection between the consumption of polyphenol-rich beverages and foods and the maintenance of oral health and the prevention of oral diseases (Abiko & Paudel, 2022; Dąbrowska et al., 2020; Esteban-Fernández et al., 2017; Guo et al., 2023; Requena et al., 2010). Hops, for instance, a key ingredient in beer, is a complex plant comprising resins, essential oils, polyphenols, cellulose, various proteins, and water. Renowned for its antimicrobial properties against bacterial growth, hops and their components are increasingly recognized for their potential contributions to human health. Extensive research has highlighted the effectiveness of hops as potent antimicrobial, antiinflammatory, and anticancer agents. The primary health benefits are attributed to three main hop components: polyphenols, bitter acids, and essential oils. Given their systemic impact on health, the influence of hop components on oral health becomes a noteworthy area of exploration (Abiko & Paudel, 2022). Studies suggest that hop components could play a role in addressing various oral diseases, including dental caries, periodontal diseases, oral lichen planus, and oral candidiasis. The antimicrobial effects of hops may contribute to preventing bacterial growth in the oral cavity, potentially reducing the risk of dental issues. Additionally, the antiinflammatory properties of hop components may have implications for managing conditions like periodontal diseases, where inflammation plays a crucial role. Overall, polyphenols exert their potent antioxidant effects through three primary mechanisms (Borowska et al., 2018; Mężyńska & Brzóska, 2019) (Table 17.1).

17.8 Phytochemicals

Phytochemicals, also known as plant chemicals, are compounds produced by plants through primary and secondary metabolism. They are found in foods such as vegetables, fruits, cereals, legumes, and nuts, and they possess various biological activities (Kumar et al., 2023). Studies have shown that phytochemical compositions, including essential oils, offer promising opportunities for addressing oral infections. Essential oils are known for their lower toxicity compared to conventional treatments, and they harbor biologically active compounds with medicinal properties capable of addressing oral health issues such as periodontitis, tooth decay, and gingivitis (Reddy, 2019). The products derived from different medicinal plants such as *Azadirachta indica, Thymus vulgaris, Asparagus racemosus, Juglans regia*, and *Ocimum sanctum* have different types of phytochemicals, and some are used in oral health-related products (Kumar et al., 2021). In this context, phyto-bioactive compounds were encapsulated with a nanocarrier to increase their biostability and solubility to protect against their degradation, with the aim of improving the absorption and prolonging the circulation of bioactive compounds in the human body to promote not only oral health but for other parts of the body (Nsairat et al., 2023).

17.8.1 Carotenoids

Carotenoids, including β-carotene and lycopene, as well as polyphenols, are antioxidants commonly found in fruits and vegetables (tomato, carrot). Scientific studies have demonstrated the effectiveness of these compounds in preventing and treating periodontal diseases (González-Aguilar et al., 2008). Specifically, a deficiency in β-carotene, a precursor of vitamin A, has been associated with periodontitis and gingivitis. Research indicates that supplementing vitamin A alongside other treatments improves outcomes in the management of periodontal diseases (Pooja, n.d.). These findings underscore the significance of adequate carotenoid intake in the prevention and treatment of periodontal diseases (Kaur et al., 2019).

TABLE 17.2 Sugar substitutes in tooth-friendly confectionery and oral care products.

Categories	Example
Hydrogenated carbohydrates (sugar alcohols)	Sorbitol, mannitol, xylitol, erythritol, Isomalt (Palatinit), lactitol, maltitol, Maltitol sirups, hydrogenated glucose sirup
Bulking agent	Polydextrose
Novel disaccharides	Leucrose, isomaltulose (Palatinose)
Noncaloric, nonnutritive, and intense sweeteners	Acesulfame K, aspartame, cyclamate, saccharin, sucralose, stevia, thaumatin

17.9 Alternative sweeteners and their impacts on tooth decay

The use of sucrose substitutes in confections is believed to have contributed to the decrease in the prevalence of dental caries in industrialized nations. Marthaler et al. (1994) explored this trend in Switzerland, a country where a wide range of confectioneries with sucrose substitutes has been accessible since 1970. Their study findings suggested that the presence of sucrose substitutes is one of the factors contributing to the decrease in dental caries prevalence in Switzerland since the 1980s. However, there is no data to support the notion that confections containing sucrose substitutes are as effective as fluoride in reducing dental caries levels. Various sugar alternatives, sweeteners, and bulking agents are employed in the formulation of drinks, sugar-free sweets, confectionery, and chewing gum, as outlined in Table 17.2. Widely used sugar alcohols (*Polyol*), such as sorbitol, isomalt, maltitol, mannitol, xylitol, lactitol, and hydrogenated starch hydrolysates along with emerging options like erythritol, offer alternatives with promising results. The relative sweetness of these sugar alcohols compared to sucrose ranges from 0.5 to 1, and studies have examined their fermentation by oral microorganisms in vitro. All sugar alcohols, which are confirmed as hypo- or nonacidogenic, demonstrate reduced or almost no production of extracellular polysaccharides. Xylitol, in particular, stands out as it not only impedes the growth of *mutans streptococci* but is also considered anticariogenic based on animal experiments (Bahador et al., 2012; Nassar et al., 2021). The idea that xylitol may diminish the caries-inducing impact on newly erupted teeth has been proposed, hinting at a possible enduring protective effect against cavities, even years after stopping the use of xylitol products (Humaid & Bamashmous, 2022; Janakiram et al., 2017; Riley et al., 2015; Havenaar, 1984). Animal experiments have led to the conclusion that xylitol possesses anticariogenic properties (Humaid & Bamashmous, 2022; Janket et al., 2019). Notably, findings indicate that children born to mothers who frequently indulge in xylitol-sweetened chewing gum show reduced colonization by mutans streptococci (Söderling, 2009). Despite the widely held belief in its superior efficacy for caries control, the clinical evidence backing this notion has been questioned and deemed weak (Twetman, 2009). In addressing this issue, van Loveren conducted a focused review on clinical studies examining the preventive and therapeutic effects of sugar alcohols on dental caries. His findings indicated that the observed effects of sugar alcohols in preventing dental caries in gums and candies are likely linked to the stimulation of salivary flow. However, there is a lack of specific evidence supporting a caries-preventive effect solely attributable to xylitol (van Loveren, 2004). Despite these challenges, the distinctive characteristics of xylitol can still be strategically utilized for marketing purposes and may positively influence dietary habits across various age groups. Novel disaccharides like isomaltulose and leucrose, characterized by very low acidogenicity and good gastrointestinal tolerance, have been developed for tooth-friendly sweets which are presently available in the market (Van Loveren et al., 2012). Intense sweeteners like stevia, acesulfame K, aspartame, cyclamate, saccharin, and sucralose, not serving as substrates for oral microorganisms, can be designated as noncariogenic. Their potent sweetness permits the use of minimal quantities. As a result, these sweeteners are predominantly employed to enhance the sweetness of beverages such as coffee, soft drinks, and tea. While light soft drinks might not directly contribute to dental caries, they may contain heightened acid levels, posing a potential risk of tooth erosion.

17.10 Customized approach to nutritional choices

Tailoring functional foods involves customizing dietary choices to address specific health needs, in this case, focusing on oral health. Customizing nutritional choices based on individual oral health needs involves a comprehensive assessment of specific concerns and the implementation of strategies to optimize the intake of functional food ingredients. The initial step in this tailored approach is evaluating an individual's dental history, including any existing issues such as cavities, gum disease, or enamel erosion. Additionally, consideration is given to overall health conditions, like diabetes or autoimmune disorders, and the impact of medication use on oral health (Beaudette et al., 2017). To tailor functional foods to individual needs, a targeted strategy is adopted. For those with a history of cavities or weakened enamel, increasing the intake of calcium and vitamin D is emphasized, with a focus on dairy or fortified plant-based alternatives. Individuals with inflammatory conditions affecting the gums benefit from incorporating omega-3 fatty acids found in fatty fish or flaxseeds (Craig & Brothers, 2021). Considering an individual's medical and dental history is crucial in tailoring functional foods. For those with a history of gum disease, a focus is placed on supporting gum health through foods rich in antioxidants and vitamin C, promoting tissue healing and resilience. In cases of weakened enamel, recommendations include foods high in calcium, phosphorus, and vitamin D to enhance enamel strength (Nishida et al., 2000a,b). Probiotics play a significant role in gut health, and tailoring functional foods involves recognizing the uniqueness of each person's gut microbiome. Recommendations for probiotic-rich foods like yogurt, kefir, and fermented vegetables are personalized based on taste preferences and individual tolerance (Dahiya & Nigam, 2022).

Taking into account dietary preferences and restrictions is another key aspect of tailoring functional foods. This involves adapting meal plans to align with vegetarian, vegan, or omnivorous dietary choices and addressing any food allergies or sensitivities by providing alternative sources to meet nutritional requirements without triggering adverse reactions (Craig & Mangels, Fresán, et al., 2021). Cultural and culinary considerations are also part of the customization process, encouraging a diverse range of functional foods that align with oral health goals. This includes exploring traditional dishes and ingredients that contribute to a rich and enjoyable eating experience. Additionally, considering different cooking methods, such as steaming, roasting, or raw consumption, based on individual preferences ensures the retention of nutritional value (Zhang et al., 2019).

Optimizing the intake of functional food ingredients involves strategic meal planning, ensuring that each meal includes a variety of food groups to provide a range of nutrients. Regular snacking on healthy options like cheese, nuts, or fruits is encouraged to maintain saliva production between meals. Adequate hydration, achieved through regular water intake, helps cleanse the mouth and maintain saliva production (Esmaeili et al., 2022). Other essential strategies include limiting the consumption of sugary and acidic foods to prevent enamel erosion and cavities. Establishing healthy oral hygiene habits, such as brushing or rinsing the mouth after meals, is crucial, especially if acidic or sugary foods are consumed. Flossing is also emphasized to remove food particles between teeth. Supplementation may be considered based on individual needs, with a recommendation to consult healthcare professionals for personalized guidance (Tungare & Paranjpe, 2023).

Lifestyle factors, such as physical activity levels and stress management, are integrated into the customization process. For individuals with higher activity levels, emphasis may be placed on adequate protein intake for muscle repair and overall health. Stress-reducing functional foods, rich in magnesium or B-vitamins, may be recommended for those facing high stress levels, recognizing the impact of stress on oral health (Bradlee et al., 2018). Based on this, 3D printing technology can be a strong tool for developing specific foods to support oral health. 3D printing represents a cutting-edge manufacturing process where objects are constructed layer by layer from a 3D computer-aided design, utilizing various printing technologies. The versatility of 3D printing technology enables the creation of unique products and structures that are unattainable through conventional methods. A primary advantage of this emerging technology lies in its capacity to customize food by tailoring nutrition, introducing novel multiflavored, colored, and textured properties, and allowing for the incorporation of a diverse range of ingredients (Javaid et al., 2022). The significance of food printing has garnered attention for its ability to craft intricate geometric structures, facilitating mass customization and offering both economic and environmental benefits. Beyond the inherent nutritional value, this innovative technology has paved the way for the concept of personalized nutrition. Integrating specific functional ingredients into adaptable food sources can have a profound impact on addressing various nutritional challenges and potentially treating chronic disorders (Eswaran et al., 2023). As research opportunities within the realm of 3D food printing continue to expand, there is a compelling case to support the idea of food customization and personalized nutrition. This transformative technology not only opens avenues for creative culinary possibilities but also holds promise in addressing individual health needs through tailored nutritional solutions (Zhu et al., 2023).

17.11 Exploring future trends in functional foods for oral health

Exploring future trends in functional foods for oral health involves delving into potential advancements in research and development that can enhance the preventive and therapeutic aspects of oral care. As technology and scientific understanding progress, several exciting trends are emerging in the realm of functional foods tailored to support and promote oral health (Ofek et al., 2012). Advances in genetics and personalized nutrition are likely to lead to the development of functional foods tailored to individuals' specific oral health needs. Precision nutrition can consider genetic predispositions and unique dietary requirements to create personalized diets that promote optimal oral well-being (Mullins et al., 2020). The realm of functional food research and development is undergoing continual evolution, presenting intriguing possibilities for advancing oral health through innovative ingredients. Speculating on potential breakthroughs involves considering emerging trends and novel compounds that could have a positive impact on oral well-being (Galanakis, 2021). One avenue of exploration lies in the potential use of prebiotics specifically tailored to nourish beneficial bacteria within the oral microbiome. This targeted approach may foster a balanced microbial environment, potentially mitigating conditions such as gum disease and cavities (Azad et al., 2020).

Researchers are increasingly exploring the potential of bioactive compounds and nutraceuticals derived from natural sources. These compounds, such as polyphenols, probiotics, and peptides, exhibit specific health-promoting properties and may play a key role in preventing and managing oral diseases. Future functional foods may harness these bioactive components for targeted oral health benefits (Arshad et al., 2021; Puri et al., 2022). As the understanding of the oral microbiome deepens, functional foods designed to modulate and maintain a healthy balance of oral bacteria are likely to emerge. Probiotics, prebiotics, and other microbiome-targeted ingredients may be incorporated into foods to support a diverse and beneficial microbial environment in the mouth (Maier, 2023).

Innovations in packaging and delivery systems can enhance the efficacy of functional foods for oral health. Smart packaging may include time-released ingredients or technologies that optimize the delivery of bioactive compounds, ensuring sustained benefits within the oral cavity (Puttasiddaiah et al., 2022). Future trends may witness increased collaboration between the oral care and nutrition industries. Joint efforts could lead to the development of functional foods that seamlessly integrate oral health benefits with nutritional advantages, addressing both systemic and oral well-being. Exploring these future trends in functional foods for oral health highlights the potential for exciting breakthroughs that could revolutionize preventive and therapeutic approaches to oral care. As research and development progress, consumers can anticipate a diverse range of innovative functional foods that contribute not only to overall health but also to the promotion of optimal oral hygiene. Extracting bioactive compounds from natural sources, such as certain plants or marine organisms, holds promise for promoting oral health. These compounds may possess antiinflammatory, antimicrobial, or antioxidative properties, providing a natural means of maintaining a healthy mouth (Lordan et al., 2011).

Envisioning a future of enzyme-enhanced functional foods raises the prospect of aiding oral health by facilitating the breakdown of food particles and promoting improved digestion. This innovative approach could contribute to reduced plaque formation and enhanced overall oral hygiene (Meyer, 2010). Advancements in nanotechnology open the door to the nanoencapsulation of essential nutrients like calcium and vitamin D. This cutting-edge technique might improve the absorption of these nutrients within the oral cavity, fostering stronger teeth and better overall dental health (Ayala-Fuentes & Chavez-Santoscoy, 2021). Customized probiotics represent another area of potential advancement, with formulations designed to address individual oral health needs. These sophisticated probiotics could target specific issues, such as gum inflammation or the prevention of harmful bacteria associated with dental problems (Sivamaruthi et al., 2020).

Innovations in functional foods with remineralization properties could revolutionize oral health. By incorporating minerals like fluoride, calcium, and phosphorus in innovative ways, these foods may contribute to rebuilding tooth enamel and preventing decay (Xu et al., 2023). While these advancements remain speculative, the ongoing research in these diverse are as holds the promise of transformative functional foods that could revolutionize oral health maintenance and contribute to comprehensive well-being. Collaborative efforts between researchers, nutritionists, and healthcare professionals will play a pivotal role in translating these innovative concepts into practical dietary solutions.

17.12 Conclusion

Caries arises from a complex interplay among oral microbes, dietary components, and their fermentation on tooth surfaces. The impact of various dietary elements on microbial fermentation is scrutinized both in controlled laboratory settings (in vitro) and within the oral environment (in situ). Numerous dietary factors have been pinpointed for their role in either exacerbating or mitigating the development of tooth decay. When combined with enhanced oral hygiene practices and the use of fluoridated toothpaste, functional food ingredients that hinder the growth of oral microflora or impede their fermentation processes play a significant role in the reduction of dental caries. Although certain products, such as sugar alcohols, have long been available on the market, ongoing research continues to reveal the beneficial effects of specific phytochemicals. Furthermore, emerging evidence suggests promising prospects for innovative concepts such as probiotics in the realm of oral caries prevention.

Guideline: WHO suggests a further reduction of the intake of free sugars to below 5% of total energy intake 2015.

References

Abiko, Y., & Paudel, D. (2022). Uehara, Hops components and oral health. *Journal of Functional Foods, 92*. Available from https://doi.org/10.1016/J.JFF.2022.1050352022.

Altabbal, S., Athamnah, K., Rahma, A., Wali, A. F., Eid, A. H., Iratni, R., & Al Dhaheri, Y. (2023). Propolis: A detailed insight of its anticancer molecular mechanisms. *MDPI, United Arab Emirates Pharmaceuticals, 16*(3). Available from https://doi.org/10.3390/ph16030450, https://www.mdpi.com/journal/pharmaceuticals.

Angarita-Díaz, Md. P., Arias, J. C., Bedoya-Correa, C., Cepeda, M. J., Arboleda, M. F., Chacón, J. M., & Leal, Y. (2020). The effect of commercial functional food with probiotics on microorganisms from early carious lesions. *Nature Research, Colombia Scientific Reports, 10*(1). Available from https://doi.org/10.1038/s41598-020-67775-z, www.nature.com/srep/index.html.

Angarita-Díaz, M. P., Forero-Escobar, D., Cerón-Bastidas, X. A., Cisneros-Hidalgo, C. A., Dávila-Narvaez, F., Bedoya-Correa, C. M., Freitas, S. C., Cabrera-Arango, C. L., & Melo-Colina, R. (2020). Effects of a functional food supplemented with probiotics on biological factors related to dental caries in children: a pilot study. *European Archives of Paediatric Dentistry, 21*(1), 161–169. Available from https://doi.org/10.1007/s40368-019-00468-y, http://rd.springer.com/journal/40368.

Arshad, R., Gulshad, L., Haq, I. U., Farooq, M. A., Al-Farga, A., Siddique, R., Manzoor, M. F., Karrar, E. (2021., Nanotechnology: A novel tool to enhance the bioavailability of micronutrients. John Wiley and Sons Inc, *Pakistan Food Science and Nutrition, 9*(6), 3354–3361. Available from onlinelibrary.wiley.com/journal/10.1002/%28ISSN%292048-7177, https://doi.org/10.1002/fsn3.2311.

Ayala-Fuentes, J. C., & Chavez-Santoscoy, R. A. (2021). Nanotechnology as a key to enhance the benefits and improve the bioavailability of flavonoids in the food industry. *MDPI, Mexico Foods, 10*((11). Available from https://doi.org/10.3390/foods10112701, https://www.mdpi.com/2304-8158/10/11/2701/pdf.

Azad, M. A. K., Gao, J., Ma, J., Li, T., Tan, B., Huang, X., & Yin, J. (2020). Opportunities of prebiotics for the intestinal health of monogastric animals. *KeAi Communications Co., China Animal Nutrition, 6*(4), 379–388. Available from https://doi.org/10.1016/j.aninu.2020.08.001, http://www.keaipublishing.com/en/journals/animal-nutrition/.

Bahador, A., Lesan, S., & Kashi, N. (2012). Effect of xylitol on cariogenic and beneficial oral streptococci: A randomized, double-blind crossover trial. *Iranian Journal of Microbiology, 4*(2), 75–81. Available from http://ijm.tums.ac.ir/index.php/ijm/article/view/446/187, Iran.

Beaudette, J. R., Fritz, P. C., Sullivan, P. J., & Ward, W. E. (2017). Oral health, nutritional choices, and dental fear and anxiety. *MDPI AG, Canada Dentistry Journal, 5*(1). Available from https://doi.org/10.3390/dj5010008, https://www.mdpi.com/2304-6767/5/1/8/pdf.

Borowska, S., Michalina Brzoska, M., & Tomczyk, M. (2018). Complexation of bioelements and toxic metals by polyphenolic compounds - Implications for Health. *Current Drug Targets, 19*(14), 1612–1638. Available from https://doi.org/10.2174/13894501196661804031015555.

Botelho, J., Machado, V., Proença, L., Delgado, A. S., & Mendes, J. J. (2020). Vitamin D deficiency and oral health: A comprehensive review. *MDPI AG, Portugal Nutrients, 12*(5). Available from https://doi.org/10.3390/nu12051471, https://www.mdpi.com/2072-6643/12/5/1471/pdf.

Bradlee, M. L., Mustafa, J., Singer, M. R., & Moore, L. L. (2018). High-protein foods and physical activity protect against age-related muscle loss and functional decline. *Journals of Gerontology - Series A Biological Sciences and Medical Sciences, 73*(1), 88–94. Available from https://doi.org/10.1093/gerona/glx070, http://biomedgerontology.oxfordjournals.org/.

Cagetti, M. G., Wolf, T. G., Tennert, C., Camoni, N., Lingström, P., & Campus, G. (2020). The role of vitamins in oral health. A systematic review and meta-analysis. MDPI AG, Italy. *International journal of environmental research and public health, 17*(3). Available from https://doi.org/10.3390/ijerph17030938, https://www.mdpi.com/1660-4601/17/3/938/pdf.

Chugh, P., Dutt, R., Sharma, A., Bhagat, N., & D, M. S. (2020). A critical appraisal of the effects of probiotics on oral health. *Journal of Functional Foods, 70*, 103985. Available from https://doi.org/10.1016/j.jff.2020.103985.

Craig, W. J., Mangels, A. R., Fresán, U., Marsh, K., Miles, F. L., Saunders, A. V., Haddad, E. H., Heskey, C. E., Johnston, P., Larson-Meyer, E., & Orlich, M. (2021). The safe and effective use of plant-based diets with guidelines for health professionals. *Nutrients, 13*(11), 4144. Available from https://doi.org/10.3390/nu13114144.

Craig, W. J., & Brothers, C. J. (2021). *Nutrients*, 2021.

Dahiya, D., & Nigam, P. S. (2022). The gut microbiota influenced by the intake of probiotics and functional foods with prebiotics can sustain wellness and alleviate certain ailments like gut-inflammation and colon-cancer. *Microorganisms, 10*(3). Available from https://doi.org/10.3390/microorganisms10030665, https://www.mdpi.com/2076-2607/10/3/665/pdf.

Dame-Teixeira, N., Parolo, C. C. F., Maltz, M., Tugnait, A., Devine, D., & Do, T. (2016). Actinomyces spp. gene expression in root caries lesions. Co-Action Publishing, Brazil. *Journal of Oral Microbiology, 8*(1). Available from https://doi.org/10.3402/jom.v8.32383, http://www.journaloforalmicrobiology.net/index.php/jom/article/download/32383/48760.

Dąbrowska, Z., Bijowski, K., Dąbrowska, E., & Pietruska, M. (2020). Effect of oxidants and antioxidants on oral health. *Medycyna Ogólna i Nauki o Zdrowiu, 26*(2), 87–93. Available from https://doi.org/10.26444/monz/122255.

Esmaeili, M., Ajami, M., Barati, M., Javanmardi, F., Houshiarrad, A., Mousavi Khaneghah, A. (2022). The significance and potential of functional food ingredients for control appetite and food intake. John Wiley and Sons Inc, *Iran Food Science and Nutrition, 10*(5), 1602–1612, Available from onlinelibrary.wiley.com/journal/10.1002/%28ISSN%292048-7177, https://doi.org/10.1002/fsn3.2783.

Esteban-Fernández, A., Zorraquín-Peña, I., González de Llano, D., Bartolomé, B., & Moreno-Arribas, M. V. (2017). *The role of wine and food polyphenols in oral health. Trends in Food Science and Technology* (69, pp. 118–130). Spain: Elsevier Ltd. Available from http://www.elsevier.com/wps/find/journaldescription.cws_home/601278/description#description, https://doi.org/10.1016/j.tifs.2017.09.008.

Eswaran, H., Ponnuswamy, R. D., & Kannapan, R. P. (2023). *Perspective approaches of 3D printed stuffs for personalized nutrition: A comprehensive review. Annals of 3D Printed Medicine* (12). India: Elsevier Inc. Available from https://www.journals.elsevier.com/annals-of-3d-printed-medicine, https://doi.org/10.1016/j.stlm.2023.100125.

Folayan, M., & Tantawi, M. E. (2023). Decarbonization of transport and oral health. *BioMed, 3*(3), 392–399. Available from https://doi.org/10.3390/biomed3030032.

Galanakis, C. M. (2021). Functionality of food components and emerging technologies. *Foods, 10*(1), 128. Available from https://doi.org/10.3390/foods10010128.

Goiana, M. L., Mattos, A. L. A., de Azeredo, H. M. C., de Freitas Rosa, M., & Fernandes, F. A. N. (2022). Influence of dielectric barrier discharge cold plasma treatment on starch, gelatin, and bacterial cellulose biodegradable polymeric films. *MDPI, Brazil Polymers, 14*(23). Available from https://doi.org/10.3390/polym14235215, http://www.mdpi.com/journal/polymers.

González-Aguilar, G., Robles-Sánchez, R. M., Martínez-Téllez, M. A., Olivas, G. I., Alvarez-Parrilla, E., & De La Rosa, L. A. (2008). Bioactive compounds in fruits: Health benefits and effect of storage conditions. *Stewart Postharvest Review, 4*(3). Available from https://doi.org/10.2212/spr.2008.3.8Mexico, http://docserver.ingentaconnect.com/deliver/connect/sphs/17459656/v4n3/s8.pdf?expires = 1214315183&id = 44820352&titleid = 75001622&accname = Elsevier&checksum = 3089B06515E0943FBB7C7C2D09C32D89.

Guo, Y., Li, Z., Chen, F., & Chai, Y. (2023). Polyphenols in oral health: Homeostasis maintenance, disease prevention, and therapeutic applications. Multidisciplinary Digital Publishing Institute (MDPI), *China Nutrients, 15*(20), Available from http://www.mdpi.com/journal/nutrients/. Available from https://doi.org/10.3390/nu15204384.

Hasler, C. M., Brown, A. C., & American Dietetic Association (2009). Position of the american dietetic association: Functional foods. *Journal of the American Dietetic Association, 109*(4), 735–746. Available from https://doi.org/10.1016/j.jada.2009.02.023

Havenaar, R. (1984). The anti-cariogenic potential of xylitol in comparison with sodium fluoride in rat caries experiments. *Journal of Dental Research, 63*(2), 120–123. Available from https://doi.org/10.1177/00220345840630020401.

How, Y.-H., & Yeo, S.-K. (2021). Oral probiotic and its delivery carriers to improve oral health: A review. *Microbiology, 167*(8). Available from https://doi.org/10.1099/mic.0.001076.

Huang, Y. Z., Jin, Z., Wang, Z. M., Qi, L. B., Song, S., Zhu, B. W., & Dong, X. P. (2021). *Marine Bioactive Compounds as Nutraceutical and Functional Food Ingredients for Potential Oral Health. Frontiers in Nutrition* (8). China: Frontiers Media S.A. Available from journal.frontiersin.org/journal/nutrition. Available from https://doi.org/10.3389/fnut.2021.686663.

Humaid, J. A. L., & Bamashmous, M. (2022). Meta-analysis on the effectiveness of xylitol in caries prevention. *Wolters Kluwer (UK) Ltd., Saudi Arabia Journal of International Society of Preventive and Community Dentistry, 12*(2), 133–138. Available from https://doi.org/10.4103/jispcd.JISPCD_164_21, www.jispcd.org/.

Jain, P., & Sharma, P. (2012). Probiotics and their efficacy in improving oral health: A review. *Journal of Applied Pharmaceutical Science, 2*(11), 151–163. Available from https://doi.org/10.7324/JAPS.2012.21128India, http://www.japsonline.com/admin/php/uploads/713_pdf.pdf.

Janakiram, C., Deepan Kumar, C. V., & Joseph, J. (2017). Xylitol in preventing dental caries: A systematic review and meta-analyses. *Journal of Natural Science, Biology and Medicine, 8*(1), 16–21. Available from https://doi.org/10.4103/0976-9668.198344, www.jnsbm.org.

Janket, S. J., Benwait, J., Isaac, P., Ackerson, L. K., & Meurman, J. H. (2019). Oral and systemic effects of xylitol consumption. *Caries Research, 53*(5), 491–501. Available from https://doi.org/10.1159/000499194, http://content.karger.com/ProdukteDB/produkte.asp?Aktion = JournalHome&ProduktNr = 224219.

Javaid, M., Haleem, A., Singh, R. P., & Suman, R. (2022). 3D printing applications for healthcare research and development. *Global Health Journal, 6*(4), 217–226. Available from https://doi.org/10.1016/j.glohj.2022.11.001, https://www.sciencedirect.com/journal/global-health-journal.

Kaur, G., Kathariya, R., Bansal, S., Singh, A., & Shahakar, D. (2016). Dietary antioxidants and their indispensable role in periodontal health. *Journal of Food and Drug Analysis, 24*(2), 239–246. Available from https://doi.org/10.1016/j.jfda.2015.11.003, http://www.elsevier.com/journals/journal-of-food-and-drug-analysis/1021-9498#.

Kaur, K., Sculley, D., Wallace, J., Turner, A., Ferraris, C., Veysey, M., Lucock, M., & Beckett, E. L. (2019). *Micronutrients and bioactive compounds in oral inflammatory diseases. Journal of Nutrition and Intermediary Metabolism* (18). Australia: Elsevier Inc. Available from http://www.journals.elsevier.com/journal-of-nutrition-and-intermediary-metabolism/, https://doi.org/10.1016/j.jnim.2019.100105.

Kim, H., Han, C. Y., Eun, S. H., Kim, M. G., Im, A. R., & Lee, B. (2023). Inhibitory effects of Bacillus velezensis ID-A01 supernatant against Streptococcus mutans. *BMC Microbiology, 23*(1). Available from https://doi.org/10.1186/s12866-023-03114-2, https://bmcmicrobiol.biomedcentral.com/.

Kim, J., Kim, M. J., & Kho, H. S. (2016). Oral manifestations in vitamin B12 deficiency patients with or without history of gastrectomy. *BMC Oral Health, 16*(1). Available from https://doi.org/10.1186/s12903-016-0215-y, http://www.biomedcentral.com/bmcoralhealth/.

Komara, I., Sopiatin, S., Hafizh, F. R., Miranda, A., & Metta, P. (2023). Oral health management through plaque control in gingivitis with autism spectrum disorder (ASD): A rapid review. *Journal of International Dental and Medical Research, 16*(1), 340–347. Available from http://www.jidmr.com/journal/archieve/.

Kostecka-Sochoń, P., Onopiuk, B. M., & Dabrowska, E. (2018). *Protective effect of increased zinc supply against oxidative damage of sublingual gland in chronic exposure to cadmium: Experimental study on rats. Oxidative Medicine and Cellular Longevity.* Poland: Hindawi Limited. Available from http://www.hindawi.com/journals/oximed/, https://doi.org/10.1155/2018/3732842.

Kumar, H., Singh, R., Dhanjal, D. S., Chopra, C., Cruz-Martins, N., Nasrallah, G. K., Majdalawieh, A. F., Manickam, S., Siddiqui, S. A., Kumar, D., Sharma, I., & Sharma, V. (2023). Impact of phytoconstituents on oral health practices: A post COVID-19 observation. *Food Science and Human Wellness*. Available from https://doi.org/10.26599/fshw.2022.9250197.

Kumar, M., Prakash, S., Radha., Kumari, N., Pundir, A., Punia, S., Saurabh, V., Choudhary, P., Changan, S., Dhumal, S., Pradhan, P. C., Alajil, O., Singh, S., Sharma, N., Ilakiya, T., Singh, S., & Mekhemar, M. (2021). Beneficial role of antioxidant secondary metabolites from medicinal plants in maintaining oral health. *Antioxidants, 10*(7). Available from https://doi.org/10.3390/antiox10071061, https://www.mdpi.com/2076-3921/10/7/1061/pdf.

Lamont, R. J., Koo, H., & Hajishengallis, G. (2018). The oral microbiota: Dynamic communities and host interactions. *Nature Reviews Microbiology, 16*(12), 745–759. Available from https://doi.org/10.1038/s41579-018-0089-x, http://www.nature.com/nrmicro/index.html.

Lordan, S., Ross, R. P., & Stanton, C. (2011). Marine bioactives as functional food ingredients: Potential to reduce the incidence of chronic diseases. *Marine Drugs, 9*(6), 1056–1100. Available from https://doi.org/10.3390/md9061056, http://www.mdpi.com/1660-3397/9/6/1056/pdf.

van Loveren, C. (2004). Sugar alcohols: What is the evidence for caries-preventive and caries-therapeutic effects. *Caries Research, 38*(3), 286–293. Available from https://doi.org/10.1159/000077768.

Van Loveren, C., Broukal, Z., & Oganessian, E. (2012). Functional foods/ingredients and dental caries. *European Journal of Nutrition, 51*(2), S15. Available from https://doi.org/10.1007/s00394-012-0323-7.

Lu, M., Xuan, S., & Wang, Z. (2019). Oral microbiota: A new view of body health. *Food Science and Human Wellness, 8*(1), 8–15. Available from https://doi.org/10.1016/j.fshw.2018.12.001.

Maier, T. (2023). Oral Microbiome in health and disease: Maintaining a healthy, balanced ecosystem and reversing dysbiosis. *Microorganisms, 11*(6). Available from https://doi.org/10.3390/microorganisms11061453, www.mdpi.com/journal/microorganisms.

Marthaler, T. M., Steiner, M., Menghini, G., & Bandi, A. (1994). Caries prevalence in Switzerland. *International Dental Journal, 44*(4), 393–401.

Matsukubo, T., & Takazoe, I. (2006). Sucrose substitutes and their role in caries prevention. *International Dental Journal, 56*(3), 119–130. Available from https://doi.org/10.1111/j.1875-595x.2006.tb00083.x.

Małgorzata, M. M. S., & Słotwińska. (2011). The teeth bleaching and environment of oral cavity. *Nowa Stomatol*, 2011.

Meyer, A. S. (2010). Enzyme technology for precision functional food ingredient processes. *Annals of the New York Academy of Sciences, 119*(1), 126–132. Available from https://doi.org/10.1111/j.1749-6632.2009.05255.x, http://www.blackwellpublishing.com/0077-8923.

Moynihan, P., & Petersen, P. E. (2004). Diet, nutrition and the prevention of dental diseases. *Public Health Nutrition. 7 (1 A)*, 201–226. Available from https://doi.org/10.1079/PHN2003589.

Mu, R., & Chen, J. (2023). *Oral bio-interfaces: Properties and functional roles of salivary multilayer in food oral processing, . Trends in Food Science and Technology* (132, pp. 121–131). China: Elsevier Ltd. Available from http://www.elsevier.com/wps/find/journaldescription.cws_home/601278/description#description, https://doi.org/10.1016/j.tifs.2023.01.003.

Mullins, V. A., Bresette, W., Johnstone, L., Hallmark, B., & Chilton, F. H. (2020). Genomics in personalized nutrition: Can you "eat for your genes"? *Nutrients, 12*(10), 1–23. Available from https://doi.org/10.3390/nu12103118, https://www.mdpi.com/2072-6643/12/10/3118/pdf.

Mężyńska, M., & Brzóska, M. M. (2019). Review of polyphenol-rich products as potential protective and therapeutic factors against cadmium hepatotoxicity. *Journal of Applied Toxicology, 39*(1), 117–145. Available from https://doi.org/10.1002/jat.3709, http://onlinelibrary.wiley.com/journal/10.1002/(ISSN)1099-1263.

Nassar, H. M., Alhazzazi, T. Y., Hazzazi, L. W., & Gregory, R. L. (2021). *The anticariogenic effect of xylitol on seven Streptococcus mutans strains*, 2021.

Nishida, M., Grossi, S. G., Dunford, R. G., Ho, A. W., Trevisan, M., & Genco, R. J. (2000a). Calcium and the risk for periodontal disease. *Journal of Periodontology, 71*(7), 1057–1066. Available from https://doi.org/10.1902/jop.2000.71.7.1057, http://www.joponline.org.

Nishida, M., Grossi, S. G., Dunford, R. G., Ho, A. W., Trevisan, M., & Genco, R. J. (2000b). Dietary vitamin C and the risk for periodontal disease. *Journal of Periodontology, 71*(8), 1215–1223. Available from https://doi.org/10.1902/jop.2000.71.8.1215, http://www.joponline.org.

Nsairat, H., Lafi, Z., Al-Sulaibi, M., Gharaibeh, L., & Alshaer, W. Impact of nanotechnology on the oral delivery of phyto-bioactive compounds. *Food Chemistry, 424*, 136438. Jordan: Elsevier Ltd. Available from www.elsevier.com/locate/foodchem, https://doi.org/10.1016/j.foodchem.2023.136438.

Ofek, I., Pruzzo, C., & Spratt, D. (2012). Functional foods: Towards improving oral health. *Journal of Biomedicine and Biotechnology, 2012*, 1–2. Available from https://doi.org/10.1155/2012/618314.

Oteiza, P. I. (2012). Zinc and the modulation of redox homeostasis. *Free Radical Biology and Medicine, 53*(9), 1748–1759. Available from https://doi.org/10.1016/j.freeradbiomed.2012.08.568.

Pooja, S. (n.d.). Antioxidants and its Role in Periodontitis-A Short Review. (n.d.).

Puri, V., Nagpal, M., Singh, I., Singh, M., Dhingra, G. A., Huanbutta, K., Dheer, D., Sharma, A., & Sangnim, T. (2022). A Comprehensive Review on Nutraceuticals: Therapy Support and Formulation Challenges. *Nutrients, 14*(21). Available from https://doi.org/10.3390/nu14214637, http://www.mdpi.com/journal/nutrients/.

Puttasiddaiah, R., Lakshminarayana, R., Somashekar, N. L., Gupta, V. K., Inbaraj, B. S., Usmani, Z., Raghavendra, V. B., Sridhar, K., & Sharma, M. (2022). Advances in nanofabrication technology for nutraceuticals: New insights and future trends. *Bioengineering*, *9*(9). Available from www.mdpi.com/journal/bioengineering, https://doi.org/10.3390/bioengineering9090478.

Qamar, Z., Alghonaim, M. F., Almohana, S. A., Almohana, A. A., & Zeeshan, T. (2021). Potential biochemical effects of honey in oral health care: A review. *International Food Research Journal*, *28*(1), 23–30. Available from https://doi.org/10.47836/ifrj.28.1.02.

Quelemes, V., Nagakubo, V. D., & Kaibori, Y. (2023). Oral microbiota: The influences and interactions of saliva. *IgA, and Dietary Factors in Health and Disease*, *11*. Available from https://doi.org/10.3390/MICROORGANISMS110923072023.

Reddy, D. N. (2019). Essential oils extracted from medicinal plants and their applications. In Natural Bio-active Compounds: Volume 1: Production and Applications. Springer Singapore, India Springer Singapore, India, 237–283. Available from https://doi.org/10.1007/978-981-13-7154-7, https://doi.org/10.1007/978-981-13-7154-7_9.

Requena, T., Monagas, M., Pozo-Bayón, M. A., Martín-Álvarez, P. J., Bartolomé, B., del Campo, R., Ávila, M., Martínez-Cuesta, M. C., Peláez, C., & Moreno-Arribas, M. V. (2010). Perspectives of the potential implications of wine polyphenols on human oral and gut microbiota. *Trends in Food Science & Technology*, *21*(7), 332–344. Available from https://doi.org/10.1016/j.tifs.2010.04.004.

Riley, P., Moore, D., Ahmed, F., Sharif, M. O., & Worthington, H. V. (2015). Xylitol-containing products for preventing dental caries in children and adults. *Cochrane Database of Systematic Reviews*, *2015*(3). Available from https://doi.org/10.1002/14651858.CD010743.pub2, http://as.wiley.com/WileyCDA/Brand/id-6.html.

Rouzi, M., Zhang, X., Jiang, Q., Long, H., Lai, W., & Li, X. (2023). Impact of Clear Aligners on Oral Health and Oral Microbiome During Orthodontic Treatment. *International Dental Journal*, *73*(5), 603–611. Available from https://doi.org/10.1016/j.identj.2023.03.012, https://www.sciencedirect.com/journal/international-dental-journal.

Santonocito, S., Giudice, A., Polizzi, A., Troiano, G., Merlo, E. M., Sclafani, R., Grosso, G., & Isola, G. (2022). A cross-talk between diet and the oral microbiome: Balance of nutrition on inflammation and immune system's response during periodontitis. *Nutrients*, *14*(12). Available from https://doi.org/10.3390/nu14122426, https://www.mdpi.com/2072-6643/14/12/2426/pdf?version = 1654938280.

Silva, A. M., Miranda, L. F. B., Araújo, A. S. M., Prado Júnior, R. R., & Mendes, R. F. (2020). Electric toothbrush for biofilm control in individuals with Down syndrome: A crossover randomized clinical trial. *Sociedade Brasileira de Hematologia e Hemoterapia, Brazil Brazilian Oral Research*, *34*, e057. Available from https://doi.org/10.1590/1807-3107BOR-2020.VOL34.0057, https://www.scielo.br/pdf/bor/v34/1807-3107-bor-34-e057.pdf.

Simone-Finstrom, M., & Spivak, M. (2010). Propolis and bee health: The natural history and significance of resin use by honey bees. *Apidologie*, *41* (3), 295–311. Available from https://doi.org/10.1051/apido/2010016.

Sivamaruthi, B. S., Kesika, P., & Chaiyasut, C. (2020). A review of the role of probiotic supplementation in dental caries. *Probiotics and Antimicrobial Proteins*, *12*(4), 1300–1309. Available from https://doi.org/10.1007/s12602-020-09652-9, http://www.springer.com/new + %26 + forthcoming + titles + %28default%29/journal/12602.

Söderling, E. M. (2009). Xylitol, Mutans Streptococci, and Dental Plaque. *Advances in Dental Research*, *21*(1), 74–78. Available from https://doi.org/10.1177/0895937409335642.

Takahashi, N., & Nyvad, B. (2011). The role of bacteria in the caries process: Ecological perspectives. *Journal of Dental Research*, *90*(3), 294–303. Available from https://doi.org/10.1177/0022034510379602.

Tungare, S., & Paranjpe, A. G. (2023). Diet and nutrition to prevent dental problems. *StatPearls*, 2023.

Twetman, S. (2009). Consistent evidence to support the use of xylitol- and sorbitol-containing chewing gum to prevent dental caries. *Evidence-based dentistry*, *10*(1), 10–11. Available from https://doi.org/10.1038/sj.ebd.6400626.

Tóthová, L., Kamodyová, N., Červenka, T., & Celec, P. (2015). Salivary markers of oxidative stress in oral diseases. *Frontiers in Cellular and Infection Microbiology*, *5*. Available from https://doi.org/10.3389/fcimb.2015.00073.

Vajawat, M., Deepika, P. C., Kumar, V., & Rajeshwari, P. (2015). A clinicomicrobiological study to evaluate the efficacy of manual and powered toothbrushes among autistic patients. *Contemporary Clinical Dentistry*, *6*(4), 500–504. Available from https://doi.org/10.4103/0976-237X.169848, http://www.contempclindent.org/.

Varela-López, A., Navarro-Hortal, M. D., Giampieri, F., Bullón, P., Battino, M., & Quiles, J. L. (2018). Nutraceuticals in periodontal health: A systematic review on the role of vitamins in periodontal health maintenance. *Molecules*, *23*(5). Available from https://doi.org/10.3390/molecules23051226, http://www.mdpi.com/1420-3049/23/5/1226/pdf.

Vikneshan, M., Ankola, A. V., Hiremath, A., Hebbal, M., & Suganya, M. (2016). Functional foods and its role in improving oral health. *Journal of Scientific Dentistry*, *6*(1), 13–19. Available from https://doi.org/10.5005/jsd-6-1-13.

Vlaicu, P. A., Untea, A. E., Saracila, M., & Oancea, A. G. (2023). Designing nutrition for health—Incorporating dietary by-products into poultry feeds to create functional foods with insights into health benefits, risks, bioactive compounds, food component functionality and safety regulations. *Foods*, *2023*. Available from https://doi.org/10.3390/FOODS122140012023.

Willis, J. R., & Gabaldón, T. (2020). The human oral microbiome in health and disease: From sequences to ecosystems. *Microorganisms*, *8*(2). Available from https://doi.org/10.3390/microorganisms8020308, https://www.mdpi.com/2076-2607/8/2/308/pdf.

World Health Organization. (2015). Guideline: sugars intake for adults and children. [cited 2024 Feb 6];59. Available from https://www.who.int/publications/i/item/9789241549028

Xu, Y., You, Y., Yi, L., Wu, X., Zhao, Y., Yu, J., Liu, H., Shen, Y., Guo, J., & Huang, C. (2023). *Dental plaque-inspired versatile nanosystem for caries prevention and tooth restoration. Bioactive Materials* (20, pp. 418–433). China: KeAi Communications Co. Available from http://www.keaipublishing.com/en/journals/bioactive-materials/, https://doi.org/10.1016/j.bioactmat.2022.06.010.

Yakubov, G. E., Macakova, L., Wilson, S., Windust, J. H. C., & Stokes, J. R. (2015). *Aqueous lubrication by fractionated salivary proteins: Synergistic interaction of mucin polymer brush with low molecular weight macromolecules. Tribology International* (89, pp. 34–45). Australia: Elsevier Ltd. Available from www.elsevier.com/inca/publications/store/3/0/4/7/4, https://doi.org/10.1016/j.triboint.2014.12.025.

Zhang, T., Chen, J., & Hu, B. (2019). Quality authenticity, loyalty, local food and sustainable tourism experience. *Sustain, 11*(2019). Available from https://doi.org/10.3390/SU11234372019.

Zhu, W., Iskandar, M. M., Baeghbali, V., & Kubow, S. (2023). Three-dimensional printing of foods: A critical review of the present state in healthcare applications, and potential risks and benefits. Multidisciplinary Digital Publishing Institute (MDPI). *Foods, 12*(17), 3287. Available from www.mdpi.com/journal/foods, https://doi.org/10.3390/foods12173287.

Zulhendri, F., Felitti, R., Fearnley, J., & Ravalia, M. (2021). The use of propolis in dentistry, oral health, and medicine: A review. *Journal of Oral Biosciences, 63*(1), 23–34. Available from https://doi.org/10.1016/j.job.2021.01.001, http://www.sciencedirect.com/science/journal/13490079.

Chapter 18

Functional foods for ocular health and vision

Busra Goz, Burcu Ersoy and Zehra Gulsunoglu-Konuskan
Faculty of Health Sciences, Department of Nutrition and Dietetics, Istanbul Aydin University, Kucukcekmece, Istanbul, Türkiye

18.1 Introduction

The World Health Organization (WHO) predicts that the global elderly population will be 2.1 billion in 2050 (WHO, 2022). As the population ages, eye diseases will become more prevalent, posing a significant public health concern (Chen et al., 2024). Eye-related diseases can greatly impact individuals' quality of life. For instance, age-related macular degeneration can affect daily activities such as driving, reading, and household chores (Koçak et al., 2014). Moreover, the economic burden of treating these diseases is substantial (Rein et al., 2022; Wittenborn et al., 2013; Yang et al., 2021). Globally, the number of people affected by blindness and/or vision impairment from cataract disease is 94 million, refractive error is 88.4 million people, age-related macular degeneration is 8 million, glaucoma is 7.7 million, and diabetic retinopathy is 3.9 million according to WHO (2023) (Fig. 18.1). Presbyopia is the leading cause of near vision impairment, affecting 826 million people.

There are many complex factors in the etiology of age-related eye diseases. Oxidative stress is known as a common cause of age-related eye diseases. It is thought that antioxidants may have potential therapeutic benefits as both a cost-effective and simple method for the prevention and/or treatment of eye diseases (Li et al., 2010; Loskutova et al., 2019; Sideri et al., 2019; Weikel et al., 2012). Studies show that there is a relationship between nutrition and eye-related diseases such as age-related macular degeneration, diabetic retinopathy, cataract, and glaucoma, and that some macro- and micronutrients can decrease the risk of these diseases (Grosso et al., 2013; Pastor-Valero, 2013; Tan et al., 2008). This chapter discusses the potential benefits of functional foods and their components for ocular health and vision.

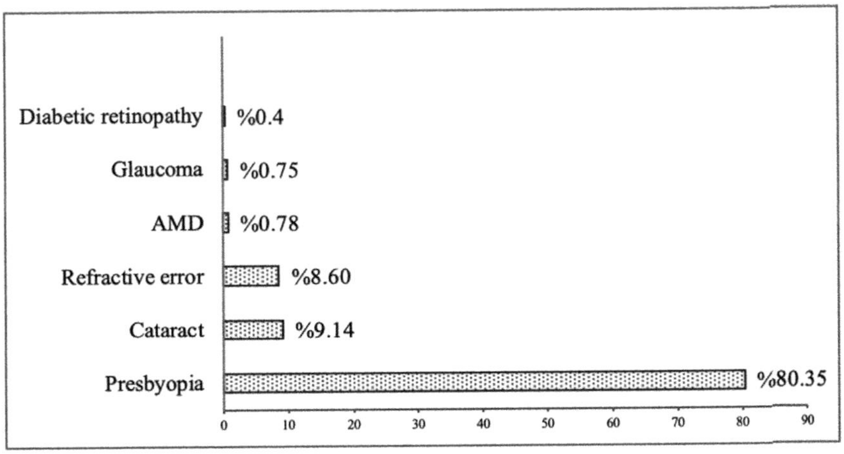

FIGURE 18.1 The major causes of vision impairment and blindness. *Data from WHO (2023).*

Unleashing the Power of Functional Foods and Novel Bioactives. DOI: https://doi.org/10.1016/B978-0-443-28862-3.00018-2

18.2 Common eye disorders that cause visual impairment

Vision stands out as the most crucial of human senses, intricately managed by the brain's complex visual pathways connecting the eyes and their components. These pathways translate neural impulses from retinal photoreceptors, located behind retinal ganglion cells, into a three-dimensional image. Light, focused by the lens and cornea onto retinal photoreceptors, triggers this process. Any disruption in this system, encompassing the eyes, brain, and their connections, results in impaired vision. Various factors, including genetic mutations, environments, lifestyles, aging, and malnutrition, contribute to vision dysfunction. Among the ocular disorders escalating in adult populations globally are refractive errors, dry eye, diabetic retinopathy, glaucoma, ocular surface dysfunction, cataracts, and age-related macular degeneration. Additionally, conditions like blepharitis, dry eyes, and allergic conjunctivitis can cause discomfort in individuals without visual dysfunction (Medori et al., 2022). Fig. 18.2 outlines the risk factors influencing eye health and Table 18.1 shows the common eye conditions amongst children and adults.

18.2.1 Diabetic retinopathy

Diabetes, aside from increasing the risk of cataracts, most commonly leads to diabetic retinopathy, a major cause of vision loss (Cheung et al., 2010; Lawler et al., 2019). It is predicted that around 160 million people will be influenced by this condition by 2045 (Teo et al., 2021). Hyperglycemia induces retinal vascular endothelial dysfunction, primarily through retinal ischemia and increased vascular permeability exacerbated by hypertension (Cheung et al., 2010). Oxidative stress in diabetic retinopathy causes the release of proinflammatory cytokines and leukocytes, damaging nucleic acids, cellular proteins, and causing loss of various retinal cells, including neuronal, pericyte, and endothelial cells, ultimately disrupting the blood–retinal barrier (Chen et al., 2009). Free radicals also enhance protein kinase C activity and affect advanced glycation end products, contributing to vascular permeability and retinal inflammation (Chen et al., 2009). Some researches suggest that antioxidant vitamins might effectively treat diabetic retinopathy by scavenging free radicals (Jariyapongskul et al., 2007; Pazdro & Burgess, 2010).

18.2.2 Age-related macular degeneration

High density of photoreceptors located in the macula provides high-resolution vision by converting light into electrical impulses sent to the brain. Age-related macular degeneration leads to photoreceptor damage in the macula, causing central visual field deterioration and potential sight loss (Lamkin-Kennard & Popovic, 2019). Age-related macular degeneration is a complex disease, with advanced age being the main risk factor (Guymer & Campbell, 2023). Photoreceptor cell loss, lipofuscin accumulation, and metabolic dysfunction of the retinal pigment epithelium are the primary causes of age-related macular degeneration (Edwards et al., 2022).

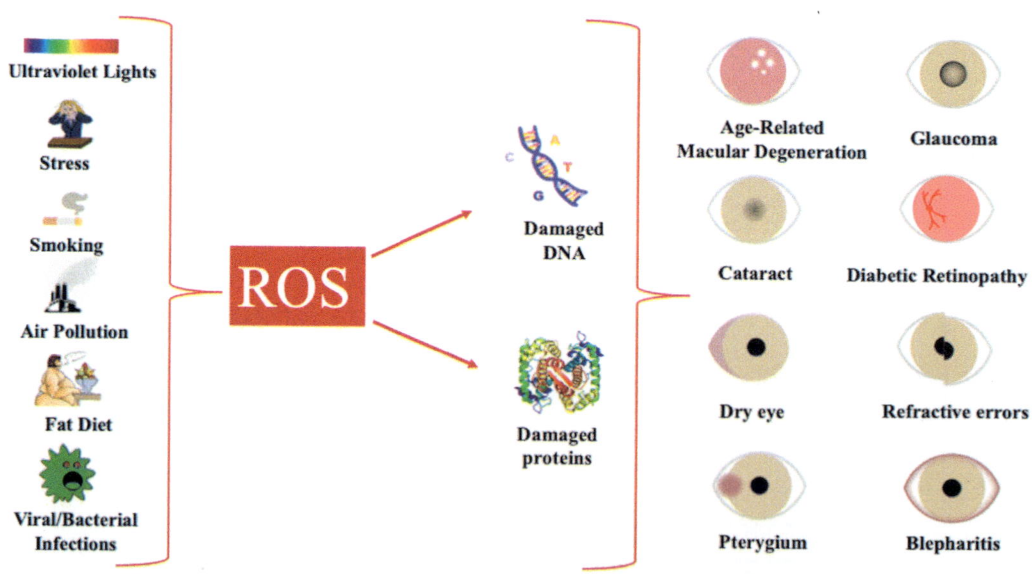

FIGURE 18.2 The risk factors affecting eye diseases. *Modified from WHO (2019) and Maiuolo et al. (2023).*

TABLE 18.1 Common Eye Conditions, Causes, Prevention and Treatment Strategies Among Children and Adults (2019).

Eye Dysfunctions	Causes	Can Cause Vision Impairment?	Prevention	Treatment
Common Conditions Among Children				
Corneal scarring	Vitamin A deficiency, Measles infection	Yes	Immunization, Treatment with high dose Vitamin A	Optical iridectomy
Corneal scarring in newborn "ophthalmia neonatorum"	*Chlamydia trachomatis* or *Neisseria gonorrhoeae* infection	Yes	Instilling an antibiotic or aseptic and cleaning the eyelids shortly after birth	Antibiotics administered topically and systemically
Retinopathy of prematurity	Abnormal development of the retinal blood vessels in preterm	Yes	Reducing the preterm birth, antenatal steroids, high-quality neonatal care	Laser treatment
Congenital and developmental cataract	Most bilateral cases are unknown. Intrauterine infections, metabolic disorders, hereditary factors, and trauma are the known causes	Yes	Rubella immunization	Cataract surgery
Common Conditions Among Adults				
Cataract	Main risk factors: UVB exposure, cigarette smoking, corticosteroid usage, diabetes	Yes	NG[a]	Surgery
Age-related macular degeneration	The main modifiable risk factor is smoking cigarettes	Yes	Quitting smoking	Agents that inhibit vascular endothelial growth factor
Glaucoma	NG	Yes	Regular eye examinations	Interventions to reduce intraocular pressure include therapeutic eye drops, laser therapy, and surgery
Diabetic retinopathy	Diabetes	Yes	Management of risk factors	Early detection, periodic screening
Pterygium	NG	In advanced cases	Wearing of sunglasses	Lubricating eye drops, surgical removal
Dry eyes	Contact lens wear, autoimmune conditions, blepharitis, lid disorders, some medications, aging	Not typically	NG	Lubricating eye drops
Blepharitis	NG	No	NG	Antibiotics, warm compresses, antiinflammatory agents, eyelid massage and cleansing
Refractive errors	NG	Yes	Presbyopia, hypermetropia, and astigmatism cannot be prevented. However, they might be delayed the onset and progression of myopia	intraocular lenses, laser refractive surgery, spectacles, or contact lenses

(*Continued*)

TABLE 18.1 (Continued)

Eye Dysfunctions	Causes	Can Cause Vision Impairment?	Prevention	Treatment
Corneal opacity due to injury	Ocular injury	Yes	Wearing of protective eyewear	In some cases, corneal transplant or shortage of corneal tissue
Trachoma	*Chlamydia trachomatis*	Yes	Antibiotic treatment, facial cleanliness, environmental improvements	Surgery
Onchocerciasis	*Onchocerca volvulus*	Yes	Infection cannot be prevented with vaccine or medication	Ivermectin treatment
Conjunctivitis	Bacterial or viral infections	Not typically	Hygiene measures	Antibiotic drops, antiinflammatory agents

The information in the table was taken from "World Report on Vision" published by WHO (2019).
[a]*NG: Not Given.*

18.2.3 Cataract

Clouding of the crystalline lens inside the eye, known as cataract, causes decreased vision, primarily due to aging but also linked to genetic predisposition, diseases, traumas, and medications (Braakhuis et al., 2019). Risk factors include smoking, corticosteroid use, diabetes, obesity, and exposure to ultraviolet light, as well as advanced glycation end products, oxidative stress, accumulation of lens proteins, genetic abnormalities, Na^{+}/K^{+}-ATPase deformation, and polyol pathways (Erdurmuş et al., 2019). Cataract surgery with intraocular lens implantation is the primary treatment, but access can be limited in developing countries and subject to long waiting lists in developed ones, with postoperative complications possible (Lim et al., 2020; Zhu et al., 2017). Due to oxidative damage leading to proteolysis and apoptosis in lens epithelial cells, antioxidant supplementation might slow cataract progression, but its preventive efficacy remains uncertain (Braakhuis et al., 2019; Dubois & Bastawrous, 2017; Nita & Grzybowski, 2016).

18.2.4 Glaucoma

Glaucoma, characterized by a distinctive structural alteration in the optic nerve head, is projected to affect around 111.8 million individuals by 2040 (Shen et al., 2004; Tham et al., 2014). This condition is typified by specific visual field losses (Allingham et al., 2004). Increased intraocular pressure poses a risk in primary open-angle glaucoma, with treatment primarily focused on reducing this pressure (Allingham et al., 2004). However, even with reduced intraocular pressure, vision loss may still progress, possibly due to oxidative stress. Reactive oxygen species (ROS) production contributes to glaucoma's etiology through oxidative damage (He et al., 2008). Elevated glutamate levels, changes in nitric oxide metabolism, ROS-induced oxidative damage, and vascular alterations are considered disease risk factors. ROS induce harmful alterations in proteins, lipids, and deoxyribonucleic acid (DNA), with lipid-rich structures like retinal ganglion cells being particularly vulnerable to oxidative damage (Tezel, 2006). Oxidative stress may harm the trabecular meshwork, leading to increased intraocular pressure and ganglion cell loss (Izzotti et al., 2006).

18.3 Functional food components

Functional foods, increasingly in the spotlight for their potential health benefits, are formulated not only for basic nutrition but also for additional health benefits when consumed regularly. These foods are rich in bioactive compounds such as probiotics, prebiotics, antioxidants, and vitamins, which can enhance overall well-being, including ocular health (Fig. 18.3) (Shaikh, 2022). Recognizing the influence of diet on ocular health, studies suggest that initiatives like improving diet quality and promoting physical activity can benefit both general health and eyesight (Table 18.2) (Burton et al., 2021). It has been found that bioactive compounds in functional foods provide effective antioxidant

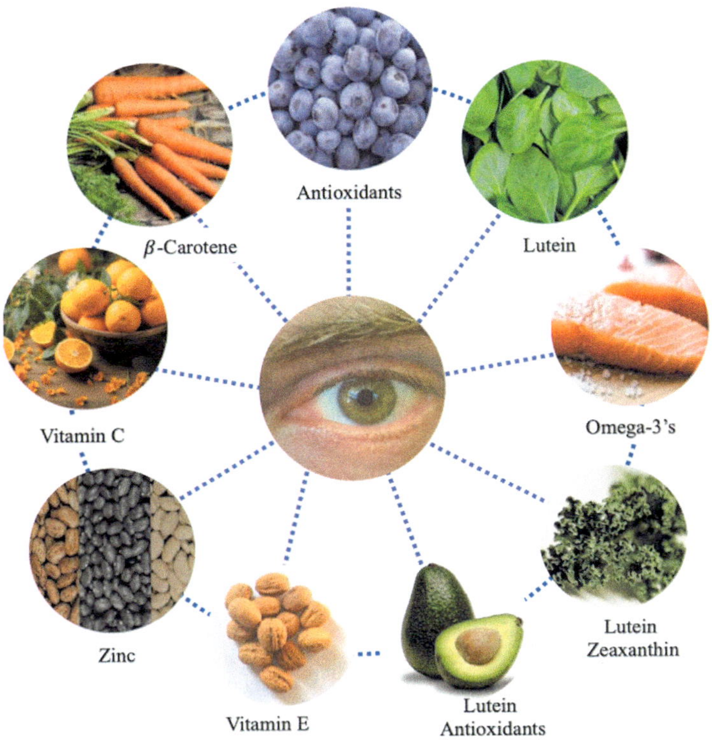

FIGURE 18.3 Functional foods and their main components in management of eye disorders.

protection for the eyes (Rossino & Casini, 2019). Considering the crucial interaction between gut microbiota and functional food components, it is vital as it influences nutrient absorption essential for healthy eyes (Laparra & Sanz, 2010). In addition, understanding the effects of food processing on the health functions of food components is critical, since new compounds may affect the health of the eyes (Zheng & Xiao, 2022). This section delves into the intricate relationship between functional food and ocular health, exploring their sources, benefits, and impact on ocular health. Through examining these components, it is aimed to provide a comprehensive overview of how dietary choices can influence ocular wellbeing and maintain healthy eyes throughout life.

18.3.1 Vitamin and mineral-rich functional foods

The consumption of vitamin and mineral rich foods has been associated with various health benefits, including the maintenance of ocular health and vision. Vegetables and fruits, in particular, are important sources of vitamins, minerals, and phytochemicals that act as antioxidants and have protective mechanisms. Vitamin A, a vital fat-soluble nutrient, is integral to immune function, growth, cellular division, and vision. In vision, 11-cis retinaldehyde (retinal) combines with opsin to form rhodopsin in photoreceptor segments, initiating the visual pathway upon light exposure. Regenerated in the retinal pigment epithelium, 11-cis retinal maintains the visual cycle while promoting conjunctival and corneal epithelial integrity (Wolf, 2001). Vitamin A deficiency predominantly affects the skin and eyes, leading to severe dry eye, Bitot's spots, and night blindness (Gilbert, 2013; Sajovic et al., 2022). Ocular surface cells undergo metaplasia and keratinization, while retinal degeneration may occur due to vitamin A deficiency (Sparrow, 2016). Vitamin A profoundly influences retinal pigment epithelial cell function and structure, modulating gene expressions of proteins and angiogenic factors (Wiseman et al., 2017). A population-based study on individuals aged 60 and over found significant inverse associations between cataracts and lutein, zeaxanthin, and retinol levels (Ravindran et al., 2011). The Recommended Dietary Allowance (RDA) for individuals aged over 18 is 700 and 900 μg in retinol activity equivalents per day for women and men, respectively (Ross et al., 2012). Rich sources of vitamin A include milk and dairy products, meat, eggs, fish, and, notably, poultry and livestock livers, which contain retinol and its ester (Carazo et al., 2021).

Vitamin C is known as a water-soluble vitamin and plays crucial roles in various biological functions. It exists in two forms: ascorbic acid and its oxidized form, dehydroascorbic acid (Figueroa-Méndez & Rivas-Arancibia, 2015). Known for its antioxidant properties, vitamin C neutralizes ROS and reactive nitrogen species (RNS) like hydrogen

TABLE 18.2 Overview of Studies Utilizing Functional Foods and Their Bioactive Components for Eye Diseases.

Functional Food	Type of Eye Diseases	Daily Dose	Type and Duration of Study	Main Findings	References
Dietary vitamin C	Nuclear, posterior subcapsular, and cortical cataracts	Q1: 10.8 mg/day; Q2: 19.6 mg/day; Q3: 28.6 mg/day; Q4: 402 mg/day; Q5: 66.4 mg/day	A cross-sectional study, By 24-hour recall	There was an inverse relationship between vitamin C intake and cataract disease	Ravindran et al. (2011)
High intake of vitamins E and C through daily fruits and vegetables	Cataract	Median intake of Vitamin C (mg/day): 67.0, 96.0, 122.6, and 173.14; Median intake of Vitamin E (μg/day): 7.14, 8.72, 9.84, and 11.66	A cross-sectional study, Semi-quantitative food frequency questionnaire	Consuming vegetables and fruits rich in vitamins E and C significantly reduced the prevalence of cataracts or cataract surgery	Pastor-Valero (2013)
Multivitamin supplements (vitamins C and E)	Cataract, Age-related macular degeneration	400 IU Vitamin E; 500 mg of vitamin C	Randomized, double-blind, placebo-controlled trial, 11.2 years	Risk of cataract ↓, No significant association with age-related macular degeneration	Christen et al. (2014)
Dietary vitamin E or dietary and supplement vitamin E	Age-related macular degeneration	9.8 mg Vitamin E (diet); 39.7 mg Vitamin E (diet + supplements); 826 μg lutein and zeaxanthin	Follow up for 5 years, 10 years, or both	Late age-related macular degeneration predicted with higher total vitamin E intake, There was an association between higher dietary intake of zeaxanthin and lutein and a reduced risk of age-related macular degeneration in the long term	Tan et al. (2008)
Vitamins C and E, β-carotene, and zinc	Age-related macular degeneration	500 mg vitamin C, 400 IU vitamin E, 15 mg β-carotene, 80 mg zinc	Follow up for 6.3 years	Risk of progression of advanced early age-related macular degeneration to late age-related macular degeneration ↓	Age-Related Eye Disease Study Research Group (2001)
Oral fish oil, oral combined fish + flaxseed oils, or ω-3 eye drops	Contact lens discomfort	900 mg/day EPA + 600 mg/day DHA; 900 mg/day EPA + 600 mg/day DHA + 900 mg/day ALA; 0.025% EPA + 0.0025% DHA eye drops four times per day	12 weeks	Contact lens discomfort ↓	Downie et al. (2018)

peroxide, superoxide radical anion, singlet oxygen, reactive nitrogen oxide, and hydroxyl radical. These effects protect organs like the brain, stomach, and eyes from oxidative stress (Barros et al., 2011). Research shows that vitamin C in the aqueous humor protects ocular tissues against oxidative damage (Barros et al., 2011).

The RDA for adults over 18 is 75 mg for women and 90 mg for men per day (Ross et al., 2012). Vitamin C is found in peppers, tomatoes, citrus fruits, leafy vegetables, kiwi, mango, and broccoli (Cahill et al., 2009). However, the vitamin content of foods may decrease with storage and heating (Lykkesfeldt et al., 2014). Although vitamin C deficiency is rare, it may occur in malnourished individuals, excessive alcohol consumers, those with malabsorption, or kidney failure. Deficiency can lead to scurvy, cardiovascular diseases, neurodegenerative diseases, and disorders in the skin, gums, and bones due to its effect on collagen synthesis. Vitamin C's antioxidant role is also implicated in ROS-related conditions such as glaucoma, age-related macular degeneration, and cataracts (Grosso et al., 2013).

Vitamin C is found in the lens and the ocular humor decreases with age (Senthilkumari et al., 2014; Shui et al., 2009). This decline may contribute to cataract severity. Supplemental vitamin C intake has been shown to increase lens vitamin C levels, protecting against oxidative damage from ultraviolet (UV) light and regenerating glutathione and vitamin E to enhance antioxidant capacity (Lim et al., 2020). It scavenges α-tocopheryl radicals, preserving the reducing powers of antioxidants like α-tocopherol (Corti et al., 2010).

A population-based cross-sectional analytical study of individuals aged 60 and over ($n = 5638$) found an inverse relationship between cataract disease and vitamin C, across all three types (nuclear cataract, posterior subcapsular cataract, and cortical cataract) (Ravindran et al., 2011). Similarly, a multicenter, cross-sectional study of 599 individuals aged 65 and over concluded that high intake of vitamins E and C from daily fruits and vegetables significantly reduced cataract prevalence (Pastor-Valero, 2013). Another study with 314 frequency-matched controls and 314 cases aged 45–85 years found significant inverse relationships between vegetable and fruit intake and cataracts, suggesting protective effects of carotene, vitamin C, and vitamin E (Theodoropoulou et al., 2014). However, a double-blind, randomized, placebo-controlled study with 11,545 US men aged ≥50 showed no significant relationship between daily vitamin C supplementation (500 mg) or alternate-day vitamin E supplementation (400 IU) and cataract risk after eight years of treatment and follow-up (Christen, Glynn, Chew, et al., 2010). Serum vitamin C levels were found to be low in normal-tension glaucoma patients (Yuki et al., 2010), and while vitamins A and E intake or serum levels were not associated with glaucoma prevalence, and vitamin C supplements were linked to reduced risk (Wang et al., 2013).

Vitamin E is known as a fat-soluble vitamin found in foods and occurs naturally in 8 chemical forms, including α, β, γ, δ-tocopherol and α, β, γ, δ-tocotrienol. Among these, α-tocopherol is the most biologically active (Szewczyk et al., 2021). It acts as an antioxidant, preventing lipid oxidation in cell membranes by attacking free radicals (Rasmussen & Johnson, 2013). Vitamin E may delay cellular damage, regulate inflammatory cytokines, and affect eye health positively by influencing enzyme and molecule activities in inflammatory cells (Edwards et al., 2022). Additionally, it improves vasodilation, inhibits platelet aggregation (Rasmussen & Johnson, 2013), and may prevent retinal neurodegeneration linked to oxidative stress (Edwards et al., 2022).

Several studies have examined the relationship between vitamin E and eye diseases. Higher total vitamin E intake predicted late age-related macular degeneration (Tan et al., 2008), and both dietary zinc and vitamin E were inversely associated with age-related macular degeneration incidence (Van Leeuwen et al., 2005). A metaanalysis found a significant relationship between high serum tocopherol levels, dietary vitamin E intake, and reduced age-related cataract risk, but no significant association with supplemental vitamin E intake (Zhang et al., 2015). However, long-term supplementation with 600 IU of natural-source vitamin E did not significantly affect the incidence of cataracts or age-related macular degeneration (Christen et al., 2008; Christen, Glynn, Chew, et al., 2010). In a study of 11,545 male physicians, alternate-day vitamin E supplementation and daily vitamin C supplementation did not significantly affect cataract risk after 8 years (Christen, Glynn, Sesso, et al., 2010). Another study with 14,236 male physicians found no significant effect of alternate-day vitamin E or daily vitamin C supplementation on age-related macular degeneration risk (Christen et al., 2012).

Zinc, highly concentrated in ocular tissues like neuroretina, cornea, and retinal pigment epithelium, plays vital roles in cellular functions. It binds tightly to proteins and functions as a cofactor for enzymes like catalase and superoxide dismutase, protecting the retina from oxidative damage (Decanini et al., 2007; Ugarte & Osborne, 2014). Additionally, zinc is crucial for DNA-binding proteins and transcriptional regulation, affecting the expression of zinc-binding proteins in the retina (Ugarte & Osborne, 2014). There is no specific zinc storage system in the body, so adequate daily intake of zinc is necessary. Zinc deficiency, often observed in the elderly due to malnutrition, can impact retinal health (Gilbert et al., 2019). Food sources rich in zinc include fish, meat, oysters, whole grains, nuts, beans, dairy products, and eggs, with oysters being the richest source. However, the bioavailability of zinc from plant sources may be reduced due to phytates (Stiles et al., 2024).

The RDA of zinc for adults over 18 is 8 mg for women and 11 mg for men per day (Ross et al., 2012). Although zinc concentrations in the retina are implicated in age-related macular degeneration, conclusive evidence on the effectiveness of zinc intake to prevent or treat this condition is lacking (Ugarte & Osborne, 2014). A research on individuals with dry age-related macular degeneration showed that supplementation of zinc-monocysteine significantly improved macular light flash recovery time, contrast sensitivity, and visual acuity over 6 months (Newsome, 2008). Another study stated a 35% decrease in the risk of age-related macular degeneration with above-average intake of vitamin C, vitamin E, β-carotene, and zinc (Van Leeuwen et al., 2005). Similarly, a population-based cohort study demonstrated the protective effects of zinc against age-related macular degeneration (Tan et al., 2008).

Selenium, a component of antioxidant enzymes like glutathione peroxidase, has an important role in protecting cells from oxidative damage. Glutathione peroxidase, dependent on selenium, helps reduce hydroperoxides within the cell and protect membrane lipids from oxidative damage (Post et al., 2018). Although selenium's antioxidant effects suggest a potential role in protecting the macula, its influence on age-related macular degeneration remains unclear (Khoo et al., 2019). However, a research based on National Health and Nutrition Examination Survey (NHANES) data from 2001 to 2008, involving 7,525 participants, reported a significant negative relationship between cataract incidence and selenium intake (Xu et al., 2023). Post et al. (2018) also stated that low selenium levels were significant predictors of cataracts (age-related, nuclear, and cortical).

18.3.2 Carotenoid-rich functional foods

Carotenoids are natural pigments categorized into two subcategories: carotenes (such as β-carotene, α-carotene) and xanthophyll carotenoids (such as lutein, zeaxanthin, and astaxanthin). The main foodstuffs of carotenoids are given in Table 18.3. Carotenoids are increasingly recognized as valuable dietary components with numerous health benefits. Beyond their roles in photosynthesis and pigmentation, they are now appreciated for their health-promoting properties (Rostamabadi et al., 2019). For instance, carotenoid-rich diets positively correlated with carotenoid depot in the retina and protection against blue light (Wegner & Khoramnia, 2011).

β-Carotene, a retinol (vitamin A) precursor found in vegetables and fruits, acts as an antioxidant, protecting DNA from free radical damage and contributing to eye health. The Age-Related Eye Disease Study (AREDS) showed that daily supplementation with antioxidative vitamins and minerals, including β-carotene, diminished the risk of advanced age-related macular degeneration by 25% over five years (Age-Related Eye Disease Study Research Group, 2001).

Zeaxanthin and lutein obtained from the diet present in dark green leafy vegetables such as kale, broccoli, and spinach and yellow and orange fruits such as carrots, papaya, and peaches. These have proven to be effective in the interception of age-related macular degeneration (Flaxman et al., 2017; Subczynski et al., 2010). Lutein carries antiinflammatory properties and behave as a significant antioxidant and is found in yellow or orange colored foods like melon, orange/yellow peppers, corn, carrots, salmon, and fish. The role of lutein in the suppression of age-related macular degeneration, which can lead to blindness, has been well documented. Studies indicated that lower consumption of fruits and green leafy vegetables may enhance the risk of this disease (Feng et al., 2019; Mitra et al., 2021). Lutein also increases macular pigment optical density, which improves visual acuity (Weigert et al., 2011). The Age-Related Eye Disease Study 2 (AREDS2) found that lutein reduces the risk of advanced age-related macular degeneration. In vitro researches have shown that it protects against cataracts by inhibiting lens cell proliferation and migration (Chew et al., 2012, 2014). Likewise, lutein consumption is associated with a lower incidence of nuclear cataracts, according to meta analyses (Babizhayev, 2016; Buscemi et al., 2018). Zeaxanthin is a vital xanthophyll carotenoid known for its potent antioxidant, prooxidant, and antiinflammatory properties. Studies indicated that zeaxanthin helps to reduce problems and suppress oxidative stress in retinal tissues, functioning alongside lutein as a macular pigment (Manikandan et al., 2016). Zeaxanthin supplementation has also been associated with a delayed cataract formation (Nakajima et al., 2014). Arnold et al. (2013) indicated the therapy of age-related macular degeneration patients with kale extract over four-week, resulting in increased lutein and zeaxanthin levels in serum, as well as improved visual functioning in age-related macular degeneration patients on account of elevated plasma xanthophyll levels.

Astaxanthin, another xanthophyll carotenoid, is a red pigment naturally present in various organisms such as phytoplankton, microalgae, and marine species like salmon, tuna, shrimp, crustaceans, lobster, and crayfish (Ambati et al., 2014). Astaxanthin treatment has been found to improve various eye diseases with studies showing its ability to avoid light-induced retinal dysfunction (Otsuka et al., 2013). After a year of treatment, a group receiving oral supplements containing astaxanthin, zeaxanthin, lutein, vitamin C, vitamin E, zinc, and copper showed a considerable rise in retinal function compared to control group (Parisi et al., 2008).

18.3.3 Functional foods rich in fatty acids

Polyunsaturated fatty acids (PUFA) are fatty acids with multiple double bonds and are crucial for nutrition and human health, with ω-3s and ω-6s being the two main classes. α-Linolenic acid (ALA) and linoleic acid (LA) are essential short-chain ω-3 and ω-6 fatty acids, respectively, required for biological functions and growth but cannot be synthesized by the human body. ALA serves as a precursor of eicosapentaenoic acid (EPA) and docosahexaenoic acid (DHA), while LA is a precursor of arachidonic acid (AA) (Britten-Jones, Craig, & Downie, 2023). The relative intake of ω-6s / ω-3s ratio determines the balance of by-products derived from their metabolism, influencing immunity, systemic inflammation, and cellular

TABLE 18.3 Main Food Sources of Carotenoids.

Carotenoids	Food Sources	Concentration (μg/g)	References
α-Carotene	Carrot	382	Ashour et al. (2017), Piyarach et al. (2020)
	Sweet potatoes	8.61	Kammona et al. (2015)
	Pumpkin	25	Piyarach et al. (2020)
	Zucchini	36	Ashour et al. (2017)
β-Carotene	Carrot	549–862	Ashour et al. (2017) Piyarach et al. (2020)
	Sweet potatoes	117–708	Kammona et al. (2015), Pritwani and Mathur (2017)
	Broccoli	10.5–68	Ashour et al. (2017), dos Reis et al. (2015)
	Pumpkin	470	Pritwani and Mathur (2017)
	Apricot	190.9	İncedayı et al. (2016)
	Mangoes	79.5	Olale et al. (2019)
	Kale	406	Piyarach et al. (2020)
	Long coriander	276	Piyarach et al. (2020)
	Spinach	43	Wen Lee et al. (2022)
	Zucchini	57	Ashour et al. (2017)
Lutein	Spinach	114	Wen Lee et al. (2022)
	Carrot	121	Ashour et al. (2017)
	Kale	126–619	Piyarach et al. (2020), Wen Lee et al. (2022)
	Broccoli	7.3–174	Ashour et al. (2017), dos Reis et al. (2015)
	Pumpkin	384	Piyarach et al. (2020)
	Long coriander	945	Piyarach et al. (2020)
	Zucchini	471	Ashour, Enssaf, and El-hamzy (2017)
Lycopene	Tomatoes	88.5–107.1	Ordoñez-Santos and Ledezma-Realpe (2013), Suwanaruang (2016)
	Watermelon	23.0–144.3	Dhakane-Lad and Kar (2021), Ordoñez-Santos and Ledezma-Realpe (2013), Suwanaruang (2016)
	Bananas	31.2	Suwanaruang (2016)
	Pink grapefruit juice	33.6–53.7	Dhakane-Lad and Kar (2021)
	Guava	36.1–54.0	Dhakane-Lad and Kar (2021), Ordoñez-Santos and Ledezma-Realpe (2013)
	Papaya	6.21–53.0	Dhakane-Lad and Kar (2021), Ordoñez-Santos and Ledezma-Realpe (2013), Suwanaruang (2016)
Zeaxanthin	Egg yolk	762	Perry et al. (2009)
	Orange	1665	Perry et al. (2009)
	Corn	202	Perry et al. (2009)
	Paprika	22	Perry et al. (2009)

signaling. ω-3 PUFAs play a crucial role in neural development and function and have been widely reported for their potential to modulate ocular and systemic inflammation (Britten-Jones, Craig, & Downie, 2023).

Dietary sources high in LA are cereals and vegetable oils made from sunflower, safflower, and corn, while ALA is found in chia seeds, flaxseed, and vegetable oils from walnuts, soya beans, and canola, as well as in green leafy vegetables (Calder, 2013; Meyer et al., 2003). EPA and DHA are plenty in fish oils and marine-based foods like salmon, mackerel, and tuna with fatty fish containing higher concentrations than lean fish (Zhang et al., 2020). ω-3 supplements, typically prepared as ethyl esters or reesterified to a glycerol (e.g., in fish oil) or phospholipid backbone (e.g., in krill oil), have demonstrated bioavailability comparable to natural triglycerides and superior to ethyl ester supplements (Schuchardt et al., 2011). In dry eye disease, ω-3 supplementation, particularly in phospholipid from like krill oil, has shown additional benefits in the reduction of ocular surface inflammation compared to placebo (Deinema et al., 2017).

An optimal ω-6 to ω-3 ratio in the diet is suggested to be 4/1, as higher proportions have been linked to cardiovascular disease and autoimmune conditions (Britten-Jones, Craig, & Downie, 2023). Studies have shown that a 15/1 ω-6 to ω-3 ratio is related to a considerably higher risk of dry eye disease compared to a 4/1 ratio (Miljanović et al., 2005). In dry eye disease, the ratio of ω-6 to ω-3 correlates with corneal epithelium and tear dysfunction (Walter et al., 2016). DHA's role in maintaining nerve integrity is of particular interest, as seen in studies where EPA derivatives like resolvin E1 have reduced corneal inflammation and promoted epithelial cell differentiation (Li et al., 2010). Clinical studies have shown that topical ω-3 PUFA therapy decreases ocular surface inflammation in dry eye diseases and contact lens discomfort, though direct evaluation of their neuroprotective effects in dry eye disease remains lacking (Downie et al., 2018; Rashid et al., 2008). Recent research has revealed a positive correlation between systemic ω-3 levels and corneal nerve parameters, suggesting that PUFA intake may affect corneal nerve structure (Britten-Jones, Craig, Anderson, et al., 2023). Supplementation with ALA, EPA, and DHA has provided significant clinical improvement in dry eye symptoms (Ng et al., 2022).

18.3.4 Antioxidant-rich functional foods

Retinal tissue is vulnerable to oxidative stress because of its high metabolic needs, leading to the of ROS (Wang et al., 2021). Oxidative stress arises from an imbalance between ROS production and elimination (Miranda & Romero, 2019), originating from various resources with the inclusion of the mitochondrial respiratory chain and enzymatic reactions in the retina and retinal pigment epithelium (Wang et al., 2021). Excessive ROS can damage DNA, proteins, and lipids, contributing to cell death, inflammation, and angiogenesis (Miranda & Romero, 2019). The retina employs antioxidants like ascorbate, catalase, vitamin E, glutathione, and others to counteract ROS, but age or certain pathologies may diminish this defense (Liang & Godley, 2003). Consequently, oxidative stress is implicated in retinal diseases like age-related macular degeneration, diabetic retinopathy, glaucoma, and retinal dystrophies, suggesting antioxidants as potential therapeutic options (Wang et al., 2021).

Anthocyanins, flavonoids abundant in plants, may influence retinal blood circulation by modulating ET-1 metabolism via the ET-1 receptor, potentially altering blood flow in the optic nerve heads (Nomi et al., 2019). In a clinical study on patients with normal tension glaucoma, oral administration of 50 mg blackcurrant anthocyanin daily for 6 days significantly altered blood flow in the optic nerve head and peripapillary retina, despite an increase in plasma ET-1 concentrations (Sato et al., 2006). Similarly, in patients with open-angle glaucoma, intake of anthocyanins from blackcurrant increased serum ET-1 levels, suggesting a potential neuroprotective effect (Ohguro et al., 2012). Nomi et al. (2019) found that anthocyanin can be a safe and effective neuroprotective therapy for open-angle glaucoma and normal tension glaucoma. Blueberry extract was shown to reduce critical flicker fusion, which reduces ocular fatigue sensations related to video imaging terminal load, including ocular pain, eye heaviness, discomfort sensation, and foreign body sensation (Ozawa et al., 2015). In a study by Ogawa et al. (2014), lingonberry extract was evaluated as an antiblue LED agent. According to the researchers, lingonberries contain high levels of anthocyanins and resveratrol, which protect retinal photoreceptor cells against the damage caused by blue LED light via the inhibition of the activation of proapoptotic proteins and ROS.

A number of bioactive compounds are present in *Crocus sativus* L., commonly known as saffron, which have strong antioxidant properties. These include crocins, crocetin, picrocrocrocrocin, and safranal, which all possess antiinflammatory and antioxidant properties. Research has shown that saffron components also possess antiinflammatory and antiapoptotic features (Nam et al., 2010; Tamaddonfard et al., 2013). Studies on saffron extract suggest its potential protective effect in glaucoma patients. Consumption of aqueous saffron extract for three weeks has been shown reducing intraocular pressure and associated neuroinflammation in primary open-angle glaucoma (Choo et al., 2022; Fernández-Albarral et al., 2019). A number of studies have evaluated the effect of oral saffron supplementation (daily dose between 20 and 50 mg) on vision-related parameters in patients with age-related macular degeneration. Despite variations in formulations, doses, intervention times, test methods, and outcome measures, both short- and long-term follow-ups have shown improvements in vision. Toxicological studies have reported the safety of saffron for human consumption, with an effective dose of 30 mg/day and toxic effects occurring at 5 g or more, and about 20 g being a lethal dose (Christodoulou et al., 2015; Mohamadpour et al., 2013).

Curcumin, a water-insoluble pigment obtained from the rhizome of *Curcuma longa* from the *Zingiberaceae* family, is a biologically active phytochemical compound with various health benefits. Curcumin extract also contains carotene, lycopene, epigallocatechin gallate, and quercetin. It is used in the suppression on and treatment of many diseases, particularly inflammatory diseases and cancer (Maiuolo et al., 2023). Curcumin reduces oxidative damage by scavenging ROS and RNS. Given that most retinal diseases involve increased ROS and decreased levels of scavenging antioxidants, curcumin is thought to have a positive effect in treating eye diseases (Magdalena Radomska-Leśniewska et al., 2017). Studies have demonstrated that curcumin can preserve human retinal epithelial cells from death (Nebbioso et al., 2021). Additionally, improvement was reported in patients with chronic uveitis who were given oral curcumin capsules (75 mg/capsule) (Chung et al., 2012).

Coenzyme Q_{10}, also called ubiquinone, is the only fat-soluble antioxidant. In its reduced form ($CoQ_{10}H_2$), it exhibits both direct and indirect antioxidant properties. Directly, it reduces the accumulation of ROS, while indirectly it regenerates a form of vitamin E (Acosta et al., 2016; Maiuolo et al., 2023). A study has shown that young individuals (30 years) have higher Coenzyme Q_{10} concentrations compared to older individuals (80 years), emphasizing the role of oxidative stress in age-related diseases such as atherosclerosis, cataracts, and Alzheimer's disease (Dusting & Triggle, 2005; Maiuolo et al., 2023). Increased ROS accumulation during aging leads to heightened cell damage mediated by apoptotic mechanisms of cell death (Maiuolo et al., 2023). In a study, plasma Coenzyme Q_{10} levels were significantly reduced in patients with age-related macular degeneration when compared with the control group, suggesting a relationship between Coenzyme Q_{10} and the pathogenesis of this disease (Bilbao-Malavé et al., 2021). Since glaucoma prevalence increases with age, there may be a possible association with the glaucoma and Coenzyme Q_{10} deficiency in the elderly. Experimental studies have also demonstrated that intravitreal administration of Coenzyme Q_{10} minimizes apoptosis in glaucoma patients (Lee et al., 2014; Miles, 2007). The normal concentration area of Coenzyme Q_{10} in human plasma is 0.8−1.2 mg/L, and in case of deficiency, adults are usually supplemented with 1.2−3 g/day (Maiuolo et al., 2023).

18.4 Future perspective

Functional foods and ocular health can improve vision and prevent eye diseases through dietary interventions. As ongoing research continues to uncover the intimate relationship between nutrition and ocular health, functional foods with specific nutrients and bioactive compounds will play an important role in maintaining optimal vision and preventing ocular diseases. One promising area of future research is functional foods that address specific ocular health needs. Among these foods may be a precise combination of nutrients known to support eye health, including antioxidants, vitamins, lutein, zeaxanthin, and ω-3 fatty acids. Supplements, snacks, and beverages fortified with these nutrients may ease the process of incorporating these nutrients into our daily diets. Moreover, advances in food technology could improve the bioavailability and efficacy of these nutrients. Nanoencapsulation could be used to improve the absorption of lipophilic compounds like lutein and zeaxanthin, ensuring that they reach target tissues at therapeutic levels (Rostamabadi et al., 2019). The release of nutrients can also be controlled over time in a novel formulation, enhancing their bioactivity and extending their effects. There is also a clear connection between gut health and eye functions that could be explored in future research, which is known as the gut−eye axis. Microbiota in the gut may affect oxidative stress and systemic inflammation, both of which can affect ocular health (Grant et al., 2022). Therefore functional foods that support a healthy gut microbiota may improve ocular health indirectly by reducing inflammation and increasing immunity. New strategies for maintaining vision and preventing eye diseases may emerge from continued research on functional foods and ocular health. Globally, eye care can be revolutionized by harnessing the power of nutrition and innovative food technologies.

18.5 Conclusion

Eye diseases globally diminished individuals' quality of life and increased healthcare costs. It is now established that a healthy diet is crucial for maintaining good vision and preventing various eye problems. Scientific research indicates that micronutrients, vitamins, and natural compounds with antioxidant and antiinflammatory properties are key in alleviating and protecting against ocular diseases. As people age, it becomes increasingly important to ensure a balanced intake of healthy fats, carbohydrates, fiber, and protein, as well as micronutrients and vitamins, to support our eye health.

References

Acosta, M. J., Vazquez Fonseca, L., Desbats, M. A., Cerqua, C., Zordan, R., Trevisson, E., & Salviati, L. (2016). Coenzyme Q biosynthesis in health and disease. *Biochimica et Biophysica Acta - Bioenergetics*, *1857*(8), 1079–1085. Available from https://doi.org/10.1016/j.bbabio.2016.03.036, http://www.elsevier.com/locate/bbabio.

Age-Related Eye Disease Study Research Group. (2001). A randomized, placebo-controlled, clinical tiral of high-dose supplementation with vitamins C and E, beta-carotene, and zinc for age-related macular degeneration and vision loss: ARDES report no. 8. *Archives of Ophthalmology*, *119*(10), 1417–1436. Available from https://doi.org/10.1001/archopht.124.8.1213-a.

Allingham, R. R., Damji, K., Freedman, S., Moroi, S., & Shafranov, G. (2004). *Archives of ophthalmology shields' textbook of glaucoma, 5th Edition Archives of Ophthalmology* (p. 1213) American Medical Association (AMA). Available from 10.1001/archopht.124.8.1213-a.

Ambati, R. R., Moi, P. S., Ravi, S., & Aswathanarayana, R. G. (2014). Astaxanthin: Sources, extraction, stability, biological activities and its commercial applications - A review. *Marine Drugs*, *12*(1), 128–152. Available from https://doi.org/10.3390/md12010128, http://www.mdpi.com/1660-3397/12/1/128/pdf.

Arnold, C., Jentsch, S., Dawczynski, J., & Böhm, V. (2013). Age-related macular degeneration: Effects of a short-term intervention with an oleaginous kale extract—A pilot study. *Nutrition (Burbank, Los Angeles County, Calif.)*, *29*(11-12), 1412–1417. Available from https://doi.org/10.1016/j.nut.2013.05.012.

Ashour, M. M. S., Enssaf, M. A., & El-hamzy. (2017). Influence of different cooking methods on physicochemical characteristics, phytochemical profile, antioxidant capacity and chromatic parameters of selected vegetables. *Middle East Journal of Applied Sciences* (04), 1127–1147.

Babizhayev, M. A. (2016). Generation of reactive oxygen species in the anterior eye segment. Synergistic codrugs of N-acetylcarnosine lubricant eye drops and mitochondria-targeted antioxidant act as a powerful therapeutic platform for the treatment of cataracts and primary open-angle glaucoma. *BBA Clinical*, *6*, 49–68. Available from https://doi.org/10.1016/j.bbacli.2016.04.004, http://www.journals.elsevier.com/bba-clinical/.

Barros, A. I. R. N. A., Nunes, F. M., Gonalves, B., Bennett, R. N., & Silva, A. P. (2011). Effect of cooking on total vitamin C contents and antioxidant activity of sweet chestnuts (Castanea sativa Mill.). *Food Chemistry*, *128*(1), 165–172. Available from https://doi.org/10.1016/j.foodchem.2011.03.013.

Bilbao-Malavé, V., González-Zamora, J., de la Puente, M., Recalde, S., Fernandez-Robredo, P., Hernandez, M., Layana, A. G., & Saenz de Viteri, M. (2021). Mitochondrial dysfunction and endoplasmic reticulum stress in age related macular degeneration, role in pathophysiology, and possible new therapeutic strategies. *Antioxidants*, *10*(8), 1170. Available from https://doi.org/10.3390/antiox10081170.

Braakhuis, A. J., Donaldson, C. I., Lim, J. C., & Donaldson, P. J. (2019). Nutritional strategies to prevent lens cataract: Current status and future strategies. *Nutrients*, *11*(5). Available from https://doi.org/10.3390/nu11051186, https://www.mdpi.com/2072-6643/11/5/1186/pdf.

Britten-Jones, A. C., Craig, J. P., Anderson, A. J., & Downie, L. E. (2023). Association between systemic omega-3 polyunsaturated fatty acid levels, and corneal nerve structure and function. *Eye (Basingstoke)*, *37*(9), 1866–1873. Available from https://doi.org/10.1038/s41433-022-02259-0, https://www.nature.com/eye/.

Britten-Jones, A. C., Craig, J. P., & Downie, L. E. (2023). Omega-3 polyunsaturated fatty acids and corneal nerve health: Current evidence and future directions. *Ocular Surface*, *27*, 1–12. Available from https://doi.org/10.1016/j.jtos.2022.10.006, http://www.elsevier.com/wps/find/authored_newsitem.cws_home/companynews05_02205.

Burton, M. J., Ramke, J., Marques, A. P., Bourne, R. R. A., Congdon, N., Jones, I., Ah Tong, B. A. M., Arunga, S., Bachani, D., Bascaran, C., Bastawrous, A., Blanchet, K., Braithwaite, T., Buchan, J. C., Cairns, J., Cama, A., Chagunda, M., Chuluunkhuu, C., Cooper, A., … Faal, H. B. (2021). The lancet global health commission on global eye health: Vision beyond 2020. *The Lancet Global Health*, *9*(4), e489. Available from https://doi.org/10.1016/S2214-109X(20)30488-5, http://www.elsevier.com/journals/the-lancet-global-health/2214-109x.

Buscemi, S., Corleo, D., Di Pace, F., Petroni, M., Satriano, A., & Marchesini, G. (2018). The effect of lutein on eye and extra-eye health. *Nutrients*, *10*(9), 1321. Available from https://doi.org/10.3390/nu10091321.

Cahill, L., Corey, P. N., & El-Sohemy, A. (2009). Vitamin C deficiency in a population of young canadian adults. *American Journal of Epidemiology*, *170*(4), 464–471. Available from https://doi.org/10.1093/aje/kwp156.

Calder, P. C. (2013). Omega-3 polyunsaturated fatty acids and inflammatory processes: Nutrition or pharmacology? *British Journal of Clinical Pharmacology*, *75*(3), 645–662. Available from https://doi.org/10.1111/j.1365-2125.2012.04374.x.

Carazo, A., Macáková, K., Matoušová, K., Krčmová, L. K., Protti, M., & Mladěnka, P. (2021). Vitamin A update: Forms, sources, kinetics, detection, function, deficiency, therapeutic use and toxicity. *Nutrients*, *13*(5), 1703. Available from https://doi.org/10.3390/nu13051703.

Chen, J., Zhu, Y., Li, Z., Chen, X., Chen, X., Huang, S., Xie, R., Zhang, Y., Ye, G., Luo, R., Shen, X., Lin, L., & Zhuo, Y. (2024). Global impact of population aging on vision loss prevalence: A population-based study. *Global Transitions*, *6*, 28–36. Available from https://doi.org/10.1016/j.glt.2023.12.003, https://www.sciencedirect.com/science/journal/25897918.

Chen, Y., Hu, Y., Zhou, T., Zhou, K. K., Mott, R., Wu, M., Boulton, M., Lyons, T. J., Gao, G., & Ma, J. X. (2009). Activation of the wnt pathway plays a pathogenic role in diabetic retinopathy in humans and animal models. *American Journal of Pathology*, *175*(6), 2676–2685. Available from https://doi.org/10.2353/ajpath.2009.080945, http://ajp.amjpathol.org/cgi/reprint/175/6/2676.

Cheung, N., Mitchell, P., & Wong, T. Y. (2010). Diabetic retinopathy. *The Lancet*, *376*(9735), 124–136, Elsevier B.V. Australia. Available from https://doi.org/10.1016/S0140-6736(09)62124-3, http://www.journals.elsevier.com/the-lancet/.

Chew, E. Y., Clemons, T., Sangiovanni, J. P., Danis, R., Domalpally, A., McBee, W., Sperduto, R., & Ferris, F. L. (2012). The age-related eye disease study 2 (AREDS2): Study design and baseline characteristics (AREDS2 Report Number 1). *Ophthalmology*, *119*(11), 2282–2289. Available from https://doi.org/10.1016/j.ophtha.2012.05.027.

Chew, E. Y., Clemons, T. E., SanGiovanni, J. P., Danis, R. P., Ferris, F. L., Elman, M. J., Antoszyk, A. N., Ruby, A. J., Orth, D., Bressler, S. B., Fish, G. E., Hubbard, G. B., Klein, M. L., Chandra, S. R., Blodi, B. A., Domalpally, A., Friberg, T., Wong, W. T., Rosenfeld, P. J., … Sperduto, R. D. (2014). Secondary analyses of the effects of lutein/zeaxanthin on age-related macular degeneration progression AREDS2 report no. 3. *JAMA Ophthalmology*, *132*(2), 142–149. Available from https://doi.org/10.1001/jamaophthalmol.2013.7376, http://archopht.jamanetwork.com/article.aspx?articleid = 1788227, United States.

Choo, P. P., Woi, P. J., Bastion, M. L. C., Omar, R., Mustapha, M., & Md Din, N. (2022). Review of evidence for the usage of antioxidants for eye aging. *BioMed Research International*, *2022*. Available from https://doi.org/10.1155/2022/5810373, http://www.hindawi.com/journals/biomed/.

Christen, W. G., Glynn, R. J., Chew, E. Y., & Buring, J. E. (2008). Vitamin E and age-related cataract in a randomized trial of women. *Ophthalmology*, *115*(5), 822. Available from https://doi.org/10.1016/j.ophtha.2007.06.040, http://www.elsevier.com/locate/ophtha.

Christen, W. G., Glynn, R. J., Chew, E. Y., & Buring, J. E. (2010). Vitamin E and age-related macular degeneration in a randomized trial of women. *Ophthalmology*, *117*(6), 1163–1168. Available from https://doi.org/10.1016/j.ophtha.2009.10.043.

Christen, W. G., Glynn, R. J., Manson, J. E., Macfadyen, J., Bubes, V., Schvartz, M., Buring, J. E., Sesso, H. D., & Gaziano, J. M. (2014). Effects of multivitamin supplement on cataract and age-related macular degeneration in a randomized trial of male physicians. *Ophthalmology*, *121*(2), 525–534. Available from https://doi.org/10.1016/j.ophtha.2013.09.038.

Christen, W. G., Glynn, R. J., Sesso, H. D., Kurth, T., MacFadyen, J., Bubes, V., Buring, J. E., Manson, J. A. E., & Gaziano, J. M. (2010). Age-related cataract in a randomized trial of vitamins E and C in men. *Archives of Ophthalmology*, *128*(11), 1397–1405. Available from https://doi.org/10.1001/archophthalmol.2010.266, http://archopht.ama-assn.org/cgi/reprint/128/11/1397, United States.

Christen, W. G., Glynn, R. J., Sesso, H. D., Kurth, T., MacFadyen, J., Bubes, V., Buring, J. E., Manson, J. E., & Gaziano, J. M. (2012). Vitamins e and C and medical record-confirmed age-related macular degeneration in a randomized trial of male physicians. *Ophthalmology*, *119*(8), 1642–1649. Available from https://doi.org/10.1016/j.ophtha.2012.01.053.

Christodoulou, E., Kadoglou, N. P., Kostomitsopoulos, N., & Valsami, G. (2015). Saffron: A natural product with potential pharmaceutical applications. *Journal of Pharmacy and Pharmacology*, *67*(12), 1634–1649. Available from https://doi.org/10.1111/jphp.12456, http://www.interscience.wiley.com/jpages/0022-3573.

Chung, S. H., Choi, S. H., Choi, J. A., Chuck, R. S., & Joo, C. K. (2012). Curcumin suppresses ovalbumin-induced allergic conjunctivitis. *Molecular Vision*, *18*, 1966–1972.

Corti, A., Casini, A. F., & Pompella, A. (2010). Cellular pathways for transport and efflux of ascorbate and dehydroascorbate. *Archives of Biochemistry and Biophysics*, *500*(2), 107–115. Available from https://doi.org/10.1016/j.abb.2010.05.014.

Decanini, A., Nordgaard, C. L., Feng, X., Ferrington, D. A., & Olsen, T. W. (2007). Changes in select redox proteins of the retinal pigment epithelium in age-related macular degeneration. *American Journal of Ophthalmology*, *143*(4), 607. Available from https://doi.org/10.1016/j.ajo.2006.12.006, http://www.elsevier.com/locate/ajo.

Deinema, L. A., Vingrys, A. J., Wong, C. Y., Jackson, D. C., Chinnery, H. R., & Downie, L. E. (2017). A randomized, double-masked, placebo-controlled clinical trial of two forms of omega-3 supplements for treating dry eye disease. *Ophthalmology*, *124*(1), 43–52. Available from https://doi.org/10.1016/j.ophtha.2016.09.023, http://www.elsevier.com/locate/ophtha.

Dhakane-Lad, J., & Kar, A. (2021). Supercritical CO2 extraction of lycopene from pink grapefruit (*Citrus paradise* Macfad) and its degradation studies during storage. *Food Chemistry*, *361*130113. Available from https://doi.org/10.1016/j.foodchem.2021.130113.

Downie, L. E., Gad, A., Wong, C. Y., Gray, J. H. V., Zeng, W., Jackson, D. C., & Vingrys, A. J. (2018). Modulating contact lens discomfort with anti-inflammatory approaches: A randomized controlled trial. *Investigative Ophthalmology and Visual Science.*, *59*(8), 3755–3766. Available from https://doi.org/10.1167/iovs.18-24758, https://iovs.arvojournals.org/.

Dubois, V. D. P., & Bastawrous, A. (2017). N-acetylcarnosine (NAC) drops for age-related cataract. *Cochrane Database of Systematic Reviews*, *2017* (2). Available from https://doi.org/10.1002/14651858.CD009493.pub2, http://as.wiley.com/WileyCDA/Brand/id-6.html.

Dusting, G. J., & Triggle, C. (2005). Are we over oxidized? Oxidative stress, cardiovascular disease, and the future of intervention studies with antioxidants. *Vascular Health and Risk Management*, *1*(2), 93–97. Available from https://doi.org/10.2147/vhrm.1.2.93.64080.

Edwards, G., Olson, C. G., Euritt, C. P., & Koulen, P. (2022). Molecular mechanisms underlying the therapeutic role of vitamin E in age-related macular degeneration. *Frontiers in Neuroscience*, *16*. Available from https://doi.org/10.3389/fnins.2022.890021, https://www.frontiersin.org/journals/neuroscience#.

Erdurmuş, M., Simavlı, H., & Aydın, B. (2019). *Cataracts: An overview* (pp. 231–244). Elsevier BV. Available from 10.1016/b978-0-12-815245-4.00014-4.

Feng, L., Nie, K., Jiang, H., & Fan, W. (2019). Effects of lutein supplementation in agerelated macular degeneration. *PLoS One*, *14*(12). Available from https://doi.org/10.1371/journal.pone.0227048, https://journals.plos.org/plosone/article/file?id = 10.1371/journal.pone.0227048&type = printable.

Fernández-Albarral, J. A., Ramírez, A. I., De Hoz, R., López-Villarín, N., Salobrar-García, E., López-Cuenca, I., Licastro, E., Inarejos-García, A. M., Almodóvar, P., Pinazo-Durán, M. D., Ramírez, J. M., & Salazar, J. J. (2019). Neuroprotective and anti-inflammatory effects of a hydrophilic saffron extract in a model of glaucoma. *International Journal of Molecular Sciences*, *20*(17). Available from https://doi.org/10.3390/ijms20174110, https://www.mdpi.com/1422-0067/20/17/4110/pdf.

Figueroa-Méndez, R., & Rivas-Arancibia, S. (2015). Vitamin C in health and disease: Its role in the metabolism of cells and redox state in the brain. *Frontiers in Physiology*, *6*. Available from https://doi.org/10.3389/fphys.2015.00397, http://journal.frontiersin.org/article/10.3389/fphys.2015.00397/full.

Flaxman, S. R., Bourne, R. R. A., Resnikoff, S., Ackland, P., Braithwaite, T., Cicinelli, M. V., Das, A., Jonas, J. B., Keeffe, J., Kempen, J., Leasher, J., Limburg, H., Naidoo, K., Pesudovs, K., Silvester, A., Stevens, G. A., Tahhan, N., Wong, T., Taylor, H., … Zheng, Y. (2017). Global causes of blindness and distance vision impairment 1990–2020: A systematic review and meta-analysis. *The Lancet Global Health*, *5*(12), e1221. Available from https://doi.org/10.1016/S2214-109X(17)30393-5, http://www.elsevier.com/journals/the-lancet-global-health/2214-109x.

Gilbert, C. (2013). The eye signs of vitamin A deficiency. *Community Eye Health Journal*, *26*(84), 66–67. Available from http://www.cehjournal.org/wp-content/uploads/the-eye-signs-of-vitamin-a-deficiency.pdf, United Kingdom.

Gilbert, R., Peto, T., Lengyel, I., & Emri, E. (2019). Zinc nutrition and inflammation in the aging retina. *Molecular Nutrition and Food Research*, *63*(15). Available from https://doi.org/10.1002/mnfr.201801049, http://onlinelibrary.wiley.com/journal/10.1002/(ISSN)1613-4133.

Grant, M. B., Bernstein, P. S., Boesze-Battaglia, K., Chew, E., Curcio, C. A., Kenney, M. C., Klaver, C., Philp, N. J., Rowan, S., Sparrow, J., Spaide, R. F., & Taylor, A. (2022). Inside out: Relations between the microbiome, nutrition, and eye health. *Experimental Eye Research*, *224*. Available from https://doi.org/10.1016/j.exer.2022.109216, http://www.elsevier.com/inca/publications/store/6/2/2/8/2/7/index.htt.

Grosso, G., Bei, R., Mistretta, A., Marventano, S., Calabrese, G., Masuelli, L., Giganti, M. G., Modesti, A., Galvano, F., & Gazzolo, D. (2013). Effects of vitamin C on health: A review of evidence. *Frontiers in Bioscience*, *18*(3), 1017–1029. Available from https://doi.org/10.2741/4160, http://www.frontbiosci.org/fbs/getfile.php?FileName = /2013/v18/af/4160/4160.pdf.

Guymer, R. H., & Campbell, T. G. (2023). Age-related macular degeneration. *The Lancet*, *401*(10386), 1459–1472. Available from https://doi.org/10.1016/S0140-6736(22)02609-5, http://www.journals.elsevier.com/the-lancet/.

He, Y., Leung, K. W., Zhang, Y. H., Duan, S., Zhong, X. F., Jiang, R. Z., Peng, Z., Tombran-Tink, J., & Ge, J. (2008). Mitochondrial complex i defect induces ROS release and degeneration in trabecular meshwork cells of POAG patients: Protection by antioxidants. *Investigative Ophthalmology and Visual Science*, *49*(4), 1447–1458. Available from https://doi.org/10.1167/iovs.07-1361, http://www.iovs.org/cgi/reprint/49/4/1447, China.

İncedayı, B., Tamer, C. E., Sınır, G. Ö., Suna, S., & Çopur, Ö. U. (2016). Impact of different drying parameters on color, β-carotene, antioxidant activity and minerals of apricot (Prunus armeniacaL.). *Food Science and Technology*, *36*(1), 171–178. Available from https://doi.org/10.1590/1678-457X.0086.

Izzotti, A., Bagnis, A., & Saccà, S. C. (2006). The role of oxidative stress in glaucoma. *Mutation Research - Reviews in Mutation Research*, *612*(2), 105–114. Available from https://doi.org/10.1016/j.mrrev.2005.11.001.

Jariyapongskul, A., Rungjaroen, T., Kasetsuwan, N., Patumraj, S., Seki, J., & Niimi, H. (2007). Long-term effects of oral vitamin C supplementation on the endothelial dysfunction in the iris microvessels of diabetic rats. *Microvascular Research*, *74*(1), 32–38. Available from https://doi.org/10.1016/j.mvr.2007.03.002.

Kammona, S., Othman, R., Jaswir, I., & Jamal, P. (2015). Characterisation of carotenoid content in diverse local sweet potato (ipomoea batatas) flesh tubers. *International Journal of Pharmacy and Pharmaceutical Sciences*, *7*(2), 347–351. Available from http://innovareacademics.in/journals/index.php/ijpps/article/download/3643/pdf_629.

Khoo, H. E., Ng, H. S., Yap, W. S., Goh, H. J. H., & Yim, H. S. (2019). Nutrients for prevention of macular degeneration and eye-related diseases. *Antioxidants*, *8*(4). Available from https://doi.org/10.3390/antiox8040085, https://www.mdpi.com/2076-3921/8/4/85/pdf.

Koçak, N., Onur, B. E., Kaya, M., Aslankara, H., Cimilli, H. C., & Kaynak, S. (2014). Glokom Hastalığı ve Yaşa Bağlı Makula Dejeneransının Yaşam Kalitesi Üzerine Etkileri. *Türk Oftalmoloji Dergisi*, *44*(2), 83–87. Available from https://doi.org/10.4274/tjo.13471.

Lamkin-Kennard, K. A., & Popovic, M. B. (2019). *Sensors: Natural and Synthetic Sensors. Biomechatronics* (pp. 81–107). Elsevier, https://www.elsevier.com/books/biomechatronics/popovic/978-0-12-812939-510.1016/B978-0-12-812939-5.00004-5.

Laparra, J. M., & Sanz, Y. (2010). Interactions of gut microbiota with functional food components and nutraceuticals. *Pharmacological Research*, *61*(3), 219–225. Available from https://doi.org/10.1016/j.phrs.2009.11.001.

Lawler, T., Liu, Y., Christensen, K., Vajaranant, T. S., & Mares, J. (2019). Dietary antioxidants, macular pigment, and glaucomatous neurodegeneration: A review of the evidence. *Nutrients*, *11*(5). Available from https://doi.org/10.3390/nu11051002, https://www.mdpi.com/2072-6643/11/5/1002/pdf.

Lee, D., Shim, M. S., Kim, K. Y., Noh, Y. H., Kim, H., Kim, S. Y., Weinreb, R. N., & Ju, W. K. (2014). Coenzyme Q10 inhibits glutamate excitotoxicity and oxidative stress-mediated mitochondrial alteration in a mouse model of glaucoma. *Investigative Ophthalmology and Visual Science.*, *55*(2), 993–1005. Available from https://doi.org/10.1167/iovs.13-12564, http://www.iovs.org/content/55/2/1006.full.pdf.

Van Leeuwen, R., Boekhoorn, S., Vingerling, J. R., Witteman, J. C. M., Klaver, C. C. W., & Hofman, A. (2005). P.T.V.M. De Jong, Dietary intake of antioxidants and risk of age-related macular degeneration. *JAMA: the Journal of the American Medical Association*, *294*(24), 3101–3107. Available from https://doi.org/10.1001/jama.294.24.3101, http://jama.ama-assn.org/cgi/reprint/294/24/3101.

Li, N., He, J., Schwartz, C. E., Gjorstrup, P., & Bazan, H. E. P. (2010). Resolvin E1 improves tear production and decreases inflammation in a dry eye mouse model. *Journal of Ocular Pharmacology and Therapeutics*, *26*(5), 431–439. Available from https://doi.org/10.1089/jop.2010.0019.

Liang, F. Q., & Godley, B. F. (2003). Oxidative stress-induced mitochondrial DNA damage in human retinal pigment epithelial cells: A possible mechanism for RPE aging and age-related macular degeneration. *Experimental Eye Research*, *76*(4), 397–403. Available from https://doi.org/10.1016/S0014-4835(03)00023-X, http://www.elsevier.com/inca/publications/store/6/2/2/8/2/7/index.htt.

Lim, J. C., Arredondo, M. C., Braakhuis, A. J., & Donaldson, P. J. (2020). Vitamin C and the lens: New insights into delaying the onset of cataract. *Nutrients*, *12*(10), 1–21. Available from https://doi.org/10.3390/nu12103142, https://www.mdpi.com/2072-6643/12/10/3142/pdf.

Loskutova, E., O'Brien, C., Loskutov, I., & Loughman, J. (2019). Nutritional supplementation in the treatment of glaucoma: A systematic review. *Survey of Ophthalmology*, *64*(2), 195–216. Available from https://doi.org/10.1016/j.survophthal.2018.09.005, http://www.sciencedirect.com/science/journal/00396257.

Lykkesfeldt, J., Michels, A. J., & Frei, B. (2014). Vitamin C. *Advances in Nutrition*, *5*(1), 16–18. Available from https://doi.org/10.3945/an.113.005157, http://advances.nutrition.org/content/5/1/16.full.pdf.

Magdalena Radomska-Leśniewska, D., Bałan, B. J., & Skopiński, P. (2017). Angiogenesis modulation by exogenous antioxidants. *Central European Journal of Immunology*, *42*(4), 370–376. Available from https://doi.org/10.5114/ceji.2017.72804.

Maiuolo, J., Bulotta, R. M., Oppedisano, F., Bosco, F., Scarano, F., Nucera, S., Guarnieri, L., Ruga, S., Macri, R., Caminiti, R., Musolino, V., Gliozzi, M., Carresi, C., Cardamone, A., Coppoletta, A., Nicita, M., Carnevali, A., Scorcia, V., & Mollace, V. (2023). Potential properties of natural nutraceuticals and antioxidants in age-related eye disorders. *Life (Chicago, Ill.: 1978)*, *13*(1). Available from https://doi.org/10.3390/life13010077, http://www.mdpi.com/journal/life/.

Manikandan, R., Thiagarajan, R., Goutham, G., Arumugam, M., Beulaja, M., Rastrelli, L., Skalicka-Woźniak, K., Habtemariam, S., Orhan, I. E., Nabavi, S. F., & Nabavi, S. M. (2016). Zeaxanthin and ocular health, from bench to bedside. *Fitoterapia*, *109*, 58–66. Available from https://doi.org/10.1016/j.fitote.2015.12.009, http://www.elsevier.com/locate/fitote.

Medori, M. C., Naureen, Z., Dhuli, K., Placidi, G., Falsini, B., & Bertelli, M. (2022). Dietary supplements in retinal diseases, glaucoma, and other ocular conditions. *Journal of Preventive Medicine and Hygiene*, *63*(2), E189. Available from https://doi.org/10.15167/2421-4248/jpmh2022.63.2S3.2760.

Meyer, B. J., Mann, N. J., Lewis, J. L., Milligan, G. C., Sinclair, A. J., & Howe, P. R. C. (2003). Dietary intakes and food sources of omega-6 and omega-3 polyunsaturated fatty acids. *Lipids*, *38*(4), 391–398, American Oil Chemists Society Australia. Available from https://doi.org/10.1007/s11745-003-1074-0, http://www.springerlink.com/content/0024-4201.

Miles, M. V. (2007). The uptake and distribution of coenzyme Q(10). *Mitochondrion*, *7*, S72. Available from https://doi.org/10.1016/j.mito.2007.02.012.

Miljanović, B., Trivedi, K. A., Dana, M. R., Gilbard, J. P., Buring, J. E., & Schaumberg, D. A. (2005). Relation between dietary n-3 and n-6 fatty acids and clinically diagnosed dry eye syndrome in women. *American Journal of Clinical Nutrition*, *82*(4), 887–893. Available from https://doi.org/10.1093/ajcn/82.4.887, http://www.ajcn.org/contents-by-date.2005.shtml.

Miranda, M., & Romero, F. J. (2019). Antioxidants and retinal diseases. *Antioxidants*, *8*(12), 604. Available from https://doi.org/10.3390/antiox8120604.

Mitra, S., Rauf, A., Tareq, A. M., Jahan, S., Emran, T. B., Shahriar, T. G., Dhama, K., Alhumaydhi, F. A., Aljohani, A. S. M., Rebezov, M., Uddin, M. S., Jeandet, P., Shah, Z. A., Shariati, M. A., & Rengasamy, K. R. R. (2021). Potential health benefits of carotenoid lutein: An updated review. *Food and Chemical Toxicology*, *154*112328. Available from https://doi.org/10.1016/j.fct.2021.112328.

Mohamadpour, A. H., Ayati, Z., Parizadeh, M. R., Rajbai, O., & Hosseinzadeh, H. (2013). Safety evaluation of crocin (a constituent of saffron) tablets in healthy volunteers. *Iranian Journal of Basic Medical Sciences*, *16*(1), 39–46. Available from http://www.mums.ac.ir/shares/basic_medical/basicmedjou/2013/saf/a4.pdf, Iran.

Nakajima, E., Hammond, K. B., Shearer, T. R., & Azuma, M. (2014). Activation of the mitochondrial caspase pathway and subsequent calpain activation in monkey RPE cells cultured under zinc depletion. *Eye (Basingstoke)*, *28*(1), 85–92. Available from https://doi.org/10.1038/eye.2013.239, http://www.nature.com/eye/index.html.

Nam, K. N., Park, Y. M., Jung, H. J., Lee, J. Y., Min, B. D., Park, S. U., Jung, W. S., Cho, K. H., Park, J. H., Kang, I., Hong, J. W., & Lee, E. H. (2010). Anti-inflammatory effects of crocin and crocetin in rat brain microglial cells. *European Journal of Pharmacology*, *648*(1-3), 110–116. Available from https://doi.org/10.1016/j.ejphar.2010.09.003.

Nebbioso, M., Franzone, F., Greco, A., Gharbiya, M., Bonfiglio, V., & Polimeni, A. (2021). Recent advances and disputes about curcumin in retinal diseases. *Clinical Ophthalmology*, *15*, 2553–2571. Available from https://doi.org/10.2147/OPTH.S306706, https://www.dovepress.com/getfile.php?fileID = 70708.

Newsome, D. A. (2008). A randomized, prospective, placebo-controlled clinical trial of a novel zinc-monocysteine compound in age-related macular degeneration. *Current Eye Research*, *33*(7), 591–598. Available from https://doi.org/10.1080/02713680802178437.

Ng, A., Woods, J., Jahn, T., Jones, L. W., & Sullivan Ritter, J. (2022). Effect of a novel omega-3 and omega-6 fatty acid supplement on dry eye disease: A 3-month randomized controlled trial. *Optometry and Vision Science*, *99*(1), 67–75. Available from https://doi.org/10.1097/opx.0000000000001826.

Nita, M., & Grzybowski, A. (2016). The role of the reactive oxygen species and oxidative stress in the pathomechanism of the age-related ocular diseases and other pathologies of the anterior and posterior eye segments in adults. *Oxidative Medicine and Cellular Longevity*, *2016*. Available from https://doi.org/10.1155/2016/3164734, http://www.hindawi.com/journals/oximed/.

Nomi., Iwasaki-Kurashige., & Matsumoto. (2019). Therapeutic effects of anthocyanins for vision and eye health. *Molecules (Basel, Switzerland)*, *24*(18), 3311. Available from https://doi.org/10.3390/molecules24183311.

Ogawa, K., Kuse, Y., Tsuruma, K., Kobayashi, S., Shimazawa, M., & Hara, H. (2014). Protective effects of bilberry and lingonberry extracts against blue light-emitting diode light-induced retinal photoreceptor cell damage in vitro. *BMC Complementary and Alternative Medicine*, *14*. Available from https://doi.org/10.1186/1472-6882-14-120, http://www.biomedcentral.com/1472-6882/14/120.

Ohguro, H., Ohguro, I., Katai, M., & Tanaka, S. (2012). Two-year randomized, placebo-controlled study of black currant anthocyanins on visual field in glaucoma. *Ophthalmologica. Journal International d'ophtalmologie. International Journal of Ophthalmology. Zeitschrift fur Augenheilkunde*, *228*(1), 26–35. Available from https://doi.org/10.1159/000335961.

Olale, K., Walyambillah, W., Mohammed, S. A., Sila, A., & Shepherd, K. (2019). FTIR-DRIFTS-based prediction of β-carotene, α-tocopherol and l-ascorbic acid in mango (Mangifera indica L.) fruit pulp. *SN Applied Sciences*, *1*(3). Available from https://doi.org/10.1007/s42452-019-0297-7, http://springer.com/snas.

Ordoñez-Santos, L. E., & Ledezma-Realpe, D. P. (2013). Lycopene concentration and physico-chemical properties of tropical fruits. *Food and Nutrition Sciences*, *04*(07), 758–762. Available from https://doi.org/10.4236/fns.2013.47097.

Otsuka, T., Shimazawa, M., Nakanishi, T., Ohno, Y., Inoue, Y., Tsuruma, K., Ishibashi, T., & Hara, H. (2013). The protective effects of a dietary carotenoid, astaxanthin, against light-induced retinal damage. *Journal of Pharmacological Sciences*, *123*(3), 209–218. Available from https://doi.org/10.1254/jphs.13066FP, https://www.jstage.jst.go.jp/article/jphs/123/3/123_13066FP/_pdf.

Ozawa, Y., Kawashima, M., Inoue, S., Inagaki, E., Suzuki, A., Ooe, E., Kobayashi, S., & Tsubota, K. (2015). Bilberry extract supplementation for preventing eye fatigue in video display terminal workers. *The Journal of nutrition, health and aging*, *19*(5), 548–554. Available from https://doi.org/10.1007/s12603-014-0573-6.

Parisi, V., Tedeschi, M., Gallinaro, G., Varano, M., Saviano, S., & Piermarocchi, S. (2008). Carotenoids and antioxidants in age-related maculopathy Italian study. Multifocal electroretinogram modifications after 1 year. *Ophthalmology*, *115*(2), 324. Available from https://doi.org/10.1016/j.ophtha.2007.05.029, http://www.elsevier.com/locate/ophtha.

Pastor-Valero, M. (2013). Fruit and vegetable intake and vitamins C and e are associated with a reduced prevalence of cataract in a Spanish Mediterranean population. *BMC Ophthalmology*, *13*(1). Available from https://doi.org/10.1186/1471-2415-13-52.

Pazdro, R., & Burgess, J. R. (2010). The role of vitamin E and oxidative stress in diabetes complications. *Mechanisms of Ageing and Development*, *131*(4), 276–286. Available from https://doi.org/10.1016/j.mad.2010.03.005.

Perry, A., Rasmussen, H., & Johnson, E. J. (2009). Xanthophyll (lutein, zeaxanthin) content in fruits, vegetables and corn and egg products. *Journal of Food Composition and Analysis*, *22*(1), 9–15. Available from https://doi.org/10.1016/j.jfca.2008.07.006.

Piyarach K. Nipawan K. Chadapon C. Daluwan S. Kunjana R. 2020 Effect of Drying on β-Carotene, α Carotene, Lutein and Zeaxanthin Content in Vegetables and Its Application for Vegetable Seasoning. E3S Web of Conferences 141 EDP Sciences Thailand http://www.e3s-conferences.org/10.1051/e3sconf/202014102007.

Post, M., Lubiński, W., Lubiński, J., Krzystolik, K., Baszuk, P., Muszyńska, M., & Marciniak, W. (2018). Serum selenium levels are associated withage-related cataract. *Annals of Agricultural and Environmental Medicine*, *25*(3), 443–448. Available from https://doi.org/10.26444/aaem/90886, http://www.aaem.pl/pdf-90886-29055?filename = Serum%20selenium%20levels%20are.pdf.

Pritwani, R., & Mathur, P. (2017). β-Carotene content of some commonly consumed vegetables and fruits available in Delhi, India. *Journal of Nutrition & Food Sciences*, *07*(05). Available from https://doi.org/10.4172/2155-9600.1000625.

Rashid, S., Jin, Y., Ecoiffier, T., Barabino, S., Schaumberg, D. A., & Dana, M. R. (2008). Topical omega-3 and omega-6 fatty acids for treatment of dry eye. *Archives of Ophthalmology*, *126*(2), 219–225. Available from https://doi.org/10.1001/archophthalmol.2007.61, http://archopht.ama-assn.org/cgi/reprint/126/2/219, United States.

Rasmussen, H. M., & Johnson, E. J. (2013). Nutrients for the aging eye. *Clinical Interventions in Aging*, *8*, 741–748. Available from https://doi.org/10.2147/CIA.S45399, http://www.dovepress.com/getfile.php?fileID = 16469, United States.

Ravindran, R. D., Vashist, P., Gupta, S. K., Young, I. S., Maraini, G., Camparini, M., Jayanthi, R., John, N., Fitzpatrick, K. E., Chakravarthy, U., Ravilla, T. D., & Fletcher, A. E. (2011). Inverse association of vitamin C with cataract in older people in India. *Ophthalmology*, *118*(10), 1958. Available from https://doi.org/10.1016/j.ophtha.2011.03.016, http://www.elsevier.com/locate/ophtha.

Rein, D. B., Wittenborn, J. S., Zhang, P., Sublett, F., Lamuda, P. A., Lundeen, E. A., & Saaddine, J. (2022). The economic burden of vision loss and blindness in the United States. *Ophthalmology*, *129*(4), 369–378. Available from https://doi.org/10.1016/j.ophtha.2021.09.010, http://www.elsevier.com/locate/ophtha.

dos Reis, L. C. R., de Oliveira, V. R., Hagen, M. E. K., Jablonski, A., FlÔres, S. H., & de Oliveira Rios, A. (2015). Carotenoids, flavonoids, chlorophylls, phenolic compounds and antioxidant activity in fresh and cooked broccoli (Brassica oleracea var. Avenger) and cauliflower (Brassica oleracea var. Alphina F1). *LWT*, *63*(1), 177–183. Available from https://doi.org/10.1016/j.lwt.2015.03.089, https://www.journals.elsevier.com/lwt.

Ross, A. C., Caballero, B., Cousins, R. J., Tucker, K. L., & Ziegler, T. R. (2012). *Modern nutrition in health and disease: Eleventh edition. Modern Nutrition in Health and Disease: Eleventh Edition* (pp. 1–1616). United States: Wolters Kluwer Health Adis (ESP). Available from http://www.lww.com/Product/9781605474618.

Rossino, M. G., & Casini, G. (2019). Nutraceuticals for the treatment of diabetic retinopathy. *Nutrients*, *11*(4). Available from https://doi.org/10.3390/nu11040771, https://www.mdpi.com/2072-6643/11/4/771/pdf.

Rostamabadi, H., Falsafi, S. R., & Jafari, S. M. (2019). Nanoencapsulation of carotenoids within lipid-based nanocarriers. *Journal of Controlled Release*, *298*, 38–67. Available from https://doi.org/10.1016/j.jconrel.2019.02.005, http://www.elsevier.com/locate/jconrel.

Sajovic, J., Meglič, A., Glavač, D., Markelj, Š., Hawlina, M., & Fakin, A. (2022). The role of vitamin A in retinal diseases. *International Journal of Molecular Sciences*, *23*(3), 1014. Available from https://doi.org/10.3390/ijms23031014.

Sato, E. A., Ohtake, Y., Shinoda, K., Mashima, Y., & Kimura, I. (2006). Decreased blood flow at neuroretinal rim of optic nerve head corresponds with visual field deficit in eyes with normal tension glaucoma. *Graefe's Archive for Clinical and Experimental Ophthalmology*, *244*(7), 795–801. Available from https://doi.org/10.1007/s00417-005-0177-2.

Schuchardt, J., Schneider, I., Meyer, H., Neubronner, J., Von Schacky, C., & Hahn, A. (2011). Incorporation of EPA and DHA into plasma phospholipids in response to different omega-3 fatty acid formulations - A comparative bioavailability study of fish oil vs. krill oil. *Lipids in Health and Disease*, *10*. Available from https://doi.org/10.1186/1476-511X-10-145.

Senthilkumari, S., Talwar, B., Dharmalingam, K., Ravindran, R. D., Jayanthi, R., Sundaresan, P., Saravanan, C., Young, I. S., Dangour, A. D., & Fletcher, A. E. (2014). Polymorphisms in sodium-dependent vitamin C transporter genes and plasma, aqueous humor and lens nucleus ascorbate concentrations in an ascorbate depleted setting. *Experimental Eye Research*, *124*, 24–30. Available from https://doi.org/10.1016/j.exer.2014.04.022, http://www.elsevier.com/inca/publications/store/6/2/2/8/2/7/index.htt.

Shaikh, S. (2022). *Sources and health benefits of functional food components*. IntechOpen. Available from 10.5772/intechopen.104091.

Shen, F., Chen, B., Danias, J., Lee, K. C., Lee, H., Su, Y., Podos, S. M., & Mittag, T. W. (2004). Glutamate-induced glutamine synthetase expression in retinal Müller cells after short-term ocular hypertension in the rat. *Investigative Ophthalmology and Visual Science*, *45*(9), 3107–3112. Available from https://doi.org/10.1167/iovs.03-0948.

Shui, Y. B., Holekamp, N. M., Kramer, B. C., Crowley, J. R., Wilkins, M. A., Chu, F., Malone, P. E., Mangers, S. J., Hou, J. H., Siegfried, C. J., & Beebe, D. C. (2009). The gel state of the vitreous and ascorbate-dependent oxygen consumption. *Archives of Ophthalmology*, *127*(4), 475–482. Available from https://doi.org/10.1001/archophthalmol.2008.621, http://archopht.ama-assn.org/cgi/reprint/127/4/475, United States.

Sideri, O., Tsaousis, K. T., Li, H. J., Viskadouraki, M., & Tsinopoulos, I. T. (2019). The potential role of nutrition on lens pathology: A systematic review and meta-analysis. *Survey of Ophthalmology*, *64*(5), 668–678. Available from https://doi.org/10.1016/j.survophthal.2019.03.003, http://www.sciencedirect.com/science/journal/00396257.

Sparrow, J. R. (2016). Vitamin A-aldehyde adducts: AMD risk and targeted therapeutics. *Proceedings of the National Academy of Sciences of the United States of America*, *113*(17), 4564–4569. Available from https://doi.org/10.1073/pnas.1600474113, http://www.pnas.org/content/113/17/4564.full.pdf.

Stiles, L. I., Ferrao, K., & Mehta, K. J. (2024). Role of zinc in health and disease. *Clinical and Experimental Medicine*, *24*(1). Available from https://doi.org/10.1007/s10238-024-01302-6, https://www.springer.com/journal/10238.

Subczynski, W. K., Wisniewska, A., & Widomska, J. (2010). Location of macular xanthophylls in the most vulnerable regions of photoreceptor outer-segment membranes. *Archives of Biochemistry and Biophysics*, *504*(1), 61–66. Available from https://doi.org/10.1016/j.abb.2010.05.015.

Suwanaruang, T. (2016). Analyzing lycopene content in fruits. *Agriculture and Agricultural Science Procedia*, *11*, 46–48. Available from https://doi.org/10.1016/j.aaspro.2016.12.008.

Szewczyk, K., Chojnacka, A., & Górnicka, M. (2021). Tocopherols and tocotrienols—bioactive dietary compounds. *International Journal of Molecular Sciences*, *22*(12).

Tamaddonfard, E., Farshid, A. A., Eghdami, K., Samadi, F., & Erfanparast, A. (2013). Comparison of the effects of crocin, safranal and diclofenac on local inflammation and inflammatory pain responses induced by carrageenan in rats. *Pharmacological Reports*, *65*(5), 1272–1280. Available from https://doi.org/10.1016/S1734-1140(13)71485-3, http://www.if-pan.krakow.pl/pjp/pdf/2013/5_1272.pdf.

Tan, J. S. L., Wang, J. J., Flood, V., Rochtchina, E., Smith, W., & Mitchell, P. (2008). Dietary antioxidants and the long-term incidence of age-related macular degeneration. The Blue Mountains Eye Study. *Ophthalmology*, *115*(2), 334–341. Available from https://doi.org/10.1016/j.ophtha.2007.03.083.

Teo, Z. L., Tham, Y. C., Yu, M., Chee, M. L., Rim, T. H., Cheung, N., Bikbov, M. M., Wang, Y. X., Tang, Y., Lu, Y., Wong, I. Y., Ting, D. S. W., Tan, G. S. W., Jonas, J. B., Sabanayagam, C., Wong, T. Y., & Cheng, C. Y. (2021). Global prevalence of diabetic retinopathy and projection of burden through 2045: Systematic review and meta-analysis. *Ophthalmology*, *128*(11), 1580–1591. Available from https://doi.org/10.1016/j.ophtha.2021.04.027, http://www.elsevier.com/locate/ophtha.

Tezel, G. (2006). Oxidative stress in glaucomatous neurodegeneration: Mechanisms and consequences. *Progress in Retinal and Eye Research*, *25*(5), 490–513. Available from https://doi.org/10.1016/j.preteyeres.2006.07.003.

Tham, Y. C., Li, X., Wong, T. Y., Quigley, H. A., Aung, T., & Cheng, C. Y. (2014). Global prevalence of glaucoma and projections of glaucoma burden through 2040: A systematic review and meta-analysis. *Ophthalmology*, *121*(11), 2081–2090. Available from https://doi.org/10.1016/j.ophtha.2014.05.013, http://www.elsevier.com/locate/ophtha.

Theodoropoulou, S., Samoli, E., Theodossiadis, P. G., Papathanassiou, M., Lagiou, A., Lagiou, P., & Tzonou, A. (2014). Diet and cataract: A case-control study. *International Ophthalmology*, *34*(1), 59–68. Available from https://doi.org/10.1007/s10792-013-9795-6, http://www.wkap.nl/journalhome.htm/0165-5701.

Ugarte, M., & Osborne, N. N. (2014). Recent advances in the understanding of the role of zinc in ocular tissues. *Metallomics*, *6*(2), 189–200. Available from https://doi.org/10.1039/c3mt00291h, United Kingdom.

Walter, S. D., Gronert, K., McClellan, A. L., Levitt, R. C., Sarantopoulos, K. D., & Galor, A. (2016). ω-3 tear film lipids correlate with clinical measures of dry eye. *Investigative Ophthalmology and Visual Science.*, *57*(6), 2472–2478. Available from https://doi.org/10.1167/iovs.16-19131, http://iovs.arvojournals.org/data/Journals/IOVS/935270/i1552-5783-57-6-2472.pdf.

Wang, P., Chin, E. K., & Almeida, D. (2021). Antioxidants for the treatment of retinal disease: Summary of recent evidence. *Clinical Ophthalmology*, *15*, 1621–1628. Available from https://doi.org/10.2147/OPTH.S307009, https://www.dovepress.com/getfile.php?fileID = 68600.

Wang, S. Y., Singh, K., & Lin, S. C. (2013). Glaucoma and vitamins A, C, and e supplement intake and serum levels in a population-based sample of the United States. *Eye (Basingstoke)*, *27*(4), 487–494. Available from https://doi.org/10.1038/eye.2013.10, http://www.nature.com/eye/index.html.

Wegner, A., & Khoramnia, R. (2011). Cataract is a self-defence reaction to protect the retina from oxidative damage. *Medical Hypotheses*, *76*(5), 741–744. Available from https://doi.org/10.1016/j.mehy.2011.02.013.

Weigert, G., Kaya, S., Pemp, B., Sacu, S., Lasta, M., Werkmeister, R. M., Dragostinoff, N., Simader, C., Garhöfer, G., Schmidt-Erfurth, U., & Schmetterer, L. (2011). Effects of lutein supplementation on macular pigment optical density and visual acuity in patients with age-related macular degeneration. *Investigative Opthalmology & Visual Science*, *52*(11), 8174. Available from https://doi.org/10.1167/iovs.11-7522.

Weikel, K. A., Chiu, C. J., & Taylor, A. (2012). Nutritional modulation of age-related macular degeneration. *Molecular Aspects of Medicine*, *33*(4), 318–375. Available from https://doi.org/10.1016/j.mam.2012.03.005.

Wen Lee, H., Bi, X., & Jeyakumar Henry, C. (2022). Carotenoids, tocopherols and phylloquinone content of 26 green leafy vegetables commonly consumed in Southeast Asia. *Food Chemistry*, *385*132729. Available from https://doi.org/10.1016/j.foodchem.2022.132729.

WHO. (2019). *World report on vision*. World Health Organization. Available from https://www.who.int/publications/i/item/world-report-on-vision.

WHO. (2022). *Ageing and health*. World Health Organization. Available from https://www.who.int/news-room/fact-sheets/detail/ageing-and-health.

WHO. (2023). *Blindness and vision impairment*. Global Data on Visual Impairments. Available from https://www.who.int/news-room/fact-sheets/detail/blindness-and-visual-impairment.

Wiseman, E. M., Bar-El Dadon, S., & Reifen, R. (2017). The vicious cycle of vitamin a deficiency: A review. *Critical Reviews in Food Science and Nutrition*, *57*(17), 3703–3714. Available from https://doi.org/10.1080/10408398.2016.1160362, http://www.tandf.co.uk/journals/titles/10408398.asp.

Wittenborn, J. S., Zhang, X., Feagan, C. W., Crouse, W. L., Shrestha, S., Kemper, A. R., Hoerger, T. J., & Saaddine, J. B. (2013). The economic burden of vision loss and eye disorders among the united states population younger than 40 years. *Ophthalmology*, *120*(9), 1728–1735. Available from https://doi.org/10.1016/j.ophtha.2013.01.068.

Wolf, G. (2001). The discovery of the visual function of vitamin A. *The Journal of Nutrition*, *131*(6), 1647–1650. Available from https://doi.org/10.1093/jn/131.6.1647.

Xu, B., Liu, Z., Zhao, J., & Yu, Z. (2023). Selenium intake help prevent age-related cataract formation: Evidence from NHANES 2001-2008. *Frontiers in Nutrition*, *10*.

Yang, X., Chen, H., Zhang, T., Yin, X., Man, J., He, Q., & Lu, M. (2021). Global, regional, and national burden of blindness and vision loss due to common eye diseases along with its attributable risk factors from 1990 to 2019: a systematic analysis from the global burden of disease study 2019. *Aging*, *13*(15), 19614–19642. Available from https://doi.org/10.18632/aging.203374, http://www.impactaging.com/index.html.

Yuki, K., Murat, D., Kimura, I., Ohtake, Y., & Tsubota, K. (2010). Reduced-serum vitamin C and increased uric acid levels in normal-tension glaucoma. *Graefe's Archive for Clinical and Experimental Ophthalmology*, *248*(2), 243–248. Available from https://doi.org/10.1007/s00417-009-1183-6.

Zhang, A. C., Singh, S., Craig, J. P., & Downie, L. E. (2020). Omega-3 fatty acids and eye health: Opinions and self-reported practice behaviors of optometrists in Australia and New Zealand. *Nutrients*, *12*(4), 1179. Available from https://doi.org/10.3390/nu12041179.

Zhang, Y., Jiang, W., Xie, Z., Wu, W., & Zhang, D. (2015). Vitamin E and risk of age-related cataract: A meta-analysis. *Public Health Nutrition*, *18*(15), 2804–2814. Available from https://doi.org/10.1017/S1368980014003115, http://journals.cambridge.org/PHN.

Zheng, J., & Xiao, H. (2022). *The effects of food processing on food components and their health functions, volume II. Frontiers Research Topics*. Frontiers Media SA. Available from 10.3389/978-2-83250-833-6.

Zhu, X., Zhang, S., Chang, R., & Lu, Y. (2017). New cataract markers: Mechanisms of disease. *Clinica Chimica Acta*, *472*, 41–45. Available from https://doi.org/10.1016/j.cca.2017.07.010, http://www.elsevier.com/locate/clinchim.

Chapter 19

Functional foods for hair loss and alopecia

Sayna Zahedinia[1], Esila Bayar[2,3], Atefeh Karimidastjerd[1] and Zakir Showkat Khan[4,5]

[1]*Yildiz Technical University, Faculty of Chemical and Metallurgical Engineering, Food Engineering Department, Istanbul, Türkiye,* [2]*Faculty of Health Sciences, Nutrition and Dietetics Department, Istanbul Aydin University, Istanbul, Türkiye,* [3]*Faculty of Health Sciences, Nutrition and Dietetics Department, Hacettepe University, Sıhhiye, Ankara, Türkiye,* [4]*Department of Food Science & Technology, Guru Nanak Dev University, Amritsar, Punjab, India,* [5]*Department of Food Technology, School of Applied and Life Sciences, Uttaranchal University, Dehradun, Uttarakhand, India*

19.1 Introduction

Alopecia, commonly referred to as hair loss, can impact individuals across various age groups and backgrounds. There exist eight primary categories of hair loss, each presenting distinctive features and underlying causes. While prevalent, numerous instances are potentially reversible through appropriate treatment and attentive care. If you are experiencing hair loss, consulting with a healthcare provider can assist in identifying the specific type and devising a tailored plan to address your needs (Fang et al., 2024; Gordon et al., 2011; Pratt et al., 2017).

Hair is composed of protein, lipids, water, and various trace elements. However, the intricate process of hair growth demands ample energy and relies on an array of essential elements, including hormones, minerals, and vitamins. Insufficient quantities of any of these elements can potentially trigger hair loss. Nutrients essential for bodily functions are acquired through the digestion of food. Upon ingestion, food travels through the digestive tract where enzymes and gut bacteria break it down into basic components for absorption and utilization. Consequently, any disruptions in digestion can indirectly impact hair health and lead to hair loss (Hart et al., 2002; Morowitz et al., 2011; Rebello et al., 2017).

Alopecia areata (AA) is a common, clinically heterogeneous, immune-mediated, nonscarring hair loss disorder (Villasante et al., 2015). Androgenetic alopecia, also known as male pattern baldness, is the most common hair loss disorder, affecting up to 80% of men and up to 40% of women with Caucasian heritage (Giordano et al., 2017). Alopecia, the loss of hair on the scalp and/or body, is experienced by millions of people worldwide and can be a very debilitating condition (Dinkins et al., 2023). Alopecia areata (AA) is the most frequent localized nonscarring hair loss that can affect any hair-bearing skin (Mustafa et al., 2021). There are three major forms of AA progression: diffused loss of hair in well-defined patches (diffuse AA), total loss of hair from the scalp (alopecia totalis, AT), and complete loss of body hair (alopecia universalis, AU) (Ahn et al., 2021).

Recent studies on bioactive compounds effects on hair health and growth showed that these compounds can treat hair loss. According to these investigations, bioactive compounds can play a crucial role in hair follicle health as well as increase hair thickness, enhance hair cell proliferation, and regulate the expression of genes associated with the hair cycle (Abelan et al., 2022; Hwang et al., 2022; Khantham et al., 2023; Ruksiriwanich et al., 2022; Tenore et al., 2018; Zhou et al., 2018).

In addition to the benefits of bioactive compounds for hair, they can also control the proliferation and differentiation of stem cells, regulate Wnt/β-catenin and BMP signaling pathways, and protect hair cells from damage (Ferdousi et al., 2022; Kruger et al., 2016; Zhang, Li et al., 2021). In addition, some compounds exhibit antiinflammatory properties, stress-resistant effect, and can stimulate keratin expression, which helps maintain healthy hair growth (Parisi et al., 2018; Tenore et al., 2018). Additionally, the potential of bioactive compounds to promote wound healing, hair cell stress tolerance, and hair follicle regrowth was investigated and These compounds have been found to activate the Wnt signaling pathway, shield hair cells from damage, and inhibit enzymes like 5α-reductase, which is implicated in hair

Unleashing the Power of Functional Foods and Novel Bioactives. DOI: https://doi.org/10.1016/B978-0-443-28862-3.00019-4

loss (Fung et al., 2023; Jung, Jung et al., 2022; Ou et al., 2009; Zamani et al., 2022; Zhang, Li et al., 2021; Zhang et al., 2024). In this chapter, the bioactive compounds of different foods like Kombucha tea extract, Fermented Carica papaya L., flax and flaxseed oil, pumpkin seeds, grape seed oil, Rooibos and white tea, seaweeds, and anthocyanins have been mentioned as well as macro- and micronutritional and gut microbiome benefits and their functions on hair health highlighted.

19.2 Bioactive compounds

Bioactive compounds represent a diverse and potent category of molecules predominantly found in natural sources such as foods, plants, and medicinal herbs, exerting significant effects on biological systems beyond basic nutritional value (Banwo et al., 2021). These compounds, derived from a myriad of sources including grains, legumes, fruits, vegetables, and medicinal plants, are recognized for their pivotal physiological and metabolic functions, contributing to health benefits that encompass the prevention of chronic diseases, inflammation, and cancer (Kussmann et al., 2023). Their efficacy, intimately tied to bioavailability, involves complex processes of gastrointestinal absorption and cellular transport, highlighting the importance of their roles in managing and preventing disease (Ferreira et al., 2017).

The scientific community classifies bioactive compounds based on their origin and structural characteristics into principal categories: lipophilic compounds, such as essential oils and carotenoids, and hydrophilic compounds, notably polyphenols (Rashidinejad & Mahdi Jafari, 2020). This classification extends to include phytochemicals, zoochemicals, and microbial-derived compounds, each possessing distinct biochemical properties and health implications. For example, phytochemicals encompass subclasses such as flavonoids, phenolic acids, and tannins, whereas zoochemicals include entities like omega-3 fatty acids, acclaimed for their cardioprotective attributes (Chhikara et al., 2022; Granado-Lorencio & Hernández-Alvarez, 2016; Kayode et al., 2023).

The academic investigation into these compounds is driven by the imperative to understand their molecular interactions and biological impacts comprehensively (Singh et al., 2019). This involves rigorous methodologies for the extraction, isolation, and analysis of these compounds, followed by in vitro and in vivo assessments of their biological activities (Singh et al., 2019). The mechanisms through which bioactive compounds exert their effects are multifaceted, involving antioxidative, antiinflammatory, antimicrobial, and enzyme inhibitory actions, among others (Favela-González et al., 2020; Zengin et al., 2019). Notably, the antioxidative properties are primarily attributed to their ability to scavenge free radicals, mitigating oxidative stress and forestalling cellular damage (Favela-González et al., 2020).

Furthermore, research has highlighted the potential of bioactive compounds in dermatological applications, particularly in promoting hair growth and preventing hair loss (Tansathien et al., 2021). This exploration of herbal extracts as alternative treatments underscores the potential of bioactive compounds in supporting hair health (Rajput & Kumar, 2020).

19.2.1 Kombucha tea extract

Kombucha tea, a fermented beverage renowned for its rich chemical composition and health-promoting properties, has been the subject of increased scientific scrutiny due to its bioactive compounds (Antolak et al., 2021). The fermentation process, essential to Kombucha's production, involves a synbiotic culture of bacteria and yeasts (SCOBY), with acetic acid bacteria and lactic acid bacteria playing pivotal roles (Villarreal-Soto et al., 2018). This process not only enriches the tea with a diverse array of bioactive components, including minerals like potassium and manganese, vitamins such as E, K, and B, amino acids, and other fermentation-formed compounds, but also enhances its therapeutic efficacy (Bortolomedi et al., 2022; Martínez Leal et al., 2018).

Recent research has illuminated the potential health benefits of Kombucha tea extracts, underscoring their anticancer, antiinflammatory, and antioxidant capacities, alongside contributions to dermatological health, particularly in hair vitality (Alboreadi et al., 2022; Villarreal-Soto et al., 2019). Components such as cinnamaldehyde, eugenol, chlorogenic acid, and quercetin have been identified as key contributors to the antioxidant activity of Kombucha, a critical feature for its health-promoting attributes (Alboreadi et al., 2022). The antioxidant properties of Kombucha tea extracts are instrumental in safeguarding hair follicles against free radical damage, thus preventing hair loss and promoting healthy hair growth (Alboreadi et al., 2022; Herman & Herman, 2023).

Moreover, the antiinflammatory effects emerging from the fermentation process contribute to scalp health by alleviating irritation and diminishing inflammation, creating an optimized environment for hair follicles that supports hair growth and contributes to overall hair health (Antolak et al., 2021). The presence of polyphenols, vitamins, and minerals in Kombucha tea extracts, enhanced through fermentation, underlines their efficacy in promoting hair growth and maintaining hair health (Antolak et al., 2021; Bortolomedi et al., 2022).

19.2.2 Fermented *Carica papaya* L.

The tropical fruit *Carica papaya* L., widely recognized for its palatability, harbors a wealth of bioactive constituents, rendering it a significant subject of scientific scrutiny for its health-promoting attributes (Canini et al., 2007; Khadam et al., 2019). These bioactive entities, especially those derived from the fermented variant of *C. papaya* L., have captivated interest due to their prospective therapeutic merits. Analytical investigations employing gas chromatography–mass spectrometry have unearthed a spectrum of phenolic compounds within *C. papaya* L. leaves, evidencing the presence of bioactive components that endow papaya leaves with antioxidant capabilities (Leitão et al., 2022). Additionally, papaya peel showed significant DPPH radical scavenging activity by removing methanol, indicating its potential as a source of antioxidants (Elegbede & Lateef, 2019; Martial-Didier et al., 2017).

C. papaya L. is a repository of diverse pharmacologically active compounds such as proteolytic enzymes (papain and chymopapain), alkaloids, flavonoids, triterpenes, and organic acids, which are implicated in its wide-ranging pharmacological actions, including antiinflammatory, antioxidant, and antimicrobial properties (Chávez-Quintal et al., 2011). These attributes are further augmented by the seed extracts of C. papaya, which exhibit commendable antioxidant capacity, thereby underlining the significance of its bioactive compounds for health enhancement (Agada et al., 2020). Additionally, the antiangiogenic potential of *C. papaya* L. leaf extract, primarily through constituents like quercetin, ascorbic acid, and lycopene, posits a novel avenue for cancer therapy by inhibiting angiogenic receptors (Tayal et al., 2019).

The therapeutic potential of *C. papaya* L. extends beyond general health benefits to specifically fostering hair health through its rich assortment of bioactive compounds, including phenolic antioxidants, flavonoids, alkaloids, saponins, and tannins (Callixte et al., 2020; Dangi et al., 2023; Farooq, 2013). These ingredients not only have antioxidant and antidiabetic properties, but also anticancer properties, which are important for scalp health (Agada et al., 2020). The incorporation of phenolic compounds and carotenoids in *C. papaya* fruit suggests its utility as a natural pigment and antioxidant source (Rivera-Pastrana & Yahia, 2010; Velasco Arango et al., 2019). Fermentation processes have been acknowledged for augmenting the bioavailability and efficacy of *C. papaya*'s bioactive compounds, enhancing its nutraceutical and antioxidant profiles (Kadiri et al., 2016; Leitão et al., 2023). This fermented preparation is linked to the reactivation of the immune system and indirectly supports hair health by improving overall health (Barot, 2017; Fujita et al., 2017). Fig. 19.1 shows important bioactive compounds of papaya that help hair growth.

19.2.3 Seeds

19.2.3.1 Flax and flaxseed oil

Flax and its derivative, flaxseed oil, are renowned for their wealth of bioactive compounds, encompassing essential fatty acids, lignans, dietary fiber, phenolic compounds, flavonoids, and cyclolinopeptides, which collectively confer a myriad of health advantages. Specifically, flaxseed is celebrated for its abundant omega-3 fatty acids, lignans such as secoisolariciresinol diglucoside (SDG), and mucilage, which are instrumental in its antioxidant and antiinflammatory properties (Alaswad & Krishnan, 2016). These compounds, alongside phenolic acids, flavonoids, and lignins, substantially bolster flaxseed's

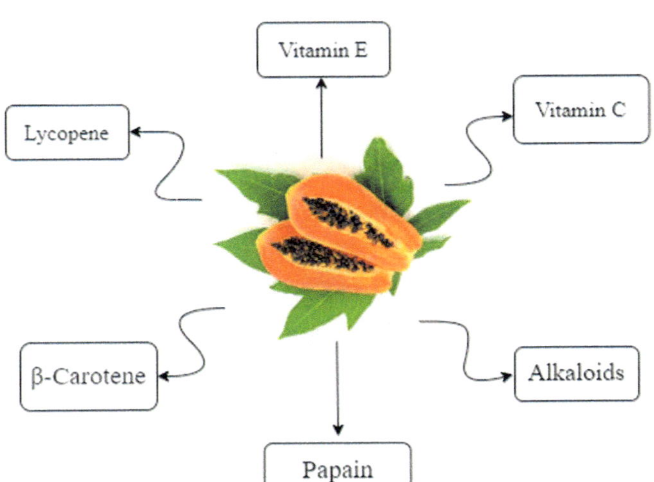

FIGURE 19.1 Bioactive compounds of papaya that help to hair growth.

antioxidant efficacy (Bhushana Daddala et al., 2022; Multescu et al., 2022), positing it as a pivotal agent in the prevention of chronic ailments, including cancer, diabetes, and cardiovascular diseases (Bhushana Daddala et al., 2022).

In parallel, flaxseed oil's bioactive components, notably alpha-linolenic acid, lignans, and proteins, have been linked to anticancer properties and the suppression of pro-inflammatory mediators, highlighting its potential in inflammation reduction (Yang et al., 2021). The antibacterial efficacy of flaxseed against pathogens like Streptococcus mutans further accentuates its health-promoting capabilities (Sultana et al., 2022). Consequently, the functional properties and health benefits of flaxseed and flaxseed oil's bioactive compounds render them highly sought-after food ingredients, with potential applications spanning food science, medicine, and materials science (Kumari et al., 2024; Waszkowiak & Mikołajczak, 2020).

Pertaining to hair health, the bioactive components of flax and flaxseed oil, rich in essential fatty acids, lignans, and dietary fiber, have been associated with various health benefits, including mitigation of cardiovascular disease, diabetes, cancer, and autoimmune disorders (Goyal et al., 2014). These benefits indirectly influence hair health by promoting overall well-being. Flaxseed oil's capacity to alleviate oxidative stress and inflammation, alongside the cardiovascular and antiinflammatory merits of alpha-linolenic acid, plays a critical role in fostering a healthy scalp environment (Fale et al., 2022). The lignans within flaxseed oil also contribute to reducing cancer risk and thwarting cellular transformations leading to cancer (Adolphe et al., 2010; Nowak & Jeziorek, 2023). Fig. 19.2 shows important bioactive compounds of flaxseed that help hair growth.

19.2.3.2 Pumpkin seeds

Pumpkin seeds are a wealthy source of bioactive compounds that offer different wellbeing benefits. These bioactive compounds incorporate tocopherols, polyunsaturated fatty acids, phytosterols, unsaturated fatty acids, carotenoids, polyphenols, and cancer prevention agents (Batool et al., 2022; Hussain, Kausar, Sehar, et al., 2022). Pumpkin seed oil, extracted from pumpkin seeds, is especially known for its utilitarian properties and potential nutraceutical applications due to its different bioactive compounds (Bardaa et al., 2016). The main sterols in pumpkin seed oil are Δ7,22,25-stigmastatrienol, Δ7,25-stigmastadienol, and spinasterol, whereas triterpenic compounds are more abundant in the alcoholic fraction (Montesano et al., 2018). Furthermore, pumpkin seed oil may be a wealthy source of unsaturated greasy acids, polyphenols, carotenoids, and other antioxidant compounds (Šamec et al., 2022; Singh & Kumar, 2023).

Among the bioactive substances found throughout different pumpkin parts that are responsible for their health benefits are carotenoids, lutein, zeaxanthin, vitamin E, ascorbic acid, phytosterols, selenium, and linoleic acid (Batool et al., 2022; Kaur et al., 2019). The bioactive compounds found in pumpkin seeds and their byproducts have antioxidant, antimicrobial, and even health-promoting qualities. Additionally, the health benefits of pumpkin seeds are attributed to the presence of phenolic compounds like quercetin, kaempferol, luteolin, caffeic acid, vanillic acid, sinapinic acid, ferulic acid, apigenin, and protocatechuic acid (Akomolafe et al., 2021; Leichtweis et al., 2022; Pateiro et al., 2023).

Pumpkin seed bioactive compounds have been linked to a variety of health-promoting effects, including the ability to heal wounds and exhibit antioxidant, antihyperglycemic, and antihyperlipidemic properties (Hussain, Kausar, Jamil, et al., 2022; Tzortzakis et al., 2018). The presence of essential fatty acids, carotenoids, tocopherols, and polyphenols in pumpkin seeds highlights their potential as functional foods with beneficial effects on human health (Lestari & Meiyanto, 2018; Rohman & Irnawati, 2019).

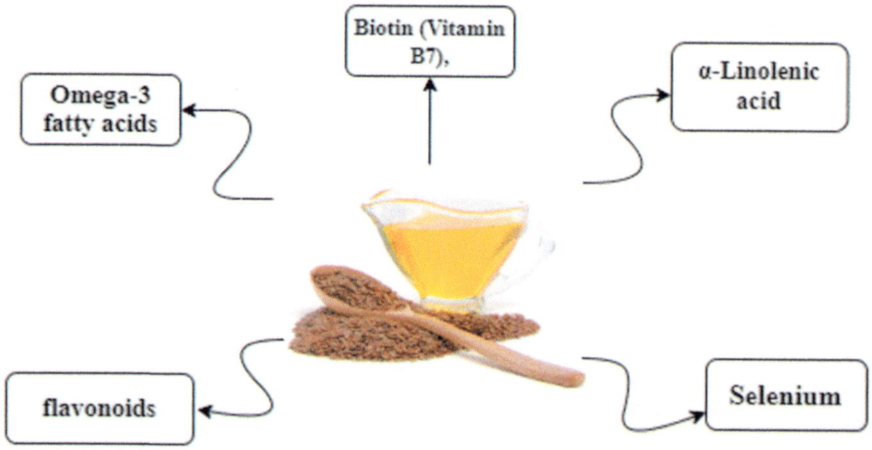

FIGURE 19.2 Bioactive compounds of flaxseed that help to hair growth.

The bioactive compounds present in pumpkin seeds offer numerous benefits for hair health. Pumpkin seeds are rich in various nutrients and bioactive components that have been associated with promoting overall well-being and potentially supporting hair health. Pumpkin seed oil, in particular, has been recognized for its health benefits, including its antioxidant properties (Šamec et al., 2022). These antioxidants can help combat oxidative stress, which is a common factor that can affect hair health. Additionally, pumpkin seeds contain essential fatty acids, proteins, and minerals that are essential for maintaining healthy hair. The high potassium content and low salt content in pumpkin seeds have been linked to substantial therapeutic benefits, including enhancing cardiovascular health and supporting cell defense mechanisms (Aziz et al., 2023). Furthermore, the presence of bioactive compounds in pumpkin seeds, such as phytosterols, may contribute to their antioxidant properties, which can help protect hair follicles from damage and promote scalp health (Rezig et al., 2022).

19.2.3.3 Grape seed oil

Grape seed oil is rich in bioactive compounds and is known for its many health benefits and functional benefits. Tocopherols, phytosterols, unsaturated fatty acids, carotenoids, phenols, and antioxidants are some of these products. Grape seed oil is especially valuable for its quality, as linoleic acid constitutes 70% of all fatty acids and unsaturated fatty acids constitute 90% (Assumpção et al., 2016; Matthäus, 2008). Tocopherols and tocotrienols, two forms of vitamin E that are abundant in grape seed oil, add to the antioxidant qualities of the oil (de Menezes et al., 2023; Wen et al., 2016). Studies have shown the presence of phenolic compounds in grape seed oil, such as gallic acid, epicatechin, catechin, proanthocyanidins, and procyanidins, which contribute to its high antioxidant capacity (Bjelica et al., 2019). Grape seed oil also contains phytosterols, known for their potential health benefits, including cholesterol-lowering effects (Crews et al., 2006). The bioactive compounds in grape seed oil have been associated with antimicrobial properties, making it a potential candidate for applications in medicine and food preservation (Garavaglia et al., 2016b).

According to recent studies, grape seed oil is an important source of bioactive compounds that have many benefits for hair (Nunes et al., 2017). Rich in phenolic compounds such as flavonoids, carotenoids, phenolic acids, tannins, and stilbenes, grape seed oil exhibits antioxidant effects that can help combat oxidative stress, a common factor affecting hair health (Gitea et al., 2023; Spinei & Oroian, 2021). These antioxidants play a crucial role in protecting hair follicles from damage and promoting scalp health. Moreover, grape seed oil has been found to possess various beneficial properties for health, including antiinflammatory, cardioprotective, antimicrobial, and anticancer effects (Garavaglia et al., 2016).

Additionally, grape seed oil is rich in unsaturated fatty acids, especially linoleic acid and oleic acid, which are beneficial for cardiovascular and general health (Ebrahimi-Mameghani et al., 2020; Garavaglia et al., 2016; Juhaimi et al., 2017) (a). These fatty acids contribute to the oil's health benefits and may indirectly support hair health by promoting a healthy scalp environment. Furthermore, grape seed oil has been associated with improving insulin resistance and metabolic syndrome, indicating its potential in addressing underlying health conditions that may impact hair health (Gasmi et al., 2023; Puri et al., 2022; Zhou et al., 2022). The oil's composition, including high levels of vitamin E, unsaturated fatty acids, and phenolic compounds, makes it a promising candidate for promoting hair health and overall well-being (Zhou et al., 2022).

19.2.4 Rooibos and white tea

Rooibos, also known as red bush tea and white tea, both offer remarkable health benefits due to their unique bioactive compounds (Joubert & de Beer, 2012; Smit et al., 2022). Rooibos, originating from the South African Aspalathus linearis plant, is rich in a diverse spectrum of phytochemicals, including polyphenols, flavonoids, chalcones, and antioxidants (Smit et al., 2022). Notably, it contains aspalathin, a unique C-linked dihydrochalcone glucoside, which plays a significant role in its health benefits (Nehme et al., 2023). This compound, along with others found in rooibos, has been shown to offer therapeutic potential in managing type 2 diabetes mellitus, oxidative stress, and metabolic syndrome (Nehme et al., 2023). Additionally, these compounds have antioxidant, antiinflammatory, and cardioprotective properties, which have been linked to improvements in glucose metabolism, insulin sensitivity, and overall energy regulation (Krafczyk et al., 2009).

White tea, derived from the Camellia sinensis plant, is known for its high content of polyphenols, catechins, theanine, gamma-aminobutyric acid (GABA), and flavonoids (Joubert & de Beer, 2012). The minimal oxidation process in its production preserves these bioactive compounds, making white tea a potent antioxidant source with antiinflammatory and antimicrobial properties (Muller et al., 2018; Orlando et al., 2019). Research has suggested that white tea can offer significant cardiometabolic health benefits, including antiobesity properties and cardioprotective effects (Abiri et al., 2023; Yıldırım et al., 2020). Similar to rooibos, it has potential impacts on bone health and metabolic syndrome, demonstrating the ability to improve bone mineral density and regulate glucose metabolism (Abiri et al., 2023).

Both rooibos and white tea, through their rich arrays of bioactive compounds, present extensive health advantages (Tiedtke & Marks, 2002). These teas have been studied for their capacity to address conditions such as diabetes, cardiovascular health, and oxidative stress, contributing significantly to metabolic and overall well-being (Ajuwon et al., 2015). The unique components found in these teas, particularly aspalathin in rooibos and the synergistic blend of catechins, theanine, and flavonoids in white tea, underscore their potential in promoting health and preventing disease (Garnier & Shahidi, 2021; Muller et al., 2022).

White Rooibos bioactive compounds have shown potential in addressing hair loss concerns. Studies have indicated that Rooibos tea extracts can inhibit osteoclast formation and activity by attenuating NF-κB activity, demonstrating antiinflammatory properties that could be beneficial for hair health (Gebashe et al., 2022; Moosa et al., 2018). Additionally, the antioxidant activity of Rooibos tea extracts has been highlighted, suggesting a role in reducing oxidative stress, which is a contributing factor to hair loss (Akinfenwa et al., 1936). Research has explored the use of Rooibos extract in enhancing antioxidant activity, indicating its potential to combat oxidative stress that may impact hair follicles (Pengilly et al., 2008). The antioxidant properties of Rooibos tea could help protect hair follicles from damage and support overall hair health. Furthermore, investigations into the use of green Rooibos extract have shown potential health benefits, indicating a growing interest in the therapeutic properties of Rooibos compounds (Joubert & de Beer, 2012). The bioactive compounds in Rooibos tea, such as chalcones and polyphenols, have been associated with various health benefits, including antiinflammatory and antioxidant effects (Moosa et al., 2018). These properties could play a role in promoting scalp health and creating a favorable environment for hair growth. Additionally, the potential enhancement of antioxidant yield with fungal enzymes in Rooibos extract suggests a method to increase the beneficial compounds that could positively impact hair health (Pengilly et al., 2008).

White tea bioactive compounds have shown promise in addressing hair loss concerns. Studies have highlighted the potential benefits of bioactive compounds found in white tea, such as catechins and flavonoids, in promoting hair growth. These compounds possess antioxidant, antiinflammatory, and stress-inhibitory properties that can positively impact hair regrowth (Parisi et al., 2018). Additionally, the presence of oleic acid in tea seed oil, a major active compound in white tea, is believed to stimulate hair growth (Riangjanapatee et al., 2022). The bioactive compounds in white tea, including catechins, proanthocyanidins, and flavonols, contribute to its antioxidant activity, making it a valuable source of functional compounds with physiological properties (Zhang et al., 2017). These compounds have been associated with various health benefits, including the potential to mitigate bone loss and reduce the risk of osteoporotic fractures (Shen et al., 2011). Furthermore, the antiinflammatory and antioxidant effects of white tea bioactive compounds have been linked to their ability to influence hair growth (Park & Lee, 2021).

19.2.5 Seaweeds

Recent research underscores the significance of seaweeds as a reservoir of diverse bioactive compounds, including phenolics, fatty acids, pigments, alkaloids, flavonoids, and polysaccharides (Gan & Baroutian, 2022; Pandey et al., 2020; Sanjayasari et al., 2021; Zhong et al., 2020). These compounds, lauded for their antioxidant, antiinflammatory, and antimicrobial activities (Lomartire & Gonçalves, 2022; Sobuj et al., 2021), have been harnessed for various therapeutic and cosmetic applications. Notably, there is a growing body of evidence supporting the utility of these seaweed-derived bioactives in mitigating hair loss, a condition affecting a significant portion of the global population (Jesumani et al., 2019; Salehi et al., 2019).

The antioxidant properties of seaweed bioactives, particularly polyphenols and flavonoids, are crucial in combating oxidative stress in hair follicles, a known factor contributing to hair loss (Lomartire et al., 2021; Salehi et al., 2019).

Furthermore, seaweeds contain essential nutrients such as proteins with vital amino acids and polyunsaturated fatty acids, which are instrumental in nourishing the scalp and hair follicles (Lomartire et al., 2021). These nutrients enhance the moisture content and elasticity of hair strands, preventing breakage and encouraging the growth of strong, healthy hair (Lomartire et al., 2021).

The antiinflammatory effects of seaweed bioactives also play a significant role in maintaining scalp health. By alleviating inflammation and soothing the scalp, these compounds create an optimal environment for hair growth, thereby addressing one of the root causes of hair loss (Pangestuti et al., 2021). Additionally, the improvement in scalp blood circulation, attributed to these bioactive compounds, ensures that essential nutrients and oxygen are efficiently delivered to hair follicles, further supporting hair growth and vitality (Pangestuti et al., 2021).

Beyond direct hair health benefits, the protective and restorative effects of seaweed compounds on overall skin health, including antiphotoaging properties, contribute to a healthier scalp environment, which is foundational for preventing hair loss and promoting hair regeneration (Pangestuti et al., 2021).

19.2.6 Anthyocyanins

Anthocyanins, potent bioactive compounds prevalent in various botanical sources, have garnered research interest for their multifaceted benefits on human health, particularly in the context of hair vitality and scalp wellness (Gonçalves et al., 2021). These naturally occurring compounds are distinguished by their profound antioxidant capabilities, which have been posited to afford protection to hair follicles against oxidative stress, which is a predominant contributory factor in the etiology of hair loss. The oxidative stress defense mechanism is crucial as it counters the cellular damage in hair follicles, potentially decelerating the hair loss process (Gonçalves et al., 2021).

Recent investigations have illuminated the potential role of anthocyanins in mitigating the proliferation of metastatic cells, thereby underscoring a prospective utility in fostering scalp health and augmenting hair regrowth (Gonçalves et al., 2021). This property is particularly noteworthy as it not only suggests a preventive approach against scalp pathologies but also underscores a broader therapeutic potential in dermatological health, specifically in enhancing the microenvironment conducive for hair growth (Gonçalves et al., 2021).

Parallel research streams have elucidated the contributory effects of anthocyanins on skin health, a factor intrinsically linked to the condition of the scalp and, consequently, hair health. By promoting a healthier scalp milieu, anthocyanins may facilitate conditions that are propitious for hair proliferation and mitigate the underlying causes of hair diminution (Horie et al., 2021). Moreover, the vasculoprotective attributes of anthocyanins delineated in recent studies signify an enhanced blood circulation, which is imperative for the nourishment and oxygenation of hair follicles, thereby fostering a robust hair growth environment (Horie et al., 2021).

Innovatively, recent research by Jung, Yoo et al. (2022) delves into the molecular dynamics facilitated by anthocyanins, particularly their role in the activation of the Wnt signaling pathway. This pathway is pivotal for hair follicle development and cyclical regeneration. The engagement of anthocyanins with this pathway, promoting the proliferation of dermal papilla cells, highlights a direct mechanistic approach through which these compounds may spur hair growth and revitalize dormant hair follicles (Jung, Jung et al., 2022).

Furthermore, the continuous ingestion of anthocyanins has been correlated with significant ameliorations in conditions like diabetic retinopathy and vasculopathy, portraying an extensive impact on vascular health (Rossino, & Dal Monte, & Casini, 2019). This broader vascular improvement posits additional benefits to scalp circulation, thereby indirectly advocating for enhanced hair follicle health and function (Dal & Sigrist, 2016; Rossino & Casini, 2019).

19.3 Macro- and micronutritional effects

The cellular activity of hair follicles is quite intense and is known to have a rapid turnover rate. To meet and maintain this intense activity, cells require macro- and micronutrients as well as energy (Rizer et al., 2015). There are many factors affecting hair loss and alopecia. Macronutrients, micronutrients, and energy intake are among these factors.

The protein in the hair structure contains keratin. Keratin is a group of proteins found especially in the skeletal structure of hair and epithelial cells. Keratin is involved in maintaining cell integrity and stability (Gropper et al., 2022). Keratin is known to be one of the main components in hair structure. Hair loss is observed in conditions associated with deficiency of protein intake (kwashiorkor, marasmus, anorexia nervosa, etc.) (Lin et al., 2016). The body in general is affected by hypometabolic conditions such as starvation, anorexia nervosa, and marasmus. In that case, hair loss from the head and lanugo-type hair on the face and arms is observed (Gropper et al., 2022). It is also known that some amino acids (e.g., taurine, methionine, and cysteine) are involved in the mechanisms associated with hair loss (Milani & Colombo, 2023).

Zinc is found in organs, tissues, and body fluids. There is a variation in the zinc content of foods. Good sources of zinc are red meat, seafood, poultry, pork, and dairy products. Whole grains and legumes also contain moderate levels of zinc. Zinc from animal sources is better absorbed in the body than zinc from plant sources. Zinc supplements are available as tablets, lozenges, sprays, and gels (Gropper et al., 2022). Zinc is a mineral with immunomodulatory effects and is responsible for the function of hair follicles. In the case of regression of hair follicles, apoptosis of the cells, which are responsible for keratin production, occurs. It is known that endonucleases are involved in this apoptosis, and zinc acts as a potential inhibitor of these endonucleases. Therefore it is thought that zinc may act as a potential inhibitor for regression of hair follicles. Due to its role in DNA stability and repair activities, zinc is thought to be an important factor in hair biology (Abdel Fattah et al., 2016). Zinc deficiency is associated with skin lesions, poor wound healing, and hair loss (Gropper et al., 2022). In a study aiming to assess zinc levels in hair and serum in individuals with chronic telogen effluvium disease, an association was found between low zinc levels and chronic telogen effluvium disease (Zufishan et al., 2024). In another study aiming to assess the state of zinc and copper minerals in hair loss, it was found that patients with hair loss had lower serum zinc levels than the control group. It was concluded that impairment in zinc metabolism could play a part in hair loss (Kil et al., 2013). Both studies seem to support each other and suggest a relationship between zinc levels and hair loss diseases.

Essential fatty acids cannot be synthesized in the body. It must be acquired from the diet. Some sources of linoleic acid are plant oils and poultry fat, and some sources of α-linolenic acid are flaxseed, soybean, and canola oil (Gropper et al., 2022). The deficiency of essential fatty acids causes depigmentation and hair loss (Lin et al., 2016). Poor growth, skin abnormalities, and raised bumps can also be seen due to deficiency of n-6 series in adults and children (Gropper et al., 2022). In a study evaluating the effect of a 6-month-specific omega-3, omega-6, and antioxidant supplement on hair loss, it was concluded that such supplementation was effective against hair loss (Le Floc'h *et al.*, 2015). In another study evaluating the effect of a nutrient complex consisting of omega-3, omega-6, omega-9, and an antioxidant over hair loss and hair health, this complex was proven to cause total 5α-reductase inhibition. And the inhibition of 5α-reductase is linked to improved hair loss and hair health. Therefore it is concluded that such complex may be effective for a healthy scalp (Zanzottera et al., 2017). According tothese studies, it is thought that supplements containing essential fatty acids as well as antioxidants can be used as an adjuvant to improve hair health.

Vitamin A is a vitamin that is soluble in fat. The source of preformed vitamin A (retinoids) is foods of animal origin (especially liver, dairy products, eggs, oily fish, etc.). On the other hand, carotenoids are fat-soluble pigments found mainly in plant foods. Provitamin A carotenoids can be converted to retinal in the body. Beta-carotene, one of these carotenoids, is found in foods such as spinach, carrots, and cabbage (Gropper et al., 2022). Retinol, retinal, and retinoic acid are derivatives of vitamin A. While retinal is vitamin A aldehyde, and retinol is known as vitamin A alcohol (Zhong et al., 2012). It is known that high levels of vitamin A can cause hair loss. While it is often caused by extreme intake of vitamin A supplements, sometimes it can also occur because of diseases such as chronic kidney disease (Lin et al., 2016). The alpha-retinoid nuclear receptor and vitamin D receptor are thought to be involved together and influence the hair cycle. In a review article aiming to assess the role of micronutrients in hair follicle cycle and their role in the treatment of hair loss, low levels of iron, zinc, and vitamin D were found to be associated with telogen effluvium and alopecia areata. Androgenetic alopecia was related to low iron and vitamin D levels. Low vitamin A levels were associated with telogen effluvium and hair breakage, while high vitamin A levels were associated with telogen effluvium (Ruiz-Tagle et al., 2018). In a study aimed at assessing the dietary habits of patients with alopecia areata, it was found that alopecia areata was related to body mass index and high retinol intake was a possible tool to predict a score representing alopecia severity (Hagino et al., 2021). In the view of these studies, it can be assumed that there is an association between low or high levels of vitamin A and hair loss diseases.

In 1931 following the finding that eating raw eggs caused hair loss, dermatitis, and various neuromuscular problems, biotin was discovered and shown to treat and prevent disease. Biotin (vitamin H) is known to be widely available in foods. Liver and eggs are particularly good sources. Other types of meat, sunflower seeds, and sweet potatoes also contain biotin, but in smaller amounts compared to liver and eggs. It is found in free form in multivitamins and supplements, and it is being used as an agent in hair and skin conditions (Gropper et al., 2022). Biotin is a vitamin that is soluble in water. Although biotin is used in cosmetics or health products for hair and skin, the scientific basis for its use in this way is not strong enough. The strongest effect exists when biotin is used to treat biotin deficiency. In this way, biotin appears to be effective in hair loss, as one of the indicators of biotin deficiency. In a study aiming to evaluate biotin deficiency in women with hair loss, biotin deficiency was found in 38% of women with hair loss. It was concluded that oral biotin supplements should not be used indiscriminately, but only when biotin is identified as the cause of hair loss (Trüeb, 2016). In a review study, the efficiency of biotin in hair and nail growth was evaluated, supporting the statement that biotin should not be used indiscriminately as stated in the previous study. It was stated that biotin supplementation may be effective in cases of biotin deficiency due to hereditary, acquired, or pathological reasons, but there is no sufficient evidence on the use of biotin supplementation in healthy persons (Patel et al., 2017). According to these studies, it is considered that biotin should be used in cases of deficiency, which may be associated with hair loss, but no definite conclusion can be made regarding supplement intake.

Chronic boron toxicity in infants (25–76 mg/kg body weight) (Gropper et al., 2022), chronic hypocalcemia (low serum calcium concentration) in patients (Kane & Prelack, 2019), and clinical selenosis (Lanham-New et al., 2011) are among the causes of hair loss. It is also known that vitamin C promotes the growth of hair follicles (Ruiz-Tagle et al., 2018). Plant-based foods (vegetables, fruits, legumes, and nuts) are good sources of boron; asparagus, broccoli, green peppers, and citrus fruits are good sources of vitamin C; dairy products are good sources of calcium; organ meats and seafood are good sources of selenium. The selenium content in foods is highly related to the composition of the soil in which they are grown (Gropper et al., 2022). Hair loss or alopecia can occur due to aging of the scalp. One of the influences on aging is reactive oxygen species. It is thought that dietary or supplemental intake of nutrients with antioxidant properties (such as vitamin E and selenium) can be a factor in interfering with reactive oxygen species reducing aging and related hair loss. Vitamin E directly interferes with free radicals, while selenium is a cofactor for enzymes that makes lipid peroxides harmless (Pincemail & Meziane, 2022). In a study aiming to evaluate the effects of a supplement containing methionine, taurine, cysteine, hydrolyzed collagen, selenium, and iron in patients with androgenic alopecia and telogen effluvium, it was found that such treatment may be effective against hair loss (Milani & Colombo, 2023).

Iron is one of the nutrients that affects hair growth. Although the mechanism is not clear yet, it is thought that iron's role as a cofactor for the enzyme ribonucleotide reductase, which limits the rate of DNA synthesis, may play a role in hair loss. In addition, genes affecting hair follicles are thought to be regulated by iron (Guo & Katta, 2017). It is thought that the iron bioavailability status of the body may be effective in the proliferation of hair follicular cells. It is also thought that the state of ferritin required by the cells may also be effective in hair growth (Ruiz-Tagle et al., 2018). Iron exists in foods as both heme iron and nonheme iron. Source of hem iron is foods of animal origin (especially meat, fish, and poultry); meanwhile, source of nonheme iron is whole grains, legumes, and nuts (Gropper et al., 2022). In a study aimed at determining the etiology of alopecia in women, seventy percent of female alopecia cases were found to be due to iron deficiency (Lin et al., 2023). In another study aiming to evaluate the iron and zinc levels in women with androgenic alopecia, lower zinc and iron levels were found in patients (Dhaher et al., 2018).

Vitamin D is involved in the proliferation and differentiation of keratinocytes (keratin-producing cells). It also has a regulatory role on genes and cell turnover. The vitamin D receptor takes a part in the process of differentiation of hair follicles and the onset of the first hair cycle (Saini & Mysore, 2021). Vitamin D is found in foods in the form of D_3 and D_2. Good sources of vitamin D_3 are fatty fish and fish oils. Also, good sources of vitamin D_2 are sun-dunder-ried mushrooms. Due to the limited number of foods containing vitamin D, food enrichment is practiced. It is known that vitamin D can be synthesized from the skin by exposure to ultraviolet sunlight. Vitamin D supplements usually contain the D_3 form of vitamin D (Gropper et al., 2022). In a study aiming to evaluate vitamin D levels and the influence of vitamin D_3 analogs in patients with alopecia areata, it was found that serum vitamin D levels were significantly lower in patients with alopecia areata. Also, D_3 analogs were found to be influential in improving hair growth (Fahim et al., 2023). In a study aiming to assess the relationship between alopecia areata and vitamin D and calcium status in the body, serum 25(OH)D deficiency was found in patients with alopecia areata (Liu et al., 2020). In another study aiming to assess the influence of vitamin D in telogen effluvium, oral vitamin D_3 therapy was applied to 40 patients, and improved hair growth was found in young women who did not use sunscreen and benefited from milk proteins (Sattar et al., 2021). In a study aimed at investigating the effectiveness of a supplement containing vitamin D_3 and some other nutrients (such as omega-3 and omega-6), on androgenetic alopecia, an improvement in hair condition was found 24 weeks after supplementation (Nichols et al., 2017). According to with these studies, serum vitamin D levels can be associated with hair loss, and vitamin D supplementation might have therapeutic effects on hair loss. Fig. 19.3 shows some micronutrients related to hair loss and alopecia. Also, Table 19.1 shows the studies investigating the effect of supplements containing various micronutrients for the treatment of hair loss and alopecia.

Energy, inadequate or excessive intake of macro and micronutrients might be related to hair loss. There are studies investigating the relation between serum levels of nutrients or intake of supplements containing nutrients and hair loss. In line with these studies, it is seen that the level of nutrients in serum or supplement intake might be related to hair loss.

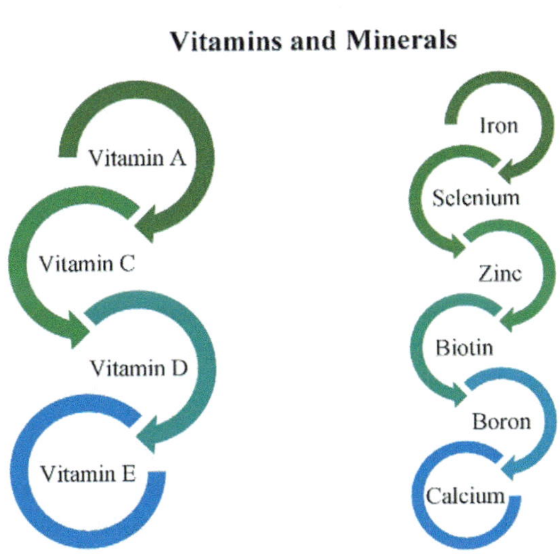

FIGURE 19.3 Some micronutrients related to hair loss and alopecia.

TABLE 19.1 Case Studies on Supplements Containing Various Micronutrients for the Treatment of Hair Loss and Alopecia.

Case Studies	Aim	Methodology and Study Population	Key Results	References
Female pattern hair loss	Evaluate the effects of a 6-month supplementation	Randomized, comparative study 120 healthy female subjects	Effective against hair loss	Le Floc'h et al. (2015)
Hair loss/Hair health	Evaluate the effect of a nutritional complex	In vitro and in vivo study Phase 1: In vitro experiment (in culture of human keratinocytes, to lower 5α-reductase activity) Phase 2: In vivo study (30 volunteers, 6 months nutritional complex treatment)	Effective against the inhibition of total 5α-reductase Effective for a healthy scalp Progress in vascularization and hair diameter Decrease in hair loss perception	Zanzottera et al. (2017)
Female pattern hair loss	Evaluate the effect of iron supplementation	Retrospective study 155 patients	Related to iron deficiency Supplementation within 6 months, better prognosis	Lin et al. (2023)
Androgenic alopecia/Chronic telogen effluvium	Evaluate the effect of oral supplementation	Prospective, randomized study 83 subjects	Effective against hair loss	Milani and Colombo (2023)
Androgenetic alopecia	Evaluate the effect of oral supplementation	Open label study	Effective against androgenetic alopecia	Nichols et al. (2017)

19.3.1 External and internal factors

Hair loss is common worldwide. Although the mechanisms underlying hair loss are not completely understood, it is known that there are many factors related to the pathogenesis of hair loss (Wang et al., 2024). Stress, drugs, immunity, genetic profile, nutritional deficiencies, chronic and endocrine disorders, sudden weight loss, and hormone levels can be mentioned as factors that can cause hair loss and alopecia (Gokce et al., 2022). In a systematic review aimed at assessing the epidemiology and burden of alopecia areata, there was no difference related to gender (such as the incidence of alopecia areata) (Villasante et al., 2015).

The hair cycle involves the cooccurrence of apoptosis and proliferation. Through this process, cells continue to renew itself. Normally, apoptosis occurs as a process for the regeneration of hair follicles, but when there is an influence of external and internal factors (e.g., chemotherapeutic drugs, UV radiation, and viruses), this leads to abnormal apoptosis of hair follicles, which in turn may cause hair damage (Wang et al., 2024).

As known, one of the main mechanisms of hair loss is gene expression. Epigenetic factors such as regimes, stress, sleep cycle, or lifestyle affect gene expression. It is reported that biological twins react to hair loss at different rates due to epigenetic factors. Cellular metabolism is also thought to play a role in genetic predisposition (Rajput, 2022). When genetic factors are considered, it has been reported that girls affected by alopecia between the ages of 6–10 years have a family history of early onset of alopecia. Also, the frequency of family history of alopecia is higher in patients with early onset of hair loss than in patients with late onset of hair loss (Ohn et al., 2022). In another review, family history is reported to be more frequent in children with alopecia areata, but, in general, it does not affect most patients with alopecia areata (Villasante et al., 2015).

Hair loss can be observed after bariatric surgery, which is associated with micronutrient deficiencies and rapid weight loss. In a study evaluating the prevalence of hair loss after bariatric surgery, the prevalence of hair loss after laparoscopic sleeve gastrectomy was found to be 56% (Katsogridaki et al., 2018). In another study evaluating nutritional symptoms and biological parameters after Roux-en-Y gastric bypass and sleeve gastrectomy, it was found that the rate of hair loss was 65% in the short term and 35% in the long term. Hair loss was recognized as one of the most prevalent nutritional symptoms after bariatric surgery (Ledoux et al., 2020). In a study on common complications after metabolic and bariatric surgery, 18 studies were evaluated, and it was found that postoperative hair loss was frequent especially in young women (Zhang, Fan et al., 2021).

Androgenetic alopecia (male pattern hair loss) is a disease influenced by hormones. Androgens are hormonal regulators of androgenetic alopecia and are related to the regulation of the hair cycle and gene expression in androgen-sensitive hair follicles. Estrogens are also related to the regulation of the hair cycle and are a potential challenger for androgens (Heilmann-Heimbach et al., 2020). Androgens, estrogens, and progesterone are thought to take a part in the hair cycle. Androgens might also play a role in inhibiting hair follicles on the scalp, which can lead to alopecia. For estrogens, it is known that increased levels may promote the anagen phase in hair follicles (Kamp et al., 2022).

Stress plays a part in the mechanism of hair loss. It causes high levels of cortisol in the blood, which leads to a decrease in hyaluronan and proteoglycan, which are related to normal hair growth. In this way, stress causes hair loss. Stress hormones also cause the release of pro-inflammatory cytokines, leading to hair loss (Salhab et al., 2022). Acute stress causes hyperactivation of the nervous systems, leading to the development of autoimmune diseases. Alopecia areata is a chronic inflammatory disease. It is thought that mechanism-wise, in this condition, immune cells cause inflammation in the hair follicles, which can lead to alopecia areata (Ahn et al., 2023).

Beta blockers, anticonvulsants, anticoagulants, and antidepressants are thought to cause telogen effluvium. It is known that the effect usually starts after 12 weeks. The changes in drug dosage can cause excessive hair loss. Conditions that cause physiological stress such as trauma, fever, and chronic diseases can cause telogen effluvium. Hyper and hypothyroidism, chronic infections, and inflammatory disorders may also be the causes of telogen hair loss (Asghar et al., 2020). In a study aiming to assess the role of nutrition and diet in alopecia, it was concluded that alopecia areata and some scarring alopecia diseases are autoimmune and given the relationship between autoimmune diseases and antiinflammatory diets, the Mediterranean diet (a diet rich in antiinflammatory nutrients) or diets rich in protein and soy may be effective in the treatment of alopecia (Pham et al., 2020). The gut microbiota is also thought to have an impact on alopecia areata. A review aiming to assess the pathogenic link between microbiota and alopecia areata concluded that there are indications of malformations in the microbiome of patients with alopecia areata, but the scientific basis is not fully supported (Sánchez-Pellicer et al., 2022). Fig. 19.4 shows some of the external and internal factors affecting hair loss and alopecia.

19.3.2 Fermented foods and gut microbiota factors

The gut–skin axis has been a topic of recent research interest, shedding light on the potential relationship between the gut microbiome and skin health and hair loss conditions such as alopecia. There has been a growth in alopecia areata and other alopecia subtypes (Sánchez-Pellicer et al., 2022). Based on revealed results, there is a correlation between gut dysbiosis, alopecia areata, and androgenetic alopecia, suggesting that changes in the gut microbiome spectrum might play a role in the development of hair loss conditions (Brzychcy et al., 2022; Hayashi et al., 2017; Xie et al., 2019). Hayashi and coworkers (2017) have illustrated that antibiotic-associated dysbiosis, specifically the proliferation of some certain probiotic bacterial species like *Lactobacillus murinus*, can damage gut flora and contribute to the beginning of alopecia. This research emphasized the potential importance of gut dysbiosis in hair loss (Hayashi et al., 2017). As well, the other survey of the scalp and gut microbiome relation to androgenetic alopecia has made it clear that there is a clear connection between microbiome composition and hair loss conditions (Jung, Yoo et al., 2022). Studies have highlighted the potential interplay between microbial dysbiosis in the gut and the pathophysiology of alopecia areata (Juhasz et al., 2020; Mahmud et al., 2022; Rudnicka & Waśkiel-Burnat, 2021; Schneider & Nelson, 2019; Xie et al., 2019). Apart from aging and genetic factors, inflammation and increasing inflammatory biomarkers in the body, unbalanced gut microbiota, chronic diseases, sleeping disorder, insufficient essential vitamins, and minerals can cause hair,

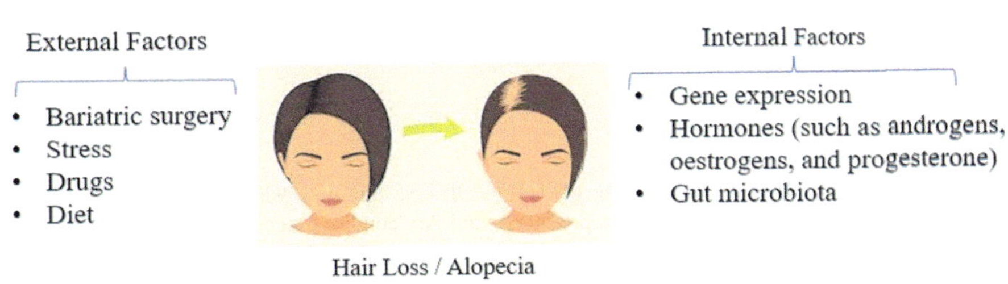

FIGURE 19.4 Some of the external and internal factors affect hair loss and alopecia.

loss which can be moderated and treated by probiotics, in over all a healthy gut−skin axis. It was reported that *Clostridium* spp. stimulate $CD^{4+}FOXP^{3+}$ regulatory T cells (Treg cells) by producing short-chain fatty acids (SCFAs). These SCFAs play a role in immune system improvements and Treg cells (Xu et al., 2023).

Research has investigated the impact of the gut microbiome on skin health through the gut−skin axis, claiming 93% improvement in terms of thickness and hair numbers after probiotic supplement consumption. Probiotic supplement was reported to lower serum glucose, insulin resistance, and improvement of most lipid markers. These actions might have improved microvascular function to regulate local blood-tissue exchange, which contributed to hair growth. Besides, a significant increase of serum biotin concentration was reported, which might be because of probiotic bacteria's ability to synthesize more B vitamins, including biotin. They indicated that a significant increase of serum interferon-gamma (IFN-γ), which act as a regulator of immune system responses and inflammation and in contrary significant reductions in the inflammation makers, including interleukin-6 (IL-6) and interleukin-31 (IL-31), make it clear that probiotic bacteria can stimulate the antiinflammatory component of the immune system of body to release cytokines and hormones that disrupt the damaging inflammatory cycle (Yu et al., 2022). Fecal microbiota transplantation as a treatment approach for the potential therapeutic implications of modulating the gut microbiome in alopecia areata has been explored, and results indicated that successful hair regrowth in patients was observed (Xu et al., 2023; Yu et al., 2022). In Fig. 19.5 the relation between gut probiotic and alopecia areata immune system response markers is shown.

Once nutrients are broken down after digestion, they pass the intestinal wall to enter either the bloodstream or the lymphatic system. The intestinal wall acts as a protective barrier when food comes from outside and contains the vast spectrum of microbial population within the gut. However, it must also allow for the passage of essential nutrients to cells by bloodstream (Rolim, 2015; Schell et al., 2022). The permeability of this barrier is the key to protection which can be influenced by various diet types, gut microbiota itself, or intestinal inflammation. While there is not a direct link between intestinal permeability and hair loss, any damage in the intestinal wall (leaky gut) can disrupt the digestive process and inhibit nutrient absorption. Consequently, insufficient nutrients can impact on the hair growth and healthy hair follicles. Providing essential nutrients from food relies on a properly functioning digestive tract and a balanced and healthy gut microbiota. Gut microbiota can synthesize some elements such as amino acids, triglycerides, and various vitamins (B1, B9, B7, B2, B5, K). Imbalances in gut bacteria have been linked to conditions like inflammatory bowel disease and overall health by protecting against harmful pathogens (Davani-Davari et al., 2019). The relationship between gut microbiota and hair loss is increasingly recognized, with studies indicating that enhancing gut health may promote hair regrowth in individuals with conditions like Alopecia areata (Hart et al., 2002; Morowitz et al., 2011; Rebello et al., 2017).

Probiotics are live microorganisms with health benefits to the host. The main probiotics are *Lactobacillus* and *Bifidobacterium* and Saccharomyces (Flesch et al., 2014; Lebaka et al., 2018). Probiotics (not only in gut microbiota but also on the skin) have been found to potentially influence hair health positively by promoting hair growth, reducing hair loss, and enhancing scalp and skin state. Also, studies suggest that probiotics can counteract the negative effects of oxidative stress on hair follicles, reduce inflammation in the skin, and promote hair growth by initiating the anagen phase in hair follicles (Park et al., 2020; Shavandi et al., 2020; Wadstein et al., 2020). Additionally, probiotics may be associated with thicker skin, improved follicular development, and increased folliculogenesis, all contributing to healthier hair growth (Ale & Binetti, 2021). Probiotics have been linked to:

1. promoting angiogenesis,
2. supplying essential nutrients for hair growth,

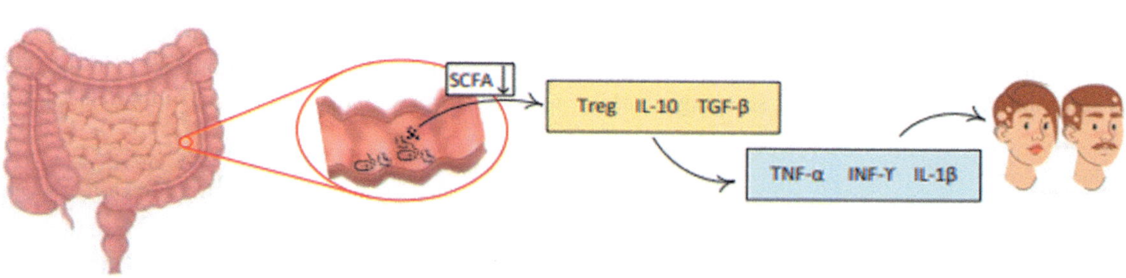

FIGURE 19.5 Gut microbiota and AA relation. As SCFAs can stimulate the release of TNF-α, IFN-γ, and IL-1 when its amount decreases, it causes an end in T_{reg} cells and makes hormonal factors such as TGF-β and IL-10 to be produced, and AA condition occurs (Xu et al., 2023). *AA*, Alopecia areata; *IFN-γ*, interferon gamma; *IL-1*, interleukin-1; *IL-10*, interleukin-10; *SCFAs*, short- chain fatty acids; *TGF-β*, transforming growth factor-β; *TNF-α*, tumor necrosis factor-alpha.

3. improving peripheral vascular blood flow, which could positively impact hair growth (Direito et al., 2021; Lee et al., 2022),
4. modulating cell cycles in hair follicles,
5. regulating the scalp microbiome,
6. inducing the production of beneficial metabolites that stimulate hair growth mechanisms (Mayer et al., 2023; Tsai et al., 2023),
7. decreasing immunomodulatory effects, activating various immune cells and cytokine production, which may aid in tissue repair and regeneration (Lukic et al., 2017),
8. inhibiting of pathogenic bacteria growth,
9. accelerating of wound healing,
10. promoting of collagen production and hair follicle formation (Polak et al., 2021),
11. associating with thicker skin,
12. improving follicular development,
13. increasing folliculogenesis that contributing to healthier hair growth (Flesch et al., 2014; Yu et al., 2022).

Prebiotics, which are known as nondigestible carbohydrates, mainly oligosaccharides like fructans, galacto-oligosaccharides, and noncarbohydrate oligosaccharides like cocoa-derived flavanols and honey (Schell et al., 2022; Davani-Davari et al., 2023), can be used to promote unique, favorable changes in the gut that confer health benefits to the host. These benefits have been associated with increased numbers of potentially beneficial microbes, including bifidobacteria and lactobacilli in the gut and/or increased production of metabolites like SCFA by gut microbes (Schell et al., 2022). The best prebiotic foods can be named vegetables, and nondigestible starch contains fruits, legumes, and also nuts such as onion, celery, chestnut, chicory roots, sweet potato, and asparagus (Rolim, 2015).

Postbiotics, mainly L-lactic acid, short-chain fatty acids (SCFAs) like acetate, propionate, and butyrate, polyamines, small metabolites such as AI-3 and histamine, or even proteins such as p45/p75 (Lee et al., 2016; Martyniak et al., 2021; Mora-Sánchez et al., 2020), which are metabolic byproducts from probiotic microorganisms, can be produced after consumption of prebiotics by probiotics. They have been suggested to have biological activity in the host (Martyniak et al., 2021; Mora-Sánchez et al., 2020). Studies have indicated that postbiotics may play a role in maintaining gut health, helping gut inflammatory conditions, preventing pathogen bacteria from adhering to intestine, and potentially impacting on skin and alopecia conditions (de Silva Vale et al., 2023; Rinaldi et al., 2020). Postbiotics are mainly obtained during fermentations by lactic acid bacteria and yeast (de Silva Vale et al., 2023). Moreover, postbiotics have been reported to exhibit pleiotropic activities in the human body (Montazeri-Najafabady et al., 2021). The use of postbiotics in cosmetic and food supplement products for the treatment of alopecia has also been explored, suggesting their efficacy in promoting hair growth and hair loss (Rinaldi et al., 2020). In Fig. 19.6 the definitions of prebiotic, probiotic, postbiotic, synbiotic, and paraprobiotic were summarized.

Synbiotic, a combination of probiotics and prebiotics, is known as a functional combination with health aspects. This mixture presents a multiplicative factor on individual actions (Flesch et al., 2014) such as beneficial effects on weight loss, gene expression, body composition, gut microbiota, and metabolic health (Kilic Yildirim et al., 2022; Lyon et al., 2023; Sergeev et al., 2020; Zeinali et al., 2020). The synergistic relationship between probiotics and prebiotics in synbiotic products can lead to improved outcomes in terms of weight management, immune system improvements, and

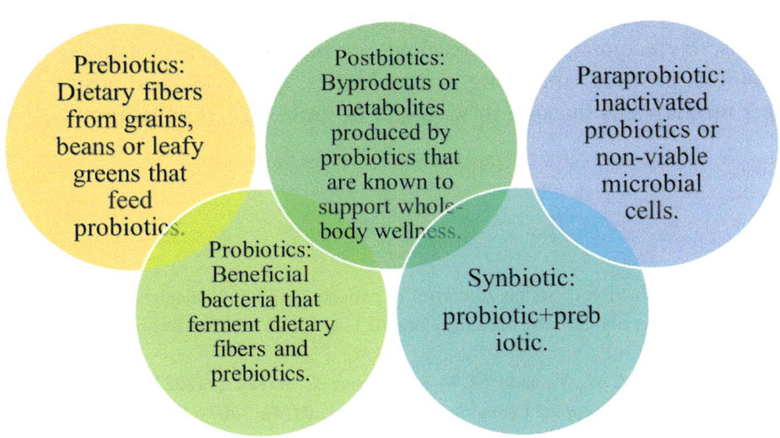

FIGURE 19.6 The definition of prebiotic, probiotic, postbiotic, synbiotic, and paraprobiotic (Cruz et al., 2010).

metabolic parameters. In addition, the potential of synbiotics in addressing conditions like hirsutism has also been explored (Lolou, 2021). Research protocols have been designed to investigate the impact of synbiotic supplementation on various health parameters, such as gut microbiome composition and inflammatory markers that can affect hair and scalp health as well (Lyon et al., 2023; Zeinali et al., 2020).

Fermented foods, like fermented milk products, kimchi, and Cheonggukjang, or any other fermented fruits like fermented papaya and fermented mangosteen (Mayer et al., 2023), have been associated with potential benefits for hair health, including addressing conditions like alopecia. Studies have shown that probiotics from fermented foods can have a positive impact on scalp and facial skin conditions, glucose, lipid metabolism, and hair health, leading to improvements in hair thickness and count (Park et al., 2020). Specifically, a clinical pilot study suggested that a probiotic product derived from kimchi and Cheonggukjang could promote hair growth and reverse hair loss (Gruskiene et al., 2021). Fermented milk products have been identified as an excellent matrix for incorporating bioactive ingredients, making them functional foods that can potentially support overall health, including hair health (Kim et al., 2021). It can be assumed that fermented foods as functional foods with physiological activities may contribute to improvements in blood circulation and intestinal regulation, which could indirectly impact hair health. Feeding probiotic microorganisms with prebiotics is recommended by researchers. For example, the prebiotic properties of *Euglena gracilis* have been investigated, showing its ability to promote the growth of beneficial bacteria like Lactobacillus and the accumulation of antioxidants (Dai et al., 2022).

More research is needed to comprehensive understand the mechanisms through which probiotics—gut microbiota—and fermented foods exert these effects, including reducing inflammation, modulating epithelial secretion of chemokines that attract immune cells, promoting angiogenesis, modulating cell cycles, improving overall scalp and skin condition, the process of dysbiosis, and enhancing tissue repair and regeneration. The mechanisms underlying this association and explore the therapeutic potential of targeting the gut microbiome in the management of alopecia (Barquero-Orias et al., 2021). In addition, the combination of probiotics and prebiotics in synbiotic products and supplements presents a promising future for promoting general health, including hair-skin health. Based on current research, postbiotics may have the potential to influence hair health and could be considered a novel approach in the management of conditions like alopecia.

In the food industry, the development and formulation of functional foods with probiotic, prebiotic, postbiotics, and synbiotic obligatorily require a comprehensive understanding of in vivo and in vitro analysis as well, the sensory aspects. For the easier storage and manufacturing conditions, paraprobiotics (nonviable probiotics) are considered nowadays (Martyniak et al., 2021). In addition to food industry and supplements, the cosmetic industry is working on the development of products that contain probiotics that can help scalp and skin (Min, 2022).

19.4 Conclusion

In conclusion, hair loss and various types of alopecia significantly affect individuals' quality of life. Multiple factors contribute to hair loss, including age, cancer treatments, hormonal imbalances, scalp infections, stress, thyroid disorders, and more. Functional foods have emerged as key alternative treatment options. While specific medical treatments are necessary for different alopecia types based on their underlying causes, general symptoms can often be alleviated by consuming functional foods. Maintaining a balance of macronutrients and micronutrients, such as protein, essential amino acids, vitamins, and minerals like zinc and vitamin D3, is highly recommended. The Mediterranean diet, rich in healthy oils, antioxidants, fiber, and B vitamins, is recognized as a particularly healthy and practical choice. Additionally, a growing variety of probiotic and prebiotic products, including paraprobiotics, synbiotics, and postbiotics, are now available on the market. Investigating their mechanisms through in vivo and in vitro studies holds promise for advancing clinical treatments.

References

Abdel Fattah, N. S. A., Atef, M. M., & Al-Qaradaghi, S. M. Q. (2016). Evaluation of serum zinc level in patients with newly diagnosed and resistant alopecia areata. *International Journal of Dermatology*, *55*(1), 24–29. Available from https://doi.org/10.1111/ijd.12769, http://onlinelibrary.wiley.com/journal/10.1111/(ISSN)1365-4632.

Abelan, U. S., de Oliveira, A. C., Cacoci, É. S. P., Martins, T. E. A., Giacon, V. M., Velasco, M. V. R., & Lima, C. R. Rd. C. (2022). Potential use of essential oils in cosmetic and dermatological hair products: A review. *Journal of Cosmetic Dermatology*, *21*(4), 1407–1418. Available from https://doi.org/10.1111/jocd.14286, http://onlinelibrary.wiley.com/journal/10.1111/(ISSN)1473-2165.

Abiri, B., Amini, S., Hejazi, M., Hosseinpanah, F., Zarghi, A., Abbaspour, F., & Valizadeh, M. (2023). Tea's anti-obesity properties, cardiometabolic health-promoting potentials, bioactive compounds, and adverse effects: A review focusing on white and green teas. *Food Science & Nutrition, 11* (10), 5818–5836. Available from https://doi.org/10.1002/fsn3.3595.

Adolphe, J. L., Whiting, S. J., Juurlink, B. H. J., Thorpe, L. U., & Alcorn, J. (2010). Health effects with consumption of the flax lignan secoisolariciresinol diglucoside. *British Journal of Nutrition, 103*(7), 929–938. Available from https://doi.org/10.1017/S0007114509992753.

Agada, R., Usman, W. A., Shehu, S., & Thagariki, D. (2020). In vitro and in vivo inhibitory effects of Carica papaya seed on α-amylase and α-glucosidase enzymes. *Heliyon, 6*(3). Available from https://doi.org/10.1016/j.heliyon.2020.e03618, http://www.journals.elsevier.com/heliyon/.

Ahn, D., Kim, H., Lee, B., & Hahm, D. H. (2023). Psychological stress-induced pathogenesis of alopecia areata: Autoimmune and apoptotic pathways. *International Journal of Molecular Sciences, 24*(14). Available from https://doi.org/10.3390/ijms241411711, http://www.mdpi.com/journal/ijms.

Ahn, H., Lee, S. Y., Lee, K. H., & Jung, W. J. (2021). Alopecia treatment using minimally manipulated human umbilical cord-derived mesenchymal stem cells: Three case reports and review of literature. *World Journal of Clinical Cases, 9*(15), 3741–3751. Available from https://doi.org/10.12998/wjcc.v9.i15.3741, https://www.wjgnet.com/2307-8960/about.htm.

Ajuwon, O. R., Marnewick, J. L., & Davids, L. M. (2015). *Rooibos (Aspalathus linearis) and its Major Flavonoids—Potential Against Oxidative Stress-Induced Conditions*. InTech. Available from 10.5772/61614.

Akinfenwa, A. O., Abdul, N. S., Marnewick, J. L., & Hussein, A. A. (1936). Protective effects of linearthin and other chalcone derivatives from Aspalathus linearis (Rooibos) against UVB induced oxidative stress and toxicity in. human skin cells. *Plants, 10*(9), 1936.

Akomolafe, S. F., Olasehinde, T. A., & Aluko, B. T. (2021). Diets supplemented with raw and roasted pumpkin (*Cucurbita pepo* L) seeds improved some biochemical parameters associated with erectile function in rats. *Journal of Food Biochemistry, 45*(2). Available from https://doi.org/10.1111/jfbc.13629, http://onlinelibrary.wiley.com/journal/10.1111/(ISSN)1745-4514.

Juhaimi, F. A., Geçgel., Gülcü, M., Hamurcu, M., & Özcan, M. M. (2017). Bioactive properties, fatty acid composition and mineral contents of grape seed and oils. *South African Journal of Enology and Viticulture, 38*(1), 103–108. Available from https://doi.org/10.21548/38-1-1042, http://www.journals.ac.za/index.php/sajev/article/download/1042/773.

Alaswad, A. A., & Krishnan, H. B. (2016). Immunological investigation for the presence of lunasin, a chemopreventive soybean peptide, in the seeds of diverse plants. *Journal of Agricultural and Food Chemistry, 64*(14), 2901–2909. Available from https://doi.org/10.1021/acs.jafc.6b00445, http://pubs.acs.org/journal/jafcau.

Alboreadi, M. A., Al-Najdawi, M. M., Jarrar, Q. B., & Moshawih, S. (2022). Evaluation of hair growth properties of Topical Kombucha tea extracts. *Advances in Traditional Medicine, 22*(1), 155–161. Available from https://doi.org/10.1007/s13596-020-00534-7, https://www.springer.com/journal/13596.

Antolak, H., Piechota, D., & Kucharska, A. (2021). Kombucha Tea—A double power of bioactive compounds from tea and symbiotic culture of bacteria and yeasts (SCOBY. *Antioxidants, 10*(10), 1541. Available from https://doi.org/10.3390/antiox10101541.

Asghar, F., Shamim, N., Farooque, U., Sheikh, H., & Aqeel, R. (2020). Telogen effluvium: A review of the literature. *Cureus*. Available from https://doi.org/10.7759/cureus.8320.

Assumpção, C. F., Nunes, I. L., Mendonça, T. A., Bortolin, R. C., Jablonski, A., Flôres, S. H., & de Oliveira Rios, A. (2016). Bioactive compounds and stability of organic and conventional Vitis labrusca grape seed oils. *Journal of the American Oil Chemists' Society, 93*(1), 115–124. Available from https://doi.org/10.1007/s11746-015-2742-0.

Aziz, A., Noreen, S., Khalid, W., Ejaz, A., Faiz ul Rasool, I., Maham, N., Munir, A., Farwa, N., Javed, M., Ercisli, S., Okcu, Z., Marc, R. A., Nayik, G. A., Ramniwas, S., & Uddin, J. (2023). Pumpkin and pumpkin byproducts: Phytochemical constitutes, food application and health benefits. *ACS Omega, 8*(26), 23346–23357. Available from https://doi.org/10.1021/acsomega.3c02176, pubs.acs.org/journal/acsodf.

Banwo, K., Olojede, A. O., Adesulu-Dahunsi, A. T., Verma, D. K., Thakur, M., Tripathy, S., Singh, S., Patel, A. R., Gupta, A. K., Aguilar, C. N., & Utama, G. L. (2021). Functional importance of bioactive compounds of foods with Potential Health Benefits: A review on recent trends. *Food Bioscience, 43*. Available from https://doi.org/10.1016/j.fbio.2021.101320, http://www.journals.elsevier.com/food-bioscience/.

Bardaa, S., Ben Halima, N., Aloui, F., Ben Mansour, R., Jabeur, H., Bouaziz, M., & Sahnoun, Z. (2016). Oil from pumpkin (*Cucurbita pepo* L.) seeds: Evaluation of its functional properties on wound healing in rats. *Lipids in Health and Disease, 15*(1). Available from https://doi.org/10.1186/s12944-016-0237-0, http://www.lipidworld.com/home/.

Barot, B. N. Therapeutic Potential of Fermented Papaya Preparation in Doxorubicin Induced Toxicity Maharaja Sayajirao University of Baroda. (2017), 2017.

Barquero-Orias, D., Muñoz Moreno-Arrones, O., & Vañó-Galván, S. (2021). Alopecia and the microbiome: A future therapeutic target? *Actas Dermo-sifiliograficas, 112*(6), 495–502. Available from https://doi.org/10.1016/j.ad.2020.12.005, http://www.doyma.es/ad/.

Batool, M., Ranjha, M. M. A. N., Roobab, U., Manzoor, M. F., Farooq, U., Nadeem, H. R., Nadeem, M., Kanwal, R., Abdelgawad, H., Al Jaouni, S. K., Selim, S., & Ibrahim, S. A. (2022). Nutritional value, phytochemical potential, and therapeutic benefits of pumpkin (Cucurbita sp.). *Plants, 11*(11). Available from https://doi.org/10.3390/plants11111394, https://www.mdpi.com/2223-7747/11/11/1394/pdf?version = 1653452349.

Bjelica, M., Vujasinović, V., Rabrenović, B., & Dimić, S. (2019). Some chemical characteristics and oxidative stability of cold pressed grape seed oils obtained from different winery waste. *European Journal of Lipid Science and Technology, 121*(8). Available from https://doi.org/10.1002/ejlt.201800416, http://onlinelibrary.wiley.com/journal/10.1002/(ISSN)1438-9312.

Bortolomedi, B. M., Paglarini, C. S., & Brod, F. C. A. (2022). Bioactive compounds in kombucha: A review of substrate effect and fermentation conditions. *Food Chemistry, 385*. Available from https://doi.org/10.1016/j.foodchem.2022.132719, www.elsevier.com/locate/foodchem.

Brzychcy, K., Dróżdż, I., Skoczylas, S., Płoszaj, T., Sobolewska-Sztychny, D., Skibińska, M., Narbutt, J., & Lesiak, A. (2022). Gut microbiota in alopecia areata. *Advances in Dermatology and Allergology, 39*(6), 1162–1170. Available from https://doi.org/10.5114/ada.2022.120453.

Callixte, C., Baptiste, N. J., & Arwati, H. (2020). Phytochemical screening and antimicrobial activities of methanolic and aqueous leaf extracts of Carica papaya Grown in Rwanda. *Molecular and Cellular Biomedical Sciences*, *4*(1), 39. Available from https://doi.org/10.21705/mcbs.v4i1.74.

Canini, A., Alesiani, D., D'Arcangelo, G., & Tagliatesta, P. (2007). Gas chromatography–mass spectrometry analysis of phenolic compounds from Carica papaya L. leaf. *Journal of Food Composition and Analysis*, *20*(7), 584–590. Available from https://doi.org/10.1016/j.jfca.2007.03.009.

Chávez-Quintal, P., González-Flores, T., Rodríguez-Buenfil, I., & Gallegos-Tintoré, S. (2011). Antifungal activity in ethanolic extracts of Carica papaya L. cv. maradol leaves and seeds. *Indian Journal of Microbiology*, *51*(1), 54–60. Available from https://doi.org/10.1007/s12088-011-0086-5.

Chhikara, N., Panghal, A., Chaudhary, G., Kumari, A., & Chhikara, N. (2022). *Food function and health benefits of functional foods. Functional Foods* (pp. 419–441). Wiley. Available from https://doi.org/10.1002/9781119776345.ch12.

Crews, C., Hough, P., Godward, J., Brereton, P., Lees, M., Guiet, S., & Winkelmann, W. (2006). Quantitation of the main constituents of some authentic grape-seed oils of different origin. *Journal of Agricultural and Food Chemistry*, *54*(17), 6261–6265. Available from https://doi.org/10.1021/jf060338y.

Cruz, A. G., Cadena, R. S., Walter, E. H. M., Mortazavian, A. M., Granato, D., Faria, J. A. F., & Bolini, H. M. A. (2010). Sensory analysis: Relevance for prebiotic, probiotic, and synbiotic product development. *Comprehensive Reviews in Food Science and Food Safety*, *9*(4), 358–373. Available from https://doi.org/10.1111/j.1541-4337.2010.00115.x.

Bhushana Daddala, G., Swaroopa Rani, A., & Kiran Kumar, A. (2022). Evaluation of antioxidant, antimicrobial activity and phytochemical screening of aqueous methanolic extract of linum usitatissimum. *Journal of Advanced Scientific Research*, *13*(01), 147–152. Available from https://doi.org/10.55218/jasr.202213115.

Dai, J., He, J., Chen, Z., Qin, H., Du, M., Lei, A., Zhao, L., & Wang, J. (2022). Euglena gracilis Promotes lactobacillus growth and antioxidants accumulation as a potential next-generation prebiotic. *Frontiers in Nutrition*, *9*. Available from https://doi.org/10.3389/fnut.2022.864565.

Dal, S., & Sigrist, S. (2016). The protective effect of antioxidants consumption on diabetes and vascular complications. *Diseases*, *4*(3), 24. Available from https://doi.org/10.3390/diseases4030024.

Dangi, I., Sahu, M., Verma, L., & Banweer, J. (2023). Hair growth stimulating effect and phytochemical evaluation hydoalcoholic extract of Carica papaya leaves. *World J. Pharm. Res*, *12*, 169–776.

da Silva Vale, A., de Melo Pereira, G. V., de Oliveira, A. C., de Carvalho Neto, D. P., Herrmann, L. W., Karp, S. G., Soccol, V. T., & Soccol, C. R. (2023). Production, formulation, and application of postbiotics in the treatment of skin conditions. *Fermentation*, *9*(3), 264. Available from https://doi.org/10.3390/fermentation9030264.

Dhaher, S. A., Yacoub, A. A., & Jacob, A. A. (2018). Estimation of zinc and iron levels in the serum and hair of women with androgenetic alopecia: Case-control study. *Indian Journal of Dermatology*, *63*(5), 369–374. Available from https://doi.org/10.4103/ijd.IJD_624_16, http://www.e-ijd.org.

Dinkins, J., Iwuala, C., Akintilo, L., Ugonabo, N., Shapiro, J., Sicco, K. L., & Adotama, P. (2023). Commonly used hair oils in the Black community: A narrative review in their use to treat androgenetic alopecia. *International Journal of Dermatology*, *62*(8), 980–985. Available from https://doi.org/10.1111/ijd.16657, http://onlinelibrary.wiley.com/journal/10.1111/(ISSN)1365-4632.

Direito, R., Rocha, J., Sepodes, B., & Eduardo-Figueira, M. (2021). From Diospyros kaki L.(persimmon) phytochemical profile and health impact to new product perspectives and waste valorization. *Nutrients*, *13*(9), 2021.

Ebrahimi-Mameghani, M., Irandoost, P., & Pourmoradian, S. (2020). The effects of grape seed oil on the cardiovascular risk factors in overweight and obese women: A double-blind randomized clinical trial. *Current Topics in Nutraceutical Research*, *18*(2), 1–6. Available from https://doi.org/10.37290/ctnr2641-452X.18:1-6, https://www.nchpjournals.com/CTNR.

Elegbede, J. A., & Lateef, A. (2019). Green synthesis of silver (Ag), gold (Au), and silver–gold (Ag–Au) alloy nanoparticles: A review on recent advances, trends, and biomedical applications. *Informa UK Limited*, 3–89. Available from https://doi.org/10.1201/9780429425660-1.

Fahim, M., Khoso, H., Hussain, A., & Bakhtiar, R. (2023). Deficiency in alopecia areata and responsiveness to vitamin D analogues: A prospective trial. *Journal of Pakistan Association of Dermatologists*, *33*(4), 1242–1248. Available from https://jpad.com.pk/index.php/jpad/atj.

Fale, S. K., Umekar, M. J., Das, R., & Alaspure, M. (2022). A comprehensive study of herbal cosmetics prepared from flaxseed. *Multidisciplinary International Research Journal of Gujarat Technological University*, *4*, 106–112, 2022.

Fang, C., Yang, H., Hui, J., Fan, D., & Deng, J. (2024). Natural bioactive compounds as potential sources for alleviation and treatment of androgenetic alopecia: A research advance. *eFood*, *5*(2). Available from https://doi.org/10.1002/efd2.138.

Farooq, T. (2013). *Phytochemical and pharmacological investigation of the leaves of Carica papaya Linn. (Doctoral dissertation, East West University).*

Favela-González, K. M., Hernández-Almanza, A. Y., & De la Fuente-Salcido, N. M. (2020). The value of bioactive compounds of cruciferous vegetables (Brassica) as antimicrobials and antioxidants: A review. *Journal of Food Biochemistry*, *44*(10). Available from https://doi.org/10.1111/jfbc.13414, http://onlinelibrary.wiley.com/journal/10.1111/(ISSN)1745-4514.

Ferdousi, F., Sasaki, K., Xu, D., Zheng, Y. W., Szele, F. G., & Isoda, H. (2022). Editorial: Directing stem cell fate using plant extracts and their bioactive compounds. *Frontiers in Cell and Developmental Biology*, *10*. Available from https://doi.org/10.3389/fcell.2022.957601, https://www.frontiersin.org/journals/cell-and-developmental-biology#.

Ferreira, I. C. F. R., Martins, N., & Barros, L. (2017). Phenolic compounds and its bioavailability: In vitro bioactive compounds or health promoters? *Advances in Food and Nutrition Research*, *82*, 1–44. Available from https://doi.org/10.1016/bs.afnr.2016.12.004, http://www.elsevier.com/wps/find/bookdescription.cws_home/704624/description#description.

Flesch, A. G. T., Poziomyck, A. K., & Damin, D. D. C. (2014). The therapeutic use of symbiotics. *ABCD. Arquivos Brasileiros de Cirurgia Digestiva (São Paulo).*, *27*(3), 206–209. Available from https://doi.org/10.1590/s0102-67202014000300012.

Fujita, Y., Tsuno, H., Nakayama, J., & Ahlenstiel, G. (2017). Fermented papaya preparation restores age-related reductions in peripheral blood mononuclear cell cytolytic activity in tube-fed patients. *PLoS One*, *12*(1)e0169240. Available from https://doi.org/10.1371/journal.pone.0169240.

Fung, E. S., Parker, J. A., & Monnot, A. D. (2023). Evaluating the impact of hair care product exposure on hair follicle and scalp health. *Alternatives to Laboratory Animals*, *51*(5), 323–334. Available from https://doi.org/10.1177/02611929231190863, https://journals.sagepub.com/home/atl.

Gan, A., & Baroutian, S. (2022). Current status and trends in extraction of bioactives from brown macroalgae using supercritical CO 2 and subcritical water. *Journal of Chemical Technology & Biotechnology*, *97*(8), 1929–1940. Available from https://doi.org/10.1002/jctb.7063.

Garavaglia, J., Markoski, M. M., Oliveira, A., & Marcadenti, A. (2016). Grape seed oil compounds: Biological and chemical actions for health. *Nutrition and Metabolic Insights*, *9*, 59–64. Available from https://doi.org/10.4137/NMI.S32910, http://www.la-press.com/redirect_file.php?fileId = 7763&filename = 5843-NMI-Grape-Seed-Oil-Compounds:-Biological-and-Chemical-Actions-for-Health.pdf&fileType = pdf.

Garnier, A., & Shahidi, F. (2021). Spices and herbs as immune enhancers and anti-inflammatory agents: A review. *Journal of Food Bioactives*, *14*. Available from https://doi.org/10.31665/jfb.2021.14266.

Gasmi, A., Mujawdiya, P. K., Beley, N., Shanaida, M., Lysiuk, R., Lenchyk, L., Noor, S., Muhammad, A., Strus, O., Piscopo, S., Komisarenko, A., Fedorovska, M., & Bjørklund, G. (2023). Natural compounds used for treating hair loss. *Current Pharmaceutical Design*, *29*(16), 1231–1244. Available from https://doi.org/10.2174/1381612829666230505100147, http://www.eurekaselect.com/606/journal/current-pharmaceutical-design.

Gebashe, F. C., Naidoo, D., Amoo, S. O., & Masondo, N. A. (2022). Cosmeceuticals: A newly expanding industry in South Africa. *Cosmetics*, *9*(4), 77. Available from https://doi.org/10.3390/cosmetics9040077, www.mdpi.com/journal/cosmetics.

Giordano, S., Romeo, M., & Lankinen, P. (2017). Platelet-rich plasma for androgenetic alopecia: Does it work? Evidence from meta analysis. *Journal of Cosmetic Dermatology*, *16*(3), 374–381. Available from https://doi.org/10.1111/jocd.12331.

Gitea, M. A., Bungau, S. G., Gitea, D., Pasca, B. M., Purza, A. L., & Radu, A.-F. (2023). Evaluation of the phytochemistry–therapeutic activity relationship for grape seeds oil. *Life (Chicago, Ill.: 1978)*, *13*(1), 2023.

Gokce, N., Basgoz, N., Kenanoglu, S., Akalin, H., Ozkul, Y., Ergoren, M. C., Beccari, T., Bertelli, M., & Dundar, M. (2022). An overview of the genetic aspects of hair loss and its connection with nutrition. *Journal of Preventive Medicine and Hygiene*, *63*(2), E228. Available from https://doi.org/10.15167/2421-4248/jpmh2022.63.2S3.2765.

Gonçalves, A. C., Nunes, A. R., Falcão, A., Alves, G., & Silva, L. R. (2021). Dietary effects of anthocyanins in human health: A comprehensive review. *Pharmaceuticals*, *14*(7). Available from https://doi.org/10.3390/ph14070690, https://www.mdpi.com/1424-8247/14/7/690/pdf.

Gordon, K., Gordon, K., & Tosti, A. (2011). Alopecia: Evaluation and treatment. *Clinical, Cosmetic and Investigational Dermatology*, 101. Available from https://doi.org/10.2147/CCID.S10182.

Goyal, A., Sharma, V., Upadhyay, N., Gill, S., & Sihag, M. (2014). Flax and flaxseed oil: An ancient medicine & modern functional food. *Journal of Food Science and Technology*, *51*(9), 1633–1653. Available from https://doi.org/10.1007/s13197-013-1247-9.

Granado-Lorencio, F., & Hernández-Alvarez, E. (2016). Functional foods and health effects: A nutritional biochemistry perspective. *Current Medicinal Chemistry*, *23*(26), 2929–2957. Available from https://doi.org/10.2174/0929867323666160615105746.

S.S. Gropper, J.L. Smith, T.P. Carr, Advanced nutrition and human metabolism. (2022), 2022.

Gruskiene, R., Bockuviene, A., & Sereikaite, J. (2021). Microencapsulation of bioactive ingredients for their delivery into fermented milk products: A review. *Molecules (Basel, Switzerland)*, *26*(15), 4601. Available from https://doi.org/10.3390/molecules26154601.

Guo, E. L., & Katta, R. (2017). Diet and hair loss: Effects of nutrient deficiency and supplement use. *Dermatology Practical & Conceptual*, 1–10. Available from https://doi.org/10.5826/dpc.0701a01.

Hagino, T., Okazaki, S., Serizawa, N., Suzuki, K., Kaga, M., Otsuka, Y., Mikami, E., Hoashi, T., Saeki, H., Matsuda, H., Mitsui, H., & Kanda, N. (2021). Dietary habits in Japanese patients with alopecia areata. *Clinical, Cosmetic and Investigational Dermatology*, *14*, 1579–1591. Available from https://doi.org/10.2147/ccid.s335440.

Hart, A. L., Stagg, A. J., Frame, M., Graffner, H., Glise, H., Falk, P., & Kamm, M. A. (2002). The role of the gut flora in health and disease, and its modification as therapy. *Alimentary Pharmacology & Therapeutics*, *16*(8), 1383–1393. Available from https://doi.org/10.1046/j.1365-2036.2002.01310.x.

Hayashi, A., Mikami, Y., Miyamoto, K., Kamada, N., Sato, T., Mizuno, S., Naganuma, M., Teratani, T., Aoki, R., Fukuda, S., Suda, W., Hattori, M., Amagai, M., Ohyama, M., & Kanai, T. (2017). Intestinal dysbiosis and biotin deprivation induce alopecia through overgrowth of *Lactobacillus murinus* in mice. *Cell Reports*, *20*(7), 1513–1524. Available from https://doi.org/10.1016/j.celrep.2017.07.057.

Heilmann-Heimbach, S., Hochfeld, L. M., Henne, S. K., & Nöthen, M. M. (2020). Hormonal regulation in male androgenetic alopecia—Sex hormones and beyond: Evidence from recent genetic studies. *Experimental Dermatology*, *29*(9), 814–827. Available from https://doi.org/10.1111/exd.14130, http://onlinelibrary.wiley.com/journal/10.1111/(ISSN)1600-0625.

Herman, A., & Herman, A. P. (2023). Biological activity of fermented plant extracts for potential dermal applications. *Pharmaceutics*, *15*(12). Available from https://doi.org/10.3390/pharmaceutics15122775, http://www.mdpi.com/journal/pharmaceutics.

Horie, K., Nanashima, N., Maeda, H., Tomisawa, T., & Oey, I. (2021). Blackcurrant (Ribes nigrum L.) extract exerts potential vasculoprotective effects in ovariectomized rats, including prevention of elastin degradation and pathological vascular remodeling. *Nutrients*, *13*(2), 560. Available from https://doi.org/10.3390/nu13020560.

Hussain, A., Kausar, T., Sehar, S., Sarwar, A., Ashraf, A. H., Jamil, M. A., Noreen, S., Rafique, A., Iftikhar, K., Quddoos, M. Y., Aslam, J., & Majeed, M. A. (2022). A Comprehensive review of functional ingredients, especially bioactive compounds present in pumpkin peel, flesh and seeds, and their health benefits. *Food Chemistry Advances*, *1*. Available from https://doi.org/10.1016/j.focha.2022.100067, https://www.journals.elsevier.com/food-chemistry-advances.

Hussain, A., Kausar, T., Jamil, M. A., Noreen, S., Iftikhar, K., Rafique, A., Iqbal, M. A., Majeed, M. A., Quddoos, M. Y., Aslam, J., & Ali, A. (2022). In vitro role of pumpkin parts as pharma-foods: Antihyperglycemic and antihyperlipidemic activities of pumpkin peel, flesh, and seed powders, in alloxan-induced diabetic rats. *International Journal of Food Science*, *2022*. Available from https://doi.org/10.1155/2022/4804408, http://www.hindawi.com/journals/ijfs/.

Hwang, S. B., Park, H. J., & Lee, B. H. (2022). Hair-growth-promoting effects of the fish collagen peptide in human dermal papilla cells and C57BL/6 mice modulating Wnt/β-Catenin and BMP Signaling Pathways. *International Journal of Molecular Sciences*, *23*(19). Available from https://doi.org/10.3390/ijms231911904, http://www.mdpi.com/journal/ijms.

Jesumani, V., Du, H., Aslam, M., Pei, P., & Huang, N. (2019). Potential use of seaweed bioactive compounds in skincare—A review. *Marine Drugs*, *17*(12), 688. Available from https://doi.org/10.3390/md17120688.

Joubert, E., & de Beer, D. (2012). Phenolic content and antioxidant activity of rooibos food ingredient extracts. *Journal of Food Composition and Analysis*, *27*(1), 45–51. Available from https://doi.org/10.1016/j.jfca.2012.03.011.

Juhasz, M., Chen, S., Khosrovi-Eghbal, A., Ekelem, C., Landaverde, Y., Baldi, P., & Atanaskova Mesinkovska, N. (2020). Characterizing the skin and gut microbiome of alopecia areata patients. *SKIN The Journal of Cutaneous Medicine*, *4*(1), 23–30. Available from https://doi.org/10.25251/skin.4.1.4.

Jung, D. R., Yoo, H. Y., Kim, M. J., Singh, V., Park, S. H., Jeong, M., Park, B. J., & Shin, J. H. (2022). Comparative analysis of scalp and gut microbiome in androgenetic alopecia: A Korean cross-sectional study. *Frontiers in Microbiology*, *13*. Available from https://doi.org/10.3389/fmicb.2022.1076242, https://www.frontiersin.org/journals/microbiology#.

Jung, H., Jung, D. M., Lee, S. S., Kim, E. M., Yoon, K., & Kim, K. K. (2022). Mangifera Indica leaf extracts promote hair growth via activation of Wnt signaling pathway in human dermal papilla cells. *Animal Cells and Systems*, *26*(3), 129–136. Available from https://doi.org/10.1080/19768354.2022.2085790, http://www.tandfonline.com/loi/tacs20.

Kadiri, O., Gbadamosi, S. O., Olawoye, B., & Akanbi, C. T. (2016). Changes in total phenolic and protein contents during production of protein isolates from Carica papaya (Pawpaw) Seeds. *Turkish Journal of Agriculture - Food Science and Technology*, *4*(11), 1006. Available from https://doi.org/10.24925/turjaf.v4i11.1006-1013.550.

Kamp, E., Ashraf, M., Musbahi, E., & DeGiovanni, C. (2022). Menopause, skin and common dermatoses. Part 1: hair disorders. *Clinical and Experimental Dermatology*, *47*(12), 2110–2116. Available from https://doi.org/10.1111/ced.15327.

Kane, K., & Prelack, K. (2019). *Medical nutrition therapy*. Burlington, MA, US: World Headquarters, Jones & Bartlett Learning, LLC.

Katsogridaki, G., Tzovaras, G., Sioka, E., Perivoliotis, K., Zachari, E., Magouliotis, D., Tasiopoulou, V., Chatedaki, C., & Zacharoulis, D. (2018). Hair loss after laparoscopic sleeve gastrectomy. *Obesity Surgery*, *28*(12), 3929–3934. Available from https://doi.org/10.1007/s11695-018-3433-3.

Kaur, S., Panghal, A., Garg, M. K., Mann, S., Khatkar, S. K., Sharma, P., & Chhikara, N. (2019). Functional and nutraceutical properties of pumpkin – A review. *Nutrition & Food Science*, *50*(2), 384–401. Available from https://doi.org/10.1108/nfs-05-2019-0143.

Kayode, O. T., Ohanaka, N. J., Kolawole, I. O., Afolabi, O. A., & Iyobhebhe, M. E. (2023). Reproductive health-promoting effects of functional foods. *Functional Food Institute, Nigeria Functional Foods in Health and Disease*, *13*(9), 448–458. Available from https://doi.org/10.31989/ffhd.v13i9.1130, https://www.ffhdj.com/index.php/ffhd/article/view/1130/1912.

Khadam, S., Afzal, U., Gul, H., Hira, S., Satti, M., Yaqub, A., Ajab, H., & Gulfraz, M. (2019). Phytochemical screening and bioactivity assessment of leaves and fruits extract of Carica papaya. *Pakistan Journal of Pharmaceutical Sciences, Pakistan Pakistan Journal of Pharmaceutical Sciences*, *32*(5), 1941–1948. Available from http://www.pjps.pk/wp-content/uploads/pdfs/32/5/Paper-4.pdf.

Khantham, C., Ruksiriwanich, W., Sringarm, K., Prom-u-thai, C., Jamjod, S., Arjin, C., Muangsanguan, A., Rachtanapun, P., Jantanasakulwong, K., Phimolsiripol, Y., Barba, F. J., Sommano, S. R., Chutoprapat, R., & Boonpisuttinant, K. (2023). Effects of bioactive composition in Oryza sativa L. cv. KDML105 Bran extract on gene expression related to hair cycle in human hair follicle dermal papilla cells. *Agronomy*, *13*(2). Available from https://doi.org/10.3390/agronomy13020295, www.mdpi.com/journal/agronomy/.

Kil, M. S., Kim, C. W., & Kim, S. S. (2013). Analysis of serum zinc and copper concentrations in hair loss. *Annals of Dermatology*, *25*(4), 405–409. Available from https://doi.org/10.5021/ad.2013.25.4.405South, http://pdf.medrang.co.kr/Aod/025/Aod025-04-02.pdf, Korea.

Kilic Yildirim, G., Dinleyici, M., Vandenplas, Y., & Dinleyici, E. C. (2022). Effects of multispecies synbiotic supplementation on anthropometric measurements, glucose and lipid parameters in children with exogenous obesity: A randomized, double blind, placebo-controlled clinical trial (probesity-2 trial). *Frontiers in Nutrition*, *9*. Available from https://doi.org/10.3389/fnut.2022.898037, journal.frontiersin.org/journal/nutrition.

Kim, I. S., Hwang, C. W., Yang, W. S., & Kim, C. H. (2021). Current perspectives on the physiological activities of fermented soybean-derived Cheonggukjang. *International Journal of Molecular Sciences*, *22*(11). Available from https://doi.org/10.3390/ijms22115746, https://www.mdpi.com/1422-0067/22/11/5746/pdf.

Krafczyk, N., Woyand, F., & Glomb, M. A. (2009). Structure-antioxidant relationship of flavonoids from fermented rooibos. *Molecular Nutrition and Food Research*, *53*(5), 635–642. Available from https://doi.org/10.1002/mnfr.200800117Germany, http://www3.interscience.wiley.com/cgi-bin/fulltext/121641922/PDFSTART.

Kruger, M., Boney, R., Ordoobadi, A. J., Sommers, T. F., Trapani, J. G., & Coffin, A. B. (2016). Natural bizbenzoquinoline derivatives protect zebrafish lateral line sensory hair cells from aminoglycoside toxicity. *Frontiers in Cellular Neuroscience*, *10*(2016). Available from https://doi.org/10.3389/fncel.2016.00083, http://journal.frontiersin.org/article/10.3389/fncel.2016.00083/pdf.

Kumari, P., Ahina, K. M., Kannan, K., Sreekumar, S., Lakra, R., Sivagnanam, U. T., & Syamala Kiran, M. (2024). In vivo soft tissue regenerative potential of flax seed mucilage self-assembled collagen aerogels. *Biomedical Materials*, *19*(2)025023. Available from https://doi.org/10.1088/1748-605x/ad1f79.

Kussmann, M., Abe Cunha, D. H., & Berciano, S. (2023). Bioactive compounds for human and planetary health. *Frontiers in Nutrition*, *10*. Available from https://doi.org/10.3389/fnut.2023.1193848, journal.frontiersin.org/journal/nutrition.

Lanham-New, S. A., Macdonald, I. A., & Roche, H. M. (2011). *Nutrition and Metabolism*. Wiley. Available from https://doi.org/10.1002/9781444327779.

Le Floc'h, C., Cheniti, A., Connétable, S., Piccardi, N., Vincenzi, C., & Tosti, A. (2015). Effect of a nutritional supplement on hair loss in women. *Journal of Cosmetic Dermatology*, *14*(1), 76–82. Available from https://doi.org/10.1111/jocd.12127.

Lebaka, V. R., Wee, Y. J., Narala, V. R., & Joshi, V. K. (2018). Development of new probiotic foods—A case study on probiotic juices. In A. M. Grumezescu, & A. M. Holban (Eds.), *Therapeutic, Probiotic, and Unconventional Foods* (pp. 55–78). Elsevier.

Ledoux, S., Flamant, M., Calabrese, D., Bogard, C., Sami, O., & Coupaye, M. (2020). What are the micronutrient deficiencies responsible for the most common nutritional symptoms after bariatric surgery? *Obesity Surgery*, *30*(5), 1891–1897. Available from https://doi.org/10.1007/s11695-020-04412-8.

Lee, H., Kim, H., Kim, J. H., Park, S. D., Shim, J. J., & Lee, J. L. (2022). Lactobacillus paracasei HY7015 and Lycopus lucidus Turcz. extract promotes human dermal papilla cell cytoprotective effect and hair regrowth rate in C57BL/6 Mice. *Molecules (Basel, Switzerland)*, *27*(23). Available from https://doi.org/10.3390/molecules27238235, http://www.mdpi.com/journal/molecules.

Lee, J., Yang, W., Hostetler, A., Schultz, N., Suckow, M. A., Stewart, K. L., Kim, D. D., & Kim, H. S. (2016). Characterization of the anti-inflammatory Lactobacillus reuteri BM36301 and its probiotic benefits on aged mice. *BMC Microbiology*, *16*(1). Available from https://doi.org/10.1186/s12866-016-0686-7, http://www.biomedcentral.com/bmcmicrobiol/.

Leichtweis, M. G., Molina, A. K., Pires, T. C. S., Dias, M. I., Calhelha, R., Bachari, K., Ziani, B. E. C., Oliveira, M. B. P. P., Pereira, C., & Barros, L. (2022). Biological activity of pumpkin byproducts: Antimicrobial and antioxidant properties. *Molecules (Basel, Switzerland)*, *27*(23). Available from https://doi.org/10.3390/molecules27238366, http://www.mdpi.com/journal/molecules.

Leitão, M., Ribeiro, T., García, P. A., Barreiros, L., & Correia, P. (2022). Benefits of fermented papaya in human health. *Foods*, *11*(4), 563. Available from https://doi.org/10.3390/foods11040563.

Leitão, M., Ferreira, B., Guedes, B., Moreira, D., García, P. A., Barreiros, L., & Correia, P. (2023). Screening of Antioxidant Effect of Spontaneous and Bioinoculated with Gluconobacter oxydans Fermented Papaya: A Comparative Study. *Fermentation*, *9*(2), 124. Available from https://doi.org/10.3390/fermentation9020124.

Lestari, B., & Meiyanto, E. (2018). A review: The emerging nutraceutical potential of pumpkin seeds. *Indonesian Journal of Cancer Chemoprevention*, *9*(2), 92. Available from https://doi.org/10.14499/indonesianjcanchemoprev9iss2pp92-101.

Lin, C. S., Chan, L. Y., Wang, J. H., & Chang, C. H. (2023). Diagnosis and treatment of female alopecia: Focusing on the iron deficiency-related alopecia. *Tzu Chi Medical Journal*, *35*(4), 322–328. Available from https://doi.org/10.4103/tcmj.tcmj_95_23, http://www.tcmjmed.com/backissues.asp.

Lin, R. L., Garibyan, L., Kimball, A. B., & Drake, L. A. (2016). Systemic causes of hair loss. *Annals of Medicine*, *48*(6), 393–402. Available from https://doi.org/10.1080/07853890.2016.1180426.

Liu, Y., Li, J., Liang, G., Cheng, C., Li, Y., & Wu, X. (2020). Association of alopecia areata with vitamin D and calcium levels: A systematic review and meta-analysis. *Dermatology and Therapy*, *10*(5), 967–983. Available from https://doi.org/10.1007/s13555-020-00433-4.

Lolou, V. (2021). The role of probiotics and synbiotics on hirsutism. *Fermentation*, *7*(1). Available from https://doi.org/10.3390/fermentation7010010, https://www.mdpi.com/2311-5637/7/1/10/pdf.

Lomartire, S., & Gonçalves, A. M. M. (2022). Antiviral activity and mechanisms of seaweeds bioactive compounds on enveloped viruses—A review. *Marine Drugs*, *20*(6). Available from https://doi.org/10.3390/md20060385, https://www.mdpi.com/1660-3397/20/6/385/pdf?version = 1654681082.

Lomartire, S., Marques, J. C., & Gonçalves, A. M. M. (2021). An overview to the health benefits of seaweeds consumption. *Marine Drugs*, *19*(6). Available from https://doi.org/10.3390/md19060341, https://www.mdpi.com/1660-3397/19/6/341.

Lukic, J., Chen, V., Strahinic, I., Begovic, J., Lev-Tov, H., Davis, S. C., Tomic-Canic, M., & Pastar, I. (2017). Probiotics or pro-healers: the role of beneficial bacteria in tissue repair. *Wound Repair and Regeneration*, *25*(6), 912–922. Available from https://doi.org/10.1111/wrr.12607, http://onlinelibrary.wiley.com/journal/10.1111/(ISSN)1524-475X.

Lyon, J., Connell, M., Chandrasekaran, K., & Srivastava, S. (2023). Effect of synbiotics on weight loss and metabolic health in adults with overweight and obesity: A randomized controlled trial. *Obesity*, *31*(8), 2009–2020. Available from https://doi.org/10.1002/oby.23801, http://onlinelibrary.wiley.com/journal/10.1002/(ISSN)1930-739X.

Mahmud, M. R., Akter, S., Tamanna, S. K., Mazumder, L., Esti, I. Z., Banerjee, S., Akter, S., Hasan, M. R., Acharjee, M., Hossain, M. S., & Pirttilä, A. M. (2022). Impact of gut microbiome on skin health: Gut-skin axis observed through the lenses of therapeutics and skin diseases. *Gut Microbes*, *14*(1). Available from https://doi.org/10.1080/19490976.2022.2096995, http://www.tandfonline.com/toc/kgmi20/current.

Martial-Didier, A. K., Hubert, K. K., Jean Parfait, K. E., & Kablan, T. (2017). Phytochemical properties and proximate composition of papaya (Carica papaya L. var solo 8) peels. *Turkish Journal of Agriculture - Food Science and Technology*, *5*(6), 676–680. Available from https://doi.org/10.24925/turjaf.v5i6.676-680.1154.

Martínez Leal, J., Valenzuela Suárez, L., Jayabalan, R., Huerta Oros, J., & Escalante-Aburto, A. (2018). A review on health benefits of kombucha nutritional compounds and metabolites. *CyTA - Journal of Food*, *16*(1), 390–399. Available from https://doi.org/10.1080/19476337.2017.1410499.

Martyniak, A., Medyńska-Przęczek, A., Wędrychowicz, A., Skoczeń, S., & Tomasik, P. J. (2021). Prebiotics, probiotics, synbiotics, paraprobiotics and postbiotic compounds in IBD. *Biomolecules*, *11*(12). Available from https://doi.org/10.3390/biom11121903, https://www.mdpi.com/2218-273X/11/12/1903/pdf.

Matthäus, B. (2008). Virgin grape seed oil: Is it really a nutritional highlight? *European Journal of Lipid Science and Technology*, *110*(7), 645–650. Available from https://doi.org/10.1002/ejlt.200700276.

Mayer, W., Weibel, M., De Luca, C., Ibragimova, G., Trakhtman, I., Kharaeva, Z., Chandler, D. L., & Korkina, L. (2023). Biomolecules of fermented tropical fruits and fermenting microbes as regulators of human hair loss, hair quality, and scalp microbiota. *Biomolecules*, *13*(4). Available from https://doi.org/10.3390/biom13040699, http://www.mdpi.com/journal/biomolecules.

de Menezes, M. L., Johann, G., Diório, A., Schuelter Boeing, J., Visentainer, J. V., Raimundini Aranha, A. C., & Curvelo Pereira, N. (2023). Comparison of the chemical composition of grape seed oil extracted by different methods and conditions. *Journal of Chemical Technology and Biotechnology*, *98*(5), 1103–1113. Available from https://doi.org/10.1002/jctb.7314, http://onlinelibrary.wiley.com/journal/10.1002/(ISSN)1097-4660.

Milani, M., & Colombo, F. (2023). Efficacy and tolerability of an oral supplement containing amino acids, iron, selenium, and marine hydrolyzed collagen in subjects with hair loss (androgenetic alopecia, AGA or FAGA or telogen effluvium). A prospective, randomized, 3-month, controlled, assessor-blinded study. *Skin Research and Technology*, *29*(6). Available from https://doi.org/10.1111/srt.13381.

Min, K.-N. (2022). Study on the efficiency of relieving hair loss of human body-derived lactobacillus combined cosmetics. *Journal of the Korea Convergence Society, 13*(5), 35–43, 2022.

Montazeri-Najafabady, N., Ghasemi, Y., Dabbaghmanesh, M. H., Ashoori, Y., Talezadeh, P., Koohpeyma, F., Abootalebi, S. N., & Gholami, A. (2021). Exploring the bone sparing effects of postbiotics in the post-menopausal rat model. *BMC Complementary Medicine and Therapies, 21*(1). Available from https://doi.org/10.1186/s12906-021-03327-w, https://link.springer.com/journal/12906/volumes-and-issues.

Montesano, D., Blasi, F., Simonetti, M. S., Santini, A., & Cossignani, L. (2018). Chemical and nutritional characterization of seed oil from *Cucurbita maxima* L. (Var. Berrettina) pumpkin. *Foods, 7*(3). Available from https://doi.org/10.3390/foods7030030, https://www.mdpi.com/2304-8158/7/3.

Moosa, S., Kasonga, A. E., Deepak, V., Marais, S., Magoshi, I. B., Bester, M. J., Kruger, M. C., & Coetzee, M. (2018). Rooibos tea extracts inhibit osteoclast formation and activity through the attenuation of NF-κB activity in RAW264.7 murine macrophages. *Food and Function, 9*(6), 3301–3312. Available from https://doi.org/10.1039/c7fo01497j, http://pubs.rsc.org/en/journals/journal/fo.

Mora-Sánchez, B., Balcázar, J. L., & Pérez-Sánchez, T. (2020). Effect of a novel postbiotic containing lactic acid bacteria on the intestinal microbiota and disease resistance of rainbow trout (Oncorhynchus mykiss. *Biotechnology Letters, 42*(10), 1957–1962. Available from https://doi.org/10.1007/s10529-020-02919-9, www.wkap.nl/journalhome.htm/0141-5492.

Morowitz, M. J., Carlisle, E. M., & Alverdy, J. C. (2011). Contributions of intestinal bacteria to nutrition and metabolism in the critically ill. *Surgical Clinics of North America, 91*(4), 771–785. Available from https://doi.org/10.1016/j.suc.2011.05.001.

Muller, C. J. F., Joubert, E., Chellan, N., Miura, Y., & Yagasaki, K. (2022). New insights into the efficacy of aspalathin and other related phytochemicals in type 2 diabetes—A review. *International Journal of Molecular Sciences, 23*(1). Available from https://doi.org/10.3390/ijms23010356, https://www.mdpi.com/1422-0067/23/1/356/pdf.

Muller, C. J. F., Malherbe, C. J., Chellan, N., Yagasaki, K., Miura, Y., & Joubert, E. (2018). Potential of rooibos, its major C-glucosyl flavonoids, and Z-2-(β-D-glucopyranosyloxy)-3-phenylpropenoic acid in prevention of metabolic syndrome. *Critical Reviews in Food Science and Nutrition, 58* (2), 227–246. Available from:. Available from https://doi.org/10.1080/10408398.2016.1157568, www.tandf.co.uk/journals/titles/10408398.asp.

Multescu, M., Marinas, I. C., Susman, I. E., & Belc, N. (2022). Byproducts (flour, meals, and groats) from the vegetable oil industry as a potential source of antioxidants. *Foods, 11*(3). Available from https://doi.org/10.3390/foods11030253, https://www.mdpi.com/2304-8158/11/3/253/pdf.

Mustafa, A. I., Khashaba, R. A., Fawzy, E., Baghdady, S. M. A. E. R., & Rezk, S. M. (2021). Cross talk between oxidative stress and inflammation in alopecia areata. *Journal of Cosmetic Dermatology, 20*(7), 2305–2310. Available from https://doi.org/10.1111/jocd.13814, http://onlinelibrary.wiley.com/journal/10.1111/(ISSN)1473-2165.

Nehme, R., Chervet, A., Decombat, C., Longechamp, L., Rossary, A., Boutin, R., Rousset, A., Senejoux, F., Vachias, C., Auxenfans, C., Fraisse, D., Guyon, J. B., Filaire, E., Berthon, J. Y., Diab-Assaf, M., Delort, L., & Caldefie-Chezet, F. (2023). Aspalathus linearis (rooibos) targets adipocytes and obesity-associated inflammation. *Nutrients, 15*(7). Available from https://doi.org/10.3390/nu15071751, http://www.mdpi.com/journal/nutrients/.

Nichols, A. J., Hughes, O. B., Canazza, A., & Zaiac, M. N. (2017). An open-label evaluator blinded study of the efficacy and safety of a new nutritional supplement in androgenetic alopecia: A pilot study. *Journal of Clinical and Aesthetic Dermatology, 10*(2), 52–56. Available from https://www.ncbi.nlm.nih.gov/pmc/articles/PMC5367873/pdf/jcad_10_2_52.pdf.

Nowak, W., & Jeziorek, M. (2023). The role of flaxseed in improving human health. *Healthcare, 11*(3), 395. Available from https://doi.org/10.3390/healthcare11030395.

Nunes, M. A., Rodrigues, F., & Oliveira, M. B. P. P. (2017). Grape processing by-products as active ingredients for cosmetic proposes. In *Handbook of grape processing by-products: Sustainable solutions*, (pp. 267–292). Elsevier Inc.

Orlando, P., Chellan, N., Louw, J., Tiano, L., Cirilli, I., Dludla, P., Joubert, E., & Muller, C. J. F. (2019). Aspalathin-rich green rooibos extract lowers LDL-cholesterol and oxidative status in high-fat diet-induced diabetic vervet monkeys. *Molecules (Basel, Switzerland), 24*(9). Available from https://doi.org/10.3390/molecules24091713, https://www.mdpi.com/1420-3049/24/9/1713/pdf.

Ou, H. C., Cunningham, L. L., Francis, S. P., Brandon, C. S., Simon, J. A., Raible, D. W., & Rubel, E. W. (2009). Identification of FDA-approved drugs and bioactives that protect hair cells in the zebrafish (Danio rerio) lateral line and mouse (Mus musculus) utricle. *Journal of the Association for Research in Otolaryngology, 10*(2), 191–203. Available from https://doi.org/10.1007/s10162-009-0158-y.

Pandey, A. K., Chauhan, O. P., & Semwal, A. D. (2020). Seaweeds. *Defence Life Science Journal, 5*(4), 315–322. Available from https://doi.org/10.14429/dlsj.5.15632.

Pangestuti, R., Shin, K. H., & Kim, S. K. (2021). Anti-photoaging and potential skin health benefits of seaweeds. *Marine Drugs, 19*(3). Available from https://doi.org/10.3390/MD19030172, https://www.mdpi.com/1660-3397/19/3/172.

Parisi, O. I., Scrivano, L., Amone, F., Malivindi, R., Ruffo, M., Vattimo, A. F., Pezzi, V., & Puoci, F. (2018). Interconnected PolymerS TeChnology (IPSTiC): An effective approach for the modulation of 5α-reductase activity in hair loss conditions. *Journal of Functional Biomaterials, 9*(3). Available from https://doi.org/10.3390/jfb9030044, http://www.mdpi.com/2079-4983/9/3/44/pdf.

Park, D. W., Lee, H. S., Shim, M. S., Yum, K. J., & Seo, J. T. (2020). Do kimchi and Cheonggukjang probiotics as a functional food improve androgenetic alopecia? A clinical pilot study. *World Journal of Men's Health, 38*(1), 95–102. Available from https://doi.org/10.5534/wjmh.180119, https://www.wjmh.org/Synapse/Data/PDFData/2074WJMH/wjmh-38-95.pdf.

Park, S., & Lee, J. (2021). Modulation of hair growth promoting effect by natural products. *Pharmaceutics, 13*(12). Available from https://doi.org/10.3390/pharmaceutics13122163, https://www.mdpi.com/1999-4923/13/12/2163.

Pateiro, M., Domínguez, R., Munekata, P. E. S., Nieto, G., Bangar, S. P., Dhama, K., & Lorenzo, J. M. (2023). Bioactive compounds from leaf vegetables as preservatives. *Foods, 12*(3). Available from:. Available from https://doi.org/10.3390/foods12030637, www.mdpi.com/journal/foods.

Patel, D. P., Swink, S. M., & Castelo-Soccio, L. (2017). A review of the use of biotin for hair loss. *Skin Appendage Disorders, 3*(3), 166–169. Available from https://doi.org/10.1159/000462981, https://www.karger.com/Journal/Home/261870.

Pengilly, M., Joubert, E., Van Zyl, W. H., Botha, A., & Bloom, M. (2008). Enhancement of Rooibos (Aspalathus linearis) aqueous extract and antioxidant yield with fungal enzymes. *Journal of Agricultural and Food Chemistry*, *56*(11), 4047–4053. Available from https://doi.org/10.1021/jf073095y.

Pham, C. T., Romero, K., Almohanna, H. M., Griggs, J., Ahmed, A., & Tosti, A. (2020). The role of diet as an adjuvant treatment in scarring and nonscarring alopecia. *Skin Appendage Disorders*, *6*(2), 88–96. Available from https://doi.org/10.1159/000504786, https://www.karger.com/Journal/Home/261870.

Pincemail, J., & Meziane, S. (2022). On the potential role of the antioxidant couple vitamin E/selenium taken by the oral route in skin and hair health. *Antioxidants*, *11*(11), 2270. Available from https://doi.org/10.3390/antiox11112270.

Polak, K., Jobbágy, A., Muszyński, T., Wojciechowska, K., Frątczak, A., Bánvölgyi, A., Bergler-Czop, B., & Kiss, N. (2021). Microbiome modulation as a therapeutic approach in chronic skin diseases. *Biomedicines*, *9*(10), 1436. Available from https://doi.org/10.3390/biomedicines9101436.

Pratt, C. H., King, L. E., Messenger, A. G., Christiano, A. M., & Sundberg, J. P. (2017). Alopecia areata. *Nature Reviews Disease Primers*, *3*. Available from https://doi.org/10.1038/nrdp.2017.11, http://www.nature.com/nrdp/.

Puri, V., Nagpal, M., Singh, I., Singh, M., Dhingra, G. A., Huanbutta, K., Dheer, D., Sharma, A., & Sangnim, T. (2022). A comprehensive review on nutraceuticals: Therapy support and formulation challenges. *Nutrients*, *14*(21), 4637. Available from https://doi.org/10.3390/nu14214637.

Rajput, M., & Kumar, N. (2020). Medicinal plants: A potential source of novel bioactive compounds showing antimicrobial efficacy against pathogens infecting hair and scalp. *Gene Reports*, *21*100879. Available from https://doi.org/10.1016/j.genrep.2020.100879.

Rajput, R. (2022). Influence of nutrition, food supplements and lifestyle in hair disorders. *Indian Dermatology Online Journal*, *13*(6), 721–724. Available from https://doi.org/10.4103/idoj.idoj_175_22, www.idoj.in/.

Rashidinejad, A., & Mahdi Jafari, S. (2020). *Nanoencapsulation of bioactive food ingredients* (pp. 279–344). Elsevier BV. Available from 10.1016/b978-0-12-815866-1.00008-x.

Rebello, D., Wang, E., Yen, E., Lio, P. A., & Kelly, C. R. (2017). Hair growth in two alopecia patients after fecal microbiota transplant. *ACG Case Reports Journal*, *4*(1). Available from https://doi.org/10.14309/CRJ.2017.107, https://journals.lww.com/acgcr/pages/default.aspx.

Rezig, L., Harzalli, Z., Gharsallah, K., Mahfoudhi, N., Chouaibi, M., Majdoub, H., & Oueslati, I. (2022). Microwave and roasting impact on pumpkin seed oil and its application in full-fat mayonnaise formula. *Foods*, *11*(18), 2732. Available from https://doi.org/10.3390/foods11182732.

Riangjanapatee, P., Khongkow, M., Treetong, A., Unger, O., Phungbun, C., Jaemsai, S., Bootsiri, C., & Okonogi, S. (2022). Development of tea seed oil nanostructured lipid carriers and in vitro studies on their applications in inducing human hair growth. *Pharmaceutics*, *14*(5), 984. Available from https://doi.org/10.3390/pharmaceutics14050984.

Rinaldi, F., Trink, A., & Pinto, D. (2020). Efficacy of postbiotics in a prp-like cosmetic product for the treatment of alopecia area celsi: A randomized double-blinded parallel-group study. *Dermatology and Therapy*, *10*(3), 483–493. Available from https://doi.org/10.1007/s13555-020-00369-9.

Rivera-Pastrana, D. M., & Yahia, E. M. (2010). G.A. González-Aguilar, Phenolic and carotenoid profiles of papaya fruit (*Carica papaya* L.) and their contents under low temperature storage. *Journal of the Science of Food and Agriculture*, *90*(14), 2358–2365. Available from https://doi.org/10.1002/jsfa.4092Mexico, http://onlinelibrary.wiley.com/doi/10.1002/jsfa.4092.

Rizer, R. L., Stephens, T. J., Herndon, J. H., Sperber, B. R., Murphy, J., & Ablon, G. R. (2015). A marine protein-based dietary supplement for subclinical hair thinning/loss: Results of a multisite, double-blind, placebo-controlled clinical trial. *International Journal of Trichology*, *7*(4), 156–166,. Available from https://doi.org/10.4103/0974-7753.171573, http://www.ijtrichology.com/.

Rohman, A., & Irnawati. (2019). Pumpkin (Cucurbita maxima) seed oil: Chemical composition, antioxidant activities and its authentication analysis. *Food Research*, *4*(3), 578–584. Available from https://doi.org/10.26656/fr.2017.4(3).242.

Rolim, P. M. (2015). Development of prebiotic food products and health benefits. *Food Science and Technology (Brazil)*, *35*(1), 3–10. Available from https://doi.org/10.1590/1678-457X.6546, http://www.scielo.br/pdf/cta/v35n1/0101-2061-cta-35-1-3.pdf.

Rossino, M. G., & Casini, G. (2019). Nutraceuticals for the treatment of diabetic retinopathy. *Nutrients*, *11*(4). Available from https://doi.org/10.3390/nu11040771, https://www.mdpi.com/2072-6643/11/4/771/pdf.

Rossino, M. G., Dal Monte, M., & Casini, G. (2019). Relationships between neurodegeneration and vascular damage in diabetic retinopathy. *Frontiers in Neuroscience*, *13*. Available from https://doi.org/10.3389/fnins.2019.01172, https://www.frontiersin.org/journals/neuroscience#.

Rudnicka, L., & Waśkiel-Burnat, A. (2021). Systemic aspects of alopecia areata Comment to the article by Lai and Sinclair. *Journal of the European Academy of Dermatology and Venereology*, *35*(3)e214. Available from https://doi.org/10.1111/jdv.16936, http://onlinelibrary.wiley.com/journal/10.1111/(ISSN)1468-3083.

Ruiz-Tagle, S. A., Figueira, M. M., Vial, V., & Espinoza-Benavides, L. (2018). M. Miteva, Micronutrients in hair loss. *Our Dermatology Online/Nasza Dermatologia Online*, *9*.

Ruksiriwanich, W., Khantham, C., Muangsanguan, A., Chittasupho, C., Rachtanapun, P., Jantanasakulwong, K., Phimolsiripol, Y., Sommano, S. R., Sringarm, K., Ferrer, E., & Barba, F. J. (2022). Phytochemical constitution, anti-inflammation, anti-androgen, and hair growth-promoting potential of shallot (*Allium ascalonicum* L.) extract. *Plants*, *11*(11). Available from https://doi.org/10.3390/plants11111499, https://www.mdpi.com/2223-7747/11/11/1499/pdf?version = 1654180705.

Saini, K., & Mysore, V. (2021). Role of vitamin D in hair loss: A short review. *Journal of Cosmetic Dermatology*, *20*(11), 3407–3414. Available from https://doi.org/10.1111/jocd.14421.

Salehi, B., Sharifi-Rad, J., Seca, A. M. L., Pinto, D. C. G. A., Michalak, I., Trincone, A., Mishra, A. P., Nigam, M., Zam, W., & Martins, N. (2019). Current trends on seaweeds: Looking at chemical composition, phytopharmacology, and cosmetic applications. *Molecules (Basel, Switzerland)*, *24*(22). Available from https://doi.org/10.3390/molecules24224182, https://www.mdpi.com/1420-3049/24/22/4182/pdf.

Salhab, O., Khayat, L., & Alaaeddine, N. (2022). Stem cell secretome as a mechanism for restoring hair loss due to stress, particularly alopecia areata: Narrative review. *Journal of Biomedical Science*, *29*(1). Available from https://doi.org/10.1186/s12929-022-00863-6.

Šamec, D., Loizzo, M. R., Gortzi, O., Çankaya, İ. T., Tundis, R., Suntar, İ., Shirooie, S., Zengin, G., Devkota, H. P., Reboredo-Rodríguez, P., Hassan, S. T. S., Manayi, A., Kashani, H. R. K., & Nabavi, S. M. (2022). The potential of pumpkin seed oil as a functional food—A comprehensive review of chemical composition, health benefits, and safety. *Comprehensive Reviews in Food Science and Food Safety*, *21*(5), 4422–4446. Available from https://doi.org/10.1111/1541-4337.13013, http://onlinelibrary.wiley.com/journal/10.1111/(ISSN)1541-4337.

Sánchez-Pellicer, P., Navarro-Moratalla, L., Núñez-Delegido, E., Agüera-Santos, J., & Navarro-López, V. (2022). How our microbiome influences the pathogenesis of alopecia areata. *Genes*, *13*(10), 1860. Available from https://doi.org/10.3390/genes13101860.

Sanjayasari, D., Meinita, M. D. N., & Winanto, T. (2021). Retention and survival optimization of juvenile green mussel (Perna viridis) by using substrate from different seaweed extracts. *Jurnal Ilmiah Perikanan dan Kelautan*, *13*(2), 193–200. Available from https://doi.org/10.20473/jipk.v13i2.23515, https://e-journal.unair.ac.id/JIPK/article/download/23515/15697.

Sattar, F., Almas, U., Ibrahim, N. A., Akhtar, A., Shazad, M. K., Akram, S., Khan, M. S. N., & Murtaza, G. (2021). Efficacy of oral vitamin D3 therapy in patients suffering from diffuse hair loss (*Telogen effluvium*). *Journal of Nutritional Science and Vitaminology*, *67*(1), 68–71. Available from https://doi.org/10.3177/jnsv.67.68, https://www.jstage.jst.go.jp/article/jnsv/67/1/67_68/_pdf/-char/en.

Schell, K. R., Fernandes, K. E., Shanahan, E., Wilson, I., Blair, S. E., Carter, D. A., & Cokcetin, N. N. (2022). The potential of honey as a prebiotic food to re-engineer the gut microbiome toward a healthy state. *Frontiers in Nutrition*, *9*. Available from https://doi.org/10.3389/fnut.2022.957932, journal.frontiersin.org/journal/nutrition.

Schneider, A. M., & Nelson, A. M. (2019). Skin microbiota: Friend or foe in pediatric skin health and skin disease. *Pediatric Dermatology*, *36*(6), 815–822. Available from https://doi.org/10.1111/pde.13955, http://onlinelibrary.wiley.com/journal/10.1111/(ISSN)1525-1470.

Sergeev, I. N., Aljutaily, T., Walton, G., & Huarte, E. (2020). Effects of synbiotic supplement on human gut microbiota, body composition and weight loss in obesity. *Nutrients*, *12*(1). Available from https://doi.org/10.3390/nu12010222, https://www.mdpi.com/2072-6643/12/1/222/pdf.

Shavandi, A., Saeedi, P., Gérard, P., Jalalvandi, E., Cannella, D., & Bekhit, A. E. D. (2020). The role of microbiota in tissue repair and regeneration. *Journal of Tissue Engineering and Regenerative Medicine*, *14*(3), 539–555. Available from https://doi.org/10.1002/term.3009, http://onlinelibrary.wiley.com/journal/10.1002/(ISSN)1932-7005.

Shen, C. L., Yeh, J. K., Cao, J. J., Chyu, M. C., & Wang, J. S. (2011). Green tea and bone health: Evidence from laboratory studies. *Pharmacological Research*, *64*(2), 155–161. Available from https://doi.org/10.1016/j.phrs.2011.03.012, http://www.elsevier.com/inca/publications/store/6/2/2/9/3/1/index.htt.

Singh, A., & Kumar, V. (2023). Phyto-chemical and bioactive compounds of pumpkin seed oil as affected by different extraction methods. *Food Chemistry Advances*, 2100211. Available from https://doi.org/10.1016/j.focha.2023.100211.

Singh, J., Metrani, R., Shivanagoudra, S. R., Jayaprakasha, G. K., & Patil, B. S. (2019). Review on Bile Acids: Effects of the Gut Microbiome, Interactions with Dietary Fiber, and Alterations in the Bioaccessibility of Bioactive Compounds. *Journal of Agricultural and Food Chemistry*, *67* (33), 9124–9138. Available from https://doi.org/10.1021/acs.jafc.8b07306, http://pubs.acs.org/journal/jafcau.

Smit, S. E., Manirafasha, C., Marais, E., Johnson, R., & Huisamen, B. (2022). Cardioprotective function of green rooibos (Aspalathus linearis) extract supplementation in ex vivo ischemic prediabetic rat hearts. *Planta Medica*, *88*(1), 62–78. Available from https://doi.org/10.1055/a-1239-9236, https://eref.thieme.de/ejournals/archive/1439-0221/;content_type = ejournal;content_ids = 1439-0221.

Sobuj, M. K. A., Islam, M. A., Islam, M. S., Islam, M. M., Mahmud, Y., & Rafiquzzaman, S. M. (2021). *Effect of Solvents on Bioactive Compounds and Antioxidant Activity of Padina Tetrastromatica and Gracilaria Tenuistipitata Seaweeds Collected From Bangladesh*. Research Square. Available from https://www.researchsquare.com/browse, 10.21203/rs.3.rs-557313/v1.

Spinei, M., & Oroian, M. (2021). The potential of grape pomace varieties as a dietary source of pectic substances. *Foods*, *10*(4), 867. Available from https://doi.org/10.3390/foods10040867.

Sultana, U., Zaidi, S. A., Iqbal, N., Quraishi, F., Khan, M. A., & Ali Baloch, F. (2022). Antibacterial activity of flax seeds extract rinse against Streptococcus mutans colonies. *Journal of Pharmaceutical Research International*, 19–24. Available from https://doi.org/10.9734/jpri/2022/v34i11b35863.

Tansathien, K., Chareanputtakhun, P., Ngawhirunpat, T., Opanasopit, P., & Rangsimawong, W. (2021). Hair growth promoting effect of bioactive extract from deer antler velvet-loaded niosomes and microspicules serum. *International Journal of Pharmaceutics*, *597*120352. Available from https://doi.org/10.1016/j.ijpharm.2021.120352.

Tayal, N., Srivastava, P., & Srivastava, N. (2019). Anti angiogenic activity of *Carica papaya* leaf extract. *Journal of Pure and Applied Microbiology*, *13*(1), 567–571. Available from https://doi.org/10.22207/jpam.13.1.64.

Tenore, G. C., Caruso, D., Buonomo, G., D'Avino, M., Santamaria, R., Irace, C., Piccolo, M., Maisto, M., & Novellino, E. (2018). Annurca apple nutraceutical formulation enhances keratin expression in a human model of skin and promotes hair growth and tropism in a randomized clinical trial. *Journal of Medicinal Food*, *21*(1), 90–103. Available from:. Available from https://doi.org/10.1089/jmf.2017.0016, www.liebertonline.com/jmf.

Tiedtke, J., & Marks, O. (2002). Rooibos-The new "white tea" for hair and skin care. *Euro Cosmetics*, *10*(6), 16–19.

Trüeb, R. M. (2016). Serum biotin levels in women complaining of hair loss. *International Journal of Trichology*, *8*(2), 73–77. Available from https://doi.org/10.4103/0974-7753.188040, http://www.ijtrichology.com/.

Tsai, W. H., Fang, Y. T., Huang, T. Y., Chiang, Y. J., Lin, C. G., & Chang, W. W. (2023). Heat-killed Lacticaseibacillus paracasei GMNL-653 ameliorates human scalp health by regulating scalp microbiome. *BMC Microbiology*, *23*(1). Available from https://doi.org/10.1186/s12866-023-02870-5, https://bmcmicrobiol.biomedcentral.com/.

Tzortzakis, N., Chrysargyris, A., & Petropoulos, S. A. (2018). Phytochemicals content and health effects of cultivated and underutilized species of the cucurbitaceae family. *Science Publishers Ltd*, 99–165. Available from https://doi.org/10.2174/9781681087399118010007.

Velasco Arango, V. A., Edwin Sotelo Barbosa, J., Eduardo Ordoñez Santos, L., & Igor Hleap Zapata, J. (2019). Characterization of functional components flour epicarp papaya (Carica papaya L) as a source of natural pigments. *Respuestas*, *24*(2), 39–48. Available from https://doi.org/10.22463/0122820x.1829.

Villarreal-Soto, S. A., Beaufort, S., Bouajila, J., Souchard, J. P., Renard, T., Rollan, S., & Taillandier, P. (2019). Impact of fermentation conditions on the production of bioactive compounds with anticancer, anti-inflammatory and antioxidant properties in kombucha tea extracts. *Process Biochemistry*, *83*, 44–54. Available from. Available from https://doi.org/10.1016/j.procbio.2019.05.004, www.elsevier.com/inca/publications/store/4/2/2/8/5/7.

Villarreal-Soto, S. A., Beaufort, S., Bouajila, J., Souchard, J. P., & Taillandier, P. (2018). Understanding kombucha tea fermentation: A review. *Journal of Food Science*, *83*(3), 580–588. Available from https://doi.org/10.1111/1750-3841.14068, http://www3.interscience.wiley.com/journal/118509799/issueyear?year = 2008.

Villasante Fricke, A. C., & Miteva, M. (2015). Epidemiology and burden of alopecia areata: A systematic review. *Clinical, Cosmetic and Investigational Dermatology*, *8*, 397–403,. Available from https://doi.org/10.2147/CCID.S53985, http://www.dovepress.com/getfile.php?fileID = 26121.

Wadstein, J., Thom, E., & Gadzhigoroeva, A. (2020). Integral roles of specific proteoglycans in hair growth and hair loss: Mechanisms behind the Bioactivity of Proteoglycan Replacement Therapy with Nourkrin® with Marilex® in Pattern Hair Loss and Telogen Effluvium. *Dermatology Research and Practice*, *2020*, 1–17. Available from https://doi.org/10.1155/2020/8125081.

Wang, W., Wang, H., Long, Y., Li, Z., & Li, J. (2024). Controlling hair loss by regulating apoptosis in hair follicles: A comprehensive overview. *Biomolecules*, *14*(1), 20. Available from https://doi.org/10.3390/biom14010020.

Waszkowiak, K., & Mikołajczak, B. (2020). The effect of roasting on the protein profile and antiradical capacity of flaxseed meal. *Foods*, *9*(10), 1383. Available from https://doi.org/10.3390/foods9101383.

Wen, X., Zhu, M., Hu, R., Zhao, J., Chen, Z., Li, J., & Ni, Y. (2016). Characterisation of seed oils from different grape cultivars grown in China. *Journal of Food Science and Technology*, *53*(7), 3129–3136. Available from https://doi.org/10.1007/s13197-016-2286-9, http://www.springerlink.com/content/121580/.

Xie, W. R., Yang, X. Y., Xia, H. H. X., Wu, L. H., & He, X. X. (2019). Hair regrowth following fecal microbiota transplantation in an elderly patient with alopecia areata: A case report and review of the literature. *World Journal of Clinical Cases*, *7*(19), 3074–3081. Available from https://doi.org/10.12998/wjcc.v7.i19.3074, https://f6publishing.blob.core.windows.net/a24d7857-08e4-4eb3-a033-10cceb5ec80e/WJCC-7-3074.pdf.

Xu, W., Wan, S., Xie, B., & Song, X. (2023). Novel potential therapeutic targets of alopecia areata. *Frontiers in Immunology*, *14*. Available from https://doi.org/10.3389/fimmu.2023.1148359.

Yang, J., Wen, C., Duan, Y., Deng, Q., Peng, D., Zhang, H., & Ma, H. (2021). The composition, extraction, analysis, bioactivities, bioavailability and applications in food system of flaxseed (Linum usitatissimum L.) oil: A review. *Trends in Food Science & Technology*, *118*, 252–260. Available from https://doi.org/10.1016/j.tifs.2021.09.025.

Yıldırım, M., Saral, S., Mercantepe, T., İskender, H., Tümkaya, L., Atak, M., & Taşçı, F. (2020). White tea reduced bone loss by suppressing the TRAP/CTX pathway in ovariectomy-induced osteoporosis model rats. *Cells, Tissues, Organs*, *209*(1), 64–74. Available from https://doi.org/10.1159/000507791.

Yu, P., Teng, X., Liu, T., Li, Y., Ni, J., Xue, S., & Wang, J. (2022). Effect of an oral probiotic formula on scalp and facial skin condition, glucose, and lipid metabolism. *Functional Foods in Health and Disease*, *12*(7), 394–409. Available from https://doi.org/10.31989/ffhd.v12i7.944, https://ffhdj.com/index.php/ffhd/article/view/944.

Zamani, P., Mokhtari, O., & Dehghanian, F. (2022). Identification of beta-sitosterol and stigmasterol as possible inhibitors of 5 alpha-reductase 1: An in-silico study. *Precision Medicine and Clinical OMICS*, *1*(1). Available from https://doi.org/10.5812/pmco.121545.

Zanzottera, F., Bizzaro, G., Michelotti, A., & Nobile, V. (2017). Efficacy of a nutritional supplement, standardized in fatty acids and phytosterols, on hair loss and hair health in both women and men. *Journal of Cosmetology & Trichology*, *03*(02). Available from https://doi.org/10.4172/2471-9323.1000121.

Zeinali, F., Aghaei Zarch, S. M., Vahidi Mehrjardi, M. Y., Kalantar, S. M., Jahan-Mihan, A., Karimi-Nazari, E., Fallahzadeh, H., Hosseinzadeh-Shamsi-Anar, M., Rahmanian, M., Fazeli, M. R., & Mozaffari-Khosravi, H. (2020). Effects of synbiotic supplementation on gut microbiome, serum level of TNF-α, and expression of microRNA-126 and microRNA-146a in patients with type 2 diabetes mellitus: study protocol for a double-blind controlled randomized clinical trial. *Trials*, *21*(1). Available from https://doi.org/10.1186/s13063-020-04236-y, http://www.trialsjournal.com/home/.

Zengin, G., Stefanucci, A., Rodrigues, M. J., Mollica, A., Custodio, L., Aumeeruddy, M. Z., & Mahomoodally, M. F. (2019). *Scrophularia lucida* L. as a valuable source of bioactive compounds for pharmaceutical applications: In vitro antioxidant, anti-inflammatory, enzyme inhibitory properties, in silico studies, and HPLC profiles. *Journal of Pharmaceutical and Biomedical Analysis*, *162*, 225–233. Available from https://doi.org/10.1016/j.jpba.2018.09.035, www.elsevier.com/locate/jpba.

Zhang, H., Jiang, Y., Lv, Y., Pan, J., Duan, Y., Huang, Y., Zhu, Y., Zhang, S., & Geng, K. (2017). Effect of water quality on the main components in Fuding white tea infusions. *Journal of Food Science and Technology*, *54*(5), 1206–1211. Available from https://doi.org/10.1007/s13197-017-2571-2, http://www.springerlink.com/content/121580/.

Zhang, W., Zhao, S., Luo, Y., Zhang, Y., Feng, Y., Tang, F., Zhou, X., Peng, S., Fan, Y., Xie, S., Li, H., Lai, Q., Fu, L., Luo, Y., Pei, S., Chen, Z., Lu, T., Tang, R., Chen, Y., & Jiao, Y. (2024). Discovery of (2S)-N-(6-Cyano-5-(trifluoromethyl)pyridin-3-yl)-3-(6-(4-cyanophenyl)-3,6-diazabicyclo[3.1.1]heptan-3-yl)-2-hydroxy-2-methylpropanamide as a Highly Potent and Selective Topical Androgen Receptor Antagonist for Androgenetic Alopecia Treatment. *Journal of Medicinal Chemistry*, *67*(1), 322–348. Available from https://doi.org/10.1021/acs.jmedchem.3c01417, http://pubs.acs.org/jmc.

Zhang, W., Fan, M., Wang, C., Mahawar, K., Parmar, C., Chen, W., & Yang, W. (2021). Hair loss after metabolic and bariatric surgery: A systematic review and meta-analysis. *Obesity Surgery*, *31*(6), 2649–2659. Available from https://doi.org/10.1007/s11695-021-05311-2, https://www.springer.com/journal/11695.

Zhang, Z., Li, W., Liu, Y., Yang, Z., Ma, L., Zhuang, H., Wang, E., Wu, C., Huan, Z., Guo, F., & Chang, J. (2021). Design of a biofluid-absorbing bioactive sandwich-structured Zn–Si bioceramic composite wound dressing for hair follicle regeneration and skin burn wound healing. *Bioactive Materials*, *6*(7), 1910–1920. Available from https://doi.org/10.1016/j.bioactmat.2020.12.006.

Zhong, B., Robinson, N. A., Warner, R. D., Barrow, C. J., Dunshea, F. R., & Suleria, H. A. R. (2020). LC-ESI-QTOF-MS/MS characterization of seaweed phenolics and their antioxidant potential. *Marine Drugs*, *18*(6). Available from https://doi.org/10.3390/md18060331, https://www.mdpi.com/1660-3397/18/6/331/pdf.

Zhong, M., Kawaguchi, R., Kassai, M., & Sun, H. (2012). Retina, Retinol, retinal and the natural history of vitamin A as a light sensor. *Nutrients*, *4*(12), 2069–2096. Available from https://doi.org/10.3390/nu4122069.

Zhou, D. D., Li, J., Xiong, R. G., Saimaiti, A., Huang, S. Y., Wu, S. X., Yang, Z. J., Shang, A., Zhao, C. N., Gan, R. Y., & Li, H. B. (2022). Bioactive compounds, health benefits and food applications of grape. *Foods*, *11*(18). Available from https://doi.org/10.3390/foods11182755, www.mdpi.com/journal/foods.

Zhou, L., Wang, H., Jing, J., Yu, L., Wu, X., & Lu, Z. (2018). Morroniside regulates hair growth and cycle transition via activation of the Wnt/β-catenin signaling pathway. *Scientific Reports*, *8*(1). Available from:. Available from https://doi.org/10.1038/s41598-018-32138-2, www.nature.com/srep/index.html.

Zufishan, S., Haque, Z., Nazar, S., Afaq, E., Aamir, E., & Rafique, S. (2024). Role of zinc in chronic telogen effluvium in serum and hair of patients with alopecia. *Journal of the Pakistan Medical Association*, *74*(2), S47. Available from https://doi.org/10.47391/JPMA-DUHS-S10, http://jpma.org.pk.

Chapter 20

The role of functional foods in diabetes management

Mahta Mirzaei[1,2], Samira Alahyaribeik[2], Niloofar Mirdamadi[3], Yan Fang[2] and Mahdieh Nadali Hazaveh[2]

[1]*Department of Food Technology, Safety and Health, Faculty of Bioscience Engineering, Ghent University, Ghent, Belgium,* [2]*Food Chemistry and Technology Research Centre, Department of Molecular Biotechnology, Environmental Technology, and Food Technology, Ghent University Global Campus, Yeonsu-gu, Incheon, South Korea,* [3]*School of Medicine, Tehran University of Medical Sciences, Tehran, Iran*

20.1 Introduction

Diabetes mellitus (DM) is a global health concern, presenting a metabolic disorder associated with persistent high blood sugar level (Irondi & Ademiluyi, 2017). Diabetes is caused by insufficient active insulin or an aberrant response to insulin, resulting in excessive blood glucose levels (hyperglycemia). Type I diabetes (T1DM) is caused by the pancreas's failure to generate insulin. Type II diabetes (T2DM), which is thought to account for 90−95% of all diabetes cases, is caused by insufficient insulin production or insulin resistance (Giri & Ohshima, 2012).

Diabetes has become a major epidemic in the previous century, made more pressing in the last few decades by the exponential development of obesity, and has become one of the top causes of death globally (Giri & Ohshima, 2012). The International Diabetes Federation (IDF) estimates that the global prevalence of diabetes in 2019 was 9.3% (463 million people), with a projected increase to 10.2% (578 million) by 2030 and 10.9% (700 million) by 2045 (Saeedi et al., 2019).

The prevalence of diabetes has been associated with a variety of factors, including age, physical activity, place of residence, education level, economic status, and employment status. For instance, low- and middle-income countries have seen faster increases in prevalence than high-income countries. Diabetes death rates by age increased by 3% between 2000 and 2019. The prevalence of diabetes is rising steadily, necessitating effective strategies for prevention and management.

While obesity and lack of physical activity have been repeatedly linked to an increased risk of diabetes, new data from epidemiological studies indicate that the composition of one's diet is also linked to the risk of developing T2DM. Data suggesting a diet high in low-glycemic index foods may help prevent diabetes, which is now becoming more widely available (Riccardi et al., 2005). In recent years, there has been a growing emphasis on incorporating foods abundant in specific bioactive compounds to prevent and/or control various chronic conditions, including T2DM. This emerging trend among T2DM patients has resulted in the use of functional foods and alternative medicine (Wang et al., 2016).

Functional foods are characterized by their inclusion of biologically active components that have been linked to promoting physiological well-being and playing a role in the prevention and management of diseases. Functional foods are designed to confer health benefits beyond basic nutritional functions, and their composition often includes bioactive compounds such as phytochemicals, polysaccharides, fibers, polyunsaturated fatty acids, vitamins, and bioactive peptides (Granato et al., 2020).

Consistency, including functional foods such as fruits, vegetables, whole grains, seaweed, probiotic, and prebiotics in the daily diet, may improve postprandial hyperglycemia and/or improve cholesterol management, attenuate oxidative stress and inflammatory processes, improve gut microflora, and subsequently prevent the development of long-term diabetes complications (Alkhatib et al., 2017; Gisbert et al., 2023; Mirmiran et al., 2014).

In this chapter, we will explore a range of bioactive compounds that have been identified for their potential in combating diabetes, with a focus on the mechanism(s) involved in their activity. Subsequently, we will delve into diverse categories of functional foods, examining their recent evidence-supported roles in antidiabetic activities.

Unleashing the Power of Functional Foods and Novel Bioactives. DOI: https://doi.org/10.1016/B978-0-443-28862-3.00020-0

20.2 The possible mechanisms underlying the antidiabetic activity of bioactive compounds

The development of diabetes is complex and may arise from a combination of genetic and environmental factors, such as an unhealthy lifestyle, gender, being overweight, and obesity, among others.

Despite decades of continuous research, the action mechanism of some natural antidiabetic compounds has not been fully elucidated. The possible mechanisms, which refer to the ability of compounds to lower the level of glucose in the blood, mainly include promotion of insulin secretion, improvement of insulin sensitivity, reducing the absorbance of glucose from the digestive system, and enhancing the uptake of glucose by cells. Other mechanisms such as decreasing oxidative stress, antiinflammatory effects, regulation of gut microbiota, and regulation of lipid metabolism may result in reducing the complications associated with diabetes.

20.2.1 Promotion of insulin secretion

Severe β-cell dysfunction and insufficient insulin secretion are the primary physio pathological mechanisms involved in the development of T2DM. β-cells are responsible for producing insulin, a critical regulator of metabolism. A series of actions in β-cells results in fusion of secretory granules and insulin secretion. While certain foods such as free fatty acids and amino acids can enhance glucose-induced insulin secretion, insulin is largely secreted in response to glucose. Furthermore, a number of hormones such as melatonin, estrogen, leptin, growth hormone, and glucagon-like peptide-1 control the insulin secretion (Fu et al., 2013). The stimulatory effect of diverse bioactive compounds in functional foods, including phenolic compounds, probiotics, and bioactive peptides on insulin secretion by the pancreas has been documented (Niibo et al., 2019; Parthsarathy et al., 2019; Saji et al., 2020).

20.2.2 Improvement of insulin resistance

Insulin resistance (IR) describes an impairment of insulin sensitivity and can be explained as the inability of a specific dose of insulin, either endogenous or exogenous, to adequately improve a person's absorption and utilization of glucose (Lebovitz, 2001).

Insulin interacts with insulin receptors (INSRs) on the plasma membrane of target cells. This interaction leads to the recruitment/phosphorylation of downstream proteins, primary insulin receptor substrate (IRS), P13-kinase (P13K), and protein kinase B (PKB/AKT) isoforms. These downstream targets are generally conserved among insulin signaling target tissues and that initiate the insulin response (Li et al., 2022b). Due to the complexity of insulin function, interference with insulin activity can occur in several different ways. Changes in genes that code for proteins involved in the insulin action cascade or environmental variables that increase circulating factors and disrupt protein—protein interactions or tyrosine phosphorylation can lead to IR (Mastrototaro & Roden, 2021).

20.2.3 Reducing absorbance of glucose from digestive system

Absorption of glucose in the small intestine physiologically contributes to the regulation of blood glucose levels and is considered a target for treatment of diabetes. Decreasing of blood glucose rise can be achieved by blunting dietary carbohydrate digestion in the gut through inhibition of digestive enzymes, including α-amylase (αA) and α-glucosidase (αG). αA and αG are two key starch digestive enzymes that breakdown carbohydrates and raise postprandial glucose levels (PPG). In diabetes, controlling postprandial hyperglycemia and lowering the risk of developing diabetes can be accomplished by inhibiting the activity of these two enzymes.

Compounds with inhibitory activity on sodium-glucose transport protein 1 (SGLT1) and glucose transporter-2 (GLUT2) also play important roles in reducing PPG elevations (Zhouyao et al., 2022). Most researchers believe that when glucose concentrations in the intestine are low, SGLT1-mediated active transport enhances glucose transport across enterocytes' apical membranes. Its subsequent release into the bloodstream is assisted by the GLUT2 transporter, which is located in the basolateral membrane (Gromova et al., 2021).

20.2.4 Improving glucose uptake by cells

Insulin resistance arises from diminished glucose utilization or impaired metabolism in peripheral insulin-sensitive tissues. The glucose transporter protein 4 (GLUT4), exclusively present in insulin-sensitive skeletal, cardiac, and adipose tissues, orchestrates glucose conversion, metabolism, and transport. The role of GLUT4 involves facilitating glucose transportation to maintain cellular functions. Reduced transport via GLUT4 contributes to insulin resistance. Elevating GLUT4 expression or translocation is a key strategy to improve glucose uptake, crucial for managing glucose homeostasis (Wu et al., 2016). Targeting glucose uptake in peripheral tissues, like skeletal muscle and adipose tissue, to lower elevated blood glucose levels in diabetic patients is a promising approach for developing novel antidiabetic drugs sourced from natural products. In addition, Glucokinase (GK), a key regulator of glucose homeostasis in vivo, is responsible for catalyzing the conversion of glucose to glucose 6-phosphate in pancreatic β-cells, hepatic hepatocytes, specific hypothalamic neurons, and intestinal epithelial cells. GK-mediated glucose phosphorylation significantly improves glucose uptake and metabolism, potentially reducing hepatic glucose output. Glucokinase activators have received widespread attention as a promising new therapeutic agent for the treatment of T2DM (Ren et al., 2022).

20.3 Biomolecules with antidiabetic activity

The incorporation of specific biomolecules into functional foods offers enormous potential for diabetes prevention and treatment. Polyphenols, omega-3 fatty acids, fiber, polysaccharides, vitamins, and bioactive peptides all have important roles in regulating glucose metabolism and insulin sensitivity. Incorporating these bioactive components into one's diet can help to promote a healthier lifestyle by reducing the consequences of metabolic problems.

20.3.1 Phytochemicals

Phytochemicals are a wide variety of nonnutritive chemical compounds found in plant foods. Flavonoids, phenolic acids, isoflavones, curcumin, isothiocyanates, and carotenoids are some familiar examples of these compounds. Several types of phytochemicals derived from natural products have received a lot of interest in recent decades due to their biological properties, including antidiabetic activity. In their 2015 work, Xiao and Hogger discussed the existing state of knowledge and future perspective for dietary polyphenols in T2DM (Xiao & Högger, 2015). Vinayagam et al. (2017) outlined the mechanisms of dietary polyphenols in the treatment and prevention of T2DM (Vinayagam et al., 2017). Rasines-Perea and Teissedre (2017) conducted a thorough assessment of the benefits of grape polyphenols consumption for DM treatment (Rasines-Perea & Teissedre, 2017), and Cao et al. (2019) comprehensively reviewed the clinical trials of dietary polyphenols for T2DM treatment (Cao et al., 2019). In a recently published review paper, most notable medicinal and dietary plants along with their isolated antidiabetic phytochemicals, as well as the mechanism involved for their antidiabetic activity, are discussed (Alam et al., 2022).

Many plant extracts, including medical herbs, fruits, and vegetables, are recognized for their content of phytochemical compounds with antidiabetic properties (Zhu et al., 2020). The biological characteristics of these phytochemical compounds exhibit variability, and the particular mechanism by which they exert antidiabetic benefits is not well known (Rahman et al., 2021).

Polyphenolic compounds, including flavonoids (e.g., anthocyanins, epigallocatechin gallate, quercetin, naringin, rutin, and kaempferol) and nonflavonoid polyphenols (e.g., resveratrol, curcumin, tannins, phenolic acids, stilbenes, and lignans), may contribute to DM management by various mechanisms, including regulating lipid and glucose metabolism, modulating intestinal microflora, scavenging reactive oxygen species (ROS), slowing the deterioration of pancreatic β-cell function caused by oxidative stress, reducinginflammation, decreasing food intake, and inhibiting starch digestive enzymes (Chen et al., 2022; Rahman et al., 2021).

Flavonoids have been the subject of several research studies, among various phenolic compounds. For example, flavonoids constitute the main components of traditional Chinese herbal medicines, *Pueraria lobata*, *Ohwi*, and *thomsonii benth*, which have demonstrated efficacy in reducing blood glucose level (Wang et al., 2022). The antidiabetic activity of flavonoids is notably associated with inhibition of digestive enzymes αA and αG (Zhu et al., 2020).

Based on molecular docking study, the inhibitory activity of flavonoids against αA and αG is aided by hydrogen bonds present between the OH-groups in ring B of flavonoid and catalytic units of enzymes, which is mostly due to binding to sites other than the active site of the enzyme to reduce catalytic activity (Pang et al., 2019). The structure–function relationship of flavonoids with inhibitory effects against αA and αG has not been thoroughly explored. The number of hydroxyl groups on ring B as well as the C2 = C3 double bond, C3–OH, and C = O at the C4 position and linkage of the B ring at the 3 position have been discovered to affect the inhibitory effect of flavonoids (Pang et al., 2019).

The ability of anthocyanins to combat diabetes is linked to their antioxidant activity which enhances antioxidant status by lowering cellular reactive oxygen species (ROS) levels and protecting pancreatic β-cells from oxidative stress. The development of T2DM appears to be closely correlated with the oxidative stress and presence of ROS in various organs and tissues. Oxidative stress can induce insulin resistance through the impairment of insulin signaling pathway.

Oxidative stress can also adversely affect the functionality of pancreatic β-cells, leading to incorrect insulin secretion and increase in apoptosis of β-cells (Ahangarpour et al., 2019; Cianciosi et al., 2018). Additionally, dietary anthocyanins exhibit notable inhibitory effects on digestive enzymes like αA and αG, or maltase, as well as modifying effects on gut microbiota (Sun et al., 2021).

Oleuropein is a phenolic secoiridoid glycoside consisting of a polyphenol and is plentiful in extra virgin olive oil (Chaari, 2020). Inhibition of amyloidosis, a protein aggregation disease, is one of the known mechanisms associated with the antidiabetic activity of oleuropein. Chaari (2020) reported the role of oleuropein in inhibition of human islet amyloid polypeptide (hIAPP) formation and consequently inhibition of amyloid deposits in pancreatic islets of T2DM patients which leads to β-cells dysfunction and loss of β-cell mass, both of which are key features of T2DM.

Other types of phytochemicals as components of plants and plant products have also been discovered to exhibit antidiabetic activity through different mechanisms, including inhibition of αA and αG activity, increasing insulin sensitivity, inhibition of DPP-4 enzyme, and increasing insulin secretion from β-cells. For example, Etsassala et al. (2022) examined phytochemicals isolated from methanolic extract of *Plectranthus ecklonii's leaves* for inhibitory effects against αA and αG. Among numerous compounds that have been isolated, parvifloron G exhibited moderate αG inhibitory activity (Etsassala et al., 2022). Teerapongpisan et al. (2022) examined 13 compounds isolated from twig and leaf extract of Uvaria rufa Blume for αA and αG inhibitory activity. Of these, uvariaruflavone showed the highest αG inhibitory activity, and ferrudiol displayed the highest αA inhibitory activity (Teerapongpisan et al., 2022).

The fundamental stage in discovering new bioactive molecules from plants is the extraction step. Traditionally, techniques like maceration, decoction, percolation, infusion, and hot continuous extraction are the standard approaches for this purpose. However, new methods such as ultrasound-assisted solvent extraction, microwave-assisted solvent extraction, and supercritical fluid extraction have gained considerable attention in recent years (Abu-Odeh et al., 2022). Following extraction, the subsequent procedure involves filtration of extract and then subjecting it to evaporation under reduced pressure. Purification of phytochemicals is typically accomplished using methods such as high-performance liquid chromatography (HPLC) and thin layer chromatography (TLC).

Several studies have employed in silico analysis approaches to predict the physicochemical and pharmacokinetic properties of phytochemicals. For example, the online software SwissADME (available at https://swissadme.ch) was utilized by Etsassala et al. (2022) to predict the physicochemical and pharmacokinetic properties of compounds isolated from plants. Molecular docking study has also been performed in various research studies to study the interaction between phytochemicals and αA and αG, sodium-glucose linked transporter-2 (SGLT-2) (Lavalle-González et al., 2013), dipeptidyl peptidase 4 (DPP-4) (Huang et al., 2019), insulin receptor tyrosine kinase (Li et al., 2022a), and glucose transporter-4 (GLUT4) (Thabah et al., 2023). The molecular docking analysis of parvifloron G, a phytochemical derived from *P. ecklonii*, against αG showed that hydrogen bond and Van der Waals interactions occurred at the enzyme's binding site. However, these interactions were found to be weaker in comparison to the interactions observed between enzyme and acarbose, a medication with αG inhibitory mechanism. Interestingly, the results also indicated that despite acarbose displaying the strongest interaction with αG, parvifloron G exhibited the highest affinity for the target molecule (Etsassala et al., 2022). The kinetic study of enzymes can explain the inhibitory mechanism of phytochemicals as well. The study of 11 gallotannins isolated from the roots of Euphorbial fischeriana exhibited the mixed inhibition type of isolates on αG (Zhang et al., 2022).

One main challenge for the usage of phytochemicals is their low bioavailability. It is essential to recognize that the polyphenols abundant in the human diet might not necessarily exhibit the highest activity in the body. This can be due to limited absorption in the intestine, extensive metabolisms, or rapid elimination (Bresciani et al., 2017). Absorption of polyphenols can be influenced by factors like the dosage and size of phenolic compounds, an individual's previous diet habit, the composition of the food matrix, gender, and variations in gut microbial populations. It is worth noting that only a small fraction, approximately 5–10% of the overall intake of dietary polyphenols, is directly absorbed in the stomach and the small intestine (Rasines-Perea & Teissedre, 2017).

20.3.2 Bioactive peptides

Bioactive peptides (BAPs) are short protein fragments obtained through enzymatic hydrolysis of food proteins such as milk, eggs, meat, fish, and cereal grains and offer substantial health benefits, including antidiabetic activity (Chelliah et al., 2021; Kitts & Weiler, 2003).

Bioactive peptides demonstrate antidiabetic effects by protection and reparation of pancreatic β-cells, improving insulin secretion in response to glucose, controlling glucose absorption and lipid metabolism, modulating insulin signaling pathways, influencing the sensitivity of cells to insulin, and inhibiting DPP-IV and glucose digestion enzymes such as αA and αG (Acquah et al., 2022). The regulatory impact on the insulin pathway can occur through various mechanisms, including upregulation of GLUT4 and insulin signaling, modulation of glucose transporters in adipocytes, and regulation of PI3K/Akt signaling pathway.

Peptides derived from sardine muscle, egg white protein, pinto beans, cumin seed protein, and whey exhibited αA and αG inhibitory activity (Iwaniak et al., 2018; Lacroix & Li-Chan, 2013; Xia et al., 2017). Patil et al. also mentioned that bioactive peptides derived from whey protein can positively impact glucose metabolism by reducing PPG levels and increasing plasma insulin concentrations in both normal and diabetic individuals (Patil et al., 2015). Plant-derived bioactive peptides also function as an inhibitory factor in enzymes like αA, αG, and DPP-IV, and glucose transporter systems involved in T2DM (Patil et al., 2020). Numerous studies have demonstrated that bioactive peptides derived from milk possess potent DPP-IV inhibiting properties (Patil et al., 2020; Power et al., 2014; Xia et al., 2017).

The capacity to suppress DPP-IV activity was also demonstrated by peptides derived from black beans, eggs, fish, amaranth, rice bran, corn, and silver carp protein (Li-Chan et al., 2012).

According to studies, active peptides derived from fish protein hydrolysates, soybeans, bean, and milk were effective in improving antioxidant status and protecting pancreatic β-cells from intracellular ROS caused by high glucose exposure. Hyperglycemia induces overproduction of free radicals, including reactive oxygen species (ROS) and nitric oxide (NO) radicals, leading to insulin resistance and various cellular dysfunctions. Protecting pancreatic β-cells from oxidative damage could be a crucial strategy to mitigate damage and reduce the development of T2DM (Fernández-Tomé et al., 2014; Han et al., 2013; Nasri et al., 2015; Oseguera Toledo et al., 2016; Xia et al., 2017).

Bioactive peptides may be potential compounds for regulating T2DM via other mechanisms such as inhibitory effects on lipid accumulation as have been reported for bean protein hydrolysate (Oseguera Toledo et al., 2016) and soybean protein hydrolysate (Martinez-Villaluenga et al., 2009) rich in bioactive peptides, as well as fermented goat whey (Hammé et al., 2010). There is a negative correlation between the proportion of adipose tissue and level of secretory adiponectin, an insulin sensitizer. This suggests that reducing fat accumulation by bioactive peptides could enhance glucose tolerance by improving insulin sensitivity (Xia et al., 2017).

A review conducted in 2020 concluded compelling evidence from in vitro and in vivo studies, demonstrating the potential of food sources to be processed into bioactive peptides with antidiabetic properties (Acquah et al., 2022). A review on plant-derived bioactive peptides concluded that certain peptide fractions showed insulin-mimetic action in animal models. Plant-derived bioactive peptides also function as an inhibitory factor against αA, αG, DPP-IV, and glucose transporter systems involved in T2DM (Patil et al., 2020). A list of most recently antidiabetic peptides is summarized in Table 20.1.

Peptides often exhibit distinct bioactivities in laboratory settings compared to real-world applications due to challenges related to bioavailability, absorption, and vulnerability to physiological enzymes that break them down into inactive components. Ensuring the effectiveness of these peptides requires resistance to gastrointestinal proteases and easy absorption into blood serum without degradation. This stability is crucial for the secure delivery of peptides, maintaining their in vitro bioactivity, and facilitating their intended impact at cellular sites of action (Bhandari et al., 2020).

The essential step in the discovery of antidiabetic peptides involves their purification to identify structures and assess activities. Peptide's purification relies on factors like molecular size, charge, polarity, solubility, and other physical chemistry properties. Meanwhile, combining multidimensional chromatography with several separation methods can yield better separation results (Lu et al., 2023). Consideration should be given to bioinformatics analyses due to their potential in identifying, characterizing, and generating bioactive peptides. Molecular docking predicts the preferred conformation of a molecule when bound to another to form a stable complex. This technique is commonly used to assess how an identified peptide can bind to an enzyme and exhibit inhibitory activity (Rivero-Pino et al., 2020).

While the complete understanding of the structure–function relationship of bioactive peptides remains elusive, certain characteristics have been identified. For example, bioactive peptides exhibiting DPP-IV inhibitory properties often possess a hydrophobic N-terminal region, preferably featuring tryptophan and having proline or alanine as the second-to-last residue at the N-terminal, or possess a low molecular mass (Rivero-Pino et al., 2020).

The αA inhibitory activity of peptides is influenced by aromatic–aromatic interactions, which involve hydrogen bonds, electrostatic interactions, and Van der Waals forces. These interactions may create a sliding barrier through hydrogen bonding with the active/substrate-binding region of the enzyme. The αA enzyme itself contains aromatic residues like phenylalanine, tryptophan, and tyrosine. Some studies suggest that peptides with branched chains (e.g., Lys, Phe, Tyr, and Trp) and cationic residues may prefer binding to αA (Gong et al., 2020; Rivero-Pino et al., 2020).

20.3.3 Polysaccharides

Polysaccharides are complex carbohydrates composed of multiple sugar units linked together. They can be broadly divided into three main groups based on their structure and functions: starch, glycogen, and dietary fibers. From a

TABLE 20.1 A List of Most Recently Identified Antidiabetic Peptides.

Origin	Identified Peptide	Production Method	Mechanism	ref.
Atlantic salmon skin gelatin and trimmings	Hydrolysates containing peptides such as GPAGAVLGPK and AVLGPQ, GPAGL	Hydrolysis by alcalase 2.4 L and flavourzyme 500 L	DPP-IV inhibitory activity; Insulin and GLP-1 secretory activity from pancreatic BRIN-BD11 and enteroendocrine GLUTag cells	Harnedy et al. (2018a)
Oat globulins	LQAFEPLR (IC50: 141.7 μM), EFLLAGNNK, and LQAFEPLR	Hydrolysis by trypsin and purification by ultrafiltration, LC-mass spectrometry	Inhibition of DPP-IV and αG in Caco-2 cells upregulation of αG, GLUT2 and GLUT5 expression in the enterocytes	Wang et al. (2018)
Tempe	VH and ALEP	Fermentation process Proteomic study	DPP-IV inhibitory activity (in silico analysis)	Tamam et al. (2019)
Camel milk	LDLWDDFKGL and MPSKPPLL	Hydrolysis by alcalase, bromelain, and papain	αA and porcine pancreatic lipase (PPL), and DPP-IV inhibitory activity	Mudgil et al. (2018)
Casein prepared from raw and boiled sheep milk	Unidentified hydrolysates	Hydrolysis by chymotrypsin	αA inhibitory activity	Jan et al. (2016)
Black bean (*Phaseolus vulgaris l.*)	EGLELLLLLLAG, AKSPLF and FEELN (DPP-IV inhibitory activity), TTGGKGGK (αG inhibitory activity), AKSPLF and MEVM (αA inhibitory activity)	Hydrolysis by alcalase, analysis by biochemical and in silico methods, purification by LC-ESI-MS/MS	DPP-IV inhibitory activity, αG Lowering SGLT1 and GLUT2 expression and	Mojica and de Mejía (2016)
Blue whiting (Micromesistius poutassou)	Unidentified hydrolysates	Hydrolysis by alcalase and flavourzyme and simulated gastrointestinal digestion	Modulating insulin and GLP-1 release, DPP-IV inhibitory activity in BRIN-BD11 and GLUTag cells	Harnedy et al. (2018b)
Spirulina platensis	Protein extract, including GVPMPNK, RNPFVFAPTLLTVAAR, and LRSELAAWSR	Protein extraction and chromatographic fractionation of peptides	αA, αG, and DPP-IV inhibitory activity, Increasing glycogen content, hexokinase and pyruvate kinase activity in insulin resistant-HepG2 cell model	Hu et al. (2019)
Arthrospira platensis	Unidentified hydrolysates	Enzymatic hydrolysis by alcalase and pepsin	αA, αG and DPP-IV inhibitory activity	Villaró et al. (2023)
Bovine and camel milk	Unidentified hydrolysates	Fermentation by probiotic strains *Lactococcus lactis* KX881782 and *Lactobacillus acidophilus* DSM9126	αA, αG inhibitory activity	Ayyash et al. (2018)

(Continued)

TABLE 20.1 (Continued)

Origin	Identified Peptide	Production Method	Mechanism	ref.
Cumin seed	FFRSKLLSDGAAAAKGALLPQYW (IC50:0.02 μM) RCMAFLLSDGAAAAQQLLPQYQYW (IC50:0.04 μM) DPAQPNYPWTAVLVFRH (IC50:0.03 μM)	Hydrolysis by Protamex, fractionation by the GELFREE® 8100 system	αA inhibitory activity	Siow and Gan (2016)
Pinto bean (Phaseolus vulgaris cv. Pinto)	PPHMLP PPMHLP PLPWGAGF GDAACCGLPLLP PPHMGGP PLPPHDLL FNPFPSPHTP	Hydrolysis by Protamex and fractionation by centrifugal ultrafiltration filters	αA inhibitory activity	Ngoh and Gan (2016)
Hard-to-cook bean (*Phaseolus vulgaris L*)	LLSL, QQEG, and NEGEAH	Hydrolysis with either alcalase® or bromelain Separation by ultrafiltration membrane system	αA and αG inhibitory activity, DPP-IV inhibitory activity, increasing glucose-stimulated insulin secretion from iNS-1E cells	Oseguera-Toledo et al. (2015)
An endophytic Aspergillus awamori	Peptide containing serine, threonine, tyrosine, and valine amino acid	Purification on Sephadex LH-20 column and semi prep HPLC	αA (IC50:3.75 μg/mL) and αG (IC50: 5.625 μg/mL) inhibitory activity	Singh and Kaur (2016)
Quinoa *(Chenopodium quinoa Willd.)*	GEHGSDGNV IQAEGGLT (DPP-IV inhibitory activity: 15.05%, 55.85% αG inhibitory activity at concentration of 250 μM) DKDYPK (22.16% αG inhibitory activity at concentration of 250 μM) GEHGSDGNV (6.86% αA inhibitory activity, 30.84% αG inhibitory activity at concentration of 250 μM)	Simulated gastrointestinal digestion	DPP-IV, αA, and αG inhibitory activity	Vilcacundo et al. (2017)
Rambutan (Nephelium lappaceum L.) and pulasan (Nephelium mutabile) seeds	20 peptides from rambutan and 31 peptides from pulasan	Hydrolysis by pepsin and/or chymotrypsin	αA inhibitory activity	Evaristus et al. (2018)
Whey	Ile-Pro-Ala	Evaluating peptides originated from B-lactoglobulin for DPP-IV inhibitory activity using BIOPET database	Inhibiting DPP-IV, reducing glucose levels, and stimulating insulin secretion	Tulipano et al. (2011)
Soybean	Peptide fractions obtained by Ultrafiltration	Digestion by pepsin and pancreatin.	DPP-IV, αA, and αG inhibitory activity	González-Montoya et al. (2018)

biologic insight, fibers can be categorized into two groups based on their plant source: edible (dietary) and nonedible. Dietary fibers further fall into subgroups distinguished by their water solubility or insolubility, each exhibiting distinct viscoelastic properties. Soluble fibers, whether viscose or non-viscose, encompass varieties such as inulin, β-glucans, psyllium, gum, pectin, and different types of prebiotics such as β-fructans. On the other hand, insoluble and nonviscous fibers include cellulose, certain hemicelluloses such as arabinoxylans, cereal, lignin, and resistant starch (Bozbulut & Sanlier, 2019; Neyrinck et al., 2018).

Polysaccharides come from a variety of natural sources, including bacteria, plants, animals, and algae. Several polysaccharide products have been used as alternative medicine to treat T2DM around the world. Notably, astragalus polysaccharides, rehmanniae radix, konjac glucomannan, ginseng polysaccharide, and pumpkin polysaccharide are well-established in China (Wang et al., 2016). Mushrooms and algae have also been identified as sources of polysaccharide with significant potential for T2DM therapy.

While extensive studies (Wang et al., 2016; Yang et al., 2024) have demonstrated the relationship between polysaccharides and T2DM, there are also conflicting evidences regarding their role in prevention and control; for example, a comprehensive analysis of prospective cohort studies and randomized controlled trials suggests that cereal fiber demonstrates protective effects against T2DM due to its potential modulation of gut microbiota, particularly through improving glucose tolerance, reducing inflammation, and altering the immune response, while fruit fiber provides comparatively limited protection (Davison & Temple, 2018). In another study, nine different dietary fibers were tested for their effects on T2DM rats using physiological, genomic, and metabolomic investigations. Supplementation with β-glucan, arabinogalactan, guar gum, apple pectin, glucomannan, and arabinoxylan significantly reduced fasting blood glucose (FBG) levels. However, carrageenan, xylan, and xanthan gum had little effect on glycemic control (Nie et al., 2021). In summary, the effects of different polysaccharides on glycemic control in T2DM rats vary, emphasizing the importance of considering specific types of polysaccharides in relation to their potential benefits for diabetes management.

The antidiabetic effects of polysaccharides may occur through various mechanisms, such as inhibition of digestive enzymes, inhibition of glucose absorption, regulating intestinal flora, regulating signaling pathways, and inhibiting β-cells apoptosis. Additionally, the antidiabetic activity of polysaccharides is linked to their antioxidant activity and their ability to regulate inflammation (Li et al., 2021b; Luo et al., 2021a; Wang et al., 2016, 2022; Yang et al., 2024).

The inhibition of αA and αG activity is one of the most proposed mechanisms for antidiabetic activity of polysaccharides. The activity of polysaccharides on αA and αG can be hindered by two potential factors. Initially, there may be certain groups or compounds such as free carboxyl groups, tannin, phytic acid, and uronic acid within the polysaccharide that act to suppress enzymes, leading to a direct reduction in their activity. Additionally, polysaccharides have the capability to be absorbed onto starch, thereby impeding the hydrolysis of starch by αA and αG (Hu et al., 2018; Jiang et al., 2019).

Hydrophilic nature and gel formation property of fibers is another aspect that explains their role in diabetes management. Hydrophilic fibers can form a gel-like substance when they come in contact with water in the small intestine. The viscous substance reduces the interaction area of nutrients with digestive enzymes, lowers digestion speed and glucose adsorption, and subsequently regulates insulin secretion (McRae, 2018; Tessari & Lante, 2017).

As an illustration, a research investigation noted a decrease in the diagnostic marker glycosylated hemoglobin A1c (HbA_{1c}) among patients with T2DM who consumed bread with high-fiber content, specifically β-glucan, and this reduction was attributed to many factors, including the hydrophilic nature of β-glucan (Tessari & Lante, 2017).

A significant reduction in PPG and insulin level was concluded in a research by using soy pectin, and it was stated that viscoelastic property could be the possible reason. Furthermore, certain research suggests that polysaccharides can bind to adsorbed glucose, thereby sustaining a lower glucose concentration in the small intestine (Karthikeyan et al., 2019).

Polysaccharides could play an important hyperglycemic effect when fermented by gut bacteria as it is well recognized that human gut microbiota play an important role in disease, such as diabetes (Hu et al., 2018). A study found that consuming a high-fiber diet improved glucose homeostasis, altered serum metabolome, reduced systemic inflammation, and alleviated psychiatric comorbidities in T2DM patients. The study found that a high-fiber diet increased the abundance of beneficial gut microorganisms while decreasing the abundance of opportunistic pathogens, implying that changes in intestinal microbiota contributed to the observed improvements in serum metabolism and mood (Chen et al., 2023a).

Polysaccharides' ability to suppress β-cell apoptosis could also be a significant improvement in the treatment of T2DM. Zhang et al. (2019) conducted research to shed light on the methods by which Angelica sinensis polysaccharide (ASP), derived from *Angelica sinensis*' root, reduced T2DM by protecting β-cells. The study found that ASP efficiently inhibited both the death receptor and mitochondrial pathways of β-cells, both in vivo and in vitro. This combined action helped to restore pancreatic islets in mice with T2DM (Zhang et al., 2019). The most recently identified polysaccharides with antidiabetic activity are listed in Table 20.2.

There is limited information on structural specifications and structure–function relationship of polysaccharides with antidiabetic activity. The αA and αG inhibitory activity of polysaccharides is closely related to their structural

TABLE 20.2 Recently Identified Polysaccharides With Antidiabetic Activity.

Source of Polysaccharide	Mechanism	Structural Property	Extraction Method	Ref.
Wheat brane	αA (IC50 = 0.40 -1.92 mg/mL) and αG (IC50 = 0.38-1.17 mg/mL) inhibitory activity	WXA-1 (MW: 193 kDa) and AXA-1 (MW: 107 kDa)	Sequential extraction with water and alkaline solution, DEAE cellulose-52 chromatography and sephacryl S-400 gel permeation chromatography	Lv et al. (2021)
Chaenomeles speciosa seeds	αA (IC50 = 6.24 mg/mL) and αG(IC50 = 4.59 mg/mL) inhibitory activity	MW: 8.65*10^6 Da was composed of Rha, GlcA, Gal, and Ara	Water at 60°C and 1500 rpm for 2 h	Deng et al. (2020)
Cyclocarya paliurus	Increasing insulin secretion due to protective effect on pancreatic islet β-cells	A heteropolysaccharide consisting of D-xylose, L-arabinose, D-glucose, D-galactose, L-rhamnose, and D-mannose, with MW of 1,167 kD	Extraction by hot water and purifying with column chromatography	Li et al. (2021a)
Green algae (Chaetomorpha linum)	Inhibition of human islet amyloid polypeptide (hIAPP) aggregation	Sulfated rhamnogalactoarabinan	Water extraction following by preparative ion-exchange and size exclusion chromatography	Qin et al. (2022)
Pueraria lobata (Willd.) Ohwi and Pueraria thomsonii	Regulating PPAR signaling pathway and regulating the structure of gut microbiota	–	Extraction by hot water and precipitation with ethanol	Wang et al. (2022)
Laminaria japonica	Preventing high-fat-diet-induced insulin resistance in mice through the regulation of gut microbiota	–	Water extraction and precipitation with ethanol, deproteinizing with chloroform and n-butanol, purifying with DEAE-cellulose column and sephacryl S-500 column	Li et al. (2021b)
Pueraria lobata root polysaccharide (PLP)	Alleviating insulin resistance via regulation of enzyme activities and gene expression related to glucose metabolism and activating insulin signaling pathways (Akt2, PI3K, and GLUT2) in mice		–	Luo et al. (2021b)
Root of Pueraria lobata	Inhibitory effect against αA (IC50 = 3.945 μmol/L)	A water-soluble polysaccharide (PL70-1-1) with main chain consisted of (1→)-linked β-D-glucose, (1→4)-linked α-D-glucose, (1→4, 6)-linked β-D-glucose, and (1→3)-linked α-D-glucose, and the branch chain consisted of (1→)-linked β-D-glucose	Water extraction followed by DEAE-cellulose 52 anion exchange column and sephacryl S-100 gel filtration column chromatography purification	Xu et al. (2018a)

(Continued)

TABLE 20.2 (Continued)

Source of Polysaccharide	Mechanism	Structural Property	Extraction Method	Ref.
Rosa roxburghii Tratt (Rosaceae) (Ci Li) fruit polysaccharide	Improving insulin resistance of diabetic mice and reversing diabetes-induced gut disorder by enhancing the abundances of beneficial bacteria	–	Extraction with water at 55°C–95°C for 3.5 h and water/material ratio of 15–35 mL/g	Wang et al. (2019a)
Mulberry fruit polysaccharide	Modulation of gut microbiota	MW: 210.10-20.84 kDa	Water extraction and precipitation with ethanol 80% (v/v) and ultrapure water	Chen et al. (2018)
Mulberry fruit polysaccharide (MFP)	Increasing insulin secretion and promoting pancreatic β cell proliferation	MW: 19.54–195.23 KDa	Refluxing with ethanol/ water (90%, v/v) at 70 °C for 4 h, removing proteins by chloroform: n-butyl alcohol (4: 1, v/v) and precipitation with dehydrated ethanol 80% (v/v)	Chen et al. (2017)
Annona squamosa	αG inhibitory activity (IC50 = 11.89 μM)	Polysaccharide (GASP3-3-I) composed of arabinose, and D-galactose, D-xylose, and D-glucose, l-rhamnose with MW of 2.28 × 10^6 Da	Extraction by hot water and ethanol	Ren et al. (2017)
Brasenia schreberi	Regulating insulin signaling pathway and gut microbiota in type 2 diabetic mice	Mw 50–100 KDa	Extraction with NaOH at 70 °C for 3 h and purification through ultrafiltration and fractionation by DEAE Sepharose Fast flow column	Liu et al. (2022a)

characteristics such as monosaccharide content, molecular weight, glycosyl linkage types, and molecular conformation. Recent research on structural properties of polysaccharides with αA and αG inhibitory activity extracted from blackcurrant fruits showed that polysaccharides with lowest molecular weight have highest inhibitory effects against αA and αG (Xu et al., 2018b). The higher amounts of arabinose or xylose residues have been reported to be related to the hypoglycemic activity of polysaccharides (Jiao et al., 2018). In a study performed by Lv et al. (2021), two distinct polysaccharide fractions were isolated from wheat bran by sequential extraction using hot water and alkaline solution. These fractions were then analyzed for structural properties and inhibitory activity against αA and αG. The findings revealed that both polysaccharide fractions were heteropolysaccharide with different backbone. Notably, the alkaline-extracted polysaccharide exerted a more potent inhibitory activity against αA and αG compared to water extracted polysaccharide. It also exhibited a competitive inhibition of αA and a mixed-type noncompetitive inhibition of αG. The higher inhibitory activity of alkaline-extracted polysaccharide was assumed to be related to its lower molecular weight, higher content of arabinose and xylose, and higher amounts of ferulic acid content (Lv et al., 2021). In another study, two polysaccharides, ATPS-PP-1 and ATPS-PP-2, were isolated from pumpkin. ATPS-PP-1 has a (1→3)-linked-Glcp backbone, a branch point at O-3 of (1→3,4)-linked-Glcp, and terminal Glcp as a side chain. ATPS-PP-2 has a backbone made up of (1→3)-linked-Galp, (1→6)-linked-Glcp, (1→3,6)-linked-Glcp, and (1→4)-linked-Glcp. ATPS-PPs inhibited NF-κB-iNOS mRNA expression, reducing oxidative stress in islet β-cells. Notably, ATPS-PP-1 outperformed ATPS-PP-2 in terms of hypoglycemic action, indicating that different types of glycosidic bond connections and molecular weights can influence polysaccharide performance (Khan et al., 2019).

20.3.4 Unsaturated fatty acid

Functional unsaturated fatty acids are a promising dietary supplement for improving glycemic homeostasis (Coelho et al., 2017). Polyunsaturated fatty acids are divided into ω-6 (including linoleic acid and arachidonic acid) and ω-3 series (comprising α-linolenic acid, eicosapentaenoic (EPA), and docosahexaenoic (DHA)) based on their double bond positions and functions. ω-3 unsaturated fatty acids, as important life-active substances in the human body, have been widely studied for their important bioactive functions such as antidiabetic, anticardiovascular disease, and antiinflammatory.

Susmita et al. concluded that the mechanisms by which ω-3 unsaturated fatty acids improve insulin sensitivity are associated with improved insulin signaling, inhibition of mitochondrial dysfunction, and endoplasmic reticulum stress, but the specific molecular processes need to be further explored (Sinha et al., 2023). In addition, ω-3 unsaturated fatty acids have been proven to modulate metabolic disorders associated with chronic diseases by altering the diversity and abundance of the intestinal microbiota and restoring the intestinal microbiota homeostasis (Jayapala & Lim, 2023).

In alternative research findings, studies have indicated interventions involving EPA and DHA in patients with T2DM. The antidiabetic effects of EPA and DHA were associated with enhanced production of the endogenous insulin sensitizer (Flachs et al., 2006) and their capacity to reverse oxidative stress in obese hypertensive rat model (Dasilva et al., 2016). Linoleic acid exerts antidiabetic effects by improving glucose uptake through activation of AMPK and Akt pathways and inhibition of protein tyrosine phosphatases associated with insulin resistance (Yoon et al., 2021). Notably, diets rich in ω-3 fatty acids may improve insulin sensitivity associated with lipotropic nutrition and prevent hepatic steatosis (Moreira et al., 2020). On the other hand, the beneficial effects of unsaturated fatty acids on insulin sensitivity have been demonstrated in many clinical trials. A clinical study demonstrated that ω-3 fatty acids can mitigate the progression of diabetes complications through interventions that reduce inflammation (Limonte et al., 2020).

Numerous epidemiological and clinical studies have shown that the unsaturated fatty acids derived from nuts, including pine (Takala et al., 2023), virgin argan (Bellahcen et al., 2012), almond (Gayathri et al., 2023), pistachio (Jamshidi et al., 2018), and walnut (Sun et al., 2020), may reduce the risk of developing T2DM. Plant seed extract is also one of the main sources of unsaturated fatty acids, such as quinoa (Chaudhary et al., 2023), chia (Tavera-Hernández et al., 2023), chickpea (Jukanti et al., 2012), sophora pachycarpa seed (Mahdavi et al., 2021), and bitter gourd (Naik et al., 2021).

Several functional foods containing unsaturated fatty acids have been developed for the management of diabetes. For instance, Song et al. investigated the functionality of fermented milk containing conjugated linoleic acid on T2DM mice model. Mice treated with fermented milk for 6 weeks had decreased body weight and glucose tolerance. Dyslipidemia, insulin sensitivity, and leptin regulation were all improved (Song et al., 2016). A wheat flour chip doped with ω-3 oil from fish viscera and gill by-products and caffeoylquinic-rich powder of artichoke bract by-products was prepared, and in vitro and in vivo experiments demonstrated that the mechanism of improvement of glycemic homeostasis was associated with inhibition of lipid peroxidation and activation of antioxidant enzymes (Benkhoud et al., 2021). In summary, a large number of studies on unsaturated fatty acids as potential nutritional supplements for the prevention and treatment of T2DM provide impetus for future clinical studies.

20.3.5 Vitamins

The link between vitamin intake and diabetes is complex and involves many factors. Several clinical studies show that deficits in specific vitamins are widespread among diabetic patients. A definitive and substantial association between vitamin consumption and diabetes indicators, as well as the mechanism(s) underlying their action, has yet to be established.

Vitamin C deficiency is a common condition among the diabetic patients. While certain studies, such as those referenced by Khodaeian et al. (2015) and Kunsongkeit et al. (2019), have not identified a significant association between vitamin C consumption and insulin resistance or other diabetes markers, several others have indicated an inverse relationship between vitamin C and diabetic markers such as FBG (Carr & Maggini, 2017; Nosratabadi et al., 2023; Pearson et al., 2017) or HbA_{1c} (Pohanka, 2021; Puvvada, 2020).

A randomized controlled trial of 937 participants in 2017 reported a controlling effect of vitamin C on glycemia and insulin indicators in diabetic patients. This effect was detectable in FBG more than insulin concentration, and according to the meta-analysis, the age, body mass index (BMI), plasma glucose level, and the duration of supplementation were effective parameters. The longer consumption and higher age resulted in larger reduction in glucose content (Ashor et al., 2017). In another study in 2019 on 31 diabetic patients, a significant reduction was observed in PPG and hyperglycemia by having 1000 mg/day ascorbic acid supplement (Mason et al., 2019).

Furthermore, a prospective, randomized controlled study in 2020 analyzed 53 diabetic patients and reported that vitamin C can reduce the FBG, alone or in combination with phytochemicals (Ragheb et al., 2020). In 2022 a study analyzed data from 25206 individuals with prediabetes or diabetic spanning the years 1999 to 2018 and reported an inverse correlation between FBG and serum vitamin C level. Furthermore, a study revealed that vitamin C may retard the start of diabetes in prediabetic people and potentially reduce the mortality rate. As a result, researchers recommended having a dose of 500–1000 milligrams of vitamin C in a day (Sun et al., 2022).

Vitamin D deficiency is also associated with the development and progression of IR and T2DM. Adequate vitamin D levels can minimize low-grade inflammation, promote cellular health, avoid hypermethylation, and regulate gene expression in insulin-sensitive tissues. While vitamin D supplementation for glucose homeostasis control has yielded inconsistent outcomes, ongoing research aims to provide more definitive answers for clinical application (Vondra & Hampl, 2021). Consequently, there has been consideration of using vitamin D supplementation as an intervention to reduce the risk of diabetes. The notion that the risk of T2DM could be influenced by the status of vitamin D is biologically feasible. This is due to the reported associations of low blood levels of 25-hydroxyvitamin D [25(OH)D], a stable form of vitamin D in bloodstream with both impaired pancreatic β-cell function and insulin resistance (Pittas et al., 2019). For example, in a prospective study involving 14,709 participants with T2DM from the UK Biobank, researchers aimed to investigate the associations between serum [25(OH)D] levels and vitamin D receptor (VDR) polymorphisms and the risk of diabetic microvascular complications. Higher blood 25(OH)D concentrations, particularly ≥ 75 nmol/L, were substantially related with a decreased risk of composite diabetes microvascular sequelae, diabetic retinopathy, diabetic nephropathy, and diabetic neuropathy over an 11.2-year median follow-up period. The findings suggest that maintaining appropriate vitamin D levels may contribute to preventing diabetic microvascular problems (Chen et al., 2023b).

Some studies have also shown that vitamin E plays a role in regulating DM and IR because of its antioxidant and antiinflammatory properties (Balbi et al., 2018; Kim et al., 2016; Zhao et al., 2016). A meta-analysis study in 2023 on a total sample of 2171 diabetes patients reported a significant decrease in HbA_{1c} and fasting insulin with vitamin E supplementation. Also, a reduction in FBG was detected in the group with vitamin E supplementation for a duration of less than 10 weeks (Asbaghi et al., 2023).

Overall, while further research is needed to gain a complete understanding, these findings indicate that some vitamins may influence diabetes indicators and could potentially act as therapies for glycemic management and prevention.

20.4 Antidiabetic potential of different categories of functional foods

The study of functional foods as prospective diabetes treatments has received a lot of attention. Several types of functional foods, such as fruits, vegetables, whole grains, probiotics and prebiotics, seaweed, and mushrooms, show potential for antidiabetic activity. These foods frequently contain bioactive substances like polyphenols, fiber, and antioxidants, which contribute to their medicinal properties. According to research, eating these functional foods on a regular basis can help control blood sugar levels, increase insulin sensitivity, and reduce diabetic complications. Incorporating a variety of these nutrient-dense foods into one's diet has the potential to help manage diabetes and improve overall health. Nonetheless, more extensive research is required to explain the specific mechanisms and appropriate dietary patterns for exploiting the antidiabetic potential of functional foods.

20.4.1 Fruit and vegetables

Fruit and vegetable-rich diets can help delay or avoid DM and its problems (Gowd et al., 2021). Fruit eating introduces bioactive elements into the human diet, including phytochemicals, fibers, and vitamins (Wojdyło et al., 2016). Fruit consumption, whether fresh, freeze-dried, juice, pomace, or extract, has been shown to improve glucose management.

Several epidemiological research, clinical studies, in vivo, and in vitro studies have shown that fruits with varied phytochemical profiles can decrease blood glucose levels. For example, a systematic review of seven randomized controlled trials on the effects of blueberry and cranberry consumption on T2DM found that daily cranberry juice consumption (240 mL) for 12 weeks and blueberry extract supplementation (9.1–9.8 mg anthocyanins) for 8–12 weeks were beneficial in controlling glucose levels in T2DM subjects (Rocha et al., 2019). An 8-week intervention trial in Finland indicated that the intake of bilberry was associated with enhancements in FBG levels and insulin secretion in individuals with metabolic syndrome (de Mello et al., 2017). In an European cohort study, a notable inverse correlation between dietary flavonoids and the onset of T2DM was observed, highlighting the importance of plant-based diets in controlling the development of T2DM (Zamora-Ros et al., 2013). Several dose-response meta-analyses and cohort studies have also demonstrated that a fruit-rich diet, particularly fruits high in flavonols, flavan-3-ols, isoflavones, and anthocyanins, has an essential role in the prevention of T2DM (Liu et al., 2014; Rienks et al., 2018; Zhou et al., 2018).

Notably, flavan-3-ol monomers, proanthocyanidin dimers and trimers, and the flavonol myricetin all demonstrated a substantial association with a lower incidence of T2DM in European populations (Zamora-Ros et al., 2014). Fig. 20.1 summarizes a list of fruits recognized for their antidiabetic activity, along with the reported mechanisms that may contribute to their potential effects.

The bioactive compounds in vegetables also linked to the decrease or reversal of T2DM typically include dietary fiber, resistant starch, vitamins C and E, carotenoids, flavonoids, thiosulfides, magnesium, selenium, chromium, and zinc. Carotenoids, including α- and β-carotene, lycopene, lutein, zeaxanthin, and β-cryptoxanthin, protect against diabetes progression by reducing oxidative stress, which interferes with glucose uptake by cells. Thiosulfides lower blood glucose levels via increasing pancreatic insulin production. Magnesium is crucial since it is required for insulin secretion and activity. Chromium is an insulin cofactor that improves insulin function. Zinc is essential for insulin production, regulating blood sugar levels and interacting with other nutrients (Upadhyay, 2017) (Fig. 20.2).

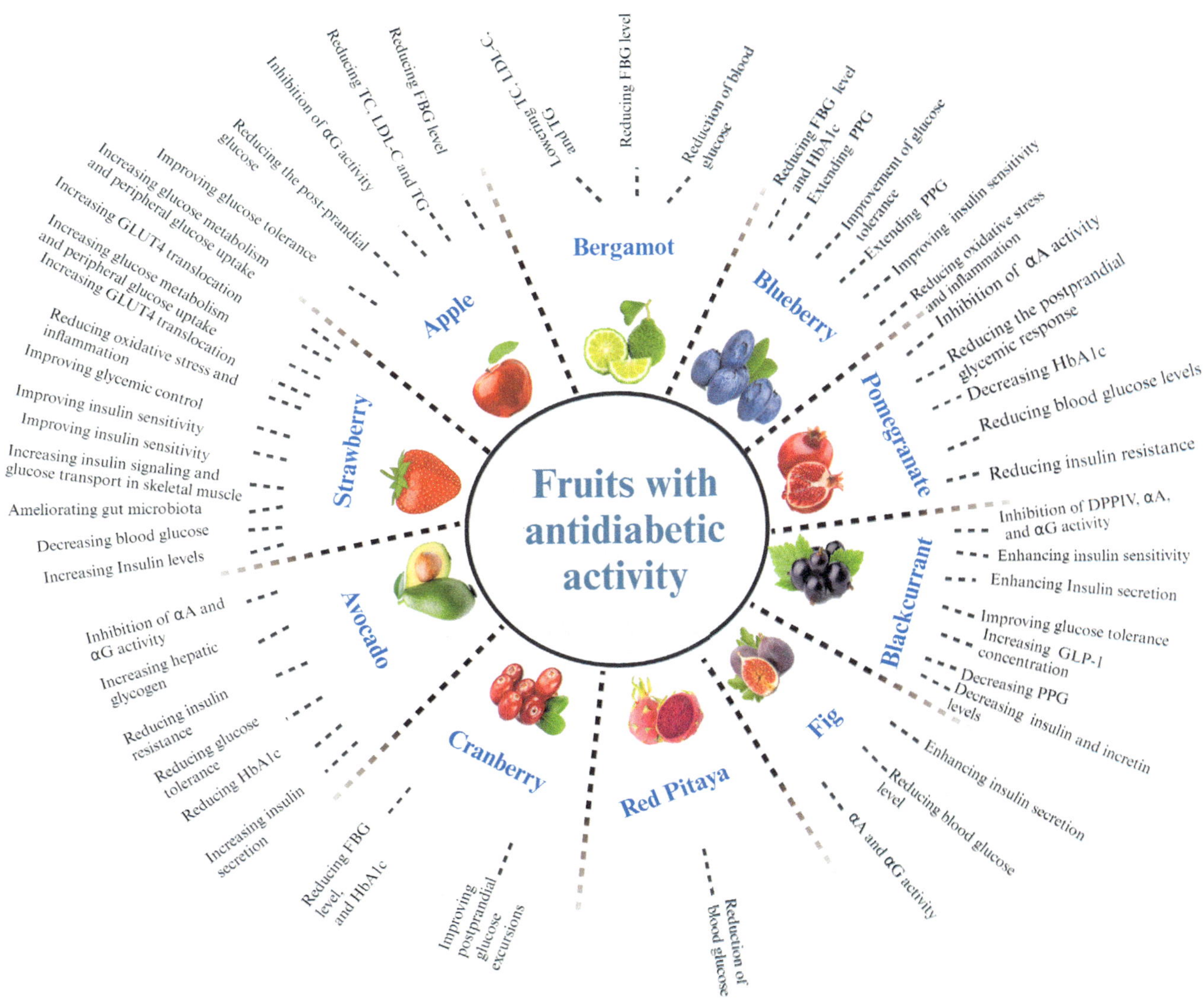

FIGURE 20.1 The list of fruits with antidiabetic action and their potential mechanisms. The graph is created using BioRender.com. (Abdulazeez & Ponnusamy, 2016; Ajani & Olanrewaju, 2014; Basu et al., 2010; Bell et al., 2017; Castro-Acosta et al., 2016; de Oliveira et al., 2022; de Oliveira Raphaelli et al., 2019; Del Toro-Equihua et al., 2016; Delpino et al., 2022; Denis et al., 2015; Di Folco et al., 2018; Farsi et al., 2014; Gazwi et al., 2023; Gondwe et al., 2008; Grabež et al., 2020; Guo et al., 2017; Iizuka et al., 2018; Irudayaraj et al., 2016; Kerimi et al., 2017; Kowalski & de Mejia, 2021; Liu et al., 2019, 2022b; Mollace et al., 2019; Nizamutdinova et al., 2009; Petersen et al., 2019; Poolsup et al.; Rao & Adinew, 2011; Saputri & Saraswati, 2021; Schell et al., 2017; Shoji et al., 2017; Sun et al., 2019; Takikawa et al., 2010; Wojdyło et al., 2016; Yang et al., 2021).

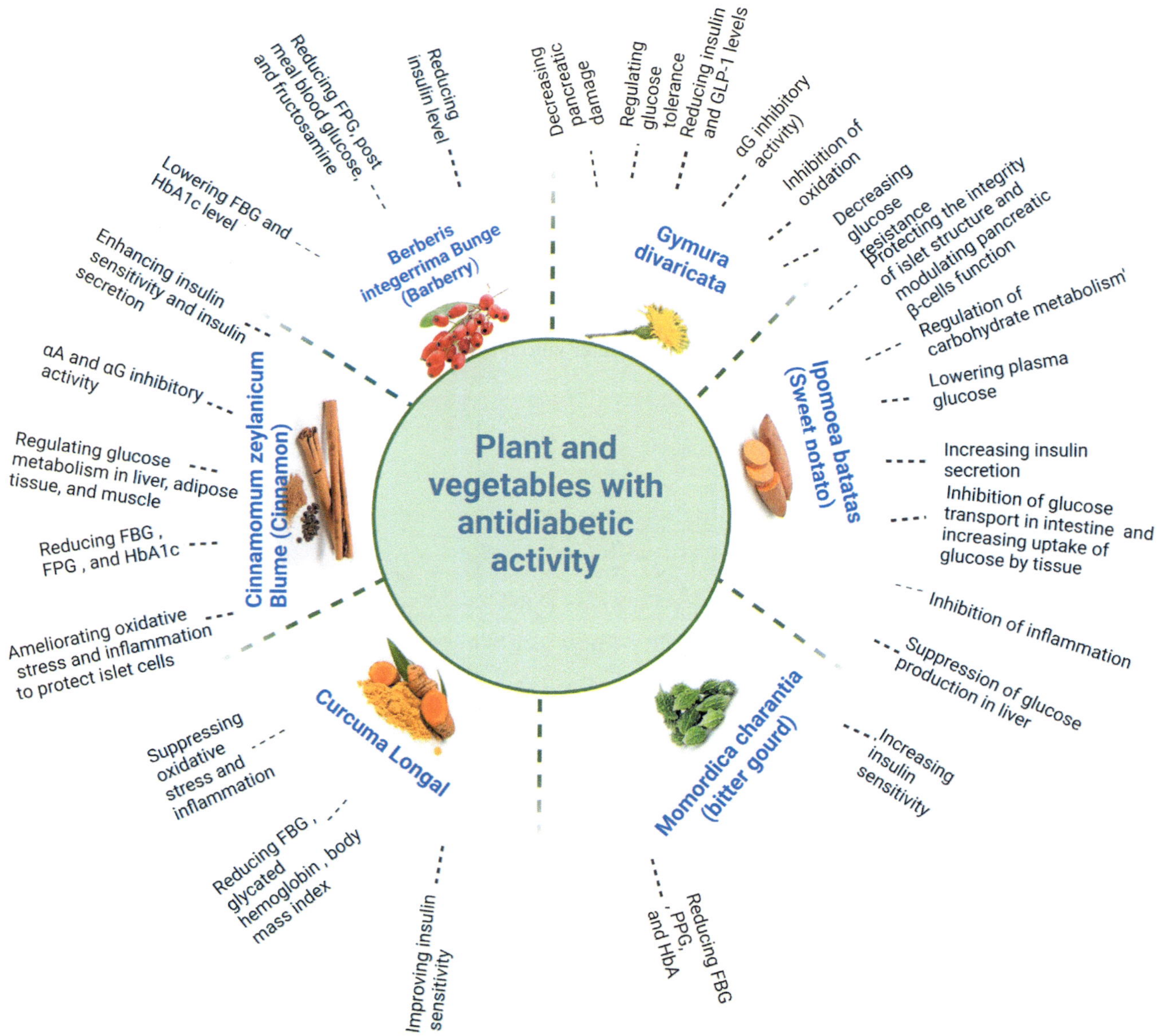

FIGURE 20.2 . The list of plants and vegetables with antidiabetic action and their potential mechanisms. The graph is created using BioRender.com (Arisanti et al., 2023; Aslam, 2017; Deyno et al., 2019; Joseph & Jini, 2013; Khaliq et al., 2015; Kim et al., 2020; Kinoshita et al., 2023; Li et al., 2018; Li, Shi, et al., 2018; Luo et al., 2021c, 2021d; Marton et al., 2021; Mishra et al., 2015; Peter et al., 2019; Pivari et al., 2019; Rashidi et al., 2018; Safari et al., 2020; Shang et al., 2021; Shih et al., 2020; Xu & Zhang, 2017; Xu et al., 2015; Yin et al., 2018; Zare et al., 2019).

Several varieties of medicinal herbs are also utilized around the world for their potential in the treatment of diabetes, including *Allium sativum* (garlic), Ginseng species, Momordica charantia (bitter melon), *Trigonella foenum-graecum* (fenugreek), Allium cepa (onion), Aloe barbadensis miller (Aloe vera), Cajanus cajan (Pigeon pea), Coccinia grandis (Ivy gourd), Caesalpinia bonducella (Kankarej), Ficus benghalensis (Banyan), ginger (Zingiber officinale) and turmeric (Curcuma longa), Gymnema sylvestre (Gurmar), Ocimum sanctum (Tulsi), Pterocarpus marsupium (Indian kino), Swertia chirayita (Bitter stick), Syzygium cumini (Jamun), Tinospora cordifolia (Giloy), Mucuna pruriens (Cattle's bean), Murraya koenigii (Curry tree), and Brassica juncea (Mustard) (Beidokhti & Jäger, 2017; Raigond et al., 2018).

20.4.2 Whole cereal grains

Whole grains (WG) are one of the main and common food categories in the human diet, which consists of starchy endosperm, germ, and bran (van der Kamp et al., 2022). The evidence from an epidemiological study (Khalid et al., 2022;

Musa-Veloso et al., 2021) and a metaanalysis study also demonstrated that the prevention and control of T2DM are associated with a higher intake of whole grains or cereal fiber (Wang et al., 2019b).

The most widely known effects of WG-based products against T2DM have been caused by functional components such as prebiotic compounds, phytochemicals, and minerals (Dalton et al., 2012). However, the impact of WG particle size on glycemic response in individuals with T2DM has been investigated, with studies indicating that larger particle size may influence glucose absorption rate because a larger particle size reduces the amount of surface area available to enzymes, resulting in a slower rate of glucose absorption (Reynolds et al., 2020). For instance, a research study conducted to evaluate the effect of consuming flour types of bread supplied with two types of flour (roller-milled and stone-ground) on the concentration of PPG in participants with T2DM aged 18–75 years indicated that consuming breads with larger flour particle size significantly decreased PPG concentration compared to all other breads (Reynolds et al., 2020). In the same manner, a randomized crossover trial was conducted to estimate the effect of whole-grain particle size on postprandial glycaemia in 31 participants (males and females) under risk factors for T2DM (Åberg et al., 2020). The findings indicated that less-processed whole-grain foods significantly improved glycemia variables such as body weight in adults with T2DM in comparison with whole-grain foods that were finely milled. In addition, consumption of less-processed whole grains for breakfast and all meals compared with finely milled grains significantly reduced PPG by 9% and 6%, respectively (Åberg et al., 2020). Therefore incorporating whole-grain foods with an appropriate particle size can be beneficial for individuals with T2DM (Reynolds et al., 2020).

Various mechanisms regarding the antidiabetic effects of WG have been mentioned in current data, but some of the most important are controlling the glycemic response, increasing insulin sensitivity, decreasing adipocyte cell size, modulating the expression of adipose tissue genes, improving pancreatic β-cell functions, increasing insulin secretion, modulation of gut microbial, and antiinflammatory activity (Zeng et al., 2020). A mouse model was used in a study to assess the nutritional value of highland barley cookies enhanced with WG. In vivo research showed that integrating WG into cookies significantly reduced the projected glycemic index (pGI) and body weight. It also helped maintain a healthy gut bacteria composition, controlled serum lipid profiles, and reduced liver damage as compared to the control group. The scientists attributed these beneficial results to the expansion of probiotics such as *Desulfovibrio*, *Veillonella*, and *Weissella*, all of which produce propionate (Guo et al., 2024).

Whole grains contain prebiotic components such as inulin, β-glucan, and fiber, which contribute to their antidiabetic properties via modulating gut microbiota and metabolic responses (Ma et al., 2019). Furthermore, the gut microbiome synthesizes several beneficial metabolites, including short-chain fatty acids (SCFAs) such as acetic acid, propionic acid, and butyric acid (Ma et al., 2019), which contribute to the improvement of T2DM. For example, in a crossover clinical trial, granola containing various amounts of cereal β-glucan (high: 6.6 g, medium: 3.2 g, and low: 0.8 g) was incorporated into low-fat milk as an evening meal of 14 healthy adults, and the levels of appetite-regulating hormones and microbiota were evaluated after 3 days (Telle-Hansen et al., 2022). The data indicated that consuming medium amounts of β-glucan significantly reduced blood glucose levels, while consumption of β-glucan regardless of its amount markedly increased the level of acetate and butyrate. Furthermore, when compared with the low β-glucan meal, both medium and high β-glucan meal remarkably increased the concentration of peptide YY. Peptide YY is a peptide hormone that plays a role in regulating appetite and food intake (Telle-Hansen et al., 2022). Another study looked into the molecular mechanism of glucose tolerance after 83 days of high β-glucan barley supplementation in diet-induced obese mice. The study found that β-glucan barley significantly increased glucose tolerance, cecal SCFA levels (acetate and propionate), GLP-1 levels in the portal vein, and cecal GLP-1 pool size when compared to the control group (Suzuki & Aoe, 2021).

Whole grains also encompass various types of phytochemicals such as phenolic acids, flavanones, carotenoids, anthocyanidins, and phytosterols (Table 20.3). These compounds might contribute to the potential of WG in managing diabetes (Okarter & Liu, 2010). According to a research paper, the presence of bound phenolics in rice bran dietary fiber could regulate glucose metabolism. This was evidenced by a reduction in FBG level in db/db mice following one-week interventions. Also, the study noted a significant increase in the expression level of GLUT4 in skeletal muscle. This increase was attributed to the activation of the insulin IRS1/AKT/GLUT4 signaling pathway and alteration of gut microbiota, especially Lachnospiraceae and Ruminococcaceae. These bacteria have a significant role in the production of butyric acid (Zhang et al., 2020b). As a result of this finding, the presence of bound phenolics in dietary fiber plays a significant role in the regulation of glucose metabolism in addition to fiber content in whole-grain diets.

Whole grains also include high levels of minerals such as phosphorus, potassium, zinc, iron, magnesium, and selenium (Laskowski et al., 2019). Minerals are primarily found in the aleurone cells at the interior of the bran and are chelated by inositol-6-phosphate (phytate) in whole grain (Bohn et al., 2007). A 6-week randomized crossover design was used to assess the effect of whole grain versus refined grain wheat meals on insulin sensitivity in obese persons. Whole-grain diets included approximately 30% more magnesium than refined diets. The results showed that a diet rich in

TABLE 20.3 Different Contents of Phenolic Acids in Cereals.

Cereals	Content in Whole Grains (μg/g)	References
Barley	1088 ± 37-828 ± 63	Horvat et al. (2020)
Maize	8962 ± 447	Das and Singh (2016)
Millet	219.96 -1658.37	Goudar et al. (2023)
Oat	1202 ± 52.9 - 1687 ± 80.2	Multari et al. (2018)
Black Rice	301- 428.7	Sumczynski et al. (2016)
Rye	984.29 ± 42.09 -3369.19 ± 53.26	Kulichová et al. (2019)
Sorghum	174.40 ± 4.09 - 1238.83 ± 31.67	Shen et al. (2018)
Wheat	654 ± 29	Horvat et al. (2020)

whole grains greatly enhanced insulin sensitivity. The authors stated that regardless of fiber's effect on insulin metabolism, magnesium may also play a role in the improvement of insulin sensitivity through decreasing inflammation and oxidative stress, endothelial dysfunction, platelet aggregation, and CVD-related diseases (Pereira et al., 2002). However, the health advantages of minerals as part of whole grain and wheat diets are less obvious, and the influence of whole-grain minerals on biomarkers related to T2DM needs greater investigation in the future (Lillioja et al., 2013).

Furthermore, whole grains may have a positive impact on diabetic patients' blood lipid profiles. For example, in a survey, consumption of whole-wheat bread for 12 weeks significantly decreased the concentration of low-density lipoprotein cholesterol (LDL-c), triglyceride, total cholesterol, HbA_{1c}, and body weight in patients with T2DM in comparison to a control group (Nazari et al., 2021).

20.4.3 Probiotics and prebiotics

Probiotics are live microbial supplements that, when ingested in proper doses, benefit the host body. *Bacillus*, *Propionibacterium*, *Lactobacillus*, *Bifidobacterium*, *Streptococcus*, *Coccobacilli*, and nonpathogenic yeasts such as *Saccharomyces* are other examples (Gomes et al., 2014). New words have recently emerged, such as parabiotics (inactivated probiotics or crude cell extracts) and postbiotics (metabolic products derived from probiotics or lysed cells) (Nataraj et al., 2020). Prebiotics are molecules that bacteria selectively use. Examples include fructooligosaccharides (FOS), galactooligosaccharides (GOS), xylooligosaccharides (XOS), inulin, resistant starch, pectin, pectin-like compounds, and β-glucans (Gibson et al., 2017; Senés-Guerrero et al., 2020). Furthermore, noncarbohydrate substances such as polyunsaturated fatty acids, minerals, and polyphenols have prebiotic action (Gibson et al., 2017).

Diets containing probiotic and prebiotic supplements facilitate the prevention and/or cure of diseases such as T2DM by modulating the gut microbiota and its homeostasis (Li et al., 2020). In Japan, a study indicated that the consumption of fermented milk containing *L. casei* strain for 16 weeks significantly reduced bacterial translocation, gut dysbiosis, and the growth of harmful bacteria such as *Blautia coccoides* and *Clostridium leptum* in patients with T2DM (Sato et al., 2017). Similarly, a study has been conducted to evaluate the antidiabetic mechanisms of fermented camel milk containing probiotics in db/db mice. The authors stated that probiotics significantly increased the amount of SCFAs, promoted GLP-1 release by upregulation of G protein-coupled receptor 43/41 (GPR43/41), enhanced insulin secretion, and inhibited apoptosis in pancreas via regulating PI3K/AKT molecular pathways (Wang et al., 2020). Studies have indicated that consumption of probiotics in both forms (parabiotics and postbiotics) could improve glucose tolerance and insulin resistance by reducing HbA_{1c} and the regulation of the gut microbiota-butyrate-inflammatory axis in diabetic mice (Li et al., 2016).

Synbiotics are known as a mixture comprising live microorganisms and substrate(s) selectively utilized by host microorganisms that confer a health benefit on the host, including T2DM management (Swanson et al., 2020). A functional yogurt enriched with whey protein, inulin, calcium, vitamin D3, and probiotic bacteria (*S. thermophilus*, *Lactobacillus delbrueckii* subsp. *bulgaricus*, and *B. lactis* Bb-12) significantly reduced triglycerides concentration, fat percentage, and body fat mass, along with improving insulin resistance in humans who suffered from metabolic syndrome (Mohammadi-Sartang et al., 2018). In the same manner, in a survey, yogurt was enriched with *B. lactis* BB-12,

L. acidophilus LA-5, inulin, and monk fruit extract to improve blood glucose regulation in animals fed with a high-fat diet. The result displayed a significant increase in SCFA levels, improvement in liver and kidney damage, and a reduction of insulin resistance and HbA_{1c} levels in comparison to regular yogurt (Ban et al., 2020). Likewise, the incorporation of soybean oligosaccharides, *S. thermophilus* CCFM218, *L. acidophilus* CCFM6, and *L. plantarum* CCFM47 into yogurt had antihyperglycemic activity by inhibiting αG and production of short-chain fatty acids (propionic and butyric acids) (Muganga et al., 2015).

A study which carried out to investigate the antidiabetic effect of four different types of synbiotic yogurt (with inulin and microencapsulated probiotics) in diabetic rats indicated that the microencapsulation significantly improved the survival of probiotics in yogurt samples in comparison to free probiotic cells, and the concentration of the glucose and total cholesterol remarkably reduced in diabetic rats fed with yogurt containing inulin, a microencapsulated *L. acidophilus* compared to the diabetic control group (Naguib et al., 2021). This underscores the importance of safeguarding probiotic cells to ensure an adequate delivery of cells into the body for exerting antidiabetic activity (Misra et al., 2022).

20.4.4 Seaweeds

The nutritional value of seaweed makes it a popular food in countries such as Korea, China, and Japan (Nicol et al., 2020). Three separate groups of algae, namely, brown algae (Ochrophyta, Phaeophyceae), red algae (Rhodophyta), and green algae (Chlorophyta), are known to date (Guiry & M, 2021). The quality and quantity of bioactive compounds in seaweed can be influenced by a variety of parameters, including harvesting period, salinity, temperature, geographical location, season, pH, water nutrient content, and herbivory (Pacheco et al., 2020). Studies have shown that seaweed-derived bioactive compounds, including polysaccharides, phytochemicals, polyunsaturated fatty acids, and minerals, have significant potential for the management of T2DM through reducing absorbance of glucose from the digestive system, improvement of insulin resistance, improving glucose uptake by cells, and regulation of lipid metabolism (Gheda et al., 2021; Peng et al., 2011; Shrestha et al., 2021). There have been some claims that integrating seaweed into food formulations increased their antidiabetic properties. For example, seaweeds (Sargassum wightii and Ulva lactuca) were mixed into bread and chapatti products to assess their glycemic index and reaction in Wistar albino mice. According to the findings, goods containing seaweed had a lower glycemic reaction than normal bread. The authors suggested that Sargassum wightii and Ulva lactuca showed antiglycemic effects via inhibiting αA, αG, and DPP-4 enzymes (Devi et al., 2022). Another in vitro study discovered that incorporating marine-derived algal food rich in astaxanthin, a carotenoid pigment, into wholemeal cookies significantly decreased the rate of glucose released during in vitro digestion while increasing the total concentration of phenolic content and antioxidant capacity of the cookies (Hossain et al., 2017). In another study, stigmasterol was extracted from the seaweed Gelidium spinosum and used to create a nanoemulsion conjugate for the manufacturing of functional biscuits (Poulose et al., 2021). In vitro and in vivo studies found that stigmasterol from the seaweed Gelidium spinosum had antioxidant and αA inhibitor capabilities, as well as reducing blood sugar, urea, and creatinine levels in streptozotocin (STZ)-induced hyperglycemic rats (Poulose et al., 2021).

20.4.5 Mushroom

Mushroom is an edible delicacy with high nutritional and functional potential, which can be used as a functional food (Yadav & Negi, 2021). Three categories of mushrooms can be considered based on their edibility, including nonpoisonous, edible (Lepiota procera), and poisonous (Lepiota margani) (Ramírez-Terrazo et al., 2021). According to the findings, 2,000 out of at least 12000 known species worldwide are placed in the edible group. Commercially, 35 species of edible mushrooms are on the market, while almost 200 wild species of mushrooms are used in medicine and pharmaceuticals (Beulah et al., 2013). Some countries such as Russia, China, Japan, and Korea have applied mushroom-derived preparations in their clinical practice (Chang & Wasser, 2012). The beneficial effect of mushrooms is related to their biological compounds, including proteins and peptides, polysaccharides, fibers, and phytochemicals (Yadav & Negi, 2021). Terpenoids, which are secondary metabolites, as well as polysaccharides, can reduce inflammatory factors, block glucosidase, and facilitate glucose uptake and lipid metabolism, resulting in glucose homeostasis with mushroom eating (Dasgupta & Acharya, 2019). Moreover, various in vitro and in vivo studies have evaluated the application of nutraceuticals derived from edible and medicinal mushrooms in food (Ma et al., 2018). For instance, it has been proven that oral administration of freeze-dried and powdered *Pleurotus ostreatus* suspension at a dose of 50 mg/kg/body weight/daily for 2 weeks in T2DM patients significantly reduced fasting plasma glucose (FPG) and PPG, as a result of increasing glucose utilization by peripheral tissues, promoting insulin secretion, inhibition of glycogen synthase kinase (GSK), and a promotion of glycogen synthesis (Jayasuriya et al., 2015). Furthermore, a diabetic rat model was used to evaluate the effects of oyster mushroom powder (OMP) on AMPK phosphorylation and GLUT4 transcription levels. The treatment of streptozotocin-induced diabetic rats with 5% OMP for 8 weeks increased gene expression of GLUT4 and P-AMPK by 6 and 1.5-fold, respectively (Asrafuzzaman et al., 2018). In another study, mushroom powder was mixed into durum wheat pasta to examine its nutritional value, in vitro glycemic response, and antioxidant potential. It was discovered that enriched pasta with mushroom powder boosted the overall phenolic content of samples as well as their antioxidant capabilities, lowered starch degradation, and the area under the curve (AUC) of reducing sugars generated during digestion (Lu et al., 2018). In addition to lowering FBG, triglycerides, serum alanine aminotransferase, and high-density lipoprotein cholesterol, mushroom consumption was also associated with a reduction in body fat and BMI (Zhang et al., 2020a). These findings support the usefulness of mushrooms as functional meals for diabetic individuals.

References

Abdulazeez, S. S., & Ponnusamy, P. (2016). Antioxidant and hypoglycemic activity of strawberry fruit extracts against alloxan induced diabetes in rats. *Pakistan Journal of Pharmaceutical Sciences, 29*(1), 255–261.

Åberg, S., et al. (2020). Whole-grain processing and glycemic control in type 2 diabetes: A randomized crossover trial. *Diabetes Care, 43*(8), 1717–1723.

Abu-Odeh, A., et al. (2022). In vitro and in vivo antidiabetic activity, phenolic content and microscopical characterization of Terfezia claveryi. *Molecules (Basel, Switzerland), 27*(15).

Acquah, C., et al. (2022). Anti-diabetic effects of bioactive peptides: recent advances and clinical implications. *Critical Reviews in Food Science and Nutrition, 62*(8), 2158–2171.

Ahangarpour, A., Sayahi, M., & Sayahi, M. (2019). The antidiabetic and antioxidant properties of some phenolic phytochemicals: A review study. *Diabetes Metab Syndr, 13*(1), 854–857.

Ajani, A., & Olanrewaju, B. O. (2014). Avocado pear fruits and leaves aqueous extracts inhibit α-amylase, α-glucosidase and snp induced lipid peroxidation—an insight into mechanisms involve in management of type 2 diabetes. *Int J Appl Nat Sci, 3*, 21–34.

Alam, S., et al. (2022). Antidiabetic phytochemicals from medicinal plants: Prospective candidates for new drug discovery and development. *Frontiers in Endocrinology (Lausanne), 13*, 800714.

Alkhatib, A., et al. (2017). Functional foods and lifestyle approaches for diabetes prevention and management. *Nutrients, 9*. Available from https://doi.org/10.3390/nu9121310.

Arisanti, C. I. S., et al. (2023). Mechanism of anti-diabetic activity from sweet potato (*Ipomoea batatas*): A systematic review. *Foods, 12*(14), 2810.

Asbaghi, O., et al. (2023). Effect of vitamin E intake on glycemic control and insulin resistance in diabetic patients: An updated systematic review and meta-analysis of randomized controlled trials. *Nutrition Journal, 22*(1), 1–22.

Ashor, A., et al. (2017). Effects of vitamin C supplementation on glycaemic control: A systematic review and meta-analysis of randomised controlled trials. *European Journal of Clinical Nutrition, 71*(12), 1371–1380.

Aslam, H. (2017). Comparison of anti-diabetic activity of berberis lycium royle stem bark (Barberry) and pioglitazone in type 2 diabetes induced mice model. *Journal of Islamabad Medical & Dental College, 6*(1), 35–39.

Asrafuzzaman, M., et al. (2018). Oyster mushroom functions as an anti-hyperglycaemic through phosphorylation of AMPK and increased expression of GLUT4 in type 2 diabetic model rats. *Journal of Taibah University medical sciences, 13*(5), 465–471.

Ayyash, M., et al. (2018). In vitro investigation of anticancer, antihypertensive, antidiabetic, and antioxidant activities of camel milk fermented with camel milk probiotic: A comparative study with fermented bovine milk. *Journal of Dairy Science, 101*(2), 900–911.

Balbi, M. E., et al. (2018). Antioxidant effects of vitamins in type 2 diabetes: A meta-analysis of randomized controlled trials. *Diabetology & Metabolic Syndrome, 10*(1), 1–12.

Ban, Q., et al. (2020). Effects of a synbiotic yogurt using monk fruit extract as sweetener on glucose regulation and gut microbiota in rats with type 2 diabetes mellitus. *Journal of Dairy Science, 103*(4), 2956–2968.

Basu, A., et al. (2010). Blueberries decrease cardiovascular risk factors in obese men and women with metabolic syndrome. *The Journal of Nutrition, 140*(9), 1582–1587.

Beidokhti, M. N., & Jäger, A. K. (2017). Review of antidiabetic fruits, vegetables, beverages, oils and spices commonly consumed in the diet. *Journal of Ethnopharmacology, 201*, 26–41.

Bell, L., et al. (2017). A study of glycaemic effects following acute anthocyanin-rich blueberry supplementation in healthy young adults. *Food & Function, 8*(9), 3104–3110.

Bellahcen, S., et al. (2012). Prevention of chemically induced diabetes mellitus in experimental animals by virgin argan oil. *Phytotherapy research, 26* (2), 180–185.

Benkhoud, H., et al. (2021). Antioxidant, antidiabetic, and antihyperlipidemic activities of wheat flour-based chips incorporated with omega-3-rich fish oil and artichoke powder. *Journal of Food Biochemistry, 45*(3), e13297.

Beulah, G., A.A. Margret, and J. Nelson. *MARVELOUS MEDICINAL MUSHROOMS*. 2013.

Bhandari, D., et al. (2020). A review on bioactive peptides: Physiological functions, bioavailability and safety. *International Journal of Peptide Research and Therapeutics, 26*(1), 139–150.

Bohn, L., et al. (2007). Quantitative analysis of phytate globoids isolated from wheat bran and characterization of their sequential dephosphorylation by wheat phytase. *Journal of Agricultural and Food Chemistry*, *55*(18), 7547–7552.

Bozbulut, R., & Sanlier, N. (2019). Promising effects of β-glucans on glyceamic control in diabetes. *Trends in Food Science & Technology*, *83*, 159–166.

Bresciani, L., et al. (2017). Absorption profile of (poly)phenolic compounds after consumption of three food supplements containing 36 different fruits, vegetables, and berries. *Nutrients*, *9*(3).

Cao, H., et al. (2019). Dietary polyphenols and type 2 diabetes: Human Study and Clinical Trial. *Critical Reviews in Food Science and Nutrition*, *59* (20), 3371–3379.

Carr, A. C., & Maggini, S. (2017). Vitamin C and immune function. *Nutrients*, *9*(11), 1211.

Castro-Acosta, M. L., et al. (2016). Drinks containing anthocyanin-rich blackcurrant extract decrease postprandial blood glucose, insulin and incretin concentrations. *The Journal of Nutritional Biochemistry*, *38*, 154–161.

Chaari, A. (2020). Inhibition of human islet amyloid polypeptide aggregation and cellular toxicity by oleuropein and derivatives from olive oil. *International Journal of Biological Macromolecules*, *162*, 284–300.

Chang, S.-T., & Wasser, S. P. (2012). The role of culinary-medicinal mushrooms on human welfare with a pyramid model for human health. *International journal of medicinal mushrooms*, *14*(2).

Chaudhary, N., Walia, S., & Kumar, R. (2023). Functional composition, physiological effect and agronomy of future food quinoa (Chenopodium quinoa Willd.): A review. *Journal of Food Composition and Analysis*105192.

Chelliah, R., et al. (2021). The role of bioactive peptides in diabetes and obesity. *Foods*, *10*(9).

Chen, C., et al. (2017). Hypoglycemic effects of a Fructus Mori polysaccharide in vitro and in vivo. *Food & function*, *8*(7), 2523–2535.

Chen, C., et al. (2018). Modulation of gut microbiota by mulberry fruit polysaccharide treatment of obese diabetic db/db mice. *Food & function*, *9*(7), 3732–3742.

Chen, L., et al. (2022). Anti-diabetic and anti-obesity: Efficacy evaluation and exploitation of polyphenols in fruits and vegetables. *Food Res Int*, *157*, 111202.

Chen, L., et al. (2023a). High-fiber diet ameliorates gut microbiota, serum metabolism and emotional mood in type 2 diabetes patients. *Front Cell Infect Microbiol*, *13*, 1069954.

Chen, X., et al. (2023b). Vitamin D status, vitamin D receptor polymorphisms, and risk of microvascular complications among individuals with type 2 diabetes: A prospective study. *Diabetes Care*, *46*(2), 270–277.

Cianciosi, D., et al. (2018). Phenolic compounds in honey and their associated health benefits: A review. *Molecules (Basel, Switzerland)*, *23*(9).

Coelho, O. G. L., et al. (2017). Polyunsaturated fatty acids and type 2 diabetes: Impact on the glycemic control mechanism. *Critical Reviews in Food Science and Nutrition*, *57*(17), 3614–3619.

Dalton, S. M. C., Tapsell, L. C., & Probst, Y. (2012). Potential health benefits of whole grain wheat components. *Nutrition Today*, *47*(4), 163–174.

Das, A. K., & Singh, V. (2016). Antioxidative free and bound phenolic constituents in botanical fractions of Indian specialty maize (*Zea mays* L.) genotypes. *Food Chemistry*, *201*, 298–306.

Dasgupta, A., & Acharya, K. (2019). Mushrooms: An emerging resource for therapeutic terpenoids. *3 Biotech*, *9*(10), 369.

Dasilva, G., et al. (2016). Lipidomics to analyze the influence of diets with different EPA: DHA ratios in the progression of Metabolic Syndrome using SHROB rats as a model. *Food Chemistry*, *205*, 196–203.

Davison, K. M., & Temple, N. J. (2018). Cereal fiber, fruit fiber, and type 2 diabetes: Explaining the paradox. *Journal of Diabetes and its Complications*, *32*(2), 240–245.

de Mello, V. D., et al. (2017). Fasting serum hippuric acid is elevated after bilberry (Vaccinium myrtillus) consumption and associates with improvement of fasting glucose levels and insulin secretion in persons at high risk of developing type 2 diabetes. *Molecular Nutrition & Food Research*, *61*(9), 1700019.

de Oliveira Raphaelli, C., et al. (2019). Apple phenolic extracts strongly inhibit α-glucosidase activity. *Plant Foods for Human Nutrition*, *74*, 430–435.

de Oliveira, M. S., et al. (2022). Blueberry consumption and changes in obesity and diabetes mellitus outcomes: A systematic review. *Metabolites*, *13* (1), 19.

Del Toro-Equihua, M., et al. (2016). Effect of an avocado oil-enhanced diet (*Persea americana*) on sucrose-induced insulin resistance in Wistar rats. *Journal of food and drug analysis*, *24*(2), 350–357.

Delpino, F. M., et al. (2022). Effects of blueberry and cranberry on type 2 diabetes parameters in individuals with or without diabetes: A systematic review and meta-analysis of randomized clinical trials. *Nutrition, Metabolism and Cardiovascular Diseases*, *32*(5), 1093–1109.

Deng, Y., et al. (2020). Novel polysaccharide from Chaenomeles speciosa seeds: Structural characterization, α-amylase and α-glucosidase inhibitory activity evaluation. *International Journal of Biological Macromolecules*, *153*, 755–766.

Denis, M.-C., et al. (2015). Prevention of oxidative stress, inflammation and mitochondrial dysfunction in the intestine by different cranberry phenolic fractions. *Clinical Science*, *128*(3), 197–212.

Devi, N.A., et al., *IN VIVO STUDY OF GLYCEMIC RESPONSE OF PRODUCTS INCORPORATED WITH SELECTED SEAWEEDS*. 2022. 11: p. 2022.

Deyno, S., et al. (2019). Efficacy and safety of cinnamon in type 2 diabetes mellitus and pre-diabetes patients: A meta-analysis and meta-regression. *Diabetes Research and Clinical Practice*, *156*, 107815.

Di Folco, U., et al. (2018). Effects of a nutraceutical multicompound including bergamot (Citrus Bergamia Risso) juice on metabolic syndrome: A pilot study. *Mediterranean Journal of Nutrition and Metabolism*, *11*, 119–126.

Etsassala, N., et al. (2022). Alpha-glucosidase and alpha-amylase inhibitory activities, molecular docking, and antioxidant capacities of *Plectranthus ecklonii* constituents. *Antioxidants (Basel), 11*(2).

Evaristus, N. A., Wan Abdullah, W. N., & Gan, C. Y. (2018). Extraction and identification of α-amylase inhibitor peptides from Nephelium lappacheum and Nephelium mutabile seed protein using gastro-digestive enzymes. *Peptides, 102*, 61–67.

Farsi, E., et al. (2014). Standardized extract of Ficus deltoidea stimulates insulin secretion and blocks hepatic glucose production by regulating the expression of glucose-metabolic genes in streptozitocin-induced diabetic rats. *BMC Complementary and Alternative Medicine, 14*(1), 1–13.

Fernández-Tomé, S., et al. (2014). In vitro chemo-protective effect of bioactive peptide lunasin against oxidative stress in human HepG2 cells. *Food Research International, 62*, 793–800.

Flachs, P., et al. (2006). Polyunsaturated fatty acids of marine origin induce adiponectin in mice fed a high-fat diet. *Diabetologia, 49*, 394–397.

Fu, Z., Gilbert, E. R., & Liu, D. (2013). Regulation of insulin synthesis and secretion and pancreatic Beta-cell dysfunction in diabetes. *Current Diabetes Reviews, 9*(1), 25–53.

Gayathri, R., et al. (2023). Effect of almond consumption on insulin sensitivity and serum lipids among Asian Indian adults with overweight and obesity—A randomized controlled trial. *Frontiers in Nutrition, 9*, 1055923.

Gazwi, H. S., et al. (2023). The hypoglycemic and hypolipidemic effects of polyphenol-rich strawberry juice on diabetic rats. *Plant Foods for Human Nutrition, 78*(3), 512–519.

Gheda, S., et al. (2021). Antidiabetic and antioxidant activity of phlorotannins extracted from the brown seaweed Cystoseira compressa in streptozotocin-induced diabetic rats. *Environmental Science and Pollution Research, 28*, 22886–22901.

Gibson, G. R., et al. (2017). Expert consensus document: The International Scientific Association for Probiotics and Prebiotics (ISAPP) consensus statement on the definition and scope of prebiotics. *Nature reviews Gastroenterology & hepatology, 14*(8), 491–502.

Giri, A., & Ohshima, T. (2012). Chapter 5 - Bioactive marine peptides: Nutraceutical value and novel approaches. In S.-K. Kim (Ed.), *Advances in food and nutrition research* (pp. 73–105). Academic Press.

Gisbert, M., et al. (2023). Antioxidant and antidiabetic properties of phlorotannins from Ascophyllum nodosum seaweed extracts. *Molecules (Basel, Switzerland), 28*. Available from https://doi.org/10.3390/molecules28134937.

Gomes, A. C., et al. (2014). Gut microbiota, probiotics and diabetes. *Nutrition Journal, 13*(1), 1–13.

Gondwe, M., et al. (2008). Effects of Persea americana Mill (Lauraceae)["Avocado"] ethanolic leaf extract on blood glucose and kidney function in streptozotocin-induced diabetic rats and on kidney cell lines of the proximal (LLCPK1) and distal tubules (MDBK). *Methods and Findings in Experimental and Clinical Pharmacology, 30*(1), 25–35.

Gong, L., et al. (2020). Inhibitors of α-amylase and α-glucosidase: Potential linkage for whole cereal foods on prevention of hyperglycemia. *Food Science & Nutrition, 8*(12), 6320–6337.

González-Montoya, M., et al. (2018). Bioactive peptides from germinated soybean with anti-diabetic potential by inhibition of dipeptidyl peptidase-IV, α-amylase, and α-glucosidase enzymes. *International Journal of Molecular Sciences, 19*(10).

Goudar, G., et al. (2023). Phenolic, nutritional and molecular interaction study among different millet varieties. *Food Chemistry Advances, 2*, 100150.

Gowd, V., et al. (2021). Multi-mechanistic antidiabetic potential of astaxanthin: An update on preclinical and clinical evidence. *Molecular Nutrition & Food Research, 65*(24), 2100252.

Grabež, M., et al. (2020). Beneficial effects of pomegranate peel extract on plasma lipid profile, fatty acids levels and blood pressure in patients with diabetes mellitus type-2: A randomized, double-blind, placebo-controlled study. *Journal of Functional Foods, 64*, 103692.

Granato, D., et al. (2020). Functional foods: Product development, technological trends, efficacy testing, and safety. *Annual Review of Food Science and Technology, 11*(1), 93–118.

Gromova, L. V., Fetissov, S. O., & Gruzdkov, A. A. (2021). Mechanisms of glucose absorption in the small intestine in health and metabolic diseases and their role in appetite regulation. *Nutrients, 13*(7).

Guiry, M.D.G., G.M., *World-wide electronic publication AlgaeBase*, in *World-wide electronic publication*. 2021: National University of Ireland, Galway.

Guo, T., et al. (2024). Whole-grain highland barley premade biscuit prepared by hot-extrusion 3D printing: Printability and nutritional assessment. *Food Chemistry, 432*, 137226.

Guo, X.-f, et al. (2017). Apple and pear consumption and type 2 diabetes mellitus risk: a meta-analysis of prospective cohort studies. *Food & function, 8*(3), 927–934.

Hammé, V., et al. (2010). Effects of lactokinins from fermented acid goat whey on lipid content and adipogenesis of immortalised human adipocytes. *International Dairy Journal, 20*(9), 642–645.

Han, D. N., et al. (2013). Protective effect of β-casomorphin-7 on cardiomyopathy of streptozotocin-induced diabetic rats via inhibition of hyperglycemia and oxidative stress. *Peptides, 44*, 120–126.

Harnedy, P. A., et al. (2018a). Atlantic salmon (Salmo salar) co-product-derived protein hydrolysates: A source of antidiabetic peptides. *Food Research International, 106*, 598–606.

Harnedy, P. A., et al. (2018b). Blue whiting (Micromesistius poutassou) muscle protein hydrolysate with in vitro and in vivo antidiabetic properties. *Journal of Functional Foods, 40*, 137–145.

Horvat, D., et al. (2020). Phenolic acid profiles and antioxidant activity of major cereal crops. *Antioxidants, 9*(6), 527.

Hossain, A. M., et al. (2017). The effect of astaxanthin-rich microalgae "Haematococcus pluvialis" and wholemeal flours incorporation in improving the physical and functional properties of cookies. *Foods, 6*(8), 57.

Hu, J.-L., Nie, S.-P., & Xie, M.-Y. (2018). Antidiabetic mechanism of dietary polysaccharides based on their gastrointestinal functions. *Journal of Agricultural and Food Chemistry, 66*(19), 4781–4786.

Hu, S., et al. (2019). Identification of anti-diabetes peptides from Spirulina platensis. *Journal of Functional Foods*, *56*, 333–341.

Huang, P. K., et al. (2019). Natural phenolic compounds potentiate hypoglycemia via inhibition of Dipeptidyl peptidase IV. *Sci Rep*, *9*(1)15585.

Iizuka, Y., et al. (2018). Blackcurrant extract ameliorates hyperglycemia in type 2 diabetic mice in association with increased basal secretion of glucagon-like peptide-1 and activation of AMP-activated protein kinase. *Journal of Nutritional Science and Vitaminology*, *64*(4), 258–264.

Irondi, E. and A. Ademiluyi, *FUNCTIONAL FOODS AND MANAGEMENT OF DIABETES*. 2017. 2-19.

Irudayaraj, S. S., et al. (2016). Antioxidant, antilipidemic and antidiabetic effects of ficusin with their effects on GLUT4 translocation and PPARγ expression in type 2 diabetic rats. *Chemico-Biological Interactions*, *256*, 85–93.

Iwaniak, A., Darewicz, M., & Minkiewicz, P. (2018). Peptides derived from foods as supportive diet components in the prevention of metabolic syndrome. *Compr Rev Food Sci Food Saf*, *17*(1), 63–81.

Jamshidi, S., et al. (2018). Wild pistachio (*Pistacia atlantica* mutica) oil improve metabolic syndrome features in rats with high fructose ingestion. *Iranian Journal of Basic Medical Sciences*, *21*(12), 1255.

Jan, F., Kumar, S., & Jha, R. (2016). Effect of boiling on the antidiabetic property of enzyme treated sheep milk casein. *Vet World*, *9*(10), 1152–1156.

Jayapala, H. P., & Lim, S. Y. (2023). N-3 polyunsaturated fatty acids and gut microbiota. *Combinatorial Chemistry & High Throughput Screening*, *26* (5), 892–905.

Jayasuriya, W. B. N., et al. (2015). Hypoglycaemic activity of culinary Pleurotus ostreatus and P. cystidiosus mushrooms in healthy volunteers and type 2 diabetic patients on diet control and the possible mechanisms of action. *Phytotherapy research*, *29*(2), 303–309.

Jiang, Z., et al. (2019). Inhibitory effects of a sulfated polysaccharide isolated from edible red alga Bangia fusco-purpurea on α-amylase and α-glucosidase. *Bioscience, Biotechnology, and Biochemistry*, *83*(11), 2065–2074.

Jiao, Y., et al. (2018). Characterization of a new heteropolysaccharide from green guava and its application as an α-glucosidase inhibitor for the treatment of type II diabetes. *Food & function*, *9*(7), 3997–4007.

Joseph, B., & Jini, D. (2013). Antidiabetic effects of Momordica charantia (bitter melon) and its medicinal potency. *Asian pacific journal of tropical disease*, *3*(2), 93–102.

Jukanti, A. K., et al. (2012). Nutritional quality and health benefits of chickpea (Cicer arietinum L.): A review. *British Journal of Nutrition*, *108*(S1), S11–S26.

Karthikeyan, J., et al., *Effect of bolus viscosity on carbohydrate digestion and glucose absorption processes: An in vitro study*. 2019. 31(11).

Kerimi, A., et al. (2017). Pomegranate juice, but not an extract, confers a lower glycemic response on a high–glycemic index food: Randomized, crossover, controlled trials in healthy subjects. *The American Journal of Clinical Nutrition*, *106*(6), 1384–1393.

Khalid, W., et al. (2022). Nutrients and bioactive compounds of Sorghum bicolor L. used to prepare functional foods: a review on the efficacy against different chronic disorders. *International Journal of Food Properties*, *25*(1), 1045–1062.

Khaliq, T., Sarfraz, M., & Ashraf, M. (2015). Recent progress for the utilization of curcuma longa, Piper nigrum and Phoenix dactylifera seeds against type 2 diabetes. *The West Indian Medical Journal*, *64*(5), 527.

Khan, B. M., Cheong, K.-L., & Liu, Y. (2019). Pumpkin polysaccharides: Purification, characterization and hypoglycemic potential. *International Journal of Biological Macromolecules*, *139*, 842–849.

Khodaeian, M., et al. (2015). Effect of vitamins C and E on insulin resistance in diabetes: a meta-analysis study. *European Journal of Clinical Investigation*, *45*(11), 1161–1174.

Kim, S. K., et al. (2020). Hypoglycemic efficacy and safety of Momordica charantia (bitter melon) in patients with type 2 diabetes mellitus. *Complementary Therapies in Medicine*, *52*, 102524.

Kim, Y., et al. (2016). Suppression of NLRP3 inflammasome by γ-tocotrienol ameliorates type 2 diabetes. *Journal of Lipid Research*, *57*(1), 66–76.

Kinoshita, A., et al. (2023). White-skinned sweet potato (*Ipomoea batatas* L.) acutely suppresses postprandial blood glucose elevation by improving insulin sensitivity in normal rats. *Heliyon*, *9*(4).

Kitts, D. D., & Weiler, K. (2003). Bioactive proteins and peptides from food sources. Applications of bioprocesses used in isolation and recovery. *Current Pharmaceutical Design*, *9*(16), 1309–1323.

Kowalski, R., & de Mejia, E. G. (2021). Phenolic composition, antioxidant capacity and physical characterization of ten blackcurrant (Ribes nigrum) cultivars, their juices, and the inhibition of type 2 diabetes and inflammation biochemical markers. *Food Chemistry*, *359*, 129889.

Kulichová, K., et al. (2019). Phenolic compounds and biological activities of rye (Secale cereale L.) grains. *Open Chemistry*, *17*(1), 988–999.

Kunsongkeit, P., et al. (2019). Effect of vitamin C as an adjunct in nonsurgical periodontal therapy in uncontrolled type 2 diabetes mellitus patients. *European journal of dentistry*, *13*(03), 444–449.

Lacroix, I. M., & Li-Chan, E. C. (2013). Inhibition of dipeptidyl peptidase (DPP)-IV and α-glucosidase activities by pepsin-treated whey proteins. *Journal of Agricultural and Food Chemistry*, *61*(31), 7500–7506.

Laskowski, W., et al. (2019). How important are cereals and cereal products in the average polish diet? *Nutrients*, *11*(3), 679.

Lavalle-González, F. J., et al. (2013). Efficacy and safety of canagliflozin compared with placebo and sitagliptin in patients with type 2 diabetes on background metformin monotherapy: a randomised trial. *Diabetologia*, *56*(12), 2582–2592.

Lebovitz, H. E. (2001). Insulin resistance: Definition and consequences. *Experimental and Clinical Endocrinology & Diabetes: Official Journal, German Society of Endocrinology [and] German Diabetes Association*, *109*(Suppl 2), S135–S148.

Li, B., et al. (2022a). Extracellular vesicles regulate the transmission of insulin resistance and redefine noncommunicable diseases. *Front Mol Biosci*, *9*, 1024786.

Li, J., et al. (2018). The aqueous extract of Gynura divaricata (L.) DC. improves glucose and lipid metabolism and ameliorates type 2 diabetes mellitus. *Evidence-Based Complementary and Alternative Medicine*, *2018*.

Li, J., Shi, Z., & Mi, Y. (2018). Purple sweet potato color attenuates high fat-induced neuroinflammation in mouse brain by inhibiting MAPK and NF-κB activation. *Molecular medicine reports*, *17*(3), 4823–4831.

Li, M., et al. (2022b). Trends in insulin resistance: Insights into mechanisms and therapeutic strategy. *Signal Transduct Target Ther*, *7*(1), 216.

Li, Q., et al. (2021a). Hypoglycemic mechanism of polysaccharide from Cyclocarya paliurus leaves in type 2 diabetic rats by gut microbiota and host metabolism alteration. *Sci China Life Sci*, *64*(1), 117–132.

Li, Q. M., et al. (2021b). Laminaria japonica polysaccharide prevents high-fat-diet-induced insulin resistance in mice via regulating gut microbiota. *Food Funct*, *12*(12), 5260–5273.

Li, W.-Z., et al. (2020). Gut microbiota and diabetes: From correlation to causality and mechanism. *World journal of diabetes*, *11*(7), 293.

Li, X., et al. (2016). A comparative study of the antidiabetic effects exerted by live and dead multi-strain probiotics in the type 2 diabetes model of mice. *Food & function*, *7*(12), 4851–4860.

Li-Chan, E. C., et al. (2012). Peptides derived from atlantic salmon skin gelatin as dipeptidyl-peptidase IV inhibitors. *Journal of Agricultural and Food Chemistry*, *60*(4), 973–978.

Lillioja, S., et al. (2013). Whole grains, type 2 diabetes, coronary heart disease, and hypertension: links to the aleurone preferred over indigestible fiber. *Biofactors (Oxford, England)*, *39*(3), 242–258.

Limonte, C., et al. (2020). 1061-P: Effects of Long-Term Vitamin D and Omega-3 Fatty Acid Supplementation on Inflammatory and Cardiac Biomarkers in Patients with Type 2 Diabetes. *Diabetes*, *69*(Supplement_1).

Liu, G., et al. (2022a). Antidiabetic potential of polysaccharides from Brasenia schreberi regulating insulin signaling pathway and gut microbiota in type 2 diabetic mice. *Current Research in Food Science*, *5*, 1465–1474.

Liu, H., et al. (2022b). Physicochemical properties of dietary fiber of bergamot and its effect on diabetic mice. *Frontiers in Nutrition*, *9*, 1040825.

Liu, W., et al. (2019). Whole blueberry protects pancreatic beta-cells in diet-induced obese mouse. *Nutrition & Metabolism*, *16*(1), 1–9.

Liu, Y.-J., et al. (2014). Dietary flavonoids intake and risk of type 2 diabetes: a meta-analysis of prospective cohort studies. *Clinical Nutrition*, *33*(1), 59–63.

Lu, H., et al. (2023). Alpha-Glucosidase Inhibitory Peptides: Sources, Preparations, Identifications, and Action Mechanisms. *Nutrients*, *15*(19).

Lu, X., et al. (2018). Addition of mushroom powder to pasta enhances the antioxidant content and modulates the predictive glycaemic response of pasta. *Food Chemistry*, *264*, 199–209.

Luo, D., et al. (2021a). Pueraria lobata root polysaccharide alleviates glucose and lipid metabolic dysfunction in diabetic db/db mice. *Le Pharmacien Biologiste*, *59*(1), 382–390.

Luo, D., et al. (2021b). Pueraria lobata root polysaccharide alleviates glucose and lipid metabolic dysfunction in diabetic db/db mice. *Pharmaceutical Biology*, *59*(1), 380–388.

Luo, D., Mu, T., & Sun, H. (2021c). Profiling of phenolic acids and flavonoids in sweet potato (Ipomoea batatas L.) leaves and evaluation of their anti-oxidant and hypoglycemic activities. *Food Bioscience*, *39*, 100801.

Luo, D., Mu, T., & Sun, H. (2021d). Sweet potato (Ipomoea batatas L.) leaf polyphenols ameliorate hyperglycemia in type 2 diabetes mellitus mice. *Food & Function*, *12*(9), 4117–4131.

Lv, Q. Q., et al. (2021). Structural characterization, α-amylase and α-glucosidase inhibitory activities of polysaccharides from wheat bran. *Food Chemistry*, *341*(Pt 1)128218.

Ma, G., et al. (2018). A critical review on the health promoting effects of mushrooms nutraceuticals. *Food Science and Human Wellness*, *7*(2), 125–133.

Ma, Q., et al. (2019). Research progress in the relationship between type 2 diabetes mellitus and intestinal flora. *Biomedicine & Pharmacotherapy*, *117*, 109138.

Mahdavi, B., et al. (2021). Antidiabetic effect of Sophora pachycarpa seeds extract in streptozotocin-induced diabetic mice: A statistical evaluation. *Journal of Investigative Medicine*, *69*(6), 1201–1207.

Martinez-Villaluenga, C., et al. (2009). Protein hydrolysates from beta-conglycinin enriched soybean genotypes inhibit lipid accumulation and inflammation in vitro. *Molecular Nutrition & Food Research*, *53*(8), 1007–1018.

Marton, L. T., et al. (2021). The effects of curcumin on diabetes mellitus: A systematic review. *Frontiers in endocrinology*, *12*, 669448.

Mason, S. A., et al. (2019). Ascorbic acid supplementation improves postprandial glycaemic control and blood pressure in individuals with type 2 diabetes: Findings of a randomized cross-over trial. *Diabetes, obesity and metabolism*, *21*(3), 674–682.

Mastrototaro, L., & Roden, M. (2021). Insulin resistance and insulin sensitizing agents. *Metabolism: Clinical and Experimental*, *125*, 154892.

McRae, M. P. (2018). Dietary fiber intake and type 2 diabetes mellitus: An umbrella review of meta-analyses. *Journal of Chiropractic Medicine*, *17* (1), 44–53.

Mirmiran, P., Bahadoran, Z., & Azizi, F. (2014). Functional foods-based diet as a novel dietary approach for management of type 2 diabetes and its complications: A review. *World J Diabetes*, *5*(3), 267–281.

Mishra, A., et al. (2015). Effect of Momordica charantia fruits on streptozotocin-induced diabetes mellitus and its associated complications. *Int. J. Pharm. Pharm. Sci*, *7*, 356–363.

Misra, S., et al. (2022). Emerging technologies and coating materials for improved probiotication in food products: A review. *Food and Bioprocess Technology*, *15*(5), 998–1039.

Mohammadi-Sartang, M., et al. (2018). The effect of daily fortified yogurt consumption on weight loss in adults with metabolic syndrome: A 10-week randomized controlled trial. *Nutrition, Metabolism and Cardiovascular Diseases*, *28*(6), 565–574.

Mojica, L., & de Mejía, E. G. (2016). Optimization of enzymatic production of anti-diabetic peptides from black bean (*Phaseolus vulgaris* L.) proteins, their characterization and biological potential. *Food Funct*, *7*(2), 713–727.

Mollace, V., et al. (2019). *Hypoglycemic and hypolipemic effects of a new lecithin formulation of bergamot polyphenolic fraction: a double blind, randomized, placebo-controlled study.* Endocrine, Metabolic & Immune Disorders-Drug Targets (Formerly Current Drug Targets-Immune. *Endocrine & Metabolic Disorders), 19*(2), 136–143.

Moreira, R. J., et al. (2020). Lipoatrophy-associated insulin resistance and hepatic steatosis are attenuated by intake of diet rich in omega 3 fatty acids. *Molecular Nutrition & Food Research, 64*(7), 1900833.

Mudgil, P., et al. (2018). Characterization and identification of novel antidiabetic and anti-obesity peptides from camel milk protein hydrolysates. *Food Chemistry, 259*, 46–54.

Muganga, L., et al. (2015). Screening for lactic acid bacteria based on antihyperglycaemic and probiotic potential and application in synbiotic set yoghurt. *Journal of Functional Foods, 16*, 125–136.

Multari, S., et al. (2018). Identification and quantification of avenanthramides and free and bound phenolic acids in eight cultivars of husked oat (Avena sativa L) from Finland. *Journal of Agricultural and Food Chemistry, 66*(11), 2900–2908.

Musa-Veloso, K., et al. (2021). A systematic review and meta-analysis of randomized controlled trials on the effects of oats and oat processing on postprandial blood glucose and insulin responses. *The Journal of Nutrition, 151*(2), 341–351.

Naguib, A.-m, et al. (2021). The potential impact of different types of yogurt fortified with inulin and/or microencapsulated probiotic bacteria on diabetic rats. *Jordan Journal of Biological Sciences. All rights reserved-Volume, 14*(4), 700.

Naik, M., et al. (2021). Extraction kinetics and quality evaluation of oil extracted from bitter gourd (*Momardica charantia* L.) seeds using emergent technologies. *Lwt, 140*, 110714.

Nasri, R., et al. (2015). Ameliorating effects of goby fish protein hydrolysates on high-fat-high-fructose diet-induced hyperglycemia, oxidative stress and deterioration of kidney function in rats. *Chemico-Biological Interactions, 242*, 71–80.

Nataraj, B. H., et al. (2020). Postbiotics-parabiotics: The new horizons in microbial biotherapy and functional foods. *Microbial Cell Factories, 19*(1), 1–22.

Nazari, J., et al. (2021). Effect of consumption of whole-wheat breads on FBS, HbA1c, and blood lipids in patients with type 2 diabetes. *Preventive nutrition and food science, 26*(3), 269.

Neyrinck, A. M., et al. (2018). Wheat-derived arabinoxylan oligosaccharides with bifidogenic properties abolishes metabolic disorders induced by western diet in mice. *Nutr Diabetes, 8*(1), 15.

Ngoh, Y. Y., & Gan, C. Y. (2016). Enzyme-assisted extraction and identification of antioxidative and α-amylase inhibitory peptides from Pinto beans (*Phaseolus vulgaris* cv. Pinto). *Food Chemistry, 190*, 331–337.

Nicol, K., et al. (2020). Using seaweed as a supplement or a food ingredient to increase iodine status in women with low habitual intake. *The Proceedings of the Nutrition Society, 79*(OCE2).

Nie, Q., et al. (2021). Bioactive dietary fibers selectively promote gut microbiota to exert antidiabetic effects. *Journal of Agricultural and Food Chemistry, 69*(25), 7000–7015.

Niibo, M., et al. (2019). Probiotic Lactobacillus gasseri SBT2055 improves insulin secretion in a diabetic rat model. *Journal of Dairy Science, 102*(2), 997–1006.

Nizamutdinova, I. T., et al. (2009). The anti-diabetic effect of anthocyanins in streptozotocin-induced diabetic rats through glucose transporter 4 regulation and prevention of insulin resistance and pancreatic apoptosis. *Molecular Nutrition & Food Research, 53*(11), 1419–1429.

Nosratabadi, S., et al. (2023). The effects of vitamin C supplementation on glycemic control in patients with type 2 diabetes: A systematic review and meta-analysis. *Diabetes & Metabolic Syndrome: Clinical Research & Reviews, 17*(8), 102824.

Okarter, N., & Liu, R. H. (2010). Health benefits of whole grain phytochemicals. *Critical Reviews in Food Science and Nutrition, 50*(3), 193–208.

Oseguera Toledo, M. E., et al. (2016). Common bean (*Phaseolus vulgaris* L.) protein-derived peptides increased insulin secretion, inhibited lipid accumulation, increased glucose uptake and reduced the phosphatase and tensin homologue activation in vitro. *Journal of Functional Foods, 27*, 160–177.

Oseguera-Toledo, M. E., Gonzalez de Mejia, E., & Amaya-Llano, S. L. (2015). Hard-to-cook bean (*Phaseolus vulgaris* L.) proteins hydrolyzed by alcalase and bromelain produced bioactive peptide fractions that inhibit targets of type-2 diabetes and oxidative stress. *Food Res Int, 76*(Pt 3)), 839–851.

Pacheco, D., et al. (2020). Invasive seaweeds in the Iberian Peninsula: A contribution for food supply. *Marine Drugs, 18*(11), 560.

Pang, G. M., et al. (2019). Herbal medicine in the treatment of patients with type 2 diabetes mellitus. *Chin Med J (Engl), 132*(1), 78–85.

Parthsarathy, V., et al. (2019). Boarfish (Capros aper) protein hydrolysate has potent insulinotropic and GLP-1 secretory activity in vitro and acute glucose lowering effects in mice. *International Journal of Food Science & Technology, 54*(1), 271–281.

Patil, P., et al. (2015). Food protein-derived bioactive peptides in management of type 2 diabetes. *European Journal of Nutrition, 54*(6), 863–880.

Patil, S. P., et al. (2020). Plant-derived bioactive peptides: A treatment to cure diabetes. *Int J Pept Res Ther, 26*(2), 955–968.

Pearson, J. F., et al. (2017). Vitamin C status correlates with markers of metabolic and cognitive health in 50-year-olds: Findings of the CHALICE cohort study. *Nutrients, 9*(8), 831.

Peng, J., et al. (2011). Fucoxanthin, a marine carotenoid present in brown seaweeds and diatoms: Metabolism and bioactivities relevant to human health. *Marine Drugs, 9*(10), 1806–1828.

Pereira, M. A., et al. (2002). Effect of whole grains on insulin sensitivity in overweight hyperinsulinemic adults. *The American Journal of Clinical Nutrition, 75*(5), 848–855.

Peter, E. L., et al. (2019). *Momordica charantia* L. lowers elevated glycaemia in type 2 diabetes mellitus patients: Systematic review and meta-analysis. *Journal of Ethnopharmacology, 231*, 311–324.

Petersen, C., et al. (2019). Dietary supplementation with strawberry induces marked changes in the composition and functional potential of the gut microbiome in diabetic mice. *The Journal of Nutritional Biochemistry, 66*, 63–69.

Pittas, A. G., et al. (2019). Vitamin D supplementation and prevention of type 2 diabetes. *New England journal of medicine, 381*(6), 520–530.

Pivari, F., et al. (2019). Curcumin and type 2 diabetes mellitus: Prevention and treatment. *Nutrients, 11*(8), 1837.

Pohanka, M. (2021). Glycated hemoglobin and methods for its point of care testing. *Biosensors, 11*(3), 70.

Poolsup, N., N.A.-O. Suksomboon, and N.J. Paw, *Effect of dragon fruit on glycemic control in prediabetes and type 2 diabetes: A systematic review and meta-analysis*. (1932-6203 (Electronic)).

Poulose, N., et al. (2021). Anti-diabetic potential of a stigmasterol from the seaweed Gelidium spinosum and its application in the formulation of nanoemulsion conjugate for the development of functional biscuits. *Frontiers in Nutrition, 8*, 694362.

Power, O., et al. (2014). Food protein hydrolysates as a source of dipeptidyl peptidase IV inhibitory peptides for the management of type 2 diabetes. *The Proceedings of the Nutrition Society, 73*(1), 34–46.

Puvvada, R. C. (2020). Association of vitamin C status in diabetes mellitus: Prevalence and predictors of vitamin C deficiency. *Future Journal of Pharmaceutical Sciences, 6*, 1–5.

Qin, L., et al. (2022). Antidiabetic-activity sulfated polysaccharide from Chaetomorpha linum: Characteristics of its structure and effects on oxidative stress and mitochondrial function. *International Journal of Biological Macromolecules, 207*, 333–345.

Ragheb, S. R., et al. (2020). Impact of Rutin and Vitamin C combination on oxidative stress and glycemic control in patients with type 2 diabetes. *Clinical nutrition ESPEN, 35*, 128–135.

Rahman, M. M., et al. (2021). Role of phenolic compounds in human disease: Current knowledge and future prospects. *Molecules (Basel, Switzerland), 27*(1).

Raigond, P., et al. (2018). Quantification of biguanide and related compounds (anti-diabetic) in vegetables and fruits. *Journal of Food Composition and Analysis, 74*, 82–88.

Ramírez-Terrazo, A., et al. (2021). Breaking the paradigms of residual categories and neglectable importance of non-used resources: The "vital" traditional knowledge of non-edible mushrooms and their substantive cultural significance. *Journal of Ethnobiology and Ethnomedicine, 17*, 1–18.

Rao, U. M., & Adinew, B. (2011). Remnant B-cell-stimulative and anti-oxidant effects of Persea americana fruit extract studied in rats introduced into streptzotocin-induced hyperglycaemic state. *African Journal of Traditional, Complementary and Alternative Medicines, 8*(3).

Rashidi, H., et al. (2018). The effects of active ingredients of barberry root (Berberine) on Glycemic control and insulin resistance in type 2 diabetic patients. *Jundishapur journal of natural pharmaceutical products, 13*(1).

Rasines-Perea, Z., & Teissedre, P. L. (2017). Grape polyphenols' effects in human cardiovascular diseases and diabetes. *Molecules (Basel, Switzerland), 22*(1).

Ren, Y., et al. (2022). Glucokinase as an emerging anti-diabetes target and recent progress in the development of its agonists. *Journal of Enzyme Inhibition and Medicinal Chemistry, 37*(1), 606–615.

Ren, Y.-y, et al. (2017). Structural characterization and inhibition on α-glucosidase activity of acidic polysaccharide from Annona squamosa. *Carbohydrate Polymers, 174*, 1–12.

Reynolds, A. N., et al. (2020). Wholegrain particle size influences postprandial glycemia in type 2 diabetes: a randomized crossover study comparing four wholegrain breads. *Diabetes Care, 43*(2), 476–479.

Riccardi, G., Capaldo, B., & Vaccaro, O. (2005). Functional foods in the management of obesity and type 2 diabetes. *Current Opinion in Clinical Nutrition & Metabolic Care, 8*(6).

Rienks, J., et al. (2018). Polyphenol exposure and risk of type 2 diabetes: Dose-response meta-analyses and systematic review of prospective cohort studies. *The American Journal of Clinical Nutrition, 108*(1), 49–61.

Rivero-Pino, F., Espejo-Carpio, F. J., & Guadix, E. M. (2020). Antidiabetic food-derived peptides for functional feeding: Production, functionality and in vivo evidences. *Foods, 9*(8).

Rocha, D. M. U. P., et al. (2019). Effects of blueberry and cranberry consumption on type 2 diabetes glycemic control: A systematic review. *Critical Reviews in Food Science and Nutrition, 59*(11), 1816–1828.

Saeedi, P., et al. (2019). Global and regional diabetes prevalence estimates for 2019 and projections for 2030 and 2045: Results from the International Diabetes Federation Diabetes Atlas, 9(th) edition. *Diabetes Research and Clinical Practice, 157*107843.

Safari, Z., et al. (2020). The effect of barberry (*Berberis vulgaris* L.) on glycemic indices: A systematic review and meta-analysis of randomized controlled trials. *Complementary Therapies in Medicine, 51*, 102414.

Saji, N., et al. (2020). Rice bran phenolic extracts modulate insulin secretion and gene expression associated with β-cell function. *Nutrients, 12*(6).

Saputri, B.Y. and I.W. Saraswati. *Red Dragon Fruit Effectiveness On Decrease Blood Glucose Levels In Patients Type II Diabetes Mellitus In Kepatihan*. in *The 3rd Joint International Conference*. 2021.

Sato, J., et al. (2017). Probiotic reduces bacterial translocation in type 2 diabetes mellitus: A randomised controlled study. *Scientific reports, 7*(1) 12115.

Schell, J., et al. (2017). Cranberries improve postprandial glucose excursions in type 2 diabetes. *Food & function, 8*(9), 3083–3090.

Senés-Guerrero, C., et al. (2020). Dietary fiber and gut microbiota. *Science and technology of fibers in food systems*, 277–298.

Shang, C., et al. (2021). Beneficial effects of cinnamon and its extracts in the management of cardiovascular diseases and diabetes. *Food & function, 12*(24), 12194–12220.

Shen, S., et al. (2018). Phenolic compositions and antioxidant activities differ significantly among sorghum grains with different applications. *Molecules (Basel, Switzerland), 23*(5), 1203.

Shih, C.-K., et al. (2020). White sweet potato ameliorates hyperglycemia and regenerates pancreatic islets in diabetic mice. *Food & Nutrition Research*, 64.

Shoji, T., et al. (2017). Chronic administration of apple polyphenols ameliorates hyperglycaemia in high-normal and borderline subjects: A randomised, placebo-controlled trial. *Diabetes Research and Clinical Practice*, *129*, 43–51.

Shrestha, S., Zhang, W., & Smid, S. (2021). Phlorotannins: A review on biosynthesis, chemistry and bioactivity. *Food Bioscience*, *39*, 100832.

Singh, B., & Kaur, A. (2016). Antidiabetic potential of a peptide isolated from an endophytic Aspergillus awamori. *Journal of Applied Microbiology*, *120*(2), 301–311.

Sinha, S., et al. (2023). The effect of omega-3 fatty acids on insulin resistance. *Life (Chicago, Ill.: 1978)*, *13*(6), 1322.

Siow, H.-L., & Gan, C.-Y. (2016). Extraction, identification, and structure–activity relationship of antioxidative and α-amylase inhibitory peptides from cumin seeds (*Cuminum cyminum*). *Journal of Functional Foods*, *22*, 1–12.

Song, K., et al. (2016). Anti-diabetic effect of fermented milk containing conjugated linoleic acid on type II diabetes mellitus. *Korean Journal for Food Science of Animal Resources*, *36*(2), 170.

Sumczynski, D., et al. (2016). Determination of contents and antioxidant activity of free and bound phenolics compounds and in vitro digestibility of commercial black and red rice (*Oryza sativa* L.) varieties. *Food Chemistry*, *211*, 339–346.

Sun, B., et al. (2020). Beneficial effects of walnut (*Juglans regia* L.) oil-derived polyunsaturated fatty acid prevents a prooxidant status and hyperlipidemia in pregnant rats with diabetes. *Nutrition & Metabolism*, *17*(1), 1–11.

Sun, C., et al. (2021). Anti-diabetic effects of natural antioxidants from fruits. *Trends in Food Science & Technology*, *117*, 3–14.

Sun, H., et al. (2022). Decreasing vitamin C intake, low serum vitamin C level and risk for us adults with diabetes. *Nutrients*, *14*(19), 3902.

Sun, Y.-L., Zhou, F.-M., & Wang, H.-R. (2019). Mechanism of pomegranate ellagic polyphenols reducing insulin resistance on gestational diabetes mellitus rats. *American Journal of Translational Research*, *11*(9), 5487.

Suzuki, S., & Aoe, S. (2021). High β-glucan barley supplementation improves glucose tolerance by increasing GLP-1 secretion in diet-induced obesity mice. *Nutrients*, *13*(2), 527.

Swanson, K. S., et al. (2020). The International Scientific Association for Probiotics and Prebiotics (ISAPP) consensus statement on the definition and scope of synbiotics. *Nature Reviews Gastroenterology & Hepatology*, *17*(11), 687–701.

Takala, R., Ramji, D. P., & Choy, E. (2023). The beneficial effects of pine nuts and its major fatty acid, pinolenic acid, on inflammation and metabolic perturbations in inflammatory disorders. *International Journal of Molecular Sciences*, *24*(2), 1171.

Takikawa, M., et al. (2010). Dietary anthocyanin-rich bilberry extract ameliorates hyperglycemia and insulin sensitivity via activation of AMP-activated protein kinase in diabetic mice. *The Journal of Nutrition*, *140*(3), 527–533.

Tamam, B., et al. (2019). Proteomic study of bioactive peptides from tempe. *Journal of Bioscience and Bioengineering*, *128*(2), 241–248.

Tavera-Hernández, R., et al. (2023). Chia (*Salvia hispanica* L.), a Pre-Hispanic Food in the treatment of diabetes mellitus: Hypoglycemic, antioxidant, anti-inflammatory, and inhibitory properties of α-glucosidase and α-amylase, and in the prevention of cardiovascular disease. *Molecules (Basel, Switzerland)*, *28*(24), 8069.

Teerapongpisan, P., et al. (2022). α-Glucosidase inhibitory and α-amylase inhibitory activities of compounds isolated from Uvaria rufa Blume. *Natural Product Research*, *36*(23), 6039–6043.

Telle-Hansen, V. H., et al. (2022). A three-day intervention with granola containing cereal beta-glucan improves glycemic response and changes the gut microbiota in healthy individuals: A crossover study. *Frontiers in Nutrition*, *9*, 796362.

Tessari, P., & Lante, A. (2017). A multifunctional bread rich in beta glucans and low in starch improves metabolic control in type 2 diabetes: A controlled trial. *Nutrients*, *9*. Available from https://doi.org/10.3390/nu9030297.

Thabah, D., et al. (2023). Potentilla fulgens upregulate GLUT4, AMPK, AKT and insulin in alloxan-induced diabetic mice: an in vivo and in silico study. *Archives of Physiology and Biochemistry*, *129*(5), 1071–1083.

Tulipano, G., et al. (2011). Whey proteins as source of dipeptidyl dipeptidase IV (dipeptidyl peptidase-4) inhibitors. *Peptides*, *32*(4), 835–838.

Upadhyay, R. K. (2017). Nutritional and therapeutic potential of Allium vegetables. *J. Nutr. Ther*, *6*(1), 18–37.

van der Kamp, J.-W., et al. (2022). Consensus, global definitions of whole grain as a food ingredient and of whole-grain foods presented on behalf of the whole grain initiative. *Nutrients*, *14*(1), 138.

Vilcacundo, R., Martínez-Villaluenga, C., & Hernández-Ledesma, B. (2017). Release of dipeptidyl peptidase IV, α-amylase and α-glucosidase inhibitory peptides from quinoa (Chenopodium quinoa Willd.) during in vitro simulated gastrointestinal digestion. *Journal of Functional Foods*, *35*, 531–539.

Villaró, S., et al. (2023). Production of enzymatic hydrolysates with in vitro antioxidant, antihypertensive, and antidiabetic properties from proteins derived from Arthrospira platensis. *Food Res Int*, *163*, 112270.

Vinayagam, R., Xiao, J., & Xu, B. (2017). An insight into anti-diabetic properties of dietary phytochemicals. *Phytochemistry Reviews*, *16*(3), 535–553.

Vondra, K., & Hampl, R. (2021). Vitamin D and new insights into pathophysiology of type 2 diabetes. *Hormone Molecular Biology and Clinical Investigation*, *42*(2), 203–208.

Wang, F., et al. (2018). Oat globulin peptides regulate antidiabetic drug targets and glucose transporters in Caco-2 cells. *Journal of Functional Foods*, *42*, 12–20.

Wang, L., et al. (2019a). Polysaccharide from Rosa roxburghii Tratt fruit attenuates hyperglycemia and hyperlipidemia and regulates colon microbiota in diabetic db/db mice. *Journal of Agricultural and Food Chemistry*, *68*(1), 147–159.

Wang, P.-C., et al. (2016). Anti-diabetic polysaccharides from natural sources: A review. *Carbohydrate Polymers*, *148*, 86–97.

Wang, Y., et al. (2019b). Whole grain and cereal fiber intake and the risk of type 2 diabetes: a meta-analysis. *International Journal of Molecular Epidemiology and Genetics*, *10*(3), 38.

Wang, Y., et al. (2020). Composite probiotics alleviate type 2 diabetes by regulating intestinal microbiota and inducing GLP-1 secretion in db/db mice. *Biomedicine & Pharmacotherapy, 125*, 109914.

Wang, Z., et al. (2022). Efficacy and mechanism of Pueraria lobata and Pueraria thomsonii polysaccharides in the treatment of type 2 diabetes. *Nutrients, 14*(19).

Wojdyło, A., et al. (2016). Phenolic compounds, antioxidant and antidiabetic activity of different cultivars of Ficus carica L. fruits. *Journal of Functional Foods, 25*, 421–432.

Wu, H., et al. (2016). PGC-1α, glucose metabolism and type 2 diabetes mellitus. *The Journal of Endocrinology, 229*(3), R99–r115.

Xia, E. Q., et al. (2017). Marine peptides as potential agents for the management of type 2 diabetes mellitus—A prospect. *Marine Drugs, 15*(4).

Xiao, J. B., & Högger, P. (2015). Dietary polyphenols and type 2 diabetes: current insights and future perspectives. *Current Medicinal Chemistry, 22* (1), 23–38.

Xu, B.-Q., Yang, P., & Zhang, Y.-Q. (2015). Hypoglycemic activities of lyophilized powder of Gynura divaricata by improving antioxidant potential and insulin signaling in type 2 diabetic mice. *Food & Nutrition Research, 59*(1), 29652.

Xu, B.-Q., & Zhang, Y.-Q. (2017). Bioactive components of Gynura divaricata and its potential use in health, food and medicine: A mini-review. *African Journal of Traditional, Complementary and Alternative Medicines, 14*(3), 113–127.

Xu, C., et al. (2018a). Isolation, purification, characterization and bioactivities of a glucan from the root of Pueraria lobata. *Food & function, 9*(5), 2644–2652.

Xu, Y., et al. (2018b). Characterization, antioxidant and hypoglycemic activities of degraded polysaccharides from blackcurrant (*Ribes nigrum* L.) fruits. *Food Chemistry, 243*, 26–35.

Yadav, D., & Negi, P. S. (2021). Bioactive components of mushrooms: Processing effects and health benefits. *Food Research International, 148*, 110599.

Yang, H.-J., et al. (2021). Aqueous blackcurrant extract improves insulin sensitivity and secretion and modulates the gut microbiome in non-obese type 2 diabetic rats. *Antioxidants, 10*(5), 756.

Yang, M.-H., et al. (2024). Advances in polysaccharides of natural source of anti-diabetes effect and mechanism. *Molecular Biology Reports, 51*(1), 101.

Yin, X.-L., Xu, B.-Q., & Zhang, Y.-Q. (2018). Gynura divaricata rich in 3, 5 – /4, 5-dicaffeoylquinic acid and chlorogenic acid reduces islet cell apoptosis and improves pancreatic function in type 2 diabetic mice. *Nutrition & Metabolism, 15*, 1–12.

Yoon, S.-Y., et al. (2021). Linoleic acid exerts antidiabetic effects by inhibiting protein tyrosine phosphatases associated with insulin resistance. *Journal of Functional Foods, 83*, 104532.

Zamora-Ros, R., et al. (2013). The association between dietary flavonoid and lignan intakes and incident type 2 diabetes in European populations: The EPIC-InterAct study. *Diabetes Care, 36*(12), 3961–3970.

Zamora-Ros, R., et al. (2014). Dietary intakes of individual flavanols and flavonols are inversely associated with incident type 2 diabetes in European populations. *The Journal of Nutrition, 144*(3), 335–343.

Zare, R., et al. (2019). Efficacy of cinnamon in patients with type II diabetes mellitus: A randomized controlled clinical trial. *Clinical nutrition, 38*(2), 549–556.

Zeng, Y., et al. (2020). Molecular mechanism of functional ingredients in barley to combat human chronic diseases. *Oxidative Medicine and Cellular Longevity, 2020.*

Zhang, J., et al. (2022). Diverse gallotannins with α-glucosidase and α-amylase inhibitory activity from the roots of Euphorbia fischeriana steud. *Phytochemistry, 202*, 113304.

Zhang, S., et al. (2020a). Association between edible mushroom intake and the prevalence of newly diagnosed non-alcoholic fatty liver disease: results from the Tianjin Chronic Low-Grade Systemic Inflammation and Health Cohort Study in China. *British Journal of Nutrition, 123*(1), 104–112.

Zhang, X., et al. (2020b). Bound phenolics ensure the antihyperglycemic effect of rice bran dietary fiber in db/db mice via activating the insulin signaling pathway in skeletal muscle and altering gut microbiota. *Journal of Agricultural and Food Chemistry, 68*(15), 4387–4398.

Zhang, Y., et al. (2019). Oral administration of Angelica sinensis polysaccharide protects against pancreatic islets failure in type 2 diabetic mice: Pancreatic β-cell apoptosis inhibition. *Journal of Functional Foods, 54*, 361–370.

Zhao, L., et al. (2016). Regulation of obesity and metabolic complications by gamma and delta tocotrienols. *Molecules (Basel, Switzerland), 21*(3), 344.

Zhou, Y., et al. (2018). Dietary intake of flavonoid subclasses and risk of type 2 diabetes in prospective cohort studies: A dose–response meta-analysis. *Clinical Nutrition, 37*(6), 2294–2298.

Zhouyao, H., et al. (2022). The inhibition of intestinal glucose absorption by oat-derived avenanthramides. *J Food Biochem, 46*(10)e14324.

Zhu, J., et al. (2020). The inhibitory effects of flavonoids on α-amylase and α-glucosidase. *Critical Reviews in Food Science and Nutrition, 60*(4), 695–708.

Chapter 21

Sustainable farming practices: nurturing the future of functional foods

Anka Trajkovska Petkoska[1], Biljana Trajkovska[2], Hyrije Koraqi[3], Nishant Kumar[4] and Anita T. Broach[5]

[1]*Faculty of Technology and Technical Sciences - Veles, University St. Kliment Ohridski - Bitola, North Macedonia,* [2]*Faculty of Biotechnical Sciences, University St. Kliment Ohrdiski, Bitola, North Macedonia,* [3]*Food Science and Biotechnology, University for Business and Technology-UBT, Prishtina, Kosovo,* [4]*National Institute of Food Technology Entrepreneurship and Management (NIFTEM), Kundli, Haryana, India,* [5]*CSI: Create.Solve.Innovate. LLC, Christiansburg, VA, United States*

21.1 Introduction

Nowadays, the food and agriculture sectors stand at a crossroads. The main issue, including hunger and lifestyle of almost 10 billion people, should be solved by 2050. Looking back, major improvements in agricultural practices and food productivity have been recorded in addition to a variety of multisectoral innovations—all focused on satisfying the food demand of the current and upcoming population. However, the progress has often come with socio-economic and environmental penalties that include soil degradation, biodiversity loss, water scarcity, or deforestation, accompanied by high levels of greenhouse gas (GHG) emissions. The planet is already stressed and overconsumed due to the degradation of natural resources, compromising the damage of the planet and insecurity of future generations.

The path to planetary well-being and prosperity should be on the to-do list for every nation; it is clearly given by many global and national initiatives for saving the planet like the 2030 UN Agenda for Sustainable Development Goals (SDGs, UN 2015) (Transforming Our World: The 2030 Agenda For Sustainable Development,30 Agenda For Sustainable Development, 2015) that provide relationship between people and the planet, prosperity, food, agriculture, and climate (Times of crisis, times of change: Science for accelerating transformations to sustainable development, 2023). To align ourselves to this agenda and overcome the current challenges, the world requires many transformations in different sectors (agricultural, food processing, digital technologies, etc.) accommodating the principles of sustainability, solving poverty and hunger, and leaving no one behind. Agricultural practices and food processing have a great potential to transform the rural regions and to bring socio-economic prosperity to countries by achieving UN Agenda for SDGs; the management of natural resources and people's living places is addressed as unity, and a future is focused not solely on the end goal but also on the way to achieve it without any environmental stresses (Transforming Food and Agriculture to Achieve The SDGs: 20 interconnected actions to guide decision-makers, 2018). Moreover, the functional food is a category of food known for its therapeutic purposes, encompassing both conventional and modified variants. Conventional functional foods comprise natural or whole-food ingredients that inherently offer functional substances. In contrast, modified functional foods involve the addition of specific ingredients for targeted health benefits (Arshad et al., 2021). These foods are often associated with various physiological advantages, including enhanced physical performance, cognitive function, organ health, emotional well-being, and even the potential to alleviate chronic illnesses (Granado-Lorencio & Hernández-Alvarez, 2016). The term "functional food" is defined differently across various sources in the literature, reflecting its multifaceted nature and broad scope (Arshad et al., 2021).

21.2 Sustainable farming practices

Sustainable agriculture embodies a holistic approach to plant and animal production according to US Code Title 7, Section 3103 (https://www.nal.usda.gov/farms-and-agricultural-production-systems/sustainable-agriculture).

Unleashing the Power of Functional Foods and Novel Bioactives. DOI: https://doi.org/10.1016/B978-0-443-28862-3.00021-2

It is a nuanced system tailored to specific sites, designed to endure over the long term. This agricultural philosophy seeks to achieve several interconnected goals. In the first place, sustainable agriculture aims to provide food along with the nutritional for human needs. It acknowledges how important agriculture is in providing these necessities for human survival. Second, the cornerstones of sustainable agriculture are natural resources and the environment, which form the foundation of the agricultural economy. Recognizing their inherent worth and influence on the planet's general well-being, it works to improve and preserve these fundamental components. The foundation of sustainability is efficiency, which seeks to maximize the utilization of nonrenewable as well as on-farm resources. To acknowledge nature's wisdom in preserving balance, natural biological cycles and their controls are integrated. Importantly, sustainable agriculture is an economic enterprise in addition to an ecological one. It is committed to ensuring the economic viability of farm operations, acknowledging that long-term sustainability requires financial stability for those working the land. Lastly, the concept of sustainable agriculture extends beyond the fields and pastures. It aspires to improve the overall quality of farmers' life and society at large. By fostering a harmonious relationship between agriculture and the broader community, it seeks to create a sustainable future that benefits everyone (https://www.nal.usda.gov/farms-and-agricultural-production-systems/sustainable-agriculture).

Sustainability in agriculture prioritizes soil health, water management, and biodiversity preservation through specific practices:

1. **Soil conservation**: Sustainable agriculture safeguards and nurtures soil by utilizing natural fertilizers like organic and green manure. This approach promotes healthier soil, benefiting plants, water, air, and overall environmental well-being.
2. **Water management**: Sustainable practices protect water resources by growing plants suited to the local ecology, utilizing methods such as green manure and mulching to retain water in the soil. Techniques like contour barriers and drip irrigation contribute to efficient water use and conservation.
3. **Biodiversity preservation**: Instead of relying on chemical controls, sustainable agriculture employs natural or integrated pest management to maintain a balance in nature. Practices like crop rotation, cultivating different agricultural products, and creating habitats for natural predators contribute to biodiversity preservation.

Sustainable agriculture is crucial in solving the challenges that world is facing in the future due to the rapid growth of global population. By embracing these practices, it ensures the long-term productivity of soil, efficient water use, and the preservation of biodiversity, thus providing multiple benefits for both the environment and agricultural sustainability (Tuğrul, 2019). In addition, multisectoral collaborations, novel ideas, and innovative practices will accomplish toward more natural way of designing the processes/technologies and delivering suitable solutions (Fig. 21.1).

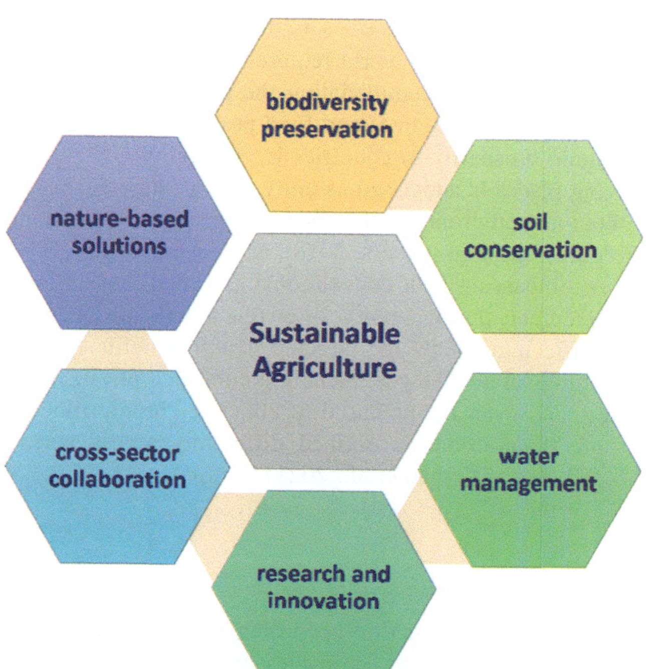

FIGURE 21.1 Functions and management of sustainable agriculture practice.

21.2.1 Organic farming

Organic farming, endorsed by the USDA, adopts a holistic approach to minimize reliance on artificial inputs, emphasizing ecological processes and organic fertilizers to sustain soil health, ecosystems, and human well-being, promoting environmentally responsible, long-term economic development by providing toxin-free food and maintaining ecological balance (Sailaja & Manohari, 2021). The positive impacts of organic farming extend across various dimensions. One significant aspect is its contribution to agroecosystem resilience in the face of climate change. Organic farming practices, such as crop rotations, utilization of crop residues, and reliance on biological systems, serve as potent and environmentally sound strategies (Murmu et al., 2022). This resilience is crucial in addressing the challenges posed by a changing climate on agricultural productivity.

Environmental sustainability is another key advantage of organic farming. By promoting sustainable eco-friendly practices, conservation efforts, and restoration activities, organic farming addresses contemporary agricultural issues. It actively reduces soil erosion, reduced bioaccumulation, and biomagnification, enhances natural resources, and supports biodiversity, contributing to a healthier overall environment (Merrigan et al., 2022). Health benefits associated with organic farming manifest through the production of nutrient-rich and pesticide-free organic products. Research indicates that organic products have a better nutritive profile as well as being free of harmful residues and additives (Hammed et al., 2019; Pandiselvi et al., 2017). Avoiding the chemical pesticides and fertilizers in the organic farming directly addresses health concerns related to conventional agricultural practices. Furthermore, organic livestock practices have an important role in supporting livestock welfare and preventing the spread of antibiotic-resistant bacteria. The prohibition of antibiotics and other drugs aligns with the broader goal of mitigating health crises associated with the overuse of antibiotics in conventional agriculture (Merrigan et al., 2022).

However, the transition to organic farming is prompted by the recognition of the negative impacts of the Green Revolution. This historical agricultural transformation, while increasing food production and self-sufficiency, resulted in adverse consequences such as soil degradation, water pollution, and various health issues (Geissen et al., 2021). In response, there is a growing emphasis on shifting toward organic farming, utilizing organic fertilizers, and sustainable practices. The objective is to restore soil fertility, maintain sustainable agriculture, and address contemporary challenges in farming (Seufert et al., 2017). Sustainable agriculture, encompassing organic farming principles, focuses on nurturing socio-economic and the environmental aspects. This approach aims to address concerns related to soil health, environmental pollution, and public health while seeking economic viability (Ebitu et al., 2021). A comparative analysis reveals significant similarities between organic and sustainable farming. Both approaches prioritize environmental stewardship, soil health, and reduced reliance on nonrenewable resources, aligning with the shared goal of ensuring the well-being of future generations along with the awareness for the environment protection (Seufert et al., 2017).

Organic agriculture spans across 187 countries, with more than 3 million farmers managing over 70 million hectares of organic farmland (Willer et al., 2021). In 2020 the worldwide sales of organic food/beverages are more than 120 billion euros. Notably, the United States leads the organic market with sales amounting to close to EUR 50 billion, followed by Germany and France (Willer et al., 2024). The contribution of organic farming to sustainable development aligns with the UN SDGs; it plays a pivotal role in reducing GHGs like methane and nitrous oxide.

21.2.1.1 Organic farming and functional food

Over the past two decades, numerous studies consistently highlight the correlation between organic farming and the production of functional foods, emphasizing higher nutritional value and lower levels of harmful substances compared to conventional methods. Notably, organic crops exhibit increased levels of nutrients and antioxidants like vitamin C, iron, and magnesium, underlining the significance of organic farming practices in prioritizing soil health, biodiversity, and ecological processes (Barański et al., 2014; Brandt et al., 2011; Fess & Benedito, 2018; Smith-Spangler et al., 2012). The evidence suggests potential health benefits linked to consuming organic produce, as it tends to show less pesticide residues or antibiotic-resistant bacteria. Moreover, the higher concentrations of phytochemicals, including phenols, flavonoids, and carotenoids, found in organic crops contribute to the functional qualities of food, potentially offering health-promoting effects (Fess & Benedito, 2018). While some studies note variations in nutrient content based on factors like crop variety and soil conditions, the overarching trend emphasizes the positive impact of organic farming on the nutritional quality of produce. The observed higher level of plant metabolites related to defense in organic vegetables further underscores the potential of organic farming to yield functional foods with enhanced bioactive compounds (Brandt et al., 2011). In contrast, conventionally grown crops consistently show higher levels of pesticide residues and heavy metals like cadmium, raising concerns about potential health risks associated with their consumption. The collective findings from various metaanalyzes affirm that opting for organically grown foods may provide consumers not only with enhanced nutritional benefits but also a reduced intake of harmful substances commonly associated with conventional farming practices (Fess & Benedito, 2018). As the demand for functional foods and healthier dietary choices continues to grow, the role of organic farming in providing nutrient-rich, safe, and environmentally sustainable food becomes increasingly significant. Embracing organic farming practices aligns with the broader goal of promoting sustainable agriculture, protecting the environment, and fostering human well-being through the production of functional foods with enhanced nutritional profiles.

Organic farming goes beyond its environmental advantages, promoting soil health through the utilization of nutrient-rich composts, minerals like rock phosphate, and the implementation of crop rotation. A key determinant, soil organic carbon (SOC) is very important for the soil health; it significantly influences various aspects of soil physical structure. This includes enhancements in water holding capacity, water infiltration, and aggregate stability. Moreover, SOC positively impacts cations exchange capacity, thereby fostering soil biological properties. These properties include an increase in nutrient composition, promotion of water cycling, reduction of specific soil pathogens, and mitigation of soil acidity (Papadopoulos et al., 2014). The adoption of organic management results in a swifter increase in SOC compared to conventional techniques, as demonstrated by studies (Bueren & Myers, 2012). Additionally, tillage practices play a pivotal role in SOC dynamics, with different systems impacting SOC at various depths (Gattinger et al., 2012). By avoiding synthetic fertilizers, organic farming contributes to an overall reduction in environmental impact. This approach addresses consumer concerns about exposure to harmful chemicals and fosters the preservation of cleaner water sources (Zhou & Ding, 2022).

However, despite these numerous advantages, organic farming faces challenges such as higher costs, time consumption, and potentially lower yields compared to conventional farming. Studies indicate that organic yields can be 25% lower, impacting profitability and sustainability (Alvarez, 2022). To address these challenges, adopting sustainable agricultural practices, including agroforestry, integrated pest management, and water conservation techniques, is crucial to ensuring a balance between environmental stewardship and economic viability. The organic farming is beneficial in the production of functional foods in terms of positive impacts on climate resilience, environmental sustainability, and human health. However, addressing challenges such as lower yields requires a strategic integration of sustainable practices to achieve a harmonious balance between ecological well-being and economic viability.

21.2.2 Precision farming for functional crops

Precision farming is a strategic management approach that involves continuous observation, measurement, and responsive adaptation to crop, field, and animal variability. Its aims include enhancing yields, improving animal performance, reducing costs, and optimizing processes for increased profitability. This methodology also promotes work safety, reduces environmental impacts, and supports overall agricultural sustainability. In precision crop farming, advanced sensing technologies provide detailed data on soil conditions, climate, fertilizer needs, water availability, and pest infestations, enabling well-informed decision-making in agricultural practices (Zhang, 2015). Therefore the soil sensors, a key subset of precision agriculture technology, play a crucial role in evaluating soil properties, offering a labor-saving and timely alternative to traditional methods (Boursianis et al., 2022). Various soil sensors, such as soil electrical conductivity (ECa) sensors, soil water content sensors (FDR or TDR), and soil moisture content sensors (including tensiometers), contribute valuable data for efficient irrigation management, nutrient availability assessment, and overall soil health monitoring (Gaikwad et al., 2015). The integration of mobile sensors, like those developed by Smolka et al. (2017), presents on-site analysis capabilities for primary plant nutrients, offering a cost-effective and time-efficient alternative to traditional laboratory soil analysis. In addition, ground-penetrating radar (GPR) and gamma-ray spectrometry (GRS) add further dimensions to soil analysis, providing insights into soil hydrology parameters and nutrient distribution (de Campos Bernardi & Perez, 2014).

In parallel, precision seeding emerges as a central focus within precision agriculture, aiming to enhance the accuracy and efficiency of the sowing process (Jianbo et al., 2014). Consistent crop emergence, influenced by precise seeding depths, significantly impacts final crop yields. Innovations like dynamic coulter depth control systems, electric seeders with optical fiber detection, and wheel mobile robots for wheat precision seeding showcase the evolving landscape of precision seeding technologies (Jin et al., 2019; Kirkegaard Nielsen et al., 2018). These advancements not only contribute to increased yield but also align with the principles of precision farming.

Smart irrigation systems, another critical component of precision agriculture, are designed to optimize water use efficiency, solving the challenges of climate change and increasing water demand from various sectors (Shi et al., 2021). Technologies such as IoT-based systems (Internet of Things), satellite data integration, and automated irrigation control offer precise water application to crops, minimizing waste and promoting sustainable agricultural development

(Goap et al., 2018). These systems empower farmers to make informed decisions about irrigation, leveraging real-time data to adapt to changing conditions.

The realm of smart fertilization systems complements precision agriculture by offering controlled and efficient nutrient supply, minimizing environmental impact (Mikula et al., 2020). UAV-based granular fertilizer spreaders by variable-rate technology (VRT), IoT-driven organic fertilizer mixing, and agricultural robots for fertilizer spraying exemplify the integration of technology into fertilization practices (Song et al., 2021). These advancements align with the principles of precision agriculture, providing targeted nutrient application and reducing resource consumption.

The integration of technology into farm machinery represents a transformative shift in agricultural practices, with auto-steered agricultural vehicles guided by GNSS (Global Navigation Satellite Systems), exemplifying the fusion of mechanics with geolocation technologies (Romano et al., 2020). The ISO 11783 (ISOBUS) further facilitates communication and data exchange between agricultural entities, ensuring interoperability in precision agriculture. Agricultural robots, or agrobots, equipped with autonomous capabilities, redefine the role of farmers, emphasizing skills in data analysis and automation (Lowenberg-DeBoer et al., 2020).

As precision agriculture advances, the symbiotic relationship between technology and farm machinery becomes increasingly evident (Fig. 21.2). This integration not only enhances efficiency and productivity but also lays the foundation for sustainable and environmentally conscious farming practices. The correlation between precision farming and the emerging field of functional food is profound, as the data-driven, resource-efficient approach of precision agriculture contributes to the production of healthier and more nutritionally valuable crops. This intersection has the potential to shape the future of agriculture, ensuring a balance between productivity, environmental stewardship, and human health.

21.2.3 Climate-smart agriculture

Climate-smart agriculture (CSA) is an approach to sustainable farming introduced by the UN Food and Agriculture Organization (FAO, 2009). It addresses the challenges posed by climate change while promoting functional food production. The primary objectives of CSA are centered on improving the efficiencies of agricultural systems and farmers' income, ensuring food security, and enhancing adaptability to climate change. (FAO, 2009) Addressing water shortages through sustainable practices is crucial for ensuring water security, which is fundamental to food security (Schlamovitz & Becker, 2021). Climate variability and change pose threats to global food production, necessitating adaptive strategies (McKinley et al., 2021). Mitigating agricultural GHG emissions requires focused measures (Pachauri & Mayer, 2014). Additionally, integrating information resources in CSA encounters challenges such as standardization, data completeness, and accuracy (Schlamovitz & Becker, 2021).

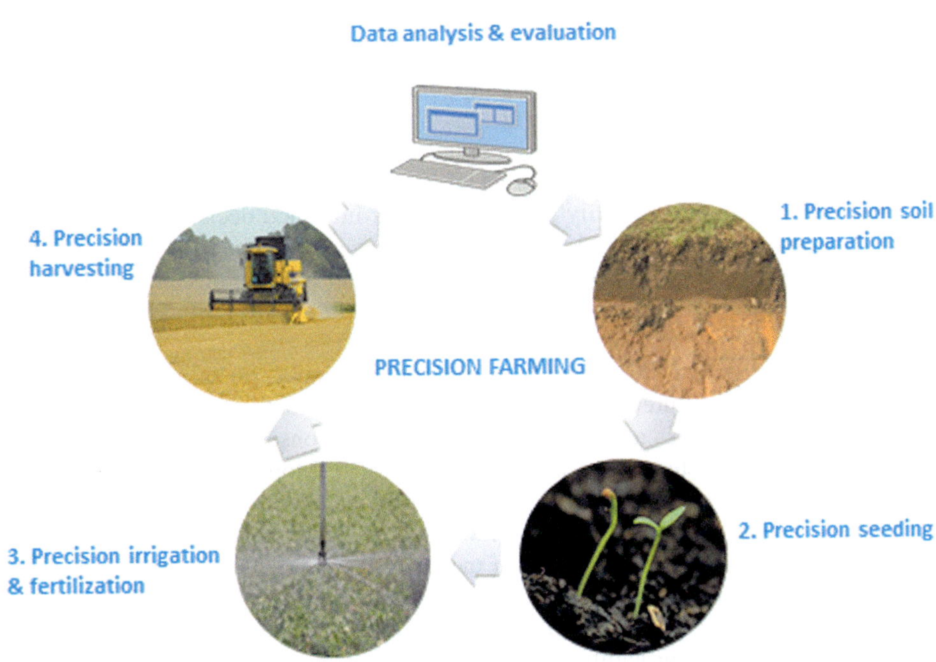

FIGURE 21.2 Precision farming of crop production.

Climate-smart agriculture (CSA) places a high priority on reducing GHG emissions and enhancing climate adaptability in the United States and other developed countries (Long et al., 2016). For example, California is actively pursuing sustainable water management and has set a target to achieve a 40% reduction in methane emissions from the dairy industry by 2030, guided by regulations like the methane law (Vechi et al., 2023). In Europe, the focus is on leveraging the service functions of agricultural systems, incorporating satellite data into precision agriculture to make informed decisions in front of uncertain weather conditions (Thornton et al., 2018). A closer examination of the environmental impact of agriculture, covering 37.6% of the global land surface, underscores its dual role as a significant source of GHGs and a sector highly susceptible to climate effects (Pachauri & Mayer, 2014).

Globally, GHG emissions from the agriculture, more particularly carbon dioxide (CO_2), methane (CH_4), and nitrous oxide (N_2O), are increasing due to anthropogenic activities (Shakoor et al., 2021). The expansion of human settlements into uninhabited areas exacerbates these environmental impacts by converting natural ecosystems into agricultural lands, resulting in the loss of soil organic carbon (SOC). SOC serves as a crucial carbon sink, storing about three times the organic carbon present in the atmosphere (Lefèvre et al., 2017). Even minor alterations in the organic carbon stock can have a substantial impact on atmospheric CO_2 concentrations. Addressing these challenges necessitates a dual approach: reducing agricultural CH_4 and N_2O emissions and increasing SOC storage in terrestrial ecosystems (Zhao et al., 2023). Effective land management practices, such as minimizing cultivation frequency and extent to reduce soil disturbance, play a pivotal role in mitigating soil carbon loss and enhancing SOC storage. While croplands experience higher percentages of SOC loss, they also offer potential for improved SOC gain through enhanced management practices. In contrast, grazing lands with lower loss in SOC may provide opportunities to increase total SOC storage due to their larger land extent.

In developing nations, CSA tailors strategies to address specific regional challenges. For instance, in Maharashtra, India, CSA practices, such as well digging, drip irrigation, and rainwater collection, address climate risks and water scarcity (Khatri-Chhetri et al., 2019; Rama Rao et al., 2013). These practices, coupled with nutrient management like farmyard manure and straw residue incorporation, enhance water and fertilizer utilization efficiency, improving agricultural productivity while reducing overall water and fertilizer consumption (Khatri-Chhetri et al., 2019). Similarly, Vietnam, Nepal, Pakistan, Zambia, Malawi, and Namibia have embraced CSA measures to enhance crop yields, cut production costs, and improve resilience to climate change.

Improving fertilizer nitrogen use efficiency (NUE) is a vital component of CSA. Strategic fertilizer application, considering type, amount, plant growth stage, and soil conditions, minimizes nitrogen loss through leaching or gaseous forms. Additionally, maintaining soil pH above 6, coapplication of animal manure and chemical fertilizers, and optimizing animal stocking rates contribute to effective NUE and fall under CSA practices (Zhao et al., 2023).

Climate-smart agriculture (CSA) stands as a critical strategy in sustainable agriculture, effectively addressing the challenges of mitigating GHG emissions and enhancing SOC storage. By implementing strategic measures in fertilizer use, land management, and soil carbon enhancement, agriculture plays a pivotal role in achieving a balance between increased productivity, climate change resilience, and environmental sustainability. This approach not only counters the adverse effects of climate change but also contributes to improved soil quality, nutrient retention, and increased agricultural productivity, aligning seamlessly with the concept of functional food.

Looking ahead, the future of CSA lies in technological advancements and innovative agricultural practices. The integration of advanced internet technologies (remote sensing, the Internet of Things (IoT), and artificial intelligence (AI)) is indispensable for ensuring agricultural information security and making well-informed decisions (Meier et al., 2020). Remote sensing provides crucial data on crop growth, yield, and disaster management, while IoT enhances data collection through sensors for improved farm management (Jusoh et al., 2021); AI, with applications in crop recognition, yield prediction, and climate adaptation, emerges as a key player in shaping the future of CSA (Hamrani et al., 2020).

Future CSA initiatives center on enhancing cropping patterns and management techniques, including practices like multiple cropping, crop diversification, and no-till agriculture, with a focus on boosting productivity and reducing GHG emissions (Datta et al., 2011). The integration of biochar as a soil additive and adopting conservation agriculture practices further promote the sustainability of agricultural systems (Purakayastha et al., 2019). Moreover, the future of CSA envisions the "Internet + Weather" service, an innovative combination of meteorological services and technological platforms tailored to effectively meet farmers' needs. Additionally, agricultural weather index-based insurance development emerges as a crucial direction for CSA, providing a risk management mechanism for agricultural producers, especially in the context of climate-related disasters (Abdi et al., 2022). In essence, the future trajectory of CSA is geared toward not only ensuring a resilient and sustainable agriculture sector but also toward supporting the production of functional foods through informed and technology-driven agricultural practices.

21.2.4 Regenerative agriculture

Regenerative agriculture is a potential sustainable alternative to traditional farming, with claims of positive environmental and social impacts. Despite its growing popularity, there is a lack of a universally accepted definition, leading to varied interpretations. Regenerative agriculture is often described as a farming approach that aims to enhance soil health, biodiversity, and ecosystem services. It is viewed as a holistic design striving to produce food efficiently while revitalizing the soil and promoting carbon sequestration. The absence of a clear and agreed-upon definition poses challenges for researchers studying its adoption and impacts. Additionally, consumers may face confusion or misinformation about products labeled as regeneratively produced. The lack of a standardized understanding could also undermine the term's credibility over time and hinder the development of supportive policies and programs (Jayasinghe et al., 2023).

21.2.5 Sustainable aquaponics and functional foods

The term "aquaponics" made its debut in 1981 when a US business magazine described the innovative functions of Disney's EPCOT theme park. EPCOT's "The Land" aimed to cultivate a variety of crops and even shrimps through aquaponics, hydroponics, and other cutting-edge farming methods. (Nation's Business: A General Magazine for Businessmen, 1981) Subsequently, Rakocy (Rakocy, 1994) introduced the term "aquaponics" in the context of an experimental station at University of the Virgin Islands, integrating vegetable hydroponics with fish culture in recirculating systems. The term is believed to originate from the combination of "aquaculture" and "hydroponics," though the exact first use remains unconfirmed (Rakocy, 1994). Aquaponics is an integrated system that combines recirculating aquaculture and hydroponics to create a closed-loop environment mirroring natural ecology. In this system, fish waste serves as nutrient for plants, and the plants filter the water for the fish. This symbiotic relationship not only enhances water quality for the fish but also reduces overall water consumption. Aquaponics is perceived as sustainable, scalable from hobby units to commercial facilities, and offers advantages such as reduced land and water requirements, faster plant growth, year-round production, operational efficiency, minimal effluents, and simultaneous cultivation of multiple crops (Pattillo, 2017).

In aquaponics, two main systems, coupled and de-coupled, are recognized in the literature. Coupled systems assume fish feed provides precise nutrients for plants, but nutrient removal by plants requires additional fish feed. Variables like feeding time, volume, fish and plant size, temperature, pH, and water chemistry affect nutrient uptake rates. De-coupled systems separate fish and plant segments, allowing individual treatment in the case of disease without compromising the entire system (Pattillo, 2017). Additionally, the FAO document considers three types of aquaponics systems:

1. Deep water culture (DWC): In these systems, plants are placed in polystyrene sheets that float in canals where air is supplied from the bottom. Common in large commercial setups, especially for growing specific crops like lettuce, salad leaves, or basil.
2. Media-filled bed (flood and drain systems): Popular for small-scale aquaponics, these units efficiently use space, are cost-effective, and are suitable for beginners. The media in the grow beds supports plant roots and serves as filtration, making it a simple yet effective design.
3. Nutrient film technique (NFT): Plastic pipes are used for this technique for horizontal growth of vegetables; water from the biofilter is pumped into each pipe, creating a shallow stream of nutrient-rich aquaponic water. Plants are placed in holes along the top of the pipe for growth (https://www.fao.org/3/br812e/br812e.pdf) (Piccolo et al., 2014).

Benefits of soilless cultures are plenty. They enhance production by precisely managing factors like nutrients, pH, oxygen, and temperature, resulting in higher yields and cost savings. Water control is optimized, using minimal water compared to traditional methods, saving time and labor. Plant nutrition is monitored meticulously, minimizing the risk of toxic substances. Controlled conditions in soilless cultures prevent weed, disease, and insect development, reducing the need for pesticides. Root surroundings are easily controlled, ensuring optimal conditions for growth. Soilless cultivation allows for quick crop turnover, increasing income, and is ideal for cultivation on unsuitable land. (Joshi et al., 2022) However, there are drawbacks. The initial setup cost is high, although it pays off in the first few years. Workforce shortage is a challenge in soilless agriculture. While open systems have low morbidity, closed systems require intensive care and sanitation to prevent pathological injuries (Joshi et al., 2022). Notably, aquaponics plays an important role in producing functional food in a sustainable and efficient way for cultivating nutrient-rich crops while minimizing environmental impact.

21.3 Food system transformations

Poor quality diets and malnutrition like stunting, wasting, obesity, vitamins and minerals deficiencies, and obesity currently affect many countries; therefore the problem of food security is a great challenge worldwide. The unsustainable food systems and unhealthy food consumptions are real treats to the global biosphere, unbalanced world, and affect the climate changes opposing the global population growth; at the same time, the world is facing multiple crises like conflicts, energy crisis, pandemic treats, and wars.

Climate changes together with the growth of global population intensify the issues related to food security. Namely, "it exists when all people, at all times, have physical and economic access to sufficient, safe and nutritious food that meets their dietary needs and food preferences for an active and healthy life" (Thakur, Prieto, et al., 2023).

Moreover, the current food system is a large emitter of GHGs; it is $\sim 30\%$ of total global emissions that causes disruption of ecosystem and biodiversity that later negatively affects the food processes. However, there is enough food quantity in the world, but due to inequitably distribution, the key nutrients remain in short supply for many people. It contributes to a range of negative outcomes, such as health problems, diseases, biodiversity loss, and consequently shortage, inaccessible, and unaffordable healthy diets (EAT–Lancet Commission 2.0: securing a just transition to healthy, environmentally sustainable diets for all, The Lancet, 2023). Therefore the changes in diet habits, as well as in global food systems, should undergo suitable transformations. All together with food waste and loss, they are all related to food security but also could be positively aligned with the global socio-economic and environmental initiatives. By now, the current linear model of the economy is the model of the constant food supply with a short useful life; it supports only an increased food production to satisfy the customer's needs without paying an attention to other social and environmental aspects (Nardella et al., 2022).

In this context, there are a lot of reports of meaning of sustainable, resilient, climate-compatible food systems as well as the healthy diets that positively contribute to the global planetary health and well-being—they are not only good for the planet but also good for people (Galanakis, 2024; Trajkovska Petkoska & Trajkovska-Broach, 2021a; Trajkovska Petkoska & Trajkovska-Broach, 2021b; Trajkovska Petkoska & Trajkovska-Broach, 2021c; Trajkovska Petkoska & Trajkovska-Broach, 2021d; Trajkovska Petkoska, 2021). They contribute to all four pillars of food security, which are availability, access, utilization, and stability, but also are in-line with the sustainability principles: health and culture as addition to social, economic, and environmental. Fig. 21.3 presents the four important dimensions of sustainability (Qu et al., 2024; Trajkovska Petkoska & Trajkovska-Broach, 2021a; Trajkovska Petkoska & Trajkovska-Broach, 2021b; Trajkovska Petkoska & Trajkovska-Broach, 2021c; Trajkovska Petkoska & Trajkovska-Broach, 2021d).

21.3.1 Sustainable food systems—planetary healthy diets

According to many scientific evidence, plant-based and less processed food categories that do not compromise the health benefits and nutrition for consumers are ranked better than other diet styles in terms of their eco-friendliness and overall well-being. Namely, a plant-based diet that includes fewer or no animal-sourced foods provides a better human health and environmental benefits. It is a "win-win" option that is good for both people and for the planet (Trajkovska Petkoska & Trajkovska-Broach, 2021a; Trajkovska Petkoska & Trajkovska-Broach, 2021b; Trajkovska Petkoska & Trajkovska-Broach, 2021c; Trajkovska Petkoska & Trajkovska-Broach, 2021d; Qu et al., 2024).

Therefore the food systems need an urgent transformation. When transformed toward sustainable, affordable, resilient, and inclusive healthy options, they become a pulling force for ending the hunger and food insecurity as well as to align with the UN SDGs concept and the Paris Agreement (EAT–Lancet Commission 2.0: securing a just transition to healthy, environmentally sustainable diets for all, The Lancet, 2023). There are many scientific reports that support

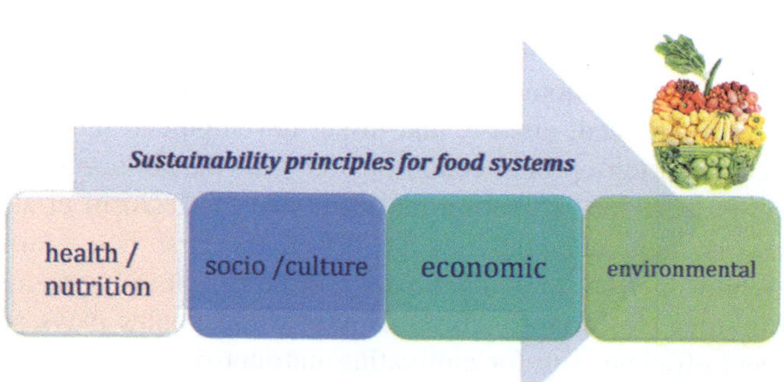

FIGURE 21.3 Main principles of sustainable food systems toward healthy diets.

sustainable food systems in terms of reduced environmental degradation such as lower impact on climate changes, biodiversity, clean water, or land-system, and proper utilization of natural resources. In addition, sustainable food systems are mostly aligned with the SDGs# 1, 2, 8 11, 12, 13 as well as in context to the statement by Willett et al. (2019): *"Transformation to healthy diets by 2050 will require substantial dietary shifts. Global consumption of fruits, vegetables, nuts and legumes will have to double, and consumption of foods such as red meat and sugar will have to be reduced by more than 50%. A diet rich in plant-based foods and with fewer animal source foods confers both improved health and environmental benefits"* (EAT–Lancet Commission 2.0: securing a just transition to healthy, environmentally sustainable diets for all, The Lancet, 2023; Willett et al., 2019).

Therefore the "universal healthy diet" emphasizes the consumption of plant-based foods while reducing the consumption of unhealthy foods; it promotes many health benefits for people (Trajkovska Petkoska & Trajkovska-Broach, 2021a; Trajkovska Petkoska & Trajkovska-Broach, 2021b). They should be aligned with the national strategies for prosperity, health, and sustainability; major gaps between them should be identified and properly addressed. In general case, they are usually like trade-offs of reaching healthy diets, especially in a transition phase from a broken to a repaired food system, or so (EAT–Lancet Commission 2.0: securing a just transition to healthy, environmentally sustainable diets for all, The Lancet, 2023). In this context, the key strategies for achieving a good food system transformation are as follows: (1) commitment to shifting to healthy diets (national/international level); (2) switching the agricultural priorities—production of healthy food instead of large food quantities; (3) intensifying the food production in a sustainable way—produce of high-quality items that are eco-sustainable and socio-economically supportive; (4) good management of land and water resources; and (5) reducing the food loss and waste (Willett et al., 2019).

In this context, the healthy dietary patterns like Mediterranean diet (MD), New Nordic diet (NND), or other territorial diets as representatives of sustainable food systems should be repositioned—not only to feed but also to nourish people worldwide. They could serve as climate-smart and resilient options that will improve human well-being, provide food security for all generations. At the same time, they promote social and economic prosperity for all. The abovementioned key strategies for food transformation (i.–iv.) will be accomplished in this way (Trajkovska Petkoska & Trajkovska-Broach, 2021a; Trajkovska Petkoska & Trajkovska-Broach, 2021b; Trajkovska Petkoska & Trajkovska-Broach, 2021c; Trajkovska Petkoska & Trajkovska-Broach, 2021d; Franchini et al., 2023; Miller et al., 2021; Peng et al., 2018; Donini & Berry, 2023).

In general, a healthy diet is a relationship between physical, mental, and social aspects—it is an optimized intake of a wide range of plant-based nutrients, but less of animal-based ones and saturated fats, sugars, or processed type of foods; this is the case of Mediterranean lifestyle and diet. There is a wide scientific portfolio that demonstrates its health benefits like prevention of noncommunicable diseases, depression, aging, then neuro-degenerative processes, etc. (Trajkovska Petkoska & Trajkovska-Broach, 2021a; Trajkovska Petkoska & Trajkovska-Broach, 2021b; Donini & Berry, 2023).

21.3.2 Food loss and waste

Decrease of the food quantity and/or quality by food suppliers in the chain is declared as food loss, while decrease in the quantity and/or quality of food made by actions of food services, shops, and consumers is food waste (Moving forward on food loss and waste reduction. Rome: Food and Agriculture Organization of the United Nations, 2019). Substantial reduction of the food loss and food waste (FLW) is essential for the sustainability aspects of the global food systems since they lead to loss of valuable resources engaged in the food (land, energy, water, workforce) as well as lead to emissions of GHGs and pollutants (EAT–Lancet Commission 2.0: securing a just transition to healthy, environmentally sustainable diets for all, The Lancet, 2023). FLW is the third largest pollutant in the world (Transforming Our World: The 2030 Agenda For Sustainable Development,30 Agenda For Sustainable Development (2015); Times of crisis, times of change: Science for accelerating transformations to sustainable development, 2023; Tuğrul, 2019).

Food businesses related to agricultural crops and food manufacturing produce huge quantities of waste biomass, in most cases, including those from plants (peels, seeds, leaves, kernels, pomace) or animal origin. Approximately more than 1 billion tons of food annually ($\sim$17% of the total food production) is wasted. It costs close to USD 2.5 trillion annually enough to feed many people who are starving worldwide. Moreover, FLW causes $\sim$ 4.4 Gtons $CO2_{eq}$ emissions which is $\sim$ 10% of the total GHGs generated by human activity (Aschemann-Witzel et al., 2023; Carnaval et al., 2024; Morganti et al., 2022). Conventional techniques for FLW treatment like landfilling and incineration are ineffective in terms of energy recovery and cause detrimental environmental effects from GHGs—they are not in-line with the global sustainability trends and principles of circular economy. However, the UN 2030 Agenda has already recognized this challenge as SDG 12 (ensure sustainable consumption and production patterns) (Huang et al., 2021; Rashwan et al., 2023; Basri et al., 2021).

Therefore the effective utilization of the biomass and by-products from agricultural and food sector by employing novel/innovative technologies will help to take care of the ***environment*** and contribute toward the sustainable food systems (Fig. 21.3). Reduced FLW provides a huge savings for consumers and operators; namely, redistribution of surplus food has an important ***social*** dimension, while the recovery of nutrients and secondary raw materials is an important ***economic*** attribute (Geissen et al., 2021; Seufert et al., 2017). It is known that agricultural wastage contains beneficial compounds such as a variety of bioactive—micro- and macronutrients, dietary fiber, carotenoids, phenolic compounds, natural pigments, and enzymes; their incorporation into food categories as extracts, powders, oils, or so can create functional—nutritive and healthy food products, or could contain valuable components important for pharma or cosmetic sector (Fig. 21.4) (Cano-Lamadrid & Artés-Hernández, 2022; Messinese et al., 2024; Minervini et al., 2022; Rashwan et al., 2023; Trombetta, 2021).

From the circular economy point, the upcycled food is a key determinant that attracts a lot of attention in the last years as a green sustainable initiative to *close the loop* in the food/agriculture sector (Aschemann-Witzel et al., 2023; Ighalo, 2024; Morganti et al., 2022; Tlais et al., 2020; Willett et al., 2019).

The food sector annually produces tons of by-products during processing, but sometimes the processing of fruits and vegetables is associated with making a lot of wastage that could not be avoided. It usually happens during the pre- and postharvesting process of during the preparation or food processing (Brandt et al., 2011; Times of crisis, times of change: Science for accelerating transformations to sustainable development, 2023). Therefore the scientists and food engineers thought about utilization of these side streams and generated biowaste and their incorporation into valuable products. This is also in context of increased consumers' awareness for natural products without synthetic additives, or with elements that provide health benefits (Fontana & Recovery, 2023). In this context, there are a lot of practical examples of extraction/isolation of useful components of biowaste from agricultural or industrial sites. In most cases, blanching, drying, homogenization, and grinding into powder are used as pretreatments of extraction techniques; extractions, like ultrasound-assisted, microwave-assisted, enzymatic-assisted, high pressure extraction, and pulsed electric

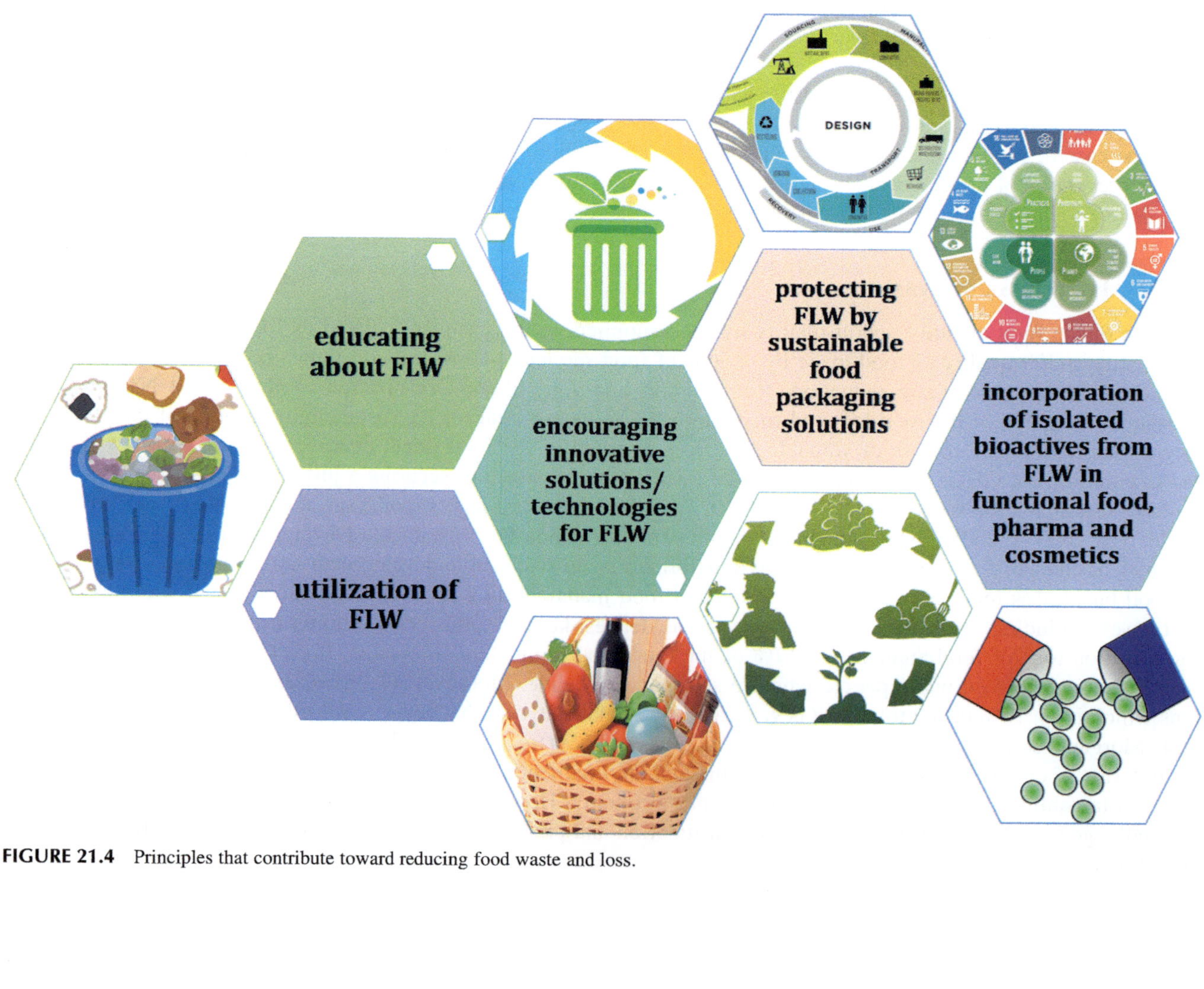
DESIGN
educating about FLW
protecting FLW by sustainable food packaging solutions
encouraging innovative solutions/ technologies for FLW
incorporation of isolated bioactives from FLW in functional food, pharma and cosmetics
utilization of FLW

FIGURE 21.4 Principles that contribute toward reducing food waste and loss.

field-assisted, are good examples of nonthermal or green technologies among the other extraction types like hot-pressurized liquid or supercritical extractions that mostly require suitable solvents or higher temperature treatments that could affect the bioactive compounds or be an energy extensive. Recovery, characterization, functionality, and application of bioactive compounds from plant-based food products and their by-products (Artés-Hernández et al., 2023; Boateng, 2023; Cano-Lamadrid & Artés-Hernández, 2022; Khan et al., n.d.; Linares & Rojas, 2022; Liu et al., 2023; Negro et al., 2016; Pai et al., 2022; Teshome et al., 2023).

Nowadays, there are many waste utilization and valorization practices that have used agro-industrial waste, for example, olive pomace derived from oil production, or grape pomace from wineries, and others refer to use of fruit/vegetable by-products derived from different food industries, for example, from apple, citrus, or other fruit processing facilities, or from potato, tomato, and carrots sites (Le et al., 2024). These by-products are rich with compounds with potential antioxidant and antimicrobial properties (carotenoids, phenolic compounds, tocopherols, phytosterols, chlorophylls, pectin, etc.) (Ebrahimi et al., 2023; Fontana & Recovery, 2023; Fotschki et al., 2023; Kumar et al., 2023; Liu et al., 2023) and could possess certain biological functions like anticancer, antiviral, antidiabetic, etc. (Fig. 21.5) (Ferreira & Gomes, & Santos, 2023; Lesmana et al., 2022; Roy et al., 2023; Sar et al., 2023). Most of them could be used for preparation of functional food due to their health benefits (Teshome et al., 2023) or to preserve the good in a natural way (Flores-Contreras et al., 2024). The extraction steps of these components are directly linked to their functionality, applicability, bioaccessibility, and bioavailability as well as synergistic/antagonist effects in the matrix where they are included (Fontana & Recovery, 2023; Günal-Köroğlu et al., 2023).

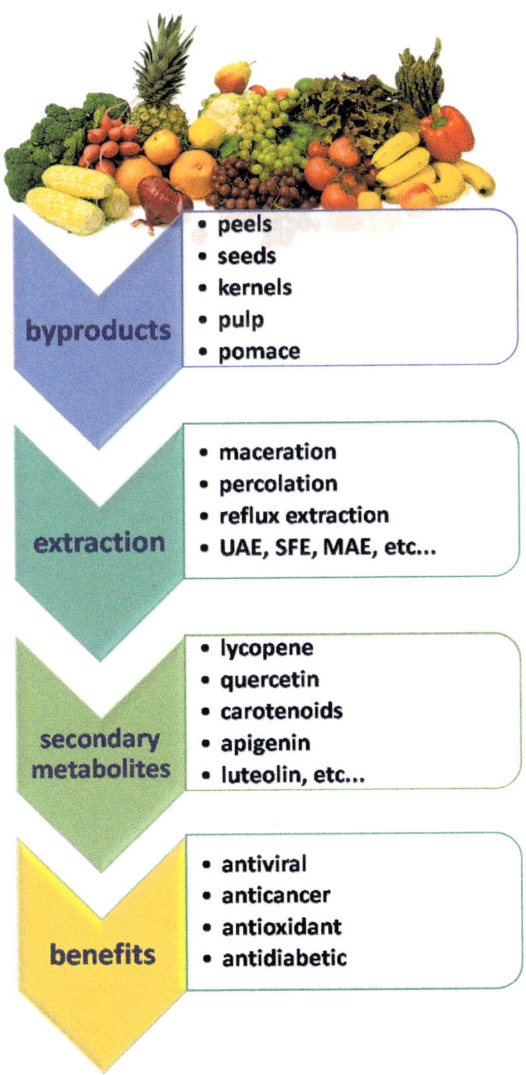

FIGURE 21.5 Waste utilization practice for harnessing of bioactive compounds.

TABLE 21.1 Utilization of Food Waste and Loss for a Variety of Applications.

Type of by-Product/ Biowaste	Application/Activity	References
Pomegranate peels	Antimicrobial, antioxidant functional additives to food; nutraceuticals for better human health; edible films/coatings	Arun et al. (2022), Ain et al. (2023), Bodana et al. (2024), Fırat et al. (2023)
Apple waste	Functional addition in food; edible coatings	Kauser et al. (2024), Salimi et al. (2024)
Blackcurrant press cake	Antioxidant activity; improved bioaccessibility and digestion	dos Santos Lima et al. (2024)
Citrus waste	Active packaging films (antioxidant, antimicrobial); Food preservation; Health benefits (antitumor, antidiabetic, antiviral); energy recovery	Das et al. (2020), Magalhães et al. (2023), Mahato et al. (2018), Negro et al. (2016), Šafranko et al. (2023), Satari and Karimi (2018), Singh et al. (2020), Yun and Liu (2022)
Date seeds/waste extracts	Biological attributes (prebiotic potential, gut microbiota modulation); active films	Rangaraj et al. (2021), Subhash et al. (2024)
Onion waste	Functional food (antioxidant phenolic compounds)	Imeneo et al. (2022)
Mango peels	Antimicrobial, antioxidant, enzymatic	Kučuk et al. (2024)
Garlic peel extracts	Multifunctional packaging film (antimicrobial, antioxidant)	Chaudhary et al. (2021)
Rice husk fibers	Antimicrobial films	Srivastava et al. (2023)
Acerola waste	Medical applications (wound healing, antioxidant, and anticancer effects)	Vega-Baudrit et al. (2023)
Apricot waste	nutrient source, emulsifier, stabilizer, functional food formulations (antioxidant, antibacterial)	Sarabandi et al. (2023)
Red beetroot and banana peels	Functional edible films (natural pigments, dopamine addition)	Šeremet et al. (2022)
Plum waste	Biocomposite films (smart indicator)	Chen et al. (2023), Sheikh et al. (2023)
Seafood by-products	Functional food (peptides, enzymes, minerals)	Siddiqui et al. (2023)
Walnut sheets	Different application (reinforcements)	Anari et al. (2024), Sultanova et al. (2023)
Winemaking-derived and grapevine by-products	Food ingredients (bioactive-phenolic, nutrients, vitamins), biodiesel, different chemical products; edible films/coatings	Bredun et al. (2023), Pinto et al. (2023), Rodrigues Machado et al. (2023), Salgado-Ramos et al. (2023)
Grape seed, green tea extract	Edible active films (antioxidants)	Ahmadzadeh et al. (2023)
Grape pomace	Films (antioxidants, antimicrobial, antiinflammatory), biofuels, cosmetics	Gubitosa et al. (2023), Kokkinomagoulos and Kandylis (2023)
Tomato by-products	Food products (carotenoids, phenolic, Tocopherols and tocotrienols, sterols, dietary fibers) and pigments; packaging	Mariño-Cortegoso et al. (2022), Moradi and Fathi (2023), Ouatmani et al. (2023)
Avocado waste	Biofuels, animal feed, natural fertilizers, food ingredients and supplements (rutin, fatty acids, kaempferol, quercetin, chlorogenic acid, chlorophyll, carotenoids)	Sandoval-Contreras et al. (2023), Siol and Sadowska (2023)
Fish/seafood waste	Functional foods and supplements (proteins and functional hydrolysates)	Balange et al. (2023)

(*Continued*)

TABLE 21.1 (Continued)

Type of by-Product/ Biowaste	Application/Activity	References
Watermelon waste	Medical use (neuroprotective, cardio-protective, kidney-protective, antidiabetic, antimicrobial); biodiesel, nutrition and food industry,	Elsayed et al. (2022), Fırat et al. (2023), Rezagholizade-shirvan et al. (2023)
Animal by-products	food and pharmaceutical sectors, packaging films (chitosan, keratin, gelatin, collagen, myofibrillar proteins, whey proteins)	Thakur, Santhosh, et al. (2023)
Ginger waste	Antimicrobial materials, environmental remediation agents, supercapacitors, bioenergy and heterogeneous catalysts (essential oil and oleoresin)	Inthalaeng et al. (2023)
Olive pomace	Film packaging (reinforcement)	Espadas-Aldana et al. (2021)

However, these by-products could be used as animal feed, or as good addition to cosmetic or pharmaceutical products, furthermore for production of biomaterials (e.g., bioplastic) (Butler et al., 2023; Frosi et al., 2023; Gautam et al., 2022; Messinese et al., 2024; Mishra et al., 2023; Karimi Sani et al., 2023), active compounds in packaging materials, edible films/coatings (Carnaval et al., 2024), natural colorants/pigments, biofuels, platforms for a variety of chemicals, waste water treatments (Boakye et al., 2022; Ighalo, 2024), and bio-fertilizers (Long et al., 2016; Shakoor et al., 2021; Song et al., 2021; Times of crisis, times of change: Science for accelerating transformations to sustainable development, 2023; Thornton et al., 2018; Vechi et al., 2023). There are many positive practices of utilization of biowaste and agro-industrial side streams and products, and some cases are presented in Table 21.1.

The research and innovation initiatives around the globe for reducing the food loss and waste and applying the principles of circular economy for turning FLW into valuable products will increase the economic benefits of food, pharma, and cosmetic industries ensuring a healthy environment for everyone. Investments in green initiatives with the power of new scientific evidence in the field of food processing, bioscience, and biotechnology will address many challenges for efficient utilization of natural resources with less pollution and emissions and better food quality (Morganti et al., 2022).

21.4 Functional foods

According to UN FAO, functional foods are those food categories that not only include nutrients but also incorporate other elements that could potentially contribute to promoting health (https://www.fao.org/faoterm/viewentry/en/?entryId = 170967). They play an important role in providing food security and nutrition for consumers. Functional foods (FF) have raised consumers' interest toward healthy diets; some of them are food items enriched with bioactive components such as carotenoids, flavonoids, lycopene, and many others, possessing potential health benefits, while others are natural products like fruits, vegetables, e.g., mushroom, flaxseed, onions, etc.—they are also rich with a variety of bioactive with beneficial health properties, like cardio-protective effect, antioxidant, antiinflammatory, antiviral, or antitumor. FF consumers have a positive contribution to own health and global well-being which is well aligned to SDG #3 (good health and well-being) (Oluwole et al., 2023).

As it was mentioned in the previous section, fruit and vegetable processing industry generates significant waste and by-products, including pomace rich in bioactive compounds. These residues, like grape and citrus peels, are high in polyphenolic compounds, offering potential as natural antioxidants in various food applications (Ben-Othman et al., 2020) and valorization of dairy products (Nakov, Trajkovska, Atanasova-Pancevska, et al., 2023; Nakov, Trajkovska, Zlatev, et al., 2023). Additionally, carrot residues yield pectin-enriched fractions with antioxidant properties, while cocoa bean shells serve as low-cost alternatives for cocoa flavoring and exhibit antioxidant activity (Rojo-Poveda et al., 2020). Extracted polyphenols or carotenoids or other valuable components from fruit/vegetable wastes have been utilized as natural preservatives extending shelf life, enhancing antioxidant capacity, or as natural coloring agents replacing the synthetic ones (Table 21.2 (Nayak & Bhushan, 2019).

TABLE 21.2 Examples of Functional Food Items With Addition of Extracts From Biowaste/biomass.

Type of Functional Food	Functional Food Item	References
Pomegranate peels	Ice cream (emulsifier); yoghurt (improved antioxidant capacity); muscle food (benefits of phenolic compounds)	Ain et al. (2023), Das et al. (2021), Fırat et al. (2023), Kennas et al. (2020)
Mango peels	Noodles (higher phenolic content and antioxidant activity; increased fiber and protein contents)	Kabir et al. (2024)
Citrus waste	Food preservation; yoghurt (multifunctional additive for the development of probiotic and synbiotic product with enhanced antioxidant and antibacterial properties); gluten free biscuits (w/ health benefits)	Fathy et al. (2022), Magalhães et al. (2023), Nuzzo et al. (2022)
Grape by-products /pomace	Crackers (high in fiber); Cookies (total dietary fiber) salmon burgers (-increased dietary fiber content and storage stability) noodle (replacement of flour) muffins (rich in antioxidant compounds and total dietary fiber)	Chen et al. (2021), Cilli et al. (2020), Kuchtová et al. (2018), Marcos et al. (2023), Troilo et al. (2022)
Brassica by-products	Fortified food	Artés-Hernández et al. (2023)
Tomato by-products (peels, seeds)	Food products—focaccia-type flatbread; (carotenoids, phenolic, tocopherols and tocotrienols, sterols, dietary fibers)	Fernandez-Pan et al. (2023)
Cocoa hull waste	Ayran (enriched with antioxidants)	Altin et al. (2018)
Red beetroot pomace	Biscuits (enriched with antioxidants)	Hidalgo et al. (2018)
Apple pomace	Yoghurt (increase in the total dietary fiber content/ antioxidant activity)	Popescu et al. (2022)
Grape and aronia pomace	Cookies (polyphenols)	Molnar et al. (2023)
Cauliflower by-products	Pizza (enriched with glucobrassicin, lutein, β-carotene, β-sitosterol); pork patties (antioxidant and antibacterial improvement); apple juice beverage (enriched with isothiocyanates);	Amofa-Diatuo et al. (2017), Nartea et al. (2023), Zhang et al. (2020)
Broccoli by-products	Beer (bioactive sulforaphane); gluten-free sponge cakes; wheat pasta (volatile organic compounds); pesto sauce (increased antioxidants)	Castillejo et al. (2021), Drabińska et al. (2022), Krupa-Kozak et al. (2019), Sánchez-Bravo et al. (2023)
By-products from chestnut shell, grape seed, and pomegranate peel	Yoghurt (antioxidant and antibacterial properties)	Ferreira and Santos (2023)
Watermelon (rind) waste	Candy (with antioxidant activity, antimicrobial effect); ice cream (pectin as natural emulsifier)	Fırat et al. (2023), Rezagholizade-shirvan et al. (2023)
Date seeds	Biscuits (enhanced antioxidant properties)	Ranasinghe et al. (2024)
Hemp press cake flour	Yoghurt (antioxidant properties)	Nakov, Trajkovska, Atanasova-Pancevska, et al. (2023), Nakov, Trajkovska, Zlatev, et al. (2023)

21.5 Challenges and future directions

Looking ahead, future research directions and innovations should aim to enhance the synergy between sustainable agriculture and functional foods (Fig. 21.6). Exploring novel farming techniques, such as agroecology and regenerative agriculture, can optimize yield while minimizing environmental impact. Integrating precision nutrition concepts into agricultural practices can lead to the cultivation of crops with enhanced nutritional profiles. Innovations in sustainable packaging, food wastage reduction, and value addition to agricultural by-products also present promising avenues. Additionally, leveraging technology for data-driven decision-making in agriculture can contribute to more efficient resource utilization. By aligning consumer education with continuous advancements in research and innovation, we can forge a path toward a sustainable and resilient future in agriculture and food processing. This journey involves not only meeting the immediate needs of our global population but doing so in a way that ensures a thriving planet for generations to come.

However, transitioning to sustainable farming practices encounters challenges that demand nuanced solutions. These challenges include resistance to change, lack of awareness, and economic constraints. To address these hurdles, comprehensive consumer education initiatives are paramount, especially for increase of awareness for sustainable farming practices, their positive impact, as well as the long-term benefits for communities. Simultaneously, industry-driven research and development instilled with innovation play a pivotal role in overcoming barriers to the adoption and scaling of sustainable farming practices. Investment in cutting-edge technologies, precision agriculture, and eco-friendly processing methods can revolutionize the sector. Furthermore, collaborations between governments, private enterprises, and research institutions can stimulate the development of sustainable solutions that are economically viable and environment-friendly.

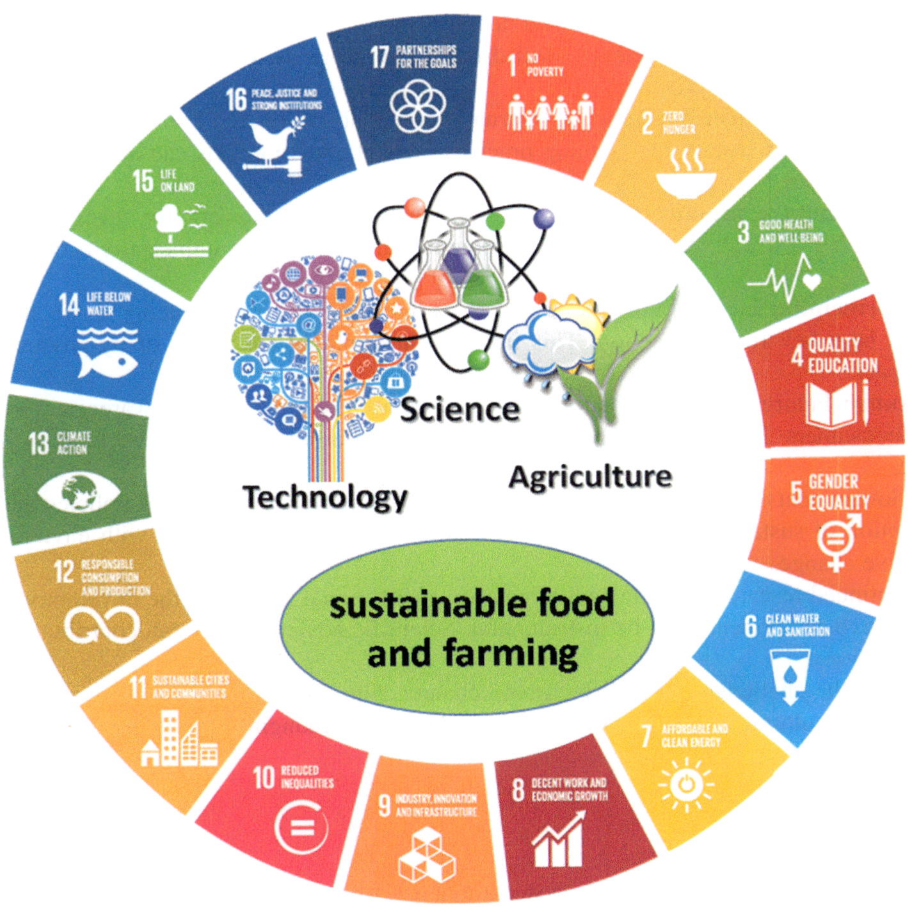

FIGURE 21.6 SDGs, sustainable food, and farming should be correlated through novel scientific findings and innovation.

21.5.1 Challenges

1. **Global adoption of sustainable practices:** Encouraging widespread adoption of sustainable farming practices poses a significant challenge. Overcoming traditional methods and promoting awareness about the benefits of sustainable agriculture is crucial.
2. **Uniform definition of regenerative agriculture:** The absence of a universally accepted definition for regenerative agriculture presents challenges in standardizing and implementing practices. Developing a cohesive framework is essential for effective adoption.
3. **Technological accessibility:** Ensuring that technology-driven farming practices, such as precision farming, are accessible to farmers globally, especially those in developing regions, remains a challenge. Bridging the technological gap is vital for widespread implementation.
4. **Policy implementation:** The successful execution of sustainable farming practices necessitates supportive policies at local and international levels. Aligning governmental policies with sustainable agriculture goals and ensuring compliance can be challenging.
5. **Consumer behavior and education:** Shifting consumer behavior toward sustainable and functional foods requires comprehensive education and awareness programs. Overcoming ingrained dietary habits and preferences poses a challenge in promoting healthier and more sustainable food choices.
6. **Economic viability:** Balancing the economic viability of sustainable farming practices with the need for affordable, nutritious food is a challenge. Ensuring that farmers can sustain their livelihoods while adopting environment-friendly practices is crucial.

21.5.2 Future directions

1. **Advancements in agricultural technology:** Continued research and development in agricultural technology, including precision farming tools and innovative cultivation methods, will drive future progress. Embracing cutting-edge technologies can enhance sustainability and productivity.
2. **Global collaboration for sustainable agriculture:** Encouraging international collaboration and knowledge-sharing platforms can facilitate the global adoption of sustainable farming practices. Collaborative efforts can address challenges collectively and promote best practices.
3. **Standardization of regenerative agriculture practices:** Establishing a standardized framework for regenerative agriculture practices is essential. Ongoing research and dialog among experts can contribute to universally accepted guidelines and principles.
4. **Integration of circular economy principles:** Incorporating these principles into food systems, reducing waste, and promoting resource efficiency will be a key future direction. This involves maximizing the utility of by-products and minimizing environmental impact.
5. **Education and awareness programs:** Future initiatives should prioritize extensive education and awareness programs targeting both farmers and consumers. Promoting the benefits of sustainable farming practices and functional foods can drive behavioral change.
6. **Policy reforms and incentives:** Governments and international organizations need to enact supportive policies and incentives that encourage the adoption of sustainable farming practices. Aligning economic benefits with environmental stewardship can drive positive change.
7. **Research on functional foods**: Continued research into the health benefits of functional foods and the development of new varieties enriched with bioactive components will be instrumental. Scientific advancements can contribute to a broader range of functional food options.
8. **Climate-resilient agriculture:** Given the challenges posed by climate change, future directions should emphasize the development of climate-resilient agricultural practices. Strategies for adapting to changing climate patterns will be crucial for long-term sustainability.

21.6 Conclusion

Innovative agricultural practices are focused on sustainable farming systems that are accompanied by sustainable principles—environment, economy, and social, in addition to health benefits, local national, and cultural aspects. They provide space for all farms in all dimensions to produce a variety of foods with a good nutritive profile adapted to local customs and markets. In most of the cases, it uses science-based and novel practices that can maximize productivity, profit, and well-being. Moreover, the food production systems become suitable to the raw materials that are locally available and easy accessible, producing food categories that are sustainable, nutritive, and affordable for people around. This approach in farming and production practices also means that the system will be also resilient to natural disaster like floods or droughts, or other impacts due to global warming and climate changes. The global or national adoption of healthy and sustainable diets is good for the people, planet, and prosperity providing well-being for all because food will be an important issue of the 21st century, and it is our responsibility to build a safe food chain. It is possible only if the policymakers and stakeholders are in agreement and compatible with research ideas, innovation, and technology in the particular areas of interest—it is the path to suitable food and agricultural transition. In addition, reducing or zeroing the food loss and waste contributes to sustainability of the food systems; the positive practices of FLW utilization are presented as novel sustainable or innovative approaches for improving quality and safety parameters in food preservation, extraction of active bioactive compounds, and their incorporation in different food products labeled as functional foods.

Furthermore, a promising trajectory for the future of functional foods is depicted by the complex tapestry created by the development of agriculture and the search for sustainable food systems. The journey through history, starting with the Neolithic Revolution and ending with modern sustainable farming methods, highlights the significant influence of agriculture on the development of societies, the world's population, and the complex relationship between health and the environment. Sustainable agricultural methods, which are sensitive to environmental issues while simultaneously promoting the development of functional foods, are at the center of the subject matter. Techniques like precision farming, organic farming, climate-smart agriculture, regenerative agriculture, and cutting-edge systems like aquaponics are examples of adaptive responses that prioritize biodiversity, soil health, and ecological balance while also helping to produce nutrient-dense, pesticide-free functional foods.

Envisioning the future of agriculture entails a compelling emphasis on sustainable and technology-driven methods, fostering a harmonious coexistence of ecological integrity, economic viability, and the production of functional foods. This forward-looking perspective aligns seamlessly with the broader objective of cultivating a resilient and balanced global food system. Furthermore, the urgency to transform food systems acts as a rallying call at the nexus of health, environmental stewardship, and societal equity. The outlined strategies, ranging from championing healthy diets to effectively reducing food loss and waste, underscore a collective commitment necessary to realize the UN sustainable development goals. Repositioning healthy dietary patterns and leveraging technology for sustainable farming practices emerge as pivotal elements in building climate-smart and resilient food systems that not only nourish people but also contribute to ecological harmony. In essence, this comprehensive discourse directs a spotlight on sustainable farming practices: Nurturing the Future of Functional Foods. The interconnectedness of human and planetary well-being within the context of food systems demands a global alliance committed to prioritizing sustainable farming practices. This collective endeavor, spanning policy changes, technological innovations, and individual choices, charts a course toward a resilient future for sustainable food systems. Through such concerted actions, we ensure the health, prosperity, and sustenance of present and future generations on a thriving planet without leaving anyone behind.

References

Abdi, M. J., Raffar., Zulkafli, Z., Nurulhuda, K., Rehan, B. M., Muharam, F. M., et al. (2022). Index-based insurance and hydroclimatic risk management in agriculture: A systematic review of index selection and yield-index modelling methods. *International Journal of Disaster Risk Reduction*, *67*.

Ahmadzadeh, S., Hettiarachchy, N., Luthra, K., Chen, J., Seo, H.-S., Atungulu, G. G., & Ubeyitogullari, A. (2023). Effects of polyphenol-rich grape seed and green tea extracts on the physicochemical properties of 3D-printed edible soy protein films. *Food Packaging and Shelf Life*, *40*, 101184. Available from https://doi.org/10.1016/j.fpsl.2023.101184.

Ain, H. B. U., Tufail, T., Bashir, S., Ijaz, N., Hussain, M., Ikram, A., Farooq, M. A., & Saewan, S. A. (2023). Nutritional importance and industrial uses of pomegranate peel: A critical review. *Food Science and Nutrition*, *11*(6), 2589–2598. Available from https://doi.org/10.1002/fsn3.3320, onlinelibrary.wiley.com/journal/10.1002/%28ISSN%292048-7177.

Altin, G., Gültekin-Özgüven, M., & Ozcelik, B. (2018). Liposomal dispersion and powder systems for delivery of cocoa hull waste phenolics via Ayran (drinking yoghurt): Comparative studies on in-vitro bioaccessibility and antioxidant capacity. *Food Hydrocolloids*, *81*, 364–370. Available from https://doi.org/10.1016/j.foodhyd.2018.02.051, https://www.journals.elsevier.com/food-hydrocolloids.

Alvarez, R. (2022). Comparing productivity of organic and conventional farming systems: A quantitative review. *Archives of Agronomy and Soil Science*, *68*(14), 1947–1958. Available from https://doi.org/10.1080/03650340.2021.1946040.

Amofa-Diatuo, T., Anang, D. M., Barba, F. J., & Tiwari, B. K. (2017). Development of new apple beverages rich in isothiocyanates by using extracts obtained from ultrasound-treated cauliflower by-products: Evaluation of physical properties and consumer acceptance. *Journal of Food*

Composition and Analysis, 61, 73–81. Available from https://doi.org/10.1016/j.jfca.2016.10.001, http://www.elsevier.com/inca/publications/store/6/2/2/8/7/8/index.htt.

Anari, E. S., Soltanizadeh, N., & Fathi, M. (2024). The potential of DBD plasma pretreatment for the isolation of micro- and nano-cellulose fibers from the walnut shells. *Carbohydrate Polymers, 327*, 121692. Available from https://doi.org/10.1016/j.carbpol.2023.121692.

Arshad, M. S., Khalid, W., Ahmad, S., Khan, K., Ahmad, H., & Safdar, M. (2021). Functional foods and human health: An overview functional. *Foods - Phytochemicals and Health Promoting Potential.*

Artés-Hernández, F., Martínez-Zamora, L., Cano-Lamadrid, M., Hashemi, S., & Castillejo, N. (2023). Genus brassica by-products revalorization with green technologies to fortify innovative foods: A scoping review. *Foods., 12*(3), 561. Available from https://doi.org/10.3390/foods12030561.

Arun, K. B., Madhavan, A., Anoopkumar, A. N., Surendhar, A., Liz Kuriakose, L., Tiwari, A., Sirohi, R., Kuddus, M., Rebello, S., Kumar Awasthi, M., Varjani, S., Reshmy, R., Mathachan Aneesh, E., Binod, P., & Sindhu, R. (2022). Integrated biorefinery development for pomegranate peel: Prospects for the production of fuel, chemicals and bioactive molecules. *Bioresource Technology, 362*, 127833. Available from https://doi.org/10.1016/j.biortech.2022.127833.

Aschemann-Witzel, J., Asioli, D., Banovic, M., Perito, M. A., Peschel, A. O., & Stancu, V. (2023). Defining upcycled food: The dual role of upcycling in reducing food loss and waste. *Trends in Food Science and Technology, 132*, 132–137. Available from https://doi.org/10.1016/j.tifs.2023.01.001, http://www.elsevier.com/wps/find/journaldescription.cws_home/601278/description#description.

Balange, M. D. S., Layana, A. K., & Naidu. (2023). *Advances in Food and Nutrition Research Harnessing value and sustainability: Fish waste valorization and the production of valuable byproducts. Advances in Food and Nutrition Research* (pp. 175–192). Elsevier. Available from https://doi.org/10.1016/bs.afnr.2023.08.001.

Barański, M., Średnicka-Tober, D., Volakakis, N., Seal, C., Sanderson, R., Stewart, G. B., Benbrook, C., Biavati, B., Markellou, E., Giotis, C., Gromadzka-Ostrowska, J., Rembiałkowska, E., Skwarło-Sońta, K., Tahvonen, R., Janovská, D., Niggli, U., Nicot, P., & Leifert, C. (2014). Higher antioxidant and lower cadmium concentrations and lower incidence of pesticide residues in organically grown crops: A systematic literature review and meta-analyses. *British Journal of Nutrition, 112*(5), 794–811. Available from https://doi.org/10.1017/S0007114514001366, http://journals.cambridge.org/BJN.

Basri, M. S. M., Shah, N. N. A. K., Sulaiman, A., Tawakkal, I. S. M. A., Nor, M. Z. M., Ariffin, S. H., Ghani, N. H. A., & Salleh, F. S. M. (2021). Progress in the valorization of fruit and vegetable wastes: Active packaging, biocomposites, by-products, and innovative technologies used for bioactive compound extraction. *Polymers, 13*(20). Available from https://doi.org/10.3390/polym13203503, https://www.mdpi.com/2073-4360/13/20/3503/pdf.

Ben-Othman, S., Jõudu, I., & Bhat, R. (2020). Bioactives from agri-food wastes: Present insights and future challenges. *Molecules (Basel, Switzerland), 25*(3), 510. Available from https://doi.org/10.3390/molecules25030510.

Boakye, P., Ohemeng-Boahen, G., Darkwah, L., Sokama-Neuyam, Y. A., Appiah-Effah, E., Oduro-Kwarteng, S., Asamoah Osei, B., Asilevi, P. J., & Woo, S. H. (2022). Waste biomass and biomaterials adsorbents for wastewater treatment. *Green Energy and Environmental Technology, 2022*, 1–25. Available from https://doi.org/10.5772/geet.05.

Boateng, I. D. (2023). Mechanisms, capabilities, limitations, and economic stability outlook for extracting phenolics from agro-byproducts using emerging thermal extraction technologies and their combinative effects. *Food and Bioprocess Technology.* Available from https://doi.org/10.1007/s11947-023-03171-5, https://www.springer.com/journal/11947.

Bodana, V., Swer, T. L., Kumar, N., Singh, A., Samtiya, M., Sari, T. P., & Babar, O. A. (2024). Development and characterization of pomegranate peel extract-functionalized jackfruit seed starch-based edible films and coatings for prolonging the shelf life of white grapes. *International Journal of Biological Macromolecules, 254*, 127234. Available from https://doi.org/10.1016/j.ijbiomac.2023.127234.

Boursianis, A. D., Papadopoulou, M. S., Diamantoulakis, P., Liopa-Tsakalidi, A., Barouchas, P., Salahas, G., Karagiannidis, G., Wan, S., & Goudos, S. K. (2022). Internet of Things (IoT) and agricultural unmanned aerial vehicles (UAVs) in smart farming: A comprehensive review. *Internet of Things, 18*, 100187. Available from https://doi.org/10.1016/j.iot.2020.100187.

Brandt, K., Leifert, C., Sanderson, R., & Seal, C. J. (2011). Agroecosystem management and nutritional quality of plant foods: The case of organic fruits and vegetables. *Critical Reviews in Plant Sciences, 30*(1-2), 177–197. Available from https://doi.org/10.1080/07352689.2011.554417.

Bredun, M. A., Prestes, A. A., Panceri, C. P., Prudêncio, E. S., & Burin, V. M. (2023). Bioactive compounds recovery by freeze concentration process from winemaking by-product. *Food Research International, 173*. Available from https://doi.org/10.1016/j.foodres.2023.113220, www.elsevier.com/inca/publications/store/4/2/2/9/7/0.

Bueren, J. R., & Myers. (2012). *Organic crop breeding* (282, p. 2012). Wiley-Blackwell.

Butler, I. P., Banta, R. A., Tyuftin, A. A., Holmes, J., Pathania, S., & Kerry, J. (2023). *Pectin as a biopolymer source for packaging films using a circular economy approach: Origins, extraction, structure and films properties, . Food Packaging and Shelf Life* (40). Elsevier Ltd. Available from https://www.sciencedirect.com/science/journal/22142894, https://doi.org/10.1016/j.fpsl.2023.101224.

de Campos Bernardi, A. C., Perez, N. B. Precision agriculture for pastures. Agricultura de precisão: resultados de um novo olhar. (2014).

Cano-Lamadrid, M., & Artés-Hernández, F. (2022). By-products revalorization with non-thermal treatments to enhance phytochemical compounds of fruit and vegetables derived products: A review. *Foods, 11*(1), 59. Available from https://doi.org/10.3390/foods11010059.

Carnaval, Ld. S. C., Jaiswal, A. K., & Jaiswal, S. (2024). Agro-food waste valorization for sustainable bio-based packaging. *Journal of Composites Science, 8*(2). Available from https://doi.org/10.3390/jcs8020041, www.mdpi.com/journal/jcs.

Castillejo, N., Martínez-Hernández, G. B., & Artés-Hernández, F. (2021). Revalorized broccoli by-products and mustard improved quality during shelf life of a kale pesto sauce. *Food Science and Technology International, 27*(8), 734–745. Available from https://doi.org/10.1177/1082013220983100, http://www.sagepub.com.

Chaudhary, B. U., Lingayat, S., Banerjee, A. N., & Kale, R. D. (2021). *Development of multifunctional food packaging films based on waste Garlic peel extract and Chitosan, . International Journal of Biological Macromolecules* (192, pp. 479–490). India: Elsevier B.V. Available from www.elsevier.com/locate/ijbiomac, https://doi.org/10.1016/j.ijbiomac.2021.10.031.

Chen, K., Li, J., Li, L., Wang, Y., Qin, Y., & Chen, H. (2023). A pH indicator film based on sodium alginate/gelatin and plum peel extract for monitoring the freshness of chicken. *Food Bioscience*, *53*, 102584. Available from https://doi.org/10.1016/j.fbio.2023.102584.

Chen, S. X., Ni, Z. J., Thakur, K., Wang, S., Zhang, J. G., Shang, Y. F., & Wei, Z. J. (2021). Effect of grape seed power on the structural and physicochemical properties of wheat gluten in noodle preparation system. *Food Chemistry*, *355*. Available from https://doi.org/10.1016/j.foodchem.2021.129500, www.elsevier.com/locate/foodchem.

Cilli, L. P., Contini, L. R. F., Sinnecker, P., Lopes, P. S., Andreo, M. A., Neiva, C. R. P., Nascimento, M. S., Yoshida, C. M. P., & Venturini, A. C. (2020). Effects of grape pomace flour on quality parameters of salmon burger. *Journal of Food Processing and Preservation*, *44*(2). Available from https://doi.org/10.1111/jfpp.14329, http://onlinelibrary.wiley.com/journal/10.1111/(ISSN)1745-4549.

Das, A. K., Nanda, P. K., Madane, P., Biswas, S., Das, A., Zhang, W., & Lorenzo, J. M. (2020). A comprehensive review on antioxidant dietary fibre enriched meat-based functional foods. *Trends in Food Science and Technology*, *99*, 323–336, India, Elsevier Ltd. Available from http://www.elsevier.com/wps/find/journaldescription.cws_home/601278/description#description, 10.1016/j.tifs.2020.03.010.

Das, A. K., Nanda, P. K., Chowdhury, N. R., Dandapat, P., Gagaoua, M., Chauhan, P., Pateiro, M., & Lorenzo, J. M. (2021). Application of pomegranate by-products in muscle foods: Oxidative indices, colour stability, shelf life and health benefits. *Molecules (Basel, Switzerland)*, *26*(2). Available from https://doi.org/10.3390/MOLECULES26020467, https://www.mdpi.com/1420-3049/26/2/467/pdf.

Datta, K. S., Rao, S. C., Santra, T. K., Mandal, T. K., & Adhya. (2011). Greenhouse gas emissions from rice based cropping systems: Economic and technologic challenges and opportunities. *Mitigation and Adaptation Strategies for Global Change*, *16*(5), 597–615. Available from https://doi.org/10.1007/s11027-011-9284-z.

Donini, L. M., & Berry, E. M. (2023). Improving adherence to the Mediterranean Diet through a bio-psycho social and sociotype approach. *Frontiers in Nutrition*, *10*. Available from https://doi.org/10.3389/fnut.2023.1232078, journal.frontiersin.org/journal/nutrition.

Drabińska, N., Nogueira, M., & Szmatowicz, B. (2022). Valorisation of broccoli by-products: Technological, sensory and flavour properties of durum pasta fortified with broccoli leaf powder. *Molecules (Basel, Switzerland)*, *27*(15), 4672. Available from https://doi.org/10.3390/molecules27154672.

EAT–Lancet Commission 2.0: securing a just transition to healthy, environmentally sustainable diets for all, The Lancet 402 (2023), 352, 2023.

Ebitu, L., Avery, H., Mourad, K. A., & Enyetu, J. (2021). Citizen science for sustainable agriculture – A systematic literature review. *Land use Policy*, *103*, 105326. Available from https://doi.org/10.1016/j.landusepol.2021.105326.

Ebrahimi, P., Shokramraji, Z., Tavakkoli, S., Mihaylova, D., & Lante, A. (2023). Chlorophylls as natural bioactive compounds existing in food by-products: A critical review. *Plants*, *12*(7), 1533. Available from https://doi.org/10.3390/plants12071533.

Elsayed, D. A., Yousof, S. M., Khalil, I. A., Kolieb, E., & Zayed, M. A. (2022). *Citrullus Lanatus (Watermelon) Wastes: Maximizing the Benefits and Saving the Environment Mediterranean Fruits Bio-wastes: Chemistry, Functionality and Technological Applications* (pp. 647–665). Egypt: Springer International Publishing. Available from https://doi.org/10.1007/978-3-030-84436-3, https://doi.org/10.1007/978-3-030-84436-3_28.

Espadas-Aldana, G., Guaygua-Amaguaña, P., Vialle, C., Belaud, J.-P., Evon, P., & Sablayrolles, C. (2021). Life cycle assessment of olive pomace as a reinforcement in polypropylene and polyethylene biocomposite materials: A new perspective for the valorization of this agricultural by-product. *Coatings*, *11*(5), 525. Available from https://doi.org/10.3390/coatings11050525.

FAO, High Level Expert Forum - How to Feed the World in 2050 (2009).

Fathy, H. M., Abd El-Maksoud, A. A., Cheng, W., & Elshaghabee, F. M. F. (2022). Value-added utilization of citrus peels in improving functional properties and probiotic viability of acidophilus-bifidus-thermophilus (ABT)-type synbiotic yoghurt during cold storage. *Foods*, *11*(17). Available from https://doi.org/10.3390/foods11172677, www.mdpi.com/journal/foods.

Fernandez-Pan, F. C., Ibañez, P., Virseda, I., Arozarena, M. J., & Beriain. (2023). Stabilization and valorization of tomato byproduct: A case study for the bakery industry. *Journal of Food Science*, *88*(11), 4483–4494. Available from https://doi.org/10.1111/1750-3841.16777, http://onlinelibrary.wiley.com/journal/10.1111/(ISSN)1750-3841.

Ferreira, S. M., & Santos, L. (2023). Incorporation of phenolic extracts from different by-products in yoghurts to create fortified and sustainable foods. *Food Bioscience*, *51*, 102293. Available from https://doi.org/10.1016/j.fbio.2022.102293.

Ferreira, S. M., Gomes, S. M., & Santos, L. (2023). *The chemistry behind biological properties of agro-industrial portuguese by-products. Waste and biomass valorization*. Springer Science and Business Media B.V. Available from https://www.springer.com/journal/12649, https://doi.org/10.1007/s12649-023-02366-3.

Fess, T., & Benedito, V. (2018). Organic versus conventional cropping sustainability: A comparative system analysis. *Sustainability*, *10*(1), 272. Available from https://doi.org/10.3390/su10010272.

Flores-Contreras, E. A., González-González, R. B., Pizaña-Aranda, J. J. P., Parra-Arroyo, L., Rodríguez-Aguayo, A. A., Iñiguez-Moreno, M., et al. (2024). *Agricultural waste as a sustainable source for nanoparticle synthesis and their antimicrobial properties for food preservation*, *6*, doi.org/10.3389/fnano.2024.1346069.

Fontana., & Recovery. (2023). Characterization, functionality and applications of bioactive compounds from food-plant products and their by-products. *Plants*, *12*, 2023.

Fotschki, J., Ogrodowczyk, A. M., Wróblewska, B., & Juśkiewicz, J. (2023). Side streams of vegetable processing and its bioactive compounds support microbiota, intestine milieu, and immune system. *Molecules (Basel, Switzerland)*, *28*(11), 4340. Available from https://doi.org/10.3390/molecules28114340.

Franchini, C., Bartolotto, F., Scazzina, C. L., Carpenter, W., & Slusser. (2023). Increasing the consumption of environmentally friendly foods in a university dining hall using menu item placement. *Nutrients, 15*(18). Available from https://doi.org/10.3390/nu15183873, http://www.mdpi.com/journal/nutrients/.

Frosi, I., Balduzzi, A., Moretto, G., Colombo, R., & Papetti, A. (2023). Towards valorization of food-waste-derived pectin: recent advances on their characterization and application. *Molecules (Basel, Switzerland), 28*(17), 6390. Available from https://doi.org/10.3390/molecules28176390.

Fırat, E., Koca, N., & Kaymak-Ertekin, F. (2023). Extraction of pectin from watermelon and pomegranate peels with different methods and its application in ice cream as an emulsifier. *Journal of Food Science, 88*(11), 4353–4374. Available from https://doi.org/10.1111/1750-3841.16752, http://onlinelibrary.wiley.com/journal/10.1111/(ISSN)1750-3841.

Gaikwad, P., Devendrachari, M. C., Thimmappa, R., Paswan, B., Raja Kottaichamy, A., Makri Nimbegondi Kotresh, H., & Thotiyl, M. O. (2015). Galvanic cell type sensor for soil moisture analysis. *Analytical Chemistry, 87*(14), 7439–7445. Available from https://doi.org/10.1021/acs.analchem.5b01653, http://pubs.acs.org/journal/ancham.

Galanakis, C. M. (2024). The future of food. *Foods, 13*, 2024.

Gattinger, A., Muller, M., Haeni, C., Skinner, A., Fliessbach, N., Buchmann, P., Mäder, M., Stolze, P., Smith, N. E. H., Scialabba, U., & Niggli. (2012). Enhanced top soil carbon stocks under organic farming. *Proceedings of the National Academy of Sciences of the United States of America, 109*(44), 18226–18231. Available from https://doi.org/10.1073/pnas.1209429109Switzerland, http://www.pnas.org/content/109/44/18226.full.pdf + html.

Gautam, K., Vishvakarma, R., Sharma, P., Singh, A., Kumar Gaur, V., Varjani, S., & Kumar Srivastava, J. (2022). Production of biopolymers from food waste: Constrains and perspectives. *Bioresource Technology, 361*, 127650. Available from https://doi.org/10.1016/j.biortech.2022.127650.

Geissen, V., Silva, V., Lwanga, E. H., Beriot, N., Oostindie, K., Bin, Z., Pyne, E., Busink, S., Zomer, P., Mol, H., & Ritsema, C. J. (2021). Cocktails of pesticide residues in conventional and organic farming systems in Europe – Legacy of the past and turning point for the future. *Environmental Pollution, 278*, 116827. Available from https://doi.org/10.1016/j.envpol.2021.116827.

Goap, D., Sharma, A. K., Shukla, C., & Rama Krishna. (2018). *An IoT based smart irrigation management system using Machine learning and open source technologies, . Computers and Electronics in Agriculture* (155, pp. 41–49). India: Elsevier B.V. Available from www.elsevier.com/inca/publications/store/5/0/3/3/0/4, https://doi.org/10.1016/j.compag.2018.09.040.

Granado-Lorencio, F., & Hernández-Alvarez, E. (2016). Functional foods and health effects: A nutritional biochemistry perspective. *Current Medicinal Chemistry, 23*(26), 2929–2957. Available from https://doi.org/10.2174/0929867323666160615105746.

Gubitosa, J., Rizzi, V., Marasciulo, C., Maggi, F., Caprioli, G., Mustafa, A. M., Fini, P., De Vietro, N., Aresta, A. M., & Cosma, P. (2023). Realizing eco-friendly water-resistant sodium-alginate-based films blended with a polyphenolic aqueous extract from grape pomace waste for potential food packaging applications. *International Journal of Molecular Sciences, 24*(14), 11462. Available from https://doi.org/10.3390/ijms241411462.

Günal-Köroğlu, E., Erskine, G., Ozkan, E., Capanoglu, T., & Esatbeyoglu. (2023). *Applications and safety aspects of bioactives obtained from by-products/wastes, . Advances in Food and Nutrition Research* (107, pp. 213–261). Turkey: Academic Press Inc. Available from http://www.elsevier.com/wps/find/bookdescription.cws_home/704624/description#description, https://doi.org/10.1016/bs.afnr.2023.07.002.

Hammed, T. B., Oloruntoba, E. O., & Ana, G. R. E. E. (2019). Enhancing growth and yield of crops with nutrient-enriched organic fertilizer at wet and dry seasons in ensuring climate-smart agriculture. *International Journal of Recycling of Organic Waste in Agriculture, 8*, 81–92, Nigeria, Springer. Available from www.springer.com/environment/pollution + and + remediation/journal/40093. 10.1007/s40093-019-0274-6.

Hamrani, A., Akbarzadeh, A., & Madramootoo, C. A. (2020). Machine learning for predicting greenhouse gas emissions from agricultural soils. *Science of The Total Environment, 741*, 140338. Available from https://doi.org/10.1016/j.scitotenv.2020.140338.

Hidalgo, A., Brandolini, J., Čanadanović-Brunet, G., Ćetković, V., & Tumbas Šaponjac. (2018). Microencapsulates and extracts from red beetroot pomace modify antioxidant capacity, heat damage and colour of pseudocereals-enriched einkorn water biscuits. *Food Chemistry, 268*, 40–48. Available from ItalyElsevier Ltd.www.elsevier.com/locate/foodchem10.1016/j.foodchem.2018.06.062.

Huang, I. Y., Manning, L., James, K. L., Grigoriadis, V., Millington, A., Wood, V., & Ward, S. (2021). Food waste management: A review of retailers' business practices and their implications for sustainable value. *Journal of Cleaner Production* (285). United Kingdom: Elsevier Ltd. Available from https://www.journals.elsevier.com/journal-of-cleaner-production, https://doi.org/10.1016/j.jclepro.2020.125484.

Ighalo, J. O. (2024). Biowastes and derived green sorbents for water decontamination: Insights on thermochemical conversion strategies. *Current Opinion in Green and Sustainable Chemistry, 45*, 100880. Available from https://doi.org/10.1016/j.cogsc.2024.100880.

Imeneo, V., De Bruno, A., Piscopo, A., Romeo, R., & Poiana, M. (2022). Valorization of 'Rossa di Tropea' onion waste through green recovery techniques of antioxidant compounds. *Sustainability, 14*(8), 4387. Available from https://doi.org/10.3390/su14084387.

Inthalaeng, N., Gao, Y., Remón, J., Dugmore, T. I. J., Ozel, M. Z., Sulaeman, A., & Matharu, A. S. (2023). Ginger waste as a potential feedstock for a zero-waste ginger biorefinery: a review. *RSC Sustainability, 1*(2), 213–223. Available from https://doi.org/10.1039/d2su00099g.

Jayasinghe, S. L., Thomas, D. T., Anderson, J. P., Chen, C., & Macdonald, B. C. T. (2023). Global application of regenerative agriculture: A review of definitions and assessment approaches. *Sustainability, 15*(22), 15941. Available from https://doi.org/10.3390/su152215941.

Jianbo, Z., Junfang, X., Yong, Z., & Shun, Z. (2014). Design and experimental study of the control system for precision seed-metering device. *International Journal of Agricultural and Biological Engineering, 7*(3). Available from https://doi.org/10.3965/j.ijabe.20140703.002.

Jin, X., Li, Q., Zhao, K., Zhao, B., He, Z., & Qiu, Z. (2019). Development and test of an electric precision seeder for small-size vegetable seeds. *International Journal of Agricultural and Biological Engineering, 12*(2), 75–81, https://doi.org/10.25165/j.ijabe.20191202.4618.

Joshi, D., Nainabasti, A., Bhandari, R., Awasthi, P., Banjade, D., Malla, S., & Subedi, B. (2022). A review on soilless cultivation: The hope of urban agriculture. *Archives of Agriculture and Environmental Science, 7*(3), 473–481. Available from https://doi.org/10.26832/24566632.2022.0703022.

Jusoh, M. F., Muttalib, M. F. A., Krishnan, K. T., & Katimon, A. (2021). An overview of the internet of things (IoT) and irrigation approach through bibliometric analysis. *IOP Conference Series: Earth and Environmental Science*, *756*(1), 012041. Available from https://doi.org/10.1088/1755-1315/756/1/012041.

Kabir, M. R., Hasan, S. M. K., Islam, M. R., & Ahmed, M. (2024). Development of functional noodles by encapsulating mango peel powder as a source of bioactive compounds. *Heliyon*, *10*(1). Available from https://doi.org/10.1016/j.heliyon.2024.e24061, https://www.sciencedirect.com/science/journal/24058440.

Karimi Sani, M., Masoudpour-Behabadi, M., Alizadeh Sani, H., Motalebinejad, A. S. M., Juma, A., Asdagh, H., Eghbaljoo, S. M., Khodaei, J. W., Rhim, F., & Mohammadi. (2023). *Value-added utilization of fruit and vegetable processing by-products for the manufacture of biodegradable food packaging films*, . *Food Chemistry* (405). Iran: Elsevier Ltd. Available from www.elsevier.com/locate/foodchem, https://doi.org/10.1016/j.foodchem.2022.134964.

Kauser, S., Murtaza, M. A., Hussain, A., Imran, M., Kabir, K., Najam, A., An, Q. U., Akram, S., Fatima, H., Batool, S. A., Shehzad, A., & Yaqub, S. (2024). Apple pomace, a bioresource of functional and nutritional components with potential of utilization in different food formulations: A review. *Food Chemistry Advances*, *4*, 100598. Available from https://doi.org/10.1016/j.focha.2023.100598.

Kennas, H., Amellal-Chibane, F., Kessal, F., & Halladj. (2020). Effect of pomegranate peel and honey fortification on physicochemical, physical, microbiological and antioxidant properties of yoghurt powder. *Journal of the Saudi Society of Agricultural Sciences*, *19*(1), 99–108. Available from https://doi.org/10.1016/j.jssas.2018.07.001, https://www.journals.elsevier.com/journal-of-the-saudi-society-of-agricultural-sciences/.

Khan, Z. S., Amir, S., Cvetnić, S., Tušek, J., Benković, Jurina, M. et al., Sustainable Isolation of Bioactive Compounds and Proteins from Plant-Based Food (and Byproducts). Plants (n.d.).

Khatri-Chhetri, A., Pant, P. K., Aggarwal, V. V., Vasireddy, A., & Yadav. (2019). Stakeholders prioritization of climate-smart agriculture interventions: Evaluation of a framework. *Agricultural Systems*, *174*, 23–31. Available from IndiaElsevier Ltd.www.elsevier.com/inca/publications/store/4/0/5/8/5/1 10.1016/j.agsy.2019.03.002.

Kirkegaard Nielsen, S., Munkholm, L. J., Lamandé, M., Nørremark, M., Edwards, G. T. C., & Green, O. (2018). Seed drill depth control system for precision seeding. *Computers and Electronics in Agriculture*, *144*, 174–180. Available from DenmarkElsevier B.V.www.elsevier.com/inca/publications/store/5/0/3/3/0/4 10.1016/j.compag.2017.12.008.

Kokkinomagoulos., & Kandylis, P. (2023). Grape pomace, an undervalued by-product: industrial reutilization within a circular economy vision. *Reviews in Environmental Science and Biotechnology*, *22*(3), 739–773. Available from https://doi.org/10.1007/s11157-023-09665-0, https://www.springer.com/journal/11157.

Krupa-Kozak, U., Drabińska, N., Rosell, C. M., Fadda, C., Anders, A., Jeliński, T., & Ostaszyk, A. (2019). Broccoli leaf powder as an attractive by-product ingredient: effect on batter behaviour, technological properties and sensory quality of gluten-free mini sponge cake. *International Journal of Food Science and Technology*, *54*(4), 1121–1129. Available from https://doi.org/10.1111/ijfs.13972, http://onlinelibrary.wiley.com/journal/10.1111/(ISSN)1365-2621.

Kuchtová, V., Kohajdová, Z., Karovičová, J., & Lauková, M. (2018). Physical, textural and sensory properties of cookies incorporated with grape skin and seed preparations. *Journal of Food and Nutrition Sciences*, *68*(4), 309–317. Available from https://doi.org/10.2478/pjfns-2018-0004, http://www.degruyter.com/view/j/pjfns.2012.62.issue-4/issue-files/pjfns.2012.62.issue-4.xml.

Kumar, S., Konwar, J., Purkayastha, M. D., Kalita, S., Mukherjee, A., & Dutta, J. (2023). Current progress in valorization of food processing waste and by-products for pectin extraction. *International Journal of Biological Macromolecules*, *239*, 124332. Available from https://doi.org/10.1016/j.ijbiomac.2023.124332.

Kučuk, N., Primožič, M., Kotnik, P., Knez, Ž., & Leitgeb, M. (2024). Mango peels as an industrial by-product: A sustainable source of compounds with antioxidant, enzymatic, and antimicrobial activity. *Foods*, *13*(4), 553. Available from https://doi.org/10.3390/foods13040553.

Le, T. D., Suttikhana, I., & Ashaolu, T. J. (2024). Exploring the potential applications of biopeptides from seaweeds, insects, and food wastes: Mechanisms, utilisation, and industry implications. *International Journal of Food Science and Technology*, *59*(3), 1260–1267. Available from https://doi.org/10.1111/ijfs.16920, http://onlinelibrary.wiley.com/journal/10.1111/(ISSN)1365-2621.

Lefèvre, C., Rekik, F., Alcantara, V., & Wiese, L. (2017). *Soil organic carbon: The hidden potential*. Food and Agriculture Organization of the United Nations.

Lesmana, Y. M., Vianney, Y. A., Goenawan, K., Natalie, J., Sukweenadhi, G., Buschle-Diller., Mukti, Y. P., Erawati, C. M., & Purwanto, M. G. M. (2022). Valorization of peel-based agro-waste flour for food products: A systematic review on proximate composition and functional properties. *ACS Food Science and Technology*, *2*(1), 3–20. Available from https://doi.org/10.1021/acsfoodscitech.1c00353, https://pubs.acs.org/page/afsthl/about.html.

Linares, M. L., & Rojas. (2022). Ultrasound-assisted extraction of natural pigments from food processing by-products: A review. *Frontiers in Nutrition*, *9*. Available fromPeruFrontiers Media S.A.journal.frontiersin.org/journal/nutrition10.3389/fnut.2022.891462.

Liu, Z., de Souza, T. S. P., Holland, B., Dunshea, F., Barrow, C., & Suleria, H. A. R. (2023). Valorization of food waste to produce value-added products based on its bioactive compounds. *Processes*, *11*(3). Available from https://doi.org/10.3390/pr11030840, http://www.mdpi.com/journal/processes.

Long, T. B., Blok, V., & Coninx, I. (2016). Barriers to the adoption and diffusion of technological innovations for climate-smart agriculture in Europe: Evidence from the Netherlands, France, Switzerland and Italy. *Journal of Cleaner Production*, *112*, 9–21. Available from https://doi.org/10.1016/j.jclepro.2015.06.044.

Lowenberg-DeBoer, J., Huang, I. Y., Grigoriadis, V., & Blackmore, S. (2020). Economics of robots and automation in field crop production. *Precision Agriculture*, *21*(2), 278–299. Available from https://doi.org/10.1007/s11119-019-09667-5, www.wkap.nl/journalhome.htm/1385-2256.

Magalhães, D., Vilas-Boas, A. A., Teixeira, P., & Pintado, M. (2023). Functional ingredients and additives from lemon by-products and their applications in food preservation: A review. *Foods, 12*(5). Available from https://doi.org/10.3390/foods12051095, www.mdpi.com/journal/foods.

Mahato, N., Sharma, K., Sinha, M., & Cho, M. H. (2018). Citrus waste derived nutra-/pharmaceuticals for health benefits: Current trends and future perspectives. *Journal of Functional Foods, 40*, 307–316. Available fromSouth KoreaElsevier Ltd.http://www.elsevier.com/wps/find/journaldescription.cws_home/717426/description#description10.1016/j.jff.2017.11.015.

Marcos, J., Carriço, R., Sousa, M. J., Palma, M. L., Pereira, P., Nunes, M. C., & Nicolai, M. (2023). Effect of Grape Pomace Flour in Savory Crackers: Technological, Nutritional and Sensory Properties. *Foods, 12*(7). Available from https://doi.org/10.3390/foods12071392, www.mdpi.com/journal/foods.

Mariño-Cortegoso, S., Stanzione, M., Andrade, M. A., Restuccia, C., Rodríguez-Bernaldo de Quirós, A., Buonocore, G. G., Barbosa, C. H., Vilarinho, F., Silva, A. S., Ramos, F., Khwaldia, K., Sendón, R., & Barbosa-Pereira, L. (2022). Development of active films utilizing antioxidant compounds obtained from tomato and lemon by-products for use in food packaging. *Food Control, 140*. Available fromSpainElsevier Ltd.https://www.journals.elsevier.com/food-control10.1016/j.foodcont.2022.109128.

McKinley, J. D., LaFrance, J. T., & Pede, V. O. (2021). Climate Change Adaptation Strategies Vary With Climatic Stress: Evidence From Three Regions of Vietnam. *Frontiers in Sustainable Food Systems* (5). Australia: Frontiers Media S.A. Available from www.frontiersin.org/journals/sustainable-food-systems#, https://doi.org/10.3389/fsufs.2021.762650.

Meier, J., Mauser, W., Hank, T., & Bach, H. (2020). Assessments on the impact of high-resolution-sensor pixel sizes for common agricultural policy and smart farming services in European regions. *Computers and Electronics in Agriculture, 169*, 105205. Available from https://doi.org/10.1016/j.compag.2019.105205.

Merrigan, K., Giraud, E. G., & Scialabba, N. E. H. (2022). *Grow Organic: the Climate, Health and Economic Case for Expanding Organic Agriculture*. Natural Resources Defence Council, Natural Resources Defence Council.

Messinese, E., Pitirollo, O., Grimaldi, M., Milanese, D., Sciancalepore, C., & Cavazza, A. (2024). By-Products as sustainable source of bioactive compounds for potential application in the field of food and new materials for packaging development. *Food and Bioprocess Technology, 17*(3), 606–627. Available from https://doi.org/10.1007/s11947-023-03158-2, https://www.springer.com/journal/11947.

Mikula, K., Izydorczyk, G., Skrzypczak, D., Mironiuk, M., Moustakas, K., Witek-Krowiak, A., & Chojnacka, K. (2020). Controlled release micronutrient fertilizers for precision agriculture – A review. *Science of The Total Environment, 712*, 136365. Available from https://doi.org/10.1016/j.scitotenv.2019.136365.

Miller, K. B., Eckberg, J. O., Decker, E. A., & Marinangeli, C. P. F. (2021). Role of food industry in promoting healthy and sustainable diets. *Nutrients, 13*(8). Available from https://doi.org/10.3390/nu13082740, https://www.mdpi.com/2072-6643/13/8/2740/pdf.

Minervini, F., Comitini, F., De Boni, A., Fiorino, G. M., Rodrigues, F., Tlais, A. Z. A., Carafa, I., & De Angelis, M. (2022). Sustainable and Health-Protecting Food Ingredients from Bioprocessed Food by-Products and Wastes. *Sustainability, 14*(22), 15283. Available from https://doi.org/10.3390/su142215283.

Mishra, Y. K., Mohanta, C. N., Reddy, S. D. M., Reddy, S. K., Mandal, R., Yadavalli, H., & Sarma. (2023). Valorization of agro-industrial biowaste to biomaterials: An innovative circular bioeconomy approach. *Circular Economy, 2*(3). Available from https://doi.org/10.1016/j.cec.2023.100050, www.sciencedirect.com/journal/circular-economy.

Molnar, D., Novotni, D., Kurek, M., Galić, K., Iveković, D., Bionda, H., & Ščetar, M. (2023). Characteristics of edible films enriched with fruit by-products and their application on cookies. *Food Hydrocolloids, 135*, 108191. Available from https://doi.org/10.1016/j.foodhyd.2022.108191.

Moradi, E., & Fathi, M. (2023). Production of cellulose nanocrystals from tomato pomace as a food waste and their application for stabilizing of Pickering emulsions. *Bioactive Carbohydrates and Dietary Fibre, 30*, 100378. Available from https://doi.org/10.1016/j.bcdf.2023.100378.

Morganti, P., Gao, X., Vukovic, N., Gagliardini, A., Lohani, A., & Morganti, G. (2022). Food loss and food waste for green cosmetics and medical devices for a cleaner planet. *Cosmetics, 9*(1), 19. Available from https://doi.org/10.3390/cosmetics9010019.

Moving forward on food loss and waste reduction. Rome: Food and Agriculture Organization of the United Nations (2019), 2019.

Murmu, K., Das, P., Sarkar, A., & Bandopadhyay, P. (2022). Organic agriculture: As a climate change adaptation and mitigation strategy. *Zeichen Journal, 8*(03).

Nakov, G., Trajkovska, B., Zlatev, Z., Jukić, M., & Lukinac, J. (2023). Quality characteristics of probiotic yoghurt enriched with honey and by-products left after the production of hemp oil by cold pressing the seeds of Cannabis sativa L. *Mljekarstvo, 73*(1), 3–11. Available from https://doi.org/10.15567/mljekarstvo.2023.0101, https://hrcak.srce.hr/file/416463.

Nakov, G., Trajkovska, B., Atanasova-Pancevska, N., Daniloski, D., Ivanova, N., Lučan Čolić, M., Jukić, M., & Lukinac, J. (2023). The Influence of the Addition of Hemp Press Cake Flour on the Properties of Bovine and Ovine Yoghurts. *Foods, 12*(5), 958. Available from https://doi.org/10.3390/foods12050958.

Nardella, S., Conte, A., & Del Nobile, M. A. (2022). State-of-art on the recycling of by-products from fruits and vegetables of Mediterranean countries to prolong food shelf life. *Foods, 11*(5), 665. Available from https://doi.org/10.3390/foods11050665.

Nartea, A., Fanesi, B., Pacetti, D., Lenti, L., Fiorini, D., Lucci, P., Frega, N. G., & Falcone, P. M. (2023). Cauliflower by-products as functional ingredient in bakery foods: Fortification of pizza with glucosinolates, carotenoids and phytosterols. *Current Research in Food Science, 6*, 100437. Available from https://doi.org/10.1016/j.crfs.2023.100437.

Nation's Business: A General Magazine for Businessmen, 1981.

Nayak., & Bhushan, B. (2019). An overview of the recent trends on the waste valorization techniques for food wastes. *Journal of Environmental Management, 233*, 352–370. Available from https://doi.org/10.1016/j.jenvman.2018.12.041, https://www.sciencedirect.com/science/journal/03014797.

Negro, V., Mancini, G., Ruggeri, B., & Fino, D. (2016). Citrus waste as feedstock for bio-based products recovery: Review on limonene case study and energy valorization. *Bioresource Technology*, *214*, 806–815. Available from https://doi.org/10.1016/j.biortech.2016.05.006.

Nuzzo, A., Scurria, P., Picone, A., & Guiducci, M. (2022). Pagliaro, Giuseppe, Pantaleo, L. Albanese, F. Meneguzzo, R. Ciriminna, A Gluten-Free Biscuit Fortified with Lemon IntegroPectin. *ChemistrySelect*, *7*(5). Available from https://doi.org/10.1002/slct.202104247, http://onlinelibrary.wiley.com/journal/10.1002/(ISSN)2365-6549.

Oluwole, O., Ibidapo, O., Arowosola, T., Raji, F., Zandonadi, R. P., Alasqah, I., Lho, L. H., Han, H., & Raposo, A. (2023). Sustainable transformation agenda for enhanced global food and nutrition security: a narrative review. *Frontiers in Nutrition*, *10*. Available from https://doi.org/10.3389/fnut.2023.1226538.

Ouatmani, T., Haddadi-Guemghar, H., Hadjal, S., Boulekbache-Makhlouf, L., & Madani, K. (2023). *Tomato by-products: A potentially promising bioresource for the recovery of bioactive compounds and nutraceuticals Nutraceutics from Agri-Food By-Products* (pp. 137–171). Wiley. Available from https://www.wiley-vch.de/de?option = com_eshop&view = product&isbn = 9781394174447, https://doi.org/10.1002/9781394174867.ch5.

Pachauri, R. K., & Mayer, l (2014). Intergovernmental panel on climate change. *Climate change 2014: synthesis report.*

Pai, S., Hebbar, A., & Selvaraj, S. (2022). A critical look at challenges and future scopes of bioactive compounds and their incorporations in the food, energy, and pharmaceutical sector. *Environmental Science and Pollution Research*, *29*(24), 35518–35541. Available from https://doi.org/10.1007/s11356-022-19423-4, https://link.springer.com/journal/11356.

Pandiselvi, T., Jeyajothi, R., & Kandeshwari, M. (2017). Organic nutrient management a way to improve soil fertility and Sustainable Agriculture - A review. *International Journal of Advanced Life Sciences*, *10*(02), 175–181. Available from https://doi.org/10.26627/IJALS/2017/10.02.0005.

Papadopoulos, N. R. A., Bird, A. P., Whitmore, S. J., & Mooney. (2014). Does organic management lead to enhanced soil physical quality? *Geoderma*, *213*, 435–443. Available from https://doi.org/10.1016/j.geoderma.2013.08.033.

Pattillo, D. A. An Overview of Aquaponic Systems: Hydroponic Components. Iowa State University Extension and Outreach,Technical Bulletin #123. (2017).

Peng, W., Dernini, S., & Berry, E. M. (2018). Coping with food insecurity using the sociotype ecological framework. *Frontiers in Nutrition*, *5*. Available fromChinaFrontiers Media S.A.journal.frontiersin.org/journal/nutrition10.3389/fnut.2018.00107.

Piccolo, A., Short, C., Sommerville, C. Aquaponics – a smart fish-based solution to growing food using limited resources and little water. Smartfish Programme, Programme For The Implementation Of A Regional Fisheries Strategy For The Eastern And Southern Africa - Indian Ocean Region. (2014).

Pinto, T., Pinto, A., & Vilela, A. (2023). Edible coatings and films for preparation of grapevine by-product infusions and in freshly processed products. *Coatings*, *13*(8). Available from https://doi.org/10.3390/coatings13081350, www.mdpi.com/journal/coatings.

Popescu, L., Ceşco, T., Gurev, A., Ghendov-Mosanu, A., Sturza, R., & Tarna. (2022). Impact of Apple Pomace Powder on the Bioactivity, and the Sensory and Textural Characteristics of Yogurt. *Foods. Foods.*, *11*(22). Available from https://doi.org/10.3390/foods11223565.

Purakayastha, T. J., Bera, T., Bhaduri, D., Sarkar, B., Mandal, S., Wade, P., Kumari, S., Biswas, S., Menon, M., Pathak, H., & Tsang, D. C. W. (2019). *A review on biochar modulated soil condition improvements and nutrient dynamics concerning crop yields: Pathways to climate change mitigation and global food security*, . *Chemosphere* (227, pp. 345–365). India: Elsevier Ltd. Available from www.elsevier.com/locate/chemosphere, https://doi.org/10.1016/j.chemosphere.2019.03.170.

Qu, B., Xiao, Z., Upadhyay, A., & Luo, Y. (2024). Perspectives on sustainable food production system: Characteristics and green technologies. *Journal of Agriculture and Food Research*, *15*, 100988. Available from https://doi.org/10.1016/j.jafr.2024.100988.

Rakocy, J. E. (1994). Caribbean Food Crops Society 30th Annual Meeting, St. Thomas, U.S. Virgin Islands 258746, July 31-August 5, 1994, St. Thomas, U.S. Virgin Islands 258746, Aquaponics: The Integration Of Fish And Vegetable Culture In Recirculating Systems. Available from https://doi.org/10.22004/ag.econ.258746.

Rama Rao, C. A., Raju, B. K., Subba Rao, A. V. M., Rao, K. V., Rao, V. U. M., Ramachandran, K., Ramachandran, B., Sikka, A. K. ATLAS on Vulnerability of Indian Agriculture to Climate Change. Central Research Institute for Dryland Agriculture, Hyderabad P 116., Central Research Institute for Dryland Agriculture, Hyderabad P 116, (2013). Available from: http://ISBN:78-93-80883-22-9.

Ranasinghe, M., Sivapragasam, N., Mostafa, H., Airouyuwa, J. O., Manikas, I., Sundarakani, B., Maqsood, S., & Stathopoulos, C. (2024). Valorizing date seeds in biscuits: A novel approach to incorporate bioactive components extracted from date seeds using microwave-assisted extraction. *Resources, Environment and Sustainability*, *15*, 100147. Available from https://doi.org/10.1016/j.resenv.2023.100147.

Rangaraj, V. M., Rambabu, K., Banat, F., & Mittal, V. (2021). Effect of date fruit waste extract as an antioxidant additive on the properties of active gelatin films. *Food Chemistry*, *355*, 129631. Available from https://doi.org/10.1016/j.foodchem.2021.129631.

Rashwan, A. K., Bai, H., Osman, A. I., Eltohamy, K. M., Chen, Z., Younis, H. A., Al-Fatesh, A., Rooney, D. W., & Yap, P. S. (2023). Recycling food and agriculture by-products to mitigate climate change: a review. *Environmental Chemistry Letters*, *21*(6), 3351–3375. Available from https://doi.org/10.1007/s10311-023-01639-6, https://www.springer.com/journal/10311.

Rezagholizade-shirvan, S., Shokri, S. M., Dadpour, M. R., & Amiryousefi. (2023). Evaluation of physicochemical, antioxidant, antibacterial activity, and sensory properties of watermelon rind candy. *Heliyon*, *9*(6). Available from https://doi.org/10.1016/j.heliyon.2023.e17300, http://www.journals.elsevier.com/heliyon/.

Rodrigues Machado, T., Atatoprak, J., Santos, E. M. C., Alexandre, M. E., Pintado, J. A. P., Paiva, J., & Nunes. (2023). Potentialities of the extraction technologies and use of bioactive compounds from winery by-products: A review from a circular bioeconomy perspective. *Applied Sciences (Switzerland)*, *13*(13). Available from https://doi.org/10.3390/app13137754, www.mdpi.com/journal/applsci/.

Rojo-Poveda, L., Barbosa-Pereira, G., Zeppa, C., & Stévigny. (2020). Cocoa bean shell—A by-product with nutritional properties and biofunctional potential. *Nutrients*, *12*(4), 2020.

Romano, E., Bisaglia, C., Calcante, A., Oberti, R., Zani, A., Vinnikov, D., Marconi, A., Vitale, E., Bracci, M., & Rapisarda, V. (2020). Assessment of comfort variation among different types of driving agricultural tractors: Traditional, satellite-assisted and semi-automatic. *International Journal of Environmental Research and Public Health*, *17*(23), 8836. Available from https://doi.org/10.3390/ijerph17238836.

Roy, S., Sarkar, T., Upadhye, V. J., & Chakraborty, R. (2023). *Comprehensive review on fruit seeds: Nutritional, phytochemical, nanotechnology, toxicity, food biochemistry, and biotechnology perspective. Applied Biochemistry and Biotechnology*. India: Springer. Available from https://www.springer.com/journal/12010, https://doi.org/10.1007/s12010-023-04674-9.

Šafranko, S., Šubarić, D., Jerković, I., & Jokić, S. (2023). Citrus by-products as a valuable source of biologically active compounds with promising pharmaceutical, biological and biomedical potential. *Pharmaceuticals*, *16*(8), 1081. Available from https://doi.org/10.3390/ph16081081.

Sailaja, P.L. Manohari, Organic Farming for Sustainable Agriculture. In: A. Sailaja, PL. Manohari, ISBN: 978-93-91668-55-6. National Institute of Agricultural Extension Management (MANAGE), Rajendranagar, Hyderabad – 500 030, Telangana State, India., National Institute of Agricultural Extension Management (MANAGE), Rajendranagar, Hyderabad – 500 030, Telangana State, India (2021).

Salgado-Ramos, M., Martí-Quijal, F. J., Huertas-Alonso, A. J., Sánchez-Verdú, M. P., Moreno, A., & Barba, F. J. (2023). Winemaking-derived by-products: In-depth characterization and sustainable, advanced pulsed electric field (PEF) processing to a zero-waste-based approach. *Journal of Environmental Chemical Engineering*, *11*(5). Available from https://doi.org/10.1016/j.jece.2023.110535, http://www.journals.elsevier.com/journal-of-environmental-chemical-engineering/.

Salimi, A., Khodaiyan, F., Askari, G., & Hosseini, S. S. (2024). A zero-waste approach towards a sustainable waste management of apple: Extraction of value-added products and their application as edible coating. *Food Hydrocolloids*, *147*, 109304. Available from https://doi.org/10.1016/j.foodhyd.2023.109304.

Sandoval-Contreras, T., González Chávez, F., Poonia, A., Iñiguez-Moreno, M., & Aguirre-Güitrón, L. (2023). Avocado waste biorefinery: Towards sustainable development. *Recycling*, *8*(5). Available from https://doi.org/10.3390/recycling8050081, www.mdpi.com/journal/recycling.

dos Santos Lima, A., Maltarollo, V. G., Araújo Vieira do Carmo, M., Cezar Pinheiro, L., Mendanha Cruz, T., Augusto Ribeiro de Barros, F., Pap, N., Granato, D., & Azevedo, L. (2024). Blackcurrant press cake by-product: Increased chemical bioaccessibility and reduced antioxidant protection after in vitro simulation of gastrointestinal digestion. *Food Research International*, *182*, 114099. Available from https://doi.org/10.1016/j.foodres.2024.114099.

Sar, T., Kiraz, P., Braho, V., Harirchi, S., & Akbas, M. Y. (2023). Novel Perspectives on Food-Based Natural Antimicrobials: A Review of Recent Findings Published since 2020. *Microorganisms*, *11*(9). Available from https://doi.org/10.3390/microorganisms11092234, www.mdpi.com/journal/microorganisms.

Sarabandi, K., Mohammadi, M., Akbarbaglu, Z., Ghorbani, M., Najafi, S., Safaeian Laein, S., & Jafari, S. M. (2023). Technological, nutritional, and biological properties of apricot kernel protein hydrolyzates affected by various commercial proteases. *Food Science and Nutrition*, *11*(9), 5078–5090. Available from https://doi.org/10.1002/fsn3.3467, onlinelibrary.wiley.com/journal/10.1002/%28ISSN%292048-7177.

Satari, K., & Karimi. (2018). Citrus processing wastes: Environmental impacts, recent advances, and future perspectives in total valorization. *Resources, Conservation and Recycling*, *129*, 153–167. Available from IranElsevier B.V.www.elsevier.com/locate/resconrec10.1016/j.resconrec.2017.10.032.

Schlamovitz, J. L., & Becker, P. (2021). Differentiated vulnerabilities and capacities for adaptation to water shortage in Gaborone, Botswana. *International Journal of Water Resources Development*, *37*(2), 278–299. Available from https://doi.org/10.1080/07900627.2020.1756752.

Šeremet, D., Durgo, K., Komljenović, A., Antolić, M., Mandura Jarić, A., Huđek Turković, A., Komes, D., & Šantek, B. (2022). Red beetroot and banana peels as value-added ingredients: Assessment of biological activity and preparation of functional edible films. *Polymers*, *14*(21), 4724. Available from https://doi.org/10.3390/polym14214724.

Seufert, V., Ramankutty, N., & Mayerhofer, T. (2017). What is this thing called organic? – How organic farming is codified in regulations. *Food Policy*, *68*, 10–20. Available from CanadaElsevier Ltd.http://www.elsevier.com/inca/publications/store/3/0/4/1/9/index.htt10.1016/j.foodpol.2016.12.009.

Shakoor, A., Shakoor, S., Rehman, A., Ashraf, F., Abdullah, M., Shahzad, S. M., Farooq, T. H., Ashraf, M., Manzoor, M. A., Altaf, M. M., & Altaf, M. A. (2021). Effect of animal manure, crop type, climate zone, and soil attributes on greenhouse gas emissions from agricultural soils—A global meta-analysis. *Journal of Cleaner Production*, *278*, 124019. Available from https://doi.org/10.1016/j.jclepro.2020.124019.

Sheikh, M. A., Saini, C. S., & Sharma, H. K. (2023). Harnessing plum (*Prunus domestica* L.) processing wastes for the fabrication of bio-composite edible films: An attempt towards a food circular bioeconomy. *Food Hydrocolloids*, *142*. Available fromIndiaElsevier B.V.https://www.journals.elsevier.com/food-hydrocolloids10.1016/j.foodhyd.2023.108790.

Shi, J., Wu, X., Zhang, M., Wang, X., Zuo, Q., Wu, X., Zhang, H., & Ben-Gal, A. (2021). Numerically scheduling plant water deficit index-based smart irrigation to optimize crop yield and water use efficiency. *Agricultural Water Management*, *248*, 106774. Available from https://doi.org/10.1016/j.agwat.2021.106774.

Siddiqui, S. A., Lakshmikanth, D., Pradhan, C., Farajinejad, Z., Castro-Muñoz, R., & Sasidharan, A. (2023). Implementing fermentation technology for comprehensive valorisation of seafood processing by-products: A critical review on recovering valuable nutrients and enhancing utilisation. *Critical Reviews in Food Science and Nutrition*, 1–28. Available from https://doi.org/10.1080/10408398.2023.2286623.

Singh, B., Singh, J. P., Kaur, A., & Singh, N. (2020). Phenolic composition, antioxidant potential and health benefits of citrus peel. *Food Research International*, *132*, 109114, https://doi.org/10.1016/j.foodres.2020.109114.

Siol, M., & Sadowska, A. (2023). Chemical composition, physicochemical and bioactive properties of avocado (*Persea americana*) seed and its potential use in functional food design. *Agriculture*, *13*(2), 316. Available from https://doi.org/10.3390/agriculture13020316.

Smith-Spangler, M. L., Brandeau, G. E., Hunter, J. C., Bavinger, M., Pearson, P. J., Eschbach, V., Sundaram, H., Liu, P., Schirmer, C., Stave, I., Olkin, D. M., & Bravata. (2012). Are organic foods safer or healthier than conventional alternatives?: A systematic review. *Annals of Internal Medicine, 157*(5), 348–366. Available from https://doi.org/10.7326/0003-4819-157-5-201209040-00007, http://annals.org/data/Journals/AIM/24808/0000605-201209040-00007.pdf.

Smolka, M., Puchberger-Enengl, D., Bipoun, M., Klasa, A., Kiczkajlo, M., Śmiechowski, W., Sowiński, P., Krutzler, C., Keplinger, F., & Vellekoop, M. J. (2017). A mobile lab-on-a-chip device for on-site soil nutrient analysis. *Precision Agriculture, 18*(2), 152–168. Available from https://doi.org/10.1007/s11119-016-9452-y, www.wkap.nl/journalhome.htm/1385-2256.

Song, C., Zhou, Z., Zang, Y., Zhao, L., Yang, W., Luo, X., Jiang, R., Ming, R., Zang, Y., Zi, L., & Zhu, Q. (2021). Variable-rate control system for UAV-based granular fertilizer spreader. *Computers and Electronics in Agriculture, 180*, 105832. Available from https://doi.org/10.1016/j.compag.2020.105832.

Srivastava, V., Singh, S., & Das, D. (2023). Rice husk fiber-reinforced starch antimicrobial biocomposite film for active food packaging. *Journal of Cleaner Production, 421*, 138525. Available from https://doi.org/10.1016/j.jclepro.2023.138525.

Subhash, J., Bamigbade, B., Ramadi, G., Kamal-Eldin, B., Gan, A., Y, R., Ranadheera, S., et al. (2024). Characterizing date seed polysaccharides: A comprehensive study on extraction, biological activities, prebiotic potential, gut microbiota modulation, and rheology using microwave-assisted deep eutectic solvent. *Food Chemistry, 444*, 2024.

Sultanova, M., Dalabayev, A., Saduakas, A., Nurysh, A., Akzhanov, N., & Yakiyayeva, M. (2023). The potential of non-traditional walnut shells waste for the production of antioxidant reach extracts intended for the food industry. *Potravinarstvo Slovak Journal of Food Sciences, 17*, 391–404. Available from https://doi.org/10.5219/1862.

Sánchez-Bravo, P., Abellán, Á., Zapata, P. J., García-Viguera, C., Domínguez-Perles, R., & Giménez, M. J. (2023). Broccoli products supplemented beers provide a sustainable source of dietary sulforaphane. *Food Bioscience, 51*, 102259. Available from https://doi.org/10.1016/j.fbio.2022.102259.

Teshome, T. A., Teka, R., Nandasiri, J. R., Rout, D. V., Harouna, T., Astatkie, M. M., & Urugo. (2023). Fruit By-Products and Their Industrial Applications for Nutritional Benefits and Health Promotion: A Comprehensive Review. *Sustainability (Switzerland), 15*(10). Available from https://doi.org/10.3390/su15107840, http://www.mdpi.com/journal/sustainability/.

Thakur, M., Prieto, M. A., & Huang, H. (2023). Editorial: Agri-food innovations in the quest for food and environmental security. *Frontiers in Nutrition, 10*. Available fromIndiaFrontiers Media SAjournal.frontiersin.org/journal/nutrition10.3389/fnut.2023.1304246.

Thakur, R., Santhosh, R., Kumar, Y., Suryavanshi, V. R., Singhi, H., Madhubabu, D., Wickramarachchi, S., Pal, K., & Sarkar, P. (2023). Characteristics and application of animal byproduct-based films and coatings in the packaging of food products. *Trends in Food Science & Technology, 140*, 104143. Available from https://doi.org/10.1016/j.tifs.2023.104143.

Thornton, P. K., Whitbread, A., Baedeker, T., Cairns, J., Claessens, L., Baethgen, W., Bunn, C., Friedmann, M., Giller, K. E., Herrero, M., Howden, M., Kilcline, K., Nangia, V., Ramirez-Villegas, J., Kumar, S., West, P. C., & Keating, B. (2018). *A framework for priority-setting in climate smart agriculture research, . Agricultural Systems* (167, pp. 161–175). Kenya: Elsevier Ltd. Available from www.elsevier.com/inca/publications/store/4/0/5/8/5/1, https://doi.org/10.1016/j.agsy.2018.09.009.

Times of crisis, times of change: Science for accelerating transformations to sustainable development. United Nations publication issued by the Department of Economic and Social Affairs, United Nations publication issued by the Department of Economic and Social Affairs, (2023).

Tlais, A. Z. A., Fiorino, G. M., Polo, A., Filannino, P., & Di Cagno, R. (2020). High-value compounds in fruit, vegetable and cereal byproducts: An overview of potential sustainable reuse and exploitation. *Molecules (Basel, Switzerland), 25*(13), 2987. Available from https://doi.org/10.3390/molecules25132987.

Trajkovska Petkoska, A. (2021). Can we solve the problem of global syndemic? Mediterranean diet as a potential solution. *Acta Scientifci Nutritional Health, 5*(2), 137–145. Available from https://doi.org/10.31080/asnh.2020.05.0819.

Trajkovska Petkoska, A., & Trajkovska-Broach. (2021a). Mediterranean diet: A nutrient-packed diet and a healthy lifestyle for a sustainable world. *Journal of the Science of Food and Agriculture, 101*(7), 2627–2633. Available from https://doi.org/10.1002/jsfa.10907, http://onlinelibrary.wiley.com/journal/10.1002/(ISSN)1097-0010.

Trajkovska Petkoska, A., & Trajkovska-Broach, A. (2021b). *Mediterranean diet—A healthy dietary pattern and lifestyle for strong immunity* (pp. 279–305). Springer Science and Business Media LLC. Available from https://doi.org/10.1007/978-981-16-2450-6_13.

Trajkovska Petkoska, A., & Trajkovska-Broach, A. (2021d). Sustainable food systems and healthy diets: The case of mediterranean diet. *Acta Horticulturae et Regiotecturae, 24*(2), 110–118. Available from https://doi.org/10.2478/ahr-2021-0032.

Trajkovska Petkoska, A., & Trajkovska-Broach, A. (2021c). *Mediterranean Way of Living as an Optimal Lifestyle and a Dietary Pattern for Healthy Gut and Strong Immunity, 2021*.

Transforming Food and Agriculture to Achieve The SDGs: 20 interconnected actions to guide decision-makers Food And Agriculture Organization of The United Nations, Rome (2018).

Transforming Our World: The 2030 Agenda For Sustainable Development. United Nations, United Nations, (2015). Available from: http://sustainable-development.un.org.

Troilo, M., Difonzo, G., Paradiso, V. M., Pasqualone, A., & Caponio, F. (2022). Grape pomace as innovative flour for the formulation of functional muffins: How particle size affects the nutritional, textural and sensory properties. *Foods, 11*(12). Available from https://doi.org/10.3390/foods11121799, https://www.mdpi.com/2304-8158/11/12/1799/pdf?version = 1655551202.

Trombetta. (2021). *The Potential of Selected Agri-Food Loss and Waste to Contribute to a Circular Economy: Applications in the Food. Cosmetic and Pharmaceutical Industries*, 2021.

Tuğrul, M. Soil Management in Sustainable Agriculture Hasanuzzaman M, Carvalho Minhoto Teixeira Filho M, Fujita M, Assis Rodrigues Nogueira T. (2019).

Vechi, N. T., Mellqvist, J., Samuelsson, J., Offerle, B., & Scheutz, C. (2023). *Ammonia and methane emissions from dairy concentrated animal feeding operations in California, using mobile optical remote sensing, . Atmospheric Environment* (293). Sweden: Elsevier Ltd. Available from www.elsevier.com/locate/atmosenv, https://doi.org/10.1016/j.atmosenv.2022.119448.

Vega-Baudrit, J. R., Camacho., Menezes., Corrales, Y., Zúñiga., Chacón., et al. (2023). Biopolymer Development from Acerola (Malpighia spp.) Waste: A Sustainable Approach to Nutraceutical. *Preprints, 2023.* Available from https://doi.org/10.20944/preprints202310.0210.v2.

Willer, H., Travnicek, J., Meier, C., Schlatter, B. The World of Organic Agriculture Statistics and Emerging Trends 2021. Research Institute of Organic Agriculture FiBL, Research Institute of Organic Agriculture FiBL, (2021). Available from: https://www.fao.org/family-farming/detail/en/c/1378841/.

Willer, H., Trávníček, J., Schlatter, B. The World of Organic Agriculture - Statistics and Emerging Trends. (2024), 2024.

Willett, W., Rockström, J., Loken, B., Springmann, M., Lang, T., Vermeulen, S., Garnett, T., Tilman, D., DeClerck, F., Wood, A., Jonell, M., Clark, M., Gordon, L. J., Fanzo, J., Hawkes, C., Zurayk, R., Rivera, J. A., De Vries, W., Majele Sibanda, L., Afshin, A., Chaudhary, A., Herrero, M., Agustina, R., Branca, F., Lartey, A., Fan, S., Crona, B., Fox, E., Bignet, V., Troell, M., Lindahl, T., Singh, S., Cornell, S. E., Srinath Reddy, K., Narain, S., Nishtar, S., & Murray, C. J. L. (2019). Food in the Anthropocene: the EAT–Lancet Commission on healthy diets from sustainable food systems. *The Lancet, 393*(10170), 447–492. Available from https://doi.org/10.1016/S0140-6736(18)31788-4, http://www.journals.elsevier.com/the-lancet/.

Yun, D., & Liu, J. (2022). Recent advances on the development of food packaging films based on citrus processing wastes: A review. *Journal of Agriculture and Food Research, 9*, 100316. Available from https://doi.org/10.1016/j.jafr.2022.100316.

Zhang, Q. (2015). *Precision Agriculture Technology for Crop Farming*. CRC Press. Available from https://doi.org/10.1201/b19336.

Zhang, Y., Liang, X., Li, H., & Kang. (2020). Antioxidant extract from cauliflower leaves effectively improve the stability of pork patties during refrigerated storage. *Journal of Food Processing and Preservation, 44*(7). Available from https://doi.org/10.1111/jfpp.14510, http://onlinelibrary.wiley.com/journal/10.1111/(ISSN)1745-4549.

Zhao, J., Liu, D., & Huang, R. (2023). A Review of Climate-Smart Agriculture: Recent Advancements, Challenges, and Future Directions. *Sustainability, 15*(4), 3404. Available from https://doi.org/10.3390/su15043404.

Zhou, X., & Ding, D. (2022). Factors influencing farmers' willingness and behaviors in organic agriculture development: An empirical analysis based on survey data of farmers in Anhui Province. *Sustainability, 14*(22), 14945. Available from https://doi.org/10.3390/su142214945.

Chapter 22

The importance of labeling and certification: ensuring quality and transparency

Muskan Kumari Gupta[1], Vinay Balodi[2], Abhishek Dutt Tripathi[3], Rizwana[4], Aparna Agarwal[1] and Nilesh Prakash Nirmal[5]

[1]Department of Food & Nutrition and Food Technology, Lady Irwin College, University of Delhi, New Delhi, Delhi, India, [2]G. B. Pant University of Agriculture and Technology, Pantnagar, Uttarakhand, India, [3]Department of Dairy Science and Food Technology, Institute of Agricultural Sciences, Banaras Hindu University, Varanasi, Uttar Pradesh, India, [4]Department of Food Technology, Bhaskaracharya College of Applied Sciences, New Delhi, Delhi, India, [5]Institute of Nutrition, Mahidol University, Salaya, Nakhon Pathom, Thailand

22.1 Introduction

The global food landscape has undergone an unpredictable transformation in recent years with consumer expectations of much more than just protein and carbohydrates from their diet. This change is driven by an increased consumer awareness of health and wellness. The high surge in lifestyle-related diseases and conditions such as obesity, diabetes, and cardiovascular diseases has reached epidemic proportions, and there is a growing demand for foods not only to provide basic nutrition but also to offer additional health benefits. Scientific studies for understanding how some components of food could promote health and reduce the risk of illness have led to the development of functional foods. These so-called functional components of food differ from more widely understood "nutritional" components of food, such as calories and protein. "Functional foods" are defined as foods that provide health benefits beyond traditional basic nutrition, which are gaining significant attention as potential solutions to enhance public health outcomes. Functional food definitions that are broader, such as foods or beverages marketed with health claims [1,2], apply to many of the products consumed by individuals. Whereas others claim that foods should be fortified with known, specific health benefits [3] (Center for Science in the Public Interest 1999). In addition, some researchers suggest that for a food to be functional, it should meet scientific criteria supporting an evidenced health claim [4] (Iowa State University, 2000). A simpler definition defines functional foods as foods that may reduce the risk of disease [5], while other definitions are more detailed and stipulate these effects must be demonstrated in quantities habitually consumed as part of a regular diet [6]. The range of definitions across such a vast spectrum illustrates how necessary an inclusive, globally acceptable definition is to communicate what can be qualified as a functional food in different circumstances and regarding broader cultural contexts [7]. The indication of functional food is important to protect consumers and help them make appropriate dietary choices. Functional foods can include a wide range of products, from those naturally rich in bioactive compounds such as fruits, vegetables, edible fungi, and herbs to processed foods fortified with vitamins, minerals, probiotics, and other health-promoting ingredients.

Amidst the proliferation of functional foods in the market, effective labeling and certification mechanisms have emerged as crucial elements to guide consumers in making informed dietary choices. Proper labeling ensures that consumers have access to vital information such as nutritional content, ingredient lists, health claims, and potential allergens. Moreover, certification from reputable organizations can further enhance consumer trust by establishing the credibility and efficacy of health claims made by food producers. This is particularly important in an era characterized by misinformation and greenwashing, where products may be labeled "healthier" without substantial evidence to support such claims. This importance of labeling and certification extends beyond consumer awareness. Regulatory agencies and industry stakeholders recognize that these mechanisms can play a vital role in promoting public health, ensuring food safety, and fostering innovation within the food industry. As such, embracing and strengthening labeling and certification processes are essential for establishing a standardized framework that can support the growth of the functional foods market.

Unleashing the Power of Functional Foods and Novel Bioactives. DOI: https://doi.org/10.1016/B978-0-443-28862-3.00022-4

Labeling of functional foods plays a vital role in consumer education and informed decision-making in an increasingly health-conscious society. As the demand for functional foods burgeons, so does the necessity for clear and accurate labeling that communicates essential information regarding the nutritional content, health benefits, and safety of these products. Labels act as a bridge between manufacturers and consumers, providing insights into the composition of functional foods, including the presence of bioactive compounds, vitamins, minerals, and other health-promoting ingredients. Moreover, consumer understanding of health claims—such as "supports immune health" or "rich in antioxidants"—is critical, as these assertions can significantly influence purchasing decisions. Consequently, regulatory frameworks governing the use of such claims must be robust, ensuring that they are substantiated by scientific evidence and not misleading. An additional element to consider is the standardization of terminology, as the nomenclature used in labeling can vary widely, potentially causing confusion among consumers. For instance, terms like "natural," "organic," and "superfood" lack universally recognized definitions, leading to varied interpretations among shoppers. Thus clear guidelines should be established to govern the use of such terms, enabling consumers to discern the authenticity of the claims made by food manufacturers. Furthermore, transparent labeling practices can help mitigate the risk of greenwashing, where products may misleadingly promote health benefits without appropriate backing. Enhancing labeling initiatives facilitates public trust and confidence in functional foods while promoting better health outcomes by enabling consumers to make choices aligned with their dietary needs and preferences. Consequently, the emphasis on accurate and informative labeling not only empowers consumers but also encourages manufacturers to uphold high standards in the development and marketing of functional foods, creating a win–win scenario for all stakeholders in the food industry.

22.2 Global prospective on health claims and regulatory compliance of functional foods

With the increasing market of functional foods, the toughest obstacle comes from the regulatory compliance sections. Most foods generally taken as functional foods are herbs or some natural origin products or products identical to these natural products (Natural Identical). The most common are active components in herbs like gingerol, myristic acid, capsaicin, curcumin, vitamins, and their precursors like lycopene, carotenoids, and other xanthophylls. Other categories include microbial and fiber products which could be fiber from *Isabgol* or citrus fruits or microbial products like functional mushrooms and other edible fungi. Despite being used as a supplement for a long period, their mechanism and effects are still under research and study for almost all products. Which makes regulatory compliance a difficult task for these products. Especially in countries like India, China, and the sub-African continents where there has been a previous history of these products in Ayurveda, Siddha, and Chinese medicines, the regulatory framework becomes complex mostly due to different regulations governing the same product. This can be understood from the fact that in India all regulations of Aayush, FSSAI, and drugs may interfere with each other. The use of certain ingredients may be approved for usage in some products but may not be allowed in other regulations which the manufacturer may use to gain advantage and mislead the consumer. Another important obstacle is the claims associated with these products. Most companies use health claims for their products, one such classic example being "Complaint" which was once advertised to increase the height in children. Although unethical, the corporate world can use these strategies to its advantage due to weak regulatory policies by the government.

Since functional foods with a history of use in Ayurveda and medicine have high faith of consumers, claims in these products are often used by most companies to mislead the consumer, which mostly includes adding claims other than those present or once that are not scientifically proven but believed by most due to traditions. One big case study for this product is where a company claimed to cure the COVID-19 pandemic with its medicine; however, when investigated and cleared by the authorities, it was stated that the license was not issued for the medicine as a cure for the disease but as a supporting measure. Later, the court even issued an order to the company for taking down the claims from its products. However, all these judicial interventions are not of no vail as people had already used the medicine for its supposed cure of the disease during the pandemic. Being such a large population, no compensation is even possible for the consumers now. This was one example of the present scenario of regulations governing the claims. However, now most authorities have woken from their deep slumber and started to issue strict guidelines to stop such heinous acts. A list of regulatory acts and agencies governing functional foods for all major countries has been provided in Table 22.1. Although the process may differ, the basis for all types of regulations remains the same. Any claim should be based on a sound scientific basis and should be proven with the help of scientific and clinical trials.

In the international markets, these initiatives were first taken by the FDA (USA) since 1990 which spurred owing to the efforts of public interest groups and the food industry to foster greater health awareness. This journey began in 1984 when the National Cancer Institute (NCI) endorsed messages about the benefits of dietary fiber for Kellogg's cereal. This was later followed by the "5 a Day for Better Health" program launched by NCI and the Produce for Better

TABLE 22.1 International Laws governing Regulatory Compliance for Functional foods.

S. No.	Country	Regulation	Agency	References
1.	United States	Dietary Supplement Health and Education Act (DSHEA) of 1994	U.S. Food and Drug Administration (FDA)	U.S. Food and Drug Administration (1994)
2.	Canada	Natural Health Products Regulations (NHPR)	Health Canada	Health Canada (2004)
3.	European Union	Regulation (EC) No 1924/2006 on nutrition and health claims made on foods	European Food Safety Authority (EFSA)	European Food Safety Authority. (2006)
4.	Japan	Food for Specified Health Uses (FOSHU) system	Ministry of Health, Labour and Welfare (MHLW)	Ministry of Health, Labour and Welfare. (1991)
5.	China	Administrative Measures on Health Food	National Health Commission (NHC)	National Health Commission. (2016)
6.	Australia	Therapeutic Goods Administration (TGA) regulations for complementary medicines	Food Standards Australia New Zealand (FSANZ)	Therapeutic Goods Administration. (2020)
7.	South Korea	Functional Health Food Act	Ministry of Food and Drug Safety (MFDS)	Ministry of Food and Drug Safety. (2020)
8.	India	Food Safety and Standards (Health Supplements, Nutraceuticals, Food for Special Dietary Uses, Foods for Special Medical Purposes, and Probiotic Foods) Regulations, 2016 *updated in 2022	Food Safety and Standards Authority of India (FSSAI)	Food Safety and Standards Authority of India. (2016)
9.	Brazil	RDC No. 24/2011, which deals with health claims and functional foods	Agência Nacional de Vigilância Sanitária (ANVISA)	Agência Nacional de Vigilância Sanitária. (2011)
10.	Mexico	NOM-051-SCFI/SSA1-2010 for labeling and health claims	Federal Commission for the Protection against Sanitary Risk (COFEPRIS)	Federal Commission for the Protection against Sanitary Risk. (2010)
11.	Taiwan	Health Food Control Act	Ministry of Health and Welfare (MOHW)	Ministry of Health and Welfare. (2013)
12.	Singapore	Health Supplements Regulations under the Sale of Food Act	Singapore Food Agency (SFA)	Singapore Food Agency. (2020)
13.	New Zealand	Dietary Supplements Regulations 1985	New Zealand Food Safety Authority	New Zealand Food Safety Authority. (1985)
14.	Russia	Federal Law No. 29-FZ on the Quality and Safety of Food Products	Federal Service for Surveillance on Consumer Rights Protection and Human Wellbeing (Rospotrebnadzor)	Federal Service for Surveillance on Consumer Rights Protection and Human Wellbeing. (2000)

Health Foundation in 1991 to encourage Americans to eat five servings a day of fruits and vegetables. Just the next year in 1992, the American Heart Association allowed the use of their red "heart check" mark on products that would meet the USFDA's regulatory requirements for making a coronary heart disease health claim. The labeling of food products regulated by the Nutrition Labeling and Education Act (NLEA) of 1990 directed the FDA to change the way that food labels were regulated earlier. Most food products now carry the revised label that provides information about saturated fat, cholesterol, and dietary fiber in a format designed to help consumers choose a more healthful and nutritious diet. The first ever food-specific health claim was approved by FDA under NLEA in January 1997 which was in response to a petition from Quaker Oats Company describing a relationship between the consumption of whole oat products and reduction in risk of coronary health diseases. The FDA accepted the claim and allowed products containing a certain minimum level of soluble fiber from oat bran per serving to carry one of the following statements, "Soluble fiber from foods such as oat bran, as part of a diet low in saturated fat and cholesterol, may reduce the risk of heart disease." or "Diets low in saturated fat and cholesterol that include soluble fiber from oatmeal may reduce the risk of heart disease." (Unnevehr & Hasler, 2000). Although the claim was made and backed by the Quaker Oats company, it should always be kept in mind that the FDA did not approve any single manufacturer to use the claim for their product; once proved, any company with a sufficient amount of whole oats can use the claim on their product, indicating the health claim to be product associated which connects indirectly with the ingredient and not with the individual product of Quaker itself. From then several diet-disease relationships have been established, and various health claims have been allowed by the FDA, including calcium and a reduced risk of osteoporosis, and sodium and an increased risk of hypertension (Kurtzweil, 1998). However, it should be noted that all claims that are allowed are supposed to be backed by strong scientific evidence.

In the USA, the regulations for functional foods are now being governed by the Dietary Supplement Health & Education Act of 1994, 1994. Accordingly, the food manufacturers exporting to the country are also mandated to register their facility separately in the Dietary Supplement Health category which is separate from the other food category. The DSHEA allows manufacturers to make certain claims and market products without obtaining the FDA's pre-approval. They must notify the FDA 30 days before marketing a product with a claim. The burden of proof to demonstrate harm from these products rests on the FDA (Unnevehr & Hasler, 2000).

Note: Every manufacturing facility outside the USA needs to register with the FDA through a US agent for exporting food products to the United States, although laws governing the food regulations in the UDA should be followed, no formal approval or certificate is provided by the FDA to any company.

Another notable country in the food business is Canada, although the process resembles that of USDA, the licensing and numbering of products provide us with an idea of how the regulations work in most of the other countries in the world other than the United States. Health Canada plays a significant role in regulating health products, including dietary supplements, under the Natural Health Products Regulations (NHPR). This certification process is designed to ensure that natural health products, which can include vitamins, minerals, herbal remedies, and other supplements, are safe, effective, and of high quality before they can be marketed to consumers in Canada. To obtain a product license, manufacturers must submit an application that includes detailed information about the product's ingredients, recommended uses, and evidence supporting its safety and efficacy [22]. The application process involves the evaluation of scientific evidence and clinical data that demonstrate the product's intended health effects. Once approved, the product is assigned a Natural Product Number (NPN) or Homeopathic Medicine Number (DIN-HM), which must appear on the product label. This mark signifies that the product has met Health Canada's strict standards for safety and effectiveness [23]. Moreover, manufacturers must adhere to Good Manufacturing Practices (GMP), ensuring consistent quality and safety throughout the manufacturing process [24]. Health Canada also emphasizes postmarket surveillance, meaning that supplements continue to be monitored for any potential adverse effects after they enter the market. Consumers can access a searchable database on the Health Canada website to verify the status of licensed natural health products, enhancing transparency and consumer confidence in the supplement industry [22]. Through these rigorous regulations, Health Canada aims to protect public health while facilitating access to effective dietary supplements that can support overall wellness.

FSSAI, the primary food safety governing body, has issued guidelines for labeling and claims of functional foods in Food Safety and Standards Authority of India. (2016). FSS (Health supplements, nutraceuticals, food for special dietary uses, foods for special medical purposes, and probiotic foods) Regulations, 2016. Retrieved from https://www.fssai.gov.in/. This regulation was further updated with the 2022 regulation with slight changes; apart from these, various updates are regularly posted on the website for further clarifications and any amends made in the act. One such notification was an advisory released by FSSAI on March 7, 2023, regarding the implementation of special enforcement drives for verifying the compliance of nutraceuticals and health supplements, this action was taken due to the sale of noncompliant nutraceutical and health supplement products in the market, as well as the false and misleading label/health claims associated with these products (https://www.foodlabelsolutions.com/). Further, for any new product, approval is required from the designated officer of the area. For the formulations containing compounds present in the sections and complying with the regulations, an SOI (Statement of Ingredients and Additives) is required to be submitted with the product in the prescribed format as stated by FSSAI (Fig. 22.1). Both the ingredients and additives have to be mentioned for the products, which should be governed by the FSSAI regulations. However, these regulations are constantly changing, and anyone needs to keep themselves undated for any advisories and changes. The food authority has strictly mentioned all the parameters which should be followed, and any claims have to be mandatorily stated in the SOI while submitting. If any claim for the product is made, these have to be proven to the authority. However, this task is much more difficult than said, and the process requires the manufacturer to provide the relevant information about the product in the prescribed format, a dossier, which is then taken for scrutiny by the scientific panel. The documents include, but are not limited to, toxicological data, the research supporting the claims (published in high-impact journals), clinical data, and

Statement of Ingredients and Additives (For Food Categories 13.3-13.6)

{To be printed on letter Head of Company/Firm}

1. Name of the Food Product:
2. Type of Food Product: Health Supplement/Nutraceutical/FSDU/FSMP other than Infants/Food with added Probiotic ingredients/Food with added Prebiotic ingredients/ Specialty Food containing plant or botanical ingredients with safe history of usage (Tick any one)
3. Food Category No.:
4. Target Group (Age and Gender):
5. Target Physiological condition:
6. Product Format: Tablet/Capsule/Syrup/Any Other ______________
7. Recommended Serving Size and No. of Recommended Serves per day:
8. Any type of Claims to be made on the label:

Ingredients:

S.No.	Ingredients [Name of the Ingredients)	Schedule under Nutraceutical Regulations in which the ingredient is permitted for use / Product Approval Copy	Quantity of Ingredient Used in the product (In addition, in case of micronutrients, percentage of RDA to be declared).	Purity Criteria adopted

Additives:

S.No.	Name of the Food Additives or Group	Schedule under Nutraceutical Regulations in which the ingredient is permitted for use (Schedule VA-VF)/ Product Approval Copy	INS No.	Level of additives in the product

FIGURE 22.1 Statement of ingredient and additive for the food product.

other documents as per the requirement. These research studies should be on par with the claims being made, and the information that has been provided in the SOI, a product intended for children and pregnant and lactating women, should have relevant data to ensure the safety of the product for these groups, and once all these claims are found to be satisfactory, then a manufacturer can use a claim for the product which can be stated on the product label itself. Along with these, irrespective of the claims made or not, the authority requires the manufacturer to provide declarations along with the ingredient list (Fig. 22.2). It should also be kept in mind that just proving a claim does not empower the manufacturer to state the food product as a medicine, and regulations in India mandate the manufacturer to specify the words not for medicinal use on the product label itself.

I declare that:

1. No hormones or steroids or psychotropic ingredients have been used in the above food product.
2. The ingredients and additives used in the food product are in accordance with the type of food product/category as mentioned in the Nutraceutical Regulations.
3. Nutrients added to the product comply with the respective Recommended Daily Allowance specified by ICMR/Codex Alimentarius Commission.
4. The product is not a mere combination of vitamins and minerals.
5. No product-led health claims are being made on the product. (In case these are being made, relevant supporting documents with a copy of label shall be submitted)
6. No claim regarding prevention, treatment or cure of any disease or referring to such properties shall be made for the said food product.
7. The product is not a Drug as defined under Drugs and Cosmetics Act, 1940.

Signature of FBO/Authorised Signatory with seal

FIGURE 22.2 Declaration from the manufacturer under the Food Safety and Standards (FSS Health Supplements, Nutraceuticals, Food for Special Dietary Uses, Foods for Special Medical Purposes, & Probiotic Foods Regulations Food Safety & Standards Authority of India, 2016).

22.3 Certification standards and processes

As the demand for functional foods grows, so does the necessity for reliable certification systems that can validate the health claims and nutritional properties associated with these products. Certification can come from various entities, including government bodies, nonprofit organizations, and industry associations, each of which may have its own set of criteria and standards. These certifications often require rigorous scientific studies, testing, and documentation to demonstrate that a product meets specific health claims and safety guidelines. Functional food certification represents a growing area within the food industry that aims to validate the health benefits associated with certain food products beyond basic nutrition. These foods, often enriched with bioactive compounds such as vitamins, minerals, probiotics, and phytochemicals, are believed to contribute positively to health and wellness when consumed as part of a regular diet [25]. The certification process typically involves rigorous scientific evaluation to substantiate claims regarding the health effects of functional foods, which may include improved digestion, enhanced immune function, or reduced risk of chronic diseases [26]. Various organizations and regulatory bodies, such as the European Food Safety Authority (EFSA) and Health Canada, have established frameworks for reviewing health claims associated with functional foods, which require producers to provide robust evidence from clinical and observational studies [27]. In the United States, the FDA does not have a specific regulatory category for "functional foods"; however, it oversees health claims on food labels through its regulations, stressing the need for substantial scientific evidence to support any claim made [28]. The rise in functional food certification is linked to increasing consumer awareness and demand for foods that promote health, leading to a market poised for growth as nutritional science continues to evolve (Lee & O'Neill, 2021). Effective labeling and certification not only empower consumers to make informed food choices but also provide manufacturers with a competitive edge in the marketplace. For instance, certifications like "Heart-Check" by the American Heart Association or "NSF Certified for Sport" assure consumers that products have undergone thorough scrutiny for nutritional integrity and safety, particularly in categories where the risk of contamination or mislabeling may be prevalent, such as dietary supplements and functional beverages. Furthermore, certification not only fosters consumer confidence but also serves as a competitive differentiator in a crowded marketplace, where credibly certified products can stand out among similar offerings. Beyond consumer protection, certification plays a crucial role in promoting industry-wide standards and encouraging manufacturers to adhere to best practices in product development and marketing. However, the certification landscape is not without challenges; the proliferation of various certification programs can sometimes lead to confusion among consumers about what each label truly signifies. Clear communication about the meaning and source of certifications is vital to ensure that consumers can make informed choices and fully understand the implications of the certifications they encounter. Moreover, with growing concerns around transparency and authenticity, the rise of third-party certifications has become increasingly important, as they typically offer impartial evaluations of functional foods that bolster consumer trust. As the functional foods industry continues to evolve, the advancement and harmonization of certification processes will be essential to ensure that they effectively meet consumer needs, promote public health, and maintain the integrity of health claims being made on functional food products. Ultimately, robust certification systems foster an environment where both consumers and producers can thrive, as they bridge the gap between scientific validation and everyday consumer experiences, establishing a foundation of trust that is vital for the growth of the functional food sector.

Certification plays a crucial role in distinguishing high-quality functional foods from those that make unverified claims. According to the World Health Organization (WHO), functional foods should be evaluated based on their health benefits, safety, and efficacy [29]. Without certification, consumers may encounter misleading information, potentially leading to health risks or wasted resources on ineffective products. Regulatory bodies often mandate labeling and certification to protect public health, ensuring that consumers receive accurate information about the nutritional and health claims made by manufacturers [30]. Studies have shown that consumers are more likely to purchase products that carry credible certifications. For instance, research conducted by [31] indicated that consumers harbor a greater level of trust towards products with nutritional and health certifications than those without. This trust can significantly influence market dynamics, pushing manufacturers to seek certification as a modality to enhance their product appeal.

22.3.1 Certification programs for functional foods

Various organizations offer certification programs for functional foods, each with its own criteria, standards, and procedures (Fig. 22.3). Notable examples include:

1. Informed Choice: https://choice.wetestyoutrust.com/
2. Informed Sports: https://sport.wetestyoutrust.com/
3. NPA GMP certified: www.npanational.org
4. Clean Label Project: https://cleanlabelproject.org/

22.3.1.1 NSF International certification for dietary supplements

NSF provides certification for dietary supplements and functional foods, focusing on transparency regarding labeling and ingredient sourcing. Their certification evaluates products for potential contaminations and verifies that they meet specified health claims [32]. NSF certifies products against NSF/ANSI 173 and is based on US standards of dietary supplements. The key points include a label claim review to certify that what's on the label is in the bottle, a toxicology review to certify product formulation, and contaminant review to ensure the product contains no undeclared ingredients or unacceptable levels of contaminants. Under this program, the supplements, especially those made for athletes, are certified separately under the NSF certified for sport which is recognized by the NFL, NFL Players Association, MLB, MLB Players Association, PGA, LPGA, and Canadian Centre for Ethics in Sports.

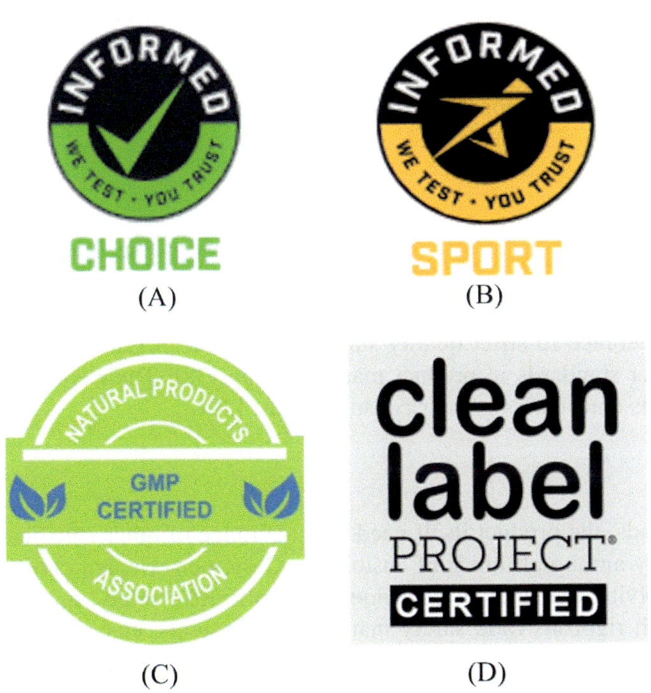

FIGURE 22.3 Certification programs for functional foods (A) Informed Choice: https://choice.wetestyoutrust.com/ (B) Informed Sports: https://sport.wetestyoutrust.com/ (C) NPA GMP certified: http://www.npanational.org (D) Clean Label Project: https://cleanlabelproject.org/.

22.3.1.2 United States Pharmacopeia Verified Mark

The United States Pharmacopeia (USP) Verified Mark is a symbol of assurance for functional foods, indicating that a product has met the high standards set by USP for quality, purity, and consistency. Products carrying this mark have undergone rigorous testing to verify that they contain the ingredients listed on the label in the correct amounts and are free from harmful contaminants. This verification is particularly important for functional foods, which are designed to provide health benefits beyond basic nutrition. By adhering to USP's stringent criteria, manufacturers demonstrate their commitment to transparency and product integrity, fostering consumer trust and ensuring the efficacy of their products (United States Pharmacopeia Dietary Supplement Verification Program, 2024; United States Pharmacopeia USP, 2024).

22.3.1.3 ConsumerLab.com

ConsumerLab.com provides an independent and highly regarded resource for evaluating functional foods, offering consumers detailed and unbiased reviews based on rigorous testing. The site conducts comprehensive analyses of functional food products to assess their ingredient quality, potency, and safety as well as to ensure that they meet label claims. By testing a wide range of products for contaminants, efficacy, and consistency, ConsumerLab.com helps consumers make informed choices and avoid misleading or substandard products. Their findings are published in detailed reports, which are accessible through a subscription model, and they often highlight which products pass their stringent quality criteria. This independent evaluation supports consumer confidence and promotes transparency in the functional food market [33,34].

22.3.1.4 Informed-Sport and Informed-Choice

Informed-Sport and Informed-Choice are certification programs that play a crucial role in ensuring the safety and integrity of functional foods, particularly for athletes and health-conscious consumers. Informed-Sport certifies that products have been tested for banned substances and contaminants, ensuring that they meet rigorous standards for sports nutrition. Similarly, Informed-Choice assures that products are free from prohibited substances and have been tested for quality and consistency. Both programs involve thorough testing by accredited laboratories and adherence to strict manufacturing practices. By obtaining certification from these programs, manufacturers demonstrate their commitment to product safety and transparency, thus fostering consumer confidence and promoting the integrity of functional foods [35,36].

22.3.1.5 Natural Products Association Good Manufacturing Practices certification

The Natural Products Association (NPA) GMP Certification is a significant quality assurance mark for functional foods, indicating that products are manufactured in compliance with stringent Good Manufacturing Practices (GMP). This certification process involves a rigorous review of a company's manufacturing facilities and practices to ensure that products are consistently produced and controlled according to quality standards. NPA GMP Certification helps guarantee that functional foods meet high standards for purity, potency, and safety, providing consumers with confidence in the products they choose. By adhering to these practices, manufacturers demonstrate their commitment to product integrity and consumer safety [37].

22.3.1.6 Clean Label Project

The Clean Label Project is a nonprofit organization dedicated to enhancing transparency and safety in the functional food industry through rigorous product testing and certification. Their certification program focuses on validating that functional foods are free from harmful contaminants, such as heavy metals, pesticides, and other environmental toxins. By conducting extensive laboratory testing and ensuring adherence to strict quality standards, the Clean Label Project helps consumers make informed choices and promotes higher standards in product manufacturing [38]. Their commitment to transparency supports the integrity of functional foods and fosters greater consumer trust [39].

22.3.2 Customer-oriented certifications

Despite programs made for the sole purpose of functional foods, the product itself needs a wide range of other certifications for a wide reach in the market and an easy acceptability among all kinds of customers. Customer-oriented certifications in the food industry are essential for meeting the evolving demands of consumers who prioritize safety, quality, and sustainability. Certifications such as ISO 22000 establish rigorous food safety management systems, ensuring that companies adhere to best practices for preventing foodborne illnesses and maintaining high hygiene standards [40]. The Global Food Safety Initiative (GFSI) benchmarks, including BRCGS (British Retail Consortium Global Standards) and

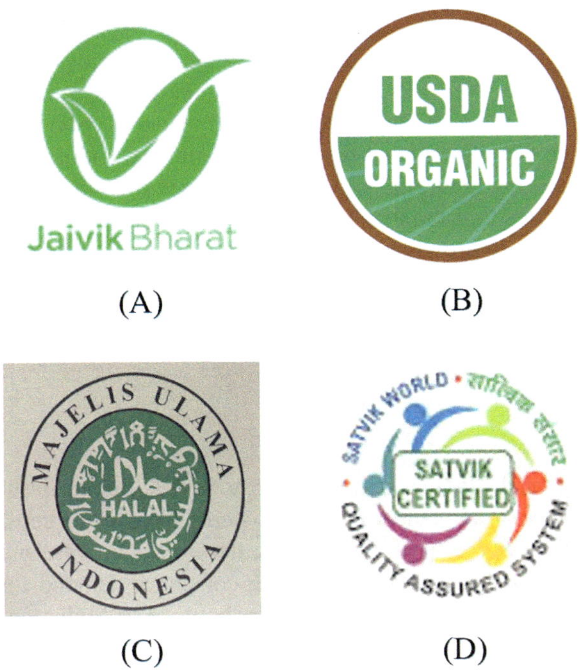

FIGURE 22.4 Customer oriented certifications (A) Jaivik Bharat: https://jaivikbharat.fssai.gov.in/ (B) USDA Organic: https://www.usda.gov/ (C) MUI Halal: https://halalmui.org/ (D) Satvik Certified: https://satvikcertification.com/.

SQF (Safe Quality Food), provide frameworks that help businesses maintain consistency in quality and traceability throughout the supply chain [41]. Additionally, certifications like Fair Trade and USDA Organic address consumer concerns about ethical sourcing and environmental impact. Fair Trade certification guarantees fair labor practices and sustainable production methods [42], while USDA Organic certifies that products are produced without synthetic pesticides or GMOs [43]. By obtaining these certifications (Fig. 22.4), companies not only enhance their credibility and build consumer trust but also align with a growing market that values both product integrity and ethical responsibility.

1. Jaivik Bharat: https://jaivikbharat.fssai.gov.in/
2. USDA Organic: https://www.usda.gov/
3. MUI Halal: https://halalmui.org/
4. Satvik Certified: https://satvikcertification.com/

22.3.2.1 Organic certification

22.3.2.1.1 APEDA Organic Certification

The organic certification in India follows a two-way approach in which the organic certification is carried out through third-party organizations for various geographical areas and products under their scope. The list of relevant certification agencies accredited by APEDA is available on the organization's website for industry retrospection. Currently, the organization is following two types of certifications: the PGS (Participatory Guarantee System) and the NPOP (National Programme for Organic Production). Both are equally recognized in India as organic programs but there has been a higher trend toward NPOP due to much more knowledge of this program among industry experts. The NPOP program is a well-suited program for both organically grown crops and lab-grown products like mushrooms and ingredients of microbial origin which are highly sought out in the functional foods industry. The system relies on the trace-net system which increases the transparency and high traceability in the industry. On critical point, differentiating these programs from other certifications is the trademarks and labeling as currently there are no trademarks provided by the APEDA for labeling organic food products, and the only legal indicators available are the scope certificates that they provided. Keeping these difficulties in labeling organic foods, FSSAI has now introduced Jaivik Bharat certification which is an extension of NPOP certification. The main objective behind the Jaivik Bharat program is to create a database for organic products for the customers but FSSAI has taken one step further by introducing the Jaivik Bharat logo (Fig. 22.4A) which can be legally used in India to distinguish organic products and provide transparency to the customers.

22.3.2.1.2 USDA Organic Certification

USDA organic certification is an essential designation for functional foods, which are defined as foods that offer health benefits beyond basic nutrition. The USDA's National Organic Program (NOP) establishes the standards that must be met for products to bear the "USDA Organic" seal, aiming to ensure that these foods are produced using environmentally sustainable practices [44]. The certification process prohibits the use of synthetic fertilizers, pesticides, and genetically modified organisms (GMOs), thus promoting a more natural growing environment that can enhance the nutritional and functional qualities of the food [45]. Furthermore, research indicates that organic foods may boast higher levels of beneficial nutrients, such as antioxidants, compared to their conventionally grown counterparts, which can contribute to better health outcomes [46]. As consumer interest in health-promoting foods rises, USDA organic certification serves as a valuable indicator of both quality and safety in the marketplace [47]. For obtaining the USDA organic certification, the industries are prescribed to first follow their origin countries organic programs. In most cases, NPOP certification (APEDA) is the first step towards obtaining an NOP certification in India.

22.3.2.2 Satvik certification

Satvik certification is a quality assurance program that verifies functional foods as compliant with Sattvik dietary principles, which emphasize purity, ethical sourcing, and adherence to vegetarian standards. Administered by various certifying bodies, Sattvik certification ensures that products are free from nonvegetarian ingredients, harmful additives, and processing methods that conflict with Sattvik principles. This certification supports the growing consumer demand for products that align with ethical and health-conscious lifestyles by promoting transparency and adherence to high standards of ingredient integrity and ethical practices. As a result, Sattvik certification helps consumers make informed choices and encourages manufacturers to uphold strict quality and ethical standards [48,49].

22.3.2.3 Halal certification

The global demand for Halal-certified products is on the rise, driven by the growing Muslim population, which is estimated to be over 1.9 billion people worldwide. Halal certification ensures that food products comply with Islamic dietary laws, making them permissible for consumption by Muslims. A halal certificate can be obtained by driving the food production process according to the Sharia law and strict avoidance of Haram ingredients in the foods. Although most countries have independent organizations providing halal certification, the most notable certification program is the MUI—Majelis Ulama Indonesia, which is accepted in almost all Islamic countries.

22.3.2.4 Kosher certification

The kosher food market generates over $12 billion annually, with a diverse consumer base that includes non-Jews seeking health benefits and food safety (Timothy & Lytton, 2012). Kosher certification for functional foods ensures that products adhere to Jewish dietary laws, which encompass specific guidelines for ingredients, preparation, and handling. This certification, provided by various certifying agencies, involves a detailed review of the product's ingredients and production processes to ensure compliance with kosher standards, which include restrictions on the types of ingredients used and the separation of dairy and meat products. Kosher certification not only assures compliance with these religious dietary laws but also often signifies adherence to high standards of quality and safety, which can enhance consumer trust. By offering kosher-certified products, manufacturers can appeal to a broader audience, including those with specific dietary restrictions or preferences [50,51]. Kosher certification is essential for accessing markets, particularly in the United States, where many ingredients require kosher status, thus expanding the market for functional foods (Joe & Regenstein, 2018). These certification programs not only protect consumers but also encourage manufacturers to adopt rigorous testing and quality control methods across the product development lifecycle.

22.4 Functional foods and its labeling

Functional foods are one of the most important topics today as they benefit health beyond basic nutrition. There are certainly several definitions that show rather the complexity of this term. The labeling requirements for functional foods as per the Food Safety and Standards Act (2006a, 2006b) include the following elements:

1. **Name of the food**: The specific name of the functional food product.
2. **List of ingredients**: A detailed list of all ingredients used in the product.
3. **Nutritional information**: Information regarding the nutritional content of the food.

4. **Vegetarian/Nonvegetarian declaration**: A declaration indicating whether the product is vegetarian or nonvegetarian.
5. **Food additives**: Information about any food additives present in the product.
6. **Manufacturer information**: The name and complete address of the manufacturer.
7. **Net quantity**: The total quantity of the product contained in the package.
8. **Lot/Code/Batch identification**: Identification details for tracking the batch of the product.
9. **Date of manufacture or packing**: The date when the product was manufactured or packed.
10. **Best before or use-by date**: The date until which the product is expected to remain safe and effective.
11. **Country of origin**: For imported food, the country where the food originates.
12. **Warnings**: Any necessary warnings related to the product.
13. **Customer care information**: Contact information for customer inquiries.
14. **Instructions for use**: Guidelines on how to use the product.

Additionally, the FSSAI logo with a license number must be imprinted on the label, along with other general label requirements (Food Safety & Standards (Packaging and Labeling) Regulation, 2011; Food Safety & Standards Authority of India, 2011). Table 22.2 provides labeling regulations for functional foods across different countries.

22.5 Transparency and mislabeling issues of functional foods

The market for functional foods that have health benefits beyond basic nutrition had very sharp growth in the past few years. Market demand for those positioned as contributing to health and wellness also continued to increase due to greater consumer interest. As a result of this market gaining popularity, it has given way to a lack of transparency and mislabeling [62]. Also, leading from these issues will be the damage to public trust, which may evoke concerns about

TABLE 22.2 Labeling Regulations for Functional Foods Across Different Countries.

Country	Regulation Act for Functional Foods	References
United States	The Food, Drug, and Cosmetic Act (FDCA) and the Dietary Supplement Health and Education Act (DSHEA)	[52]. *Food, Drug, and Cosmetic Act.* US Food and Drug Administration. Retrieved from https://www.fda.gov
European Union	Regulation (EU) No 1169/2011 for general food labeling and Regulation (EU) No 432/2012 for health claims	[53]. *Regulation (EU) No 1169/2011 on the provision of food information to consumers.* Retrieved from https://eur-lex.europa.eu
Canada	The Food and Drugs Act along with Natural Health Products Regulations (NHPR)	[54]. *Food and Drugs Act.* Government of Canada. Retrieved from https://www.canada.ca
Australia	Australia New Zealand Food Standards Code, specifically Standard 1.2.7 for health and nutrition claims	[55]. *Australia New Zealand Food Standards Code.* Food Standards Australia New Zealand. Retrieved from https://www.foodstandards.gov.au
Japan	Food Labeling Act, which includes rules for health claims and functional foods	[56]. *Food Labeling Act.* Ministry of Agriculture, Forestry and Fisheries of Japan. Retrieved from https://www.maff.go.jp
India	Food Safety & Standards Packaging and Labeling Regulations, 2011b, and Health Supplements & Nutraceuticals Regulations. Food Safety and Standards Authority of India, 2020	[57]. *Food Safety and Standards (Packaging and Labeling) Regulations.* Food Safety and Standards Authority of India. Retrieved from https://www.fssai.gov.in[58]. *Health Supplements and Nutraceuticals Regulations.* Food Safety and Standards Authority of India. Retrieved from https://www.fssai.gov.in
China	National Food Safety Standard GB 28050-2011 for nutrition labeling and GB 7718-2011 for food labeling	[59]. *Food Safety Law.* National Medical Products Administration. Retrieved from https://www.nmpa.gov.cn
Brazil	Labeling regulations under the Ministry of Agriculture, Livestock, and Supply (MAPA), covering functional foods and health claims	[60]. *Brazilian Labeling Regulations.* Ministry of Agriculture, Livestock, and Supply. Retrieved from https://www.gov.br/mapa
South Africa	SANS, (SANS) 10330:2014, which includes guidelines for functional foods and health claims	[61]. SANS,330:2014. South African Bureau of Standards. Retrieved from https://www.sabs.co.za

the efficacy of functional foods at work, and it could even cause threats to the safety of functional foods itself [63]. This section highlights the challenges of transparency and misinformation in the functional food industry, providing a reason for regulatory control of the industry and a way to increase awareness among consumers.

22.5.1 Transparency in functional food labeling

The identification of functional food ingredients in the labeling is necessary as consumers will be able to know the nutritional value and healthful ingredients that are present in those products. Open labeling includes fully disclosed ingredient lists, truthful nutritional facts, and unexaggerated health benefits. Yet, getting to this level of transparency is difficult because functional foods are multicomponent, and multiple bioactive compounds contribute jointly to their health effects [64]. The top topic surrounding transparency is health claim communication. To clarify, regulatory bodies like the US Food and Drug Administration (FDA) have created guidelines to ensure that health claims for functional foods are supported by credible scientific evidence about a relationship between a specific food product and its claimed benefits (EFSA 2011a) [52]. Despite these oversights and regulations, the disconnect between what a product's label claims it can do versus actual scientific support remains large. Functional food labels lack transparency as far as the ingredient list is concerned. Proprietary blends are used by some manufacturers that include a range of bioactive but do not divulge the specific amounts in each part. This tactic confuses the consumer regarding the efficiency of the product [65]. In addition, the use of less specific names like "natural flavors" or generic ingredients such as herbal extracts might make someone unaware of the presence of allergens that may harm them (Codex) [66]. These practices are not only counterproductive to expect transparency but also present safety risks for someone being allergic to or having dietary restrictions [64].

22.5.2 Mislabeling in the functional food industry

Functional foods also suffer from endemic mislabeling, yielding an invitation to deceive consumers who might be easily swayed by exaggerated health claims. This can be done in a variety of ways, including exaggerating health benefits, misrepresenting amounts of ingredients, or failing to disclose the presence of certain allergens in additives [63]. Manufacturers sometimes provide "clinically proven" type labels without adequate information regarding the nature or quality of the evidence [64]. Mislabeling is also a major problem where the amount of ingredients included in the product might be different than stated on the package. The health benefits of functional foods are usually related to the presence of nutrients or nonnutrients specific to vitamins, minerals, probiotics, and omega-3 fatty acids also known as bioactive compounds. However, these ingredients may be present in insufficient quantity in the product to have an effect, or the label might also lie [65]. There are many cases in which products have been mislabeled when they were marketed as natural or organic but did not meet the standards to make these claims. The use of these labels can be deceptive, especially in cases where food is associated with better health or purchase. Indeed, the meaning of the terms "natural" and "organic" can greatly differ; besides, they are not subject to strict control [67].

22.5.3 Regulatory and consumer education solutions

Regarding functional foods, solutions for transparency and mislabeling issues include stricter regulations, improved enforcement of existing rules in place (e.g., DSHEA), and greater consumer education [63]. This requires that regulatory bodies enforce substantiation of all health claims by rigorous scientific evidence and correct labeling regarding the product. This may include increased levels of inspections, stronger penalties for non-compliance, and more intensive scrutiny around marketing practices (EFSA 2011). With strict regulations, it should be ensured that consumers receive education regarding how to read functional food labels. The claims may be exaggerated so consumers need to realize if a health claim is true or false and know that third-party certifications or scientific backing on the products they buy are important [64]. Two of the major problems within the functional food industry are transparency and mislabeling; these would have much greater implications for consumer confidence and product efficacy. Although regulatory frameworks are in place to address the emerging challenges in the industry, this remains a lingering problem due to the existing gap in enforcement as well as in consumer comprehension. To protect the consumers' interests and ensure responsible growth in this category of food, more stringent regulations, increased transparency, and proper education for consumption are required. If all these issues are addressed properly, the industry can realize its full potential and make a positive contribution to improving the health of the public.

22.6 Third-party certification and its importance for labeling of functional foods

With the growth in the functional food market comes increased complexity in the products and health claims being made. The consumer landscape is daunting: poorly equipped to understand or validate many of the health claims or ingredient safety. Third-party certification emerged as an important mechanism that provides visibility and confidence in the labeling of functional foods. The contribution of third-party certification in functional food is the focus of this section, emphasizing how it would create greater assurance amongst consumers and improve compliance with regulatory standards to raise the quality of products.

22.6.1 The role of third-party certification

Third-party certification describes the process in which a neutral organization examines a product to make sure that the product has met the standards or claims that might be on its label. Unlike first-party claims, where the manufacturer claims to be doing this or that, third-party certification is far more reliable, as their claims are verified by nonbiased entities that do not have a direct stake in the product under consideration [64,65]. These can vary widely from nutritional content and safety to organic or non-GMO status, even down to specific health benefits claimed by the product. For example, products that are claimed to be "heart-healthy" may undergo rigorous evaluation to ensure that they contain the necessary level of essential nutrients responsible for maintaining heart health [68]. Certification by such recognized bodies (e.g., American Heart Association, NSF International) suggests to consumers that the claims associated with a given product have been tested appropriately and upheld in the well-respected scientific literature [69]. In addition to verifying the health claim, a third-party certification is extremely important for the assurance of the safety of functional foods. For products that include bioactive ingredients or that are marketed to address a specific health need, such protection might be essential [64]. These certification bodies thoroughly examine and analyze these products for potentially toxic pollutants, confirming their ingredient lists as well as having the factories they are produced in by following good manufacturing practices [63,66] (Codex). Overall, this type of third-party certification helps to minimize risks associated with the consumption of functional foods and cranberries safety for consumers [68].

22.6.2 Importance of third-party certification to consumer confidence

With a larger number of products making their claims on health and food products increasingly complicated, consumer trust is such a big factor in the success of the functional food market. External validation of the claims is required. According to [67], third-party certification proves to be effective in bridging this gap of trust of the consumers regarding the claims of functional foods regarding health benefits. The products having the certification logo on the packaging will most likely be trusted by a consumer, who uses these symbols as proof that the product is quality and reliable [64,69]. Third-party certification has the added virtue of giving consumers peace of mind about the ethical and environmental considerations of the products they purchase. Organic USDA, non-GMO Project Verified, or Fair Trade Certified—these certifications assure consumers that such products address certain standards set related to sustainability, ethical sourcing, and environmental impact [66,67] (Codex). This is of special importance in the marketplace where health, environmental, and social impacts of food are the greatest concerns of consumers interest [69]. Third-party certification can also be used in the protection of consumers against false labels. Mislabeling is a huge problem in the functional food industry, with most products exaggerating their health value or making claims for which there is a lack of scientific evidence to support them [63]. To avoid these practices, some certifying bodies have set very strict criteria that must be followed by products before being certified [68] (Williams, 2005).

22.6.3 Compliance with regulatory standards

Third-party certification also provides an added dimension of assurance as far as regulatory standards compliance is concerned. The FDA in the United States and the EFSA in the European Union have developed guidelines on the labeling and marketing of functional foods. However, due to the high variety of such products circulating in the market, it becomes very difficult for these agencies to effectively monitor these products for compliance [63]. Third-party certification bodies have bridged the gap through independent assessment of whether the product meets the requirements (Williams, 2005). It can also serve as a form of risk management for manufacturers especially in the case of third-party certification, since such standards reduce potential litigation related to false advertising or noncompliance with regulations on advertising [69]. Alternatively, the certification logo could also serve as a marketing tool in which products bearing such labels are perceived by consumers to be of higher quality and more trustworthy [64,67].

22.6.4 Improving product quality through certification

Certification with a third party also provides confidence in consumer trust and regulatory compliance, making quality improvement have value. The tough requirements set by a certifying body make it easier for manufacturers to defy the temptation of cutting corners in terms of product formulation, sources, and procedures [63,65]. This can result in safe foods that are commercially successful and help to meet the evolving demands of health-conscious consumers, which also fits into the trend [68]. Besides, the process of certification in most cases is followed by monitoring and reevaluation with the aim that certified products retain their quality over time. Such ongoing oversight can help to avoid degradation of quality and promise that consumers will continue to get benefits from the product [66,69] (Codex). Therefore such third-party certification develops within the functional food market integrity and sustainability. Functional food calls for third-party certification in the same way that everyone wants: another set of eyes to create transparency and consumer trust, or better yet, regulation enforcement. Consumers are saved from false notions attached as health claims or from receiving subquality products due to misleading and unethical practices by the certification bodies working for independent verifications. This process is critical for the market as this one continues to grow, and also in terms of credible quality products relying upon health, a confident third-party certification will be more important than ever.

22.6.5 Certification

Certification can be defined as a process by which a third party provides a written assurance that a product, process, or service meets certain standards (ISO, 1996). It may be viewed as a form of communication down the supply chain. The fact that the certificate is from a third party may be more convincing than if the supplier provided assurance. The certification body or certifier is the organization performing the certification. The certification body might perform the actual inspection itself or subcontract the inspection to an inspector or inspection body. The certification decision, that is, the granting of the written assurance or "certificate," is based on the inspection report, possibly complemented by other sources. Certification is always done by a third party. The verification by an entity not having a direct interest in the economic relationship between supplier and buyer assures unbiasedness. Internal control is a first-party verification. Verification by a buyer of whether the supplier adheres to a standard would be a second-party verification. Third-party verification in no way guarantees neutrality or the absence of conflicting interests. To begin with, any of the parties can set standards. Where the setting of standards is done by the producer or the first party, standards are likely to reflect the interests of the producers. Similarly, where it is set by the buyer or the second party, business interests will be represented in the standard. Second, there are also potential conflicts of interest in case the standard-setting and certification bodies happen to be the same body. The standard-setting body would like to see high implementation rates of its standard or have ideological reasons for being biased against some type of producer, which may affect the certification decision. Third, another conflict of interest might arise depending on who pays for the certification costs. Commercial certification bodies operate in competition with other bodies and, if they are too demanding in their requirements, may lose their customers.

22.7 Consumer education and awareness regarding labeling of functional foods

The major consumption has been by the way of nutrition, but their popularity over time kept increasing for the huge health benefits they deliver. They are sold and advertised as a boost in health, an ability to lower your chances of illness and improve overall wellness. However, their use is generally established on accurate packet labeling and precise interpretation by the consumers. The purpose of the review is to emphasize the position of consumers in consumer education and awareness regarding the labeling of functional food [70].

22.7.1 Importance of functional food labeling

A large portion of the customer base recognizes the potential health benefits associated with consuming functional foods, especially those that are supported by scientific evidence such as probiotics or prebiotics. An important factor in whether customers notice these functionalities is the presence or absence of appropriate labeling [71]. Such labeling is critical because it can inform consumers about the potential different physiological effects these foods may have on their bodies, which will enable them to choose more intelligently based on various health claims attributed to this kind of product [72].

22.7.2 Current labeling practices

Labeling practices for functional foods also vary greatly from country to country. The European Food Safety Authority (EFSA) regulates health claims in the European Union and ensures that the basis for claims is scientifically substantiated [73]. In the United States, the Food and Drug Administration (FDA) oversees health claims but is accused of allowing too many claims that are not strictly evidence-based [74]. Without standardization, consumer comprehension and awareness may vary widely.

22.7.3 Consumer understanding and misconceptions

With greater awareness of health issues among the population, consumers increasingly show interest in such products as people want to feel better about their overall health through better nutrition.

22.7.3.1 Consumer interest and acceptance

There is sufficient evidence that consumer interest in buying functional foods increases significantly with the making of health claims. For example, in a study conducted by [75], as consumers are exposed to functional claims, their preference for enriched products surges from almost 10% in traditional products to 30% in cases where health claims are permitted. That would imply that functional foods are more likely to gain acceptance if consumers perceive some direct health benefit.

22.7.3.2 Information and misinterpretation

While increasing the amount of information about functional foods can widen consumer interest in them, it also increases the risks of misuse and misinterpretation of that information [76]. It is further elucidated in the document that much of this misunderstanding is possibly derived from a lack of knowledge on the part of the creators of these labeling schemes about how human communication works effectively; such may be responsible for the ensuing confusion about the actual benefits of these products by an inability of consumers to process complex information relating to health claims and functional attributes.

22.7.3.3 Credibility and trust

There should be credibility in consumer communication regarding functional foods. This report, therefore, points out that most consumers find producers less credible. Hence, collaboration between producers and public authorities as well as NGOs is necessary to enhance the credibility of the information delivered [77]. The nature of these alliances can, in turn, affect consumer perceptions of trusting information related to functional foods since consumers are likely to take as trusted any information that comes from many credible sources.

22.7.3.4 Need for further research

The complexity of issues surrounding consumer perceptions about functional foods calls for further research in terms of information transmission and interpretation. This report postulates that looking into the way diverse communication strategies can enhance consumer understanding and minimize misconceptions concerning the health benefits of functional foods is important [78]. It also explores the role of risk communication in times of crisis and how this could influence consumer behavior and perceptions.

22.7.4 The role of education in enhancing awareness

Food education is going to be very instrumental in the consumers' understanding and education on functional food labeling. Programs aimed at educating consumers in reading and interpreting food

IFT and other organizations call for the implementation of educational programs that will increase consumer knowledge about functional foods. The consumer-oriented description of functional foods is a major provision that aims to guarantee the selection for health consciousness. Current practices leading to correct labeling are haphazard at best and nearly unintelligible for many consumers. Education initiatives for standardization would educate consumers and reduce some of the misconceptions. It signals a dedication to enhancing transparency for stakeholders and delivering transparent evidence-based messaging that will enable consumers to easier navigate functional foods.

22.8 Challenges and future prospective in labeling and certification of functional foods

Despite the importance of certification, several challenges exist. The multitude of certification programs can create confusion among consumers. Without a standardized approach to functional food certification, consumers may struggle to comprehend the significance of different certifications, leading to skepticism [79]. Additionally, the lack of universal definitions for terms such as "functional" and "healthy" can complicate the certification landscape, as various organizations may interpret these terms differently [80].

Moreover, certification processes can be time-consuming and costly for manufacturers, especially smaller companies that may have fewer resources. As a result, some manufacturers may choose to forgo certification altogether, potentially jeopardizing consumer safety [81]. Thus balancing the rigor of the certification process with accessibility for manufacturers, especially small and medium enterprises (SMEs), is vital for fostering a sustainable market for functional foods. The future of functional food certification is promising, especially with advancements in technology. Digital tools can enhance transparency and simplify access to certification information. For instance, blockchain technology has been proposed as a method to provide traceable certifications, ensuring that consumers can verify a product's authenticity and the integrity of its supply chain [82]. Collaboration between industry stakeholders, regulatory bodies, and academia can also help address gaps in the current certification landscape. A harmonized approach to certification could streamline processes and enhance efficiency without compromising safety or efficacy [83]. Furthermore, public education campaigns focusing on the importance of certifications can help consumers make better informed decisions about their food choices.

22.9 Conclusion

The market for functional foods has seen a significant expansion over the last decade, driven by increasing consumer awareness and interest in health-endorsing food products beyond basic nutrition. Such implications have been brought about by growing health awareness and the increasing demand for functional foods in response to a rise in diet-based diseases. The increased consumer demand for functional foods in the market highlights now more than ever why accurate and firm certification is key. Consumers are the healthiest in history and are concerned about how much they consume in their diet. An honest, informative label teaches the consumer and allows an informed choice between health goals or dietary preferences. But as we know, functional foods are complex and include several bioactive compounds—often novel ingredients. Label issues in this kind of scenario are quite clear. Health claims must be supported by sound scientific research, and information should be available in a manner that is both easy to understand and accurate. In this regard, organizations like the FSSAI as well as their international counterparts can go a long way by providing certain directions to manufacturers on how food must be manufactured according to specific laid-down norms and standards. However, the effectiveness lies in how well these rules have been enforced and whether they have been done uniformly or not. The smallest laxity in regulation or enforcement could result in misleading labels flooding the markets, confidence among consumers eroding, and harm probably caused. It is this context of uncertainty that makes one recognize the importance of third-party certification as a means to give some guarantee about whether functional food will work. When a product is certified, it means that someone else has examined the products and attested to their meeting certain standards (e.g., organic, non-GMO, or other health-promoting composition). It is hoped that these new certifications will now become trust signals in the marketplace jungle, that is, consumers can feel assured they are buying a specific standard of product and feel safe, and it meets their expectations for quality and safety. Such credible certification generally enhances the credibility of brands and consequently opens up greater possibilities for manufacturers in newer virgin territories. However, the changing face of functional foods indicates the necessity for consumers to continually learn more. It requires the consumer to be prepared for when new products and new health claims start hitting the market. They will need education in trying to understand exactly what the meanings of various labels and certifications are, what the meanings of health claims are, and how to spot a product with substantial scientific evidence supporting it.

Acknowledgment

This research work was supported by Mahidol University.

References

Dietary Supplement Health and Education Act of 1994. (1994),

Dietary Supplements Regulations. New Zealand Food Safety Authority. (1985),

Food Safety and Standards Act. 2006a. https://fssai.gov.in/home/fss-legislation/food-safety-and-standardsact.html.

Food Safety and Standards Act, Reward Scheme for Whistle Blowers. 2006b. https://fssai.gov.in/home/fsslegislation/food-safety-and-standards-act.html.

Food Safety and Standards Authority of India. (2011). *Food safety and standards (Packaging and Labeling) regulations.* FSSAI.

Food Safety and Standards (Packaging and Labeling) Regulation. 2011a. https://fssai.gov.in/home/fsslegislation/fss-regulations.html.

Food Safety and Standards (Packaging and Labeling) Regulations. Food Safety and Standards Authority of India. (2011b),

FSS (Health Supplements, Nutraceuticals, Food for Special Dietary Uses, Foods for Special Medical Purposes, and Probiotic Foods) Regulations Food Safety and Standards Authority of India. (2016),

Health Supplements and Nutraceuticals Regulations. Food Safety and Standards Authority of India. (2020),

Iowa State University. (2000). *What you need to know about new food words – phytochemicals, functional foods, and nutraceuticals,* . Information leaflet. *Iowa State University* (2). IA: Ames.

Joe, M., Regenstein. (2018). (2) Kosher and halal regulations for nutraceutical and functional foods. doi: 10.1016/B978-0-12-816467-9.00036-8

Lee, S. H., & O'Neill, C. E. (2021). Global trends in functional food consumption and healthy eating: Implications for public health promotion. *Journal of Nutritional Science*, *10*e34.

RDC No. 24. (2011),

Regulation (EC) No 1924/2006 on nutrition and health claims made on foods. European Commission. (2012),

SANS, SANS 10330:2014. South African Bureau of Standards. (2014),

Timothy, D., Lytton. (2012). (3) Kosher Certification as a Model of Private Regulation: Third-Party Certification Has Benefits Over Both Government Regulation and Unregulated Markets.

United States Pharmacopeia Dietary Supplement Verification Program. (2024). Guidelines and Standards. Retrieved from https://www.usp.org/

United States Pharmacopeia (USP). (2024). USP Verified Mark. Retrieved from https://www.usp.org/

L.J. Unnevehr and C. Hasler - Health Claims &Labeling Regulation of Functional Foods AgBioForum – Volume 3, Number 1 –2000 – Pages 10-13

Chapter 23

Educating consumers: making informed choices for better health impact

Sofiane Boudalia[1,2], Abderrahmane Aït-Kaddour[3,4], Maria Perez-Jimenez[5], Fernando Capela e Silva[5,6], Anissa Zergui[7,8] and Elsa Lamy[5]

[1]*Université 8 Mai 1945, Département d'Écologie et Génie de l'Environnement, Guelma, Algeria,* [2]*Laboratoire de Biologie, Eau et Environnement, Université 8 Mai 1945 Guelma BP 4010, Guelma, Algeria,* [3]*Université Clermont Auvergne, INRAE, VetAgro Sup, UMRF, Lempdes, France,* [4]*Department of Food Industrial Technology, Universitas Padjadjaran, Bandung, Indonesia,* [5]*MED-Mediterranean Institute for Agriculture, Environment and Development & CHANGE-Global Change and Sustainability Institute, Pólo da Mitra, University of Évora, Apartado 94, Évora, Portugal,* [6]*Department of Medical and Health Sciences, School of Health and Human Development, University of Évora, Évora, Portugal,* [7]*Department of Toxicology, University Hospital of Oran, Oran, Algeria,* [8]*Department of Pharmacy, Faculty of Medicine, University of Oran 1 Ahmed Ben Bella, Oran, Algeria*

23.1 Introduction

In recent years, with the collective awareness regarding the climate emergency and the introduction and execution of 17 interconnected Sustainable Development Goals (SDGs), where four of them are closely related to food systems and nutrition: SGD 1 (no poverty), SGD 2 (zero hunger), SGD 3 (healthy lives and promote well-being), and SGD 12 (responsible consumption and production) (Hassoun et al., 2022; Vermeulen et al., 2020), the consumer has seen their demands and expectations evolve considerably, reflecting a growing desire for a healthier diet, sustainably produced, processed and distributed, deemed safe, natural, fresh, and with high nutritional value (Granato et al., 2020; Topolska et al., 2021).

According to Granato et al. (2017), functional foods are industrially produced or natural foods that, when consistently included in a varied diet and taken in effective quantities, may offer health benefits that go beyond basic nutrition. They can come from traditional and indigenous knowledge (Gok, 2023; Rastogi et al., 2016) or be developed using experimental protocols and clinical trials to establish scientific-based evidences (Assmann et al., 2014; Venkatakrishnan et al., 2019).

From an industrial point of view, the development of functional foods goes through several stages, from conception, design, and optimization to the maturation of different formulations (Granato et al., 2020). Thereby, the incorporation of functional ingredients such as bioactive compounds (phytosterols, antioxidants, omega-3 and other polyunsaturated fatty acids, etc.), probiotics (live microorganisms, when ingested in adequate amounts, provide health advantages to the host) (Plaza-Diaz et al., 2019), prebiotics (specific substrates that nourish and support the growth of beneficial microorganisms in the host's gut) (Zahid et al., 2021), and symbiotics (mixtures of probiotics and prebiotics) (Cukkemane et al., 2020), to the developed functional food requires the use of conventional methods and technologies such as the thermal processing, or other alternative food-processing to improve extraction, protect, and improve bioavailability of bioactive compounds (e.g., supercritical fluids, pulsed electric fields, high hydrostatic pressure, microwaves, ultrasounds) (Granato et al., 2020). More recently, with the emergence of Industry 4.0 technologies, automation, and digitalization have accelerated the discovery and development of functional foods. These technologies also improved manufacturing, productivity, efficiencies, safety, traceability, and quality of functional foods (Hassoun et al., 2022). On the other hand, information technologies, associated particularly with artificial intelligence (AI), are prepared to increase the characterized functional food components available to consumers, discovering and systematically characterizing these natural, effective, and safe bioactive components that respond to specific health needs (Doherty et al., 2021; Kennedy et al., 2020). Consequently, the functional foods market, which had a valuation of USD 145.5 billion in 2022,

Unleashing the Power of Functional Foods and Novel Bioactives. DOI: https://doi.org/10.1016/B978-0-443-28862-3.00023-6

is expected to experience significant growth in the coming years. Projections suggest that by 2029, it will reach a substantial value of USD 223.2 billion, which represents a compound annual growth rate (CAGR) of 6.2% during the forecast period 2023–29 (Industry Research Biz, 2023).

From the literature, several studies reported an increase in acceptance but also awareness of functional foods (Büyükkaragöz et al., 2014; Dolgopolova et al., 2015; Pienwisetkaew et al., 2022), and several factors (drivers and barriers) were reported, such as product characteristics, physical, psychological, sociodemographic, and behavioral consumer characteristics (Baker et al., 2022a). For example, 52% of consumers surveyed in Slovakia are more skeptical and agree on the risks associated with functional foods but not on their benefits. Moreover, gender, education, and income levels appear as determinants that can influence functional food choices (Horská et al., 2023). In Vietnam, a survey was conducted to assess consumer preferences for functional milk powder. The study revealed that participants believed in the benefits of functional food and prioritized products with quality stamps from international certification bodies. However, these preferences were influenced by age and education (Phan et al., 2020). (Zanchini et al., 2022) reported that sociodemographic characteristics, such as education level and gender, as well as lifestyle variables, particularly physical activity, influence consumer behavior. Additionally, the study found that women show a greater interest in and willingness to pay for functional foods.

Therefore education level and the presence of label claims have been identified as two significant factors influencing the choice and consumption of functional foods (Ali & Rahut, 2019; Ballco & De Magistris, 2019). Consequently, to improve human health, providing clear and precise information, along with consumer education, appears to be the most effective strategies to assist, guide, and support consumers in their decision-making process. To the best of our knowledge, this chapter aims to discuss for the first time the determinants (drivers and barriers) documented in the existing literature that can influence consumer choice regarding functional foods. Then, it outlines the strategy for educating consumers to empower them to make informed choices that enhance their overall health and well-being.

23.2 Determinants (drivers and barriers) in functional food choice

23.2.1 Physiology and sensory determinants

Despite the high interest that functional foods have gained, different aspects influence their acceptance by consumers. A review of studies about consumer acceptance of functional foods has been presented (Baker et al., 2022a), from which the authors listed five groups of factors that affect the acquisition/intake of these foods: (1) product characteristics, (2) sociodemographic characteristics, (3) psychological characteristics, (4) behavioral characteristics, and (5) physical characteristics. In the group of product characteristics, overall taste and oral perception appear as one important aspect. Different studies show that most consumers are not willing to sacrifice food taste because of the potential beneficial health effects of these products. There are different examples showing this. In functional bakery products, taste appeared as the factor with the highest importance for acceptance, followed by health effects (Bruschi et al., 2015; Thunström & Nordström, 2015). Similar findings were obtained for dairy products, for example, probiotics-enriched yogurts, for which sensory aspects (including texture and flavor) were reported to be more important than nutritional and health-related aspects (Ávila et al., 2020). Even when increasing the functionality of products where the functional compounds are not usually present, such as chewing gums, the taste still appeared as the main predictor of acceptance (Jung et al., 2020).

The relevance of taste for acceptance of functional food products seems transversal to different countries/regions, based on equivalent conclusions reported in studies made in Sri Lanka (Narayana et al., 2020), India (Jain et al., 2014), or Europe (Annunziata & Vecchio, 2011). But despite food sensory quality being essential for acceptance, the effects of each particular sensory attribute may not be the same for all individuals. For example, for taste and smell, it is known that sensitivity to these sensory aspects varies among individuals, and this different sensitivity may contribute to the diverse responses and levels of acceptance among different consumers. Although most studies about the role of interindividual differences in taste (and other food sensory characteristics) sensitivity have been performed for foods in general and not particularly for functional foods, factors at the personal level may be of interest considering the diversity of compounds considered functional. The role of individual variation in sensory perception will be subsequently summarized.

As it will be detailed in the next section of this chapter, phytonutrients are usually present in the so-called functional foods. Most of these compounds are polyphenols, flavonoids, isoflavones, terpenes, and glucosinolates, which have the shortcoming of providing bitterness, sour taste, astringency, or even other off-flavors to these products, limiting their acceptance (Drewnowski & Gomez-Carneros, 2000). Interindividual variation in bitter taste sensitivity has been studied for roughly one century ago, having been discovered almost by chance when some powders of phenyl-thiocarbamide (PTC) were released in the air, being perceived as intensely bitter by some people in the lab, moderately bitter, or even not bitter at all by others (Guo & Reed, 2001).

This opened the door for subsequent studies using PTC, or 6-n-propyl thiouracil (PROP), resulting in the classification of individuals as supertasters, medium-tasters, or nontasters and linking this with identified polymorphisms in bitter taste receptors (Tepper, 2008).

The link between bitter taste sensitivity and food preferences was suggested in some studies, for example, by observing higher bitter taste sensitivity resulting in lower vegetable acceptance and intake during childhood and adolescence (Dinehart et al., 2006), or in the adult population (Sandell et al., 2014). Nevertheless, this is not consensual, and some authors failed to observe this relationship (De Toffoli et al., 2019; Mohd Nor et al., 2021; Yousaf & Tepper, 2022). In fact, a meta-analysis made some years ago did not find an association between PROP taste sensitivity and food choices, at least in adolescents (Bawajeeh et al., 2020).

Astringency is one of the oral sensory characteristics present in foods that are functional due to the increased levels of polyphenols (particularly tannins). This sensation, usually defined as dry, puckering sensation, leads to food rejection when sensed at high levels. In this case, and as previously reported for bitterness, individuals are not all equal in sensitivity. This different sensitivity has been reported as influencing the liking for phenol-containing foods, with high-sensitive individuals having lower liking levels for these foods (Dinnella et al., 2011). Nevertheless, and similarly to the relationship between bitter taste sensitivity and food acceptance, studies do not show all the same level of association, showing the need for deeper research on this issue.

The difficulty in establishing a linear association between the sensitivity for one particular sensory characteristic and food acceptance/preference may come from the interplay between different oral sensations, which may modulate global food oral perception and acceptance. The interindividual variation in sweet taste sensitivity appears to not affect only preference for sweet foods but is also a factor affecting the preference for bitter/sour foods, such as vegetables, with observations of higher preference for these by individuals more sensitive to sweetness (Louro et al., 2021; Rodrigues et al., 2020). In fact, it appears that acceptance of bitter/sour foods can be linked to the combined sensitivities to bitterness and sweetness (Ervina et al., 2021).

Furthermore, consumers typically hesitate to sacrifice the taste of their food, regardless of any potential health or environmental advantages it may offer. Spirulina is disadvantaged by its distinctive color, which is difficult to conceal when incorporated into food items. The addition of spirulina often results in a blue or greenish hue in the food, which may deter consumer appeal (Moons et al., 2018). Torri et al. (2015) reported that color can negatively affect consumers' acceptability of fiber- and polyphenol-enriched functional tomato purees. On the other hand, the color of the packaging, along with the inclusion of images, can also influence the purchase intention and consumption of functional foods (Ares et al., 2010).

In summary, to better counteract sensory aspects of functional foods, which may appear as a barrier to their acceptance, a better knowledge about how individuals' characteristics in terms of sensory sensitivity can be valuable.

23.2.2 Sociodemographic, lifestyle, and psychological determinants

In the literature, other determinants, such as sociodemographic, psychological, and lifestyle-related drivers, can influence the consumption of functional food (Kraus et al., 2017; Topolska et al., 2021; Zanchini et al., 2022).

Sociodemographic aspects appear to play a key role in the choice and consumption of functional foods. Kraus et al. (2017) reported that gender, age, and education can influence motives for purchasing and consuming functional foods based on quality and organoleptic attributes, packaging and labeling, healthful properties, and functional components. For example, older women between the ages of 35 and 60 with a university education tend to prioritize naturalness, nutritional value, freshness, food safety, and quality. However, young men typically prefer meat products as functional foods. In Vietnam, among consumers buying functional foods online, women represent 76.1% and men represent 23.9% (Quan et al., 2020). Similar findings were observed in Turkey (Gok & Ulu, 2019), Brazil, where women showed higher interest in consuming organic foods enriched with functional properties compared to men (Martins et al., 2020), and also in Germany, where the acceptance of iron-enriched vegetables was associated with the female gender (Welk et al., 2023). There are very few studies instead showing a preference of men for functional food consumption. In Canada, Arenna et al. (2019) reported that male consumers are more interested in pork enhanced with carnosine, which exhibits antiaging properties, compared to women. This gender difference observed in functional food consumption is likely due to females being associated with weight management behaviors (Bryant et al., 2023) and having a higher participation rate in weight control programs compared to men (Elliott et al., 2020; Pagoto et al., 2012), as well as their role in purchasing and preparing food within their household (Bech-Larsen & Scholderer, 2007).

Age also serves as a significant determinant in the selection and consumption of functional foods. Among older individuals (aged 35–60 years), safety, good health, and longevity emerge as primary motivators for consuming functional foods (Kraus et al., 2017). Furthermore, older people pay more attention to health concerns than younger people do (Büyükkaragöz et al., 2014). Viscecchia et al. (2019) reported that young consumers were neither purchasers nor aware of functional mozzarella cheese with health benefits such as reduced fat and enrichment in omega-3. In other previous studies, younger people aged 25 and below seem to be more interested in functional food, which is probably due to their willingness to try new foods and their open-mindedness (Çakiroğlu & Uçar, 2018; Carrillo et al., 2013). In contrast, other studies have indicated that age either has no significant effect or exhibits a negative effect, suggesting that older consumers may not be interested in functional foods (Annunziata & Mariani, 2019; Arenna et al., 2019). Regarding income, Szakály et al. (2019) reported that in Hungary, income and education positively influence the willingness to pay for foods enriched with vitamins or minerals (e.g., vitamin C), such as muesli, and probiotic products containing live flora (e.g., yogurt and kefir). Furthermore, higher income levels are associated with a greater interest in enhanced pork for carnosine (Arenna et al., 2019). Moreover, Italian unmarried female consumers' with higher income showed more willingness to pay for eggs enriched with omega-3 fatty acids (Palmieri et al., 2022), likely due to the increased purchasing power afforded by higher income (Carrillo et al., 2013). In line, findings from a web-based survey, conducted on 342 consumers, reported that the higher income and educational levels of respondents play important roles in the willingness to pay for functional pasta (Palmieri et al., 2021). In Slovakia, Horská et al. (2023) reported that skeptical consumers attach more importance to price and price discounts when buying functional foods. The "level of education" significantly influences the acceptability and consumption of functional foods among Pakistani consumers. The positive and highly significant coefficient of respondents' years of education suggests that educated individuals are more aware and inclined to consume a greater variety of functional foods. However, the presence of children within the family seems to decrease functional foods consumption (Ali & Rahut, 2019). Other studies in other regions across the globe have confirmed these results (Çakiroğlu and Uçar, 2018; Kraus et al., 2017; Szakály et al., 2019).

The *origin* and the *geographic location* can indeed influence the willingness to pay for and consumption of functional food. Variations in willingness to pay for functional bread rolls and biscuit bakery products were documented between Moscow and Irkutsk (Bruschi et al., 2015). Similar findings were reported between consumers from Coastal Croatia and Continental Croatia areas (Gajdoš Kljusuric et al., 2015), as well as between Chinese and German consumers regarding functional yogurt and soup (Siegrist et al., 2015).

Lifestyle and health aspects can significantly influence consumer behavior toward the consumption of functional food. Melbye et al. (2015) reported that physical body size has a positive effect on the purchase intentions of functional energy drinks. Moreover, sports activities and body mass index were found to be positively correlated with the willingness to pay for functional probiotics-catechin-yogurt (Moro et al., 2015). However, in another study, sports consumers reported a lower willingness to pay for functional bread rolls and biscuit bakery products (Bruschi et al., 2015). Other factors may also influence the willingness to pay for and the consumption of functional food include marital status and smoking status (Baker et al., 2022a; Moro et al., 2015).

Psychological aspects can influence consumer behavior toward functional food (Baker et al., 2022b). According to previous studies, a good level of *knowledge* regarding functional foods can increase the attitude toward these products positively (Szakály et al., 2019). Moreover, nutritional knowledge stands out as the most critical factor influencing consumer acceptance of such products (Topolska et al., 2021). In Italy, Viscecchia et al. (2019) reported that informed purchasers (with knowledge) consume more functional food than apathetic consumers.

Beliefs is another psychological determinant that may drive functional food consumption. Previous studies have shown that consumers who perceive functional foods as capable of enhancing their well-being and quality of life are more likely to accept them. For example, the willingness to pay for enriched mozzarella cheese is highly related to self-efficacy beliefs and the potential expectations from omega-3 consumption (Vecchio et al., 2016). Furthermore, in Hungary, a strong relationship between attitudes toward functional foods (e.g., willingness to pay for) and beliefs (e.g., protecting health effects) was reported (Szakály et al., 2019).

23.2.3 Nutritional and health benefits determinants

Functional foods provide a spectrum of health benefits that extend beyond their nutritional properties. These health benefits are one of the drivers for consumers (Topolska et al., 2021), who are more health conscious and who seek not just sustenance but enhanced well-being. Additionally, as it has been previously mentioned, the higher the consumers' nutritional knowledge about functional foods, the higher their acceptance (Baker et al., 2022b). Therefore understanding the benefits of functional foods is crucial to make them more attractive to consumers.

The beneficial impact of functional foods is due to the bioactive compounds they contain. These bioactive compounds can interact with body cells, tissues, or bacteria through different mechanisms, resulting in a positive effect on body health (improvement of well-being and/or reduction of disease risk) (Jaime & Santoyo, 2021). One bioactive compound can act at different levels in the organism, thus providing a variety of potential effects. While one functional food can contain various bioactive compounds, thus presenting more than one beneficial impact on human well-being (Serrano et al., 2015). However, to obtain the nutritional and health benefits of bioactive compounds, they must be regularly consumed in the quantities found in normal food rations and included in a varied diet (Jaime & Santoyo, 2021).

Bioactive compounds are molecules and microorganisms of great diversity, including vitamins, minerals, nitrogen compounds, bioactive peptides, carotenoids, phenolic compounds, bioactive lipids, sulfur compounds, phytosterols, prebiotics, and probiotics, among others (Mallhi et al., 2020; Riccardi, 2022). Natural sources of bioactive compounds are legumes, fruits, meat, fish, eggs, fungi, algae, or fermented products, among others (Câmara et al., 2021). Despite all these known sources, novel bioactive compounds are still being identified in potential food products from different origins (e.g., microalgae) (Ghosh et al., 2022; Hassan et al., 2022). Bioactive compounds can also be isolated or synthesized, then used as bioactive ingredients by incorporating them into ultra-processed food products (which do not contain functional properties themselves), thus turning them into functional foods with a positive health influence. In this regard, ultra-processed foods supplemented with bioactive ingredients that do not occur in them but that match with the food product (e.g., muesli bar with linseed) are better perceived by consumers, which can determine their purchase intention (Temesi et al., 2019).

On the other hand, as has been previously detailed, one of their main barriers to the acceptance of functional foods by consumers is the expected sensory characteristics associated with them. Indeed, some studies revealed that taste can be more relevant for consumers than the health benefits of functional foods, since consumers are unwilling to sacrifice taste for the positive impact of functional foods (Baker et al., 2022a). The undesirable flavor of some functional foods might be related to the presence of bioactive compounds that are associated with disagreeable sensory characteristics (e.g., bitterness). Despite being combined with other ingredients, the sensory properties of some bioactive compounds may determine the perception of food, thus causing their rejection or acceptance by consumers. In Table 23.1, some examples of bioactive compounds, their health and nutritional benefits, and their related sensory properties are shown.

23.2.4 Nutrition labeling legislation and regulations determinants

Nutritional labeling is a strong factor influencing consumers' purchase decisions toward food products. In the case of functional foods, in addition to nutritional labeling, health-related claims can also appear on the label. These health-related claims are the link with consumers, as they provide information about the relationship between health and diet. Some studies showed that the appearance of health claims could have a positive influence on consumer purchase decisions, even more than the proper packaging, and increase the interest in buying a food product (Domínguez Díaz et al., 2020; Hieke et al., 2016). In addition to that, health-related claims encourage consumers to make better food choices, potentially improving their eating patterns (Domínguez Díaz et al., 2020; Hieke et al., 2016). These claims are, therefore, drivers for consumers to buy functional foods.

Regarding health-related claims, consumers prefer those that are short, include qualifying words (e.g., reduce), and have positive connotations (Domínguez Díaz et al., 2020; Hieke et al., 2016). Additionally, more understandable claims and referring to generally known nutrients or ingredients are considered more truthful and reliable, thus increasing consumers' purchase intentions. While those claims referring to nutrients or ingredients too familiar for consumers decrease their interest and purchase intention (EUFIC, 2017).

As these claims seem to influence consumer choices, specific regulations must control them. Although various entities and countries have provided definitions of functional foods, there is still no official definition agreed upon by all authorities to define what a functional food is (Temple, 2022). The lack of unanimity in global regulation has led to discrepancies among countries in both the concept of functional foods and their approval processes.

As an example, Fig. 23.1 shows an overview of the regulatory frameworks (entities and laws/acts) of functional foods in Japan, the United States, and the European Union (EU), and the types of nutrition and health claims in foods approved by each jurisdiction. These have been selected as one representative country with available regulation of the three continents: North America, Asia, and Europe.

Looking at this scheme (Fig. 23.1) can be seen that, although food claims are similar in part among these countries (Japan, United States, and the EU), the approval process, the use, and the regulatory framework and entities are quite

TABLE 23.1 Examples of bioactive compounds, health/nutritional benefits, related sensory properties, and examples of both low/medium and ultra-processed foods in which the bioactive compounds can be found.

Family	Bioactive compounds	Health benefits	Sensory characteristic	Unprocessed or minimally processed foods and processed culinary ingredients[a]	Processed and ultra-processed foods[a]	References
Vitamins	Thiamin (B_1) Riboflavin (B_2) Niacin (B_3) Pantothenic acid (B_5) Pyridoxine (B_6) Biotin (B_8) Folic acid (B_9) Cyanocobalamin (B_{12}) Vitamin A Vitamin C Vitamin D Vitamin E Vitamin K	Cellular function Antioxidant Immune response Bone growth Absorption and Metabolism of nutrients	B_1: sour-bitter, burning and pungent B_2: bitter, dry, minerally, and stale B_3: bitter B_5: sweetish taste and slightly bitter aftertaste B_6: slightly bitter saline taste and acid B_8: no info B_9: tasteless B_{12}: tasteless, dry, thick and flat Vitamin A: stale chemical tasting Vitamin C: sour, tingling and sharp Vitamin D: tasteless, dry, thick and flat Vitamin E: fatty, undesirable tasting Vitamin K: moderately sweet	Fruits, seeds, roots, fungi, nuts, fish, meat, eggs, milk, etc.	Canned vegetables, legumes, cured meats and fish (processed) Breakfast cereals or biscuits fortified with B vitamins, Margarine fortified with vitamin E, A, or D (ultra-processed)	(Uribe et al., 2017)
Minerals	Calcium (Ca) Iron (Fe) Sodium (Na) Magnesium (Mg) Phosphorus (P) Potassium (K) Iodine (I) Selenium (Se) Copper (Cu) Zinc (Zn) Manganese (Mn)	Bone health Nervous system function Digestion Metabolism Cell growth	Sodium chloride: salty Potassium chloride: salty, bitter, metallic Calcium chloride: bitter, salty Magnesium chloride: bitter Lithium chloride: salty, sour Sodium sulfate: salty, bitter Calcium sulfate: salty, bitter Ferrous sulfate: metallic Copper sulfate: bitter, astringent, metallic Sodium nitrate: untasty Calcium nitrate: salty, bitter	Fruits, seeds, roots, fungi, nuts, fish, meat, eggs, milk, etc.	Bread (processed) Plant-based milks fortified with Calcium, Iron (ultra-processed)	(Delompré et al., 2019; (Gebregewergis et al., 2020)
Nitrogen compounds and non-essential bioactive peptides	Amino acids Nucleotides, Caseins, Whey proteins, Lactoferrin, Lactoglobulins, Albumin, Lactoalbumins, Seroalbumin, Growth factors, Nisine, Lysozyme, Ovalbumin, Ovotransferrin	Immune system support Antihypertensive Antithrombotic Antioxidant Opioid activity	L-Alanine: sweet L-Asparagine: bitter L-Aspartic acid: umami, sour L-Arginine: bitter L-Cysteine: sulfurous L-Glutamic acid: umami, salty L-Glycine: sweet L-Proline: sweet L-Tyrosine: bitter L-Serine: sweet	Eggs, legumes, nuts, milk, fish, meat, yogurt, etc.	Cheese (processed) Whey protein powder shakes supplemented with proteins or peptides, Infant formulas (ultra processed)	(Delompré et al., 2019; Mirzapour-Kouhdasht et al., 2023; Zaky et al., 2022)

Phenolic compounds	Phenolic acids Flavonoids (Anthocyanidins, Flavanones, Flavones, Isoflavones, Flavan-3-ols, Flavonols) Tannins Stilbenes Lignans	Antioxidant Antiinflammatory Cardiovascular health Metabolic syndrome Osteoporosis Diabetes Brain-related diseases	Benzoic acids: bitter, astringent Hydroxycinnamic acids: bitter, sweet, astringent, cinnamon Stilbenes (resveratrol): bitter, astringent Flavan-3-ols: bitter, astringent Isoflavones, flavonones, flavonols, flvanones: bitter Anthocyanidins: purple, blue, Anthocyanins: red Flavones, flavonols: brown, white	Berries, citrus fruits, red grapes, nuts, tea, coffee, herbs and spices, etc.	Fruit juices without sugar (processed) Dark chocolate, snack bars fortified with phenolic-rich sources (ultra-processed)	(Matsumura et al., 2023; Sharma et al., 2021)
Carotenoids	β-Carotene α-Carotene Lycopene Lutein Astaxanthin Zeaxanthin Capsanthin	Antioxidant Ocular health Skin protection and sun sensitivity Regulate gene transcription	β-Carotene: red, orange α-Carotene, lutein, zeaxanthin: yellow, orange Lycopene: red	Carrots, sweet potatoes, spinach, kale, bell peppers, tomatoes, mangoes, papayas, etc.	Pureed vegetables, fresh vegetable juices (processed) Smoothies fortified with carotenoid-rich extracts (ultra-processed)	(Cooperstone & Schwartz, 2016)
Non-carotenoid terpenes	Terpenes Terpenoids Phenylpropanoids	Antiinflammatory Antioxidant Antibacterial Anticancer	Aromas related to citrus, floral, herb, and green notes.	Citrus fruits, ginger, Herbs, spices, mint, herbal teas, vegetable oils, etc.	Bread, fruit in syrup (processed) Sausages, minced beef fortified with flavorings (ultra-processed)	(Masyita et al., 2022)
Bioactive lipids	Monounsaturated Fatty Acids: oleic acid. Polyunsaturated Fatty Acids: linoleic acid, α-linolenic acid, eicosapentaenoic acid (EPA), docosahexaenoic acid (DHA), linoleic acid, arachidonic acid, conjugated linoleic acid (CLA)	Cardiovascular health Antiinflammatory Antioxidative stress Improve lipid profile and cholesterol	Oleic acid: metallic, astringent, bitter α-Linoleic acid: irritant, metallic bitter Provide a smooth texture Fish taste	Salmon, sardines, avocado, nuts, eggs, vegetable oils, whole grains, etc.	Canned fish or meat in olive oil (processed) Margarines, milk, biscuits fortified with unsaturated fatty acids (ultra-processed)	(Delompré et al., 2019; Liu et al., 2023)
Sulfur compounds	Glucosinolates (aliphatic, indole, and aromatic derivatives) Organosulfur compounds (alliin, allicin, diallyl sulfide derivatives, cysteine sulfoxide derivatives)	Anticancer Antioxidant Antiinflammatory Cardiovascular health Immune system modulation Central nervous system protection	Sulfurous aroma/odor The earthy and musky aroma Pungent Bitter taste Slightly sweet (e.g., onions) Lachrymatory (induce tearing or irritation to the eyes)	Cauliflower, garlic, onions, broccoli, brussels sprouts, cabbage, kale, black truffles, etc.	Garlic oil, canned or bottled cruciferous (processed) Condiments and sauces containing sulfur compounds (ultra-processed)	(Miękus et al., 2020)

(Continued)

TABLE 23.1 (Continued)

Family	Bioactive compounds	Health benefits	Sensory characteristic	Unprocessed or minimally processed foods and processed culinary ingredients[a]	Processed and ultra-processed foods[a]	References
Phytosterols	β-sitosterol, Campesterol, Stigmasterol, Brassicasterol, campestanol, β-sitostanol	Cholesterol reduction Maintain heart health Antiinflammatory Antioxidant	Chalky taste Undesirable flavors	Almonds, walnuts, sunflower seeds, whole grains, vegetable oils, etc.	Almond, sunflower seeds with salt (processed) Margarines and dairy alternatives (e.g., plant-based milk) fortified with phytosterols (ultra-processed)	(Hu et al., 2022; (Uddin et al., 2018); Tolve et al., 2020)
Prebiotics	Inulin Fructooligosaccharides (FOS) Galactooligosaccharides Resistant Starch Glucose-derived oligosaccharides Pectic oligosaccharide	Improved gut health, Modulate the composition, population, and function of gut microbiota	Texturising, gelling agents (used as fat substitutes) Sweeteners (less than sucrose) Inulin: neutral to sweet taste FOS: fruity smell	Asparagus, sugar beet, garlic, chicory root, onion, wheat, honey, banana, barley, tomato, rye, soybean, peas, beans, chickpeas, lentils, and whole grains	Bread (low processed) Breakfast cereals fortified with dietary fiber, sausages, ice creams, and processed meats with inulin as a substitute of fat (ultra-processed)	(Davani-Davari et al., 2019)
Probiotics	Lactobacillus: *L. acidophilus, L.casei, L. plantarum.* Bifidobacterium: *B. bifidum, B. longum, B. breve* *Saccharomyces boulardii*: A yeast commonly used as a probiotic; not a bacterium. Others: *B. subtilis, B. licheniformis, E. faecalis, E. faecium, L. lactis*, etc.	Enhanced gut health Balancing gut microbiota Supporting digestive health Enhancing immune function Modulating inflammation	Probiotics themselves do not have distinctive flavors. However, the addition of probiotics may alter the taste and aroma of the final food product due to the production of different metabolites (e.g., organic acids, and aldehyde) during fermentation and extended storage.	Yogurt, kéfir, pickles, sauerkraut, etc.	Cheese, buttermilk (processed) Kombucha, fermented soy products (miso, tempeh) (ultra-processed)	(Das et al., 2022; Terpou et al., 2019)

[a]*Foods classified in minimally, processed, or ultrapocessed according to NOVA classification system (Monteiro et al., 2019).*

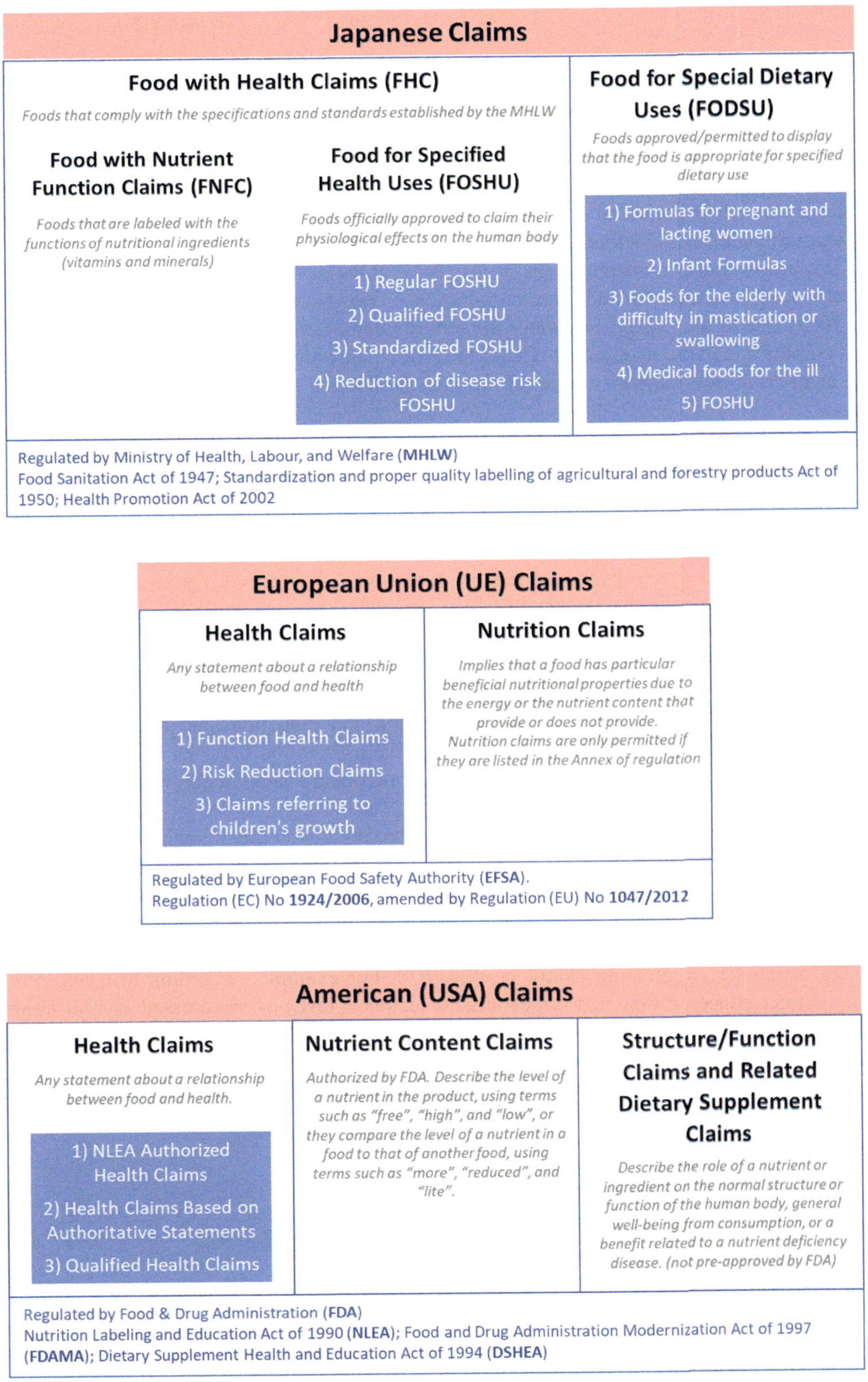

FIGURE 23.1 Overview of the type of food claims approved in Japan, the European Union (EU), and the United States (EFSA) (FDA) (MHLW).

different. As a result, there are different approval periods and processes, which are more or less strict and delayed depending on the law in each area. These variations in regulations can influence how health-related information is communicated to consumers and can increase the difficulty of the food industry in marketing functional food products internationally. Therefore, the differences in the regulatory framework can be a barrier for consumers in their choice of functional foods.

23.2.5 Sustainability and environmental impacts determinants

Given the climate crisis and the progress of science, consumers are increasingly seeking products that are healthy and are also showing a heightened concern for the environmental impact of these products (Hélias et al., 2022; Michell et al., 2020). Furthermore, exploring new categories of functional foods would not only meet the annually rising demand but also offer an ecological rationale for the adoption of the most environmentally friendly production technologies (Miniakhmetova et al., 2022). In this context, current areas of interest involve the production of functional foods using fewer inputs, the utilization of food by-products, and the incorporation of Eco-Scores on packaging to guide consumer choices (De Bauw et al., 2022; Lee et al., 2021). To assess the environmental impacts and resources utilized in food production, research studies employ life cycle assessment (LCA) to analyze the value chain throughout a product's life. This analysis encompasses stages from raw material extraction through production and extends to product use and disposal (Nemecek et al., 2024).

The environmental impact weight in both conventional and functional food choices remains poorly studied. While a few studies indicate more pro-environmental food choices resulting from Eco-Scores alone, a survey in a Belgian supermarket reveals that the adoption of an easily interpretable environmental information label enhances the overall eco-friendliness of consumers' food consumption by approximately 5.3% (Vlaeminck et al., 2014). In China, men tend to be more responsive to calorie labels, whereas they are less steered by environmental labels compared to women (Sun et al., 2024). Grunert et al. (2014) reported a low level of sustainability label use (e.g., Carbon Footprint, Fair Trade, Animal Welfare, and Rainforest Alliance) in France, the United Kingdom, Poland, Germany, Sweden, and Spain using an online survey with 4408 respondents.

In Italy, consumers of table grapes displayed a stronger inclination toward health-related properties over sustainability features. These features encompass organic production, sustainable packaging, reduced pesticide and chemical inputs, environmental certification, locally sourced products, waste valorization and reduction, and fair remuneration for workers (Seccia et al., 2019). Pappalardo & Lusk (2016) reported a negative association between beliefs regarding the environmental impact of functional foods and the willingness to pay for functional snacks made with white lupine and citrus fiber.

Innovation in production processes is also considered a crucial factor, as interventions in this domain can yield beneficial effects on the environment. The utilization of subcritical water extraction, pressurized hot water extraction, and supercritical fluid extraction can eliminate the need for organic solvents in extract production, thereby reducing the environmental impact associated with the manufacturing of functional foods (Leo and Ong). Moreover, numerous phenolic compounds have been successfully synthesized and optimized in model organisms, such as *Escherichia coli* and *Saccharomyces cerevisiae*, through metabolic engineering (Mark et al., 2019). For example, according to Chen et al. (2017), the optimization of yeast extract concentration in a triacetic acid lactone (TAL)-overexpressed *E. coli* strain resulted in the production of 475.4 ± 19.9 mg/L of *p*-Coumaric acid. In another study, the environmental impacts of obtaining 1 g of extracted polyphenols, used as an ingredient in functional food, from seaweed using ultrasound-assisted extraction were evaluated. The findings indicate that this method has significantly lower impacts compared to the conventional solvent-based method (Priyadarshini et al., 2022).

23.3 Educating consumers in functional food choice

In the last two decades, the interest of consumers in having more information about food, nutrition, and health has increased dramatically. Different aspects, like obesity epidemics, preoccupation with getting a "perfect body" through a "perfect diet," and constant communication about the health benefits of foods or food components, resulted in more awareness among consumers about healthy eating (Toner & Pitman, 2004). The demand for health-enhanced foods, such as foods with fiber-added, probiotics, and organic foods, increased. However, the information people get from different sources (media, social media, influencers, etc.) is not always translated into real knowledge and can create myths, such as the case of "clean" eating, resulting in unbalanced diets with potentially negative health outcomes (Ambwani et al., 2020).

Some studies showed that social media is an important source of nutritional and health information nowadays. Facebook, Instagram, or X (former Twitter) are good examples of web places that people recognize as sources of inspiration and connections for healthy food habits (Mete et al., 2019). But, if this can be advantageous for food and health practitioners to share their message and educate people, this can also have a dark side, which, if not well filtered by the reader, may result in health problems related to body image and food choices (Rounsefell et al., 2020). Nutritional labeling is current, nowadays, in most products, but this is not necessarily linked to healthier food choices since we still face health problems related to bad eating habits (Miller et al., 2022). Despite the lack of a consensual definition, food literacy can be considered as a concept referring to the ability to obtain, process, and understand information about food and the competence to use that information in ways that positively impact health and well-being (Palumbo, 2016). Food literacy can be an important aspect of informed food choices (Fernandez et al., 2019; Wijayaratne et al., 2018), as well as education (e.g., school level and study of scientific areas). Gao et al. (2023), observed that food literacy differs among people with different demographics but also depends on academic performance and whether they receive nutritional education or not. This link of food literacy to a specific education in nutritional sciences was also observed in other studies (e.g., Trieste et al., 2021), supporting the thought that higher education levels, although generally linked to healthier food patterns (e.g., Azizi Fard et al., 2021) cannot be assumed for all scientific areas and that more efforts need to be put into guaranteeing higher food literacy for the population in general. The observation that individuals with higher educational levels eat healthier (e.g., lower levels of total carbohydrates, including simple sugars) (Azizi Fard et al., 2021) cannot exclude the possibility of an effect of economic condition since higher education is, in general, associated with higher economic capacity. It is important to note that retail prices of functional foods are typically higher compared to conventional foods, which is a key factor influencing consumer behavior associated with these food products (Huang et al., 2019; Jaeger, 2006).

Concerning functional foods, labels have been shown to influence acceptance (Oliveira et al., 2016), despite the influence of labels being dependent on individuals' attitudes (psychological variables). A more positive attitude toward functional foods positively influences health claim valuation by individuals (Contini et al., 2023). Moreover, consumers with higher nutritional knowledge and food literacy were observed to be more positive toward functional foods (Ares et al., 2008; Žeželj et al., 2012). In a meta-analysis, Baker et al. (2022b) reported the existence of a small positive relationship between the level of food and nutritional knowledge and functional food acceptance. As well, these authors related that most of the individuals studied so far had low nutrition-related knowledge associated with consuming functional foods.

Altogether, the existing literature points to the relevance that providing education and enhancing knowledge appear to be the most effective strategies to assist, guide, and support consumers in their decision-making process regarding functional food (Alongi & Anese, 2021). On the other hand, dissemination represents the act of sharing knowledge among different stakeholders to enhance efficiency and perennialization. Concerning functional food, several studies have reported that an uninformed consumer becomes more suspicious and fearful and is less likely to consume new foods developed using new technologies (Giordano et al., 2018). Consequently, newly developed scientific evidence communicated during various scientific meetings can contribute to the promotion of innovative functional foods within the scientific community. Moreover, educating consumers is crucial to increasing their actual knowledge and making informed choices regarding newly developed functional foods and their health benefits (Deborah et al., 2021). In this regard, schools appear to be an effective platform for promoting the consumption of functional foods. Students can gain early exposure to the concepts surrounding functional foods, fostering a culture of understanding and acceptance from a young age. In Portugal, (Oliveira et al., 2023) reported that food education sessions improved the perception of functional food in 70% of enrolled students. Finally, it is important to note that engagement with policymakers is necessary to advocate for policies that promote consumer awareness and facilitate the integration of functional foods into dietary guidelines and public health initiatives (Domínguez Díaz et al., 2020).

23.4 Final remarks and future perspectives

Over the past decades, functional foods have undergone rapid development, and today they hold a significant place in our diet (Bigliardi & Galati, 2013). According to Granato et al. (2020), the creation and development of functional foods require strong interaction among food scientists, technologists, and clinicians. Above all, it also requires a battery of tests to support any health claims. However, it is very important to note that its acceptance by the consumer is also important during its development (Zanchini et al., 2022). This acceptance is subjected to several determinants, such as physiological, sociodemographic, lifestyle, health, and environmental labeling, that can drive or hinder consumer choices (Fig. 23.2.

Currently, to ensure its sustainable development, it is essential to understand these determinants. The use of vegetable waste as an alternative to traditional protein sources should increase functional food development (Pattnaik et al., 2021). Moreover, the introduction of Industry 4.0 technologies, such as Big Data (BD), deep learning, and AI

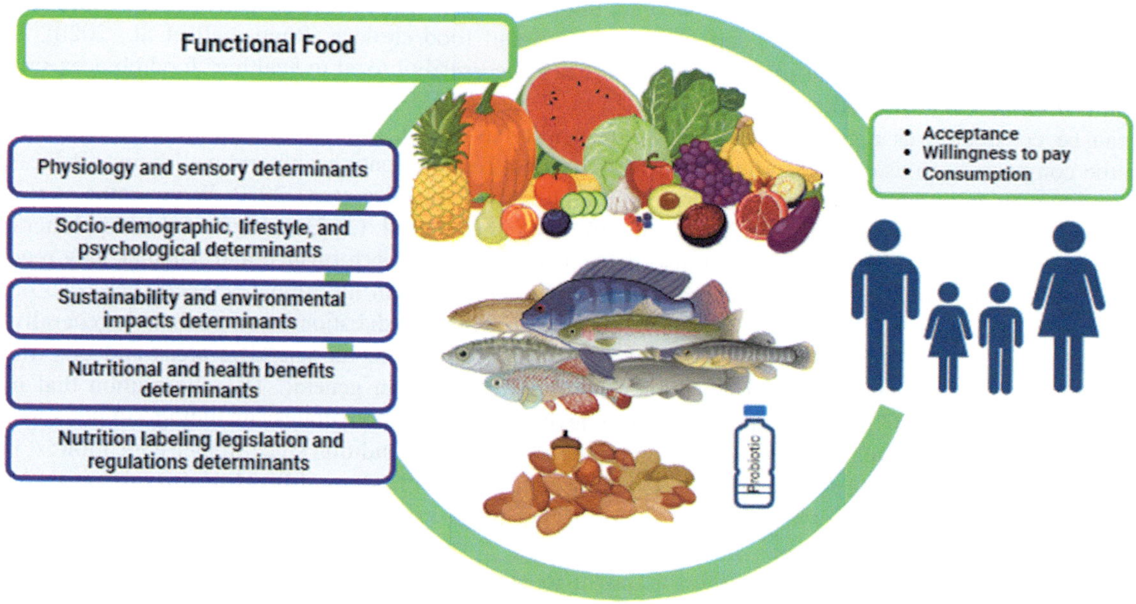

FIGURE 23.2 Determinants (drivers and barriers) in functional food choice.

technologies, can be used to evaluate data produced at all stages of the supply chain. For example, the incorporation of AI into the natural bioactive discovery and characterization process enables the prediction of bioactive molecules with predefined health benefits. It also facilitates the selection of the most appropriate source rich in these bioactives (Doherty et al., 2021). (Rein et al., 2019) reported that using deep learning models and molecular docking simulations, it is possible to predict and unlock inflammation-modulating peptides from Asian rice proteins. In another study, the Internet of Things (IoT) and AI were used to optimize the production and extraction of algal protein during functional food processing (Neo et al., 2023).

23.5 Conclusion

This chapter critically synthesized the determinants (drivers and barriers) that can influence, guide, and support consumers in their choices regarding functional food perception, acceptance, buying, and consumption. Furthermore, it outlines the strategy for educating consumers to empower them to make informed choices that enhance their overall health and well-being. Pushing functional food success requires a deep understanding of key determinants that shape consumer acceptance. Through the examined studies, these determinants have been categorized into distinct domains: physiology and sensory perception; sociodemographic, lifestyle, and psychological; nutritional and health benefits; nutrition labeling, legislation, and regulations; sustainability and environmental impacts determinants.

On the other hand, educating consumers and enhancing their knowledge appear to be the most effective strategies to improve their decision-making process regarding functional food. Dissemination and perennialization of adequate knowledge and evidence-based communication among different stakeholders seem to be the most promising ways to increase consumers' interest in these kinds of products. Achieving this objective requires the development of diverse programs implemented at school levels, scientific seminars, and engagements with policymakers. Finally, extensive research is required to overcome the challenges involved in the adoption of new technologies during the development of functional food.

Acknowledgments

The authors would like to express their sincere gratitude to Professor Aissam BOUSBIA for his valuable comments and insights on the manuscript.

Funding

This research received no specific grant from any funding agency in the public, commercial, or not-for-profit sectors.

Conflicts of Interest

The authors have stated that they have no conflicts of interest to declare.

Author Contributions

Sofiane Boudalia, Abderrahmane Aït-Kaddour, Maria Perez-Jimenez, Fernando Capela e Silva, Anissa Zergui, and Elsa Lamy: supervision, conceptualization, investigation, writing original draft, review, and editing. All authors have thoroughly reviewed and provided their consent to the final version of the manuscript for publication.

Data availability

The manuscript includes all the necessary data, which are presented in the body of the text, tables, and figures.

Ethical statement

None to be declared.

References

Ali, A., & Rahut, D. B. (2019). Healthy foods as proxy for functional foods: Consumers' awareness, perception, and demand for natural functional foods in Pakistan. *International Journal of Food Science, 2019*. Available from https://doi.org/10.1155/2019/6390650, http://www.hindawi.com/journals/ijfs/.

Alongi, M., & Anese, M. (2021). Re-thinking functional food development through a holistic approach. *Journal of Functional Foods, 81*, 104466. Available from https://doi.org/10.1016/j.jff.2021.104466.

Ambwani, S., Sellinger, G., Rose, K. L., Richmond, T. K., & Sonneville, K. R. (2020). It's healthy because it's natural." Perceptions of "clean" eating among U.S. adolescents and emerging adults. *Nutrients, 12*(6), 1–11. Available from https://doi.org/10.3390/nu12061708, https://www.mdpi.com/2072-6643/12/6/1708/pdf.

Annunziata, A., & Mariani, A. (2019). Do consumers care about nutrition and health claims? Some evidence from Italy. *Nutrients, 11*(11), 2735. Available from https://doi.org/10.3390/nu11112735.

Annunziata, A., & Vecchio, R. (2011). Factors affecting Italian consumer attitudes toward functional foods. *AgBioForum, 14*(1), 20–32. Available from: http://www.agbioforum.org/v14n1/v14n1a03-annunziata.pdf.

Arenna, E., Goddard, V., & Muringai. (2019). Consumer purchase intentions for pork with enhanced carnosine–A functional food. *Canadian Journal of Agricultural Economics/Revue canadienne d'agroeconomie, 67*(2), 151–169. Available from https://doi.org/10.1111/cjag.12190.

Ares, G., Besio, M., Giménez, A., & Deliza, R. (2010). Relationship between involvement and functional milk desserts intention to purchase. Influence on attitude towards packaging characteristics. *Appetite, 55*(2), 298–304. Available from https://doi.org/10.1016/j.appet.2010.06.016.

Ares, G., Giménez, A., & Gámbaro, A. (2008). Influence of nutritional knowledge on perceived healthiness and willingness to try functional foods. *Appetite, 51*, 663–668. Available from https://doi.org/10.1016/j.appet.2008.05.061.

Assmann, G., Buono, P., Daniele, A., Della Valle, E., Farinaro, E., Ferns, G., Krogh, V., Kromhout, D., Masana, L., Merino, J., Misciagna, G., Panico, S., Riccardi, G., Rivellese, A. A., Rozza, F., Salvatore, F., Salvatore, V., Stranges, S., Trevisan, M., ... Vetrani, C. (2014). Functional foods and cardiometabolic diseases. International Task Force for Prevention of Cardiometabolic Diseases. *Nutrition, Metabolism, and Cardiovascular Diseases, 24*(12), 1272–1300. Available from https://doi.org/10.1016/j.numecd.2014.10.010, http://www.elsevier.com/wps/find/journaldescription.cws_home/704955/description#description.

Ávila, B. P., da Rosa, P. P., Fernandes, T. A., Chesini, R. G., Sedrez, P. A., de Oliveira, A. P. T., Mota, G. N., Gularte, M. A., & Roll, V. F. B. (2020). Analysis of the perception and behaviour of consumers regarding probiotic dairy products. *International Dairy Journal, 106*. Available from https://doi.org/10.1016/j.idairyj.2020.104703, www.elsevier.com/inca/publications/store/4/0/5/8/6/0/index.htt.

Azizi Fard, N., De Francisci Morales, G., Mejova, Y., & Schifanella, R. (2021). On the interplay between educational attainment and nutrition: A spatially-aware perspective. *EPJ Data Science, 10*(1). Available from https://doi.org/10.1140/epjds/s13688-021-00273-y, http://www.epjdatascience.com/about.

Baker, M. T., Lu, P., Parrella, J. A., & Leggette, H. R. (2022a). Consumer acceptance toward functional foods: A scoping review. *International journal of environmental research and public health, 19*(3). Available from https://doi.org/10.3390/ijerph19031217, https://www.mdpi.com/1660-4601/19/3/1217/pdf.

Baker, M. T., Lu, P., Parrella, J. A., & Leggette, H. R. (2022b). Investigating the effect of consumers' knowledge on their acceptance of functional foods: A systematic review and meta-analysis. *Foods, 11*(8). Available from https://doi.org/10.3390/foods11081135, https://www.mdpi.com/2304-8158/11/8/1135/pdf.

Ballco, P., & De Magistris, T. (2019). Spanish consumer purchase behaviour and stated preferences for yoghurts with nutritional and health claims. *Nutrients, 11*(11), 2742. Available from https://doi.org/10.3390/nu11112742.

Bawajeeh, A. O., Albar, S. A., Zhang, H., Zulyniak, M. A., Evans, C. E. L., & Cade, J. E. (2020). Impact of taste on food choices in adolescence—Systematic review and meta-analysis. *Nutrients, 12*(7), 1–17. Available from https://doi.org/10.3390/nu12071985, https://www.mdpi.com/2072-6643/12/7/1985/pdf.

Bech-Larsen, T., & Scholderer, J. (2007). Functional foods in Europe: Consumer research, market experiences and regulatory aspects. *Trends in Food Science and Technology, 18*(4), 231–234. Available from https://doi.org/10.1016/j.tifs.2006.12.006, http://www.elsevier.com/wps/find/journaldescription.cws_home/601278/description#description.

Bigliardi, B., & Galati, F. (2013). Innovation trends in the food industry: The case of functional foods. *Trends in Food Science and Technology, 31*(2), 118–129. Available from https://doi.org/10.1016/j.tifs.2013.03.006.

Bruschi, V., Teuber, R., & Dolgopolova, I. (2015). Acceptance and willingness to pay for health-enhancing bakery products - Empirical evidence for young urban Russian consumers. *Food Quality and Preference, 46*, 79–91. Available from https://doi.org/10.1016/j.foodqual.2015.07.008.

Bryant, B. L., Wang, C. H., & Monaghan, M. (2023). Weight management behaviors are associated with elevated glycemic outcomes in adolescents and young adults with type 1 diabetes. *Journal of clinical psychology in medical settings, 30*(4), 876–883. Available from https://doi.org/10.1007/s10880-023-09936-6, https://www.springer.com/journal/10880.

Büyükkaragöz, A., Bas, M., Sağlam, D., & Cengiz, Ş. E. (2014). Consumers' awareness, acceptance and attitudes towards functional foods in Turkey. *International Journal of Consumer Studies, 38*(6), 628–635. Available from https://doi.org/10.1111/ijcs.12134, http://onlinelibrary.wiley.com/journal/10.1111/(ISSN)1470-6431.

Çakiroğlu, F. P., & Uçar, A. (2018). Consumer attitudes towards purchasing functional products. *Mattioli 1885, Turkey Progress in Nutrition, 20*(2), 257–262. Available from https://doi.org/10.23751/pn.v20i2.5859, http://www.mattioli1885journals.com/index.php/progressinnutrition/article/download/5859/4830.

Câmara, J. S., Albuquerque, B. R., Aguiar, J., Corrêa, R. C. G., Gonçalves, J. L., Granato, D., Pereira, J. A. M., Barros, L., & Ferreira, I. C. F. R. (2021). Food bioactive compounds and emerging techniques for their extraction: Polyphenols as a case study. *Foods, 10*(1). Available from https://doi.org/10.3390/foods10010037, https://www.mdpi.com/2304-8158/10/1/37/pdf.

Carrillo, E., Prado-Gascó, V., Fiszman, S., & Varela, P. (2013). Why buying functional foods? Understanding spending behaviour through structural equation modelling. *Food Research International, 50*(1), 361–368. Available from https://doi.org/10.1016/j.foodres.2012.10.045.

Chen, Z., Sun, X., Li, Y., Yan, Y., & Yuan, Q. (2017). Metabolic engineering of Escherichia coli for microbial synthesis of monolignols. *Metabolic Engineering, 39*, 102–109. Available from https://doi.org/10.1016/j.ymben.2016.10.021.

Contini, C., Grunert, K., Nyland Christensen, R., Boncinelli, F., Scozzafava, G., & Casini, L. (2023). Does attitude moderate the effect of labelling information when choosing functional foods? *Food Quality and Preference, 106*, 104795. Available from https://doi.org/10.1016/j.foodqual.2022.104795.

Cooperstone, J. L., & Schwartz, S. J. (2016). *Recent Insights Into Health Benefits of Carotenoids* (pp. 473–497). Elsevier BV. Available from 10.1016/b978-0-08-100371-8.00020-8.

Cukkemane, A., Kumar, P., & Sathyamoorthy, B. (2020). A metabolomics footprint approach to understanding the benefits of synbiotics in functional foods and dietary therapeutics for health, communicable and non-communicable diseases. *Food Research International, 128*, 108679. Available from https://doi.org/10.1016/j.foodres.2019.108679.

Das, T. K., Pradhan, S., Chakrabarti, S., Mondal, K. C., & Ghosh, K. (2022). Current status of probiotic and related health benefits. *Applied Food Research, 2*(2). Available from https://doi.org/10.1016/j.afres.2022.100185, https://www.journals.elsevier.com/applied-food-research.

Davani-Davari, D., Negahdaripour, M., Karimzadeh, I., Seifan, M., Mohkam, M., Masoumi, S. J., Berenjian, A., & Ghasemi, Y. (2019). Prebiotics: Definition, types, sources, mechanisms, and clinical applications. *Foods, 8*(3). Available from https://doi.org/10.3390/foods8030092, https://www.mdpi.com/2304-8158/8/3.

Deborah, B., Rotordam, M., Giacomo, S., Giulia, C., & Adele, F. (2021). Understanding consumption choices of innovative products: An outlook on the Italian functional food market. *AIMS Agriculture and Food, 6*(3), 818–837. Available from https://doi.org/10.3934/agrfood.2021050.

Delompré, T., Guichard, E., Briand, L., & Salles, C. (2019). Taste perception of nutrients found in nutritional supplements: A review. *Nutrients, 11*(9), 2050. Available from https://doi.org/10.3390/nu11092050.

De Bauw, M., De La Revilla, L. S., Poppe, V., Matthys, C., & Vranken, L. (2022). Digital nudges to stimulate healthy and pro-environmental food choices in E-groceries. *Appetite, 172*. Available from https://doi.org/10.1016/j.appet.2022.105971, http://www.elsevier.com/inca/publications/store/6/2/2/7/8/5/index.htt.

De Toffoli, A., Spinelli, S., Monteleone, E., Arena, E., Di Monaco, R., Endrizzi, I., Gallina Toschi, T., Laureati, M., Napolitano, F., Torri, L., & Dinnella, C. (2019). Influences of psychological traits and PROP Taster status on familiarity with and choice of phenol-rich foods and beverages. *Nutrients, 11*(6), 1329. Available from https://doi.org/10.3390/nu11061329.

Dinehart, M. E., Hayes, J. E., Bartoshuk, L. M., Lanier, S. L., & Duffy, V. B. (2006). Bitter taste markers explain variability in vegetable sweetness, bitterness, and intake. *Physiology & Behavior, 87*(2), 304–313. Available from https://doi.org/10.1016/j.physbeh.2005.10.018.

Dinnella, C., Recchia, A., Tuorila, H., & Monteleone, E. (2011). Individual astringency responsiveness affects the acceptance of phenol-rich foods. *Appetite, 56*(3), 633–642. Available from https://doi.org/10.1016/j.appet.2011.02.017.

Doherty, A., Wall, A., Khaldi, N., & Kussmann, M. (2021). Artificial intelligence in functional food ingredient discovery and characterisation: A focus on bioactive plant and food peptides. *Frontiers in Genetics, 12*. Available from https://doi.org/10.3389/fgene.2021.768979, https://www.frontiersin.org/journals/genetics#.

Dolgopolova, I., Teuber, R., & Bruschi, V. (2015). Consumers' perceptions of functional foods: Trust and food-neophobia in a cross-cultural context. *International Journal of Consumer Studies, 39*(6), 708–715. Available from https://doi.org/10.1111/ijcs.12184Germany, http://onlinelibrary.wiley.com/journal/10.1111/(ISSN)1470-6431.

Domínguez Díaz, L., Fernández-Ruiz, V., & Cámara, M. (2020). An international regulatory review of food health-related claims in functional food products labeling. *Journal of Functional Foods, 68*, 103896. Available from https://doi.org/10.1016/j.jff.2020.103896.

Drewnowski, A., & Gomez-Carneros, C. (2000). Bitter taste, phytonutrients, and the consumer: A review. *American Journal of Clinical Nutrition, 72* (6), 1424–1435. Available from https://doi.org/10.1093/ajcn/72.6.1424, http://www.ajcn.org/contents-by-date.2005.shtml.

Elliott, M., Gillison, F., & Barnett, J. (2020). Exploring the influences on men's engagement with weight loss services: A qualitative study. *BMC public health, 20*(1). Available from https://doi.org/10.1186/s12889-020-8252-5, http://www.biomedcentral.com/bmcpublichealth.

Ervina, E., Almli, V. L., Berget, I., Spinelli, S., Sick, J., & Dinnella, C. (2021). Does responsiveness to basic tastes influence preadolescents' food liking? Investigating taste responsiveness segment on bitter-sour-sweet and salty-umami model food samples. *Nutrients, 13*(8). Available from https://doi.org/10.3390/nu13082721, https://www.mdpi.com/2072-6643/13/8/2721/pdf.

EUFIC. (2017). Final Report Summary - CLYMBOL (Role of health-related claims and symbols in consumer behaviour). *CORDIS, EU Research Results* Role of health-related claims and symbols in consumer behaviour. *European Food Information Council (EUFIC)*. Available from https://cordis.europa.eu/project/id/311963/reporting.

Fernandez, M. A., Desroches, S., Marquis, M., Lebel, A., Turcotte, M., & Provencher, V. (2019). Which food literacy dimensions are associated with diet quality among Canadian parents? *British Food Journal, 121*(8), 1670–1685. Available from https://doi.org/10.1108/BFJ-11-2018-0724, https://www.emeraldinsight.com/loi/bfj.

Gajdoš Kljusuric, J., Čačić, J., Misir, A., & Čačić, D. (2015). Geographical region as a factor influencing consumers' perception of functional food – case of Croatia. *British Food Journal, 117*(3), 1017–1031. Available from https://doi.org/10.1108/bfj-12-2013-0282.

Gao, T., Duan, Y., Qi, Q., Mo, G., Han, S., Liu, H., & Zhang, M. (2023). Nutrition literacy differs based on demographics among University students in Bengbu, China. *Frontiers in Public Health, 11*. Available from https://doi.org/10.3389/fpubh.2023.1113211.

Gebregewergis, A., Chandravanshi, B. S., & Redi-Abshiro, M. (2020). Levels of selected metals in teff grain samples collected from three different areas of Ethiopia by microwave plasma-atomic emission spectroscopy. *Bulletin of the Chemical Society of Ethiopia, 34*, 449–462. Available from https://doi.org/10.4314/bcse.v34i3.2.

Ghosh, S., Sarkar, T., Pati, S., Kari, Z. A., Edinur, H. A., & Chakraborty, R. (2022). Novel bioactive compounds from marine sources as a tool for functional food development. *Frontiers in Marine Science, 9*. Available from https://doi.org/10.3389/fmars.2022.832957, https://www.frontiersin.org/journals/marine-science#.

Giordano, S., Clodoveo, M. L., Gennaro, B. D., & Corbo, F. (2018). Factors determining neophobia and neophilia with regard to new technologies applied to the food sector: A systematic review. *International Journal of Gastronomy and Food Science, 11*, 1–19. Available from https://doi.org/10.1016/j.ijgfs.2017.10.001, www.journals.elsevier.com/international-journal-of-gastronomy-and-food-science.

Gok, I. (2023). Functional potential of several Turkish fermented traditional foods: Biotic properties, bioactive compounds, and health benefits. *Food Reviews International, 39*(5), 2568–2593. Available from https://doi.org/10.1080/87559129.2021.1962340.

Gok, I., & Ulu, E. K. (2019). Functional foods in Turkey: Marketing, consumer awareness and regulatory aspects. *Nutrition & Food Science, 49*(4), 668–686. Available from https://doi.org/10.1108/nfs-07-2018-0198.

Granato, D., Barba, F. J., Bursać Kovačević, D., Lorenzo, J. M., Cruz, A. G., & Putnik, P. (2020). Functional foods: Product development, technological trends, efficacy testing, and safety. *Annual Review of Food Science and Technology, 11*, 93–118. Available from https://doi.org/10.1146/annurev-food-032519-051708, http://www.annualreviews.org/journal/food.

Granato, D., Nunes, D. S., & Barba, F. J. (2017). An integrated strategy between food chemistry, biology, nutrition, pharmacology, and statistics in the development of functional foods: A proposal. *Trends in Food Science & Technology, 62*, 13–22. Available from https://doi.org/10.1016/j.tifs.2016.12.010.

Grunert, K. G., Hieke, S, & Wills, J (2014). Sustainability labels on food products: Consumer motivation, understanding and use. *Food Policy, 44*, 177–189. Available from https://doi.org/10.1016/j.foodpol.2013.12.001.

Guo, S. W., & Reed, D. R. (2001). The genetics of phenylthiocarbamide perception. *Annals of Human Biology, 28*(2), 111–142. Available from https://doi.org/10.1080/03014460151056310.

Hassan, S., Meenatchi, R., Pachillu, K., Bansal, S., Brindangnanam, P., Arockiaraj, J., Kiran, G. S., & Selvin, J. (2022). Identification and characterization of the novel bioactive compounds from microalgae and cyanobacteria for pharmaceutical and nutraceutical applications. *Journal of Basic Microbiology, 62*(9), 999–1029. Available from https://doi.org/10.1002/jobm.202100477, http://onlinelibrary.wiley.com/journal/10.1002/(ISSN)1521-4028.

Hassoun, A., Prieto, M. A., Carpena, M., Bouzembrak, Y., Marvin, H. J. P., Pallarés, N., Barba, F. J., Punia Bangar, S., Chaudhary, V., Ibrahim, S., & Bono, G. (2022). Exploring the role of green and Industry 4.0 technologies in achieving sustainable development goals in food sectors. *Food Research International, 162*. Available from https://doi.org/10.1016/j.foodres.2022.112068, www.elsevier.com/inca/publications/store/4/2/2/9/7/0.

Hélias, A., van der Werf, H. M. G., Soler, L. G., Aggeri, F., Dourmad, J. Y., Julia, C., Nabec, L., Pellerin, S., Ruffieux, B., & Trystram, G. (2022). Implementing environmental labelling of food products in France. *International Journal of Life Cycle Assessment, 27*(7), 926–931. Available from https://doi.org/10.1007/s11367-022-02071-8, http://www.springerlink.com/content/0948-3349.

Hieke, S., Cascanette, T., Pravst, I., Kaur, A., Van Trijp, H., Verbeke, W., & Grunert, K. G. (2016). The role of health-related claims and symbols in consumer behaviour: The CLYMBOL project. *Agro Food Industry Hi-Tech*, *27*(3), 26–29. Available from http://www.teknoscienze.com/Contents/Riviste/Sfogliatore/AF3_2016/files/assets/common/downloads/AF3_2016.pdf.

Horská, E., Predanócyová, K., Šedík, P., Grunert, K. G., & Hupková, D. (2023). Consumer perception of functional foods and determinants of functional foods consumption in the Slovak Republic. *British Food Journal*, *125*(7), 2478–2492. Available from https://doi.org/10.1108/BFJ-07-2022-0656, https://www.emeraldinsight.com/loi/bfj.

Huang, L., Bai, L., Zhang, X., & Gong, S. (2019). Re-understanding the antecedents of functional foods purchase: Mediating effect of purchase attitude and moderating effect of food neophobia. *Food Quality and Preference*, *73*, 266–275. Available from https://doi.org/10.1016/j.foodqual.2018.11.001.

Hu, Y., Ma, C., Chen, X., Bai, G., & Guo, S. (2022). Hydrophilic phytosterol derivatives: A short review on structural modifications, cholesterol-lowering activity and safety. *Grain and Oil Science and Technology*, *5*(3), 146–155. Available from https://doi.org/10.1016/j.gaost.2022.02.001, https://www.sciencedirect.com/journal/grain-and-oil-science-and-technology.

Industry Research Biz. (2023). 2030 Forecast: Functional Foods and Drinks Market. *Global Opportunities & Innovations*. Available from https://www.industryresearch.biz/.

Jaeger, S. R. (2006). Non-sensory factors in sensory science research. *Food Quality and Preference*, *17*(1-2), 132–144. Available from https://doi.org/10.1016/j.foodqual.2005.03.004.

Jaime, L., & Santoyo, S. (2021). The health benefits of the bioactive compounds in foods. *Foods*, *10*(2), 325. Available from https://doi.org/10.3390/foods10020325.

Jain, S., Sharma, K., & Khadke, M. (2014). Consumer behavior towards functional foods in India-A study of market drivers and challenges. *IOSR Journal of Business and Management*, *2014*, 33–40.

Jung, S. E., Shin, Y. H., Severt, K., & Crowe-White, K. M. (2020). Determinants of a consumer's intention to consume antioxidant-infused sugar-free chewing gum: Measuring taste, attitude, and health consciousness. *Journal of Food Products Marketing*, *26*(1), 38–54. Available from https://doi.org/10.1080/10454446.2020.1717712, http://www.tandfonline.com/toc/wfpm20/current.

Kennedy, K., Keogh, B., Lopez, C., Adelfio, A., Molloy, B., Kerr, A., Wall, A. M., Jalowicki, G., Holton, T. A., & Khaldi, N. (2020). An artificial intelligence characterised functional ingredient, derived from rice, inhibits TNF-α and significantly improves physical strength in an inflammaging population. *Foods*, *9*(9). Available from https://doi.org/10.3390/foods9091147, https://www.mdpi.com/2304-8158/9/9/1147.

Kraus, A., Annunziata, A., & Vecchio, R. (2017). Sociodemographic factors differentiating the consumer and the motivations for functional food consumption. *Journal of the American College of Nutrition*, *36*(2), 116–126. Available from https://doi.org/10.1080/07315724.2016.1228489, http://www.tandfonline.com/toc/uacn20/current.

Lee, A., Wang, Y., & Lo, S. F. (2021). Life cycle assessment of functional food: Improving sustainability in the biotechnology industry through transparency. *Processes*, *9*(12). Available from https://doi.org/10.3390/pr9122130, https://www.mdpi.com/2227-9717/9/12/2130/pdf.

Liu, Y., Shen, N., Xin, H., Yu, L., Xu, Q., & Cui, Y. (2023). Unsaturated fatty acids in natural edible resources, a systematic review of classification, resources, biosynthesis, biological activities and application. *Food Bioscience*, *53*, 102790. Available from https://doi.org/10.1016/j.fbio.2023.102790.

Louro, T., Simões, C., Castelo, P. M., Capela E Silva, F., Luis, H., Moreira, P., & Lamy, E. (2021). How individual variations in the perception of basic tastes and astringency relate with dietary intake and preferences for fruits and vegetables. *Foods*, *10*(8). Available from https://doi.org/10.3390/foods10081961, https://www.mdpi.com/2304-8158/10/8/1961/pdf.

Mallhi, T. H., Rasheed, M., Khan, Y. H., Alzarea, A. I., & Raja, A. A. (2020). *Bioactive Compounds for the Treatment of Metabolic Disorders* (pp. 489–505). Springer Science and Business Media LLC. Available from https://doi.org/10.1007/978-3-030-45923-9_28.

Mark, R., Lyu, X., Lee, J. J. L., Parra-Saldívar, R., & Chen, W. N. (2019). Sustainable production of natural phenolics for functional food applications. *Journal of Functional Foods*, *57*, 233–254. Available from https://doi.org/10.1016/j.jff.2019.04.008, http://www.elsevier.com/wps/find/journaldescription.cws_home/717426/description#description.

Martins, A. P. de O., Bezerra, M. de F., Marques Júnior, S., Brito, A. F., Andrade Neto, J. C. de, Bezerra Galvão Júnior, J. G., Lima Júnior, D. M. de, & Rangel, A. H. do N. (2020). Consumer behavior of organic and functional foods in Brazil. *Food Science and Technology*, *40*(2), 469–475. Available from https://doi.org/10.1590/fst.03519.

Masyita, A., Mustika Sari, R., Dwi Astuti, A., Yasir, B., Rahma Rumata, N., Emran, T. B., Nainu, F., & Simal-Gandara, J. (2022). Terpenes and terpenoids as main bioactive compounds of essential oils, their roles in human health and potential application as natural food preservatives. *Food Chemistry: X*, *13*. Available from https://doi.org/10.1016/j.fochx.2022.100217, https://www.journals.elsevier.com/food-chemistry-x.

Matsumura, Y., Kitabatake, M., Kayano, S. I., & Ito, T. (2023). Dietary phenolic compounds: Their health benefits and association with the gut microbiota. *Antioxidants*, *12*(4). Available from https://doi.org/10.3390/antiox12040880, www.mdpi.com/journal/antioxidants.

Melbye, E. L., Hansen, H., & Onozaka, Y. (2015). Advertising functional foods: The effects of physical body size and appeal type on ad credibility and purchase intentions. *Journal of International Food and Agribusiness Marketing*, *27*(2), 142–154. Available from https://doi.org/10.1080/08974438.2014.918916, http://www.tandfonline.com/toc/wifa20/current.

Mete, R., Shield, A., Murray, K., Bacon, R., & Kellett, J. (2019). What is healthy eating? A qualitative exploration. *Public Health Nutrition*, *22*(13), 2408–2418. Available from https://doi.org/10.1017/S1368980019001046, http://journals.cambridge.org/PHN.

Michell, K. A., Isweiri, H., Newman, S. E., Bunning, M., Bellows, L. L., Dinges, M. M., Grabos, L. E., Rao, S., Foster, M. T., Heuberger, A. L., Prenni, J. E., Thompson, H. J., Uchanski, M. E., Weir, T. L., & Johnson, S. A. (2020). Microgreens: Consumer sensory perception and acceptance of an emerging functional food crop. *Journal of Food Science, 85*(4), 926–935. Available from https://doi.org/10.1111/1750-3841.15075, http://onlinelibrary.wiley.com/journal/10.1111/(ISSN)1750-3841.

Miękus, N., Marszałek, K., Podlacha, M., Iqbal, A., Puchalski, C., & Świergiel, A. H. (2020). Health benefits of plant-derived sulfur compounds, glucosinolates, and organosulfur compounds. *Molecules, 25*(17), 3804. Available from https://doi.org/10.3390/molecules25173804.

Miller, V., Webb, P., Cudhea, F., Shi, P., Zhang, J., Reedy, J., Erndt-Marino, J., Coates, J., Mozaffarian, D., Bas, M., Ali, J. H., Abumweis, S., Krishnan, A., Misra, P., Hwalla, N. C., Janakiram, C., Liputo, N. I., Musaiger, A., Pourfarzi, F., . . . Hakeems, R. (2022). Global dietary quality in 185 countries from 1990 to 2018 show wide differences by nation, age, education, and urbanicity. *Nature Food, 3*(9), 694–702. Available from https://doi.org/10.1038/s43016-022-00594-9.

Miniakhmetova, A. V., Sergienko, O. I., Ilina, V. S., Lepeshkin, A. I., & Baranenko, D. A. (2022). A comparative life cycle assessment of phytosterol and meadowsweet (Filipendula ulmaria) oncoprotective functional food ingredients. *Food Bioscience, 50*. Available from https://doi.org/10.1016/j.fbio.2022.102076, http://www.journals.elsevier.com/food-bioscience/.

Mirzapour-Kouhdasht, A., McClements, D. J., Taghizadeh, M. S., Niazi, A., & Garcia-Vaquero, M. (2023). Strategies for oral delivery of bioactive peptides with focus on debittering and masking. *npj Science of Food, 7*(1). Available from https://doi.org/10.1038/s41538-023-00198-y, https://www.nature.com/npjscifood/about.

Mohd Nor, N. D., Houston-Price, C., Harvey, K., & Methven, L. (2021). The effects of taste sensitivity and repeated taste exposure on children's intake and liking of turnip (Brassica rapa subsp. rapa); a bitter Brassica vegetable. *Appetite, 157*. Available from https://doi.org/10.1016/j.appet.2020.104991, http://www.elsevier.com/inca/publications/store/6/2/2/7/8/5/index.htt.

Monteiro, C. A., Cannon, G., Lawrence, M., Louzada., & Machado, P. (2019). *Ultra-processed foods, diet quality, and health using the NOVA classification system, 2019*.

Moons, I., Barbarossa, C., & De Pelsmacker, P. (2018). The determinants of the adoption intention of eco-friendly functional food in different market segments. *Ecological Economics, 151*, 151–161. Available from https://doi.org/10.1016/j.ecolecon.2018.05.012, www.elsevier.com/inca/publications/store/5/0/3/3/0/5.

Moro, D., Veneziani, M., Sckokai, P., & Castellari, E. (2015). Consumer willingness to pay for catechin-enriched yogurt: Evidence from a stated choice experiment. *Agribusiness, 31*(2), 243–258. Available from https://doi.org/10.1002/agr.21401, http://www3.interscience.wiley.com/journal/35917/home.

Narayana, M. N. K., Narayana, S., Fernando, G., & Chandima, S. (2020). Awareness and attitude towards functional dairy products among consumers in western province of Sri Lanka. *Turkish Journal of Agriculture - Food Science and Technology, 8*(6), 1308–1314. Available from https://doi.org/10.24925/turjaf.v8i6.1308-1314.3326.

Nemecek, T., Roesch, A., Bystricky, M., Jeanneret, P., Lansche, J., Stüssi, M., & Gaillard, G. (2024). Swiss Agricultural Life Cycle Assessment: A method to assess the emissions and environmental impacts of agricultural systems and products. *International Journal of Life Cycle Assessment, 29*(3), 433–455. Available from https://doi.org/10.1007/s11367-023-02255-w, https://www.springer.com/journal/11367.

Neo, Y. T., Chia, W. Y., Lim, S. S., Ngan, C. L., Kurniawan, T. A., & Chew, K. W. (2023). Smart systems in producing algae-based protein to improve functional food ingredients industries. *Food Research International, 165*. Available from https://doi.org/10.1016/j.foodres.2023.112480, www.elsevier.com/inca/publications/store/4/2/2/9/7/0.

Oliveira, D., Machín, L., Deliza, R., Rosenthal, A., Walter, E. H., Giménez, A., & Ares, G. (2016). Consumers' attention to functional food labels: Insights from eye-tracking and change detection in a case study with probiotic milk. *LWT - Food Science and Technology, 68*, 160–167. Available from https://doi.org/10.1016/j.lwt.2015.11.066.

Oliveira, L., Sousa, F., & Silveira, M. G. D. (2023). Promotion of functional foods in a school context: Evaluation of food education sessions involving cooking skills. *Journal of Culinary Science & Technology*, 1–13. Available from https://doi.org/10.1080/15428052.2023.2191877.

Pagoto, S. L., Schneider, K. L., Oleski, J. L., Luciani, J. M., Bodenlos, J. S., & Whited, M. C. (2012). Male inclusion in randomized controlled trials of lifestyle weight loss interventions. *Obesity, 20*(6), 1234–1239. Available from https://doi.org/10.1038/oby.2011.140.

Palmieri, N., Stefanoni, W., Latterini, F., & Pari, L. (2021). An Italian explorative study of willingness to pay for a new functional pasta featuring Opuntia ficus indica. *Agriculture, 11*(8), 701. Available from https://doi.org/10.3390/agriculture11080701.

Palmieri, N., Stefanoni, W., Latterini, F., & Pari, L. (2022). Factors influencing Italian consumers' willingness to pay for eggs enriched with omega-3-fatty acids. *Foods, 11*(4), 545. Available from https://doi.org/10.3390/foods11040545.

Palumbo, R. (2016). Sustainability of well-being through literacy. The effects of food literacy on sustainability of well-being. *Agriculture and Agricultural Science Procedia, 8*, 99–106. Available from https://doi.org/10.1016/j.aaspro.2016.02.013.

Pappalardo, G., & Lusk, J. L. (2016). The role of beliefs in purchasing process of functional foods. *Food Quality and Preference*, 151–158. Available from https://doi.org/10.1016/j.foodqual.2016.06.009.

Pattnaik, M., Pandey, P., Martin, G. J. O., Mishra, H. N., & Ashokkumar, M. (2021). Innovative technologies for extraction and microencapsulation of bioactives from plant-based food waste and their applications in functional food development. *Foods, 10*(2), 1–30. Available from https://doi.org/10.3390/foods10020279, https://www.mdpi.com/2304-8158/10/2/279/pdf.

Phan, T., Bremer, P., & Mirosa, M. (2020). Vietnamese consumers' preferences for functional milk powder attributes: A segmentation-based conjoint study with educated consumers. *Sustainability, 12*(13), 5258. Available from https://doi.org/10.3390/su12135258.

Pienwisetkaew, T., Wongthahan, P., Naruetharadhol, P., Wongsaichia, S., Vonganunsuntree, C., Padthar, S., Nee, S., He, P., & Ketkaew, C. (2022). Consumers' intention to purchase functional non-dairy milk and gender-based market segmentation. *Sustainability, 14*(19), 11957. Available from https://doi.org/10.3390/su141911957.

Plaza-Diaz J. Ruiz-Ojeda F.J. Gil-Campos M. Gil A. 2019 1 1 2019/01/01 Advances in Nutrition. Oxford University Press Spain Mechanisms of Action of Probiotics. Available from https://doi.org/10.1093/advances/nmy063, http://advances.nutrition.org/, 21565376 S49-S66S49.

Priyadarshini, A., Tiwari, B. K., & Rajauria, G. (2022). Assessing the environmental and economic sustainability of functional food ingredient production process. *Processes*, *10*(3). Available from https://doi.org/10.3390/pr10030445, https://www.mdpi.com/2227-9717/10/3/445/pdf.

Quan, N. H. K., Yen, N. T. N., & Chung, D. D. (2020). Functional food in Viet Nam: Trends consumer online shopping in Ho Chi Minh city. *IOP Conference Series: Materials Science and Engineering*, *991*(1), 012037. Available from https://doi.org/10.1088/1757-899x/991/1/012037.

Rastogi, S., Pandey, M. M., & Rawat, A. K. S. (2016). Traditional herbs: A remedy for cardiovascular disorders. *Phytomedicine*, *23*(11), 1082–1089. Available from https://doi.org/10.1016/j.phymed.2015.10.012, www.urbanfischer.de/journals/phytomed.

Rein, D., Ternes, P., Demin, R., Gierke, J., Helgason, T., & Schön, C. (2019). Artificial intelligence identified peptides modulate inflammation in healthy adults. *Food & Function*, *10*, 6030–6041. Available from https://doi.org/10.1039/C9FO01398A.

Riccardi, B. (2022). From bioactive molecules to their nutritional effect, biodynamic interpretation between productional and functional aspects of nutrients. *Recent Progress in Nutrition*, *02*(04), 1–16. Available from https://doi.org/10.21926/rpn.2204023.

Rodrigues, L., Silverio, R., Costa, A. R., Antunes, C., Pomar, C., Infante, P., Conceição, C., Amado, F., & Lamy, E. (2020). Taste sensitivity and lifestyle are associated with food preferences and BMI in children. *International Journal of Food Sciences and Nutrition*, *71*(7), 875–883. Available from https://doi.org/10.1080/09637486.2020.1738354, http://www.tandfonline.com/loi/iijf20.

Rounsefell, K., Gibson, S., McLean, S., Blair, M., Molenaar, A., Brennan, L., Truby, H., & McCaffrey, T. A. (2020). Social media, body image and food choices in healthy young adults: A mixed methods systematic review. *Nutrition & Dietetics*, *77*(1), 19–40. Available from https://doi.org/10.1111/1747-0080.12581.

Sandell, M., Hoppu, U., Mikkilä, V., Mononen, N., Kähönen, M., Männistö, S., Rönnemaa, T., Viikari, J., Lehtimäki, T., & Raitakari, O. T. (2014). Genetic variation in the hTAS2R38 taste receptor and food consumption among Finnish adults. *Genes and Nutrition*, *9*(6), 1–8. Available from https://doi.org/10.1007/s12263-014-0433-3, http://www.springerlink.com/content/1555-8932.

Seccia, A., Viscecchia, R., Nardone, G., & Roca, P. (2019). Table grapes as functional food: Consumer preferences for health and environmental attributes. *BIO Web of Conferences*, *15*, 03011. Available from https://doi.org/10.1051/bioconf/20191503011.

Serrano, J. C. E., Jove, M., Gonzalo, H., Pamplona, R., & Portero-Otin, M. (2015). Nutridynamics: Mechanism(s) of action of bioactive compounds and their effects. *International Journal of Food Sciences and Nutrition*, *66*, S22. Available from https://doi.org/10.3109/09637486.2015.1035231.

Sharma, S., Katoch, V., Kumar, S., & Chatterjee, S. (2021). Functional relationship of vegetable colors and bioactive compounds: Implications in human health. *The Journal of Nutritional Biochemistry*, *92*, 108615. Available from https://doi.org/10.1016/j.jnutbio.2021.108615.

Siegrist, M., Shi, J., Giusto, A., & Hartmann, C. (2015). Worlds apart. Consumer acceptance of functional foods and beverages in Germany and China. *Appetite*, *92*, 87–93. Available from https://doi.org/10.1016/j.appet.2015.05.017, http://www.elsevier.com/inca/publications/store/6/2/2/7/8/5/index.htt.

Sun, X., Wang, R., He, P., & Liu, B. (2024). Effects of environmental and nutritional labels on the dietary choices of consumers: Evidence from China. *Environmental Impact Assessment Review*, *105*, 107407. Available from https://doi.org/10.1016/j.eiar.2023.107407.

Szakály, Z., Kovács, S., Pető, K., Huszka, P., & Kiss, M. (2019). A modified model of the willingness to pay for functional foods. *Appetite*, *138*, 94–101. Available from https://doi.org/10.1016/j.appet.2019.03.020, http://www.elsevier.com/inca/publications/store/6/2/2/7/8/5/index.htt.

Temesi, Á., Bacsó, Á., Grunert, K. G., & Lakner, Z. (2019). Perceived correspondence of health effects as a new determinant influencing purchase intention for functional food. *Nutrients*, *11*(4). Available from https://doi.org/10.3390/nu11040740, https://www.mdpi.com/2072-6643/11/4/740/pdf.

Temple, N. J. (2022). A rational definition for functional foods: A perspective. *Frontiers in Nutrition*, *9*. Available from https://doi.org/10.3389/fnut.2022.957516, journal.frontiersin.org/journal/nutrition.

Tepper, B. J. (2008). Nutritional implications of genetic taste variation: The role of PROP sensitivity and other taste phenotypes. *Annual Review of Nutrition*, *28*, 367–388. Available from https://doi.org/10.1146/annurev.nutr.28.061807.155458.

Terpou, A., Papadaki, A., Lappa, I. K., Kachrimanidou, V., Bosnea, L. A., & Kopsahelis, N. (2019). Probiotics in food systems: Significance and emerging strategies towards improved viability and delivery of enhanced beneficial value. *Nutrients*, *11*(7). Available from https://doi.org/10.3390/nu11071591, https://www.mdpi.com/2072-6643/11/7/1591/pdf.

Thunström, L., & Nordström, J. (2015). Determinants of food demand and the experienced taste effect of healthy labels - An experiment on potato chips and bread. *Journal of Behavioral and Experimental Economics*, *56*, 13–20. Available from https://doi.org/10.1016/j.socec.2015.02.004, http://www.journals.elsevier.com/journal-of-behavioral-and-experimental-economics/.

Tolve, R., Cela, N., Condelli, N., Di Cairano, M., Caruso, M. C., & Galgano, F. (2020). Microencapsulation as a tool for the formulation of functional foods: The phytosterols' case study. *Foods*, *9*(4). Available from https://doi.org/10.3390/foods9040470, https://www.mdpi.com/2304-8158/9/4/470.

Toner, C., & Pitman, S. (2004). Functional foods. *Topics in clinical nutrition*, *19*(1), 71–78. Available from https://doi.org/10.1097/00008486-200401000-00011.

Topolska, K., Florkiewicz, A., & Filipiak-Florkiewicz, A. (2021). Functional food—Consumer motivations and expectations. *International journal of environmental research and public health*, *18*(10), 5327. Available from https://doi.org/10.3390/ijerph18105327.

Torri, L., Piochi, M., Lavelli, V., & Monteleone, E. (2015). Descriptive sensory analysis and consumers' preference for dietary fibre- and polyphenol-enriched tomato purees obtained using winery by-products. *LWT - Food Science and Technology*, *62*(1), 294–300. Available from https://doi.org/10.1016/j.lwt.2014.12.059.

Trieste, L., Bazzani, A., Amato, A., Faraguna, U., & Turchetti, G. (2021). Food literacy and food choice – a survey-based psychometric profiling of consumer behaviour. *British Food Journal, 123*(13), 124–141. Available from https://doi.org/10.1108/BFJ-09-2020-0845, https://www.emeraldinsight.com/loi/bfj.

Uddin, M. S., Ferdosh, S., Haque Akanda, M. J., Ghafoor, K., Rukshana, A. H., Ali, M. E., Kamaruzzaman, B. Y., Fauzi, M. B., Hadijah, S., Shaarani, S., & Islam Sarker, M. Z. (2018). Techniques for the extraction of phytosterols and their benefits in human health: A review. *Separation Science and Technology, 53*(14), 2206–2223. Available from https://doi.org/10.1080/01496395.2018.1454472.

Uribe, N. G., García-Galbis, M. R., & Espinosa, R. M. M. (2017). New advances about the effect of vitamins on human health: vitamins supplements and nutritional aspects. *Functional food-improve health through adequate food*, 57–75. Available from https://doi.org/10.5772/intechopen.69122.

Vecchio, R., Lombardi, A., Cembalo, L., Caracciolo, F., Cicia, G., Masucci, F., & Di Francia, A. (2016). Consumers' willingness to pay and drivers of motivation to consume omega-3 enriched mozzarella cheese. *British Food Journal, 118*(10), 2404–2419. Available from https://doi.org/10.1108/BFJ-01-2016-0013, http://www.emeraldinsight.com/info/journals/bfj/bfj.jsp.

Venkatakrishnan, K., Chiu, H. F., & Wang, C. K. (2019). Popular functional foods and herbs for the management of type-2-diabetes mellitus: A comprehensive review with special reference to clinical trials and its proposed mechanism. *Journal of Functional Foods, 57*, 425–438. Available from https://doi.org/10.1016/j.jff.2019.04.039, http://www.elsevier.com/wps/find/journaldescription.cws_home/717426/description#description.

Vermeulen, S. J., Park, T., Khoury, C. K., & Béné, C. (2020). Changing diets and the transformation of the global food system. *Annals of the New York Academy of Sciences, 1478*(1), 3–17. Available from https://doi.org/10.1111/nyas.14446, http://onlinelibrary.wiley.com/journal/10.1111/(ISSN)1749-6632.

Viscecchia, R., Nocella, G., De Devitiis, B., Bimbo, F., Carlucci, D., Seccia, A., & Nardone, G. (2019). Consumers' trade-off between nutrition and health claims under regulation 1924/2006: Insights from a choice experiment analysis. *Nutrients, 11*(12), 2881. Available from https://doi.org/10.3390/nu11122881.

Vlaeminck, P., Jiang, T., & Vranken, L. (2014). Food labeling and eco-friendly consumption: Experimental evidence from a Belgian supermarket. *Ecological Economics, 108*, 180–190. Available from https://doi.org/10.1016/j.ecolecon.2014.10.019, www.elsevier.com/inca/publications/store/5/0/3/3/0/5.

Welk, A. K., Mehlhose, C., Daum, D., & Enneking, U. (2023). Vegetables with enhanced iron bioavailability—German consumers' perceptions of a new approach to improve dietary iron supply. *Nutrients, 15*(10). Available from https://doi.org/10.3390/nu15102291, http://www.mdpi.com/journal/nutrients/.

Wijayaratne, S. P., Reid, M., Westberg, K., Worsley, A., & Mavondo, F. (2018). Food literacy, healthy eating barriers and household diet. *European Journal of Marketing, 52*(12), 2449–2477. Available from https://doi.org/10.1108/EJM-10-2017-0760, http://www.emeraldinsight.com/info/journals/ejm/ejm.jsp.

Yousaf, N. Y., & Tepper, B. J. (2022). The effects of cranberry polyphenol extract (CPE) supplementation on astringency and flavor perception as a function of PROP taster status and other individual factors. *International journal of environmental research and public health, 19*(19). Available from https://doi.org/10.3390/ijerph191911995, http://www.mdpi.com/journal/ijerph.

Zahid, H. F., Ranadheera, C. S., Fang, Z., & Ajlouni, S. (2021). Utilization of mango, apple and banana fruit peels as prebiotics and functional ingredients. *Agriculture, 11*(7), 584. Available from https://doi.org/10.3390/agriculture11070584.

Zaky, A. A., Simal-Gandara, J., Eun, J. B., Shim, J. H., & Abd El-Aty, A. M. (2022). Bioactivities, applications, safety, and health benefits of bioactive peptides from food and by-products: A review. *Frontiers in Nutrition, 8*. Available from https://doi.org/10.3389/fnut.2021.815640, journal.frontiersin.org/journal/nutrition.

Zanchini, R., Di Vita, G., & Brun, F. (2022). Lifestyle, psychological and socio-demographic drivers in functional food choice: A systematic literature review based on bibliometric and network analysis. *International Journal of Food Sciences and Nutrition, 73*(6), 709–725. Available from https://doi.org/10.1080/09637486.2022.2048361, http://www.tandfonline.com/loi/iijf20.

Žeželj, I., Milošević, J., Stojanović, Ž., & Ognjanov, G. (2012). The motivational and informational basis of attitudes toward foods with health claims. *Appetite, 59*(3), 960–967. Available from https://doi.org/10.1016/j.appet.2012.09.008.

Chapter 24

The future of functional foods: innovations and advancements on the horizon

Loleny Tavares[1,2,3], Eduarda Silva de Azevedo[4], Liliana R. Sousa[1,2,3], Jorge Luís[1,2,3], Caciano Pelayo Zapata Noreña[4] and J.M. Oliveira[1,2,3]

[1]*School of Design, Management and Production Technologies Northern Aveiro, University of Aveiro, Estrada do Cercal, 449, 3720-511, Oliveira de Azeméis, Portugal,* [2]*EMaRT Group—Emerging Materials, Research, Technology, University of Aveiro, Aveiro, Portugal,* [3]*CICECO Aveiro—Institute of Materials, University of Aveiro, Campus Universitário de Santiago, Aveiro, Portugal,* [4]*Institute of Food Science and Technology, Federal University of Rio Grande do Sul, Av. Bento Gonçalves, Porto Alegre, RS, Brazil*

24.1 Introduction

In the past year, a notable increase in societal interest toward consuming healthy foods and a rising demand for nutritious products have emerged as prominent trends. This phenomenon is catalyzing a significant shift toward healthier lifestyles and fostering better eating habits toward a focus on the health benefits of specific foods and their ingredients (Baker et al., 2022; Fernandes et al., 2019). The concept of functional foods was first introduced in Japan in the 1980s. Foods for Specific Health Use was established in 1991, referring to foods that demonstrated physiological benefits or reduced disease risks, in addition to performing their normal basic functions (Aguiar et al., 2019). The European Commission Concerted Action on Functional Food Science in Europe proposed a working definition of functional food: a food that beneficially affects one or more target functions in the body beyond adequate nutritional effects in a way that is relevant to either an improved state of health and well-being and/or reduction of risk of disease. It is consumed as part of a normal food pattern. It is not a pill, a capsule or any form of dietary supplement. The American Dietetic Association defined functional foods, including "whole foods and fortified, enriched, or enhanced foods" that have a "potentially beneficial effect on health when consumed as part of a varied diet on a regular basis, at effective levels"(Position of the American Dietetic Association: Functional Foods, 2012). According to the European Commission, advancing functional foods presents several key research challenges, which include discovering novel ingredients and ensuring consumer acceptance. More specifically, researchers must (1) Identify potential functional ingredients that offer health benefits; (2) Understand individual biological responses to these foods; (3) Determine the bioavailability of functional food ingredients; (4) Develop reliable biomarkers for assessing functional outcomes; (5) Explore the application of advanced technologies such as nutrigenomics, bioinformatics, and nanotechnology in functional food development; (6) Anticipate the demand for personalized nutrition and the role of functional foods; (7) Ensure the stability of these ingredients during manufacturing and digestion; and (8) Establish Dietary Reference Intakes (DRIs) for a broader range of nutrients to support commercialization.

Consumer acceptance of functional foods can be influenced by product characteristics (combination of carriers and ingredients, price, taste, brand, and health information), socio-demographic characteristics (included age, gender, educational level, household characteristics, geography and nationality, and marital status), psychological characteristics (health consciousness, motivations, perceptions, beliefs, attitudes, trust and food neophobia, and nutrition knowledge) (Baker et al., 2022). The global market for functional foods, defined as those containing ingredients with added health benefits is estimated to be at least US$33 billion (Ahire et al., 2022). Emergence of other food trends and higher consumer interest and engagement in the transition toward sustainable food development and innovative green strategies are expected to occur in the future (Hassoun et al., 2024). The emerging food trends include fortified and functional

Unleashing the Power of Functional Foods and Novel Bioactives. DOI: https://doi.org/10.1016/B978-0-443-28862-3.00024-8

foods, additive manufacturing (AM) technologies, cultured meat, precision fermentation, and personalized food and their interrelation (Guo et al., 2024; Hassoun et al., 2024).

AM technologies and cultured meat have gained significant attention from consumers and businesses due to its potential to provide abundant nutrition and biological activities while being environmentally friendly and widely available. AM technologies, commonly known as "3D printing," have advanced and developed to a stage where they offer significant freedom in design, manufacturing, and innovation across various fields, including food engineering (Krujatz et al., 2017). The global 3D food printing industry was valued at $226.2 million in 2021, and by 2031, that number is expected to globally grow up to $15.1 billion (Yang et al., 2024). Therefore, AM technology not only has an exceptional potential for producing customized, nutritious, and visually appealing foods, it also allows catering to consumer preferences (Escalante-Aburto et al., 2021). Cell-based meat is also referred to as cultured meat, clean meat, synthetic, lab-grown or in vitro meat and is a complex food product comprised in vitro cultivated animal cells (Broucke et al., 2023). Lab-grown meat (LGM) presents a possible alternative to conventional meat products and may be used to address growing food demands attributable to global population growth (Barbosa et al., 2023). In addition, the main advantages of LGM described in the literature originates from animal welfare improvement and the reduction of greenhouse emissions point of view (Broucke et al., 2023).

In this context, this chapter explores two emerging areas with significant potential for the future of functional foods: AM and LGM to produce food products. These innovative technologies are transforming the food industry by offering health benefits that extend beyond traditional nutrition. Lab-grown foods, developed through advanced cellular agriculture, aim to reduce environmental impact while providing high-quality, customizable nutrition. On the other hand, 3D-printed food products offer unique solutions for personalized diets, capable of addressing specific nutritional needs and preferences. This chapter explores the science behind these developments and their potential to enhance both human health and food sustainability.

24.2 Additive manufacturing for food production

ISO/ASTM 52900 defines AM as the general term for those technologies that successively join material to create physical objects as specified by 3D model data (ASTM ISO/ASTM52900-15 standard terminology for additive manufacturing—General principles—Terminology,900-15 standard terminology for additive manufacturing—General principles—Terminology, 2015). More specifically, AM is defined as the process of joining materials to make parts from 3D model data, usually layer upon layer, as opposed to subtractive manufacturing and formative manufacturing methodologies. ISO/ASTM 52900 and ASTM F2792 categorize AM technologies into seven distinct groups based on their unique processes, namely vat photopolymerization, sheet lamination, powder bed fusion, material extrusion, binder jetting, direct energy deposition and material jetting (ASTM ISO/ASTM52900-15 standard terminology for additive manufacturing—General principles—Terminology,900-15 standard terminology for additive manufacturing—General principles—Terminology, 2015). Food 3D printing is an emerging food processing technology that has been extensively studied in the food sector in the past decade due to the advantages of functionalization, customization, personalized nutrition design, simplified supply chain and broadening existing food materials (He et al., 2020).

The digital workflow of 3D food printing begins with a virtual 3D model (Fig. 24.1). Creating 3D food designs can be achieved using various open-source platforms and software applications, which usually need to be converted in.stl (standard tessellation language) to be interpreted by slicer softwares. Popular options include user-friendly tools like Tinkercad for beginners or more advanced software like AutoCAD and Meshmixer (all by Autodesk, Inc., San Rafael, CA) (Guo et al., 2019). In addition, 3D scanning real objects and converting them into digital models is another approach. Once a design is complete, slicing software is necessary to convert the.stl into instructions understood by the 3D printer (g-code). Commonly used slicers include Repetier-Host (Hot-World GmbH & Co. KG, Willich, Germany), Slic3r (developed independently and often bundled with other software), Cura (Ultimaker B.V., The Netherlands), and Rhino 3D (Robert McNeel & Associates) (Guo et al., 2019). These instructions include printing parameters, like temperature, nozzle size, speed, layer height, and material flow rate (Kewuyemi et al., 2022). Once the g-code file is loaded, the 3D printer initiates the programmed deposition process, building the desired object layer-by-layer. The completed structure can be used immediately, undergo post-processing like cooling or heating, or require additional finishing steps depending on the material and application. Alternatively, the printed structure can be stored at refrigerated or freezing temperatures for later consumption. In some cases, additional post-processing steps like frying, steaming, or baking might be needed, especially for cold-extruded foods. The comprehensive workflow for creating 3D printed food involves several stages: conceptualization and design, slicing and G-code generation, pre-printing preparations, 3D

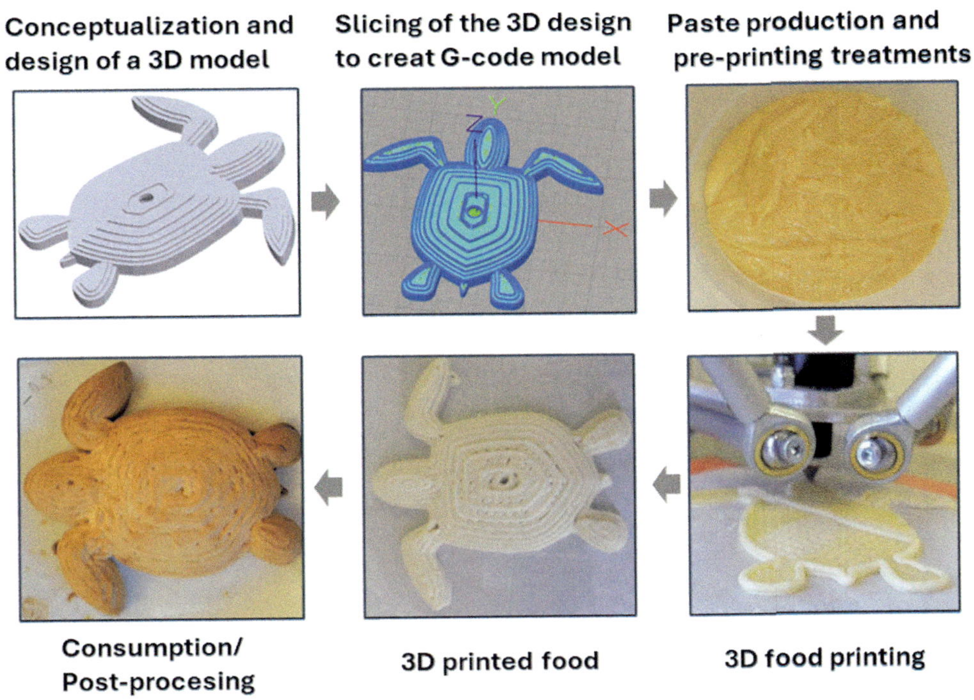

FIGURE 24.1 A comprehensive overview of the 3D food printing process using a turtle as a personalized and customized 3D printing example. Photographs kindly provided by Emart group.

printing execution, creation of the 3D printed food, and consumption or post-processing. For example, this process can be illustrated by designing a personalized turtle-shaped 3D model to produce custom cookies (Fig. 24.1).

3D food printing is still a poorly explored field, since most AM technologies are either unsuitable for food processing, they either use extremely high heat, produce adverse photopolymerization by products or have inadequate material sources. Market research suggests that 3D printers for functional fruit products should have the following characteristics (Tomašević et al., 2021): (1) Easy cleaning and refilling capabilities, enabling the use of diverse raw materials; (2) Compatibility with self-produced ingredients and adjustable printing parameters; (3) The ability to complete prints as swiftly as possible; (4) Interchangeable nozzles with different diameters to accommodate various materials and optimize printing; (5) Thermally controlled, high-capacity tanks and build plates that facilitate simultaneous cooking and printing; (6) Multi-material printing capabilities, which, while not critical, significantly enhance food design by improving nutritional value, taste, and aesthetics.

Table 24.1 presents a comprehensive overview of commercially available 3D printers for professional and consumer markets, highlighting their key features and specifications (Lee, 2021; Nachal et al., 2019; Pallottino et al., 2016; Sun et al., 2015; Yang et al., 2017). The commercial AM equipment for food printing highlights a diverse range of devices across various countries, showcasing different capabilities, technologies, and market applications, notable contributions are from countries like the United States, China, and several European nations. These food printers predominantly handle pastes, reflecting a focus on semi-solid foods that are easily extruded by AM material extrusion technology. Common materials include chocolate, cookie dough, and vegetable purées, as seen in devices like the byFlow Focus and Felix Food 3D Printer. The print area is a critical factor in determining the scale and scope of a food printer's applications. Larger print areas, such as those offered by the Lincsolution MonoPure Food (300 × 300 × 50 mm) and the Felix Food 3D Printer (220 × 195 × 170 mm), are suited for creating high quantities at the same time larger or more intricate designs. These devices are likely beneficial for commercial kitchens or culinary artists looking to produce detailed food sculptures or complex dishes. Conversely, smaller print areas like those found in the Wiiboox Sweetin (100 × 100 × 70 mm) and Print2Taste mycusini 2.0 (90 × 90 × 46 mm) are ideal for producing personalized food items such as customized chocolates and small pastries. These compact devices are perfect for use in home kitchens or small businesses looking to offer unique, bespoke food products.

The number of print heads on a food printer significantly influences its capability to handle complex tasks and diverse materials. Single-head printers, such as the Cocoa Press and Natural Machines Foodini, are generally easier to operate and maintain, making them suitable for specific applications like printing chocolate. In contrast, multihead printers like the Lincsolution MonoPure Food and Foodbot D2, which feature two print heads, and the Desktophealth

TABLE 24.1 Commercial Additive manufacturing equipment's for food printing.

Brand	Model	country	Print area (mm)	Heads	Price US$	AM Technology	Material state	Marketed Material
Lincsolution	MonoPure Food	South Korea	300 × 300 × 50	2	Upon request	MEX	Paste	Cellulse, alginate, chitosan, Agarose, gelatine, hyaluronic acid
Cocoa Press	Cocoa Press	United States	140 × 150 × 150	1	3995	MEX	Solid (heated and processed into paste)	Material: cocoa powder and vegetable oil Couverture chocolate: cocoa butter and chocolate liquor
Wiiboox	Sweetin	China	100 × 100 × 70	1	3875	MEX	Paste	Chocolate, cookie dough, potato paste, jelly
La Patisserie Numerique	Patiss3	France	unknown	1	Rent from 510 a month	MEX	Paste	Chocolate, meringue, tomato mixture, cream cheese, vegan lemon meringue,
Print4Taste	Procusini 5.0	Germany	unknown	1	3824	MEX	Paste	Chocolate
Natural Machines	Foodini	Spain	250 × 165 × 120	1	4000	MEX	Paste	Chocolate, Meringue
Print2Taste	mycusini 2.0	Germany	90 × 90 × 46	1	745	MEX	Paste	Chocolate
Foodbot	S2	China	150 x 150 x 70	1	2500	MEX	Paste	Chocolate
Foodbot	D2	China	150 x 150 x 70	2	7000	MEX	Paste	Chocolate
Wiiboox	LuckyBot + DIY kit	China	200 × 200 × 160	1	179 + 600	MEX	Paste	Chocolate, Chocolate, cookie dough, potato paste, jelly, candy
Felix Food	Felix Food 3D Printer	Netherlands	220 × 195 × 170	2	3600	MEX	Paste	Vegetable purees, fruit purees, doughs, sugars, and fats
byFlow	byFlow Focus	Netherlands	208 x 228 x 150	1	4000	MEX	Paste	Chocolate ganache, meringue, savory dips, fruit, cookie dough, meat, celery-hazelnut, marzipan, royal icing.
Delta	WASP 2040 Clay + Paste kit	Italy	200 × 200 × 40	1	3300 + 759	MEX	Paste	Cookie dough

3DBioplotter, which supports up to five heads, allow for more complex and multi-material printing. This capability is crucial for creating layered food items or combining different ingredients in a single print job. Multi-head printers are ideal for professional kitchens or research institutions where more sophisticated food printing tasks are required. The diverse price range of food printers, from budget-friendly options like the Print2Taste mycusini 2.0 at under $1,000 to premium models such as the Desktophealth 3DBioplotter exceeding $100,000, reflects the varying complexity and capabilities tailored for both casual or enthusiast users and professional markets. Therefore, AM technology offers new venues for creativity, customization, and sustainability in food production, making it an exciting field with significant implications for the future of food and cooking.

24.3 Additive manufacturing for production of functional food

AM technology have gained significant attention in recent years for their potential to revolutionize the food industry. By enabling precise control over the composition and structure of food products, AM can easy facilitate the creation of foods with tailored nutritional and functional properties. AM technology allows for the incorporation of bioactive molecules, probiotics, nutrient-rich substrates, and other actives ingredients into complex food matrices (Kewuyemi et al., 2022). Four primary AM technologies are currently employed in 3D food printing for both commercial applications and research purposes: material extrusion (MEX), selective laser sintering (SLS), binder jetting (BJT), and material jetting (MJT) (Sun et al., 2015; Tomašević et al., 2021).

A comprehensive review of relevant research, focusing on the intersection of functional foods and AM technologies was conducted using international databases and encompassing studies published between 2019 and 2024, with the findings summarized in Table 24.2, detailing the technologies, printers, parameters, materials, and key insights. MEX utilizes a continuous filament of extruded food material. This material is fed through a heated/cold nozzle and deposited in a controlled manner, layer-by-layer, to build the desired 3D structure of the food object. SLS utilizes powdered food materials. These materials are deposited in thin layers and then selectively heated to induce localized sintering. This process involves sintering of sugars or fats within the powders, causing them to fuse and form the desired 3D structure of the object. Similarly, BJT employs a different approach. Here, liquid binders are precisely deposited through tiny nozzles onto a powder bed, selectively binding the food particles together to create the 3D object. Finally, MJT relies on low-viscosity food materials. These materials are jetted as a stream of droplets that solidify rapidly to build up the object layer-by-layer according to a pre-defined design (He et al., 2020).

MEX technology has made a significant advancement in food printing by enabling the production of probiotic-rich edible products. The byFlow Focus printer, equipped with nozzles of 1.2 mm and 1.6 mm diameter, has been utilized to print cereal flour-based dough enriched with non-dairy probiotics like *Lactobacillusplantarum* and calcium caseinate (Zhang et al., 2018). These products maintain their geometry well after baking and provide the health benefits associated with probiotics, although lower moisture content in the dough resulted in brittleness and reduced stickiness. Another significant development is the creation of fortified cookies using MEX technology. By incorporating A. *platensis*, which is rich in antioxidants, into traditional dough ingredients such as wheat flour, butter, and powdered sugar, researchers have successfully enhanced the nutritional value of cookies (Vieira et al., 2020). The antioxidant encapsulation process has improved the product's overall health benefits while maintaining simple geometric designs suitable for MEX. The development of fiber-enriched snacks from mushrooms using a self-built delta MEX system represents another key achievement (Keerthana et al., 2020). This approach involved printing with wheat flour dough and white button mushrooms, resulting in snacks that are high in dietary fiber. The use of microwave cooking for these snacks has received good sensory acceptance, indicating that the printed products could be well-received by consumers. The FOODBOT-MF printer has been used to produce protein-based composite fruits, combining various protein isolates such as peanut protein, whey protein, and pea protein with fruit components (Chen et al., 2021). MEX technology has also facilitated the creation of reduced-fat 3D printed objects using casein-based inks, where Mycusini® and Procusini printers were employed to print foods from sodium caseinate, canola oil, and other stabilizers, resulting in highly porous structures with desirable sensory profiles, including a higher creamy sensation and greater stability against freezing (Shahbazi, Jäger, & Ettelaie, 2021). These printed fruits, particularly those using peanut protein isolate, have demonstrated good printability and nutritional benefits, showcasing the versatility of MEX technology in creating protein-rich foods. In another example, the byFlow printer has been used to produce cookies enriched with polyphenols (Oliveira et al., 2021). By incorporating encapsulated polyphenols into wheat flour-based dough, researchers have enhanced the bioactivity and total phenolic content of the cookies with faster cooking rate and less thermal degradation, demonstrating the potential of AM to improve the overall nutritional quality of food products. The Controlled Additive-Manufacturing Robotic Kit (CARK) has been employed to create nutrient-dense cookies from broken wheat and grape

TABLE 24.2 Production and customization of functional foods using additive manufacturing technologies (2019–2024).

AM Technology	AM printer	Parameters	Base Material	Achievements	Drawbacks	References
MEX	byFlow Focus	Nozzle: 1.2 mm or 1.6 mm. Speed: of 5 mm/s.	Cereal floor (with gluten) and probiotics: non-dairy (*Lactobacillus plantarum*) calcium caseinate.	During baking, the geometry of the 3D-printed structures containing probiotic bacteria was well-preserved. Production of probiotic rich edible products. Pastes with lower moisture content were more brittle, harder and less sticky.	Low resolution prints. Thin objects. Decreased survivability of probiotics with temperature.	Zhang et al. (2018)
MEX	Focus, Byflow	Nozzle: 1.6 mm, Speed: of 10 mm/s, layer height: 1.12 mm.	Wheat flour, butter, powdered sugar, milk and xanthan gum, microalga *A. platensis* (rich in C-phycocyanin, carotenoids and antioxidant compound)	The encapsulation of the antioxidant extract was capable of improving the antioxidant activity and colour stability along the storage time when compared to all other formulations. Dough formulations suitable for MEX. Cookies had water activity values low enough to be microbiologically stable, and the texture remained constant after 30 days of storage.	Simple geometries. The growth in the product's thickness.	Vieira et al. (2020)
MEX	Self-build delta system	Speed: 200, 400, 600, 800, and 1000 mm/min Nozzle 0.82 and 1.28 mm. Layer height: 25, 50 and 100% nozzle diameter.	Wheat flour, white button mushrooms.	Fiber-enriched snacks from mushroom Sensory attributes of the spiced 3D printed snack were more acceptable than sweet-flavored counterparts. The spice flavor better suited the 3D printed mushroom-based snack.	In plane vertical print. Difficult Infill during print. Small incorporation of additive.	Keerthana et al. (2020)
MEX	FOODBOT-MF	Speed: 1200 mm/min Nozzle 0.8 mm	Peanut protein isolate, whey protein isolate, pea protein, casein and wheat hydrolyzed protein. Sodium alginate, Guar gum, hawthorn, lemon, spinach and potato flour.	The ink based on peanut protein can be well accepted by consumers. The composite fruit and vegetable ink based on peanut isolate protein has stable and better printing properties.	Too high cohesiveness and hardness are not suitable for printing, and that would make the extrusion process in printing more difficult.Printing with ink of insufficient hardness resulted in poor printability.	Chen et al. (2021)

MEX	Mycusini®, Procusini	layer height was set at 1 mm 1 mm (slicer) 1.1 mm after the deposition of each layer Speed 15 mm/s	Sodium caseinate, canola oil, acetylated microcrystalline cellulose, cheese flavor agent and sodium azide.	Excellent sensory sensations. Production of high-quality reduced-fat 3D printed cheese. Reduced-fat 3D printed samples showed a desired sensory profile with a higher creamy sensation.	In plane vertical print. Poor shape resolution. Changes in the topographies.	Shahbazi, Jäger, and Ettelaie (2021)
MEX	byFlow	Nozzle diameter of 1.6 mm, layer height of 1.12 mm.	Wheat fine flour unsalted butter powdered sugar whole milk (xanthan gum, encapsulated polyphenols.	The bioactivity and total phenolic content improved. Total pores allow fast cooking and decrease thermal degradation.	In plane vertical print Poor shape resolution. Changes in the topographies.	Oliveira et al. (2021)
MEX	CARK (Controlled Additive-manufacturing Robotic Kit	Nozzle diameters (0.84 mm and 1.28 mm), printing speeds (400 mm/min, 600 mm/min, and 800 mm/min).	Broken wheat, fresh, ripe grapes, grape pomace Powder, grape pomace powder.	The developed product was rich in proteins and dietary fiber. Cookies with grape pomace powder received the highest preference during sensory evaluation. Enhancing the grape content led to a higher viscosity, which in turn allowed for a reduction in print speed and extrusion rate, thereby improving the printability.	Decrease in brightness and yellowness could be attributed to Maillard reaction, caramelization, and enzymatic browning effects. Sensory evaluation indicated a decrease in consumer acceptability beyond a 10% grape pomace incorporation level.	Jagadiswaran et al. (2021)
MEX	Foodini	Print speed: 2200 mm/min Nozzle height, 3 mm.	Dried guava, sugar, dried whole milk, cocoa powder, cricket flour, dried amaranth leaves, dried orange peel.	The printability evaluation showed that formulations with 6% and 8% of pregelatinized starch were more suitable for printing than the one with 10%.	Properties such as the yield stress, need to be correlated with printability tests to determine the optimum values for the rheological characteristics of a specific formulation.	Maldonado-Rosas et al. (2022)
MEX	Foodini	Nozzle diameter of 4 mm speed of 8000 or 14,000 mm/min; line thickness of 3.5 mm or 3.4 mm, flow rate of 1.4 or 1.65, nozzle height of the first layer of 6 mm or 4.5 mm.	*Arbutus unedo* L. fruits, corn starch and wheat starch.	The printed products were found to be a good source of polyphenols, namely condensed tannins. Good antimicrobial agent against pathogenic *S. aureus* and *E. coli* K-12 MG1655. High survival rate of probiotic *L. fermentum*.	Optimize the 3DP process in addition to the bioactive composition to obtain a product with desirable rheological properties. Three-layer plane print.	Markovinović et al. (2024)

(*Continued*)

TABLE 24.2 (Continued)

AM Technology	AM printer	Parameters	Base Material	Achievements	Drawbacks	References
MEX	Foodini	Nozzle diameter of 4 mm speed of 8000 or 14,000 mm/min; line thickness of 3.5 mm or 3.4 mm, flow rate of 1.4 or 1.6, nozzle height of the first layer of 6 mm or 4.5 mm	Strawberry juice (Fragaria x ananassa duch., cv. 'Albion'), corn starch, wheat starch	The production of strawberry-based functional snacks with 3D printing technology had favorable effects on the retention and stability of the bioactive components and antioxidant capacity. Corn starch resulted in a higher level of hydroxycinnamic acids, flavanols, total flavonoids, and antioxidant capacity as determined by the DPPH method heat starch had higher levels of total phenols, anthocyanins, condensed tannins, and antioxidant capacity	Lack of accuracy, poor resolution and single layer print	Bebek Markovinović et al. (2023)
MEX	Wiiboox Sweetin	Nozzle size: 0.84 mm. Print speed: 25 mm/min layer thickness: 0.4 mm	Vegetable powder (carrot) and protein powders (whey, soy, sericin and spirulina) and xanthan Gum	The optimization method demonstrated in this study is generalizable wherein other food ingredients and response of the food inks may be included for optimization	Some formulations lack definition and accuracy; smaller nozzle diameter generally translates to higher print accuracy with smooth extrusion.	Y. Zhang et al. (2022)
BJ	Spectrum Z510	Layer height 0.1 mm and core:Shell saturation 1:2.	Calcium Caseinate, medium-chain triglycerides, Tween 20 solution and wheat starch.	Increasing binder content in printed foods always led to a more cohesive sample Protein content in dry powder mixtures greatly influenced the springiness of the final product. Protein-rich foods with customized shape, texture, color, and unconventional mouthfeel	Simple model prints. Swelling during printing.	Zhu et al. (2022)
SLS	TNO powder bed printer	Velocity of 60 mm/s. Hatch distance of 0.2 mm Layer thickness of 0.3 mm Power 2.04 and 4.09 W	Palm oil, wheat starch Maltodextrin	Printing with higher area energy density decreased the ductility and increased the stiffness of the geometry distortion. Warpage was reduced by firstly printing support structures and subsequently printing the product with a successive checkerboard strategy. Printing a larger volume fraction of the product with high energy density resulted in stiffer and more brittle products	Simple model prints. Crack growth occurred along the interfaces of the unit cells, which were weakened through the printing checkerboard strategy.	Jonkers et al. (2022)

pomace powder (Jagadiswaran et al., 2021). These cookies, rich in proteins and dietary fibers, received high preference during sensory evaluations, highlighting the ability of AM to produce foods with enhanced nutritional profiles and consumer appeal. The Foodini printer has been used to produce functional snacks from dried fruits and starches (Maldonado-Rosas et al., 2022). Formulations incorporating strawberry juice, corn starch, and wheat starch have been shown to retain and stabilize bioactive components, leading to snacks with improved antioxidant capacity and nutritional benefits. Using the Foodini printer, researchers have also created polyphenol-rich products from *Arbutus unedo* L. fruits, corn starch, and wheat starch (Bebek Markovinović et al., 2024). These printed foods are effective antimicrobial agents and provide a high survival rate for probiotics like *Lactobacillus fermentum*, underscoring the potential of AM technology to produce health-promoting foods. In other study, a larger nozzle diameter of 4 mm, with print speeds of 8000 to 14,000 mm/min and a layer thickness of around 3.5 mm, was used for 3D Printing of functional strawberry snacks (Bebek Markovinović et al., 2023). These parameters are chosen to facilitate the rapid extrusion of food materials, making the system suitable for producing larger quantities of food or items with simpler geometries at high production rates. Tested materials include strawberry juice, corn starch, and wheat starch. All food samples exhibited good textural properties, a high degree of stability and minimal geometric deviations. Wiiboox Sweetin successfully printed foods with a combination of vegetable powders, protein powders, and xanthan gum. The same printer processed fruit puree (strawberry juice), starches (corn and wheat), which highlights the potential for various food ingredients to be printed (Zhang et al., 2022). These parameters are tailored for detailed printing, which is critical when working with delicate food materials. The study highlights that the optimization methods applied are adaptable to other food ingredients and can be generalized across various food inks. This is significant as it demonstrates the system's flexibility in adjusting extrusion parameters to achieve desired textures and structures in different food formulations.

BJT technology has been explored for producing customized protein-rich foods. The Spectrum Z510 printer has been used to create foods from calcium caseinate and wheat starch, resulting in products with customizable textures and unique mouthfeel, though swelling during printing remains a challenge. SLS with the TNO powder bed printer has shown promise for controlling the structure of printed foods. By printing with higher area energy density, researchers have reduced warping and increased the stiffness of the printed products, although issues with brittleness and crack growth persist. In SLS for instance, besides the adequate powder rheology, the food materials also need to sinter without degrading with heat. Also, velocity, hatch distance, layer thickness and laser power directly affect the energy density for the construction making it difficult to have a product that is not dry and brittle (Jonkers et al., 2022; Liu et al., 2017).

Analysis of Table 24.2 reveals that MEX deposition emerges as a user-friendly AM approach compared to other 3D food printing technologies. This accessibility can be attributed to its similarity to traditional manual paste deposition, a familiar technique for many cooks around the world. In contrast, others AM technologies present various limitations, where some technologies are cost-prohibitive, while others necessitate specific requirements such as compatible binders for powder beds while maintaining the powder bed's stability throughout the process, or when using thermal energy instead. The typical parameters studied in MEX food printing are usually related with the geometrical features of the prints and the capabilities and limitations of the available equipment, namely nozzle diameter, deposition rate, printing speed, layer height, and distance to the build plate. The range values differ from machine to machine, paste to paste and the relation with the material properties and the machine (Sundarsingh et al., 2023; Wang et al., 2022). Although MJT has been utilized in the food industry, no references were found regarding its application in functional foods. Therefore, it is not included, as it does not meet the research criteria for inclusion in Table 24.2.

24.4 Lab-grown foods

Global animal food production has become a critical driver of both environmental and societal dynamics, exerting profound impacts on ecosystems, climate change, and human health. With an estimated population of 10 billion in 2050 and the continuing rise in demand for meat, dairy, and other animal-derived products, the consequences of large-scale livestock farming are becoming increasingly apparent (Alexandratos & Bruinsma, 2012). The intricate web of interconnected effects encompasses deforestation, water pollution, greenhouse gas emissions, and biodiversity loss. This raises concerns about the sustainability and long-term viability of current production systems, particularly considering their occupation of more than 30% of arable land, 8% of freshwater resources, and the emission of 18% of greenhouse gases (Cai et al., 2024). Moreover, the ethical dimensions of factory farming practices and the welfare of animals involved in food production have prompted calls for a revaluation of our relationship with and approach to animal agriculture. Certainly, lab-grown foods, also known as cultured or cell-based foods, represent an innovative and evolving area of

TABLE 24.3 Examples of lab-grown foods currently in development.

Product	Cell Source	Production method	References
Steak	Primary bovine myoblasts and primary bovine adipose-derived mesenchymal stem cells	Gelatin/alginate-based hydrogel scaffold	Lee, Park, et al. (2024)
Poultry meat	Satellite cells from skeletal muscle samples of broiler chickens	Deposition in cell culture flask (T75)	Joo et al. (2022)
Salmon	Pacific salmon stem cells	Plant-based scaffolds	Wildtype and Salmon (2016)
Bovine milk ingredients	Lactating cells from cows	Cell culturing in a medium that signals the secretion of fat molecules from milk	Wilk (2024)
Honey	Plant-cell based	Cell engineering and precision fermentation to replace honeybees with microorganisms as a medium for honey production.	Melibio (2023)
Non-Conventional Food Plants (PANCs)	Cells from the callus tissues of *Tessaria absinthioides*	Cell lines propagation into solid medium cultures to obtain biomass	Martinez et al. (2023)

food technology, particularly in the development of functional foods. Cellular agriculture involves the use of single-cell organisms, cell cultures, and bioreactors for the industrial production of food and food ingredients (Zhang et al., 2020). It provides an alternative to current agricultural practices and food production systems, enabling the use of animal and plant cells to obtain cellular and acellular products, such as cultured meat and microbial biomass, as well as proteins, lipids, and food additives, respectively (Behm et al., 2022). Moreover, lab-grown foods offer precise control over the nutritional content and flavour of the final product. This level of customization can result in healthier and tastier options for consumers. In this context, bioprinting stands out as a technology facilitating the precise arrangement of cellular and acellular components within biomaterials to create 3D functional living tissues (Handral et al., 2022).

Since the initial research in the early 2000s, methods for producing food through cellular cultivation have been extensively studied and are now poised to transition from laboratories to large-scale production facilities (FAO, 2022). A significant milestone occurred in 2013 with the introduction of the first beef burger created using this technology (Post & Hocquette, 2017). Subsequently, in December 2020, regulatory approval was granted for the first cell-based chicken nuggets in Singapore. Up until 2021, a global count reveals that at least 107 companies are actively involved in developing similar products (Lee, Lee, et al., 2024). Various products and commodities, spanning meats, poultry, fish, aquatic items, dairy, and eggs, are in the pipeline for future commercialization (Waltz, 2022). The "cell-culturing" technique utilizes both plant and animal cells as sources and has the potential to generate acellular products like milk, proteins, or fats (Table 24.3).

24.4.1 Lab-grown meat as a novel functional food

The Lab-Grown foods can be derived from either animal or non-animal sources, including bovine and horse serum (Bhat et al., 2014; Sergelidis, 2019), or hydrolysed cyanobacteria known as blue-green algae and Maitake mushroom extract (Tuomisto & Teixeira De Mattos, 2011). In LGM, cells (scaffold methods) or tissues (self-organizing techniques) are cultured in vitro on a customizable and controlled platform. The straightforward and accurate manipulation of the cell microenvironment may be employed to fine-tune meat characteristics (Ben-Arye & Levenberg, 2019; Bhat et al., 2015). To cultivate muscle tissue and potentially other meat components such as fat and connective tissue, three essential components are necessary: tissue-specific cells with replicative capacity, a biomaterial temporarily maintaining cells in a tissue configuration, and a bioreactor to feed the tissue and provide mechanical and biochemical stimuli for optimal differentiation. Meat primarily comprises skeletal muscle cells, and as mature skeletal muscle cells no longer proliferate, stem cells are the only source of replication-competent precursors (Post, 2012).

LGM could serve as an excellent functional food as it is adaptable to modifications in essential amino acids and fats, enabling enrichment in vitamins, minerals, and bioactive compounds (Orzechowski, 2015). This not only allows it to match the proportionate amounts found in natural meat but also surpass them, addressing specific dietary needs for individuals with various ailments (Sergelidis, 2019). In comparison to regular meat, LGM can be engineered to be healthier and more functional by manipulating the composition of the culture medium, which might undergo certain modifications. By maintaining basic homeostatic parameters (isoionia, isoosmia, isohydria) within acceptable limits, it becomes possible to introduce changes in composition determinants of nutritional value, including minerals, vitamins, fat content, and more (Sergelidis, 2019). For instance, the ratio of saturated to polyunsaturated fatty acids could be more effectively regulated. Omega-3 presents itself as an excellent alternative to replace saturated fats, although the potential risk of higher rancidity requires careful regulation. In recent times, techniques have emerged to augment the quantity of omega-3 fatty acids in meat. Omega-3 has been shown to mitigate risk factors associated with heart disease, such as triglycerides and blood pressure, potentially influencing positively the sales of cell-based meat in the future (Roy et al., 2021). Addressing the absence of myoglobin protein in its composition, which is responsible for the red color of meat from animal origin, could be remedied by incorporating pigmented biocompounds, natural pigments like anthocyanins and betalains (Siddiqui et al., 2022). In addition to their color properties, these compounds might also serve as preservatives (da Silva et al., 2019). Furthermore, meat is a vital source of minerals, including iron. Therefore, supplementing the cell culture medium with additional iron raises the iron level in cultured meat (Rubio et al., 2019). Iron exists as a component of heme in myoglobin or in combination with ferritin. From a nutritional perspective, absorption is more effective in the non-heme form (Roy et al., 2021). Hence, LGM enriched with extra myoglobin content proves advantageous, not only in terms of its texture and taste but also nutritionally.

Examining the prolonged impact of growth factors on humans is crucial (Roy et al., 2021). As a result, potential hazards and risks could be unintentionally introduced at any phase of LGM production. It is imperative that these aspects undergo comprehensive scrutiny and receive approval from the regulations or legislation of the respective jurisdictions before introducing the product to the market (Gu et al., 2023). Regrettably, LGM often faces the perception of being unnatural among consumers globally (Bryant & Sanctorum, 2021; Siegrist & Hartmann, 2020). Nevertheless, with the rise of functional and fortified foods, consumers are increasingly open to trying products that have been modified to exhibit specific functional and nutritional characteristics (Siddiqui et al., 2022). Hence, it is imperative to enhance functionality and sensory quality to boost consumer acceptance by emphasizing the positive aspects of the technology.

Life cycle assessment studies have revealed that the production process of LGM would occupy almost negligible arable land and freshwater. Additionally, it would lead to a substantial reduction in energy consumption and greenhouse gas emissions compared to traditional meat production methods (Tuomisto et al., 2015). Furthermore, LGM offers various sustainability advantages, encompassing health and safety benefits, resource conservation, and improved animal welfare. The strictly controlled ingredients added to the culture medium and the execution of key production processes, such as seeded cell extraction, cell proliferation, and differentiation in a sterile environment LGM to effectively mitigate the risks associated with various traditional food-borne diseases, and reduce the transmission risk of animal illnesses (Cai et al., 2024). In this manner, LGM could serve as an efficient solution to balance animal protein production and environmental protection.

In recent years, various food industries have prioritized the research and development of meat analogy products, using non-meat ingredients (Han et al., 2023). These formulations typically consist of proteins, carbohydrates, water, fats, salt, and spices (Kyriakopoulou et al., 2021). When proteins are derived from vegetables like soybeans, peas, or fava beans, these products are commonly referred to as plant-based meat substitutes (McClements & Grossmann, 2021). Other potential alternatives include proteins sourced from algae, microbes, edible fungi, microalgae, and insects (Zhang et al., 2022). Proteins, as primary biomolecules, play a crucial role in shaping the gel network and forming meat-like fiber structures (Chen, Li, et al., 2023). They also contribute to water binding and stabilize emulsions and gels (Kyriakopoulou et al., 2021). Carbohydrates, on the other hand, facilitate protein cross-linking, acting as thickeners, fillers, and binders (Chen et al., 2022). Oils add sensory attributes such as tenderness, juiciness, flavor, and nutritional value to plant-based meat analog products (McClements & Grossmann, 2021). The juiciness is also closely associated with water-holding capacity (Kyriakopoulou et al., 2021). Furthermore, molecular interactions among lipids, proteins, water, and carbohydrates have significant effects on functional performance and textural characteristics (Chen, Li, et al., 2023; Chen, Zhang, et al., 2023). Emulgels and oleogels are employed as animal fat substitutes, providing health benefits by replacing saturated fat (Guo et al., 2023). During cooking, the melted fat and released water contribute to juiciness, necessitating fat substitutes with melting points closer to animal fats (Guo et al., 2023). To replicate the juiciness of meat fat, Han, Wang, Guo, Wang and Yang (Han et al., 2023) proposed creating oils from oleogel and emulgel structures using soy and whey protein isolate, soybean oil, and transglutaminase. Conversely, the substitution of canola oil with dodecenyl succinylated inulin and hydroxyethyl cellulose, used as surfactants in reduced-fat meat analogs by 3D printing, exhibited high printability and the development of fibrous soy protein and anisotropic structures (Shahbazi, Jäger & Chen, & Ettelaie, 2021). Various unit operations, including 3D printing, extrusion, shear cell, electrospinning, wet spinning, and freeze structuring, are employed in the production of meat analogs (Lima et al., n.d.). For plant-based meat for functional foods development, challenges include achieving the appropriate texture and juiciness for creating meat mimics. Until this obstacle is overcome, these technologies are more suitable for producing products like minced beef for hamburgers, franks, nuggets, and meatballs, among others. However, numerous opportunities arise for formulating enriched analog meat with micronutrients (such as vitamins and minerals), essential amino acids, bioactive compounds, and natural dyes. Additionally, there are possibilities for innovation to manufacture dishes mimicking the tender texture of meat for elderly individuals and people with swallowing difficulties.

24.4.2 Lab-grown meat products via 3D bioprinting

The shape of LGM plays a crucial role in consumer acceptance. According to a recent survey, 58 % of respondents express an interest in paying a premium for LMG. On average, 37% of respondents are willing to consider the price of regular meat for CM (Rolland et al., 2020). Currently, CM products lack the desired texture for a genuine chewing experience. Achieving highly structured and organized tissues would necessitate the engineering of highly perfused scaffolds (Stephens et al., 2018). In this context, various scaffolding technologies, such as electrospinning, electrospray, and prominently 3D bioprinting, have been proposed to fabricate 3D structures with suitable biological, structural, and mechanical characteristics (Levi et al., 2022). 3D bioprinting is an innovative process that involves arranging cellular and acellular components, precisely positioning biomaterials with cells to construct complex 3D functional living tissues (Handral et al., 2022). The three major bioprinting techniques widely utilized are inkjet, laser-assisted (LA), and extrusion-based bioprinting (EB) (Handral et al., 2022; Levi et al., 2022). Fig. 24.2 illustrates examples of cultured food production using inkjet, laser-assisted, and extrusion-based 3D bioprinting techniques.

In MJT, small-sized droplets of liquid ink are produced and deposited onto the desired location on the substrate (Li et al., 2020). This 3D bioprinting approach is considered versatile and affordable, offering precision with the ability to

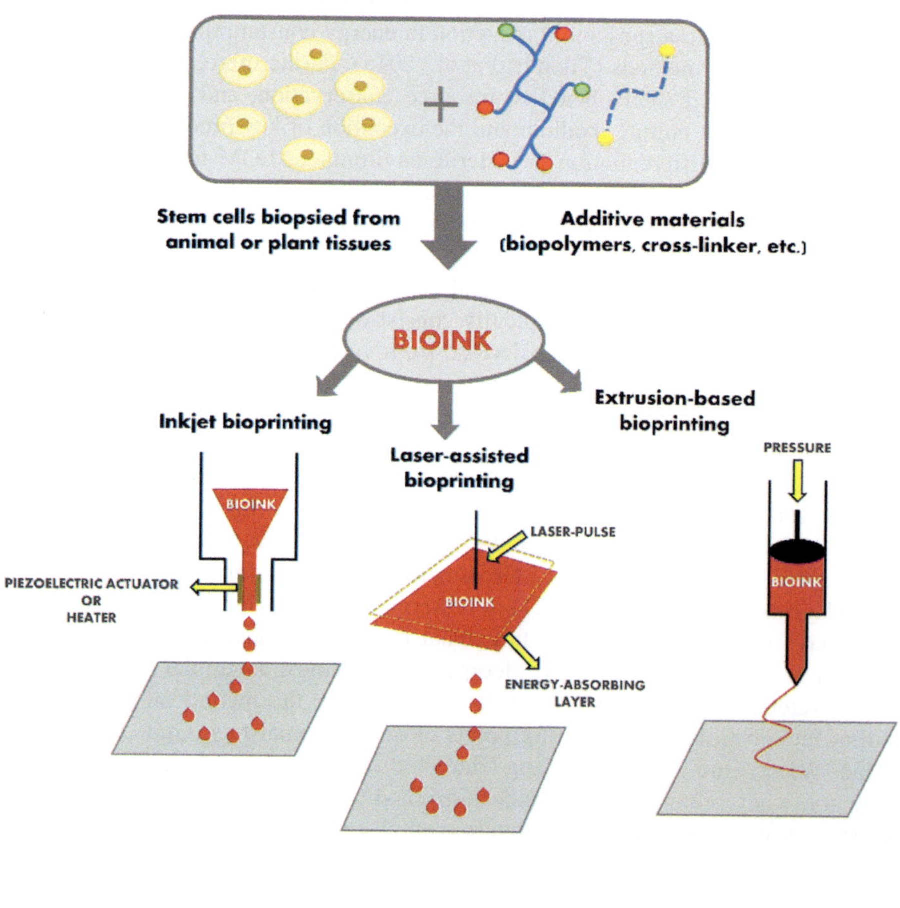

FIGURE 24.2 Inkjet, laser-assisted, and extrusion-based 3D bioprinting of cultured foods. Image provided by the authors.

achieve high printing resolutions and 70 to 96% cell viability (Levi et al., 2022). However, there are limitations to the bioinks used in this method. In addition to low viscosity, it is crucial for bioinks to have a pre-established crosslinking mechanism to stabilize the printed structure (Murphy & Atala, 2014). Additionally, the small nozzle is prone to clogging and difficult to clean, impeding production efficiency for large-scale manufacturing (Levi et al., 2022).

The LA bioprinting involves depositing a liquid bioink onto a metal-coated ribbon, followed by laser-induced cavitation, creating micro-droplets of bioink (Hakobyan et al., 2020). LA can maintain high cellular viability (over 95%), is compatible with various bioink viscosities (1 – 300 mPa/s), and the nozzle-free deposition avoids clogging issues (Murphy & Atala, 2014). However, the laser sources are costly, and laser control poses challenges (Wang et al., 2015). Furthermore, the presence of metallic residues in the final product raises safety concerns for food systems, limiting the use of LA in the commercial production of LGM (Levi et al., 2022).

One of the most prevalent 3D bioprinting approaches for LGM production is EB primarily due to its versatile nature, simplicity, and low cost, allowing for commercialization and application in various fields. In EB, the bioink is dispensed by a computer-controlled robotic system, resulting in the precise and continuous deposition of cylindrical filaments (fibers) (Cui et al., 2020; Murphy & Atala, 2014). However, printing time is relatively slow and may lead to lower cell viability (40 – 86%) compared to other methods due to shear stress on the cells during extrusion (Levi et al., 2022). EB can be achieved through various techniques, with direct ink writing being the simplest, accomplished through shear thinning of the selected bioink (Cui et al., 2020). The extruded hydrogel often spreads after deposition, requiring a fixation method to ensure the stability of the printed structure, such as photo-curing (Yirmibesoglu et al., 2021), or immersing the printed construct in a solution of a crosslinking agent (Yuan et al., 2021). Co-axial extrusion can also be employed, where the bioink and its crosslinker are printed using an assembly of co-axial needles (Costantini et al., 2019). Sacrificial writing into functional tissue (SWIFT) may also be used for patterning perfusable channels within a cellularized matrix (Skylar-Scott et al., n.d.).

Various 3D bioprinting methods necessitate the development of appropriate bioinks, carefully designed to ensure the printed scaffold's high shape fidelity while maintaining cell viability. EB relies on non-Newtonian bioinks with shear-thinning properties, typically achieved through hydrogel-based formulations (Schwab et al., 2020). Additionally, the EB bioink should display a minimal Barus effect, ensuring that the fluid does not expand after being ejected from the nozzle (Jammalamadaka & Tappa, 2018). Food-grade bioinks may comprise biopolymers like gelatin (Wang et al., 2017), cellulose (Armstrong et al., 2022), alginate (Axpe & Oyen, 2016), along with plant proteins such as zein (Tavares-Negrete et al., 2021). These biopolymers feature established food-grade crosslinking mechanisms, facilitating the formation of a stable hydrogel within the printed construct, while the bioink maintains its desired fluidic properties (Levi et al., 2022).

Bioprinted CM differs significantly from traditional CM, as it involves the printing of muscle cells, fat cells, and extracellular matrix supportive cells within a scaffold that fosters cell growth and proliferation (Handral et al., 2022). The bioink, composed of cells and biomaterials, plays a crucial role in this process by creating scaffold structures where muscle fibers are formed, eventually becoming meat. Following the printing, the meat undergoes further maturation, often with the assistance of bioreactors that facilitate nutrient transport (Singh et al., 2023). In contrast, traditional CM is produced by propagating muscle cells, attaching them to a scaffold or carrier, and then transferring them to a suitable bioreactor with growth media (Sharma et al., 2015). However, this method has inherent limitations, particularly in producing highly structured meats like steaks (Gaydhane et al., 2018). Conventional 3D cell culture, when combined with scaffolds, lacks precision in regulating cell positioning between scaffold layers, leading to challenges in tissue maturation and potentially resulting in poor nutritional and organoleptic profiles for CM (Handral et al., 2022). The 3D bioprinting process addresses these limitations by allowing precise regulation of cell-cell ratios, cell positioning, and even cell densities of specific types. This promises to achieve LGM without compromising texture and its meat-like profile. To create 3D bioprinted LGM, a biomimetic composition of edible materials that supports cell survivability and growth is essential. Key factors for successful 3D printing of LGM include the rheological properties of meat-ink, post-printing deposition, and the stability of the 3D printed scaffold during cooking (Handral et al., 2022; Levi et al., 2022).

Certainly, the versatility, precision, and reproducibility of 3D bioprinting make it a promising tool for the production of LGM. The commercialization potential of this approach has already been recognized by several companies actively developing 3D printed LGM platforms. Some of these companies include the Israeli MeaTech (specializing in beef and poultry), Aleph Farms (focused on beef), and Future Meat (offering multiple species), along with the American BlueNalu (specializing in fish and seafood) (Elemoso et al., 2020). Moreover, 3D bioprinting of LGM undeniably offers flexibility to meat products, enabling them to be crafted with distinctive textures and shapes, as well as with nutritional value and functional properties tailored for specific consumer preferences.

24.5 Perspective and future challenges on functional food

The rising healthcare costs have spurred governments, researchers, healthcare professionals, and the food industry to explore effective solutions for managing these financial pressures. Key drivers of the growing functional foods market include increasing rates of obesity and diabetes, heightened concerns about eye health, a surge in cardiovascular disease cases, changing dietary habits in developing regions, and a growing preference for preventive health measures (Daliri & Lee, 2015). Functional foods have emerged as a critical strategy in this context.

The future of functional foods is promising, with the potential to significantly impact public health and nutrition. However, addressing the challenges related to scientific validation, consumer education, regulatory compliance, economic accessibility, and sustainability is crucial for the continued growth and success of the functional food industry. The stability, formulation, and utilization of health functional foods significantly impact their actual efficacy and user experience with these products (Su et al., 2023). Furthermore, establishing clear dose-response relationships is crucial for determining the precise amount of functional ingredients necessary for optimal efficacy and to prevent potential adverse effects. Addressing factors such as variability in bioavailability, accessibility across different populations, and the necessity for standardized regulatory frameworks are also essential steps toward ensuring consistent quality and safety in the functional foods industry. By understanding these factors, researchers and food manufacturers can develop functional foods that are not only rich in beneficial ingredients but also deliver them in a form that maximizes their health impact. In addition, food industries are actively seeking alternatives to develop foods with functional properties and pharmacological attributes. Therefore, there is a growing demand to find solutions that offer high productivity while ensuring adequate quality in final food products.

The major challenge in using enriched food products lies in producing stable products and maintaining their integrity and functional properties throughout preparation, processing, transportation, and storage until they reach the consumer. The functional foods contain bioactive substances primarily including phenolic compounds, flavonoids (such as flavanols, flavones, flavanols, and flavanones), alkaloids, as well as food pigments like β-carotene, lycopene, lutein, and curcumin (Su et al., 2023). These compounds in humans are linked to a wide array of health benefits due to their bioactive properties, including anti-inflammatory, anticancer, anti-aging, cardiovascular protection, neuroprotection, immunomodulation, antidiabetic, antibacterial, antiparasitic, and antiviral effects (Dias et al., 2021). However, exposure to harsh environmental conditions can render these compounds chemically unstable, making them susceptible to degradation, volatilization, and oxidation (Tavares et al., 2021; Tavares, Smaoui, et al., 2022). In this sense, encapsulation technology have been employed as promising technology to protect and maintain the biological activities of the bioactive compounds during the processing and development of novel, enriched food products for industrial application (Tavares, Zapata Noreña, et al., 2022).

Personalized functional food products, crafted from lab-grown cells and printed with precision to deliver targeted nutrients and functionalities, signify a leap forward in advanced food innovation. These innovations not only cater to personalized nutrition needs but also hold promise for improving health outcomes and promoting sustainability in the food system. Lab-grown foods, such as meat and other items cultivated from animal cells in controlled environments, are revolutionizing food production. Similarly, AM technology is transforming food production by enabling the creation of intricate three-dimensional structures using edible materials. Personalized functional food products, developed from lab-grown cells and printed with precision to deliver targeted nutrients and functionalities, represent a major stride in advanced food innovation. The challenges for these technologies include scaling production, ensuring safety and regulatory compliance, and optimizing cost-effectiveness to make personalized functional foods accessible to a broader consumer base. Overcoming these challenges will be important in unlocking the full potential of lab-grown foods and 3D-printed food products to revolutionize the functional food industries on a global scale.

24.6 Conclusion

The development of functional food products is undergoing a profound transformation, driven by innovative advancements in lab-grown foods and 3D-printed food products. These emerging technologies offer compelling opportunities for nutrient customization, enhanced functionality, and the advancement of personalized nutrition. Leveraging the potential of lab-grown cells and additive manufacturing, the functional food industry is poised to revolutionize dietary preferences, optimize health outcomes, and contribute to a more ecologically sustainable food system. Despite these promising advances, the development of new functional food presents certain challenges, including regulatory compliance, consumer acceptance, the selection of appropriate biomaterials, and the challenge of achieving a texture and nutritional value like those of conventional product. Therefore, it is essential to ensure that consumer acceptance is maintained, and regulatory approval processes will be required to enable further development of the sector.

Acknowledgments

J. M. Oliveira acknowledges the financial support of CICECO – Aveiro Institute of Materials, UIDB/50011/2020 (DOI 10.54499/UIDB/50011/2020), UIDP/50011/2020 (DOI 10.54499/UIDP/50011/2020), and LA/P/0006/2020 (DOI 10.54499/LA/P/0006/2020), financed by national funds through the FCT/MCTES (PIDDAC). C.P.Z. Noreña acknowledges the financial support from The Brazilian National Council for Scientific and Technological Development (CNPq, proc. 308566/2022-0). LT thanks FCT for the Junior Researcher contract awarded under the 6th Edition of the Individual Call to Scientific Employment Stimulus (Ref: 2023.09409.CEECIND). LRS thanks FCT for the PhD grant (Ref: 2023.02457.BDANA).

References

Aguiar, L. M., Geraldi, M. V., Betim Cazarin, C. B., & Maróstica Junior, M. R. (2019). *Functional Food Consumption and Its Physiological Effects. Bioactive Compounds: Health Benefits and Potential Applications* (pp. 205–225). Brazil: Elsevier. Available from https://www.sciencedirect.com/book/9780128147740, https://doi.org/10.1016/B978-0-12-814774-0.00011-6.

Ahire, E. D., Sharma, N., Gupta, P. C., Khairnar, S., Surana, K., Ahire, B., Sonawane, V., Laddha, U., Sonkamble, S., Sabale, R., & Kshirsagar, S. (2022). *Developing formulations of prebiotics and probiotics. Prebiotics and Probiotics in Disease Regulation and Management* (pp. 271–290). India: Wiley. Available from https://www.wiley.com/en-us/Prebiotics + and + Probiotics + in + Disease + Regulation + and + Management-p-9781394166275, https://doi.org/10.1002/9781394167227.ch10.

Alexandratos, N., & Bruinsma, J. (2012), 2012.

Armstrong, C. D., Yue, L., Deng, Y., & Qi, H. J. (2022). Enabling direct ink write edible 3D printing of food purees with cellulose nanocrystals. *Journal of Food Engineering*, *330*. Available from https://doi.org/10.1016/j.jfoodeng.2022.111086, http://www.sciencedirect.com/science/journal/02608774.

ASTM ISO/ASTM52900-15 standard terminology for additive manufacturing—General principles—Terminology. (2015), 2015.

Axpe, E., & Oyen, M. L. (2016). Applications of alginate-based bioinks in 3D bioprinting. *International Journal of Molecular Sciences*, *17*(12). Available from https://doi.org/10.3390/ijms17121976, http://www.mdpi.com/1422-0067/17/12/1976/pdf.

Baker, M. T., Lu, P., Parrella, J. A., & Leggette, H. R. (2022). Consumer Acceptance toward Functional Foods: A Scoping Review. *International Journal of Environmental Research and Public Health*, *19*(3). Available from https://doi.org/10.3390/ijerph19031217, https://www.mdpi.com/1660-4601/19/3/1217/pdf.

Barbosa, W., Correia, P., Vieira, J., Leal, I., Rodrigues, L., Nery, T., Barbosa, J., & Soares, M. (2023). Trends and Technological Challenges of 3D Bioprinting in Cultured Meat: Technological Prospection. *Applied Sciences*, *13*(22), 12158. Available from https://doi.org/10.3390/app132212158.

Bebek Markovinović, A., Putnik, P., Bosiljkov, T., Kostelac, D., Frece, J., Markov, K., Žigolić, A., Kaurinović, J., Pavlić, B., Duralija, B., Zavadlav, S., & Bursać Kovačević, D. (2023). 3D Printing of Functional Strawberry Snacks: Food Design, Texture, Antioxidant Bioactive Compounds, and Microbial Stability. *Antioxidants*, *12*(2). Available from https://doi.org/10.3390/antiox12020436, www.mdpi.com/journal/antioxidants.

Behm, K., Nappa, M., Aro, N., Welman, A., Ledgard, S., Suomalainen, M., & Hill, J. (2022). Comparison of carbon footprint and water scarcity footprint of milk protein produced by cellular agriculture and the dairy industry. *The International Journal of Life Cycle Assessment*, *27*(8), 1017–1034. Available from https://doi.org/10.1007/s11367-022-02087-0.

Ben-Arye, T., & Levenberg, S. (2019). Tissue Engineering for Clean Meat Production. *Frontiers in Sustainable Food Systems*, *3*. Available from https://doi.org/10.3389/fsufs.2019.00046, www.frontiersin.org/journals/sustainable-food-systems#.

Bhat, Z. F., Bhat, H., & Pathak, V. (2014). *Prospects for In Vitro Cultured Meat – A Future Harvest* (pp. 1663–1683). Elsevier BV. Available from https://doi.org/10.1016/b978-0-12-398358-9.00079-3.

Bhat, Z. F., Kumar, S., & Fayaz, H. (2015). In vitro meat production: Challenges and benefits over conventional meat production. *Editorial Department of Scientia Agricultura Sinica, India Journal of Integrative Agriculture*, *14*(2), 241–248. Available from https://doi.org/10.1016/S2095-3119(14)60887-X, http://www.elsevier.com/journals/journal-of-integrative-agriculture/2095-3119.

Broucke, K., Pamel, E. V., Coillie, E. V., Herman, L., & Royen, G. V. (2023). Cultured meat and challenges ahead: A review on nutritional, technofunctional and sensorial properties, safety and legislation. *Meat Science*, *195*, 109006. Available from https://doi.org/10.1016/j.meatsci.2022.109006.

Bryant, C., & Sanctorum, H. (2021). Alternative proteins, evolving attitudes: Comparing consumer attitudes to plant-based and cultured meat in Belgium in two consecutive years. *Appetite*, *161*, 105161. Available from https://doi.org/10.1016/j.appet.2021.105161.

Cai, J., Wang, S., Li, Y., Dong, S., Liang, J., Liu, Y., & Li, S. (2024). Industrialization progress and challenges of cultivated meat. *Journal of Future Foods*, *4*(2), 119–127. Available from https://doi.org/10.1016/j.jfutfo.2023.06.002, https://www.sciencedirect.com/journal/journal-of-future-foods.

Chen, Q., Zhang, J., Zhang, Y., Kaplan, D. L., & Wang, Q. (2022). Protein-amylose/amylopectin molecular interactions during high-moisture extruded texturization toward plant-based meat substitutes applications. *Food Hydrocolloids*, *127*, 107559. Available from https://doi.org/10.1016/j.foodhyd.2022.107559.

Chen, Q., Zhang, J., Zhang, Y., Liu, H., Li, T., Wang, Q., & Kaplan, D. L. (2023). Microscopic insight into the interactions between pea protein and fatty acids during high-moisture extrusion processing. *Food Chemistry*, *404*, 134176. Available from https://doi.org/10.1016/j.foodchem.2022.134176.

Chen, Y., Li, L., Chen, L., Shao, W., Chen, X., Fan, X., Liu, Y., Ding, S., Xu, X., Zhou, G., & Feng, X. (2023). Gellan gum-gelatin scaffolds with Ca2 + crosslinking for constructing a structured cell cultured meat model. *Biomaterials*, *299*, 122176. Available from https://doi.org/10.1016/j.biomaterials.2023.122176.

Chen, Y., Zhang, M., & Phuhongsung, P. (2021). 3D printing of protein-based composite fruit and vegetable gel system. *LWT*, *141*, 110978. Available from https://doi.org/10.1016/j.lwt.2021.110978.

Costantini, M., Colosi, C., Święszkowski, W., & Barbetta, A. (2019). Co-axial wet-spinning in 3D bioprinting: state of the art and future perspective of microfluidic integration. *Biofabrication*, *11*(1), 012001. Available from https://doi.org/10.1088/1758-5090/aae605.

Cui, X., Li, J., Hartanto, Y., Durham, M., Tang, J., Zhang, H., Hooper, G., Lim, K., & Woodfield, T. (2020). Advances in Extrusion 3D Bioprinting: A Focus on Multicomponent Hydrogel-Based Bioinks. *Advanced Healthcare Materials*, *9*(15). Available from https://doi.org/10.1002/adhm.201901648, http://onlinelibrary.wiley.com/journal/10.1002/(ISSN)2192-2659.

Daliri, E. B.-M., & Lee, B. H. (2015). *Current Trends and Future Perspectives on Functional Foods and Nutraceuticals* (pp. 221–244). Springer Science and Business Media LLC. Available from https://doi.org/10.1007/978-3-319-23177-8_10.

Dias, M. C., Pinto, D. C. G. A., & Silva, A. M. S. (2021). Plant flavonoids: Chemical characteristics and biological activity. *Molecules (Basel, Switzerland)*, *26*(17). Available from https://doi.org/10.3390/molecules26175377, https://www.mdpi.com/1420-3049/26/17/5377/pdf.

Elemoso, A., Shalunov, G., Balakhovsky, Y. M., Ostrovskiy, A. Y., & Khesuani, Y. D. (2020). Bioprinting, The Roller Coaster Ride to Commercialization. *Int J Bioprint*, *6*(3), 2020.

Escalante-Aburto, A., Trujillo-de Santiago, G., Álvarez, M. M., & Chuck-Hernández, C. (2021). Advances and prospective applications of 3D food printing for health improvement and personalized nutrition. *Comprehensive Reviews in Food Science and Food Safety*, *20*(6), 5722–5741. Available from https://doi.org/10.1111/1541-4337.12849, http://onlinelibrary.wiley.com/journal/10.1111/(ISSN)1541-4337.

FAO, Thinking about the Future of Food Safety: A Foresight Report, Food and Agriculture Organization of the United Nations 2022.

Fernandes, S. S., Coelho, M. S., & Salas-Mellado, MdlM. (2019). *Bioactive Compounds as Ingredients of Functional Foods Bioactive Compounds: Health Benefits and Potential Applications* (pp. 129–142). Brazil: Elsevier. Available from https://www.sciencedirect.com/book/9780128147740, https://doi.org/10.1016/B978-0-12-814774-0.00007-4.

Gaydhane, M. K., Mahanta, U., Sharma, C. S., Khandelwal, M., & Ramakrishna, S. (2018). Cultured meat: state of the art and future. *Biomanufacturing Reviews*, *3*(1). Available from https://doi.org/10.1007/s40898-018-0005-1.

Gu, Y., Li, X., & Chan, E. C. Y. (2023). Risk assessment of cultured meat. *Trends in Food Science and Technology*, *138*, 491–499. Available from https://doi.org/10.1016/j.tifs.2023.06.037, http://www.elsevier.com/wps/find/journaldescription.cws_home/601278/description#description.

Guo, C., Zhang, M., & Bhandari, B. (2019). Model Building and Slicing in Food 3D Printing Processes: A Review. *Comprehensive Reviews in Food Science and Food Safety*, *18*(4), 1052–1069. Available from https://doi.org/10.1111/1541-4337.12443, http://onlinelibrary.wiley.com/journal/10.1111/(ISSN)1541-4337.

Guo, J., Cui, L., & Meng, Z. (2023). Oleogels/emulsion gels as novel saturated fat replacers in meat products: A review. *Food Hydrocolloids*, *137*, 108313. Available from https://doi.org/10.1016/j.foodhyd.2022.108313.

Guo, Q., Zhang, M., Mujumdar, A. S., & Yu, D. (2024). Drying technologies of novel food resources for future foods: Progress, challenges and application prospects. *Food Bioscience*, *60*. Available from https://doi.org/10.1016/j.fbio.2024.104490, https://www.sciencedirect.com/science/journal/22124292.

Hakobyan, D., Médina, C., Dusserre, N., Stachowicz, M. L., Handschin, C., Fricain, J. C., Guillermet-Guibert, J., & Oliveira, H. (2020). Laser-assisted 3D bioprinting of exocrine pancreas spheroid models for cancer initiation study. *Biofabrication*, *12*(3). Available from https://doi.org/10.1088/1758-5090/ab7cb8, https://iopscience.iop.org/article/10.1088/1758-5090/ab7cb8.

Han, C., Wang, G., Guo, J., Wang, J., & Yang, X. (2023). Oral oil release improves lubrication and sensory properties of meat analogs with protein-stabilized oleogel. *Food Hydrocolloids*, *142*, 108788. Available from https://doi.org/10.1016/j.foodhyd.2023.108788.

Handral, H. K., Hua Tay, S., Wan Chan, W., & Choudhury, D. (2022). 3D Printing of cultured meat products. *Critical Reviews in Food Science and Nutrition*, *62*(1), 272–281. Available from https://doi.org/10.1080/10408398.2020.1815172. https://www.tandfonline.com/loi/bfsn20.

Hassoun, A., Bekhit, A. E. D., Jambrak, A. R., Regenstein, J. M., Chemat, F., Morton, J. D., Gudjónsdóttir, M., Carpena, M., Prieto, M. A., Varela, P., Arshad, R. N., Aadil, R. M., Bhat, Z., & Ueland, Ø. (2024). The fourth industrial revolution in the food industry—part II: Emerging food trends. *Critical Reviews in Food Science and Nutrition*, *64*(2), 407–437. Available from https://doi.org/10.1080/10408398.2022.2106472, https://www.tandfonline.com/loi/bfsn20.

He, C., Zhang, M., & Fang, Z. (2020). 3D printing of food: pretreatment and post-treatment of materials. *Critical Reviews in Food Science and Nutrition*, *60*(14), 2379–2392. Available from https://doi.org/10.1080/10408398.2019.1641065, https://www.tandfonline.com/loi/bfsn20.

Jagadiswaran, B., Alagarasan, V., Palanivelu, P., Theagarajan, R., Moses, J. A., & Anandharamakrishnan, C. (2021). Valorization of food industry waste and by-products using 3D printing: A study on the development of value-added functional cookies. *Future Foods*, *4*, 100036. Available from https://doi.org/10.1016/j.fufo.2021.100036.

Jammalamadaka, U., & Tappa, K. (2018). Recent Advances in Biomaterials for 3D Printing and Tissue Engineering. *Journal of Functional Biomaterials*, *9*(1), 22. Available from https://doi.org/10.3390/jfb9010022.

Jonkers, N., van Dommelen, J. A. W., & Geers, M. G. D. (2022). Selective Laser Sintered food: A unit cell approach to design mechanical properties. *Journal of Food Engineering*, *335*, 111183. Available from https://doi.org/10.1016/j.jfoodeng.2022.111183.

Joo, S. T., Choi, J. S., Hur, S. J., Kim, G. D., Kim, C. J., Lee, E. Y., Bakhsh, A., & Hwang, Y. H. (2022). A Comparative Study on the Taste Characteristics of Satellite Cell Cultured Meat Derived from Chicken and Cattle Muscles. *Food Science of Animal Resources, 42*(1), 175–185. Available from https://doi.org/10.5851/kosfa.2021.e72, http://www.kosfaj.org/archive/view_article?doi = 10.5851/kosfa.2021.e72.

Keerthana, K., Anukiruthika, T., Moses, J. A., & Anandharamakrishnan, C. (2020). Development of fiber-enriched 3D printed snacks from alternative foods: A study on button mushroom. *Journal of Food Engineering, 287*, 110116. Available from https://doi.org/10.1016/j.jfoodeng.2020.110116.

Kewuyemi, Y. O., Kesa, H., & Adebo, O. A. (2022). Trends in functional food development with three-dimensional (3D) food printing technology: prospects for value-added traditionally processed food products. *Critical Reviews in Food Science and Nutrition, 62*(28), 7866–7904. Available from https://doi.org/10.1080/10408398.2021.1920569, https://www.tandfonline.com/loi/bfsn20.

Krujatz, F., Lode, A., Seidel, J., Bley, T., Gelinsky, M., & Steingroewer, J. (2017). Additive Biotech—Chances, challenges, and recent applications of additive manufacturing technologies in biotechnology. *New Biotechnology, 39*, 222–231. Available from https://doi.org/10.1016/j.nbt.2017.09.001, http://www.elsevier.com.

Kyriakopoulou, K., Keppler, J. K., & van der Goot, A. J. (2021). Functionality of ingredients and additives in plant-based meat analogues. *Foods, 10*(3). Available from https://doi.org/10.3390/foods10030600, https://www.mdpi.com/2304-8158/10/3/600/pdf.

Lee, J. (2021). A 3D Food Printing Process for the New Normal Era: A Review. *Processes, 2021*.

Lee, M., Park, S., Choi, B., Choi, W., Lee, H., Lee, J. M., Lee, S. T., Yoo, K. H., Han, D., Bang, G., Hwang, H., Koh, W. G., Lee, S., & Hong, J. (2024). Cultured meat with enriched organoleptic properties by regulating cell differentiation. *Nature Communications, 15*(1). Available from https://doi.org/10.1038/s41467-023-44359-9, https://www.nature.com/ncomms/.

Lee, S. Y., Lee, D. Y., Yun, S. H., Lee, J., Mariano, E., Park, J., Choi, Y., Han, D., Kim, J. S., & Hur, S. J. (2024). Current technology and industrialization status of cell-cultivated meat. *Journal of Animal Science and Technology, 66*(1), 2–30. Available from https://doi.org/10.5187/jast.2023.e107, https://www.ejast.org/archive/view_article?pid = jast-66-1-1.

Levi, S., Yen, F. C., Baruch, L., & Machluf, M. (2022). Scaffolding technologies for the engineering of cultured meat: Towards a safe, sustainable, and scalable production. *Trends in Food Science and Technology, 126*, 13–25. Available from https://doi.org/10.1016/j.tifs.2022.05.011, http://www.elsevier.com/wps/find/journaldescription.cws_home/601278/description#description.

Li, X., Liu, B., Pei, B., Chen, J., Zhou, D., Peng, J., Zhang, X., Jia, W., & Xu, T. (2020). Inkjet Bioprinting of Biomaterials. *Chemical Reviews, 120*(19), 10793–10833. Available from https://doi.org/10.1021/acs.chemrev.0c00008, http://pubs.acs.org/journal/chreay.

Lima, M., Costa, R., Rodrigues, I., Lameiras, J., Botelho, G. (n.d.). A Narrative Review of Alternative Protein Sources: Highlights on Meat, Fish, Egg and Dairy Analogues.

Liu, Z., Zhang, M., Bhandari, B., & Wang, Y. (2017). 3D printing: Printing precision and application in food sector. *Trends in Food Science and Technology, 69*, 83–94. Available from https://doi.org/10.1016/j.tifs.2017.08.018, http://www.elsevier.com/wps/find/journaldescription.cws_home/601278/description#description.

Maldonado-Rosas, R., Tejada-Ortigoza, V., Cuan-Urquizo, E., Mendoza-Cachú, D., Morales-de la Peña, M., Alvarado-Orozco, J. M., & Campanella, O. H. (2022). Evaluation of rheology and printability of 3D printing nutritious food with complex formulations. *Additive Manufacturing, 58*. Available from https://doi.org/10.1016/j.addma.2022.103030, https://www.journals.elsevier.com/additive-manufacturing.

Markovinović, A. B., Brdar, D., Putnik, P., Bosiljkov, T., Durgo, K., Turković, A. H., Karačonji, I. B., Jurica, K., Pavlić, B., & Granato, D. (2024). Danijela Bursać Kovačević, Strawberry tree fruits (Arbutus unedo L.): Bioactive composition, cellular antioxidant activity, and 3D printing of functional foods. *Food Chemistry, 433*, 137287. Available from https://doi.org/10.1016/j.foodchem.2023.137287.

Martinez, A. A., Panuska, C., Kurina-Sanz, M., Rinaldoni, A. N., & Orden, A. A. (2023). Undifferentiated Cells of Tessaria absinthioides with High Nutritional Value and Health-Promoting Phytochemicals. An Approach Based on Plant Cellular Agriculture. *Plant Foods for Human Nutrition, 78*(4), 742–747. Available from https://doi.org/10.1007/s11130-023-01105-2, https://www.springer.com/journal/11130.

McClements, D. J., & Grossmann, L. (2021). A brief review of the science behind the design of healthy and sustainable plant-based foods. *npj Science of Food, 5*(1). Available from https://doi.org/10.1038/s41538-021-00099-y, https://www.nature.com/npjscifood/about.

Melibio, M. Plant-Based Honey Launches at Expo West. (2023), 2023.

Murphy, S. V., & Atala, A. (2014). 3D bioprinting of tissues and organs. *Nature Biotechnology, 32*(8), 773–785. Available from https://doi.org/10.1038/nbt.2958, http://www.nature.com/nbt/index.html.

Nachal, N., Moses, J. A., Karthik, P., & Anandharamakrishnan, C. (2019). Applications of 3D Printing in Food Processing. *Food Engineering Reviews, 11*(3), 123–141. Available from https://doi.org/10.1007/s12393-019-09199-8.

Rolland, N. C. M., Rob Markus, C., Post, M. J., & Sakai, N. (2020). The effect of information content on acceptance of cultured meat in a tasting context. *PLoS One, 15*(4), e0231176. Available from https://doi.org/10.1371/journal.pone.0231176.

Oliveira, S. M., Gruppi, A., Vieira, M. V., Matos, G. S., Vicente, A. A., Teixeira, J. A. C., Fuciños, P., Spigno, G., & Pastrana, L. M. (2021). How additive manufacturing can boost the bioactivity of baked functional foods. *Journal of Food Engineering, 294*. Available from https://doi.org/10.1016/j.jfoodeng.2020.110394, http://www.sciencedirect.com/science/journal/02608774.

Orzechowski, A. (2015). Artificial meat? Feasible approach based on the experience from cell culture studies. *Journal of Integrative Agriculture, 14*(2), 217–221. Available from https://doi.org/10.1016/S2095-3119(14)60882-0, http://www.elsevier.com/journals/journal-of-integrative-agriculture/2095-3119.

Pallottino, F., Hakola, L., Costa, C., Antonucci, F., Figorilli, S., Seisto, A., & Menesatti, P. (2016). Printing on Food or Food Printing: a Review. *Food and Bioprocess Technology, 9*(5), 725–733. Available from https://doi.org/10.1007/s11947-016-1692-3.

Position of the American Dietetic Association: Functional Foods. (2004). *Journal of the American Dietetic Association, 104*(5), 814–826. Available from https://doi.org/10.1016/j.jada.2004.03.015.

Post, M. J. (2012). Cultured meat from stem cells: Challenges and prospects. *Meat Science*, *92*(3), 297–301. Available from https://doi.org/10.1016/j.meatsci.2012.04.008.

Post, M. J., & Hocquette, J. F. (2017). *New Sources of Animal Proteins: Cultured Meat. New Aspects of Meat Quality: From Genes to Ethics* (pp. 425–441). Netherlands: Elsevier. Available from https://www.sciencedirect.com/book/9780081005934, 10.1016/B978-0-08-100593-4.00017-5.

Roy, B., Hagappa, A., Ramalingam, Y. D., & Mahalingam, N. (2021). A review on lab-grown meat: Advantages and disadvantages. *Quest International Journal of Medical and Health Sciences*, *4*(1), 19–24, 2021.

Rubio, N. R., Fish, K. D., Trimmer, B. A., & Kaplan, D. L. (2019). In Vitro Insect Muscle for Tissue Engineering Applications. *ACS Biomaterials Science and Engineering*, *5*(2), 1071–1082. Available from https://doi.org/10.1021/acsbiomaterials.8b01261, http://pubs.acs.org/journal/abseba.

Schwab, A., Levato, R., D'Este, M., Piluso, S., Eglin, D., & Malda, J. (2020). Printability and Shape Fidelity of Bioinks in 3D Bioprinting. *Chemical Reviews*, *120*(19), 11028–11055. Available from https://doi.org/10.1021/acs.chemrev.0c00084, http://pubs.acs.org/journal/chreay.

Sergelidis, D. (2019). Lab Grown Meat: The Future Sustainable Alternative to Meat or a Novel Functional Food? *Biomedical Journal of Scientific & Technical Research*, *17*(1). Available from https://doi.org/10.26717/bjstr.2019.17.002930.

Shahbazi, M., Jäger, H., Chen, J., & Ettelaie, R. (2021). Construction of 3D printed reduced-fat meat analogue by emulsion gels. Part II: Printing performance, thermal, tribological, and dynamic sensory characterization of printed objects. *Food Hydrocolloids*, *121*. Available from https://doi.org/10.1016/j.foodhyd.2021.107054, https://www.sciencedirect.com/science/journal/0268005X.

Shahbazi, M., Jäger, H., & Ettelaie, R. (2021). Application of Pickering emulsions in 3D printing of personalized nutrition. Part I: Development of reduced-fat printable casein-based ink. *Colloids and Surfaces A: Physicochemical and Engineering Aspects*, *622*. Available from https://doi.org/10.1016/j.colsurfa.2021.126641, www.elsevier.com/locate/colsurfa.

Sharma, S., Thind, S. S., & Kaur, A. (2015). In vitro meat production system: why and how. *Journal of Food Science and Technology*, *52*(12), 7599–7607. Available from https://doi.org/10.1007/s13197-015-1972-3, http://www.springerlink.com/content/121580/.

Siddiqui, S. A., Bahmid, N. A., Karim, I., Mehany, T., Gvozdenko, A. A., Blinov, A. V., Nagdalian, A. A., Arsyad, M., & Lorenzo, J. M. (2022). Cultured meat: Processing, packaging, shelf life, and consumer acceptance. *LWT*, *172*. Available from https://doi.org/10.1016/j.lwt.2022.114192, https://www.journals.elsevier.com/lwt.

Siegrist, M., & Hartmann, C. (2020). Perceived naturalness, disgust, trust and food neophobia as predictors of cultured meat acceptance in ten countries. *Appetite*, *155*, 104814. Available from https://doi.org/10.1016/j.appet.2020.104814.

da Silva, D. V. T., Baião., e De Oliveira., Silva, G., Alves, D., Perrone, E., Aguila., & Paschoalin, F. (2019). Betanin, a Natural Food Additive: Stability, Bioavailability, Antioxidant and Preservative Ability Assessments. *Molecules (Basel, Switzerland)*, 2019.

Singh, A., Kumar, V., Singh, S. K., Gupta, J., Kumar, M., Sarma, D. K., & Verma, V. (2023). Recent advances in bioengineered scaffold for in vitro meat production. *Cell and Tissue Research*, *391*(2), 235–247. Available from https://doi.org/10.1007/s00441-022-03718-6, https://www.springer.com/journal/441.

Skylar-Scott, M. A., Uzel, S. G. M., Nam, L. L., Ahrens, J. H., Truby, R. L., Damaraju, S., Lewis, J. A. (n.d.). Biomanufacturing of organ-specific tissues with high cellular density and embedded vascular channels. *Science Advances*, *5*(9).

Stephens, N., Di Silvio, L., Dunsford, I., Ellis, M., Glencross, A., & Sexton, A. (2018). Bringing cultured meat to market: Technical, socio-political, and regulatory challenges in cellular agriculture. *Trends in Food Science and Technology*, *78*, 155–166. Available from https://doi.org/10.1016/j.tifs.2018.04.010, http://www.elsevier.com/wps/find/journaldescription.cws_home/601278/description#description.

Su, Q., Zhao, X., Zhang, X., Wang, Y., Zeng, Z., Cui, H., & Wang, C. (2023). Nano Functional Food: Opportunities, Development, and Future Perspectives. *International Journal of Molecular Sciences*, *24*(1). Available from https://doi.org/10.3390/ijms24010234, http://www.mdpi.com/journal/ijms.

Sun, J., Zhou, W., Huang, D., Fuh, J. Y. H., & Hong, G. S. (2015). An Overview of 3D Printing Technologies for Food Fabrication. *Food and Bioprocess Technology*, *8*(8), 1605–1615. Available from https://doi.org/10.1007/s11947-015-1528-6, http://www.springer.com/life + sci/food + science/journal/11947.

Sundarsingh, A., Zhang, M., Mujumdar, A. S., & Li, J. (2023). Research Progress in Printing Formulation for 3D Printing of Healthy Future Foods. *Food and Bioprocess Technology*. Available from https://doi.org/10.1007/s11947-023-03265-0, https://www.springer.com/journal/11947.

Tavares, L., Santos, L., & Noreña, C. P. Z. (2021). Bioactive compounds of garlic: A comprehensive review of encapsulation technologies, characterization of the encapsulated garlic compounds and their industrial applicability. *Trends in Food Science and Technology*, *114*, 232–244. Available from https://doi.org/10.1016/j.tifs.2021.05.019, http://www.elsevier.com/wps/find/journaldescription.cws_home/601278/description#description.

Tavares, L., Smaoui, S., Pinilla, C. M. B., Ben Hlima, H., & Lopes Barros, H. (2022). Ginger: A systematic review of clinical trials and recent advances in encapsulation of its bioactive compounds. *Food and Function*, *13*(3), 1078–1091. Available from https://doi.org/10.1039/d1fo02998c, http://pubs.rsc.org/en/journals/journal/fo.

Tavares, L., Zapata Noreña, C. P., Barros, H. L., Smaoui, S., Lima, P. S., & Marques de Oliveira, M. (2022). Rheological and structural trends on encapsulation of bioactive compounds of essential oils: A global systematic review of recent research. *Food Hydrocolloids*, *129*. Available from https://doi.org/10.1016/j.foodhyd.2022.107628, https://www.journals.elsevier.com/food-hydrocolloids.

Tavares-Negrete, J. A., Aceves-Colin, A. E., Rivera-Flores, D. C., Díaz-Armas, G. G., Mertgen, A. S., Trinidad-Calderón, P. A., Olmos-Cordero, J. M., Gómez-López, E. G., Pérez-Carrillo, E., Escobedo-Avellaneda, Z. J., Tamayol, A., Alvarez, M. M., & Trujillo-De Santiago, G. (2021). Three-Dimensional Printing Using a Maize Protein: Zein-Based Inks in Biomedical Applications. *ACS Biomaterials Science and Engineering*, *7*(8), 3964–3979. Available from https://doi.org/10.1021/acsbiomaterials.1c00544, http://pubs.acs.org/journal/abseba.

Tomašević, I., Putnik, P., Valjak, F., Pavlić, B., Šojić, B., Bebek Markovinović, A., & Bursać Kovačević, D. (2021). 3D printing as novel tool for fruit-based functional food production. *Current Opinion in Food Science*, *41*, 138–145. Available from https://doi.org/10.1016/j.cofs.2021.03.015, http://www.journals.elsevier.com/current-opinion-in-food-science/.

Tuomisto, H. L., Ellis, M. J., & Haastrup, P. (2015). Environmental impacts of cultured meat: alternative production scenarios. *EU Sci. Hub-Eur. Comm, EU Sci. Hub-Eur. Comm, 2015*.

Tuomisto, H. L., & Teixeira De Mattos, M. J. (2011). Environmental impacts of cultured meat production. *Environmental Science and Technology*, *45* (14), 6117–6123. Available from https://doi.org/10.1021/es200130u.

Vieira, M. V., Oliveira, S. M., Amado, I. R., Fasolin, L. H., Vicente, A. A., Pastrana, L. M., & Fuciños, P. (2020). 3D printed functional cookies fortified with Arthrospira platensis: Evaluation of its antioxidant potential and physical-chemical characterization. *Food Hydrocolloids*, *107*. Available from https://doi.org/10.1016/j.foodhyd.2020.105893, https://www.journals.elsevier.com/food-hydrocolloids.

Waltz, E. (2022). Cow-less milk: the rising tide of animal-free dairy attracts big players. *Nature Biotechnology*, *40*(11), 1534–1536. Available from https://doi.org/10.1038/s41587-022-01548-z.

Wang, M., Li, D., Zang, Z., Sun, X., Tan, H., Si, X., Tian, J., Teng, W., Wang, J., Liang, Q., Bao, Y., Li, B., & Liu, R. (2022). 3D food printing: Applications of plant-based materials in extrusion-based food printing. *Critical Reviews in Food Science and Nutrition*, *62*(26), 7184–7198. Available from https://doi.org/10.1080/10408398.2021.1911929, https://www.tandfonline.com/loi/bfsn20.

Wang, X., Ao, Q., Tian, X., Fan, J., Tong, H., Hou, W., & Bai, S. (2017). Gelatin-Based Hydrogels for Organ 3D Bioprinting. *Polymers*, *9*(9), 401. Available from https://doi.org/10.3390/polym9090401.

Wang, Z., Abdulla, R., Parker, B., Samanipour, R., Ghosh, S., & Kim, K. (2015). A simple and high-resolution stereolithography-based 3D bioprinting system using visible light crosslinkable bioinks. *Biofabrication*, *7*(4), 045009. Available from https://doi.org/10.1088/1758-5090/7/4/045009.

O. Wildtype, Salmon, The World's First Cultivated Seafood. (2016), 2016.

Wilk, Wilk Presents World's First Cell-based Yogurt Produced With Cultured Milk Fat. (2024), 2024.

Yang, F., Zhang, M., & Bhandari, B. (2017). Recent development in 3D food printing. *Critical Reviews in Food Science and Nutrition*, *57*(14), 3145–3153. Available from https://doi.org/10.1080/10408398.2015.1094732, www.tandf.co.uk/journals/titles/10408398.asp.

Yang, M., Gao, J., Yang, Q., Al Mamun, A., Masukujjaman, M., & Hoque, M. E. (2024). Modeling the intention to consume and willingness to pay premium price for 3D-printed food in an emerging economy. *Humanities and Social Sciences Communications*, *11*(1). Available from https://doi.org/10.1057/s41599-024-02776-1, https://www.nature.com/palcomms/.

Yirmibesoglu, O. D., Simonsen, L. E., Manson, R., Davidson, J., Healy, K., Menguc, Y., & Wallin, T. (2021). Multi-material direct ink writing of photocurable elastomeric foams. *Communications Materials*, *2*(1). Available from https://doi.org/10.1038/s43246-021-00186-3, https://www.nature.com/commsmat/.

Yuan, J., Yi, C., Jiang, H., Liu, F., & Cheng, G. J. (2021). Direct Ink Writing of Hierarchically Porous Cellulose/Alginate Monolithic Hydrogel as a Highly Effective Adsorbent for Environmental Applications. *ACS Applied Polymer Materials*, *3*(2), 699–709. Available from https://doi.org/10.1021/acsapm.0c01002, pubs.acs.org/journal/aapmcd.

Zhang, C., Guan, X., Yu, S., Zhou, J., & Chen, J. (2022). Production of meat alternatives using live cells, cultures and plant proteins. *Current Opinion in Food Science*, *43*, 43–52. Available from https://doi.org/10.1016/j.cofs.2021.11.002, http://www.journals.elsevier.com/current-opinion-in-food-science/.

Zhang, G., Zhao, X., Li, X., Du, G., Zhou, J., & Chen, J. (2020). Challenges and possibilities for bio-manufacturing cultured meat. *Trends in Food Science and Technology*, *97*, 443–450. Available from https://doi.org/10.1016/j.tifs.2020.01.026, http://www.elsevier.com/wps/find/journaldescription.cws_home/601278/description#description.

Zhang, L., Lou, Y., & Schutyser, M. A. I. (2018). 3D printing of cereal-based food structures containing probiotics. *Food Structure*, *18*, 14–22. Available from https://doi.org/10.1016/j.foostr.2018.10.002, http://www.journals.elsevier.com/food-structure/.

Zhang, Y., Lee, A. Y., Pojchanun, K., Lee, C. P., Zhou, A., An, J., Hashimoto, M., Tan, U. X., Leo, C. H., Wong, G., Chua, C. K., & Pant, A. (2022). Systematic Engineering approach for optimization of multi-component alternative protein-fortified 3D printing food Ink. *Food Hydrocolloids*, *131*. Available from https://doi.org/10.1016/j.foodhyd.2022.107803, https://www.journals.elsevier.com/food-hydrocolloids.

Zhu, S., Vazquez Ramos, P., Heckert, O. R., Stieger, M., van der Goot, A. J., & Schutyser, M. (2022). Creating protein-rich snack foods using binder jet 3D printing. *Journal of Food Engineering*, *332*. Available from https://doi.org/10.1016/j.jfoodeng.2022.111124, http://www.sciencedirect.com/science/journal/02608774.

Index

Note: Page numbers followed by "*f*" and "*t*" refer to figures and tables, respectively.

D

E

F

T

U

V

W

Y

Z

9780443288623